INTERVENTIONAL ONCOLOGY

INTERVENTIONAL ONCOLOGY has joined surgical, radiation and medical oncology as the fourth pillar of cancer care. Advances in imaging and image guidance for the detection, characterization, targeting and therapy of cancer now allow for minimally invasive image-guided treatment of many solid tumors without the morbidity of open surgery or the toxicity of chemotherapy and radiation. In *Interventional Oncology: Principles and Practice*, Jean-Francois Geschwind and Michael Soulen have brought together the accrued experience of pioneers and leaders in image-guided cancer therapy from around the globe to create the first comprehensive text for this emerging field. Covering the biology, techniques, clinical applications and outcomes of interventional oncologic procedures for the treatment and palliation of solid tumors throughout the body, this practical reference will be indispensable for physicians across specialties who seek to provide collaborative, leading-edge care to cancer patients.

primarily on subjects dealing with cardiac magnetic resonance imaging and oncology, and he is also the recipient of numerous national and international awards and grants for his research in the field of liver cancer. Geschwind is a member of the editorial board of the *Journal of Vascular and Interventional Radiology*, *Techniques in Vascular and Interventional Radiology* and the *World Journal of Gastroenterology* and a reviewer for numerous radiology and oncology journals. He is a member of the Hepatobiliary Task Force of the National Cancer Institute and has been a board member of the Society of Interventional Radiology Research Foundation since 2006. Geschwind is an active member of the American Association for Cancer Research, the American Society of Clinical Oncology, the International Liver Cancer Association, the American Roentgen Ray Society, the Radiological Society of North America, the Society of Interventional Radiology (SIR) and the Cardiovascular and Interventional Radiology Society of Europe (CIRSE).

Jean-Francois H. Geschwind, MD, originally from Paris, France, pursued his undergraduate studies at the University of Pennsylvania before receiving his medical degree in 1991 from Boston University School of Medicine. He completed his diagnostic radiology residency training at the University of California, San Francisco and trained in cardiovascular and interventional radiology at Johns Hopkins University School of Medicine, where he became a faculty member in 1998. In 2002, Geschwind was promoted to the rank of associate professor and appointed director of cardiovascular and interventional radiology. He is the author or co-author of more than 200 published manuscripts and abstracts,

Michael C. Soulen, MD, received his undergraduate degree from Yale and his medical degree from the University of Pennsylvania, then trained in radiology at Johns Hopkins. After clinical and research fellowships in vascular and interventional radiology at Thomas Jefferson University, he started the interventional oncology program at the University of Pennsylvania, where he is currently professor of radiology and surgery. Soulen has written 140 publications with more than 1,500 ISI citations and has given more than 100 presentations around the world. He served on the board of the SIR for nine years and as director of research education for the SIR Foundation for four years. He is a Fellow of the SIR and of the CIRSE.

INTERVENTIONAL ONCOLOGY

Principles and Practice

EDITED BY

Jean-Francois H. Geschwind

Johns Hopkins University School of Medicine

and

Michael C. Soulen

University of Pennsylvania

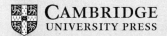
CAMBRIDGE
UNIVERSITY PRESS

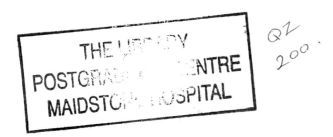
CAMBRIDGE UNIVERSITY PRESS
Cambridge, New York, Melbourne, Madrid, Cape Town, Singapore, São Paulo, Delhi

Cambridge University Press
32 Avenue of the Americas, New York, NY 10013-2473, USA

www.cambridge.org
Information on this title: www.cambridge.org/9780521864138

© Cambridge University Press 2008

This publication is in copyright. Subject to statutory exception
and to the provisions of relevant collective licensing agreements,
no reproduction of any part may take place without
the written permission of Cambridge University Press.

First published 2008

Printed in the United States of America

A catalog record for this publication is available from the British Library.

Library of Congress Cataloging in Publication Data
Interventional oncology : principles and practice / [edited by] Jean-Francois H. Geschwind, Michael C. Soulen.
p. ; cm.
Includes bibliographical references and index.
ISBN 978-0-521-86413-8 (hardback)
1. Cancer – Surgery. 2. Computer-assisted surgery. 3. Image-guided radiation therapy.   I. Geschwind, Jean-Francois H., 1963- II. Soulen, Michael C., 1958- III. Title.
[DNLM: 1. Neoplasms – surgery. 2. Neoplasms – diagnosis. 3. Radiography, Interventional – methods. 4. Surgery, Computer-Assisted – methods. QZ 268 I62 2008]

RD651.I58 2008
616.99′4059–dc22   2008017804

ISBN 978-0-521-86413-8 hardback

Cambridge University Press has no responsibility for the persistence or accuracy of URLs for external or third-party Internet Web sites referred to in this publication and does not guarantee that any content on such Web sites is, or will remain, accurate or appropriate.

Every effort has been made in preparing this publication to provide accurate and up-to-date information that is in accord with accepted standards and practice at the time of publication. Nevertheless, the authors, editors and publisher can make no warranties that the information contained herein is totally free from error, not least because clinical standards are constantly changing through research and regulation. The authors, editors and publisher therefore disclaim all liability for direct or consequential damages resulting from the use of material contained in this publication. Readers are strongly advised to pay careful attention to information provided by the manufacturer of any drugs or equipment that they plan to use.

Contents

Foreword

I AM VERY PLEASED to have been asked by Drs. Geschwind and Soulen to write a foreword for this book, *Interventional Oncology: Principles and Practice*. I suspect that I have been asked to do this for two reasons. The first is that I am editor-in-chief of the *Journal of Clinical Oncology* and therefore am very privileged to see the widest possible array of manuscripts and publications each day. Therefore, I can easily see the evolution of oncology from single disciplines to a multidisciplinary approach for patients. Indeed, more important than the proliferation of new drugs or techniques has been the evolution of the care of patients by teams of individuals, each of whom contributes special expertise, with a common endpoint of superior patient care. The second reason I was asked to write this foreword relates to this observation: Dr. Soulen and I have been colleagues for many years, and our own relationship in the care of patients has also evolved. In contrast with the time when radiology was simply a tool for clinicians to use in decision making, radiologists now take an active part in the care of many patients with cancer. As I have learned the benefits and limitations of interventional radiology from Dr. Soulen, I hope that he has also learned from me – throughout more than 30 years of practice in an

academic medical center – the aspects of oncology that aid him in helping our mutual patients.

I was very excited to see the table of contents of this new book, which I believe should be mandatory reading for all interventional radiologists and oncologists who work with them. I do hope that oncologists, in particular, read specific chapters related to techniques of interventional oncology. Likewise, I hope also that interventional oncologists read the chapters that may not directly relate to their day-to-day practices, especially in the biology of cancer and in nonradiologic approaches. In this way, radiologists and nonradiologists alike will gain more information about their colleagues' disciplines, ultimately leading to improvement in patient care.

Needless to say, all of the authors are internationally known experts in their respective fields of oncology.

It is entirely appropriate that the book begins with a chapter on tumor biology. Without this knowledge, no rational decision can be made about either systemic or local therapies. The ultimate result of tumor biology is the natural history of cancer, in either a population of patients or an individual patient. The applicability of relatively localized treatments, which is the general purview of interventional oncology, is highly affected by the natural history of the patient's tumor. Without this knowledge, localized therapies may be very effective in local control; however, if the patient's outcome is driven primarily by systemic disease, then such local control may not contribute dramatically to the patient's length or quality of life.

I found the chapter on the evaluation of the cancer patient to be particularly useful for both interventional oncologists and all other oncologists treating patients with cancer. This chapter essentially outlines the rules of practice upon which everyone must agree, so that we are all speaking the same language when discussing a patient and when evolving a mutually agreed-upon plan. Similarly, it is important that not only medical oncologists understand the principles and practice of chemotherapy; interventional oncologists and other physicians involved in the care of cancer patients must also know the mechanisms of actions of various chemotherapy agents, as well as the toxicity profiles associated with these drugs. In many settings, interventional oncologists are already administering chemotherapy in the form of chemoembolization, but there is a need for other disciplines to be aware of the toxicity profiles of standard chemotherapeutic agents. For example, surgeons who perform hepatic sections need to be aware of the toxicities of drugs such as 5-fluorouracil, oxaliplatin and irinotecan. Overtreatment with each of these drugs can lead to fatty liver and increased morbidity from surgery.

Part II, dedicated to the principles of image-guided therapies, is an extremely important section of this book. Interventional oncologists rely heavily on both standard and evolving radiographic techniques to assess not only the size and location of tumors but also the effects of both locoregional therapies and systemic therapies.

Part III is dedicated to the treatment of specific malignancies. There is potentially no more exciting and controversial topic than the treatment of primary liver cancers. Hepatocellular carcinomas represent a heterogeneous group of tumors, with differing liver substrates and differing causation. Although some tumors are found when they are small, typically by screening, and are amenable to surgical resection, most tumors in the United States are larger, multifocal and frequently metastatic. Primary liver cancer certainly represents the epitome of multidisciplinary care, with gastroenterologists, surgeons, medical oncologists and interventional radiologists all providing treatment. In addition to improved surgical techniques and liver transplant techniques, the systemic management of hepatocellular carcinoma has significantly changed recently with the introduction of the drug sorafenib, which has been shown to extend survival compared to a placebo in a large, randomized trial. This drug is now being added to surgical resection and transarterial chemoembolization (TACE) in an adjuvant fashion. Certainly, the combination of both an effective local therapy and an effective systemic therapy may lead to improvement in survival for patients with this common malignancy.

This book deals quite well with the evolution of treatment of metastases from colorectal cancer. Once considered a death sentence for a patient, this situation now is considered one that is curative in many patients, particularly with a multidisciplinary care team. The management of these patients may range from palliative therapy with systemic chemotherapy alone to multi-disciplinary treatments, including systemic chemotherapy, surgical resection and either radiofrequency ablation or TACE. Given the limited number of institutions in which all of these treatments are represented equally in quality, it goes without saying that treatment of these patients is best delivered in a setting in which treatment is not delivered only by availability of a particular technique. Many other tumors are also dealt with in a detailed and comprehensive fashion, including cholangiocarcinoma, melanoma, renal cell carcinoma and neuroendocrine tumors. The breadth of discussion for these tumors is not to be seen as a shopping list, but as an example of how broad the applicability of interventional oncology is to all disciplines of oncology.

There are excellent chapters on specific palliative techniques, including pain control, stenting and techniques of vascular access that allow medical oncologists to administer chemotherapeutic agents. Finally, the book ends with a very important chapter on potential complications of interventional oncology. This chapter is particularly important for caregivers who are not directly involved in interventional oncology, as they are frequently the ones to be called about symptoms or signs in the patient post-intervention. Thus, consciousness must be raised for post-embolization syndromes, infections and other potential complications of interventional treatments.

The need for this book is obvious. With the evolution of better systemic therapies, better surgical techniques and interventional oncology techniques, many new treatments can be offered to patients with cancer. No single caregiver or group of caregivers can treat a single patient without the help of other members of a team. Without awareness of the capabilities and limitations of partners in care, it is virtually impossible to offer patients optimal care. Drs. Geschwind and Soulen have done an admirable job of addressing a real need, frequently overlooked in existing standard textbooks. I hope that both interventional oncologists and others involved in the care of cancer patients read this book and take these messages home to their colleagues.

Daniel Haller, MD
Hospital of the University of Pennsylvania

Acknowledgments

To my mentors, Drs. Charles B. Higgins, Elias A. Zerhouni and Floyd A. Osterman, for their leadership and generous advice throughout my career. To the other numerous people who helped me along the way, to my clinical and research colleagues whose passion, creativity and sense of humor make the workplace the joy that it is. To my parents for allowing me to fulfill my dream of a research career in the United States, and to my wife, Meg and two wonderful boys, David and Marc, whose presence is my greatest source of confidence and strength.

Jean-Francois H. Geschwind, MD
Baltimore, Maryland
July 2008

The discipline of interventional oncology owes its origins to two intersecting phenomena: the evolution of interventional radiologists from procedural technicians into clinical specialists and innovations in image-guided therapy for cancer. I was fortunate to come to this crossroad early in my training under the tutelage of outstanding mentors. Foremost was Robert I. White Jr., chief of interventional radiology at Johns Hopkins University in the 1980s when I was a medical student and resident. Dr. White was a prescient champion for the clinical practice of interventional radiology and an icon for the primary role interventional radiologists could take in delivering patient care. During my clinical and research fellowships at Thomas Jefferson University, Joe Bonn and Marcelle Shapiro, with prior training in surgery and internal medicine, respectively, continued the model of the clinician-interventionist; Geoff Gardiner was a patient yet demanding master of catheter skills and Kevin Sullivan and Mack Consigny were mentors for clinical and animal research.

The origins of the interventional oncology practice at the University of Pennsylvania benefited from the wisdom and experience of leaders in interventional radiology and oncology. Stanley Baum, Constantin Cope and Michael Pentecost were sage counselors for the young faculty at the university in the 1990s. Daniel Haller, then chief of gastrointestinal oncology, was of invaluable assistance in crafting an interventional oncology program worthy of the respect of our medical and surgical colleagues.

The success of any academic clinical enterprise depends upon the teamwork and dedication of many people. A score of former and current University of

Pennsylvania faculty contributed to outstanding and innovative oncologic care and research. Too many to name individually here, my heartfelt appreciation goes to each and every one of you. More than 100 Fellows supported the clinical service during their training and went on to perpetuate the model throughout the country and the world. The nurse practitioners, physician assistants, technologists, nurses, schedulers and secretaries are the backbone that allows us to provide high-quality care.

Finally, no measure of success was achieved without the love, support and guidance of my family. From my father, Richard, the scientist, I learned the values of rigorous inquiry, open-mindedness, fairness and integrity. My mother, Renate, one of the first interventional radiologists in the country, embodies the academic clinician-teacher-researcher. A steadfast champion, she taught me perseverance and to smile in the face of adversity. My wife, Terri, brings balance to my life and keeps me engaged in the joy of home, family and friends. My children, Justin and Sarah, are far more wonderful than I could ever describe, and they think it is pretty cool that their dad edited a book.

Michael C. Soulen
Philadelphia, 2008

Contributors

EDITORS

Jean-Francois H. Geschwind, MD, FSIR
Professor of Radiology, Surgery and Oncology
Director, Cardiovascular and Interventional Radiology
Section Chief, Interventional Radiology
Director, Interventional Radiology Research
Russell H. Morgan Department of Radiology and
    Radiological Science
Johns Hopkins University School of Medicine
Baltimore, MD

Michael C. Soulen, MD, FSIR
Professor of Radiology and Surgery
Division of Interventional Radiology
University of Pennsylvania
Philadelphia, PA

CONTRIBUTORS

**Andy Adam, MD, FRCP, FRCR, FRCS, FFR
RCSI (Hon.), FRANZCR (Hon.), FMedSci**
Professor
Department of Radiology
St. Thomas' Hospital
London, UK

Kamran Ahrar, MD
Associate Professor
M.D. Anderson Cancer Center
University of Texas
Houston, TX

Bassel Atassi, MD
Research Associate
Department of Radiology
Section of Interventional Radiology
Robert H. Lurie Comprehensive Cancer
    Center
Northwestern Memorial Hospital
Chicago, IL

Anjali Avadhani, MD
Instructor
Division of Medical Oncology
University of Pennsylvania
Philadelphia, PA

Brian D. Badgwell, MD
Surgical Oncology Fellow
Department of Surgical Oncology
M.D. Anderson Cancer Center
University of Texas
Houston, TX

Todd H. Baron, MD, FASGE
Professor of Medicine
Division of Gastroenterology and Hepatology
Mayo Clinic
Rochester, MN

José I. Bilbao, MD, PhD
Servicio de Radiología
Clínica Universitaria de Navarra
Universidad de Navarra
Pamplona, Spain

Debashish Bose, MD, PhD
Assistant Professor
Department of Surgery
Johns Hopkins University School of Medicine
Baltimore, MD

Robert Bristow, MD
Associate Professor
Department of Radiation Oncology and Medical
    Biophysics
Princess Margaret Hospital
Toronto, Ontario, Canada

Manon Buijs, MD
Postdoctoral Research Fellow
Interventional Radiology Division
Johns Hopkins University School of Medicine
Baltimore, MD

Matthew R. Callstrom, MD, PhD
Assistant Professor of Radiology
Mayo Clinic
Rochester, MN

J. William Charboneau, MD
Professor of Radiology
Mayo Clinic
Rochester, MN

Michael A. Choti, MD, MBA, FACS
Professor
Department of Surgery
Johns Hopkins University School of Medicine
Baltimore, MD

Jin Wook Chung, MD
Associate Professor
Department of Radiology
Seoul National University Hospital
Seoul, Korea

Dania Cioni, MD
Professor of Radiology
University of Pisa
Pisa, Italy

Laura Crocetti, MD, PhD
Assistant Professor of Radiology
University of Pisa
Pisa, Italy

Steven C. Cunningham, MD
Postdoctoral Research Fellow
Sidney Kimmel Comprehensive Cancer Center
Johns Hopkins University School of Medicine
Baltimore, MD

Thierry de Baère, MD
Professor
Department of Interventional Radiology
Institut Gustave Roussy
Villejuif, France

Clotilde Della Pina, MD
Professor of Radiology
Division of Diagnostic and Interventional Radiology
University of Pisa
Pisa, Italy

Eric Desruennes, MD
Department of Interventional Radiology
Institut Gustave Roussy
Villejuif, France

Thomas DiPetrillo, MD
Associate Professor
Brown School of Medicine
Vice Chairman, Department of Radiation Oncology
Brown University Hospital
Providence, RI

Damian E. Dupuy, MD
Director of Tumor Ablation
Rhode Island Hospital
Professor of Diagnostic Imaging
Brown Medical School
Brown University Hospital
Providence, RI

Sydney M. Evans, VMD
Professor of Radiation Oncology
University of Pennsylvania
Philadelphia, PA

Robert Gatenby, MD, PhD
Professor of Radiology and Applied Mathematics
Vice Chairman of Clinical Research
Co-Director of the Arizona Cancer Center's
    Cancer Imaging and Technology Team
University of Arizona
Tucson, AZ

Christos S. Georgiades, MD, PhD
Assistant Professor
Russell H. Morgan Department of Radiology and
    Radiological Science
Division of Cardiovascular and Interventional
    Radiology
Johns Hopkins University School of Medicine
Baltimore, MD

Debra Gervais, MD
Associate Professor of Radiology
Massachusetts General Hospital
Boston, MA

S. Nahum Goldberg, MD
Professor in Radiology
Harvard Medical School
Director, MRI
Department of Radiology
Beth Israel Deaconess Medical Center
Boston, MA

Tiffany V. Goolsby, PharmD
Clinical Pharmacist
Johns Hopkins Pharmacy
Baltimore, MD

Manpreet Singh Gulati, DNB, MD, FRCR
Consultant Radiologist
Queen Elizabeth Hospital
Honorary Consultant
Guy's and St. Thomas' NHS Foundation Trust
London, UK

James P. Hamilton, MD
Assistant Professor
Department of Gastroenterology
Johns Hopkins University School of Medicine
Baltimore, MD

Mary J. Hendrix, PhD
Professor
Northwestern University Feinberg School of
    Medicine
Chicago, IL

Christopher Herzog, MD
Assistant Professor of Radiology
University of Frankfurt
Frankfurt, Germany

Mihkail C. S. S. Higgins, BS
Wake Forest University School of Medicine
Winston-Salem, NC

Richard Hill, PhD
Professor
Department of Medical Biophysics and Radiation
    Oncology
University of Toronto
Princess Margaret Hospital
Toronto, Ontario, Canada

Andrew Hines-Peralta, MD
Radiologist
Beth Israel Deaconess Medical Center
Department of Radiology
Boston, MA

Kelvin Hong, MD
Assistant Professor
Russell H. Morgan Department of Radiology and
    Radiological Science
Division of Cardiovascular and Interventional
    Radiology
Johns Hopkins University School of Medicine
Baltimore, MD

Fidel David Huitzil Melendez, MD
Gastrointestinal Oncology Fellow
Memorial Sloan-Kettering Cancer Center
New York, NY

Robert W. Hurst, MD
Professor of Radiology
Division of Interventional Neuroradiology
University of Pennsylvania
Philadelphia, PA

Saad Ibrahim, MD
Research Fellow
Robert H. Lurie Comprehensive Cancer Center
Northwestern Memorial Hospital
Chicago, IL

Sanaz Javadi, MD
Research Intern
M.D. Anderson Cancer Center
University of Texas
Houston, TX

Philip Johnson, MD
Professor of Oncology and Translational Research
Director of the Clinical Trials Unit Cancer Research
UK Institute for Cancer Studies
University of Birmingham
Birmingham, UK

Ihab R. Kamel, MD, PhD
Associate Professor of Radiology and Radiological
    Science
Johns Hopkins University School of Medicine
Baltimore, MD

Nancy Kemeny, MD
Attending Physician
Memorial Sloan-Kettering Cancer Center
Professor of Medicine
Weill Medical College of Cornell University
New York, NY

Michelle Kang Kim, MD
Assistant Professor of Medicine
Mount Sinai School of Medicine
New York, NY

William M.-F. Lee
Associate Professor of Medicine
Department of Medicine
Hematology/Oncology Division
University of Pennsylvania
Philadelphia, PA

Riccardo Lencioni, MD
Professor
Division of Diagnostic and Interventional Radiology
University of Pisa
Pisa, Italy

Robert J. Lewandowski, MD
Assistant Professor
Department of Radiology
Section of Interventional Radiology
Robert H. Lurie Comprehensive Cancer Center
Northwestern Memorial Hospital
Chicago, IL

Eleni Liapi, MD
Postdoctoral Research Fellow
Department of Radiology and Radiological Science
Interventional Radiology Division
Russell H. Morgan Department of Radiology and
    Radiological Science
Division of Cardiovascular and Interventional
    Radiology
Johns Hopkins University School of Medicine
Baltimore, MD

Sebastian Lindemayr, MD
Radiologist
University of Frankfurt
Frankfurt, Germany

Wen W. Ma, MD
Clinical Fellow
Gastrointestinal Oncology Program, Division of
    Medical Oncology
Sidney Kimmel Comprehensive Cancer Center
Johns Hopkins University School of Medicine
Baltimore, MD

David C. Madoff, MD, FSIR
Associate Professor
Interventional Radiology Section
Division of Diagnostic Imaging
M.D. Anderson Cancer Center
University of Texas
Houston, TX

Armeen Mahvash, MD
Assistant Professor
Interventional Radiology Section
M.D. Anderson Cancer Center
University of Texas
Houston, TX

Surena F. Matin, MD, FACS
Associate Professor
Department of Urology
M.D. Anderson Cancer Center
University of Texas
Houston, TX

Ryan A. McTaggart, MD
Radiology Resident
Brown University Hospital
Providence, RI

Wells A. Messersmith, MD
Assistant Professor
Sidney Kimmel Comprehensive Cancer Center
Johns Hopkins University School of Medicine
Baltimore, MD

James M. Metz, MD
Assistant Professor of Radiation Oncology
Abramson Cancer Center
University of Pennsylvania
Philadelphia, PA

Peter R. Mueller, MD, FSIR
Professor of Radiology
Director, Abdominal Imaging
Massachusetts General Hospital
Boston, MA

José J. Noguera, MD
Servicio de Radiología
Clínica Universitaria de Navarra
Universidad de Navarra
Pamplona, Spain

Gary Onik, MD
Director, Surgical Imaging
Florida Hospital
Celebration, FL

Daniel Palmer, MD
Clinician Scientist
Cancer Research, UK Institute for Cancer Studies
University of Birmingham
Birmingham, UK

Pankit Parikh, MD
Research Assistant
Northwestern Memorial Hospital
Chicago, IL

Jae Hyung Park, MD
Professor
Department of Radiology
Seoul National University College of Medicine
Seoul, Korea

Timothy M. Pawlik, MD, MPH
Assistant Professor
Department of Surgery
Johns Hopkins University School of Medicine
Baltimore, MD

Dario Ribero, MD
Clinical Fellow
M.D. Anderson Cancer Center
University of Texas
Houston, TX

William S. Rilling, MD, FSIR
Professor of Radiology and Surgery
Director, Section of Vascular/Interventional
    Radiology
Medical College of Wisconsin
Milwaukee, WI

Drew A. Rosielle, MD
Assistant Professor of Medicine
Palliative Care Program
Medical College of Wisconsin
Milwaukee, WI

Robert K. Ryu, MD, FSIR
Associate Professor
Department of Radiology
Northwestern Memorial Hospital
Chicago, IL

Tarun Sabharwal, FRCSI, FRCR
Consultant Radiologist
Department of Radiology
St. Thomas' Hospital
London, UK

Mansi A. Saksena, MD
Radiologist
Division of Abdominal Imaging and Intervention
Department of Radiology
Massachusetts General Hospital
Boston, MA

Riad Salem, MD, MBA, FSIR
Associate Professor
Department of Radiology
Robert H. Lurie Comprehensive Cancer Center
Northwestern Memorial Hospital
Chicago, IL

Kent T. Sato, MD
Assistant Professor
Department of Radiology
Northwestern Memorial Hospital
Chicago, IL

Richard D. Schulick, MD, FACS
Associate Professor of Surgery and Oncology
Department of Surgery
Sidney Kimmel Comprehensive Cancer Center
Johns Hopkins University School of Medicine
Baltimore, MD

Rowena Schwartz, PharmD, BCOP
Director of Oncology Pharmacy
Johns Hopkins University School of Medicine
Baltimore, MD

Eric T. Shinohara, MD
Clinical Resident
Department of Radiology Oncology
Abramson Cancer Center
University of Pennsylvania
Philadelphia, PA

Luigi Solbiati, MD
Chairman, Department of Diagnostic Imaging
Department of Radiology
General Hospital
Busto Arsizio, Italy

Stephen B. Solomon, MD
Associate Attending Physician
Co-Director, Center for Image-guided Intervention
Memorial Sloan-Kettering Cancer Center
New York, NY

Kevin L. Sullivan, MD, FSIR
Associate Professor
Department of Radiology
Thomas Jefferson University Hospital
Philadelphia, PA

Weijing Sun, MD
Associate Professor of Medicine
Director of Gastrointestinal Medical Oncology
    Program
Abramson Cancer Center
University of Pennsylvania
Philadelphia, PA

Paul J. Thuluvath, MD, FRCP
Associate Professor
Department of Medicine
Johns Hopkins University School of Medicine
Baltimore, MD

Catherine M. Tuite, MD
Assistant Professor of Radiology
University of Pennsylvania Medical Center
Philadelphia, PA

Jean-Nicolas Vauthey, MD
Professor of Surgery and Chief of the Liver Service
Department of Surgical Oncology
M.D. Anderson Cancer Center
University of Texas
Houston, TX

Thomas J. Vogl, MD
Professor
Department of Diagnostic and Interventional
    Radiology
University of Frankfurt
Frankfurt, Germany

Josephina A. Vossen, MD
Postdoctoral Research Fellow
Interventional Radiology Division
Johns Hopkins University School of Medicine
Baltimore, MD

Richard R. P. Warner, MD
Professor of Medicine
Mount Sinai School of Medicine
New York, NY

John B. Weigele, MD, PhD
Assistant Professor
Division of Interventional Neuroradiology
University of Pennsylvania
Philadelphia, PA

David E. Weissman, MD
Director of the Palliative Medicine Program
Professor of Medicine in the Division of Neoplastic
    Diseases and Related Disorders
Co-Director of End of Life Palliative Education
    Resource Center
Medical College of Wisconsin
Milwaukee, WI

Rex Yung, MD
Assistant Professor of Medicine and
    Oncology
Director of Pulmonary Oncology and
    Bronchology
Sidney Kimmel Comprehensive Cancer Center
Johns Hopkins University School of Medicine
Baltimore, MD

Stefan Zangos, MD
Radiologist
University of Frankfurt
Frankfurt, Germany

PART I

PRINCIPLES OF ONCOLOGY

Chapter 1

BIOLOGY OF CANCER

Sydney M. Evans

Robert Bristow

Robert Gatenby

Mary J. Hendrix

Richard Hill

William M.-F. Lee

"The science of today is the technology of tomorrow."
Edward Teller

Interventional radiology (IR) techniques play an important role in cancer therapy by accessing and treating tumors via image-guided methods. These methods involve both local and regional therapies, with thermal ablative technology comprising the former and intra-arterial embolization with radioactive particles the latter. Combined with systemic chemotherapy, these techniques result in increased patient survival. A more recent approach for cancer therapy involves the use of drugs that specifically target molecular, biological or physiological processes. Examples of such targets include epithelial growth factor receptor (EGFR), vascular endothelial growth factor (VEGF), protein kinases, hypoxia inducible factor (HIF), cell cycle checkpoints, apoptosis, hypoxia and angiogenesis. Drugs specific to each of these targets are currently available or are in development; some of these agents may be applicable to interventional delivery. The purpose of this chapter is to review important aspects of tumor biology that may be targeted via an interventional approach.

The clinical behavior of a tumor results from a complex set of interactions between neoplastic and non-neoplastic cells, blood vessels, blood and interstitial fluids using intercellular communication. These interactions define the **tumor microenvironment**, which continues to be extensively studied because there is evidence that it substantially influences tumor behavior and patient outcome (1, 2). This chapter begins with a review of the components and clinical/biological effects of hypoxia, pH, and glucose, discussed by Evans and Gatenby. These factors affect the tumor cell's ability to proliferate vs. die, addressed by Bristow, and the tumor's ability to develop new blood vessels (angiogenesis), discussed by Lee. Hendrix discusses a unique type of angiogenesis wherein tumor cells respond to the tumor microenvironment by undergoing phenotypic changes to vasculogenic-like networks. The balance of angiogenesis and vasculogenesis vs. cell proliferation and cell death ultimately determines the tumor's growth, invasion and metastasis; these concepts are reviewed by Hill. By understanding the mechanisms involved in the complexities of tumor biology, better therapies delivered by interventional radiology may be developed.

HYPOXIA

In the 1950s, Thomlinson and Grey first proposed that hypoxia was present in human cancer (3). They examined histopathological sections of bronchial carcinomas and noted that the distance from blood vessels to the occurrence of necrosis was constant approximately $100\mu m$. Irrespective of the size of the tumor cord, only the size of the necrotic center changed; the viable rim width remained unchanged. Viable but hypoxic cells were hypothesized to be present adjacent to the region of necrosis, and these cells were thought to be the cause of hypoxic cell resistance. The pattern of vessel → oxic tumor cells → viable hypoxic cells → necrosis is referred to as **chronic or diffusion-limited hypoxia** because it depends on the cellular respiration rate. The actual distance between blood vessels and necrosis varies between tumors depending on the rate of cellular respiration, with rapidly metabolizing tumors having more hypoxic cells. In the late 1970s, Brown et al. (4) predicted the presence of transient changes in hypoxia within tumors. This process, referred to as **perfusion-limited or acute hypoxia**, was thought to result from temporal changes in blood flow. Within 10 years, Chaplin et al. identified its presence in rodent tumors. The characteristic pattern of hypoxia adjacent to blood vessels can be demonstrated using a hypoxia-marking agent (discussed subsequently; 5). Dewhirst et al. showed that this pattern could also occur as a result of longitudinal gradients of oxygen utilization (6).

The presence of chronic and acute hypoxia is considered to be extremely important because studies as early as 1921 suggested that hypoxic cells required up to 3 times greater radiation doses to kill cells than those that were oxic (7). Studies in rodent and human cells confirmed that severely hypoxic cells ($pO2 \leq 0.1\%$) confirmed this finding (8). The effect of hypoxia is at the level of radiation-produced free radicals (molecules with an unpaired electron). Although free radicals are short-lived, they cause breakage of chemical bonds that eventually lead to cellular damage. In the absence of oxygen, deoxyribonucleic acids (DNA) damage can be repaired and cancer cells can survive. If oxygen is present in the system, it reacts with free radicals, forming organic peroxides that are nonrestorable forms of the target tissue (DNA). Thus, oxygen is said to "fix" (make permanent) DNA damage. Because the amount of radiation prescribed to a patient is limited by the tolerance of normal tissue, hypoxia is considered to be a substantial obstacle to tumor control. It is often impossible to deliver a curative radiation dose without causing unacceptable normal tissue complications. The amount of DNA damage produced depends on the partial pressure of oxygen in the cell. The radiation effect is unchanged between 21% (normal air) and 2% oxygen. When oxygen levels are very close to 0% (with enough oxygen present, however, to keep cells viable), maximal radiation survival is seen. However, even the addition of 0.25% oxygen causes substantial radiosensitization; this increase moves the survival level halfway back to the fully aerated condition (8).

In the years since the importance of hypoxia was realized, numerous techniques to overcome hypoxic cell radioresistance have been developed and tested; examples include drugs to sensitize (9–11) and kill (12, 13) hypoxic cells. The efficacy of any of these agents has been difficult to prove, and most of these reports suggest that the chosen treatments were not effective. These studies may have failed to show efficacy for reasons other than the lack of inherent drug effectiveness. Alternative explanations include the inability to deliver the appropriate drug dose because of dose-limiting toxicity and a mismatch between tissue pO2 and the optimal pO2 at which the given drug is activated. However, another important factor in the "failure" of hypoxic cell sensitizers is that most studies were very small (as discussed subsequently) and diagnostic techniques to select patients with hypoxic tumors were not performed. It is estimated that if 50% of patients in a study had hypoxic tumors [a reasonable estimate based on published reports (2)], 1000 patients would be needed to demonstrate that any treatment was effective; all of the trials using misonidazole as a radiosensitizer included fewer than 300 patients. Therefore, the ability to identify those patients with "hypoxic" tumors in advance of using investigational therapies is critical in designing such clinical trials.

In contrast to the trials just discussed, larger multi-institutional studies, meta-analyses and multivariate analyses have successfully identified subsets of tumor types that respond to hypoxic cell sensitization (14). For example, in Denmark, nimorazole is used in patients with head and neck squamous cell cancer (HNSCC); this therapy is based upon the results of a Phase III trial involving 422 patients with pharynx and supraglottic larynx carcinoma treated with nimorazole vs. placebo plus radiation (14). A significant benefit of nimorazole was observed for locoregional control and cancer-related deaths (52% vs. 41%, p = 0.002), although the survival in the control group was quite low (16%). Another approach to sensitize hypoxic tumor regions is accelerated radiation with carbogen breathing and nicotinamide (ARCON). This technique was proposed to improve tumor cell death by combining accelerated radiotherapy to counteract tumor repopulation, with carbogen breathing and nicotinamide to reduce chronic and acute hypoxia, respectively. ARCON has been shown to yield high locoregional control rates in advanced HNSCC; compliance was found to be satisfactory and morbidity acceptable. The local control rate of 80% for T3 and T4 larynx carcinomas offers excellent possibilities for organ preservation (15). Other "anti-hypoxia" therapies, including hyperbaric oxygen (HBO; 16, 17) and radiation plus hyperthermia (18) have been tested in only small groups of patients, and randomized trials will be necessary to determine their efficacy.

The ability to measure hypoxia in human tumors, and thus identify those patients who would benefit most from hypoxia-targeted therapies, has become an important goal in the past 20 years especially in light of the "failure" of the misonidazole studies. Many approaches are being developed and investigated internationally; they can generally be divided into invasive and non-invasive methods. Although there are numerous invasive methods for measurement of hypoxia, we will concentrate on the use of needle electrodes, exogenously administered markers and endogenous markers; we will not discuss the many non-invasive imaging techniques for measuring blood oxygenation, blood flow and/or perfusion.

The earliest data demonstrating the presence and significance of hypoxia in human cancer were obtained using needle electrodes. Initial measurements were performed by Gatenby et al. using a relatively large-gauge electrode (19, 20) in enlarged lymph nodes from HNSCC. Shortly thereafter, the Eppendorf electrode became available and hypoxia was demonstrated to be present and predictive of patient outcome in several cancer types [for review see (2)]. This technique is limited by the cost and availability of the probe, the need for a skilled operator and the situation that some tumors are not physically accessible to needle placement.

As early as 1981, Chapman observed that 2-nitroimidazole drugs, previously tested as hypoxic cell sensitizers, could be used in much lower concentrations as markers of hypoxic cells. Relying upon immunohistochemical (IHC) and flow cytometric (FCM) techniques, studies were performed in vitro and in vivo in animal tissues. A number of agents were used preclinically, but currently only EF5 and pimonidazole are used in humans for the purpose of measuring hypoxia (21–23). One advantage of IHC-based techniques over needle electrodes is that the spatial distribution of hypoxic cells can be studied in tissue sections. EF5 has been developed such that the binding can be quantified and oxygen maps can be generated from images of binding (24) (Figure 1.1).

In 1992, Semenza described a transcriptional complex, hypoxia inducible factor 1 alpha (HIF-1α; 25). In the ensuing years, HIF-1 and other members of the HIF family have been found to be required for the maintenance of oxygen homeostasis in physiological development, tumor growth and other pathophysiological processes (26). HIF-1 has emerged as an important mediator of gene expression patterns in tumors. More than 100 proteins are known to be regulated by HIF (27) including Glut-1, matrix metalloproteinases (MMP9), vascular endothelial growth factor (VEGF) and carbonic anhydrase 9 (CA-9). These molecules have been identified using IHC techniques and the resulting patterns used as surrogate markers for the presence of hypoxia (28, 29). Although this technique is straightforward when tissue is obtained for diagnostic or therapeutic purposes, there are some limitations to this approach. The most critical is that cellular production of each of these markers may be influenced by factors in addition to hypoxia (30, 31).

Because hypoxia has been identified as both a prognostic factor and a cause of treatment resistance (2), there has been considerable interest in performing non-invasive hypoxia measurements, particularly using positron emission tomography (PET) imaging. Representative imaging isotopes and clinically available PET agents have recently been reviewed (32). As early as 1991, ^{18}F-Fluoromisonidazole was described as an agent for non-invasive hypoxia imaging for human cancers (33). More recently, agents including [123]IAZA, [123]IAZGP, [60,62,64]Cu-ATSM and ^{18}F-EF5 have been used to detect hypoxia in various tumor types. EF5 is unique in this group of agents because it is the exact same molecule as in ^{18}F-EF5, so validation studies of 18F-EF5 PET studies using EF5 IHC are possible (Figure 1.2).

The established role of hypoxia in determining therapy response and modulating tumor physiology

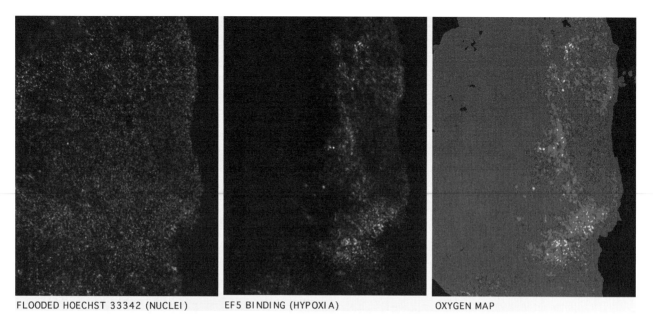

FLOODED HOECHST 33342 (NUCLEI)   EF5 BINDING (HYPOXIA)   OXYGEN MAP

FIGURE 1.1.   Generation of an oxygen map. These images represent the EF5 binding pattern and resultant oxygen map from a human extremity sarcoma. The image on the left demonstrates the location of all nuclei in the sample. Areas that are black on the EF5 image (*central image*) can represent absence of tissue, presence of oxic cells or presence of necrotic tissue. Comparison of the EF5 and Hoechst image allow these possibilities to be distinguished from each other. In the oxygen map (*right image*), areas that are green–blue represent oxic regions, red–orange represent mild to moderate hypoxia and yellow–white represent severe hypoxia. The methods used to generate oxygen maps have been previously described in detail (24). See Color Plate 1.

T1, Gd-enhanced MRI   **18F-EF5 PET**   **MRI-PET Fusion**

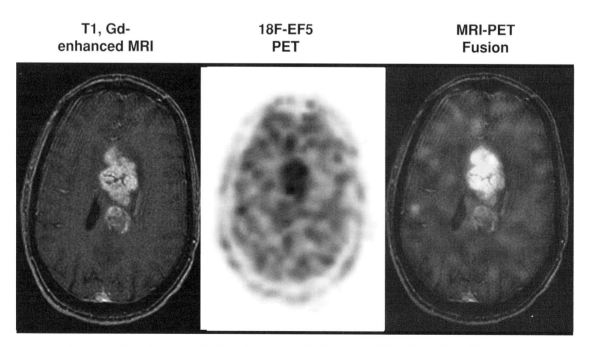

FIGURE 1.2.   Non-invasive imaging of hypoxia. MRI (T1, Gd-enhanced) and ^{18}F-EF5 PET scans from a patient with a glioblastoma multiforme (GBM). The MRI image demonstrates that this patient's tumor is contrast enhancing, compatible with the diagnosis of a GBM. There is EF5 binding in only a portion of the enhancing regions, demonstrating hypoxic heterogeneity within this mass. See Color Plate 2.

has positioned it as a critical endpoint to understand, image and treat.

GLUCOSE AND pH

Malignant cells exhibit remarkable genetic and phenotypic heterogeneity due to accumulation of large numbers of random mutations during carcinogenesis, progression and the metastatic cascade (34, 35). In fact, cancer cell genomes typically exhibit hundreds of thousands of genetic mutations (36). Studies of breast and renal cancers have found that the tumor populations in different individuals exhibit a novel set of genetic mutations (37, 38). Thus, no prototypical cancer cell genotype exists, and each invasive cancer population appears to be the result of a unique genetic pathway traveled during carcinogenesis. Yet, as pointed out by Hanahan and Weinberg, cancers have several traits ("hallmarks") in common, the most important of which is progressive invasion and destruction of normal tissue leading to the death of the host. Experimental and clinical observations have demonstrated that a second widely prevalent cancer trait is increased glucose utilization. This is, in part, due to regions of acute and chronic hypoxia in the tumor microenvironment, forcing the cells to utilize less efficient glycolytic pathways for adenosine triphosphatase (ATP) production. However, a significant contributor to increased glucose flux is aerobic glycolysis, also known as the **Warburg effect**.

In the 1920s, Warburg first noted that tumors consistently relied on anaerobic metabolic pathways, converting glucose to lactic acid even in the presence of abundant oxygen (39). Because anaerobic metabolism of glucose is substantially less efficient than oxidation to CO_2 and H_2O (2 moles of ATP per mole of glucose vs. about 36 moles of ATP per mole of glucose metabolized aerobically), tumor cells maintain ATP production by increasing glucose flux. This increased demand for glucose is the basis for tumor imaging with fluorodeoxyglucose (FDG)-PET (40–43), which is widely used in the diagnosis and treatment of human cancers. These studies show that the vast majority (perhaps all) of primary and metastatic tumors that are large enough to be imaged demonstrate substantially increased glucose uptake compared with normal tissue. Interestingly, FDG-PET imaging has also demonstrated a general correlation between tumor aggressiveness and the rate of glucose consumption (40, 41).

An important consequence of this altered metabolism is increased acid production by tumor cells. Initially it was assumed that the lactic acid produced by anaerobic metabolism would result in an acidic intracellular pH. However, studies with magnetic resonance spectroscopy (MRS) have now consistently demonstrated that the intracellular pH of tumors is the same or slightly alkaline compared with normal cells (44). This was followed by the observation that tumor cells excrete the excess protons produced by upregulated glycolyis through upregulation of the Na^+/H^+ antiport and other membrane transporters. As a result, the extracellular pH (pH_e) of tumor cells is substantially lower (usually by about 0.5 pH unit) than normal, whereas the intracellular pH remains relatively constant (45–47).

The potential consequences of extracellular acidosis are considerable. Generally, a persistent pH_e below about 7.1 results in death of normal cells due to a *p53*-dependent apoptosis pathway triggered by increased caspase activity (31, 48). Interestingly, tumor cells are relatively resistant to acidic pH_e, presumably due to mutations in *p53* or other components of the apoptotic pathway. In fact, tumor cells typically exhibit a maximum proliferation rate in relatively acidic medium (i.e., pH 6.8) (49–51).

The consistent adoption of aerobic glycolysis in cancer cells seems at odds with the commonly held view of carcinogenesis as a Darwinian process (52, 53). That is, the transition of normal cells through a sequence of premalignant lesions to cancer is usually described as somatic evolution because it is driven by mutations and environmental selection. These evolutionary forces represent an optimization process, selecting phenotypic traits that confer increased fitness. Observations that cancer cells typically exhibit aerobic glycolysis, with its inefficient energy extraction and production of a toxic, acidic environment, seems inconsistent with the maxim that evolution selects for the fittest phenotypes.

This paradox has led to the **acid-mediated tumor invasion hypothesis** (Figure 1.3) (54, 55). According to this theory, tumor cells are at an adaptive advantage because they undergo aerobic glycolysis and create an acidic microenvironment. The general concept is that tumor cells increase their own fitness relative to other populations by creating an environment that is toxic to their competitor but relatively harmless to themselves (36–42, 56).

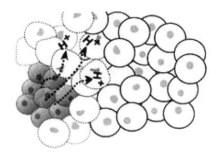

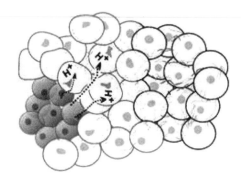

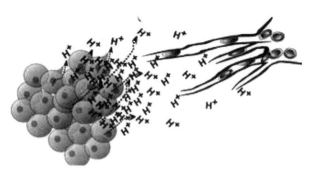

FIGURE 1.3. Proposed mechanisms for acid-mediated tumor invasion. Increased acid in the tumor extracellular space due to glycolytic metabolism causes diffusion of H$^+$ along concentration gradients from the tumor (dark cells) into peritumoral normal tissues (light cells). The resulting decrease in the extracellular pH causes normal cell death due to increased caspase activity, which triggers apoptosis via a *p53*-dependent pathway (*top panel*). In addition, the increased H$^+$ concentration results in extracellular matrix degradation due to release of cathepsin B and other proteolytic enzymes (*middle panel*) and induction of angiogenesis through release of IL-8 and VEGF (*lower panel*). See Color Plate 3.

Specifically, the model proposes the following sequence:

1. Aerobic glycolysis leads to increased acid excretion, which, in turn,

2. Creates a microenvironment with substantially reduced extratumoral pH$_e$ (54, 55).

3. H+ ions within the tumor microenvironment, likely carried by a buffering species, diffuse along concentration gradients into adjacent normal tissues.

4. As shown in Figure 1.3, acidification of the peritumoral normal tissue leads to acid-induced cell death of normal tissues with simultaneous degradation of the extracellular matrix. This results from a combination of caspase-mediated activation of *p53*-dependent apoptosis pathways (31, 48) and extracellular matrix degradation by acid-induced release of proteolytic enzymes such as cathepsin B (57).

5. Tumor growth is promoted by increased angiogenesis through acid-induced release of VEGF and interleukin-8 (IL-8) (48, 57).

6. The acidic extracellular environment also serves to inhibit proper immune function in the peritumoral tissue. Thus, by evading immune surveillance, tumor growth is further promoted (58).

As noted earlier, tumor cells have an optimal pH$_e$ substantially lower than that of normal cells (49, 50) and can continue to proliferate under conditions that are toxic to the surrounding tissue. This tolerance to the harsh environment allows cancer cells to invade into the adjacent, damaged normal tissue.

Although much of the initial evaluation of the acid-mediated tumor invasion hypothesis was performed through in-silico simulations from mathematical models, supportive experimental data have been obtained using tumors implanted in a window chamber surgically placed in SCID mice (Figure 1.4A) (59). Measurements of pH$_e$ using fluorescent ratio magnetic resonance (MR) imaging demonstrated a substantial pH gradient extending into peritumoral normal tissue. Based on these gradients, expected acid flow from the tumor into adjacent normal tissue is demonstrated by the vectors in Figure 1.4B.

In summary, the tumor edge can be envisioned as a traveling wave extending into normal tissue. This wave is preceded by a parallel traveling wave of increased microenvironmental acidity, which promotes invasion by destroying normal tissue, blunting the host immune response and stimulating angiogenesis (52). The acid-mediated tumor invasion model provides a biological mechanism by which aerobic glycolysis can confer a proliferative advantage to cancer cells. The results are consistent with clinical observations that increased glucose uptake and increased lactate concentrations correlate with

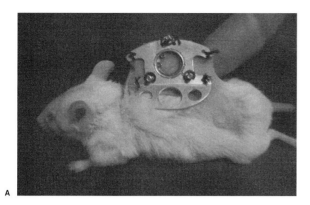

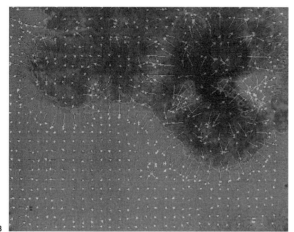

FIGURE 1.4. Fluorescence imaging in a wound chamber tumor model. (A) demonstrates the dorsal wound chamber surgically implanted in a SCID mouse. GFP-transfected tumors implanted in the chamber can be continuously observed microscopically. Regional variations in pH$_e$ can be measured using fluorescent ratio imaging. (B) demonstrates the tumor–host interface defined by the irregular line. Because the tumor cells are GFP transfected, the tumor border can be precisely defined. The vectors demonstrate the flow of acid from the tumor into normal tissue based on gradients of pH$_e$ measurement. See Color Plate 4.

increased tumor virulence and a poor clinical prognosis.

Apoptosis, Mitotic Catastrophe and Terminal Growth Arrest (Senescence)

Advances in targeted chemotherapy and radiotherapy have allowed for the use of novel molecular-targeted agents to increase tumor cell death in a tissue-specific manner. A "new" target of cancer therapy is a sub-population of cells within the tumor called tumor stem cells, which are capable of indefinite division and make up approximately 0.1% to 10% of an individual human tumor. Many types of cells do not show morphological evidence of cell damage until they attempt to divide. A cell that has lost its ability to generate a "clone" post-treatment is regarded as hav-

ing been killed, even though it may undergo a few divisions or remain intact for an extended period. Following DNA damage, the morphology of a cell at the time of cell death can be either apoptotic or necrotic. Lethally damaged cells may (1) undergo cell death secondary to **apoptosis**, (2) undergo up to four abortive mitotic cycles and then finally undergo cell lysis as a result of **mitotic catastrophe** or (3) undergo a **terminal growth arrest** (**tumor senescence**) such as that observed in irradiated normal human fibroblasts (60). The relative levels of apoptosis, mitotic catastrophe and terminal growth arrest will determine the final number of surviving tumor stem cells (i.e., **clonogenic cell kill**) following cancer therapy. More recently, apophagy (discussed subsequently), has been described.

Mitotic catastrophe and terminal growth arrest are responsible for the majority of cell kill during therapy for common epithelial tumors (e.g., prostate, breast, lung). In contrast, more treatment-sensitive tumors (e.g., lymphomas or germ cell tumors) commonly undergo apoptosis. Targeting apoptotic, cell cycle checkpoint, hypoxia and/or DNA repair pathways may augment cell kill and is relevant to any interventional radiology technique that delivers local treatment (60).

Success in cancer therapy depends on the killing of clonogenic tumor cells. For that reason, strategies that target the aforementioned pathways in order to increase tumor clonogenic kill are candidates for novel therapies. The **clonogenic cell survival assay** is widely used to quantify the survival of stem cells (clonogens). Following drug or radiation treatment, cells are incubated for a predetermined period based on their proliferative rate (usually 7–14 days). Those cells that retain unlimited proliferative capacity will divide to form discrete colonies of cells containing more than 50 cells (i.e., they are capable of at least six divisions following irradiation). The ratio of the number of colonies formed to the number of individual cells initially plated in the untreated vs. treated dishes determines the surviving cell fraction.

There are also non-clonogenic assays that can be used to estimate the relative sensitivity of cells. For example, apoptosis can be quantified by several assays, including morphologic analysis and annexin-V [or terminal deoxynucleotidyl transferase dUTP nick-end labeling (TUNEL)] staining of cultures or IHC of tissue sections. The extent of cells within the sub-G1 fraction can be assessed using FCM, relative

DNA fragmentation patterns, activation of apoptotic pathways such as caspase-3 activation or cleavage of the poly (ADP-ribose) polymerase (PARP) protein. Another non-clonogenic assay is the methyl-thiazole-tetrazolium (MTT) assay, which measures relative cell growth in control vs. treated populations over a 3- to 5-day period following radiation exposure. However, the results of these assays do not always correlate with the clonogenic survival assay of the same cell line, which remains the gold-standard assay in experimental cancer studies because it represents the cumulative cell killing as a result of the sum of all types of cell death (61, 62).

In highly treatment-sensitive cells (e.g., lymphocytes, spermatocytes, thymocytes and salivary gland epithelium and the cancers that arise from them), cancer therapies will lead to **classical apoptosis** (i.e., **Type I programmed cell death**) associated with cell membrane blebbing, the formation of nuclear apoptotic bodies and DNA laddering. A second type of programmed cell death is **autophagy** (**Type II programmed cell death**), characterized by autophagic vacuoles in the cytoplasm and engorged endoplasmic reticula and Golgi complexes. Depending on the cell type, the intracellular target(s) for the induction of the apoptotic response can be the plasma membrane, DNA or both (63). Some cell types undergo extensive apoptosis within a few hours after treatment; others undergo apoptosis over a more prolonged period. This difference may be related to the relative expression and function of proteins activated within the **extrinsic or intrinsic pathways of apoptosis**. The extrinsic apoptotic pathway is initiated by tumor necrosis factor-alpha-related apoptosis-inducing ligand (TRAIL), a member of the tumor necrosis factor (TNF) superfamily. TRAIL induces apoptosis in response to external stimuli through clustering of receptors, DR4 and DR5 in the plasma membrane, thereby forming the death-inducing signaling complex (DISC). Subsequent recruitment of the adaptor molecule FADD and activation of caspases 8 and 10 lead to caspase 3–mediated cleavage of death-effector proteins [reviewed in (64)]. The intrinsic mitochondrial-based pathway can initiate apoptosis in response to radiation-induced DNA strand breaks, checkpoint defects, hypoxia and membrane damage. Both nuclear (e.g., ATM-*p53*) and membrane (e.g., ceramide) signals can activate this pathway. Following pro-apoptotic activation of BAX (a member of the *Bcl-2* gene superfamily), the mitochondrial membrane releases cytochrome c into the cytosol. Cytochrome c then binds to the adaptor protein APAF-1, forming an "apoptosome" that activates the apoptosis-initiating protease, caspase 9, which further activates caspases 3, 6, 7 and 8, thus contributing to the final morphology of apoptosis.

Many cancer therapies upregulate the expression of pro-apoptotic genes, such as *Fas*, *Bax* and enzymes such as caspase-3, and downregulate anti-apoptotic genes, such as *Bcl-2*. These apoptosis-related genes may be useful targets for improving therapy when used in combination with drug and radiation treatments. For example, altered BAX-to-*Bcl-2* protein ratios are associated with increased apoptosis and improved clinical responses in rectal, bladder and prostate cancers (65). The level of treatment-induced apoptosis varies between tumor and normal tissues and may be superceded by *p53*-mediated tumor cell growth-arrest. However, in highly radiosensitive tumor cells such as lymphoma, a wild type *p53* genotype predicts for increased radiation-induced apoptosis and decreased clonogenic cell survival. Tumor cells expressing mutant *p53* should therefore acquire relative radioresistance. However, radiation-induced apoptosis is *p53* independent in other tissues or tumors (66). *P53*-related clinical radiosensitization and prognostic studies using apoptosis as a target or endpoint are therefore reasonable if such strategies also focus on clonogenic cell kill.

Mitotic catastrophe is the failure of mammalian cells to properly undergo mitosis after DNA damage as a result of defective DNA repair and cell cycle checkpoint control. This leads to the formation of chromosome aberrations and abnormalities (tetraploidy or aneuploidy) as well as micronuclei due to erroneous chromosomal segregation. Cells have aberrant G2 checkpoint control due to deficient activation of the ataxia telangiectasia mutated (ATM) gene, ataxia telangiectasia and Rad3-related (ATR) gene, *p53* checkpoint kinases (CHK)1/2, polo-like kinase (PLK)1, survivin and/or 14–3-3σ signaling pathways. These pathways are prone to radiation-induced mitotic catastrophe due to an uncoupling of DNA repair and G2 phase cell cycle progression. Increased mitotic catastrophe in tumor cells can also be achieved by inhibiting or decreasing the duration of DNA repair during the G2 phase. These proteins are therefore novel targets for new molecular agents to sensitize tumors to radiotherapy and/or chemotherapy.

Finally, the concept of **cellular senescence** was first described in 1961 by Hayflick and Moorhead (67). These authors observed a finite life span for human diploid cells growing in culture and a resulting terminal growth arrest or "replicative senescence." Senescent cells acquire an enlarged, flattened shape with increased cytoplasmic and nuclear granularity and express the marker senescence-associated β-galactosidase (SA-β-gal) (68). Replicative senescence is associated with increased expression of several cyclin-dependent kinase (CDK) inhibitors, including p21$^{WAF1/CIP1}$ and p16^{INK4a} (69). Although senescent cells have lost their ability to divide, they remain metabolically active for an extended period before undergoing necrosis. A phenotype very similar to that of replicative senescence can also be induced in many cell types following exposure to DNA-damaging agents, including cisplatin, cyclophosphamide, doxorubicin and ionizing radiation. This terminal growth arrest has been variously called senescence-like growth arrest, accelerated, or premature senescence. Terminal arrest of tumor cells may explain the relatively slow resolution, yet ultimate cure of some tumors following chemotherapy or radiotherapy. If this is true, treatments that differentially enhance accelerated senescence in tumor cells may be useful adjuncts to conformal radiotherapy. For example, differentiation agents (e.g., retinoids), or histone deacetylase (HDAC) inhibitors have been used to induce a senescence-like phenotype and sensitize breast, prostate, glioma and head and neck cancer cells, both in vitro and in vivo [for review see (70, 71)].

Finally, recent publications have suggested that cells can undergo autophagy following DNA damage. These cells form an "autophagosome" that encapsulates cytoplasm and organelles leading to the degradation of organelle contents. Whether autophagy induced by cancer therapy contributes to tumor cell death or represents a mechanism of resistance to radiotherapy or chemotherapy is actively being investigated (72, 73).

In order to predict individual patient response to therapy, it is important to measure disparate mechanisms of cell death using intra- or post-treatment biopsies or non-invasive imaging. Non-invasive imaging (PET or SPECT scans) may become increasingly powerful as a means to quantify apoptosis or terminal growth arrest. The resulting improved understanding of cell death will optimize the rational selection of novel molecular agents and, ultimately, the cancer therapeutic ratio.

Tumor Angiogenesis

Sustained growth of tumors depends on the development of neovasculature because tumors need an efficient method for delivery of oxygen and nutrients and effective removal of metabolic wastes. Without a vascular supply and associated blood perfusion, tumor growth is constrained by slow oxygen delivery mediated by the processes of diffusion and convection, coupled with oxygen consumption by cells nearer the supply. The subsequent development of hypoxia, reduced glucose supply and microenvironmental acidification (hallmarks of ischemia) results in cell death. Depending on their oxygen requirement, cells may not thrive when they are separated by more than a few cells, or as little as 100 microns from the nearest capillary. Increased cell death at the supply periphery may balance cell proliferation, resulting in tumor growth stasis [reviewed in (74)].

Cells adapt to hypoxia largely by activating a transcriptional program mediated by members of the HIF family of transcription factors. HIFs activate transcription of many genes that help cells, tissues and the intact organism adapt to reduced oxygen levels. Genes encoding glucose transporters and glycolytic enzymes are among those upregulated, increasing the capacity of cells to generate ATP by anaerobic means. Genes encoding vasculogenic growth factors such as VEGF are upregulated, helping tissues reoxygenate by inducing neovascularization and increasing perfusion. The gene encoding erythropoietin may also be upregulated, helping the organism increase the oxygen-carrying capacity of blood by increasing erythrocyte production. Cell death is a potential outcome of nutrient deprivation, including oxygen, and HIFs and *p53* have been shown to participate in this cellular decision [reviewed in (74)].

New vessels can form by a variety of mechanisms; **angiogenesis** and **vasculogenesis** are the best understood [reviewed in (75)]. Vasculogenesis involves the migration of endothelial precursor cells from distant sites (e.g., bone marrow) to sites of new vessel formation. This is the process by which the very first vascular channels form early in embryogenesis. Angiogenesis involves formation of new vessels from cellular elements of nearby preexisting vessels and resembles the process of sprouting. Subsequent to the formation of the first vascular channels in embryogenesis, all vessels are believed to arise by angiogenic mechanisms. Indeed, angiogenesis is believed to be the primary mechanism giving rise to tumor vessels. In the past few years, vasculogenesis has been shown to contribute to tumor neovascularization, but the extent and circumstances of this contribution are poorly defined at present. Vasculogenic mimicry, a phenomenon seen in a number of aggressive tumor types, is discussed subsequently.

Once organisms reach adult size and growth stops, the physiological need for new blood vessels abates and angiogenesis ceases except during ovulation, the menstrual cycle and in healing wounds. Normal tissues are non-angiogenic because endogenous inhibitors are present and there are few, if any, stimuli for production of promoters. Even in non-cancerous situations, gratuitous angiogenesis can be pathogenic (e.g., diabetic retinopathy), so preventing this process is an important goal.

When tumors become angiogenic, the normal balance between anti- and pro-angiogenic factors (that normally favors the former) is altered to favor the latter. This can occur via increased production of pro-angiogenic factors (e.g., VEGF), decreased production of anti-angiogenic factors (e.g., thrombospondin-1) or a combination of both mechanisms. This so-called angiogenic switch (76) is a critical step in tumor progression because progressive tumor growth, invasion of surrounding tissues, and metastasis can occur only after the "switch" has occurred. Several occurrences during tumor progression may be responsible for this event. Activation of oncogenes and inactivation of tumor suppressor genes have been shown to enhance tumor cell production of VEGF and/or decrease tumor cell production of angiogenesis inhibitors. In addition, the presence of tumor hypoxia, common in many solid tumors, causes both neoplastic and stromal cells to upregulate VEGF production.

The dependency of tumor growth on neovascularization led Judah Folkman to first postulate that inhibiting new vessel formation would be an effective way to control tumor growth (77). Proponents have argued that there are conceptual advantages of this approach to cancer therapy. These benefits include 1) the expectation that all tumor types should respond to anti-angiogenic treatment; 2) treatment resistance should not develop because non-neoplastic endothelial cells are the targets of therapy and 3) treatment should be less toxic than conventional chemotherapeutic drugs and radiation. It was anticipated that

angiogenesis inhibition should not be used in situations in which physiologic angiogenesis is active (e.g., pregnancy and surgical wound healing). In addition, successful therapy might produce tumor stasis or slowed growth rather than frank regression and therefore may require administration over a prolonged period. As clinical experience with angiogenesis inhibitors has increased, some expectations of this therapy have had to be revised. Also, side effects that had not been anticipated have been encountered (e.g., hypertension, thromboembolism).

Many strategies are being explored in the massive effort by biotechnology and pharmaceutical companies to find effective angiogenesis inhibitors. Recombinant and synthetic forms of endogenous angiogenesis inhibitors, integrin antagonists and matrix metalloproteinase (MMP) inhibitors are among the agents being developed. However, the most common approach has been VEGF-VEGF receptor activity inhibition. This angiogenic signaling axis is a favored therapy target because VEGF is close to being a "universal" tumor angiogenesis factor; oncogenesis-related and hypoxia-induced VEGF overexpression is present in most, if not all, tumors. Inhibitors of VEGF action include antagonistic antibodies to VEGF and its receptors, decoy VEGF receptors and small molecule inhibitors of VEGF receptor kinase (which include two FDA-approved agents, sorafenib and sunitinib).

A humanized neutralizing antibody to VEGF, bevacizumab, was the first FDA-approved agent designed to inhibit angiogenesis. Randomized clinical trials of combination chemotherapy with or without bevacizumab in patients with metastatic colorectal carcinoma showed that drug treatment significantly improved tumor response and prolonged overall survival (78). Combining anti-angiogenic agents with chemotherapy has rationale in preclinical studies. Tumors overexpressing VEGF often have dilated, tortuous vessels that are extremely permeable (VEGF was initially named vascular permeability factor or VPF, because of its ability to induce vessel leakiness). These vessel abnormalities predispose to intermittent interruptions in regional tumor blood flow and high tumor interstitial fluid pressures, factors that adversely affect drug delivery to tumor cells. Therapy with VEGF antagonists has been shown to rapidly reverse these vascular abnormalities in mouse tumors, and some believe that the resultant improvement in chemotherapy delivery is responsible for improvements in therapeutic efficacy (79). Other complementary explanations for the benefits of combining anti-angiogenic and chemotherapy agents have been proposed as well but will not be discussed here. Whatever the basis of the interaction, this therapeutic paradigm is one that is likely to continue to be investigated (80).

Perhaps the major difficulty confronting clinical use of angiogenesis inhibitors is the issue of monitoring their effects and determining therapeutic efficacy. Standard clinical criteria used to evaluate efficacy of cytotoxic agents such as tumor regression are not useful for evaluating the efficacy of anti-angiogenic agents because they rarely induce tumor regression. The best result is often tumor stabilization or slowed growth, but these effects are often difficult to measure. Currently, there are no imaging modalities that reliably measure tumor angiogenic activity so imaging of tumor vascularity, perfusion and/or oxygenation are used as alternatives. Reversal of VEGF effects on vascular permeability may offer another way to image therapy with VEGF antagonists. Efforts are also underway to develop serologic and cellular biomarkers of angiogenic activity. At this time, even histology does not offer a satisfactory solution to the challenge. Besides the need for invasive procedures to obtain tumor tissue for study, only tumor vascularity (measured as mean vessel density, microvessel density or MVD) and not angiogenic activity can be evaluated histologically, and correlation between these two measures is often poor (81). Rational development and use of angiogenesis inhibitors is likely to depend on finding a reliable way to monitor the effects and efficacy of these emerging therapeutic agents. Although anti-angiogenic agents are gaining a place in clinical cancer therapy, this therapeutic strategy is still in its infancy and its role and uses have yet to be fully defined.

VASCULOGENIC MIMICRY

Cancer is a disease of the tumor-host microenvironment consisting of a complex, dynamic relationship that remains enigmatic. Similarly confounding is the expression of multiple cellular phenotypes by aggressive tumor cells such as melanoma, contributing to their "plasticity." The overarching hypothesis guiding the work in the Hendrix lab is that metastatic melanoma cells express a plastic, dedifferentiated phenotype capable of adapting to various microenvironments. One of the classic examples of tumor cell plasticity is the novel concept of vascu-

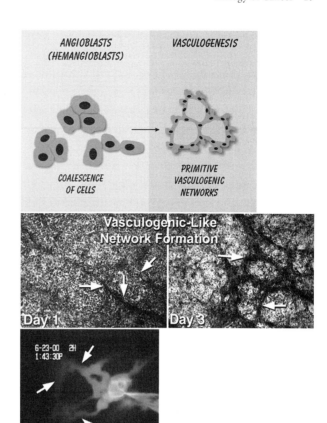

FIGURE 1.5. Schematic overview of vasculogenesis. *Upper panel*: Schematic overview of vasculogenesis, showing how endothelial cell precursors (angioblasts and hemangioblasts) coalesce and differentiate into endothelial cells that form primitive vasculogenic networks (vasculogenesis). Remodeling of these networks occurs through angiogenesis. *Lower panel*: The unique ability of aggressive melanoma cells to form vasculogenic-like networks (*arrows*) in 3-D collagen I in vitro while simultaneously expressing genes associated with an endothelial-like cell type – called vasculogenic mimicry. The ECM-rich networks are perfusable (with a fluorescent dye) by day 14. See Color Plate 5.

logenic mimicry, the unique ability of aggressive melanoma cells to express an endothelial-like cell phenotype and to form vasculogenic-like networks in 3-D culture. These processes "mimic" the pattern of embryonic vasculogenic networks, recapitulate the patterned networks seen in aggressive human tumors, and correlate with a poor prognosis (Figure 1.5).

To further understand the molecular underpinnings of vasculogenic mimicry, particularly endothelial transdifferentiation of the aggressive melanoma phenotype, the molecular signature(s) of various human melanoma cell lines isolated from poorly aggressive and aggressive tumors has been deciphered. Comparative global gene analyses of these cell lines, which were isogenically matched, revealed an unexpected finding. The aggressive tumor cells express genes (and proteins) associated with multiple cellular phenotypes and their respective precursor stem cells, including endothelial, epithelial, pericyte, fibroblast, hematopoietic, kidney, neuronal, muscle, and several other cell types (82–84). These intriguing findings support the premise that aggressive melanoma cells can acquire a multipotent, plastic phenotype. This is a concept that challenges our current thinking of how to target tumor cells that can masquerade as other cell types, particularly with embryonic stem cell–like properties.

The most significantly upregulated genes by aggressive melanoma cells include those that are involved in angiogenesis and vasculogenesis, such as the genes encoding vascular endothelial (VE)-cadherin, erythropoietin-producing hepatocellular carcinoma-A2 (EphA2), MMPs and laminin $5\gamma2$ chain (LAMC2). These molecules, with their binding partners, are a few of the factors that are required for the formation and maintenance of blood vessels and vasculogenic mimicry. Vasculogenic mimicry has been confirmed by other investigators in melanoma as well as in breast carcinoma, prostatic carcinoma, ovarian carcinoma, lung carcinoma, *Drosophila* tumors (large tumor suppressor gene, lats-negative), synoviosarcoma, rhabdomyosarcoma, pheochromocytoma, Ewing sarcoma, and cytotrophoblasts forming the placenta (85, 86). Recent data indicate an evolution in the concept of melanoma vasculogenic mimicry to that of a melanoma fluid-conducting extracellular matrix (ECM) meshwork. Work has begun on elucidating the functional relevance of this extravascular, fluid-conducting ECM meshwork that provides a site for nutritional exchange for aggressive tumors and might therefore prevent tumor necrosis (Figure 1.6). Further microdissection of the complex geometry of the melanoma-formed ECM meshwork found laminin to be a key component of this feature. The networks encase nests of tumor cells, which are hypothesized to form a suppressive shield against immune surveillance.

Studies on the molecular dissection of the physiological mechanisms critical to the function of the fluid-conducting meshwork revealed the biological relevance of the upregulated expression of tissue factor pathway–associated genes. They are essential for the anticoagulation properties of the intratumoral, ECM-rich extravascular fluid–conducting pathway. Specifically, subcutaneous injection of nude (immunodeficient) mice with fluorescently tagged

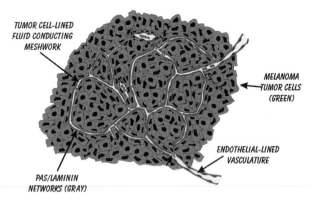

FIGURE 1.6. The biological implications of melanoma vasculogenic mimicry have evolved to a "tumor cell–lined, fluid-conducting meshwork" corresponding to periodic acid-Schiff (PAS) and laminin-positive, patterned networks. This diagram represents the current interpretation of data generated from several studies involving the use of tracers and perfusion analyses of mice containing aggressive melanoma cells (green) during tumor development. The endothelial-lined vasculature is closely apposed to the tumor cell–formed fluid-conducting meshwork, and it is suggested that as the tumor remodels, the vasculature becomes leaky, resulting in the extravascular conduction of plasma. There is also evidence of a physiological connection between the endothelial-lined vasculature and the extravascular melanoma perfusion meshwork. See Color Plate 6.

human aggressive cutaneous melanoma cells allowed the study of the blood supply to primary tumors (85). Using confocal microscopic imaging, perfusion of the mouse vasculature with a fluorescent tag and microbeads during tumor development revealed the close association of tumor-cell–lined networks with angiogenic mouse vessels at the human-mouse interface. The delivery of microbeads from the endothelium-lined mouse vasculature to the tumor-cell–lined networks indicated a physiological connection between the two compartments. Further invasive growth of melanoma into the vasculature led to the observation of erythrocytes and plasma in the tumor-cell–lined, fluid-conducting meshwork. As a follow up to these initial studies, the Hendrix lab uncovered the mechanism(s) underlying the physiological blood flow of human melanoma xenografts using color Doppler imaging (87). On the basis of gene profiling, protein detection and IHC validation, aggressive melanoma showed upregulation of tissue factor (TF), TF pathway inhibitor 1 (TFPI-1) and TFPI-2 compared with less aggressive tumors; these are critical genes that initiate and regulate the coagulation pathways. These data further illustrate that melanoma exhibits endothelial cell–like

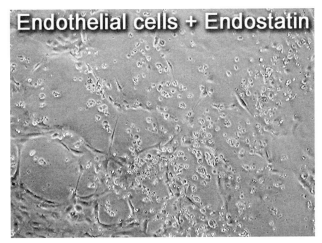

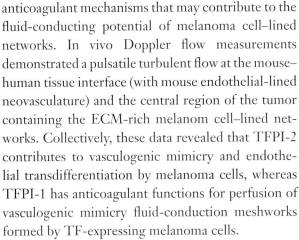

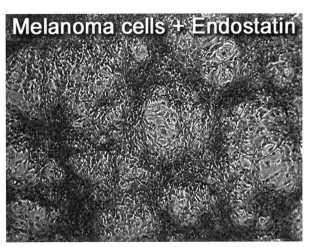

Angiogenesis is inhibited

VM is unaffected

FIGURE 1.7. Phase contrast microscopy of human microvascular endothelial cells. This image shows inhibition of angiogenesis in cells treated with endostatin (*left panel*) vs. human aggressive melanoma cells treated similarly (*right panel*), where vasculogenic mimicry (VM) and network formation are unaffected.

anticoagulant mechanisms that may contribute to the fluid-conducting potential of melanoma cell–lined networks. In vivo Doppler flow measurements demonstrated a pulsatile turbulent flow at the mouse–human tissue interface (with mouse endothelial-lined neovasculature) and the central region of the tumor containing the ECM-rich melanom cell–lined networks. Collectively, these data revealed that TFPI-2 contributes to vasculogenic mimicry and endothelial transdifferentiation by melanoma cells, whereas TFPI-1 has anticoagulant functions for perfusion of vasculogenic mimicry fluid-conduction meshworks formed by TF-expressing melanoma cells.

Additional studies have addressed the possible clinical implications of the properties shared in common by aggressive melanoma cells and endothelial cells. These include the expression of endothelial cell-specific genes and the ability of both cell types to form vascular networks. The effects of specific angiogenesis inhibitors (i.e., anginex, TNP-470 and endostatin) on melanoma cells were examined to determine whether they would have an inhibitory effect on vasculogenic mimicry in a manner similar to their inhibition of endothelial cell–driven angiogenesis (88). Anginex, TNP-470 and endostatin markedly inhibited vascular cord and tube formation by endothelial cells *in vitro*, whereas tubular network formation by melanoma cells was relatively unaffected (Figure 1.7). Endothelial cells expressed higher mRNA and protein levels for two putative endostatin receptors, α_5 integrin and heparin sulfate proteogly-

can 2, compared with melanoma cells, illuminating a mechanistic basis for the differential response of the two cell types to angiogenesis inhibitors. These findings may contribute to the development of new anti-vascular therapeutic agents that target both angiogenesis and tumor cell vasculogenic mimicry.

The Tumor Pathophysiologic Microenvironment in Progression and Metastasis

The blood vasculature that develops as solid tumors grow is characterized by severe structural and functional abnormalities and a lack of functional lymphatics resulting in a unique pathophysiological microenvironment. Most tumors have high interstitial fluid pressure (IFP), low glucose concentrations, pH_e and regions of chronic hypoxia and regions where oxygen concentration fluctuates significantly (89, 90). The microenvironment in tumors is heterogeneous within and between individual tumors – even among those of the same histopathologic type (Figure 1.8). Studies in a number of different human tumor types have demonstrated that measured levels of hypoxia are predictive of treatment failure both locally and distantly, and data from cervix cancers indicate that high IFP levels are similarly predictive, independent of the level of tumor hypoxia (91).

In the context of approaches to improve treatment for solid tumors, these findings raise two inter-related issues. First, what are the mechanisms by which the pathophysiologic environment contributes to the development of more aggressive disease and

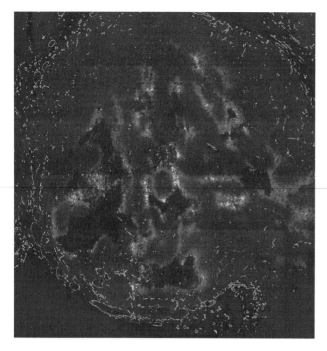 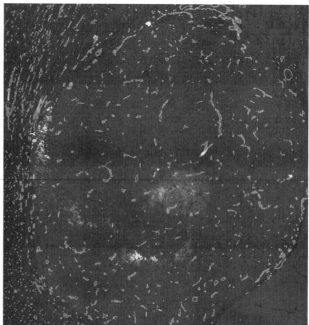

←——— 2mm ———→   ←——— 1mm ———→

FIGURE 1.8. Tumor heterogeneity. Images of two individual xenografts of human SiHa cervix cancer stained with fluorescent markers for hypoxia (EF5 – red), blood vessels (CD31 – green) and perfusion (Hoechst 33342 dye – blue). These tumors show considerable heterogeneity in these markers even though they were transplanted with cells from the same cell suspension into identical sites in two SCID mice. (From Vukovic V, Nicklee T, and Hedley DW. Multiparameter fluorescence mapping of nonprotein sulfhydryl status in relation to blood vessels and hypoxia in cervical carcinoma xenografts. Int J Radiat Oncol Biol Phys, 2002; 52: 837–843, with permission.) See Color Plate 7.

metastasis? Second, how can current methods of assessing the tumor microenvironment in human cancers be improved? Of particular interest are non-invasive approaches that can be used to measure both spatial and temporal changes prior to and during treatment. Such measurements would allow assessment of whether microenvironmental features could act as biomarkers to monitor treatment success. This is particularly applicable to new treatment strategies targeted at specific aspects of the tumor microenvironment, such as blood vasculature.

The most widely accepted hypothesis to explain why tumors tend to progress to more aggressive phenotypes as they grow, including ability to metastasize, is that the tumor cells have acquired genetic instability. This results in accumulation of both genetic and epigenetic changes that enhance the tumor's ability to resist mechanisms that would normally induce cell death (e.g., apoptosis) and to grow independently of normal growth controls. Examples of how the tumor microenvironment can be involved in this process include observations that exposure to hypoxia can impair the ability of cells to repair DNA damage,

cause mutations and both select for and induce gene expression changes causing resistance to apoptosis (92–94).

Metastasis is a complex process (Figure 1.9) involving a number of sequential steps: 1) escape (intravasation) of tumor cells from the primary tumor mass into either the blood or lymphatic circulation; 2) survival in the circulation and arrest at a new distant site (blood-borne cells) or in adjacent lymph nodes (cells in the lymphatic system); 3) escape (extravasation) from the vessels into the interstitial space at the new location; 4) initiation of growth at the new site to form a new tumor mass and 5) induction of angiogenesis to provide new blood vessels to supply nutrients to the growing tumor mass. Tumor cells that form successful metastases must be able to complete all these steps either individually or in cooperation with local stromal cells. The vast majority of tumor cells that reach the circulation fail to complete the later steps; metastasis is recognized as a very inefficient process. This inefficiency has made it difficult to monitor cells undergoing the processes of metastasis. However, the recent application of intravital

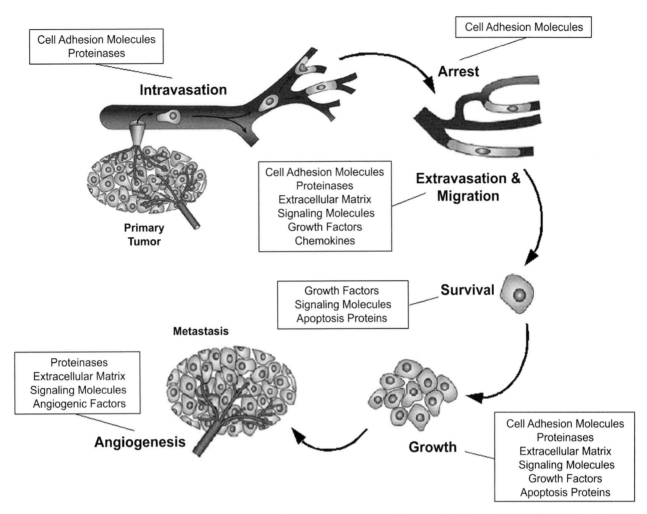

FIGURE 1.9. Metastasis Diagram. Schematic diagram illustrating the various stages of the metastatic process. (Modified from Khokha R, Voura E, and Hill RP. Tumor progression and metastasis: Cellular, molecular, and microenvironmental factors. In: Tannock IF, Hill RP, Bristow RG, et al. (eds.), The Basic Science of Oncology, 4th edition, pp. 205–230. New York: McGraw Hill, 2005, with permission.)

videomicroscopy (IVVM) has allowed tracking of fluorescence-labeled cells through these processes. Studies using IVVM have indicated the importance of the later "initiation of growth" stage for effective metastasis (step 4) (95). The development of fluorescent labels that can be genetically incorporated into cells (e.g., enhanced green fluorescent protein, DsRed, luciferase) has enhanced the ability to track tumor cells in vivo because these can often be viewed non-invasively [Figure 1.10 and (96)].

There is substantial evidence that metastatic cells express specific phenotypes that enhance their ability to form a metastasis (97). Furthermore, it is well recognized that there is a preference for tumor cells of certain histopathologic types to metastasize to specific organs (e.g., mammary and prostate cancers to bone, lung cancers and melanomas to brain) as well as to the common sites of lymph nodes, lungs and liver.

These observations provide support for a hypothesis regarding metastasis formation that was postulated more than 100 years ago (98, 99). The so-called soil and seed hypothesis was based on the idea that tumor cell–host organ interactions are critical in determining a tumor's metastatic potential. The preference of specific tumors for metastasis to specific organs reflects the concept that specific organs provide a more suitable environment for both arrest and growth of cells of a particular tumor type. For example, studies have linked the expression of a specific chemokine receptor (CXCR4) on mammary tumor cells to increased ability to home to and grow in bone (100). However, the propensity of many tumors to form lung or liver metastases may also reflect the fact that cells released into the circulation will tend to be arrested in the first-pass organ, thus producing a high cell burden there. There is also evidence that

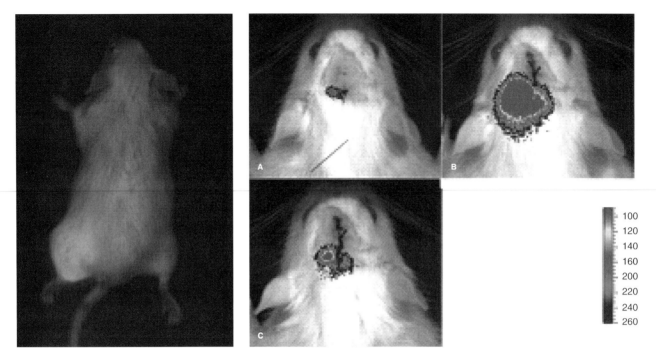

FIGURE 1.10. Examples of fluorescence imaging of tumors and bioluminescence imaging of gene activity. The left panel illustrates a tumor labeled with green fluorescent protein, imaged with a charge couple device (CCD) camera. The right group of panels illustrate a tumor growing from cells containing a luciferase gene driven by a hypoxia-sensitive promoter implanted into the brain of a rat. Injecting luciferin into the rat allows the luciferase protein to produce a burst of light that can be imaged with a CCD camera. The animal was imaged prior to treatment with pho-todynamic therapy (PDT) and then at 4 and 24 hours. (A) Prior to treatment, there is little signal because the extent of hypoxia is limited. (B) The image at 4 hours demonstrates that hypoxia, induced by the PDT caused the production of luciferase, which was able to produce light. (C) By 24 hours, hypoxia was decreased and much of the luciferase protein had been degraded, resulting in a reduced signal. (Courtesy of Drs. Wilson and Moriyama, Ontario Cancer Institute.) See Color Plate 8.

increased resistance to apoptosis may play an important role in lung metastasis (94, 101).

Exposure of cells to certain conditions in the tumor microenvironment, such as hypoxia and acid pH, has been reported to enhance their metastatic ability (102–104). The mechanisms involved are believed to result from changes in gene expression associated with exposure to stress conditions. Hypoxia, in particular, has been estimated to cause expression changes in hundreds of genes, many of which are required for survival under such conditions. Some of these gene expression changes have been demonstrated (in animal tumor models) to be capable of modifying the ability of tumor cells to form metastases. Examples include the increased expression of 1) the angiogenesis-associated proteins, such as VEGF and IL-8, 2) proteins involved in degradation of tissue matrix and invasion such as plasminogen activation receptor (uPAR), certain MMPs and lysyl oxidase (LOX), 3) proteins involved in control of apoptosis such as Fas or mdm-2 through the *p53* pathway, 4) cellular growth receptors such as c-met or the chemokine receptor CXCR4 and 5) extracellular matrix proteins such as osteopontin (OPN) that may enhance cellular adhesion or invasive properties of cells (94, 103, 104). Similarly, acidity has been reported to enhance the invasive ability of tumor cells by upregulating the activity of proteolytic enzymes [see earlier discussion and (59)]. Recently, developments in molecular imaging suggest that it may soon be possible to track changes in the expression of such genes in vivo during tumor growth [see Figure 1.10 and (105)].

Many of the studies measuring tumor oxygenation, acidity and IFP in tumors have relied on invasive needle probes that limit the measurements to accessible tumors and the extent to which monitoring over time is possible. For measurements of tumor oxygenation, a wide range of other techniques have been developed, including use of both exogenous and endogenous markers that are bound or expressed specifically in hypoxic cells (see earlier discussion and Figure 1.8). To date, these markers have largely been assessed using IHC, and a number of these studies have demonstrated a correlation between the extent of expression of these hypoxia markers in a tumor and more aggressive disease (1, 106). A variety of non-invasive approaches are currently being developed, including PET and SPECT imaging (107). Both functional MR and computed tomographic (CT) imaging are being used to assess features of tumor blood flow and tissue perfusion [e.g., (108, 109)] and recent work has also reported the use of MR imaging to assess tissue fluid flow and pHe (110). These characteristics contribute to increased IFP (111). The further development of these non-invasive techniques should allow an assessment of whether features of the microenvironment can act as biomarkers to monitor the success of new treatment strategies targeted at specific aspects of the tumor microenvironment.

REFERENCES

1. Bussink J, Kaanders JH, and van der Kogel AJ. Tumor hypoxia at the micro-regional level: Clinical relevance and predictive value of exogenous and endogenous hypoxic cell markers. Radiother Oncol 2003;67:3–15.

2. Evans S and Koch C. Prognostic significance of tumor oxygenation in humans. Cancer Lett 2003;195:1–16.

3. Thomlinson RH and Gray LH. The histological structure of some human lung cancers and the possible implications for radiotherapy. Br J Cancer 1955;9:539–579.

4. Brown JM. Evidence for acutely hypoxic cells in mouse tumours, and a possible mechanism of reoxygenation. British Journal of Radiology 1979;52:650–656.

5. Chaplin DJ, Durand RE, and Olive PL. Acute hypoxia in tumors: Implications for modifiers of radiation effects. International Journal of Radiation Oncology, Biology, Physics, 1986;12:1279–1282.

6. Dewhirst MW, Ong ET, Braun RD, et al. Quantification of longitudinal tissue pO2 gradients in window chamber tumours: Impact on tumour hypoxia. Br J Cancer 1999;79:1717–1722.

7. Holthusen H. Beitrage zur biologie der strahlenwirkung: Undersuchungen an ascarideneiern. Arch Ges Physiol 1921;187:1–24.

8. Hall EJ. Radiobiology for the Radiologist, 5th edition. New York: Harper and Row 2000.

9. Chapman JD, Gillespie CJ, Reuvers AP, et al. The inactivation of Chinese hamster cells by X-rays: The effect of chemical modifiers on single and double events. Radiat Res 1975;64:365–375.

10. Dische S. Keynote address: hypoxic cell sensitizers: Clinical developments. International Journal of Radiation Oncology, Biology, Physics 1989;16:1057–1060.

11. Urtasun RC, Coleman CN, Wasserman TH, et al. Clinical trials with hypoxic cell sensitizers: Time to retrench or time to push forward? International Journal of Radiation Oncology, Biology, Physics, 1984;10:1691–1696.

12. Brown JM. SR 4233 (tirapazamine): A new anticancer drug exploiting hypoxia in solid tumours. Br J Cancer 1993;67:1163–1170.

13. Del Rowe J, Scott C, Werner-Wasik M, et al. Single-arm, open-label phase II study of intravenously administered tirapazamine and radiation therapy for glioblastoma multiforme. J Clin Oncol 2000;18:1254–1259.

14. Overgaard J, Hansen HS, Overgaard M, et al. A randomized double-blind phase III study of nimorazole as a hypoxic radiosensitizer of primary radiotherapy in supraglottic larynx and pharynx carcinoma. Results of the Danish Head and Neck Cancer Study (DAHANCA) Protocol 5–85. Radiother Oncol 1998;46:135–146.

15. Kaanders JH, Pop LA, Marres HA, et al. ARCON: Experience in 215 patients with advanced head-and-neck cancer. International Journal of Radiation Oncology, Biology, Physics 2002;52: 769–778.

16. Becker A, Kuhnt T, Liedtke H, et al. Oxygenation measurements in head and neck cancers during hyperbaric oxygenation. Strahlentherapie und Onkologie 2002;178:105–108.

17. Brizel DM, Lin S, Johnson JL, et al. The mechanisms by which hyperbaric oxygen and carbogen improve tumour oxygenation. Br J Cancer 1995;72:1120–1124.

18. Brizel DM, Scully SP, Harrelson JM, et al. Radiation therapy and hyperthermia improve the oxygenation of human soft tissue sarcomas. Cancer Res 1996;56:5347–5350.

19. Gatenby RA, Coia LR, Richter MP, et al. Oxygen tension in human tumors: In vivo mapping using CT-guided probes. Radiology 1985;156:211–214.

20. Gatenby RA, Kessler HB, Rosenblum JS, et al. Oxygen distribution in squamous cell carcinoma metastases and its relationship to outcome of radiation therapy. International Journal of Radiation Oncology, Biology, Physics 1988;14:831–838.

21. Evans SM, Hahn SM, Magarelli DP, et al. Hypoxia in human intraperitoneal and extremity sarcomas. International Journal of Radiation Oncology, Biology, Physics 2001;49:587–596.

22. Evans SM, Judy KD, Dunphy I, et al. Hypoxia is important in the biology and aggression of human glial brain tumors [see comment]. Clin Cancer Res 2004;10:8177–8184.

23. Nordsmark M, Loncaster J, Chou SC, et al. Invasive oxygen measurements and pimonidazole labeling in human cervix carcinoma. International Journal of Radiation Oncology, Biology, Physics 2001;49:581–586.

24. Evans SM, Judy KD, Dunphy I, et al. Comparative measurements of hypoxia in human brain tumors using needle electrodes and EF5 binding. Cancer Res 2004;64:1886–1892.

25. Semenza GL and Wang GL. A nuclear factor induced by hypoxia via de novo protein synthesis binds to the human erythropoietin gene enhancer at a site required for transcriptional activation. Mol Cell Biol 1992;12:5447–5454.

26. Lahiri S, Roy A, Baby SM, et al. Oxygen sensing in the body. Progr Biophys Mol Biol 2006;91:249–286.

27. Walmsley SR, McGovern NN, Whyte MK, et al. The HIF/VHL pathway: From oxygen sensing to innate immunity. American Journal of Respiratory Cell & Molecular Biology 2008;38:251–255.

28. Hoskin PJ, Sibtain A, Daley FM, et al. GLUT1 and CAIX as intrinsic markers of hypoxia in bladder cancer: Relationship with vascularity and proliferation as

predictors of outcome of ARCON. Br J Cancer 2003;89:1290–1297.

29. Koukourakis MI, Bentzen SM, Giatromanolaki A, et al. Endogenous markers of two separate hypoxia response pathways (hypoxia inducible factor 2 alpha and carbonic anhydrase 9) are associated with radiotherapy failure in head and neck cancer patients recruited in the CHART randomized trial. J Clin Oncol 2006; 24: 727–735. Epub Jan 17, 2006.

30. Sorensen BS, Hao J, Overgaard J, et al. Influence of oxygen concentration and pH on expression of hypoxia-induced genes. Radiother Oncol 2005;76:187–193.

31. Williams AC, Collard TJ, and Paraskeva C. An acidic environment leads to p53 dependent induction of apoptosis in human adenoma and carcinoma cell lines: Implications for clonal selection during colorectal carcinogenesis. Oncogene 1999;18:3199–3204.

32. Ballinger JR. Imaging hypoxia in tumors. Semin Nucl Med 2001;31:321–329.

33. Prekeges JL, Rasey JS, Grunbaum Z, et al. Reduction of fluoromisonidazole, a new imaging agent for hypoxia. Biochem Pharmacol 1991;42:2387–2395.

34. Loeb LA. Mutator phenotype may be required for multistage carcinogenesis. Cancer Res 1991;51:3075–3079.

35. Rabinovitch PS, Reid BJ, Haggitt RC, et al. Progression to cancer in Barrett's esophagus is associated with genomic instability. Laboratory Investigation 1989;60:65–71.

36. Peinado MA, Malkhosyan S, Velazquez A, et al. Isolation and characterization of allelic losses and gains in colorectal tumors by arbitrarily primed polymerase chain reaction. Proceedings of the National Academy of Sciences of the United States of America 1992;89:10065–10069.

37. Jiang F, Desper R, Papadimitriou CH, et al. Construction of evolutionary tree models for renal cell carcinoma from comparative genomic hybridization data. Cancer Res 2000;60:6503–6509.

38. Kerangueven F, Noguchi T, Coulier F, et al. Genome-wide search for loss of heterozygosity shows extensive genetic diversity of human breast carcinomas. Cancer Res 1997;57:5469–5474.

39. Warburg O, Wind F, and Negelein E. On the metabolism of tumors in the body. In The Metabolism of Tumors, pp. 256, Ch. 215. London: Constable and Co 1930.

40. Di Chiro G, Hatazawa J, Katz DA, et al. Glucose utilization by intracranial meningiomas as an index of tumor aggressivity and probability of recurrence: A PET study. Radiology 1987;164:521–526.

41. Haberkorn U, Strauss LG, Reisser C, et al. Glucose uptake, perfusion, and cell proliferation in head and neck tumors: Relation of positron emission tomography to flow cytometry [see comment]. J Nucl Med 1991;32:1548–1555.

42. Hawkins RA, Hoh C, Glaspy J, et al. The role of positron emission tomography in oncology and other whole-body applications. Semin Nucl Med 1992;22:268–284.

43. Yonekura Y, Benua RS, Brill AB, et al. Increased accumulation of 2-deoxy-2-[18F]fluoro-D-glucose in liver metastases from colon carcinoma. J Nucl Med 1982;23:1133–1137.

44. Griffiths JR. Are cancer cells acidic? Br J Cancer 1991;64:425–427.

45. Gillies RJ, Liu Z, and Bhujwalla Z. 31P-MRS measurements of extracellular pH of tumors using 3-aminopropylphosphonate. Am J Physiol 1994;267: C195–203.

46. Martin GR and Jain RK. Noninvasive measurement of interstitial pH profiles in normal and neoplastic tissue using fluorescence ratio imaging microscopy. Cancer Res 1994;54:5670–5674.

47. Stubbs M, Rodrigues L, Howe FA, et al. Metabolic consequences of a reversed pH gradient in rat tumors. Cancer Res 1994;54:4011–4016.

48. Park HJ, Lyons JC, Ohtsubo T, et al. Acidic environment causes apoptosis by increasing caspase activity. Br J Cancer 1999;80:1892–1897.

49. Casciari JJ, Sotirchos SV, and Sutherland RM. Variations in tumor cell growth rates and metabolism with oxygen concentration, glucose concentration, and extracellular pH. J Cell Physiol 1992;151:386–394.

50. Dairkee SH, Deng G, Stampfer MR, et al. Selective cell culture of primary breast carcinoma. Cancer Res 1995;55:2516–2519.

51. Rubin H. pH and population density in the regulation of animal cell multiplication. J Cell Biol 1971;51:686–702.

52. Gatenby RA and Gillies RJ. Why do cancers have high aerobic glycolysis? Nature Reviews. Cancer 2004;4: 891–899.

53. Gatenby RA and Vincent TL. An evolutionary model of carcinogenesis. Cancer Res 2003;63:6212–6220.

54. Gatenby RA. The potential role of transformation-induced metabolic changes in tumor-host interaction. Cancer Res 1995;55:4151–4156.

55. Gatenby RA and Gawlinski ET. A reaction-diffusion model of cancer invasion. Cancer Res 1996;56:5745–5753.

56. Patz EF Jr, Lowe VJ, Hoffman JM, et al. Persistent or recurrent bronchogenic carcinoma: Detection with PET and 2-[F-18]-2-deoxy-D-glucose. Radiology 1994;191:379–382.

57. Rozhin J, Sameni M, Ziegler G, et al. Pericellular pH affects distribution and secretion of cathepsin B in malignant cells. Cancer Res 1994;54:6517–6525.

58. Lardner A. The effects of extracellular pH on immune function. Journal of Leukocyte Biology 2001;69:522–530.

59. Gatenby RA, Gawlinski ET, Gmitro AF, et al. Acid-mediated tumor invasion: A multidisciplinary study. Cancer Res 2006;66:5216–5223.

60. Bristow R and Hill R. Molecular and Cellular Basis of Radiotherapy. In: Basic Science of Oncology New York City: McGraw Hill Publishers 1998.

61. Bromfield GP, Meng A, Warde P, et al. Cell death in irradiated prostate epithelial cells: Role of apoptotic and clonogenic cell kill. Prostate Cancer & Prostatic Diseases 2003;6:73–85.

62. Brown JM and Wouters BG. Apoptosis: Mediator or mode of cell killing by anticancer agents?[comment]. Drug Resistance Updates 2001;4:135–136.

63. Abend M. Reasons to reconsider the significance of apoptosis for cancer therapy. Int J Radiat Biol 2003;79:927–941.

64. Shankar S, Singh TR, and Srivastava RK. Ionizing radiation enhances the therapeutic potential of TRAIL in

prostate cancer in vitro and in vivo: Intracellular mechanisms. Prostate 2004;61:35–49.

65. Mackey TJ, Borkowski A, Amin P, et al. bcl-2/bax ratio as a predictive marker for therapeutic response to radiotherapy in patients with prostate cancer. Urology 1998;52:1085–1090.

66. Cuddihy AR and Bristow RG. The p53 protein family and radiation sensitivity: Yes or no? Cancer & Metastasis Reviews 2004;23:237–257.

67. Hayflick L and Moorehead P. The serial cultivation of human diploid cell strains. Experimental Cell Research 1961;25:585–561.

68. Dimri GP, Lee X, Basile G, et al. A biomarker that identifies senescent human cells in culture and in aging skin in vivo. Proceedings of the National Academy of Sciences of the United States of America 1995;92:9363–9367.

69. Sedelnikova OA, Horikawa I, Zimonjic DB, et al. Senescing human cells and ageing mice accumulate DNA lesions with unrepairable double-strand breaks. Nature Cell Biology 2004;6:168–170.

70. Biade S, Stobbe CC, Boyd JT, et al. Chemical agents that promote chromatin compaction radiosensitize tumour cells. Int J Radiat Biol 2001;77:1033–1042.

71. Camphausen K, Burgan W, Cerra M, et al. Enhanced radiation-induced cell killing and prolongation of gammaH2AX foci expression by the histone deacetylase inhibitor MS-275. Cancer Res 2004;64:316–321.

72. Apel A, Herr I, Schwarz H, et al. Blocked autophagy sensitizes resistant carcinoma cells to radiation therapy. Cancer Res 2008;68:1485–1494.

73. Galluzzi L, Miguel J, Kepp V, et al. To die or not to die: That is the autophagic question. Curr Mol Med 2008;8:78–91.

74. Carmeliet P and Jain RK. Angiogenesis in cancer and other diseases. Nature 2000;407:249–257.

75. Risau W. Mechanisms of angiogenesis. Nature 1997;386:671–674.

76. Hanahan D and Folkman J. Patterns and emerging mechanisms of the angiogenic switch during tumorigenesis. Cell 1996;86:353–364.

77. Folkman J. Tumor angiogenesis: Therapeutic implications. N Engl J Med 1971;285:1182–1186.

78. Hurwitz H, Fehrenbacher L, Novotny W, et al. Bevacizumab plus irinotecan, fluorouracil, and leucovorin for metastatic colorectal cancer [see comment]. N Engl J Med 2004;350:2335–2342.

79. Jain RK. Normalization of tumor vasculature: An emerging concept in antiangiogenic therapy. Science 2005;307:58–62.

80. Kerbel RS. Antiangiogenic therapy: a universal chemosensitization strategy for cancer? Science 2006;312:1171–1175.

81. Hlatky L, Hahnfeldt P, and Folkman J. Clinical application of antiangiogenic therapy: Microvessel density, what it does and doesn't tell us [see comment]. J Natl Cancer Inst 2002;94:883–893.

82. Hendrix MJ, Seftor EA, Hess AR, et al. Molecular plasticity of human melanoma cells. Oncogene 2003;22:3070–3075.

83. Seftor EA, Meltzer PS, Kirschmann DA, et al. Molecular determinants of human uveal melanoma invasion and metastasis. Clinical & Experimental Metastasis 2002;19:233–246.

84. Seftor EA, Meltzer PS, Schatteman GC, et al. Expression of multiple molecular phenotypes by aggressive melanoma tumor cells: Role in vasculogenic mimicry. Crit Rev Oncol Hematol 2002;44:17–27.

85. Hendrix M, Seftor E, Meltzer P, et al. The stem cell plasticity of aggressive melanoma cells. In: Sell E (ed.), Germinal Stem Cells, Vol. 1, pp. 297–306. USA: Humana Press 2003.

86. van der Schaft DW, Hillen F, Pauwels P, et al. Tumor cell plasticity in Ewing sarcoma, an alternative circulatory system stimulated by hypoxia. Cancer Res 2005;65:11520–11528.

87. Ruf W, Seftor EA, Petrovan RJ, et al. Differential role of tissue factor pathway inhibitors 1 and 2 in melanoma vasculogenic mimicry. Cancer Res 2003;63:5381–5389.

88. van der Schaft DW, Seftor RE, Seftor EA, et al. Effects of angiogenesis inhibitors on vascular network formation by human endothelial and melanoma cells. J Natl Cancer Inst 2004;96:1473–1477.

89. Dewhirst MW. Mechanisms underlying hypoxia development in tumors. Adv Exp Med Biol 2003;510:51–56.

90. Vaupel P, Kelleher DK, and Hockel M. Oxygen status of malignant tumors: Pathogenesis of hypoxia and significance for tumor therapy. Semin Oncol 2001;28:29–35.

91. Milosevic M, Fyles A, Hedley D, et al. The human tumor microenvironment: invasive (needle) measurement of oxygen and interstitial fluid pressure. Semin Radiat Oncol 2004;14:249–258.

92. Bindra RS and Glazer PM. Genetic instability and the tumor microenvironment: Towards the concept of microenvironment-induced mutagenesis. Mutation Research 2005;569:75–85.

93. Graeber TG, Osmanian C, Jacks T, et al. Hypoxia-mediated selection of cells with diminished apoptotic potential in solid tumours [see comment]. Nature 1996;379:88–91.

94. Zhang L and Hill RP. Hypoxia enhances metastatic efficiency by up-regulating Mdm2 in KHT cells and increasing resistance to apoptosis. Cancer Res 2004;64:4180–4189.

95. Chambers AF, Groom AC, and MacDonald IC. Dissemination and growth of cancer cells in metastatic sites. Nature Reviews. Cancer 2002;2:563–572.

96. Hoffman RM. The multiple uses of fluorescent proteins to visualize cancer in vivo. Nature Reviews. Cancer 2005;5:796–806.

97. Khokha R, Voura E, and Hill R. Tumor progression and metastasis: Cellular, molecular, and microenvironmental factors. In: Tannock RH IF, Bristow RG, et al. (ed.), The Basic Science of Oncology, 4 edition, pp. 205–230. New York: McGraw Hill 2005.

98. Paget S. The distribution of secondary growths in cancer of the breast. Lancet 1889;1:571–573.

99. Fidler IJ. The pathogenesis of cancer metastasis: The 'seed and soil' hypothesis revisited. Nature Reviews. Cancer 2003;3:453–458.

100. Kucia M, Reca R, Miekus K, et al. Trafficking of normal stem cells and metastasis of cancer stem cells involve similar mechanisms: pivotal role of the SDF-1-CXCR4 axis. Stem Cells 2005;23:879–894.

101. Wong CW, Lee A, Shientag L, et al. Apoptosis: An early event in metastatic inefficiency. Cancer Res 2001;61: 333–338.

102. Hill RP., De Jaeger K, Jang A, et al. pH, hypoxia and metastasis. Novartis Foundation Symposium 2001;240:154–165; discussion 165–158.

103. Rofstad EK. Microenvironment-induced cancer metastasis. Int J Radiat Biol 2000;76:589–605.

104. Subarsky P and Hill RP. The hypoxic tumour microenvironment and metastatic progression. Clinical & Experimental Metastasis 2003;20:237–250.

105. Gross S and Piwnica-Worms D. Spying on cancer: Molecular imaging in vivo with genetically encoded reporters. Cancer Cell 2005;7:5–15.

106. Harris AL. Hypoxia–a key regulatory factor in tumour growth. Nature Reviews. Cancer 2002;2:38–47.

107. Koch CJ and Evans SM. Non-invasive PET and SPECT imaging of tissue hypoxia using isotopically labeled 2-nitroimidazoles. Adv Exp Med Biol 2003;510:285–292.

108. Gillies RJ, Raghunand N, Karczmar GS, et al. MRI of the tumor microenvironment. [erratum appears in J Magn Reson Imaging 2002 Dec;16(6):751]. J Magn Reson Imaging 2002;16:430–450.

109. Haider MA, Milosevic M, Fyles A, et al. Assessment of the tumor microenvironment in cervix cancer using dynamic contrast enhanced CT, interstitial fluid pressure and oxygen measurements. Int J Radiat Oncol, Biology, Physics 2005;62:1100–1107.

110. Pathak AP, Artemov D, Neeman M, et al. Lymph node metastasis in breast cancer xenografts is associated with increased regions of extravascular drain, lymphatic vessel area, and invasive phenotype. Cancer Res 2006;66:5151–5158.

111. Hassid Y, Furman-Haran E, Margalit R, et al. Non-invasive magnetic resonance imaging of transport and interstitial fluid pressure in ectopic human lung tumors. Cancer Res 2006;66:4159–4166.

Chapter 2

EVALUATION OF THE CANCER PATIENT

Anjali Avadhani

Catherine M. Tuite

Weijing Sun

The practice of oncology is truly a multidisciplinary, team-based endeavor. Combining the efforts of medical, radiation, surgical and interventional oncologists is crucial to optimizing the overall care of the cancer patient, and communication among these physicians is essential to formulate treatment plans for patients who typically have complicated medical issues. Interventional oncologists require the ability to conduct a thorough and comprehensive assessment of patients with a variety of malignancies and a range of associated medical problems. These basic assessment skills also promote smoother interactions among the various physicians who comprise the multidisciplinary team, and therefore will allow the interventional oncologist to play a key role in management of these patients. Evaluation of the cancer patient is composed of several fundamental principles, including medical history, physical examination, performance status grading, quality of life assessment, laboratory and data review and, ultimately, in-depth patient discussion on choices of treatment plans (1).

The physician should first elicit information regarding the patients' symptomatology, yielding as much information as possible on the progression of these symptoms and comparing current status with their initial presentation. Other components of the medical history that will be discussed in detail include history of present illness (HPI), review of systems,

pertinent listing of previous medical and surgical details, review of records, hereditary and environmental factors and use of drugs and medications. Subsequently, the physician performs a relevant physical examination to obtain insight on organ dysfunction, and this provides access to obtaining additional medical history in an extremely targeted fashion. The history and physical examination should be cohesive and similarly structured (2), in order to provide a background upon which further diagnostic information from laboratory and ancillary data can build.

MEDICAL HISTORY

A complete history and physical exam, even in the current time of technology-driven medicine, provide the most vital basis for any resulting diagnosis or treatment plan.

History of Present Illness

The HPI is the chronological sequence of symptomatic events and includes detailed descriptions of each associated symptom. This is the characterization, in much greater detail, of the "chief complaint" or the major health problem for which the patient is undergoing evaluation. The HPI should include information regarding the patient's initial cancer diagnosis, presenting symptoms at that time and any progression or changes since then. Any radiographic or laboratory data that are pertinent to the diagnosis should also be reviewed, and detailed medical records are typically the most accurate sources of this information. All subsequent symptomatic, diagnostic and related work-up details since time of initial presentation should then be noted in a sequential manner. The HPI should include a comprehensive list of all systemic chemotherapies given, any previous radiation therapy and all other systemic and local treatments. Particular attention should be given to total lifetime anthracycline dose; doxorubicin, for example, is associated with a dose-dependent cumulative cardiomyopathy (3), and is used often in the setting of chemoembolization for hepatocellular carcinoma (HCC). Many chemotherapeutic drugs are characterized by significant hepatic metabolism and therefore would raise concerns in patients with pre-existing liver dysfunction from their primary tumors or sites of metastatic disease. Finally, a detailed review of adverse treatment-related events and symptomatology, as well as any treatment complications, should be elicited (1).

Review of Systems

Review of systems is a vital component of the thorough medical history. All symptoms associated with the primary diagnosis, as well as secondary effects of the tumor, should be explored in detail. Systemic complaints such as fatigue, weight loss, anorexia, fever and night sweats are extremely common. For patients with primary HCC or liver metastases from other primary tumors, gastrointestinal symptoms may range from early to late effects of tumor growth. These include right upper quadrant pain from mechanical tumor effects, abdominal distension and, rarely, jaundice in the setting of biliary obstruction or severe liver dysfunction. Other gastrointestinal symptoms may include constipation, diarrhea, melena, early satiety, nausea and vomiting. Occasionally, carcinoid tumors can cause systemic symptoms based on their point of origin; flushing and diarrhea are associated with small bowel carcinoids, whereas shortness of breath, bronchospasm, palpitations, and heart failure can result from non-gastrointestinal carcinoids. Other symptoms to review include oropharyngeal soreness, chest pain, hemoptysis, flank and back pain, hematuria and enlarged lymph nodes (4). Skeletal metastases typically lead to severe bony pain, either isolated to the thoracolumbar spine or diffuse in nature (ribs, shoulders, hips). Neurological symptoms such as bowel or bladder incontinence, saddle anesthesia, gait instability and back pain should raise concern for cord compression, requiring emergent work-up and intervention. Pain is commonly associated with a variety of malignancies, and a verbally administered pain scale of 0 to 10 is useful, particularly for assessment of symptoms in older adults (5).

Past Medical History

Past medical history includes major current comorbidities, ongoing illness, and previous surgical procedures. Any co-existing medical problems that may impact the primary oncologic diagnosis and influence choice and impact of certain therapies should be elicited. For example, such chronic medical problems may include diabetes mellitus, hypertension, cardiovascular disease [including congestive heart failure (CHF) and coronary artery disease (CAD)], previous myocardial infarction (MI), chronic obstructive pulmonary disease (COPD), emphysema, peripheral vascular disease (PVD) and chronic renal insufficiency (CRF). Patients who are being considered for procedures such as chemoembolization should be asked about existing chronic liver disease, hepatitis B and C status, human immunodeficiency virus (HIV) and transfusion history. Also, any pre-existing psychological disorders, including depression and anxiety, should be ascertained in order to facilitate patient discussions in the future, and to note any anxiolytic/anti-depressant medications that may have significant hepatic metabolism. Surgical history must address resection of primary cancer, previous liver resection, and placement of hepatic arterial infusion pump (1). Finally, a complete list of any prior malignancies and their treatments should be obtained, as this may influence subsequent therapeutic options. For example, previous use of anthracyclines or mantle field radiotherapy may have lifetime dose limitations that warrant cautious review for the future.

Family History, Social History and Medications

A detailed description of family history is essential for most common malignancies. Often, a family history significant for multiple first-degree relatives with similar cancers can generate referrals for genetic counseling, in order to ascertain risk to unaffected individuals. For example, multiple first-degree family members with early diagnoses of colon cancers, or detection of numerous colonic adenomas, may be consistent with a pattern of familial adenomatous polyposis (FAP) or hereditary nonpolyposis colon cancer (HNPCC) (6).

Social history is an additional component of the complete medical evaluation of the cancer patient, yielding information regarding occupational or environmental exposures and links to malignancies (4). This segment of the history taking should include an in-depth assessment of a patient's alcohol and tobacco use (both current and previous), illegal/intravenous drug use, and any possible risk factors for hepatitis, including tattoos, incarceration and blood or blood product transfusion history. Social history should entail a comprehensive review of social support, home environment and functional status, particularly for elderly patients. These details can have enormous influence on choice of management, and can affect compliance with therapies, ability to follow up, and capacity to cope with side effects and toxicities at home. Questions regarding home environment, ability to work, availability of family and friends, driving capabilities and performance of activities of daily living (ADLs) are crucial (7). Finally, a complete list of current medications and doses should be compiled. As most patients typically use multiple medications that have some elements of hepatic metabolism, it is essential to avoid concurrent use of hepatotoxic drugs. Any drug allergies, particularly to antibiotics, should be noted.

PHYSICAL EXAMINATION

A comprehensive physical examination should be performed on every patient. During the initial office visit, a full systems approach should be used in order to obtain a detailed evaluation of the general health of the individual, whereas during subsequent follow up visits, the physical exam may become more focused and correlate with the patient's specific tumor type and extent of disease. Patients with HCC or metastatic disease to the liver often present with several physical exam findings not limited to the abdominal exam. Initial assessment of the patient should include a general evaluation of body habitus; descriptions of cachexia, bitemporal wasting and skin tenting should be provided. This should be followed by specific observations of skin. Dry mucous membranes and decreased skin turgor can indicate volume depletion in patients who have challenges with maintaining adequate oral intake. General pallor, as well as pale

sclerae, can signify the presence of anemia (4). Jaundice of the skin, sclerae and mucous membranes is frequently a late-presenting finding in patients with advanced metastatic cancer or HCC. Staining of the skin by bile pigments, jaundice is typically caused by accumulation of the conjugated form of bilirubin (2), which is most often associated with clinical scenarios of biliary dilatation and obstruction or liver failure. Jaundice may not be observed if the serum bilirubin level is below 3 mg/dl (8). Enlarged lymph nodes should be evaluated, with specific attention to cervical, supraclavicular, axillary and inguinal regions. Pathologically enlarged lymph nodes are typically detected by palpation when they are located in anatomically superficial areas. Lymph nodes that are too deep to palpate may be detected by multiple imaging modalities, including computerized tomography, magnetic resonance imagine, ultrasonography and positron emission tomography (2). Detection of pathologic enlargement of lymph nodes should always be followed by biopsy (4).

The general approach to the abdominal examination should include detection of ascites, hepatic and/or splenic enlargement, abdominal masses, abdominal fullness and nodules. Most often, patients with liver metastases or HCC present with physical exam features of enlarged, firm and irregular livers on palpation. Palpation of the liver edge within the right upper quadrant usually correlates to presence of hepatomegaly. The normal liver may be palpated as low as 4 cm to 5 cm below the right costal margin, but usually is not detected within the epigastric area (8). Presence of cirrhosis is usually detected by a nodular, small liver. Patients often have complaints of tenderness within the right upper quadrant with abdominal palpation and sometimes with percussion. Occasionally, a vascular bruit can be audible over the liver because of increased vascularity from the tumor (9). Portal vein involvement by tumor, a common feature of advanced HCC, can lead to portal hypertension and may effectively decrease blood flow to the liver (9). In addition, advanced liver disease and cirrhosis can present with massive ascites, splenomegaly, portal hypertension, proximal muscle wasting, testicular atrophy, spider angiomas (commonly found on the anterior chest and trunk), palmar erythema and lower extremity edema. Splenomegaly is detected by movement during inspiration, as enlarged spleens typically are present just beneath the abdominal wall (2). Placement in the supine position, as well as lying on the right side with flexion of the left knee, can help in identification of splenomegaly on physical exam.

Finally, a thorough cardiovascular and chest examination should be performed, particularly in patients receiving any type of anesthesia or intra-arterial therapies. In addition to evaluation of cardiac rate and rhythm, and auscultation for murmurs, peripheral pulses should be fully assessed. For patients with pulmonary involvement of their disease, physical exam findings can often include decreased unilateral breath sounds and dullness to percussion due to pleural effusion and/or lobar collapse and atelectasis. Pulse oximetry should be added to the standard set of vital signs in this subset of patients.

PERFORMANCE STATUS ASSESSMENT

Medical oncologists have traditionally used several parameters to assess performance status (PS), which is the global evaluation of patients' practical functional level and ability to care for themselves (10). PS is a correlate for the clinical health and overall well-being of the cancer patient. It is a critical tool used to determine whether a patient is a candidate for a particular mode of therapy, and is similarly used in the surveillance of the cancer patient during a therapeutic window. For example, PS has been used to determine survival and estimate prognosis, to measure treatment efficacy, and to help in selection of patients for clinical trials. Two of the most commonly used scales for PS assessment are the Karnofsky's Scale of Performance Status (KPS), and the Eastern Cooperative Oncology Group Scale of Performance Status (ECOG PS) (7). The KPS, an older scale initially used in the 1940s, rates PS from a scale of 0 to 100 in increments of 10, and incorporates information on ability to do normal activity versus need for assistance. Using this scale, a score of 100 correlates to completely normal functioning, whereas a score of 0 signifies death. The ECOG PS emerged in the 1960s and provided an alternative 5-point scale rather than the 11-point KPS. The ECOG PS score of 0 correlates to full activity without restriction, whereas a score of 5 indicates death (11). Although both scales are commonly used by medical oncologists, the ECOG scale has shown improved predictive value over the KPS, specifically in terms of patient prognosis (10). In addition to assessment of performance status, quality of life can be an important indicator of treatment effect and overall impact of disease. Evaluation of quality of life can be particularly relevant for older patients, as this population is typically most concerned about changes in quality of life rather than disease progression and death (12). Questions pertaining to ADLs and instrumental activities of daily living (IADL) are useful quality of life indices. ADL questions typically refer to basic functioning within the home, such as bathing and dressing, whereas IADL assessments focus on community activities, including driving, shopping and handling of finances (13).

LABORATORY

Routine laboratory evaluation in cancer patients is essential for diagnosis and critical in assessing eligibility for treatment and palliative procedures. Basic laboratory tests should include complete blood count (CBC) with differential of white blood cell (WBC), liver function and kidney functions. Prothrombin time (PT) and partial thromboplastin time (PTT) should also be tested, especially in patients undergoing anti-coagulation therapy such as warfarin.

TUMOR MARKERS

Some serum tests may be valuable as "surrogate makers" in disease diagnosis and as monitors of results of treatment – for example, alpha-fetoprotein (AFP), carcinoembryonic antigen (CEA), cancer antigen 19–9 (CA19–9) and chromogranin A. Those with known half-lives can be used to estimate treatment response by comparing the rate of decline to the expected decrease if there were 100% response. Tumor markers should be evaluated with caution as they can fluctuate substantially, and different laboratories may use different assays with widely variant normal ranges. Single levels do not correlate closely with actual tumor burden; trends over serial measurements are more useful reflections of disease response or progression. Patients should be educated not to focus on individual readings. Tumor markers often rise months before disease recurrence becomes evident on imaging; persistently rising markers without evidence of local recurrence should prompt a repeat metastatic work-up.

IMAGING

Cross-sectional imaging of the target organ and appropriate metastatic work-up are necessary to plan image-guided therapies. The images must be personally reviewed by the treating physician because written reports rarely provide sufficient information. Baseline images should be obtained within 1 month of planned treatment so the disease assessment is accurate, and to avoid underestimation of response because of disease progression prior to therapy. Size, number and location of tumors; anatomy and patency of relevant arteries and veins; evidence of organ obstruction; alterations due to surgery or stenting; critical adjacent structures; and presence of substantial amounts of disease outside the target organ are all considered when formulating a treatment plan and judging its risks and benefits. Similarly, post-treatment images should be personally reviewed, as many diagnostic radiologists will not be aware of the nature of the therapy performed, the expected imaging appearance or how to appropriately report imaging outcomes.

THE INITIAL CONSULTATION

The interventional oncologist's expertise in image-guided therapy must be integrated into an overall multi-disciplinary care plan for each cancer patient. Patients should understand that these procedures are not expected to be curative, and must be provided with a global overview of their disease and prognosis, expected outcomes without and with therapy, and reasonable expectations for risk, toxicity and disruption of quality of life. When appropriate, other treatment modalities should be disclosed and expert referrals offered. Expectations and resources for end of life care should be provided.

Image-guided therapy has a major role in the treatment of many solid tumors. For interventional oncologists to participate effectively, evaluation of cancer patients requires a comprehensive systematic approach to optimize the assessment and management of patient care.

REFERENCES

1. Tuite CM, Sun W, and Soulen MC. General assessment of the patient with cancer for the interventional oncologist. J Vasc Interv Radiol 2006;17:753–758.
2. Lichtman MA, Beutler E, Kipps TJ, et al. Initial Approach to the Patient: History and Physical Examination. Williams Hematology, 7th edition, pp. 3–9. New York: McGraw-Hill 2006.
3. Lefrak EA, Pitha J, and Rosenbaum S. A clinico-pathologic analysis of adriamycin cardiotoxicity. Cancer 1973;32:302–314.
4. Bitran JD. Establishing a Diagnosis, pp. 23–28. Expert Guide to Oncology, ACP Expert Guides Series, Philadelphia: American College of Physicians 2000.
5. Chen CCH, Kenefick AL, Tang ST, et al. Utilization of comprehensive geriatric assessment in cancer patients. Crit Rev Oncol Hematol 2004;29:53–67.
6. Trowbridge B and Burt RW. Colorectal cancer screening. Surg Clini North Am 2002;82:943–57.
7. Garman KS and Cohen HJ. Functional status and the elderly cancer patient. Crit Rev Oncol Hematol 2002;43:191–208.
8. Bickley LS and Szilagyi PG. Bates Guide to Physical Examination and History Taking, 8th edition. Philadelphia: Lippincott Williams & Wilkins 2002.
9. DiBisceglie AM. Epidemiology and clinical presentation of hepatocellular carcinoma. J Vasc Interv Radiol 2002;13:S169–S171.
10. Buccheri G, Ferrigno D, and Tamburini M. Karnofsky and ECOG performance status scoring in lung cancer: a prospective, longitudinal study of 536 patients from a single institution. Europ J Cancer 1996;32A:1135–1141.
11. Sorenson JB, Klee M, Palshof T, et al. Performance status assessment in cancer patients: an inter-observer variability study. Br J Cancer 1993;67:773–775.
12. Orr ST and Aisner J. Performance status assessment among oncology patients: a review. Cancer Treatment Reports 1986;70:1423–1429.
13. Enelow AJ, Forde DL, and Brummel-Smith K. Interviewing and Patient Care, 4th edition. Oxford: Oxford University Press 1996.

Chapter 3

PRINCIPLES OF CHEMOTHERAPY

Rowena Schwartz

Tiffany V. Goolsby

Wells A. Messersmith

ANTI-NEOPLASTIC AGENTS

The pharmacological approach to chemotherapy encompasses a wide number and many types of medications. Classically, cytotoxic agents that target rapidly dividing cancer cells have been the mainstay of treatment. More recently, the use of agents that target the immune system (immunotherapy), the biological pathways of malignant cells (targeted therapy) and the hormonal environment of the cancer (endocrine therapy) have been developed to use as single agents and in combination with other anti-neoplastic agents. This chapter overviews the common classes of antineoplastic agents and discusses some of the most common related toxicities. A more extensive review of these agents is available in many texts (1–3) and in published reviews. A quick reference list of toxicities for specific agents is available (4) and delineates between acute and delayed toxicities.

Agents used as cancer therapy are commonly categorized by mechanism (e.g., anti-metabolite or tyrosine kinase inhibitor) or origin (e.g., vinca alkaloid). Within a specific class of agents, the drugs differ significantly in pharmacology, activity and clinical application. Toxicities are often unique to an agent within a class, and the manifestation of a drug-induced side effect may vary significantly based on the drug dose, schedule, route of administration and drug therapy combination. Additionally, the tolerability of most drugs used in the treatment of cancer depends upon numerous aspects of an individual. Factors such as disease, organ function (e.g., renal function, liver function), comorbidities and concomitant medications impact toxicities and pharmacology of many agents.

Historically, many of the cytotoxic agents used for cancer treatment have been dosed based on weight (e.g., milligram per kilogram) or body surface area (e.g., milligram per square meter, or mg/m^2). The rationale for this dosing strategy is based on the narrow therapeutic window for many chemotherapy agents, and the perceived benefit of extrapolating doses used in animal species for initial human studies. At this time, there are many anti-cancer agents that are dosed as a fixed-dose regimen (milligram per dose), although these "standardized" doses may need to be modified on patient-specific factors (e.g., renal or liver dysfunction).

Clinical pharmacokinetics (PK) and pharmacodynamics (PD) are increasingly being used to optimize the dosing of individual cancer agents for specific patients or patient populations (e.g., older patients). PK, "what the body does to the drug," is the discipline that describes the absorption, distribution, metabolism and elimination of drugs. Pharmacokinetic models are used to predict serum concentrations of drug and to estimate volume of distribution, clearance half-life and metabolites of medications. PD, "what the drug does to the body," is the study of drug effects on both target and non-target tissues;

this includes desired and unwanted responses. Issues such as drug interactions with the PK/PD of specific agents are very important considerations for the use of anti-cancer agents in multi-drug cancer treatments, or with the concurrent use of medications for other chronic diseases.

ALKYLATING AGENTS

Alkylating agents (Table 3.1) are anti-tumor drugs that act through the covalent bonding of alkyl group (one or more saturated carbon atoms) to cellular molecules. There are many classes of alkylating agents, differing in their PK, chemical properties and activity, that share a common molecular mechanism of action. For example, the nitrosoureas have a high liphophilic character and are able to cross the blood–brain barrier. Although cross-resistance is not seen with all alkylating agents, it can be seen between some agents. Therapy with alkylating agents is often limited by their high level of toxicity to tissue and their lack of tumor selectivity.

The usual dose-limiting toxicity of alkylating agents is hematologic, clinically manifesting in bone marrow suppression (BMS), resulting in neutropenia, thrombocytopenia and anemia. The degree and duration of the myelosuppression vary among alkylating agents. Nausea and vomiting are often associated with this class of agents but, again, the degree and pattern vary depending upon the agent. Alkylating

agents are not selective for cancer cells, and damage to other tissues may result in a variety of organ toxicities. For example, cyclophosphamide and ifosfamide are associated with hemorrhagic cystitis secondary to the effect of a toxic metabolite, acrolein, on tissues of the bladder wall. Busulfan, in addition to other alkylating agents, has been associated with interstitial pneumonitis and pulmonary fibrosis. Alopecia is a common effect seen with most of these agents. Long-term complications with alkylating agents include gonadal atrophy, infertility and increased risk of secondary cancers.

Of note, many of these agents demonstrate a dose–response effect and are used at very high doses as part of the preparative regimens preceding stem cell transplantation. The side-effect profile for specific agents may be slightly different when used in high-dose regimens as compared with conventional dosing regimens.

NON-CLASSICAL ALKYLATING AGENTS

A group of cytotoxic agents often referred to as non-classical alkylating agents have diverse chemical structures and are able to covalently bind to biologic macromolecules in a manner similar to alkylating agents. The structure of non-classic alkylating agents does not include the classic alkylating chloroethyl group seen with alkylating agents. These agents are prodrugs and must undergo metabolic transformation to active intermediates. The drugs within this classification of agents are very diverse, ranging from platinum agents to the monoamine oxidase inhibitor, procarbazine.

Platinum-Containing Compounds

A group of agents based on the inclusion of elemental platinum (Table 3.2) is among the most widely used anti-neoplastic agents. The biologic actions of Pt(II) complexes are attributable to displacement reactions in which platinum binds to DNA, RNA, proteins and

TABLE 3.1 Alkylating Agents and Nonclassic Alkylating Agents

Nitrogen mustards	Cyclophosphamide (Cytoxan)
	Ifosfamide (Ifex)
	Mechlorethamine (Mustargen)
	Melphalan (Alkeran)
	Chlorambucil (Leukeran)
Azuiridines	Thiotepa (Thioplex)
	Altretamine (Hexalen)
Alkyl alkane sulfonates	Busulfan (Myleran)
Nitrosoureas	Carmustine (BCNU, BiCNU)
	Carmustine, local implant (Gliadel)
	Lomustine (CCNU, CeeNU)
	Semustine (methyl-CCNU)
	Streptozocin (Zanosar)
Non-classical alkylating agents	Procarbazine (Matulane)
	Dacarbazine (DTIC)
	Temozolomide (Temodar)
	Cisplatin (Platinol)
	Carboplatin (Paraplatin)
	Oxaliplatin (Eloxatin)

TABLE 3.2 Platinum-containing Compounds

Agent	Dose-limiting Toxicity
Cisplatin (Platinol)	Nephrotoxicity Neurotoxicity
Carboplatin (Paraplatin)	Hematologic toxicity
Oxaliplatin (Eloxatin)	Neurotoxicity

other biomolecules. Through successive displacement, these agents form a complex, similar to alkylating agents, inducing cell damage and apoptosis.

Cisplatin, carboplatin and oxaliplatin are the three commercially available platinum agents. The toxicity profile of each agent is unique, but there are some shared adverse effects. Cisplatin is associated with significant acute and delayed nausea and vomiting, which is at least partially prevented with aggressive prophylactic antiemetics. Renal toxicity, manifesting in tubular damage and associated electrolyte wasting, can be dose limiting. Carboplatin, developed with the intent to avoid the problematic nephrotoxicity of cisplatin, is associated with hematologic toxicity. Oxaliplatin, the most recent agent widely used in the treatment of colorectal cancer, has significant neurotoxicity. The neurotoxicity may manifest as a chronic peripheral neuropathy, also seen with cisplatin and carboplatin, or a unique sensory neuropathy manifested by cold sensitivity (e.g., a burning sensation when touching cold objects). In most patients, the neurotoxicity is reversible upon discontinuation of oxaliplatin.

ANTI-METABOLITES

The anti-metabolites (Table 3.3) are drugs that are structurally related to naturally occurring compounds involved in cellular production. Initially developed to be falsely substituted into the DNA during cell division, new agents appear to exert their cytotoxic effects through other cellular mechanisms. Historically, these agents were most effective against rapidly dividing cells, as many of the individual agents are active during cell cycle. Many of the more recently developed anti-metabolites have effects on resting cells (e.g., gemcitabine), or even on other cellular process (e.g., azacytadine).

Pyrimidine Analogs

Fluorinated Pyrimidines

The 5-fluoropyrimidines were originally synthesized based on the rationale that cancer cells utilized uracil more rapidly than do non-malignant cells. 5-fluorouracil (5FU) is an analog of uracil with a fluorine atom substituted for hydrogen at the carbon-5 position of the pyrimidine ring. The cytotoxic mechanism of action appears to be through inhibition of thymidylate synthetase (TS), ultimately inhibiting both DNA and RNA synthesis. The presence of a reduced-folate cofactor is required for tight binding of the active metabolite to TS, and the addition of leucovorin (a reduced folate) has been incorporated into regimens with 5FU to optimize cell kill. Capecitabine is a widely used oral precursor converted to 5FU via a three-step enzymatic process.

The main toxicities of the 5-fluoropyrimidines are based on the disruption to rapidly dividing cells; primarily manifesting as damage to the gastrointestinal tract (e.g., mucositis and diarrhea) and bone marrow suppression. The spectrum of toxicity associated with these agents is very dependent upon dose, schedule and route of administration. Toxicities seen with chronic exposure, such as a daily dosing regimen used with oral capecitabine or a continuous infusion regimen, are often associated with damage to the gastrointestinal tract. Regimens that include bolus dosing of anti-metabolites are more commonly associated with bone marrow suppression.

Cytidine Analogs

Nucleoside analogs compete with their physiologic counterpart for incorporation into nucleic acids and eventually interfere with cell division. Cytarabine has long been a cornerstone for the treatment of acute myelogenous leukemia (AML), but its action is limited secondary to development of drug resistance. The search for similarly effective alternative agents has led to the development of a number of agents that have found their utility in other diseases.

The toxicity profile of cytarabine, similar to other anti-metabolites, is dependent upon dose and schedule. Lower doses administered as a continuous

TABLE 3.3 Anti-metabolites, Anti-cancer Agents

Pyrimidines analogs	Fluorouracil (5FU)
	Floxuridine (FUDR)
	Capecitabine (Xeloda)
	Cytarabine (ara C, Cytosar)
	Gemcitabine (Gemzar)
Folate antagonists	Methotrexate
	Trimetrexate (Neutrexin)
	Pemetrexed (Alimta)
Purine analogs	Mercaptopurine (6-MP, Purinethol)
	Thioguanine (6-TG)
	Cladribine (2-cda, Leustatin)
	Clofarabine (Clolar)
	Fludarabine (Fludara)
	Nelarabine (Arranon)
	Pentostatin (Nipent)

infusion result in gastrointestinal and hematologic toxicity. Higher doses given as intermittent bolus infusions are associated with additional toxicities such as neurotoxicity and ocular toxicity.

Gemcitabine is a difluorinated analog of deoxycytidine. It was initially developed as an alternative for cytarabine for AML, but is now most commonly used in a number of solid tumors (e.g., pancreatic, lung and breast cancer). The dose-limiting toxicity is hematologic. Of note, patients often experience a mild, but distressing, flu-like syndrome following gemcitabine. Gemcitabine is also a powerful radiosensitizer.

Purine Anti-metabolites

Guanine Analogs

Some of the oldest anti-cancer agents are synthetic analogues to naturally accruing guanine. 6-Mercaptopurine (6-MP) and thioguanine, the 2-amino analog of 6MP, are both rapidly converted to ribonucleotides that ultimately inhibit purine biosynthesis. Cross resistance occurs between the two agents.

Both agents are generally well tolerated. Gastrointestinal toxicity and bone marrow suppression are the most common toxicities. 6-MP is associated with hepatotoxicity with chronic administration.

Adenosine Analogs

Many of the currently available analogs of adenosine were initially developed as an alternative to cytarabine. Fludarabine, unlike cytarabine, is incorporated into RNA, resulting in inhibition of transcription. Ultimately, the drug has found a place in the management of lymphoid malignancies and has significant immunosuppressive effects. Toxicities include myleosuppression, immunosuppression and, at higher doses, cerebellar toxicities. Cladrabine, another agent initially developed for AML, demonstrated activity in both dividing and resting cells. Similar to fludarabine, myelosuppression and immunosuppression occur.

Folate Antagonists (5)

Folate is an essential cofactor in many reactions for the synthesis of DNA; therefore, agents that inhibit the availability of cellular folate have been developed as cytotoxic agents. Dietary folates, dihydrofolates, are reduced to their biologically active tetrahydrofolate form to be utilized in the biosynthesis of DNA. Methotrexate is a folic acid analogue that inhibits dihydrofolate reductase, the enzyme that reduces dietary folic acid to the biologically active folinic acid. Methotrexate is used in a variety of doses and schedules for both cancer and autoimmune disease. High dose regimens ($>500\,mg/m^2$) are often followed within 24 hours with the reduced folate (folinic acid) leucovorin as "rescue."

Toxicities of methotrexate, similar to other antimetabolites, include bone marrow suppression and gastrointestinal toxicities. High dose methotrexate can precipitate in the renal tubule and result in renal dysfunction. Preventive strategies, including alkalinization of the urine and vigorous hydration, can help minimize precipitation of drug in the kidneys and subsequent nephrotoxicity. Chronic administration of low dose methotrexate, used to treat autoimmune disorders, may result in hepatotoxicity.

Pemetrexed is a relatively new multi-targeted antifolate analog that targets a number of enzymes involved in folate metabolism, including, but not limited to, thymidine synthetase and dihydrofolate reductase. The main toxicities include dose-limiting myelosuppression, mucositis and rash. Toxicities are decreased with supplementation of folic acid and vitamin B12.

ANTIMICROTUBULE AGENTS (6, 7)

A strategic cellular target for anti-cancer therapy is the microtubules, as they are known to play such an important role in mitosis as well in the maintenance of cell shape, scaffolding and function. Antimicrotubule agents (Table 3.4) are often naturally occurring or semisynthetic compounds.

Vinca Alkaloids

Vinca alkaloids are naturally occurring or semisynthetic nitrogenous bases that interact with tubulin and disrupt microtubule assembly, ultimately inducing metaphase arrest in dividing cells. The principal

TABLE 3.4 Anti-microtubule Agents

Vinca alkaloids	Vinblastine (Velban)
	Vincristine (Oncovin)
	Vinorelbine (Navelbine)
Taxanes	Docetaxel (Taxotere)
	Paclitaxel (Taxol)
	Paclitaxel, protein bound (Abraxane)
Podophyllotoxin derivatives	Etoposide (VP-16, Vepesid)
	Tenoposide (VM-26, Vumon)

toxicities of the vinca alkaloids differ despite structural and pharmacologic similarities. The toxicities of vincristine are primarily peripheral neurotoxicity, and limit the dosing of the drug. Myelosuppression is the dose-limiting toxicity of vinblastine, although neurotoxicity can be seen. Vindesine's dose-limiting toxicities are hematologic and neurologic. Vinorelbine also has dose-limiting hematologic toxicity. Of note, all these agents can cause significant tissue damage if extravasation occurs.

Taxanes

Taxanes (8) also exert their cytotoxic effect on microtubules, but through a different mechanism. By stabilizing microtubules against depolymerization, taxanes prevent disassembly and ultimately inhibit the dynamic reorganization of the microtubule network.

The primary toxicity of the agents in this class is myelosuppression. Paclitaxel has a high incidence of major hypersensivity reactions thought to be secondary to the diluent of Cremophor EL, which is necessary for solubility. Paclitaxel requires premedication with histamine antagonists and corticosteroids. Docetaxel is formulated in polysorbate 80 and has significantly fewer infusion-related reactions. Unique to docetaxel is a cumulative fluid-retention syndrome characterized by edema, weight gain and pleural effusions. Premedication with dexamethasone (and continued post therapy for 3 to 5 days) have helped ameliorate this toxicity. Docetaxel also has significant dermatologic effects, including rash and onychodystrophy. Alopecia is severe with these agents, and peripheral neuropathy can be dose limiting in some patients.

Nab-paclitaxel is a novel albumin-bound (nab) particle form of paclitaxel designed to circumvent the need for solvents and utilize the properties of albumin to increase intratumor concentrations of the paclitaxel (9). Nab-paclitaxel is dosed differently from paclitaxel, administered as a shorter infusion without the requirement for corticosteroid and anti-histamine premedication.

TOPOISOMERASE INHIBITORS (TABLE 3.5)

The DNA topoisomerases are key enzymes required for DNA replication, as they are responsible for relaxing the torsional stress that occurs during the unwinding of DNA double helix during cell division.

TABLE 3.5 Topoisomerase Inhibitors

Camptothecins	Irinotecan (Camptosar)
	Topotecan (Hycamptin)
Anthracycline antibiotics	Daunorubicin (Cerubidine)
	Doxorubicin (Adriamycin)
	Liposomal doxorubicin (Doxil)
	Epirubicin (Ellence)
	Idarubicin (Idamycin)
	Valrubicin (Valstar)
Anthracenedione	Mitoxantrone (Novantrone)
Podophyllotoxin derivatives	Etoposide (VP-16, Vepesid)
	Tenoposide (VM-26, Vumon)

Topoisomerase I and II can relax supercoiled DNA. Topoisomerase II enzymes can also decatenate intertwined DNA strands.

Camptothecins (10)

The camptothecins are a group of anti-cancer agents that target the nuclear DNA topoisomerase I (TOP1) enzyme. Irinotecan and topotecan interface the TOP1-DNA complex, reversibly trapping macromolecular complexes. Toxicities of these agents depend upon the agent. Irinotecan is associated with myelosuppression and diarrhea. Topotecan is predominantly associated with bone marrow suppression.

Epipodophyllotoxin Derivatives

Podophyllotoxins have long been known to inhibit microtubule formation and block mitosis in rapidly dividing cells, but, more recently, their interaction with topoisomerase II enzymes has been postulated to be the mechanism of cytotoxicity. Etoposide and teniposide are large molecular weight podophyllotoxin derivatives that are poorly water soluble, requiring use of complex vehicles. The major dose-limiting toxicity is myelosuppression, but toxicities such as alopecia, mucositis and hypersensitivity can also occur.

Anthracyline Derivatives

The anthracycline antibiotics are natural products derived from actinobacteria. Traditionally, these agents have been thought to exert a cytotoxic effect via intercalation into the DNA, resulting in DNA strand breaks. More recently, the ability of these agents to complex topoisomerase II and to form free radical products with oxygen has indicated that there is likely more than one mechanism for cytotoxicity.

The toxicity of these agents include myelosuppression, nausea and vomiting and gastrointestinal damage resulting in diarrhea and/or mucositis. Dose-limiting toxicity appears to be cardiotoxicity. Cardiotoxicity with anthracylines maybe seen with any administration, but the cardiomyopathy associated with tissue damage is thought to be based on damage to the tissue of the heart over time seen with cumulative doses >400 mg/m^2.

HORMONAL AGENTS (TABLE 3.6)

Selective Estrogen Receptor Modulators (11)

Selective estrogen receptor modulators (SERMs), historically called anti-estrogens, bind to estrogen receptors. These agents may act as estrogen receptor agonists in some tissues while acting as an antagonist in others based on conformational changes of the receptors. Tamoxifen, an estrogen receptor antagonist in breast tissue, is the first clinically identified compound with noticeable SERM activity. Fulvestrant is a steroidal estrogen receptor antagonist administered intramuscularly monthly.

Side effects associated with use of SERMs are often extensions of their physiologic activity (e.g., masculinization) or their action as estrogenic agents (e.g., increased risk of uterine cancer and thrombosis). Efforts to determine the application of SERMs with benefits such as anti-estrogen on breast tissue, but without the complications of effects on the endometrial tissue, are currently being explored.

TABLE 3.6 Hormonal Agents

Aromatase inhibitor/ inactivator	Aminoglutethimide (Cytadren) Anastrozole (Arimedex) Exemestane (Aromasin) Letrozole (Femara)
Anti-androgen	Bicalutamide (Casodex) Flutamide (Eulexin) Nilutamide (Nilandron)
Luteinizing hormone releasing hormone (LHRH) agonist	Leuprolide (Lupron) Goserelin (Zoladex) Triptorelin (Trelstar)
Luteinizing hormone releasing hormone (LHRH) antagonist	Abarelix (Plenaxis)
Selective estrogen receptor modulator (SERM)	Raloxifene (Evista) Tamoxifen (Nolvadex) Toremifene (Fareston)
Androgen	Fluoxymesterone (Halotestin)
Anti-estrogen	Fulvestrant (Faslodex)
Progestational agent	Megestrol (Megace)

Aromatase Inhibitors (12)

The source of estrogen in women post-menopause, and in men, is from the enzymatic conversion of adrenal androgens to estrogen in peripheral tissues via aromatase. Aromatase inhibitors (AI) are classified by generation, chemistry and type of binding. Aminoglutethimide, an older nonspecific AI, results in decreased production of mineralocorticoids and glucocorticoids as well as androgens and estrogens (i.e., medical adrenalectomy). Third-generation AIs such as letrozole and anastrazole are specific for inhibition of aromatase in estrogen synthesis. Exemestane is a third-generation AI but is unique in that it is an inactivator of the enzyme, versus an inhibitor. Side effects of AI include arthralgia and decreases in bone density. The impact on bone density has manifested as increased fractures and osteoporosis.

Luteinizing Hormone-releasing Hormone Agonist and Antagonists

Luteinizing hormone-releasing hormone (LHRH) is important in the biologic pathways of androgens and estrogens (13). The use of *LHRH agonists* is based on the continuous binding to the LHRH receptor (LHRH-R) on the gonadotrope cells of the pituitary, which initially stimulate LH release, over time down-regulate LHRH-R, thereby suppressing serum LH, testosterone levels and 5 alpha-dihydrotestosterone levels in males and estrogens in females. Because the initial surge of LH and hormone (e.g., testosterone) can cause adverse consequences, the "flare syndrome" may be blocked with an anti-androgen in men with prostate cancer. Results of initial therapeutic trials of LHRH agonists led to the development of sustained-release depot formulations. Abarelix (14), a gonadotropin-releasing hormone *antagonist* more recently approved, does not cause a surge of testosterone that can precipitate the flare phenomena.

Anti-androgens

Currently, there are three nonsteroidal anti-androgen agents (15) that prevent binding of dihydrotestosterone to the receptor, blocking the androgenic effects of testosterone. Flutamide was the first anti-androgen available, but bicalutamide is more often used today due to a more convenient daily dosing schedule and less toxicity (e.g., diarrhea). Nilutamide has unique toxicities (e.g., night blindness) and is not as widely used. The common side effect for this class of agent is feminization due to blocking androgen effects (e.g., gynecomastia).

TYROSINE KINASE INHIBITORS (TABLE 3.7)

Human protein tyrosine kinases are important in human carcinogenesis and have emerged as the promising new targets for anti-cancer therapy in many malignancies. Several approaches to inhibit tyrosine kinase have been developed (16). The success of BCR-ABL tyrosine kinase inhibitor (TKI) imatinib in the treatment of chronic myeloid leukemia has particularly stimulated intense research in this field. Many of the agents initially developed were used based on the targeting of one specific tyrosine kinase, although it is increasingly apparent that these molecules often target multiple kinases and have a broader application than initially determined. Additionally, it is becoming more clear that blocking one single target in a cancer may have limited effect long term, and that a more effective strategy may be to use a multi-targeted approach. Side effects of TKIs are often related to the target(s) blocked, and are unique to each agent or related agents. For example, the TKI agents such as gefitinib and erlotinib target TK involved with the epidermal growth factor receptor (EGFR), and are

TABLE 3.7 Tyrosine Kinase Inhibitors

Drug	Target(s)
Dasatinib (Sprycel)	ABL oncoproteins (including mutations resistant to imatanib), SRC family
Erlotinib (Tarceva)	EGFR
Gefitinib (Iressa)	EGFR
Imatanib (Gleevec)	ABL oncoproteins, cKIT, PDGFR
Lapatinib (Tykerb)	HER 1, HER 2
Sorafenib (Nexavar)	VEGFR-2,3, PDGFRβ, RAF
Sunitinib (Sutent)	VEGFR-1,2,3, PDGFRα and β, cKIT, FLT3
Temsirolimus	mTOR

ABL, protein tyrosine kinase that phosphorylate tyrosine residues (Abelson murine leukemia); cKIT, protooncogene; EGFR, epidermal growth factor receptor; HER, epidermal growth factor receptor (EGFR); mTOR, mammalian target of rapamycin; PDGFR, platelet-derived growth factor receptor; RAF, protein serine-threonine kinases that phosphorylate serine or threonine; SRC, protein tyrosine kinase (Rous avian sarcoma); VEGFR, vascular endothelial growth factor receptor

associated with significant rashes and gastrointestinal side effects.

BIOTHERAPY (TABLE 3.8)

Interferon

The interferons (IFN) (17) are a group of proteins with diverse immunomodulatory and anti-angiogenic properties. IFN-alpha are pleiotropic cytokines belonging to type I IFNs, extensively used in the treatment of patients with certain cancers and viral diseases. IFN-alpha can affect tumor cell functions by multiple mechanisms. In addition, these cytokines can promote the differentiation and activity of host immune cells. There is a pegylated interferon that is currently used in for treatment of hepatitis and is being evaluated in a variety of oncology settings. Side effects of IFNs are significant and can range from constitutional symptoms that are often referred to as a flu-like syndrome to hepatotoxicity. Side effects are often most severe with high dose regimens, intravenous (vs subcutaneous) administration and with initiation of therapy.

Interleukin

Interleukin-2 (IL-2), a glycoprotein produced by activated lymphocytes, is used for the treatment of melanoma and renal cell cancer (18). The precise mechanism of cytotoxicity of IL-2 is unknown; high concentrations of IL-2 have not been shown to have a direct anti-tumor effect on cancer cells in vitro. In vitro and in vivo, IL-2 stimulates the production and release of many secondary monocyte-derived and T-cell–derived cytokines, including IL-4, IL-5, IL-6, IL-8, tumor necrosis factor-α (TNFα), granulocyte macrophage-colony stimulating factor, and IFN-γ, which may have direct or indirect anti-tumor activity. In addition, IL-2 appears to stimulate the cytotoxic activities of natural killer cells, monocytes,

TABLE 3.8 Biotherapy

Interferon	Interferon α2a (Roferon-A)
	Interferon α2b (Intron)
	Interferon β-1b (Betaseron)
	Interferon γ (Actimmune)
	Peginterferon α-2a (PEG-Intron)
Interleukin-2	Aldesleukin (IL-2, Proleukin)
Immunostimulant	Levamisole (Ergamisol)

lymphokine-activated killer (LAK) cells and cytotoxic T lymphocytes (CTLs). Aldesleukin, the commercially available brand of IL-2, is associated with significant side effects that are dose and regimen dependent. High dose IL-2 is associated with capillary leak syndrome, which requires aggressive monitoring and management in an inpatient setting.

Monoclonal Antibodies (Table 3.9) (19, 20)

Antibodies and peptides play a variety of roles in cancer therapy: monoclonal antibodies (MoAbs) and peptides are directly used in anti-cancer therapy and also as targeting moieties. The mechanism for antibody-based therapy can be broadly divided into unconjugated and conjugated antibodies. Unconjugated antibodies can alter cellular function via manipulation of cell surface proteins and/or evoke immune responses against targeted cells by activating antibody-dependent cellular cytotoxicity (ADCC) and complement. Conjugated antibodies deliver toxic compounds to the tumor, such as with gemtuzumab ozogamicin or radioimmunotherapy. Radioimmunotherapy (RIT) (20) uses radiolabeled MoAbs directed against tumor-associated antigens.

Toxicities associated with MoAb therapy include infusion-related reactions such as hypersensitivity-related symptoms of dyspnea and bronchospasm. Additionally, the toxicity of the MoAb may be related to the manipulation of the target via the antibody. For example, bevacizumab targets vascular endothelial growth factor (VEGF) and angiogenesis, which may impact tissue healing and repair after surgery. Individual MoAbs have unique toxicities determined by their targets.

TABLE 3.9 Monoclonal Antibodies (MoAb)

Unconjugated MoAb	Target
Alemtuzumab (Campath)	CD52
Bevacizumab (Avastin)	VEGF
Cetuximab (Erbitux)	EGFR
Rituximab (Rituxan)	CD20
Panitumumab (Vectibix)	EGFR
Trastuzumab (Herceptin)	HER 2 neu
Conjugated MoAb	
Ibritumomab tiuxetan (Zevalin)	CD20
Tositumomab, Iodine I-131 (Bexxar)	CD20
Gemtuzumab ozogamicin (Mylotarg)	CD33

EGFR, epidermal growth factor receptor; HER, epidermal growth factor receptor; VEGF, vascular endothelial growth factor

MISCELLANOUS CYTOTOXIC AGENTS (TABLE 3.10)

A variety of agents or classes of drugs is used in the management of cancer. Although some of these agents are unique (e.g., bleomycin) in mechanism of action, several groups of drugs (e.g., histone deacetylase inhibitors) are emerging as entirely new methods of treating cancer. As the biology of cancer cell development and progression is further understood, it is anticipated that new targets and consequently new strategies of drug therapies will be identified. Of note with these new strategies is the introduction of new toxicities and the need to further evaluate the best way to optimize treatment without negatively impacting quality of life. Additionally, as new drugs are added to conventional treatment, there is a potential to broaden the scope of toxicities in an individual patient.

Immunomodulatory Drugs (21)

Thalidomide and the analogue lenalidomide belong to the family of immunomodulatory drugs (IMiDs). These agents have anti-angiogenic properties, modulate TNFα and IL-2 secretion, co-stimulate T cells, increase NK cell toxicity and have direct anti-tumor effects. Toxicities for these agents include neurotoxicity, increased thrombosis risk and, for select agents, myelosuppression. Lenalidomide is a more powerful inhibitor of TNFα and has, aside from myelosuppression, fewer side effects than thalidomide. One of the

TABLE 3.10 Miscellaneous Agents

Arsenic trioxide (Trisenox)
Asparaginase (Elspar)
Pegasparagase (Oncaspar)
Bacillus Calmette-Guérin (BCG, TheraCys, Tice)
Bexarotene (Targretin)
Bortezomib (Velcade)
Denileukin diftitox (Ontak)

IMiDs
Thalidomide (Thalomid)
Lenalidomide (Revlimid)

Retinoid acids
Tretinoin (Vesanoid)

Histone deacetylase (HDAC) inhibitors
Vorinostat (Zolinza)

DNA methyltransferase inhibitors
Azactidine (Vidaza)
Decitabine (Dacogen)

major concerns with thalidomide is the teratogenicity associated with this agent, and a registration program is required for prescribing.

Retinoids

Through its various metabolites, vitamin A controls essential physiological functions. Both naturally occurring metabolites and novel retinoid analogues have shown activity in both premalignant conditions (e.g., actinic keratosis) and cancers (e.g., acute promyelocytic leukemia or APL). Tretinoin is an oral retinoid, all-transretinoic acid (ATRA) that is one of the cornerstones of APL treatments. Side effects include headache, xerosis, cheilitis and rash. Retinoic acid syndrome is a group of symptoms including fever, dyspnea associated with pulmonary infiltrate, edema and hypotension.

Proteasome Inhibitors

Bortezomib is a reversible inhibitor of the 26S, which is a multi-catalytic threonine protease responsible for intracellular protein turnover in eukaryotic cells (22). This includes the processing and degradation of several proteins involved in cell cycle control and the regulation of apoptosis. Inhibition of the 26S proteasome prevents this targeted proteolysis, thereby affecting multiple signaling cascades within the cell. This disruption of normal homeostatic mechanisms can lead to cell death. Preclinical trials demonstrate this agent has a wide range of biological effects that result in decreased proliferation, induction of apoptosis and sensitization of tumor cells to conventional chemotherapeutic agents and irradiation. Toxicities associated with bortezomib include fatigue, neuropathy and thrombocytopenia. The side effect profile may differ dependent on drug therapy combination and patient factors such as extent of pretreatment.

Histone Deacetylase Inhibitors

Vorinostat is the first of the new class of antineoplastic agents referred to as histone deacetylase (HDAC) inhibitors. Histone acetylation is a dynamic process of cellular gene regulation that is "epigenetic," that is, not heritable in the germline. Histones are DNA-binding proteins that allow for the compaction of large amounts of DNA, yet comprise a highly dynamic process that permits efficient transcriptional regulation. HDAC inhibitors modify gene expression in cancer cells without altering gene sequences, and cause expression of genes (often tumor suppressors) that have been inappropriately

turned off during the oncogenic process. Vorinostat is available for the treatment of cutaneous T-cell lymphoma.

DNA Methyltransferase Inhibitors

Aberrant DNA methylation patterns, including hypermethylation of tumor suppressor genes, have been described in many human cancers (23). These epigenetic mutations can be reversed by DNA methyltransferase inhibitors. Decitabine and azacytine are two agents, used in the treatment of myelodysplastic syndrome, that are believed to exert a cytotoxic effect through this mechanism.

REFERENCES

1. Abeloff MD, Armitage JO, Niederhuber JE, et al. Clinical Oncology, 3rd edition. Philadelphia: Elsevier Churchill Livingstone 2004.
2. Devita VT, Hellman S, Rosenberg SA, eds. Cancer: Principles and Practices of Oncology, 7th edition. Philadelphia: Lippincott-Raven 2005.
3. Chabner BA, Longo DL, eds. Cancer Chemotherapy and Biotherapy: Principles and Practices, 3rd edition. Philadelphia: Lippincott Williams & Wilkins 2001.
4. Drugs of Choice for Cancer. Treatment Guidelines from the Medical Letter. 2003;1:41–52.
5. McGuire JJ. Anticancer antifolates: Current status and future directions. Curr Pharm Des 2003;9:2593–2613.
6. Nagle A, Hur W, Gray NS. Antimitotic agents of natural origin. Curr Drug Targets 2006;7:305–326.
7. Kiselyov A, Balakin KV, Tkachenko SE, et al. Recent progress in discovery and development of antimitotic agents. Anticancer Agents Med Chem 2007;7:189–208.
8. Kingston DG, Newman DJ. Taxoids: Cancer-fighting compounds from nature. Curr Opin Drug Discov Devel 2007 Mar;10:130–144.
9. Socinski M. Update on nanoparticle albumin-bound paclitaxel. Clin Adv Hematol Oncol [review] 2006 Oct;4(10):745–746.
10. Pommier Y. Topoisomerase I inhibitors: Camptothecins and beyond. Nat Rev Cancer 2006;6:789–802.
11. Musa MA, Khan MO, Cooperwood JS. Medicinal chemistry and emerging strategies applied to the development of selective estrogen receptor modulators. Curr Med Chem 2007;14:1249–1261.
12. Toi M, Bando H, Saji S. Aromatase and aromatase inhibitors. Breast Cancer 2001;8:329–332.
13. Moreau JP, Delavult P, Blumberg J. Luteinizing hormone-releasing hormone agonists in the treatment of prostate cancer: A review of their discovery, development, and place in therapy. Clin Ther 2006;28:1485–1508.
14. Debruyne F, Bhat G, Garnick MB. Abarelix for injectable suspension: First-in-class gonadotropin-releasing hormone antagonist for prostate cancer. Future Oncol 2006;2:677–696.
15. Wirth MP, Hakenberg OW, Froehner M. Antiandrogens in the treatment of prostate cancer. Eur Urol 2007;51:306–313.

16. Madhusudan S, Ganesan TS. Tyrosine kinase inhibitors and cancer therapy. Recent Result Cancer Res 2007;172:25–44.

17. Ferrantini M, Capone I, Belardelli F. Interferon-alpha and cancer: Mechanisms of action and new perspectives of clinical use. Biochimie 2007 Jun-Jul;89:884–893.

18. Atkins MB. Interleukin-2: Clinical applications. Semin Oncol 2002;29(Suppl 7):12–17.

19. Khandare JJ, Minko T. Antibodies and peptides in cancer therapy. Crit Rev Ther Drug Carrier Syst 2006;23:401–435.

20. Boerman OC, Koppe MJ, Postema EJ, et al. Radionuclide therapy of cancer with radiolabeled antibodies. Anticancer Agents Med Chem 2007;7:335–343.

21. Raje N, Hideshima T, Anderson KC. Therapeutics uses of immunomodulatory drugs in the treatment of multiple myeloma. Expert Rev Anticancer Ther 2006;6:1239–1247.

22. Zavrski I, Jakob C, Kaiser M, et al. Molecular and clinical aspects of proteosome inhibition in treatment of cancer. Recent Result Cancer Res 2007;176:165–176.

23. Brueckner B, Kuck D, Lyko E. DNA methyltransferase inhibitors for cancer treatment. Cancer J 2007;13:17–22.

Chapter 4

PHARMACOLOGIC PRINCIPLES OF REGIONAL THERAPY IN THE TREATMENT OF LIVER METASTASES OR PRIMARY LIVER TUMORS

Fidel David Huitzil Melendez

Nancy Kemeny

The rationale for regional chemotherapy is to maximize drug concentrations and tumor drug uptake in the target organ and minimize systemic toxicity (1). For regional drug delivery to successfully impact relevant outcomes, several important principles regarding tumor biology, drug pharmacology and delivery systems must be fulfilled (2). The model of liver metastasis from colorectal cancer complies with these principles, as colorectal cancer has a regional pattern of dissemination, with the liver being the only site of metastatic disease for long periods in some cases (3). Other salient features include the selective supply of blood to liver metastases by the hepatic artery (4) and availability of active drugs with suitable pharmacokinetic properties (5).

In this chapter, pharmacological concepts of regional therapy will be reviewed. Desirable pharmacokinetic and pharmacodynamic characteristics of drugs considered for evaluation in the hepatic arterial infusion (HAI) model of regional drug delivery will be discussed, using floxuridine (FUDR) as a model, in the context of patients with colorectal liver-only metastases (CRLM). Also, an evaluation of the pharmacology of currently approved agents for the treatment of metastatic colon cancer and their hypothetical value for regional drug delivery will be preformed. Results of Phase I and Phase II trials of HAI with these drugs, if available, will be explained in terms of the previously established pharmacologic rationale. Finally, for active drugs not already tested, a critical analysis will be done of the available pharmacokinetics data to determine the likelihood of successful incorporation of these drugs to HAI-based therapeutics. We provide an appendix with basic pharmacology definitions to enhance comprehension for the reader not familiar with these concepts.

PHARMACOLOGIC CONCEPTS USEFUL IN UNDERSTANDING AND EVALUATING POTENTIAL ADVANTAGES OF REGIONAL DELIVERY FOR SPECIFIC DRUGS

The ultimate goal of regional therapy is to improve the therapeutic index by increasing efficacy and decreasing systemic toxicity. Hepatic arterial therapy relies on two important assumptions:

1. Regional delivery of the drug leads to increased local concentration and therefore increased therapeutic response.

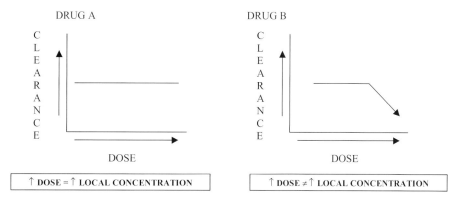

FIGURE 4.1. Regional delivery of drug A (first-order kinetics, constant clearance despite the dose) can result in increased local concentrations compared with systemic concentrations. Regional delivery of drug B (zero-order kinetics; clearance decreases after a certain dose level) will not result in increased local concentrations if the drug is administered at high doses, limiting the potential advantage of increased dose.

2. Regional delivery of the drug leads to decreased systemic exposure and reduced systemic toxicity.

The suitability of any specific drug for regional therapy can be evaluated by the extent to which it fulfills these assumptions.

Regional Delivery of the Drug Leads to Increased Local Concentrations

As described by Collins (1), increased local concentrations depend on the ratio of total body clearance for a particular drug (CL_{TB}) to the regional exchange (Q) for a particular body compartment: CL_{TB}/Q. In the model of hepatic artery drug delivery, as the regional exchange rate is constant (100 to 1000 ml/min), the local concentration for a particular drug depends upon its total body clearance. Higher CL_{TB} results in higher local concentrations. Therefore, there are two possible scenarios: drugs with clearance exhibiting first-order kinetics even at much higher doses than those normally used for systemic treatment and drugs that exhibit zero-order kinetics when an attempt to increase the dose is made. Only the first ones will fulfill the assumption that regional delivery of the drug will result in increased local concentrations (Figure 4.1).

Increased Local Concentration Leads to Increased Therapeutic Response

The paradigm that increased dose will result in increased biologic effect has been challenged by the recent development of targeted agents active against cancer (6). Most cytotoxic drugs act on DNA or tubulin and exhibit a sigmoidal steep dose-response curve, and dose selection is based on maximal tolerated dose. However, for targeted therapies, more is not necessarily better. Pharmacodynamic effect is thought to be the result of receptor occupancy and saturation. Optimal target inhibition occurs at a specific drug concentration, and increasing the dose will not increase the effect. Furthermore, at useful drug concentrations, the maximum tolerated dose may have not been reached. As this has been recognized, the need for new strategies to define the clinically active dose level for this kind of drugs is evident. The traditional Phase I trial, useful for cytotoxic drug dose selection, does not accomplish the goal for targeted agents. Other parameters, including pharmacokinetic endpoints such as achieving a predefined target plasma level or direct measurement of target inhibition, may be more relevant.

Therefore, the potential benefit for increased therapeutic response through increased local concentrations is relevant for cytotoxic drugs, but may not be as important for targeted agents (Figure 4.2).

Regional Delivery of a Drug Leads to Decreased Systemic Exposure

Decreased systemic exposure to the drug depends on the extent of metabolism or elimination of the drug during first-pass effect. In the case of HAI therapy, the hepatic extraction ratio can be estimated from the [hepatic arterial (HA) level of a drug – hepatic venous (HV) level of a drug]/hepatic arterial (HA) level. Only drugs with high hepatic extraction will potentially result in decreased systemic exposure. If hepatic extraction exhibits linear pharmacokinetics even at high doses, this may allow dose escalation

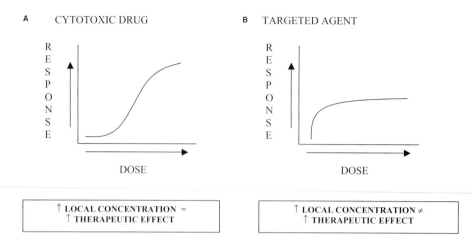

FIGURE 4.2.   (A) For drugs exhibiting steep-dose response curve, an advantage in therapeutic effect can be obtained by increasing local concentrations of the drug. (B) For drugs that exert their optimal biological effect at a specific drug concentration, no advantage in therapeutic effect can be expected by increasing local concentrations.

in the search for a greater therapeutic benefit. However, if hepatic extraction exhibits non-linear pharmacokinetics, dose escalation will result in decreased hepatic extraction ratio, with loss of the advantage of decreased systemic exposure (7). Additionally, for some drugs, first-pass metabolism results in generation of active metabolites. No decreased systemic exposure to active metabolites can be expected for these drugs (Figure 4.3).

Although the potential advantages of increased local concentration and decreased systemic exposure depend on different variables and are therefore independent, the combined advantage of regional therapy can be expressed with Collins formula:

$$\text{Advantage} = 1 + \frac{\text{Total body clearance of the drug}}{(\text{HA flow rate [1-fraction of drug extracted across liver])}}$$

Finally, effective regional drug delivery requires other drug properties to be considered, such as stability at body temperature, high solubility in order to be infused in small volumes and compatibility with titanium, stainless steel, silicone rubber and polyurethane (7).

PHARMACOLOGICAL SUITABILITY FOR HEPATIC ARTERIAL INFUSION OF DIFFERENT ACTIVE DRUGS IN COLORECTAL CANCER

Floxuridine (5-fluoro-2′-deoxyuridine)

Fluoropyrimidines are active in colorectal cancer through inhibition of thymidylate synthase (8).

FUDR, after uptake by a facilitated diffusion transport system, undergoes phosphorylation into the active nucleotide FdUMP by the enzyme thymidine kinase at the intracellular level. Negatively charged nucleotides cannot leave the cell and accumulation of the active drug within the cell occurs. FdUMP and 5,10-methylenetetrahydrofolate form a stable ternary complex with thymidylate synthetase (TS), inhibiting the transformation of dUMP into dTMP, a key step for de novo pyrimidine synthesis.

In vitro studies in multiple human colorectal cancer cell lines have shown that FUDR is more effective than 5FU, as shown by a high ratio of the half maximal inhibitory concentration (IC$_{50}$) of 5FU over FUDR on a molar basis. The dose-effect curve is sigmoidal, and potentiation of FUDR by leucovorin was more pronounced. In accordance with cell cycle specificity, prolonged exposure of human cell lines to FUDR greatly enhances growth inhibition. However, when the duration of exposure is prolonged, the influence of leucovorin modulation is decreased (8).

Animal tumor models have shown that FUDR yields better therapeutic efficacy than 5FU when studied in various schedules and in different colon tumors (8).

Early clinical trials comparing systemic FUDR and 5FU showed mixed results in terms of response rates. Overall, they were considered equivalent. A comparison of the mode of administration of FUDR showed that the rapid intravenous injection was superior to the 24-h constant infusion, with significantly higher response rates. A distinct toxicity pattern was observed with each mode of administration, with

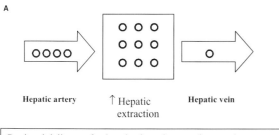

Regional delivery of a drug leads to decreased systemic exposure

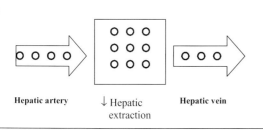

Regional delivery of a drug does not lead to decreased systemic exposure

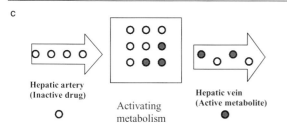

Regional delivery of inactive drug does not prevent systemic exposure to active metabolite.

FIGURE 4.3. In the HAI model, decreased systemic exposure to an active agent depends on the hepatic extraction ratio for that particular drug. (A) Drugs with high hepatic extraction will result in decreased systemic exposure and potentially less systemic toxicity. If hepatic extraction exhibits linear pharmacokinetics, and the effect is dose dependent, dose can be increased looking for a combined benefit of increased efficacy and decreased systemic exposure. (B) Drugs with low hepatic extraction will not result in decreased systemic exposure. If the drug exhibits non-linear pharmacokinetics when administered at high doses, the advantage of decreased systemic exposure will decrease as the dose is escalated. (C) If the drug is activated in the liver, decreased systemic exposure to active metabolites cannot be expected.

more mucocutaneous toxicity and diarrhea observed with the prolonged infusion and more leukopenia observed with the bolus (8).

In vitro studies have shown a sigmoidal dose-response curve to FUDR (9) and the pharmacokinetics of FUDR is linear and not saturated even at dose rates greater than used clinically (5). The CL_{TB} for FUDR has been estimated between 15,000 and 25,000 ml/min. The hepatic extraction ratio of FUDR ranges from 0.69 to 0.92 when the dose is administered intravenously as determined by HA levels – HV levels/HA levels. However, with HAI, FUDR hepatic extraction is 0.94 to 0.99. Systemic FUDR concentrations during hepatic arterial infusions were only 25% of corresponding systemic levels with peripheral venous administration (Table 4.1) (5).

Not surprisingly, with this pharmacokinetic profile, hepatic arterial infusion of FUDR in patients with liver metastases from colorectal cancer has consistently resulted in higher response rates when compared with systemic administration of either FUDR or 5FU. In randomized studies comparing HAI to intravenous delivery of fluoropyrimidines, increased median survival was also observed with HAI therapy, if crossover was not allowed. Using Collins formula, the calculated advantage for FUDR administration by hepatic arterial infusion is 1200-fold in terms of drug exposure than by systemic administration (7).

5-Fluorouracil

As a fluorinated pyrimidine, 5FU has proven activity in colorectal cancer and shares the mechanism of action with FUDR, inhibiting thymidylate synthase through the formation of FdUMP (8). However, the metabolic route is somewhat different. The predominant activation step for 5FU is its phosphoribosylation to 5-fluoridine-5'-monophospate (FUMP), a reaction catalyzed by the enzyme orotate

TABLE 4.1 Comparison of the Pharmacokinetic Profile of FUDR and 5FU in Regard to Suitability for Regional Therapy

	CL_{TB} (L/min)	Hepatic Extraction after IV Dose	Hepatic Extraction after HAI Dose	Systemic Concentration after HAI/Systemic Concentration after IV	Linear PK	Advantage of Regional Therapy
FUDR	15–25	0.69–0.92	0.95	0.25	Yes	1200-fold
5FU*	2		0.8		No	40
5FU†	0.5		0.1		No	2.2

FUDR, floxuridine

*20 mg/kg/d as a constant infusion.

†270 mg/kg/d short infusion.

Data from refs. 5, 7, and 10.

phosphoribosyl transferase (OPRT), requiring the phospate-donor 5-phosporibosyl-1-pyrophosphate as a cosubstrate. FUMP is subsequently converted to 5-fluorouridine-5'-diphosphate FUDP by a pyrimidine nucleoside monophosphate kinase. From here, FUDP can be further converted into 5-fluorouridine-5'-triphosphate (FUTP), capable of RNA incorporation and responsible for 5FU toxicity. On the other hand, FUDP can be converted to 5-fluoro-2'-deoxyuridine-5'-diphosphate (FdUDP) by ribonucleotide reductase and ultimately to 5-fluoro-2'-deoxyuridine-5'-monophosphate (FdUMP). Active metabolites can be converted back to 5FU and free 5FU can be degraded by dihydropyrimidine dehydrogenase (DPD), the level of expression of which can alter toxicity, but not anti-tumor activity.

5FU has demonstrated anti-tumor activity in vitro, in tumor models and clinical trials. This anti-tumor activity is potentiated by leucovorin. The drug is active in multiple different schedules, including bolus administration and continuous infusion administration. FU has demonstrated increased survival in the adjuvant setting (11). In metastatic disease, numerous studies show increased survival over best supportive care.

Similar to FUDR, in vitro studies have shown a sigmoidal dose-response curve. However, converse to what is observed with FUDR, 5FU does have significant saturable, nonlinear pharmacokinetics, and therefore total body clearance and hepatic extraction decrease at high dose rates (10). At a dose rate of 20 mg/kg/d as a continuous infusion, total body clearance is approximately 2000 ml/min. At a dose rate of 270 mg/kg/d, total body clearance is approximately 500 ml/min. It has been observed that clearance after IV administration depends on the mode of infusion. Higher total body clearance values ranging from 5.41 L/min to 57.9 L/min were observed with continuous venous infusion of 750 mg to 1000 mg over 8 h. Hepatic extraction at dose rate of 20 mg/kg/d as a continuous infusion is 80% but it is decreased to 10% at a dose rate of 270 mg/kg/d. Others have estimated an extraction ratio ranging from 0.22 to 0.45 after peripheral intravenous administration and a hepatic extraction ranging from 19% to 51% with HAI (5). Systemic 5FU concentrations during HAI were only 59% of corresponding systemic levels with peripheral venous administration. Of note, extraction ratios may also differ according to the mode of administra-tion. Bolus administration of 1000 mg of 5FU via the hepatic artery results in 0.11 extraction ratio while a 5-day infusion of 500 to 900 mg/m²/day results in 0.93 extraction rate. When the infusion rate is increased to 900 to 1500 mg/m²/day, the extraction ratio decreases to 0.44 (12).

Overall, 5FU pharmacokinetics is not as suitable as FUDR pharmacokinetics for HAI. The regional advantage of HAI over systemic administration of 5FU is only about six- to two-fold [10]. A comparison of the resultant area under the plasma 5FU concentration after intrahepatic arterial bolus injection and intravenous administration did not show any difference (13). Results from a randomized clinical trial comparing HAI vs. systemic administration of 5FU did not show a significant difference in terms of response rate, time to progression, duration of the response and survival rate (14).

Irinotecan

Irinotecan (CPT-11) inhibits DNA synthesis by inhibiting topoisomerase I activity, an enzyme over-expressed in colorectal cancer (15). CPT-11 undergoes sequential metabolism to SN-38 by tissue and serum carboxyl esterase and to SN-38G by hepatic uridine diphosphate glucuronosyltransferases. SN-38 is the active metabolite of CPT-11, with 100- to 1000-fold greater anti-tumor activity than CPT-11. SN-38G is the inactive metabolite. SN-38 and SN-38G undergo significant biliary excretion and entero-hepatic circulation. SN-38G may be deconjugated to form SN-38 by intestinal β-glucuronidase. The cytochrome P450 3A4 (CYP3A4) is also involved in the metabolism of CPT-11, resulting in the formation of APC, a metabolite 500-fold less potent than SN-38 in terms of anti-tumor activity. Finally, CPT-11, SN-38 and SN-38G can exist as a lactone form (intact lactone ring, active) and as a carboxylate form (open ring, inactive). When administered orally, the molar ratio of SN-38 AUC/CPT-11 is at least three-fold greater than after intravenous administration, indicating a higher exposure of SN-38 due to first-pass metabolism (15).

CPT-11 exhibits non-linear pharmacokinetics. The molar ratio of SN-38/CPT-11 decreases at higher doses, possibly due to saturation of conversion of irinotecan to SN-38. The metabolic ratio of SN-38/CPT-11 has also been shown to be significantly higher after a low-dose continuous infusion of CPT-11 than after a high-dose, short infusion of CPT-11.

Non-linear pharmacokinetics can be explained by the saturation of carboxylesterase and glucuronidation pathways (15).

The pharmacokinetics of CPT-11 has been reported for a variety of dosages and schedules.

As a result of nonlinear pharmacokinetics, clearance depends on dose and mode of administration. Dose escalation from 100 to 750 mg/m^2 administered by the intravenous route resulted in approximately 50% reduction in CPT-11 clearance, from 26 to 12 L/m^2/h (16). For multiple dosages and schedules using 30- to 90-min intravenous infusions, the clearance ranges from 232 to 352 ml/min/m^2. The administration of a low-dose continuous intravenous infusion over 14 days every 3 weeks at a dose rate ranging from 7.5 to 17.5 mg/m^2/d resulted in a clearance of 28.2 L/h (17). A second study of 5-day intravenous continuous infusion of CPT-11 at doses ranging from 25 to 40 mg/m^2/day resulted in clearance ranging from 47.4 to 101.6 L/h. This increase in clearance with lower doses administered as a continuous infusion is in agreement with non-linear pharmacokinetics (18).

Regarding hepatic extraction, no formal studies measuring levels at the hepatic veins and hepatic artery have been done. The fact that hepatic metabolism of CPT-11 results in an active compound makes hepatic extraction of the drug difficult to incorporate into the assessment of regional delivery advantage. The non-linear pharmacokinetics predicts that with higher dose rates, the clearance of the drug is actually diminished, preventing any advantage. Also, the first-pass metabolism results in an active metabolite. Therefore, a high hepatic extraction may paradoxically be deleterious for any advantage of regional therapy as it results in increased systemic exposure to the active metabolite.

Investigators have tried to overcome the non-linear pharmacokinetics pitfall by using the continuous administration of CPT-11 by HAI at low doses over 5 days. They also hypothesized increased anti-tumoral activity as a result of an increased active metabolite that is primarily active in the S-phase of the cell cycle. In a Phase I trial, patients with liver metastases from solid tumors received HAI of CPT-11 at 15 to 25 mg/m^2/day for 5 days every 3 weeks by continuous HAI (19). Patients received one cycle of intravenous CPT-11 first. Total body clearance of CPT-11 was significantly higher with HAI than with intravenous administration (11.3 vs. 8.7 l/h/m^2, p

= 0.008); the metabolic ratio ([SN-38 total/CPT-11 total] × 100) was increased with HAI compared with intravenous administration (16.2 vs. 11.3, p = 0.015). During intravenous administration, the steady-state concentrations of CPT-11 increased linearly with the dose (r, 0.536, p = 0.032), whereas the steady-state concentrations of SN-38 did not significantly increase with the dose. The opposite was true for HAI: the steady-state concentration of CPT-11 did not increase with the dose, whereas the steady-state concentrations of SN-38 showed a significant linear correlation with the dose (r, 0.566, p = 0.035). Total body clearance was independent of the dose infused. The dose-limiting toxicities were diarrhea and neutropenia at a dose level of 25 mg/m^2/day. In order to determine the efficacy of this schedule in a Phase II trial, 25 pretreated patients with colorectal cancer metastatic to the liver were treated with HAI CPT-11 at 20 mg/m^2 for 5 days (20). Partial response rate was 13.6%. Major toxicities were vomiting and diarrhea, without significant hematological toxicity. The authors discussed that systemic distribution of the metabolite SN38 and failure of entrapment into the liver metastases were responsible for the lack of superiority of the HAI approach.

Oxaliplatin

Oxaliplatin is a platinum analog with anti-tumoral activity in advanced colorectal cancer. It was first synthesized in Japan as a diaminociclohexane (DACH) oxalatoplatinum compound (21).

Oxaliplatin is a prodrug that is activated by conversion to monochloro-, dichloro- and diaquo-compounds by non-enzymatic hydrolysis, resulting in displacement of the oxalate group. The aquated derivatives of oxaliplatin are considered to be the biologically active species, capable of adduct formation with various sulfide and amino groups.

The cytotoxic activity of oxaliplatin is initiated by formation of a DNA adduct between the aquated oxaliplatin derivative and a DNA base. Initially, only monoadducts are formed but eventually oxaliplatin attaches simultaneously to two different nucleotide bases, resulting in DNA intrastrand cross-links. The modification of the three-dimensional structure of DNA will result in inhibition of DNA polymerization. On the other hand, after DNA-adduct formation, tumor cells will activate cellular repair mechanism. These mechanisms involve enzymes containing several amino and sulfur groups. Oxaliplatin can be covalently bound to these repair enzymes and can therefore impair their function. Ultimately, the combination of inhibition of DNA polymerization and inhibition of DNA repair will result in substantial DNA damage, activation of apoptotic pathways and cell death. Cellular detoxification processes competing with DNA-adduct formation include conjugation of the aquated compound to glutathione (GSH), methionine (Met) and cysteine (Cys). The conjugated products are subsequently excreted from the cell and eliminated from the body. In addition, after a 2-h infusion of oxaliplatin, 70% of the drug is bound to plasma proteins (mostly albumin), thereby losing its anti-tumor potential, and 5 days after a single infusion, this fraction increases to about 95% (22).

Preclinical evidence suggests a steep dose-response curve to oxaliplatin in human colon carcinoma cells. Freshly explanted tumor specimens from patients with isolated liver metastasis from colorectal origin were exposed to 0.1, 1, 10 and 100 μg/ml of oxaliplatin for 2 h. All tumor specimens showed significant concentration-response effects (23).

The clinical activity of oxaliplatin in advanced colorectal cancer has been demonstrated in several settings (24). As a single agent, the objective response rate to oxaliplatin is 20% to 24% in untreated patients and 10% in 5FU-pretreated patients. With oxaliplatin in combination with 5FU, the objective response rate is 51% in untreated patients. In patients with advanced colorectal cancer refractory to 5FU, the combination of 5FU/leucovorin (LV)/oxaliplatin yields a response rate of 21% to 25%. After tumor progression on 5FU/LV/CPT-11, the response rate is 9.9% or 15% (25, 26).

Regarding pharmacokinetics, discrimination between bound and free platinum in blood and plasma usually occurs. Ultrafilterable platinum (comprising non-protein bound drug and biotransformation products in plasma water) is thought to represent all the platinum species with anti-tumor and toxic properties in the circulation. Therefore, plasma ultra-filtrate represents the most relevant matrix when considering pharmacological activity.

The PKs of platinum in ultra-filtrate are triexponential, characterized by short initial α and β distribution phases (0.28 and 16.3 h, respectively) followed by a long terminal γ phase (273 h). The short initial α and β phases likely represent the rapid clearance of intact oxaliplatin and the reactive dichloro-, monochloro-, and diaquo-DACH platin intermedi-

ates into tissues and/or removal from the systemic circulation via glomerular filtration. The long terminal half-life of unbound platinum in plasma ultra-filtrate probably reflects the slow release of low molecular weight platinum conjugates. Given that the platinum in the terminal elimination phase comprises almost entirely inactive platinum conjugates, α and β phases represent the clinically relevant $t_{1/2}$ values of active platinum. No accumulation has been observed in plasma ultra-filtrate after 130 mg/m^2 every 3 weeks or 85 mg/m^2 every 2 weeks (27).

The clearance of ultra-filterable platinum decreases from 18.5 ± 4.71 L/h at 85 mg/m^2 every 2 weeks to 9.34 ± 2.85 to 10.1 ± 3.07 L/h at 130 mg/m^2 every 3 weeks. Oxaliplatin appears to be cleared equally by tissue distribution and glomerular filtration. No formal study of hepatic extraction of oxaliplatin has been conducted.

Hepatic arterial infusion of oxaliplatin has been tested in Phase I and Phase II trials.

An initial Phase I study by Kern et al. (28) on 21 patients with isolated hepatic metastases from colorectal cancer reported a maximum tolerated dose of 150 mg/m^2 every 3 weeks in combination with folinic acid 200 mg/m^2 and 5FU 600 mg/m^2 for five consecutive days. The dose-limiting toxicity consisted of leukopenia, obliteration of the hepatic artery and acute pancreatitis. Overall, toxicity consisted of nausea/vomiting (16 of 21), anemia (16 of 21), upper abdominal pain (15 of 21), sensory neuropathy (10 of 21), diarrhea (9 of 21) and thrombocytopenia (9 of 21). However, severe toxicity mainly consisted of leukopenia (4 of 21), thrombocytopenia (2 of 21), hyperbilirubinemia (2 of 21), pain (2 of 21) and diarrhea (1 of 21). Response rate was 59% in these chemonaive patients. The recommended dose for Phase II studies was 125 mg/m^2.

On a subsequent Phase II study by Guthoff et al. (29), five patients with isolated non-resectable colorectal liver metastases received HAI treatment with oxaliplatin at 130 mg/m^2 on day 1, in combination with 5FU (480 mg/m^2) and LV (140 mg/m^2) from day 1 to 5 and mitomycin C (7 mg/m^2) on day 5 every 35 days. A liver extraction ratio of 0.47 for oxaliplatin was determined by comparing the area under the plasma-concentration curve (AUC) values in venous blood observed in the present study after administration of oxaliplatin via HAI to the AUC values obtained after intravenous administration of oxaliplatin in historical controls. Mancuso et al. (30) reported on 17 patients

TABLE 4.2 Comparison of Pharmacologic Characteristics of Chemotherapy Agents Active in Colon Cancer in Regard to Suitability for Regional Therapy

	FUDR	5FU	Irinotecan	Oxaliplatin
Active in colon cancer	+	+	+	+
Steep dose-response curve	+	+	+	+
Linear pharmacokinetics	+	−	−	−
High clearance	+	−	−	−
Hepatic extraction	+++	+	−*	+

FUDR, floxuridine
*First-pass metabolism generates active metabolites.

with pretreated metastatic colorectal cancer to the liver. Oxaliplatin 20 mg/m²/day by hepatic arterial continuous infusion (HACI) for 5 days every 3 weeks was given as a single agent, as opposed to prior studies, therefore allowing accurate evaluation of the toxicity profile. Severe abdominal pain was observed in 30% of the patients and was the dose-limiting toxicity. Four of 17 patients developed hepatic toxicity defined by elevation of serum bilirubin and/or alkaline phosphatase more than twice the baseline level. Grade 3 toxicities included asthenia (1 of 17) and nausea (1 of 17). Catheter and hepatic artery thrombosis was observed in one patient as an immediate complication and as a secondary complication, arterial thrombosis was observed in seven patients, leading to definitive interruption of HAI chemotherapy. Response rate was 46%. Fiorentini et al. (31) reported on 12 patients who had evidence of progression of disease on previous regimens and were treated with HAI oxaliplatin every 3 weeks. Dose-limiting toxicity consisted of obliteration of hepatic artery, abdominal pain and severe hypotension and was observed at 175 mg/m². Therefore, the recommended dose was 150 mg/m². Ducreux et al. (32) treated 28 patients chemotherapy naïve with HAI-oxaliplatin at 100 mg/m² combined with intravenous FU/LV. Response rate was 64%. Neurotoxicity was observed in 69% of patients. Only one patient experienced grade 3 neurotoxicity. The authors stated that perhaps HAI oxaliplatin may decrease the appearance of neuropathy.

Overall, the pharmacokinetics profile of FUDR is not shared by any other active cytotoxic drug in colorectal cancer. If oxaliplatin hepatic extraction is confirmed in studies not using historical controls, oxaliplatin administration by HAI may be of some value in terms of reduced neuropathy. However, given the lack of linear pharmacokinetics, no increase in local concentrations or activity can be expected. Populations suitable for research include patients with liver-only metastases from colorectal cancer who have shown response on systemic oxaliplatin, but cannot tolerate further treatments as a result of neuropathy. Phase II comparative trials are needed to better define the real advantage of HAI of oxaliplatin.

THERAPEUTIC MONOCLONAL ANTIBODIES

Antibodies EGFR (cetuximab and panitumumab) and vascular endothelial growth factor (VEGF, bevacizumab) have been proven to be useful in metastatic colorectal cancer.

Bevacizumab is a humanized monoclonal antibody against VEGF, an important regulator of physiologic and pathologic angiogenesis. Early studies demonstrated that antibody-mediated inhibition of VEGF resulted in tumor growth inhibition in vivo (33). Improvement in the delivery of chemotherapy by altering tumor vasculature and decreasing the elevated interstitial pressure has also been postulated as a second mechanism of action (34). Results from a randomized Phase II trial demonstrated that the addition of bevacizumab to FU/LV resulted in increased response rates, time to progression and overall survival. Interestingly, a low-dose regimen of bevacizumab (5 mg/kg/every 2 weeks) was more effective than a high-dose regimen (10 mg/kg/every 2 weeks) in terms of response rate (40% vs. 24%) and survival (21.5 vs. 16.1 months). An increased risk of bleeding, hypertension, thrombosis and proteinuria was observed among patients treated with bevacizumab. No correlation with the dose used was noticed (35). Bevacizumab has also demonstrated to improve outcomes when added to a combination of irinotecan, bolus FU/LV (IFL) in a Phase III trial. Overall response rate was 44.8% and 34.8% and median survival was 20.3 and 15.6 months in the IFL

+ bevacizumab and IFL + placebo arms, respectively. Bevacizumab was associated with an increased risk (11% vs 2.3%) of grade 3 hypertension (requiring treatment) in this trial (36). Pharmacokinetic studies in 52 cancer patients receiving intravenous infusions of bevacizumab at doses ranging from 0.1 to 10 mg/kg over a 4- to 24-week period as a single agent or in combination with antineoplastic agents reveled clearance was 239 ml/day, with an initial and terminal half-life of 1.85 and 18.6 days, respectively (37). A second study (38) evaluated the pharmacokinetics of the combination of bevacizumab at 15 mg/kg and erlotinib at 150 mg/day. No pharmacokinetic interaction was noticed and reported clearance was 3.18 ml/kg/day, consistent with previous findings. No study of hepatic extraction has been done.

Cetuximab is a chimeric immunoglobulin-G1 (IgG1) monoclonal antibody that binds to EGFR with high specificity and with a higher affinity than either epidermal growth factor (EGF) or tumor growth factor-alpha (TGF-α) (39), thus blocking ligand-induced phosphorylation of EGFR, the initial step of a cascade of intracellular events related to tumor cell proliferation (40). Initial studies with C225 showed a sigmoid dose-response curve, with growth inhibition of cultured A431 cells achieving a plateau at 35%. Also, the capacity of C225 to inhibit the growth of established A431 xenografts in nude mice was demonstrated. Interestingly, as the initial dose tested was effective, the authors looked at the lowest dose of antibody retaining biologic activity. This is in contrast to what usually occurs with cytotoxic agents, in which the opposite pathway of defining the maximum tolerated dose usually occurs (41). Phase I trials (42) with escalating weekly doses of C225 revealed non-linear pharmacokinetics, with antibody doses in the range of 200 to 400 mg/m^2 being associated with complete saturation of systemic clearance. A sharp decline in systemic clearance (mL/h/kg) was observed with increasing doses: 3.09 at 20 mg/m^2, 1.16 at 50 mg/m^2, 0.811 at 100 mg/m^2, 0.433 at 200 mg/m^2 and 0.374 at 400 mg/m^2. Drug accumulation was noticed at 400 mg/m^2 but not at 200 mg/m^2. No correlation of dose and response was possible. Subsequent Phase II and Phase III trials were designed using an initial dose of 400 mg/m^2 followed by weekly infusions of 250 mg/m^2. In patients with colorectal cancer whose tumors expressed EGFR, cetuximab as a single agent showed 9% response rate after progression on an irinotecan-based regimen in a Phase II trial

(43). Grade 3 to 4 adverse events included skin rash (18%), fatigue (9%) and allergic reactions (3.5%). These results were confirmed in a subsequent phase III trial in irinotecan-refractory metastatic colorectal cancer patients. The addition of cetuximab to irinotecan in this population resulted in increased response rate (22.9% vs. 10.8%) for the combination of irinotecan and cetuximab over cetuximab as a single agent, but not increased median survival (8.6 vs. 6.9 months, $p = 0.48$) (44).

Panitumumab is a fully human monoclonal IgG2 to EGFR (45). Like cetuximab, it is directed against the extracellular ligand-binding domain of the EGFR. However, panitumumab has shown higher affinity and substantially lower 50% inhibitory concentration compared with cetuximab. Phase I trials have been conducted in renal cell cancer patients testing escalating doses of 1, 1.5, 2 or 2.5 mg/kg weekly with no loading dose (46). Skin rash was present in 100% of patients at the 2.5 mg/kg dose level. Panitumumab PKs fit a model that incorporates both linear and saturable EFGR-mediated CL mechanisms. Panitumumab concentrations increased non-linearly with the dose, which was most likely due to progressive saturation of a fixed EGFR sink. EFGR-mediated CL requires occupancy of the EGFR by panitumumab before internalization. The mean estimates for linear CL and volume of distribution were 2.59 ml/d/kg and 41.8 ml/kg, respectively. The parameters characterizing non-linear clearance were estimated at 165 μg/d/kg. The half-life averaged 15.9 days. At the 2.5-mg/kg dose, the clearance of panitumumab was close to the typical CL range of human antibodies that are not subject to an antigen sink of 1–4 mL/d/kg, but are cleared via the reticuloendothelial system.

Phase II studies in patients with metastatic colorectal cancer who had received prior treatment with fluoropyrimidine in 100% of cases, irinotecan in 96% of cases and oxaliplatin in 49% of cases, showed 9% partial response (PR) and 29% stable disease (SD) according to Response Evaluation Criteria in Solid Tumors (RECIST). At least 62% of those with a grade 2 or greater rash had either a PR or SD (47).

A subsequent Phase II trial tested panitumumab in combination with either IFL or infusional FU/LV/irinotecan (FOLFIRI) as first-line therapy for metastatic colorectal cancer. Partial response was observed in 33% of patients and stable disease in 46% of patients (48).

A Phase III trial compared panitumumab monotherapy versus best supportive care in patients

TABLE 4.3 Comparison of Pharmacologic Characteristics of Targeted Agents Active in Colon Cancer in Regard to Suitability for Regional Therapy

	Cetuximab	Bevacizumab	Panitumumab
Active in colon cancer	+	+	+
Steep dose-response curve	–	–	–
Linear pharmacokinetics	–	–	–
High clearance	–	–	–
Hepatic extraction	?	?	?

with pretreated metastatic CRC. Response rate was 36% vs. 10% in the panitumumab and in the control arm, respectively. A risk reduction of 46% in progression-free survival was noticed. Overall survival was similar, but crossover was allowed (49).

Regarding regional therapy, although therapeutic monoclonal antibodies may differ in their binding target, presumed mechanism of action and main toxicity, all of them share general pharmacokinetic and pharmacodynamic properties: of note, non-linear pharmacokinetics, very low systemic clearance and receptor mediated-mechanism of action (50). Therefore, increased local concentrations with HAI over intravenous administration are not expected. Furthermore, even if achieved, greater concentrations may not result in increased therapeutic effect. However, regional therapy may be useful to decrease systemic toxicity, if hepatic extraction is demonstrated. At normally administered doses of therapeutic antibodies, non-linear pharmacokinetics would prevent hepatic extraction. Low doses of therapeutic antibodies will exhibit linear pharmacokinetics and may enable hepatic extraction and decreased systemic toxicity when administered through HAI (Figure 4.4). Subjects suitable for research include those with liver-only metastases who cannot tolerate systemic antibodies, despite clinical response. This approach may result in continued benefit without experiencing the disturbing side effect of skin rash.

REGIONAL THERAPY PHARMACOLOGY APPENDIX

Increased local concentrations and decreased systemic exposure are two different advantages pursued with regional therapies. It is important to realize that even when both characteristics can be integrated and summarized in a single expression called **overall selectivity (Rd)**, each of these advantages is independent from the other, as they are determined by different variables (1, 7).

Increased local concentrations at the target site depend upon whether or not the drug is metabolized or eliminated by the target tissue. If there is no metabolism or elimination of drug by the target tissue, target site concentration advantage of intraarterial delivery (R_{target}) depends on the ratio of the total body clearance (CL_{TB}) to the regional exchange rate (Q).

$$R_{target} = C_{target}(IA)/C_{target}(IV) = 1 + \frac{CL_{TB}}{Q}$$

where:

$C_{target}(IA)$ = target concentrations for intraarterial delivery

$C_{target}(IV)$ = target concentrations for intravenous delivery

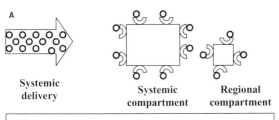

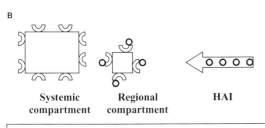

FIGURE 4.4. (A) Therapeutic antibodies administered systemically at regular doses saturate regional and systemic receptors and exhibit non-linear pharmacokinetics. (B) Therapeutic antibodies administered at low doses through HAI may exhibit linear pharmacokinetics, saturate regional receptors preferentially and result in decreased systemic toxicity.

The regional exchange rate of the liver (250 to 1000 ml/min) is not as favorable for increased local concentrations as the exchange rate of, for example, the peritoneum (5 to 25 ml/min) or the arachnoid space (0.5 to 5 ml/min). Nevertheless, it can be assumed to be constant and therefore, on a particular patient, increased local concentrations depend only on the high CL_{TB} of the drug.

When the target tissue is the exclusive route of elimination for a drug, however, no increase in concentration can be achieved if the same dose is given regionally compared with systemically:

$$R_{target} = \frac{C_{target}(reg)}{C_{target}(IV)} = 1$$

Decreased systemic exposure to the drug depends on the extent of metabolism or elimination of the drug during first-pass effect. It implies biotransformation to less active products and/or excretion by the hepatobiliary system. In the case of HAI, the fraction extracted during the first pass, also called hepatic extraction ratio, can be estimated from the hepatic arterial level – hepatic venous level/hepatic arterial level.

$$\text{Hepatic extraction ratio} = \frac{\begin{array}{c}\text{hepatic arterial level} -\\ \text{hepatic venous level}\end{array}}{\text{hepatic arterial level}}$$

Therefore, the decreased systemic concentration advantage for intraarterial delivery ($R_{systemic}$) can be expressed in terms of the fraction extracted during the first pass

$$R_{systemic} = \frac{C_{systemic}(IA)}{C_{systemic}(IV)} = 1 - E$$

Overall selectivity (Rd) summarizes the combined advantage of increased local concentrations and decreased systemic exposure:

$$Rd = \frac{R_{target}}{R_{systemic}} = \frac{C_{target}(reg)/C_{target}(IV)}{C_{systemic}(reg)/C_{systemic}(IV)}$$
$$= 1 + \frac{CL_{TB}}{Q(1-E)}$$

When the target tissue is the exclusive route of elimination for a drug, no increase in local concentrations can be achieved, and the advantage is limited to decreased systemic exposure.

$$Rd = \frac{1}{1-E}$$

Advantage of regional therapy stands only as long as the dose rate used does not saturate either CL_{TB} or

hepatic extraction. This is a potential problem with drugs that exhibit non-linear pharmacokinetics. With higher dose rates, the CL_{TB} and the hepatic extraction actually diminish and the advantage is lost.

Drugs that must be activated at a site other than the arterial infusion site have no regional delivery advantage.

Finally, it should be noted that although pharmacokinetic parameters may allow a selective increase in hepatic tumor exposure, the crucial target effect of a particular drug (e.g., DNA incorporation of a thymidine analogue) might also exhibit non-linear kinetics. In this case, the impact on what actually is most important – the drug effect – rather than the increased drug concentration, might be less selective at high than at low dose rates. This is the concept of tissue-related pharmacokinetics and takes into account not only saturating pharmacokinetics in the tumor but also in systemic tissues. If at high dose rates, the plateau for the effect is higher in systemic tissues than for the tumor itself, loss of regional selectivity is observed.

PHARMACOLOGY APPENDIX (51–54)

Pharmacokinetics refers to the mathematical analysis of the time course of drug concentrations in the body. Its importance lies on the assumption that the magnitude of a pharmacologic effect of a given drug depends on its concentration at its site of action. Therefore, factors determining drug concentration at its site of action such as absorption, distribution, metabolism and elimination are within the field of study of pharmacokinetics.

Kinetic models are useful for the purpose of the study of pharmacokinetics. The body is conceived as consisting of several interrelated compartments. A central compartment consisting of ECF space and well-perfused organs (e.g., liver, kidneys) is commonly distinguished from a peripheral or tissue compartment consisting of poorly perfused organs and tissues (e.g., muscle or fat). After a single-dose intravenous injection of a drug, a two-compartment kinetic model will depict concentrations declining in two phases: an initial rapid (alpha) distribution phase and a terminal slower (beta) elimination phase. The alpha phase is dominated by distribution of drug from the central to the peripheral compartment and terminates when there is equilibrium between the two compartments. For most drugs, distribution occurs much more rapidly than elimination, and therefore the distribution term becomes zero after only a small portion of the dose is eliminated. The beta phase is dominated by elimination of drug from the central compartment. Elimination refers to the *removal* of drug from the body. There are two processes involved in elimination: metabolism (mainly by the liver) and excretion (mainly by the kidneys). The plasma-drug concentrations over time relationships can be described using arithmetic or logarithmic scale plots. In the natural logarithmic plot, if the distribution phase is neglected, the decrease in concentration during the terminal elimination phase is near linear. This implies that a **constant fraction** of drug dose remaining in the body is eliminated per unit time (first-order kinetics). The rate constant for the elimination phase K_E can be calculated for any drug. However, if a drug is given in a dose large enough to exceed the capacity of enzyme systems to eliminate a constant proportion of the drug, the result is that a constant amount per unit of time is eliminated rather than a constant fraction (zero-order kinetics). In this case, the rate is independent of the concentration.

Metabolism refers to the disappearance of a drug when it is changed chemically into another compound, called metabolite. Drug metabolism involves the alteration of the chemical structure of the drug, commonly by an enzyme. The change generally involves conversion into a more polar form that can be more readily excreted in the urine. For some drugs, metabolism means conversion into an active species. Metabolic reactions are commonly classified as phase I or phase II. Phase I reactions include oxidations, reductions and hydrolytic reactions. Many drug oxidation reactions are catalyzed by the cytochrome P450-dependent mixed-function oxidase system. Phase II reactions involve conjugations that take place by coupling the drug molecule to an endogenous substituent group, so the resulting product will have greater water solubility or other modifications that lead to enhanced renal or biliary elimination. Conjugation may occur with glucuronate, activated glycine, acetate, sulfate and other groups. The metabolic rate of reaction is dependent on the relation of the maximum rate of reaction (V_{max}), the concentration of the drug (S) and the Michaelis constant. This relationship is described by the equation:

$$V \text{ (rate of reaction)} = \frac{V_{max}(S)}{Km + (S)}$$

Of note, during zero-order kinetics, when enzyme systems are saturated, $V = V_{max}$ and therefore the rate becomes constant.

Excretion refers to the removal of a drug from the body without chemical changes. Elimination occurs primarily by renal mechanisms into the urine.

Pharmacokinetic parameters summarize the pharmacokinetics of a drug, integrating information on metabolism, excretion, distribution, and expressing them in a standardized form to allow comparisons between drugs. Important pharmacokinetic parameters include clearance, volume of distribution, bioavailability and half-life. Ultimately, pharmacokinetic parameters of a given drug are used to calculate dosing regimens.

Drug clearance is defined as the volume of blood cleared of drug per unit time (e.g., ml/min) and describes the efficiency of elimination of a drug from the body. Total body clearance of a drug is simply the sum of clearances across the organs of elimination, either by metabolism or by excretion. Therefore, total clearance = renal clearance + hepatic clearance. Clearance relates the rate of elimination of drug (mg/min) to the plasma concentration of drug (mg/ml) and, therefore, is expressed as volume per unit time (ml/min).

$$CLp = \frac{\text{rate of elimination of drug (mg/min)}}{\text{plasma concentration of drug (mg/ml)}}$$

Clearance is an independent pharmacokinetic parameter. It does not depend on the volume of distribution, half-life, or bioavailability and is constant for a particular drug in a specific patient. The clinical utility of clearance is the calculation of a maintenance dose rate, according to the formula:

Maintenance dose rate (mg/h) =
  target concentration (mg/L) × clearance (L/h).

At first-order kinetics, every drug has one only clearance value, independent of the plasma concentration of that drug. However, during zero-order process, when the enzyme systems are saturated, the rate of elimination becomes constant. According to the formula, therefore, with a constant rate of elimination and increasing plasma concentrations of the drug, the clearance actually decreases. This concept is relevant to understand why the advantage of regional therapy is lost during zero-order kinetics. As the advantage is directly dependent on clearance of drug, increasing doses result in reduced clearance and, therefore, reduced advantage.

Volume of distribution is an independent pharmacokinetic parameter that replaces the determination of the actual volume in which drug molecules are distributed within the body, as this cannot be measured. Thus, the apparent volume of distribution (V_d) is defined as the proportionality factor between the concentration of drug in blood or plasma (mg/L) and the total amount of drug in the body (mg) and it is expressed in volume units.

Vd can be calculated from the time zero concentration (Co) after intravenous injection and the dose (D):

$$Co = D/Vd$$

The clinical utility derives from the comparison of the apparent V_d with typical body water volumes. Plasma estimated volume is 3 L, extracellular compartment estimated volume is 15 L and total body estimated volume is 45 L. When a drug bounds extensively to plasma albumin, Vd approximates the normal plasma volume. If a drug is extensively bound to tissue sites but weakly to plasma proteins, the Vd can achieve values as high as 15,000 L or 40,000 L. Provided that sampling to determine Vd is limited to plasma, Vd values can greatly exceed the total body volume.

Additional clinical utility of the Vd is the calculation of a loading dose according to the formula:

$$\text{Loading dose (mg)} = Css \text{ (mg/L)} \times Vd \text{ (L)}$$

Vd is independent of clearance, half-life or bioavailability.

Half-life ($t_{1/2}$) is defined as the time it takes for the concentration of drug to decrease by half. There are several ways in which $t_{1/2}$ can be determined. It can be read directly from the graph of log C(t) versus time. Its value can also be determined from the slope of the log Cp over time plot:

$$t_{1/2} = 0.693/Kel$$

As a dependent pharmacokinetic parameter, its value is directly proportional to the Vd and inversely proportional to clearance:

$$t_{1/2} = (0.693 \times Vd)/Cl$$

The clinical utility of half-life is multiple: calculation of the duration of a drug effect, dose-intervals, time required to eliminate the drug and time required to achieve "plateau" concentrations during repeated or maintenance dosing with a drug.

Pharmacodynamics refers to the study of the biological effect of any drug, including mechanisms of action at physiological, biochemical and molecular levels.

Concentration response relationships refer to the quantification of the amount of drug necessary to produce a given response and are usually expressed as arithmetic or logarithmic curves. Concentration assumes the steady-state drug level achieved during a constant infusion. When the drug is given as a bolus, then concentration should be interpreted as the area under the concentration (as opposed to peak concentrations) versus time curve, or C × T. Additionally, as one rarely knows the concentration of drug at the active site, it is usually necessary to work with dose-response relationships.

Receptor theory explains the concept of receptors as sites of action, a concept that is critical to understanding dose-response curves. For almost all drugs, the magnitude of the pharmacological effect depends on the concentrations of both drug and receptors at the target tissue. It assumes that at higher drug concentrations, a higher extent of receptor occupancy occurs. In addition, the extent of receptor occupancy determines the extent of pharmacological effect in a manner depicted by an S-shaped curve. At the middle of the curve, the magnitude of response increases in a nearly linear manner with progressive increases in drug concentration and receptor occupancy. At the right extreme of the curve, where the maximal effect is achieved, even large increases in drug concentration result in minor increases of the pharmacologic effect. The same phenomenon is observed at the left side of the curve, near the minimal effect zone, where relatively large increases in drug concentration produce only a modest increase of the pharmacologic effect.

Occupation of a receptor by a drug is determined by the concentration of the drug [D] and its affinity constant [K_D], and it is independent of the total receptor number [R_T]. The affinity constant is a fixed parameter and represents the concentration of drug at which half of the receptors are occupied. Low K_D means high affinity and high K_D means low affinity. Therefore, the proportion of drug bound, relative to the maximum proportion that could be bound (fractional occupancy), can be estimated with the following formula:

$$\frac{DR}{[R_T]} = \frac{[D]}{[D] + K_D}$$

DR = drug-receptor complex

R_T = total number of receptors

$[DR]/[R_T]$ = fractional occupancy

[D] = drug concentration

K_D = affinity constant

The concept of antagonists is also derived from the receptor theory. Competitive antagonists will compete for the same binding site on a given receptor. When both drugs are present and competing, the agonist occupancy is determined by the formula:

$$\frac{[DR]}{[R_T]} = \frac{[D]}{[D] + K_D(1 + [B]/K_B)}$$

Ultimately, it is implicit from the formula that competitive antagonism is surmountable. With two drugs competing for the same binding site, the drug with the higher concentration relative to its affinity constant will dominate.

Other important concepts derived from the receptor theory include partial agonists, spare receptors (signal amplification) and receptor desensitization and supersensitivity.

REFERENCES

1. Collins JM. Pharmacologic rationale for regional drug delivery. J Clin Oncol 1984; 2: 498–504.
2. Kemeny NE, D'Angelica M, and Saldinger PF. Intra-arterial chemotherapy for liver tumors. In: L.H. Blumgart (ed.), Surgery of the Liver, Biliary Tract and Pancreas, pp. 1321–1337. Elsevier Mosby: Philadelphia 2007.
3. Weiss L, et al. Haematogenous metastatic patterns in colonic carcinoma: an analysis of 1541 necropsies. J Pathol 1986; 150(3): 195–203.
4. Sigurdson ER, et al. Tumor and liver drug uptake following hepatic artery and portal vein infusion. J Clin Oncol 1987; 5(11): 1836–1840.
5. Ensminger WD, et al. A clinical-pharmacological evaluation of hepatic arterial infusions of 5-fluoro-2′-deoxyuridine and 5-fluorouracil. Cancer Res 1978; 38(11 Pt 1): 3784–3792.
6. Arteaga CL and Baselga J. Clinical trial design and end points for epidermal growth factor receptor-targeted therapies: Implications for drug development and practice. Clin Cancer Res 2003; 9(5): 1579–1589.
7. Ensminger WD. Intrahepatic arterial infusion of chemotherapy: pharmacologic principles. Semin Oncol 2002; 29(2): 119–15.

8. van Laar JA, et al. Comparison of 5-fluoro-2′-deoxyuridine with 5-fluorouracil and their role in the treatment of colorectal cancer. Eur J Cancer 1998; 34(3): 296–306.
9. Park JG, et al. Enhancement of fluorinated pyrimidine-induced cytotoxicity by leucovorin in human colorectal carcinoma cell lines. J Natl Cancer Inst 1988; 80(19): 1560–1564.
10. Wagner JG, et al. Steady-state nonlinear pharmacokinetics of 5-fluorouracil during hepatic arterial and intravenous infusions in cancer patients. Cancer Res 1986; 46(3): 1499–1506.
11. Ragnhammar P, et al. A systematic overview of chemotherapy effects in colorectal cancer. Acta Oncol 2001; 40(2–3): 282–308.
12. Boublil JL, et al. Continuous 5-day regional chemotherapy by 5-fluorouracil in colon carcinoma: Pharmacokinetic evaluation. Br J Cancer 1985; 52(1): 15–20.
13. Goldberg JA, et al. Pharmacokinetics and pharmacodynamics of locoregional 5 fluorouracil (5FU) in advanced colorectal liver metastases. Br J Cancer 1988; 57(2): 186–189.
14. Grage T, et al. Results of a prospective randomized study of hepatic artery infusion with 5-fluorourcail vs intravenous 5-fluorouracil in patients with hepatic metastases from colorectal cancer: A Central Oncology Group study. Surgery 1979; 86: 550–555.
15. Iyer L and Ratain MJ. Clinical pharmacology of camptothecins. Cancer Chemother Pharmacol 1998; 42(Suppl): S31–S43.
16. Abigerges D, et al. Phase I and pharmacologic studies of the camptothecin analog irinotecan administered every 3 weeks in cancer patients. J Clin Oncol 1995; 13(1): 210–221.
17. Herben VM, et al. Phase I and pharmacokinetic study of irinotecan administered as a low-dose, continuous intravenous infusion over 14 days in patients with malignant solid tumors. J Clin Oncol 1999; 17(6): 1897–1905.
18. Ohe Y, et al. Phase I study and pharmacokinetics of CPT-11 with 5-day continuous infusion. J Natl Cancer Inst 1992; 84(12): 972–974.
19. van Riel JM, et al. Continuous administration of irinotecan by hepatic arterial infusion: a phase I and pharmacokinetic study. Clin Cancer Res 2002; 8: 408–412.
20. van Riel JM, et al. Continuous infusion of hepatic arterial irinotecan in pretreated patients with colorectal cancer metastatic to the liver. Ann Oncol 2004; 15(1): 59–63.
21. Desoize B and Madoulet C. Particular aspects of platinum compounds used at present in cancer treatment. Crit Rev Oncol Hematol 2002; 42(3): 317–325.
22. Kweekel DM, Gelderblom H, and Guchelaar HJ. Pharmacology of oxaliplatin and the use of pharmacogenomics to individualize therapy. Cancer Treatment Reviews 2005; 31(2): 90–105.
23. Kornmann M, et al. Oxaliplatin exerts potent in vitro cytotoxicity in colorectal and pancreatic cancer cell lines and liver metastases. Anticancer Res 2000; 20(5A): 3259–3264.
24. Raymond E, et al. Oxaliplatin: A review of preclinical and clinical studies. Ann Oncol 1998; 9(10): 1053–1071.
25. Rothenberg MI, et al. Superiority of oxaliplatin and fluorouracil-leucovorin compared with either therapy

alone in patients with progressive colorectal cancer after irinotecan and fluorouracil-leucovorin: Interim results of a phase III trial. J Clin Oncol 2003; 21: 2059–2069.

26. Tournigand C, et al. FOLFIRI followed by FOLFOX6 or the reverse sequence in advanced colorectal cancer: A randomized GERCOR study. J Clin Oncol 2004; 22(2): 229–237.

27. Graham MA, et al. Clinical pharmacokinetics of oxaliplatin: A critical review. Clin Cancer Res 2000; 6(4): 1205–1218.

28. Kern W, et al. Phase I and pharmacokinetic study of hepatic arterial infusion with oxaliplatin in combination with folinic acid and 5-fluorouracil in patients with hepatic metastases from colorectal cancer. Ann Oncol 2001; 12(5): 599–603.

29. Guthoff I, et al. Hepatic artery infusion using oxaliplatin in combination with 5-fluorouracil, folinic acid and mitomycin C: Oxaliplatin pharmacokinetics and feasibility. Anticancer Res 2003; 23(6D): 5203–5208.

30. Mancuso A, et al. Hepatic arterial continuous infusion (HACI) of oxaliplatin in patients with unresectable liver metastases from colorectal cancer. Anticancer Res 2003; 23(2C): 1917–1922.

31. Fiorentini G, et al. Oxaliplatin hepatic arterial infusion chemotherapy for hepatic metastases from colorectal cancer: A phase I–II clinical study. Anticancer Res 2004; 24(3b): 2093–2096.

32. Ducreux M, et al. Hepatic arterial oxaliplatin infusion plus intravenous chemotherapy in colorectal cancer with inoperable hepatic metastases: A trial of the gastrointestinal group of the Federation Nationale des Centres de Lutte Contre le Cancer. J Clin Oncol 2005; 23(22): 4881–4887.

33. Kim KJ, et al. Inhibition of vascular endothelial growth factor-induced angiogenesis suppresses tumour growth in vivo. Nature 1993; 362(6423): 841–844.

34. Jain RK. Normalizing tumor vasculature with anti-angiogenic therapy: A new paradigm for combination therapy. Nat Med 2001; 7(9): 987–989.

35. Kabbinavar F, et al. Phase II, randomized trial comparing bevacizumab plus fluorouracil (FU)/leucovorin (LV) with FU/LV alone in patients with metastatic colorectal cancer. J Clin Oncol 2003; 21(1): 60–65.

36. Hurwitz H, et al. Bevacizumab plus irinotecan, fluorouracil, and leucovorin for metastatic colorectal cancer. N Engl J Med 2004; 350(23): 2335–2342.

37. Hsei VC, et al. Population pharmacokinetic (PK) analysis of bevacizumab (BV) in cancer subjects. In ASCO Annual Meeting 2001.

38. Herbst RS, et al. Phase I/II trial evaluating the anti-vascular endothelial growth factor monoclonal antibody bevacizumab in combination with the HER-1/epidermal growth factor receptor tyrosine kinase inhibitor erlotinib for patients with recurrent non-small-cell lung cancer. J Clin Oncol 2005; 23(11): 2544–2555.

39. Chung KY, et al. Cetuximab shows activity in colorectal cancer patients with tumors that do not express the epi-

dermal growth factor receptor by immunohistochemistry. J Clin Oncol 2005; 23(9): 1803–1810.

40. Scaltriti M and Baselga J. The epidermal growth factor receptor pathway: A model for targeted therapy. Clin Cancer Res 2006; 12(18): 5268–5272.

41. Goldstein NI, et al. Biological efficacy of a chimeric antibody to the epidermal growth factor receptor in a human tumor xenograft model. Clin Cancer Res 1995; 1(11): 1311–1318.

42. Baselga J, et al. Phase I studies of anti-epidermal growth factor receptor chimeric antibody C225 alone and in combination with cisplatin. J Clin Oncol 2000; 18(4): 904–914.

43. Saltz LB, et al. Phase II trial of cetuximab in patients with refractory colorectal cancer that expresses the epidermal growth factor receptor. J Clin Oncol 2004; 22(7): 1201–1208.

44. Cunningham D, et al. Cetuximab monotherapy and cetuximab plus irinotecan in irinotecan-refractory metastatic colorectal cancer. N Engl J Med 2004; 351(4): 337–345.

45. Cohenuram M and Saif MW. Panitumumab, the first fully human monoclonal antibody: From the bench to the clinic. Anticancer Drugs 2007; 18(1): 7–15.

46. Rowinsky EK, et al. Safety, pharmacokinetics, and activity of ABX-EGF, a fully human anti-epidermal growth factor receptor monoclonal antibody in patients with metastatic renal cell cancer. J Clin Oncol 2004; 22(15): 3003–3015.

47. Hecht JP, et al. ABX-EGF monotherapy in patients (pts) with metastatic colorectal cancer (mCRC): An updated analysis. In ASCO Annual Meeting 2004.

48. Hecht JP, et al. Panitumumab in combination with 5-fluorouracil, leucovorin, and irinotecan (IFL) or FOLFIRI for first-line treatment of metastatic colorectal cancer (mCRC). In Gastrointestinal Cancers Symposium. 2006. San Francisco.

49. Peeters M, et al. A Phase 3, multicenter, randomized controlled trial of panitumumab plus best supportive care (BSC) vs. BSC alone in patients with metastatic colorectal cancer. In American Association for Cancer Research Annual Meeting 2006.

50. Lobo ED, Hansen RJ, and Balthasar JP. Antibody pharmacokinetics and pharmacodynamics. J Pharm Sci 2004; 93(11): 2645–2668.

51. Brody T. Introductions and definitions. In: K Minneman (ed.), Brody's Human Pharmacology, pp. 3–8. Philadelphia: Elsevier-Mosby, 2005.

52. Somogyi A. Clinical pharmacokinetics and issues in therapeutics. In: K Minneman (ed.), Brody's Human Pharmacology, pp. 41–56. Philadelphia: Elsevier-Mosby, 2005.

53. Hollenberg P. Absorption, distribution, metabolism, and elimination. In: K Minneman (ed.), Brody's Human Pharmacology, pp. 27–39. Philadelphia: Elsevier-Mosby, 2005.

54. Minneman KP. Receptors and concentration-response relationships. In: K Minneman (ed.), Brody's Human Pharmacology, pp. 9–25. Philadelphia: Elsevier-Mosby, 2005.

PART II

PRINCIPLES OF IMAGE-GUIDED THERAPIES

Chapter 5

IMAGE-GUIDED INTERVENTIONS: FUNDAMENTALS OF RADIOFREQUENCY TUMOR ABLATION

Andrew Hines-Peralta

S. Nahum Goldberg

KEY POINTS

- Radiofrequency (RF) ablation is a viable alternative for the treatment of many solid focal malignancies, especially in the non-surgical candidate.

- Benefits of RF ablation include low morbidity and mortality, low cost, non-surgical patient inclusion, and same-day discharge.

- Successful treatment is a balance between complete tumor destruction and minimizing damage to surrounding normal parenchyma and adjacent structures.

- The bio-heat equation states: *coagulation necrosis = energy deposited × local tissue interactions – heat loss*. This forms the foundation of RF ablation.

- Widespread adoption of RF ablation will rely upon improving and increasing tumor ablation volume. Adjuvant therapies such as antiangiogenetics, chemotherapeutics, embolization, and radiation in this capacity hold great promise.

INTRODUCTION

Minimally invasive RF ablation continues to gain attention as a viable option for the treatment of multiple solid malignancies given continued favorable outcome studies coupled with scarce complications (1–4). Advantages of RF ablation include a wider spectrum of patients, including non-surgical candidates and outpatients, along with lower immediate morbidity and mortality, and lower cost (5–6). For these reasons and impressive initial outcomes, the indications continue to broaden to include multiple tumor types, multiple locations and ever-expanding patient selection criteria. Currently, the most commonly ablated tumor worldwide is focal hepatic cell carcinoma (HCC), but rapid acceptance of renal cell carcinoma (RCC) has been shown in many parts of the world, including the United States (7–12). Despite the numerous benefits, RF has not gained ubiquitous acceptance, likely secondary not only to limited clinical data but also to limitations in the size of ablation, the time it takes to perform ablation, and the predictability of ablation outcome, which can vary 5 to 10 mm per application (13–14). However, intense interest in this area is already resulting in improved tumor ablation, much of which is based upon adjuvant therapies such as concomitant antiangiogenics (15–16), chemotherapeutics (17–20), chemoembolization (21–29), radiation (30–34) and others (35–40).

Additionally, many of these issues can be addressed with improved knowledge of the basic principles behind RF ablation and the biophysiology of in vivo tissue heating, for which a fundamental knowledge is required to optimally perform RF ablation. It is likely that the future of RF ablation will involve multiple concomitant minimally invasive therapies for optimal success.

The goal of RF tumor ablation encompasses two specific objectives. First and foremost, the objective is to kill all viable malignant cells within a designated area. In addition, based upon studies examining tumor progression for patients undergoing surgical resection that often demonstrate the presence of viable malignant cells beyond visible tumor boundaries, conservative tumor ablation therapy will often attempt to ablate a 5- to 10-mm margin of surrounding tissue, similar to standard 1.0-cm "surgical margins" (41–42). In fact, however, this has been extrapolated for RF ablation, and it is not specifically known whether an "ablative margin" is necessary, or how large one needs to be.

The second goal of RF ablation relates specifically to one of its primary advantages, and that is the ability to minimize destruction to surrounding normal tissues. Thus, specificity and accuracy of therapy are also paramount for treatment success. For example, in RCC in a single kidney, maintaining functional renal parenchyma is a primary concern to minimize the risk for dialysis. In primary liver tumors, functional hepatic reserve is a primary predictive factor in long-term patient survival outcomes, and RF tumor ablation therapies have documented success in minimizing iatrogenic damage to cirrhotic parenchyma surrounding focal malignancies (43–44). This applies to numerous other examples and has partially fueled the rapid acceptance of this technique.

Therefore, the ultimate goal of RF ablation and all tumor ablation therapies is to achieve a balance between adequate tumor destruction and minimal damage to normal tissue and surrounding structures. Achieving this balance involves the interaction of three key components – the *technology* (i.e., the RF generator and electrodes selected), the *biology* of the tumor and background tissue and *operator* factors (Figure 5.1). In this chapter, we discuss the interaction of these three components to achieve successful tumor ablation.

THERMAL COAGULATION NECROSIS

RF ablation mediates cell death via direct effects of heat. The heat from RF ablation is produced via tissue

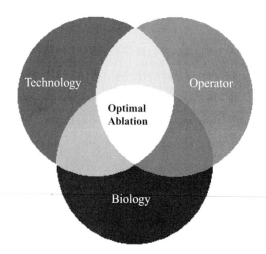

FIGURE 5.1. Conceptualization of the key components necessary to achieve optimal ablation. The three key components for achieving successful RF ablation include *technology* (i.e., the RF generator and electrodes selected), the *biology* of the tumor and background tissue; and *operator* factors. Interfaces between technology and biology include *adjuvant therapies* that modulate these two factors. *Technique* defines the interface between technology and operator, whereas *patient selection* represents the operator interacting with tumor biology. See Color Plate 9.

resistance to the transmittance of RF energy, and this resistive energy is converted to heat, analogous to heat production from an electrical resister in an electrical circuit. The cellular death that occurs from the intolerable accumulation of heat is termed **thermal coagulation necrosis** (45). Therefore, generated temperatures and their pattern of distribution within treated tissues determine the amount of tumor destruction.

Research prior to the development of RF ablation has shown that cellular homeostatic mechanisms can accommodate slight increases in temperature (to 40°C). Though increased susceptibility to damage by other mechanisms (radiation, chemotherapy) is seen at hyperthermic temperatures between 42°C and 45°C, cell function and tumor growth continue even after prolonged exposure to these temperatures (46–47). In general, irreversible cellular injury occurs when cells are heated to 46°C for 60 minutes and occurs more rapidly as temperature rises (48). However, the optimal desired temperatures for ablation are usually less than 100°C because temperatures above 105°C can result in tissue vaporization that results in total RF energy impedance (49).

However, the exact temperature at which cell death occurs is multifactorial and tissue specific. We have recently shown that depending on time and tissue, maximum temperatures at the edge of ablation known as the "critical temperature" ranged 30°C, from 46°C to 77°C for normal tissues and from 41°C to 64°C for tumor models (a 23°C difference). Likewise, the total amount of heat known as the thermal dose will also vary significantly (50).

Regardless of temperature, the basis for immediate cellular damage centers on protein coagulation of cytosolic and mitochondrial enzymes, and nucleic acid-histone protein complexes (48, 51). Damage triggers cellular death over the course of several days. "Thermal coagulation necrosis" is used to describe this thermal damage, though this can be a misnomer as the irreversible cellular injury may not fulfill strict histopathology criteria of coagulative necrosis. This is important to consider as histopathologic interpretation of coagulation necrosis, a usual indicator from standard H and E staining, may not be a reliable measure of RF ablation (51). In our laboratory and others, we utilize irreversible mitochondrial energy, which can be measured by compounds such as TTC (2,3,5-triphenyl tetrazolium chloride), as a more reliable indicator of the irreversible cell death from RF ablation (52). Visually, core ablation is white, corresponding to coagulated tissue, followed by a surrounding hyperemic "red" zone composed of partial necrosis and inflammation. This "red" zone is thought responsible for post-procedure pain.

THE BIO-HEAT EQUATION

The key biologic factors for RF ablation include blood perfusion, electrical and thermal conductivity, as well as sensitivity to heat and other adjuvant therapies. A rubric for trying to understand how these complex dynamics interact was first described by Pennes et al., now referred to as the bio-heat equation (53). This equation states:

$$\rho_t c_t \partial T(r, t)/\partial t = \nabla(k_t \nabla T) - c_b \rho_b m \rho_t(T - T_b)$$
$$+ Q_p(r, t) + Q_m(r, t)$$

where

ρ_t, ρ_b = density of tissue, blood (kg/m^3)

c_t, c_b = specific heat of tissue, blood (W s/kg C)

k_t = thermal conductivity of tissue

m = perfusion (blood flow rate/unit mass tissue) (m^3/kg s)

Q_p = power absorbed/unit volume of tissue

Q_m = metabolic heating/unit volume of tissues

T = temperature of tissue

T_b = temperature of blood

d = derivative

∇ = change

kg = kilogram

m = meter

W = watt

s = sec

C = Celsius

(r, t) = variables (place, time)

A reasonable approximation of this equation that we have previously used to describe the basic relationship guiding coagulation necrosis is "coagulation necrosis = energy deposited × local tissue interactions – heat loss."

This equation is fundamental to RF ablation in the clinical setting as well as the research setting. First, the accuracy and specificity needed to balance between total tumor destruction and minimal functional tissue loss, the ultimate objective of RF ablation, necessitate a firm understanding of heat loss and tissue interactions that will affect the extent and completeness of ablation. Secondly, as RF struggles with larger tumors, this equation outlines the three potential research arenas for improvement: (1) increasing energy deposition, (2) understanding and manipulating tissue interactions and (3) minimizing heat loss.

PART I: ENERGY DEPOSITED – TECHNOLOGY

The first component of the bio-heat equation states that cell death is determined by energy deposition, and it is no surprise that multiple methods have been developed to increase and improve energy deposition. This can be accomplished via the two major components of RF ablation, the power generator and applicator. Multiple companies have FDA approval for their RF ablation devices, but none has yet shown definitive superiority, and multiple new devices continue to be developed (55–58). Applicator design can be varied in attempts to improve energy deposition depth and distribution, and generators can be altered to deliver a complex algorithm of differing magnitudes and spectrums of RF energy (Table 5.1).

Power Generators and Energy Delivery Algorithms

Each of the three major commercially available RF generator systems relies on a different algorithm to optimally match energy delivery to tissue characteristics and uses different endpoints. It is important to

TABLE 5.1 Commercially Available Generator Algorithms and Endpoints per Manufacturer

Electrode		Algorithm	Endpoint
ValleyLab	Internally cooled	Pulsed	Time
RITA	Multi-tined	Tine extension/temperature	Stepped power
Radiotherapeutics	Multi-tined	Power/time	Impedance

mention that none of these endpoints and algorithms has been fully evaluated at this time over the wide spectrum of biologic tissues that are currently ablated. Given this paucity of "science," there is much "art" to performing RF ablation, with technique clearly playing a role in outcome. The ValleyLab system utilizes the pulse algorithm with a single defined time endpoint of 12 minutes for conventional ablation and 16 minutes for switching technology. This is likely to be refined on a tissue-by-tissue and application-by-application basis in the future. The multi-tined application system of RITA relies on a stepped power algorithm with incremental extension of tines often accompanied by a small amount of perfusion of normal saline. The end point for this algorithm is a combination of achieving defined tissue temperatures for a given amount of time. Again, given varied tissue thermal sensitivity, further refinement is anticipated. The Radiotherapeutics devices of Boston Scientific have a ramped algorithm based upon incremental increases of power for given times and rely on the uncontrolled rise in impedance (i.e., so-called roll-off) to determine adequacy of ablation. Here, too, further refinement is anticipated.

Multi-applicator Arrays

The easiest way to increase the volume of coagulation is to lengthen the exposure of the RF applicator tip, but this results in a cylindrical lesion shape that does not correspond well with the spherical geometry of most tumors. One method to create more spherical ablation is to manually move a single applicator between multiple treatments (56, 59–60). However, this is time-consuming and complicated, and for complete ablation, this requires multiple overlapping treatments in a contiguous fashion to adequately treat tumors. Hence, the time and effort required for this usually make it impractical for use in a clinical setting.

Several conventional monopolar RF applicators can simultaneously be used to increase ablation without prolonging treatment time (56, 60). Spacing no greater than 1.5 cm between individual applicators can produce uniform and reproducible tissue coagulation, with simultaneous application of RF energy producing more necrosis than sequential application. Coagulation shape is further dependent on spacing and the number of probes and most often corresponds to the array shape. This improvement in RF application results in a significant increase in ablated tumor volume of up to 800% over RF application with a single conventional probe with similar tip exposure (60).

Multi-tine Applicators

Working to overcome the technical challenges of multiprobe application, which requires multiple puncture sites, multi-tined expandable RF electrodes have been developed. These systems involve the deployment of a varying number of multiple thin, curved tines in the shape of an umbrella or more complex geometries from a central cannula (54, 55, 61). This surmounts earlier difficulties by allowing easy placement of multiple probes to create large, reproducible volumes of necrosis, such as 3.5 cm in diameter in in vivo porcine liver (55, 61).

Bipolar Arrays

Several groups have worked with bipolar arrays to increase the volume of coagulation created by RF application compared with the conventional monopolar system (57, 63). In these systems, applied RF current runs from an active electrode to a second grounding electrode in place of a grounding pad, theoretically utilizing twice as much heat for ablation. This also eliminates the need for surface grounding pads and the risk of grounding pad burns. However, the heat generated around both electrodes creates elliptical lesions, and while this results in an overall increase in coagulation volume, the shape of necrosis is generally unsuitable for tumors that are usually spherical, making the gains in coagulation less clinically significant. Some experimental applicators have utilized a combination of cryoablation and RF in an attempt to create more spherical lesions while also utilizing the proposed benefits of a bipolar system (64). Lastly, two multi-tined electrodes have been used as active and return to increase coagulation during bipolar RF ablation while also switching the applicators between active and ground to increase ablation efficiency (65).

Internally Cooled Electrodes

One of the limitations to greater RF energy deposition has been overheating surrounding the active electrode, leading to tissue charring, rising impedance and RF circuit interruption. To address this, internally cooled electrodes have been developed that are capable of greater coagulation compared with conventional monopolar RF electrodes (55–56, 58, 66–68). These electrodes contain two hollow lumens that permit continuous internal cooling of the tip with a chilled perfusate, and the removal of warmed effluent to a collection unit outside of the body. This reduces heating directly around the electrode, tissue charring and rising impedance, allowing greater RF energy deposition. With this technique, RF energy deposited into tissue and resultant coagulation necrosis were significantly greater ($p < 0.001$) than those achieved without electrode cooling (66–67).

Cluster RF

Based upon success in inducing greater volumes of necrosis by using both multiprobe arrays and cooling, one standard system now involves three 2-cm tip internally cooled applicators spaced 0.5 cm apart, producing reproducible ablation greater than 3 cm in perfused liver (68). This is one of the more popular ablation devices currently used in the clinical setting, with much reported literature (1–5, 13).

Perfused Electrodes

Perfusion electrodes have also been developed, which have small apertures at the active tip, allowing fluids (i.e., normal or hypertonic saline) to be infused or injected into the tissue before, during or after the ablation procedure. This may improve heat diffusion and electrical and thermal conduction of the tissue (69–72). At least one system clinically utilizes this technique to improve the quality of ablation produced by their applicator (69–71). Sodium chloride (NaCl) will alter the tissue characteristics in a manner more favorable for ablation through multiple fac-

tors. First, NaCl increases the electrical conductivity, which increases ablation per the bio-heat equation, as we discuss in more depth later. Also, NaCl potentially improves the thermal conduction if the flow rate is high by aiding the diffusion of heat from the central electrode (72). There is also a reduction in charring as well the "flushing" of bubbles from the electrode tract, which form during RF ablation and are known to limit electrical conductance. Lastly, hypertonic NaCl solutions have a mild toxic tumoricidal quality when injected alone (72).

Pulsed RF Application

Pulsing of energy is another strategy that has been used with RF and other energy sources such as laser to increase the mean intensity of energy deposition. When pulsing is used, periods of high energy deposition are rapidly alternated with periods of low energy deposition. If a proper balance between high and low energy deposition is achieved, preferential tissue cooling occurs adjacent to the electrode during periods of minimal energy deposition without significantly decreasing heating deeper in the tissue. Thus, even greater energy can be applied during periods of high energy deposition, thereby enabling deeper heat penetration and greater tissue coagulation (73). Synergy between a combination of both internal cooling and pulsing has resulted in greater coagulation necrosis and tumor destruction than either method alone (73).

Switching RF Applicator Energy

Several RF generator systems that enable switching among three electrically independent applicators have been created that generate significantly larger ablation than simultaneous use (74–75). This relies upon switching energy to applicators during the impedance spikes of the remaining applicators, during which time the system would typically be applying no energy to recuperate. One proposed theory is because of electrical interference between electrodes, the simultaneous method leads to less heating at the center than rapid switching when only a single electrode is active at a single point (74–75).

Comparison to Other Thermal Sources

Thermal ablation can be achieved with multiple other heat sources, including microwave (76–77), light in the form of laser energy (78) and sound in the form of focused ultrasound (79). Furthermore, cold can destroy tumors, as is well documented by the cryoablation literature (80). In the past, RF has received the lion's share of industrial support and attention given the fact that it is a very adaptable technology. Nevertheless, direct comparisons to other technologies, particularly microwave, with its reported faster and higher temperature heating, and ultrasound, which has the advantage of requiring no applicator, will be required in the future. Yet it is important to acknowledge that this must be done in a well-controlled manner given the fact that other factors such as the operator and tissue biology can potentially impact results. It is also important to stress that tumor cells, patients suffering from cancer and physicians really should not care which energy source produces cyto-toxic heat. A key facet for competitive technologies will be the ability to ablate the desired volume of tissue in a reproducible and predictable fashion. Yet, depending on the circumstances, most devices can really only achieve 3 to 5 cm of predictable coagulation (1–5). Furthermore, it must be noted that greater variability is seen with all technologies when bigger volumes of coagulation are attempted.

PART II: BIOLOGY AND TISSUE INTERACTIONS

The second of the three principal factors for successful RF ablation is the tumor biology and tissue interaction of the surroundings tissues and tumor. The adapted bio-heat equation dictates how tissue characteristics and heat loss substantially impact RF-induced thermal coagulation. These tissue characteristics include the electrical and thermal conductivity in not only the tumor, but the surrounding tissue. To this end, strategies to improve RF ablation involve the administration of adjuvant therapies to modulate the biology to better match the RF technology, including (1) minimizing heat loss, (2) maximizing heat deposition and (3) using concomitant tumoricidal therapies that can kill cells directly or increase their susceptibility to injury by heat (Table 5.2).

Effect of Tumor and Background Tissue Characteristics

There is marked heterogeneity in the inner tumor and surrounding background tissue characteristics of various tumors currently treated with RF ablation. For example, the tissue environment is very different in liver parenchyma surrounding colorectal metastases

TABLE 5.2 Adjuvant Strategies to Improve RF Ablation

1. Modulate bio-heat equation parameters to increase RF energy deposition
   a. Perfusion (heat loss)
   b. Electrical conductivity
   c. Thermal conductivity
2. Use of synergistic tumoricidal therapies with thermal ablation
   a. Chemoembolization
   b. Chemotherapy (liposomal)
   c. Radiation
   d. Antiangiogenics
   e. Other therapies such as ethanol injection

(normal liver) compared with hepatocellular carcinoma (cirrhotic liver). The time required to achieve complete ablation depends upon both inner tumor and outer background tissue perfusion (81). In experiments using two-compartment agar phantom models and computer modeling, the amount of fat in the background tissue results in significantly increased temperatures within the "tumor" core, whereas lower temperatures are observed in the background fatty tissue (82). Extrapolation with computer modeling based upon the bio-heat equation confirms lower thermal conductivity of background tissues significantly increases temperatures within a defined ablation target. Findings such as these provide insight into the "oven effect" (i.e., increased heating efficacy for tumors surrounded by cirrhotic liver or fat) and highlight the importance of both the tumor and the surrounding tissue characteristics when contemplating RF ablation efficacy. However, these results currently remain confined to an experimental setting, and caution must therefore be extended to ensure that there is no overinterpretation of positive or negative data from one clinical scenario carried to another.

Electrical Conductivity

Experimental and clinical studies have demonstrated that alteration of tissue electrical conductivity with injection of adjuvant saline around the electrode can increase RF heating (69–72, 83). Although increased tumor coagulation can be achieved by administering adjuvant pretreatment saline around the RF electrode, or using electrodes that administer continuous infusion of saline during RF application, there continues to be heterogeneity and variability in coagulation depending upon the distribution of saline in the tumor tissue, and difficulty in overall result reproducibility (83).

Decreasing Tissue Perfusion

As the bio-heat equation states, one of the impediments to cell death is heat loss, and one of the most important sources of heat loss is blood perfusion within the tumor and surrounding tissues that acts as a heat-sink to draw head energy away from the ablation site (84–86). In order to fully understand this effect, computer simulation has shown initial promise in modeling various clinical scenarios and predicting ablation under various ablation algorithms (87). In addition to tissue perfusion, larger vessels can markedly distort and limit tumor ablation. Invagination of enhancing tissue between vessel and RF lesion is observed in the vast majority of cases in which vessels are greater than 4 mm (86,88). If these larger vessels are occluded, this effect is negated, supporting the negative impact of blood flow within these vessels (88–89).

Several strategies have been used successfully to reduce the negative effect of tissue perfusion on RF heating, for instance, vascular occlusion such as the Pringle maneuver, but this often requires an open procedure and obviates the purported benefits of percutaneous treatment (89). Selective angiographic balloon occlusion and/or injection of embolization material (gelfoam or lipiodol) have also been utilized successfully and should be considered in these difficult cases. The downside is the extra technical experience that is necessary and prolonged treatment time (88–89).

Another strategy to reduce perfusion-related tissue cooling has been to employ pharmacologic agents, such as halothane and arsenic trioxide, to modulate tissue perfusion. In animal models, arsenic trioxide has demonstrated antivascular effects, and when combined with RF ablation, can potentially increase RF heating and coagulation (15–16). Recently, less toxic antiangiogenic agents have become standard therapies in the treatment of a wide range of malignancies, including RCC, by decreasing tumor vasculature and may also be used as potential adjuvants with thermal ablation. Recent studies have demonstrated that modification of tumor vessel density using antiangiogenic agents such as sorafenib to increase RF coagulation (15). In one study, the administration of sorafenib prior to RF ablation markedly decreased microvascular density and led to significantly larger zones

of RF-induced coagulation necrosis (15). Although these methods are still in their investigational phase, there is promise for their rapid acceptance and adoption in standard clinical practice.

Combining Adjuvant Cytotoxic Therapies

Although thermal ablation therapies have demonstrated efficacy in treating focal small tumors, combining these with other adjuvant cytotoxic therapies such as chemotherapy may increase treatment efficacy in larger tumors and improve overall completeness of treatment and tumor destruction. In one pilot clinical study by Goldberg et al., RF ablation combined with adjuvant intravenous liposomal doxorubicin resulted in more complete tumor treatment and ablative margin (17–20, 90). Additionally, combined RF and adjuvant liposomal chemotherapy can potentially overcome limitations imposed by tumor or organ environment, such as blood flow.

Performing transcatheter arterial chemoembolization before RF ablation for HCC has demonstrated superior outcomes over either modality alone, and is becoming a popular treatment alternative for qualifying patients (21–29, 91–92). Combined therapy for these typically non-early HCCs have shown a relatively high complete local response (especially for tumors <5 cm in diameter) with promising mid-term follow-up. The quality of life as determined by socio-family well-being and functional well-being scores are also superior in patients receiving both chemoembolization and RF ablation, a reflection of liver function, tumor recurrence and complications (93).

As of January, 2007, at least 21 studies totaling nearly 1,500 patients had been published that support a combined therapy approach (15–40, 91–104). Many of these combined either RF ablation and/or alcohol chemical ablation with chemoembolization. Yet, it is important to stress that only three of these studies were randomized prospective studies, and these contained only 114 patients. Furthermore only five studies, fewer than 100 patients in total, had 5-year follow-up. Likewise, heterogeneous patient populations regarding tumor and stage, heterogeneous therapies, including the types of ablation in adjuvants and heterogeneous follow-up limit the conclusions that can be drawn from these studies. Thus, the best size and stage for a specific combination therapy to prevent over- or undertreatment, the best window between therapies, and the best composition of chemoembolization (i.e., bland or containing specified chemotherapeutics) are unknown at this time. Thus, there are insufficient data to advocate in favor of one particular combination therapy and therefore therapies will need to be tailored on a patient-by-patient basis at this time.

Combining RF Ablation with Radiation

Recent studies have demonstrated increased tumor destruction with combination RF ablation and adjuvant radiation therapy, including initial animal research with mammary adenocarcinoma treated with combined RF ablation and radiation therapy (30). More recently, clinical studies combining RF ablation with adjuvant radiation therapy for primary lung tumors have demonstrated preliminary efficacy (31–34). Intermediate follow-up (24 to 36 months) demonstrated low complication rates and suggested outcomes greater than RF or radiation alone (31–34).

PART III: OPERATOR AND TECHNIQUE

It is well established that there are different approaches to the treatment of ablation, including who performs ablation, how it is performed, and the imaging guidance devices used (13, 105). All of these will have substantial impact on the ultimate results. In addition to interventional radiologists, many surgical specialties and other medical specialties are advocating to perform ablation. For colorectal metastases, surgical technique often involves multiple repetitive ablations at a single operation. By contrast, image-guided interventional technique enables multiple repeat treatments. The type of imaging guidance used, be it ultrasound (with or without contrast where available), computed tomography and/or magnetic resonance, will likely influence outcome (13, 105–106). Additionally, many advocate the use of multiple imaging modalities. Furthermore, multiple investigators are working on refining methods for fusing images and robotic surgery, which will undoubtedly alter outcomes due to improved targeting and monitoring technique.

Choice of Applicator

An important decision for the operator involves the choice of applicator. Proper geometric coverage that involves complete tumor destruction while minimizing normal tissue is partially dependent upon choice of single or multiple applicators (1, 13, 55). Choice of multi-tine applicator involves when to use a cluster cooled electrode versus a given multi-tined applicator. Thus, there are also many variations in technique described (or practiced) as to how to adequately, but efficiently, coagulate a tumor.

Overlapping Techniques

It is not uncommon that tumor burden exceeds the size of ablation than can be reproducibly created by a single ablative session, and for this reason, multiple treatments are often necessary during a RF ablation session for adequate treatment, as previously stated. This requires readjustment of the applicators into untreated tumor tissues between sessions. The goal of multiple treatments is to create a large contiguous spherical ablative volume, usually with a 5- to 10-mm "abative margin." However, given the geometry of trying to obtain a large complete spherical ablative zone with smaller spheres, significant overlap of previous zones is necessary for complete ablation (13, 105). Alternatively, aligning ablations "end-to-end" would result in multiple areas of untreated tumor.

Patient Selection

Perhaps the most important variable to have the greatest impact on results is the interplay between operator and patient selection. Multiple studies have shown excellent results for small tumors less than 3 cm, but difficulty has been described in treating larger tumors (1–13). Thus, for larger tumors, successful treatment is contingent upon careful patient selection with consideration of multiple variables such as tumor biology, location and number of treatment sessions.

CONCLUSION

There is no one right way to perform RF ablation, yet a fundamental knowledge of the basic principles behind RF ablation and the biophysiology of in vivo tissue heating are required to avoid the many potential pitfalls in performing optimal thermal ablation. We have provided a basic overview of the basic principles of RF ablation, focused on the three main elements, including: (1) RF technology, (2) tumor biology and (3) operator expertise. At the foundation of these three intersecting elements is the bio-heat equation that influences the extent of RF ablation. Successful tumor ablation is a balance between obtaining complete tumor destruction while minimizing damage to surrounding normal parenchyma, and is embedded in appreciation and understanding of these three interweaving elements.

Despite the numerous benefits of RF ablation, RF ablation has not yet gained ubiquitous acceptance in part because of the inability to reliably achieve large zones of coagulation for larger tumor sizes (1). Here, again, the three key elements described in this chapter dictate the potential arenas for improvement. Although multiple modifications have already been developed within the technology of RF ablation, future directions will emphasize a better understanding of tumor biology in order to alter local tissue interactions and minimize heat loss coupled with adjuvant therapies such as antiangiogenetics, embolization, chemotherapeutics and radiation.

REFERENCES

1. Dupuy D, Goldberg S. Image-guided radiofrequency tumor ablation: Challenges and opportunities – Part II. J Vasc Interv Radiol 2001; 12: 1135–1148.

2. Lencioni R, et al. Early-stage hepatocellular carcinoma in patients with cirrhosis: Long-term results of percutaneous image-guided radiofrequency ablation. Radiology 2005; 234: 961–967.

3. Dodd GD, 3rd, et al. Minimally invasive treatment of malignant hepatic tumors: At the threshold of a major breakthrough. Radiographics 2000; 20(1): 9–27.

4. Lencioni R, et al. Early stage hepatocellular carcinoma in patients with cirrhosis: Long-term results of percutaneous image-guided radiofrequency ablation. Radiology 2005; 234(3): 961–967.

5. Kim YK, et al. Radiofrequency ablation of hepatocellular carcinoma in patients with decompensated cirrhosis: Evaluation of therapeutic efficacy and safety. AJR Am J Roentgenol 2006; 186(5 Suppl): S261–268.

6. Colella G, et al. Hepatocellular carcinoma: Comparison between liver transplantation, resective surgery, ethanol injection, and chemoembolization. Transpl Int 1998; 11(Suppl 1): S193–196.

7. Gervais DA, et al. Radiofrequency ablation of renal cell carcinoma: Part 1; Indications, results, and role in patient management over a 6-year period and ablation of 100 tumors. AJR Am J Roentgenol 2005; 185(1): 64–71.

8. Pavlovich CP, et al. Percutaneous radio frequency ablation of small renal tumors: Initial results. J Urol 2002; 167(1): 10–15.

9. Gervais DA, et al. Radiofrequency ablation of renal cell carcinoma: Part 2, Lessons learned with ablation of 100 tumors. AJR Am J Roentgenol 2005; 185(1): 72–80.

10. Pautler SE, et al. Retroperitoneoscopic-guided radiofrequency ablation of renal tumors. Can J Urol 2001; 8: 1330–1333.

11. Arzola J, Baughman SM, Hernandez J, et al. Computed tomography-guided, resistance-based, percutaneous radiofrequency ablation of renal malignancies under conscious sedation at two years of follow-up. Urology 2006 Nov; 68(5): 983–987.

12. Gervais DA, Arellano RS, and Mueller PR. Percutaneous radiofrequency ablation of renal cell carcinoma. Eur Radiol 2005; 15(5): 960–967.

13. Goldberg SN and Dupuy EE. Image-guided radiofrequency tumor ablation: Challenges and opportunities – Part I. J Vasc Interv Radiol 2001; 12: 1021–1032.

14. Montgomery RS, et al. Radiofrequency ablation of hepatic tumors: variability of lesion size using a single ablation device. AJR Am J Roentgenol 2004; 182(3): 657–661.

15. Hakime A, Hines-Peralta AU, Peddy H, et al. Combination of radiofrequency ablation with antiangiogenic therapy for tumor ablation efficacy: Study in mice. Radiology. 2007 Aug; 244(2): 464–470.

16. Hines-Peralta A, Sukhatme V, Atkins M, et al. Arsenic trioxide and radiofrequency ablation: Improved tumor destruction in three animal models. Radiology 2006 Jul; 240(1): 82–89.

17. Ahmed M, Liu Z, Lukyanov AN, et al. Combination radiofrequency ablation with intratumoral liposomal doxorubicin: Effect on drug accumulation and coagulation in multiple tissues and tumor types in animals. Radiology 2005 May; 235(2): 469–477.

18. Goldberg SN, Kamel IR, Kruskal JB, et al. Radiofrequency ablation of hepatic tumors: Increased tumor destruction with adjuvant liposomal doxorubicin therapy. AJR Am J Roentgenol 2002 Jul; 179(1): 93–101.

19. Goldberg SN, et al. Percutaneous tumor ablation: Increased necrosis with combined radio-frequency ablation and intravenous liposomal doxorubicin in a rat breast tumor model. Radiology 2002; 222(3): 797–804.

20. Goldberg SN, et al. Percutaneous tumor ablation: increased coagulation necrosis with combined radiofrequency and percutaneous doxorubicin injection. Radiology 2001; 220: 420–427.

21. Veltri A, Moretto P, Doriguzzi A, et al. Radiofrequency thermal ablation (RFA) after transarterial chemoembolization (TACE) as a combined therapy for unresectable non-early hepatocellular carcinoma (HCC). Eur Radiol 2006 Mar; 16(3): 661–669.

22. Buscarini L, Buscarini E, Di Stasi M, et al. Percutaneous radiofrequency thermal ablation combined with transcatheter arterial embolization in the treatment of large hepatocellular carcinoma. Ultraschall Med 1999 Apr; 20(2): 47–53.

23. Inoue Y, Miki C, Hiro J, et al. Improved survival using multi-modality therapy in patients with lung metastases from colorectal cancer: A preliminary study. Oncol Rep 2005 Dec; 14(6): 1571–1576.

24. Qian J, Feng GS, and Vogl T. Combined interventional therapies of hepatocellular carcinoma. World J Gastroenterol 2003 Sep; 9(9): 1885–1891.

25. Kitamoto M, Imagawa M, Yamada H, et al. Radiofrequency ablation in the treatment of small hepatocellular carcinomas: Comparison of the radiofrequency effect with and without chemoembolization. AJR Am J Roentgenol 2003 Oct; 181(4): 997–1003.

26. Shen SQ, Xiang JJ, Xiong CL, et al. Intraoperative radiofrequency thermal ablation combined with portal

vein infusion chemotherapy and transarterial chemoembolization for unresectable HCC. Hepatogastroenterology 2005 Sep-Oct; 52(65): 1403–1407.

27. Yamakado K, Nakatsuka A, Akeboshi M, et al. Combination therapy with radiofrequency ablation and transcatheter chemoembolization for the treatment of hepatocellular carcinoma: Short-term recurrences and survival. Oncol Rep 2004 Jan; 11(1): 105–109.

28. Yamakado K, Nakatsuka A, Ohmori S, et al. Radiofrequency ablation combined with chemoembolization in hepatocellular carcinoma: Treatment response based on tumor size and morphology. J Vasc Interv Radiol 2002 Dec; 13(12): 1225–1232.

29. Bloomston M, Binitie O, Fraiji E, et al. Transcatheter arterial chemoembolization with or without radiofrequency ablation in the management of patients with advanced hepatic malignancy. Am Surg 2002 Sep; 68(9): 827–831.

30. Horkan C, et al. Reduced tumor growth with combined radiofrequency ablation and radiation therapy in a rat breast tumor model. Radiology 2005; 235(1): 81–8.

31. Jain SK, et al. Percutaneous radiofrequency ablation of pulmonary malignancies: Combined treatment with brachytherapy. AJR Am J Roentgenol 2003; 181(3): 711–715.

32. Grieco CA, et al. Percutaneous image-guided thermal ablation and radiation therapy: Outcomes of combined treatment for 41 patients with inoperable stage I/II non-small-cell lung cancer. J Vasc Interv Radiol 2006; 17(7): 1117–1124.

33. Dupuy DE, et al. Radiofrequency ablation followed by conventional radiotherapy for medically inoperable stage I non-small-cell lung cancer. Chest 2006; 129(3): 738–745.

34. Ricke J, Wust P, Stohlmann A, et al. CT-guided interstitial brachytherapy of liver malignancies alone or in combination with thermal ablation: Phase I-II results of a novel technique. Int J Radiat Oncol Biol Phys 2004 Apr 1; 58(5): 1496–1505.

35. Kurokohchi K, et al. Comparison between combination therapy of percutaneous ethanol injection and radiofrequency ablation and radiofrequency ablation alone for patients with hepatocellular carcinoma. World J Gastroenterol 2005; 11(10): 1426–1432.

36. Shankar S, vanSonnenberg E, Morrison PR, et al. Combined radiofrequency and alcohol injection for percutaneous hepatic tumor ablation. AJR Am J Roentgenol 2004 Nov; 183(5): 1425–1429.

37. Kurokohchi K, Watanabe S, Masaki T, et al. Combined use of percutaneous ethanol injection and radiofrequency ablation for the effective treatment of hepatocelluar carcinoma. Int J Oncol 2002 Oct; 21(4): 841–846.

38. Watanabe S, et al. Enlargement of thermal ablation zone by the combination of ethanol injection and radiofrequency ablation in excised bovine liver. Int J Oncol 2004; 24(2): 279–284.

39. Luo BM, Wen YL, Yang HY, et al. Percutaneous ethanol injection, radiofrequency and their combination in treatment of hepatocellular carcinoma. World J Gastroenterol 2005 Oct 28; 11(40): 6277–6280.

40. Sakaguchi Y, Kudo M, Fukunaga T, et al. Low-dose, long-term, intermittent interferon-alpha-2b therapy after radical treatment by radiofrequency ablation delays clinical recurrence in patients with hepatitis C virus-related hepatocellular carcinoma. Intervirology 2005 Jan–Feb; 48(1): 64–70.

41. Goldberg SN, Gazelle GS, and Mueller PR. Thermal ablation therapy for focal malignancy: A unified approach to underlying principles, technqiues, and diagnostic imaging guidance. Am J Radiol 2000; 174: 323–331.

42. Ahmed M and Goldberg SN. Thermal ablation therapy for hepatocellular carcinoma. J Vasc Interv Radiol 2002; 13(9 Suppl): S231–244.

43. Giorgio A, et al. Complications after percutaneous saline-enhanced radiofrequency ablation of liver tumors: 3-year experience with 336 patients at a single center. AJR Am J Roentgenol 2005; 184(1): 207–211.

44. Kim YK, et al. Radiofrequency ablation of hepatocellular carcinoma in patients with decompensated cirrhosis: Evaluation of therapeutic efficacy and safety. AJR Am J Roentgenol 2006; 186(5 Suppl): S261–268.

45. Zevas N and Kuwayama A. Pathologic analysis of experimental thermal lesions: Comparison of induction heating and radiofrequency electrocoagulation. J Neurosurg 1972; 37: 418–422.

46. Seegenschmiedt M, Brady L, and Sauer R. Interstitial thermoradiotherapy: Review on technical and clinical aspects. Am J Clin Oncol 1990; 13: 352–363.

47. van der Zee J, Dutch Deep Hyperthermia Group. et al., Comparison of radiotherapy alone with radiotherapy plus hyperthermia in locally advanced pelvic tumours: A prospective, randomised, multicentre trial. Lancet 2000; 355(9210): 1119–1125.

48. Trembley B, Ryan T, and Strohbehn J. "Interstitial hyperthermia: Physics, biology, and clinical aspects." In Hyperthermia and Oncology, Vol. 3 Utrecht: VSP 1992, pp. 11–98.

49. Gazelle GS, et al., Tumor ablation with radiofrequency energy. Radiology 2000; 217: 6333–6346.

50. Mertyna P, Hines-Peralta A, Liu Z, et al. Radiofrequency ablation: Variability in heat sensitivity in tumors and tissues. J Vasc Interv Radiol. 2007 May; 18(5): 647–654.

51. Goldberg SN, Gazelle GS, Compton CC, et al. Treatment of intrahepatic malignancy with radiofrequency ablation: Radiologic-pathologic correlation. Cancer 2000; 88: 2452–2463.

52. Liszczak TM, Hedley-Whyte ET, Adams JF, et al. Limitations of tetrazolium salts in delineating infracted brain. Acta Neuropathol (Berl) 1984; 65: 150–157.

53. Pennes H. Analysis of tissue and arterial blood temperatures in the resting human forearm. J Appl Physiol 1948:93–122.

54. Rossi S, Buscarini E, and Garbagnati F. Percutaneous treatment of small hepatic tumors by an expandable RF needle electrode. AJR Am J Roentgenol 1998; 170: 1015–1022.

55. de Baere T, et al. Radiofrequency liver ablation: Experimental comparative study of water-cooled versus expandable systems. AJR Am J Roentgenol 2001; 176(1): 187–192.

56. Haemmerich DG, et al., A device that allows for multiple simultaneous radiofrequency (RF) ablations in separated areas of the liver with impedance-controlled

cool-tip probes: An ex-vivo feasibility study [abstract]. Radiology 2002; 225(p): 242.

57. Desinger K, et al. Interstitial bipolar RF-thermotherapy therapy by planning by computer simulation and MRI-monitoring – a new concept for minimally invasive procedures. Proc SPIE 1999; 3249: 147–160.

58. Miao Y, et al. A comparative study on validation of a novel cooled-wet electrode for radiofrequency liver ablation. Invest Radiol 2000; 35(7): 438–444.

59. Solbiati L, Ierace T, Goldberg SN. Percutaneous US-guided RF tissue ablation of liver metastases: Long-term follow-up. Radiology 1997; 202: 195–203.

60. Goldberg SN, Gazelle GS, Dawson SL, et al. Tissue ablation with radiofrequency using multiprobe arrays. Acad Radiol 1995; 2: 670–674.

61. Miao Y, Ni Y, Yu J, et al. An ex vivo study on radiofrequency tissue ablation: Increased lesion size by using an "expandable-wet" electrode. Eur Radiol 2001; 11: 1841–1847.

62. Berber E, et al. Use of CT Hounsfield unit density to identify ablated tumor after laparoscopic radiofrequency ablation of hepatic tumors. Surg Endosc 2000; 14(9): 799–804.

63. Ritz JP, Lehmann KS, Isbert C, et al. In-vivo evaluation of a novel bipolar radiofrequency device for interstitial thermotherapy of liver tumors during normal and interrupted hepatic perfusion. J Surg Res 2006 Jun 15; 133(2): 176–184.

64. Hines-Peralta A, Hollander CY, Solazzo S, et al. Hybrid radiofrequency and cryoablation device: Preliminary results in an animal model. J Vasc Interv Radiol. 2004 Oct; 15(10): 1111–1120.

65. Haemmerich DG, Lee FTJ, Chachati L, et al. A device that allows for multiple simultaneous radiofrequency (RF) ablations in separated areas of the liver with impedance-controlled cool-tip probes: An ex vivo feasibility study. Radiology 2002; 225: 242.

66. Goldberg SN, Gazelle GS, Solbiati L, et al. Radiofrequency tissue ablation: Increased lesion diameter with a perfusion electrode. Acad Radiol 1996; 3: 636–644.

67. Lorentzen T. A cooled needle electrode for radiofrequency tissue ablation: Thermodynamic aspects of improved performance compared with conventional needle design. Acad Radiol 1996; 3: 556–563.

68. Goldberg SN, Solbiati L, Hahn PF, et al. Large-volume tissue ablation with radiofrequency by using a clustered, internally-cooled electrode technique: Laboratory and clinical experience in liver metastases. Radiology 1998; 209: 371–379.

69. Curley MG, Hamilton PS. Creation of large thermal lesions in liver using saline-enhanced RF ablation. Proc 19th International Conference IEEE/EMBS 1997: 2516–2519.

70. Livraghi T, Goldberg SN, Monti F, et al. Saline-enhanced radiofrequency tissue ablation in the treatment of liver metastases. Radiology 1997; 202: 205–210.

71. Miao Y, et al. An ex vivo study on radiofrequency tissue ablation: Increased lesion size by using an "expandable-wet" electrode. Eur Radiol 2001; 11(9): 1841–1847.

72. Ahmed M, Lobo SM, Weinstein J, et al. Improved coagulation with saline solution pretreatment during radiofrequency tumor ablation in a canine model. J Vasc Interv Radiol 2002; 12: 717–724.

73. Goldberg SN, Stein M, Gazelle GS, et al. Percutaneous radiofrequency tissue ablation: Optimization of pulsed-RF technique to increase coagulation necrosis. JVIR 1999; 10: 907–916.

74. Haemmerich DG, Lee FTJ, Mahvi DM, et al. Multiple probe radiofrequency: Rapid switching versus simultaneous power application in a computer model. Radiology 2002; 225(p): 639.

75. Lee FT Jr., Haemmerich D, Wright AS, et al. Multiple probe radiofrequency ablation: Pilot study in an animal model. J Vasc Interv Radiol 2003 Nov; 14(11): 1437–1442.

76. Brace CL, et al. Microwave ablation with a single small-gauge triaxial antenna: In vivo porcine liver model. Radiology 2007; 242(2): 435–440.

77. Dong B, et al. Percutaneous sonographically guided microwave coagulation therapy for hepatocellular carcinoma: Results in 234 patients. Am J Roentgenol 2003; 180: 1547–1555.

78. Dachman AH, et al. US-guided percutaneous laser ablation of liver tissue in a chronic pig model. Radiology 1990; 176: 129–133.

79. Jolesz FA and Hynynen K. Magnetic resonance image-guided focused ultrasound surgery. Cancer 2002; 8(Suppl 1): S100–112.

80. Hoffmann NE and Bischof JC. The cryobiology of cryosurgical injury. Urology 2002; 60: 40–49.

81. Ahmed M, et al. Radiofrequency ablation: Effect of surrounding tissue composition on coagulation necrosis in a canine tumor model. Radiology 2004; 230(3): 761–767.

82. Solazzo SA, et al. Radiofrequency ablation: importance of background tissue electrical conductivity – an agar phantom and computer modeling study. Radiology 2005; 236(2): 495–502.

83. Goldberg SN, Ahmed M, Gazelle GS, et al. Radiofrequency thermal ablation with adjuvant saline injection: Effect of electrical conductivity on tissue heating and coagulation. Radiology 2001; 219: 157–165.

84. Goldberg SN, et al. Percutaneous radiofrequency tissue ablation: Does perfusion-mediated tissue cooling limit coagulation necrosis? J Vasc Interv Radiol 1998; 9(1 Pt 1): 101–111.

85. Patterson EJ, et al. Radiofrequency ablation of porcine liver in vivo: Effects of blood flow and treatment time on lesion size. Ann Surg 1998; 227(4): 559–565.

86. Lu DS, Raman SS, Vodopich DJ, et al. Effect of vessel size on creation of hepatic radiofrequency lesions in pigs: Assessment of the "heat sink" effect. AJR 2002; 178: 47–51.

87. Liu Z, Ahmed M, Weinstein Y, et al. Characterization of the RF ablation-induced 'oven effect': The importance of background tissue thermal conductivity on tissue heating. Int J Hyperthermia 2006 Jun; 22(4): 327–342.

88. Yamasaki T, Kimura T, Kurokawa F, et al. Percutaneous radiofrequency ablation with cooled electrodes combined with hepatic arterial balloon occlusion in hepatocellular carcinoma. J Gastroenterol 2005 Feb; 40(2): 171–178.

89. Rossi S, Garbagnati F, Lencioni R, et al. Percutaneous radiofrequency thermal ablation of nonresectable hepatocellular carcinoma after occlusion of tumor blood supply. Radiology 2000; 217: 119–126.

90. Frich L, Mala T, Gladhaug IP. Hepatic radiofrequency ablation using perfusion electrodes in a pig model: Effect of the Pringle manoeuvre. Eur J Surg Oncol 2006 Jun; 32(5): 527–532.

91. Shen SQ, Xiang JJ, Xiong CL, et al. Intraoperative radiofrequency thermal ablation combined with portal vein infusion chemotherapy and transarterial chemoembolization for unresectable HCC. Hepatogastroenterology 2005 Sep-Oct; 52(65): 1403–1407.

92. Gasparini D, Sponza M, Marzio A, et al. Combined treatment, TACE and RF ablation, in HCC: Preliminary results. Radiol Med 2002 Nov–Dec; 104(5–6): 412–420.

93. Wang YB, Chen MH, Yan K, et al. Quality of life after radiofrequency ablation combined with transcatheter arterial chemoembolization for hepatocellular carcinoma: Comparison with transcatheter arterial chemoembolization alone. Qual Life Res 2007 Apr; 16(3): 389–397; Epub 2006 Nov 17.

94. Kurokohchi K, Hosomi N, Yoshitake A, et al. Successful treatment of large-size advanced hepatocellular carcinoma by transarterial chemoembolization followed by the combination therapy of percutaneous ethanol-lipiodol injection and radiofrequency ablation. Oncol Rep 2006 Nov; 16(5): 1067–1070.

95. Pacella CM, Bizzarri G, Cecconi P, et al. Hepatocellular carcinoma: Long-term results of combined treatment with laser thermal ablation and transcatheter arterial chemoembolization. Radiology 2001 Jun; 219(3): 669–678.

96. Bilchik AJ, Wood TF, Chawla SP, et al. Systemic irinotecan or regional floxuridine chemotherapy prolongs survival after hepatic cryosurgery in patients with metastatic colon cancer refractory to 5-fluorouracil. Clin Colorectal Cancer 2001 May; 1(1): 36–42.

97. Becker G, Soezgen T, Olschewski M, et al. Combined TACE and PEI for palliative treatment of unresectable hepatocellular carcinoma. World J Gastroenterol 2005 Oct 21; 11(39): 6104–6109.

98. Li YH, Wang CS, Liao LY, et al. Long-term survival of Taiwanese patients with hepatocellular carcinoma after combination therapy with transcatheter arterial chemoembolization and percutaneous ethanol injection. J Formos Med Assoc 2003 Mar; 102(3): 141–146.

99. Kamada K, Kitamoto M, Aikata H, et al. Combination of transcatheter arterial chemoembolization using cisplatin-lipiodol suspension and percutaneous ethanol injection for treatment of advanced small hepatocellular carcinoma. Am J Surg 2002 Sep; 184(3): 284–290.

100. Koda M, Murawaki Y, Mitsuda A, et al. Combination therapy with transcatheter arterial chemoembolization and percutaneous ethanol injection compared with percutaneous ethanol injection alone for patients with small hepatocellular carcinoma: A randomized control study. Cancer 2001 Sep 15; 92(6): 1516–1524.

101. Allgaier HP, Deibert P, Olschewski M, et al. Survival benefit of patients with inoperable hepatocellular carcinoma treated by a combination of transarterial chemoembolization and percutaneous ethanol injection – a single-center analysis including 132 patients. Int J Cancer 1998 Dec 18; 79(6): 601–605.

102. Tanaka K, Nakamura S, Numata K, et al. The long-term efficacy of combined transcatheter arterial embolization and percutaneous ethanol injection in the treatment of patients with large hepatocellular carcinoma and cirrhosis. Cancer 1998 Jan 1; 82(1): 78–85.

103. Lencioni R, Paolicchi A, Moretti M, et al. Combined transcatheter arterial chemoembolization and percutaneous ethanol injection for the treatment of large hepatocellular carcinoma: Local therapeutic effect and long-term survival rate. Eur Radiol 1998; 8(3): 439–444.

104. Grieco CA, Simon CJ, Mayo-Smith WW, et al. Percutaneous image-guided thermal ablation and radiation therapy: Outcomes of combined treatment for 41 patients with inoperable stage I/II non-small-cell lung cancer. J Vasc Interv Radiol 2006 Jul; 17(7): 1117–4424.

105. Kim SK, Rhim H, Kim YS, et al. Radiofrequency thermal ablation of hepatic tumors: Pitfalls and challenges. Abdom Imaging 2005 Nov–Dec; 30(6): 727–733.

106. Kawamoto S, Permpongkosol S, Bluemke DA, et al. Sequential changes after radiofrequency ablation and cryoablation of renal neoplasms: Role of CT and MR imaging. Radiographics 2007 Mar–Apr; 27(2): 343–355.

107. Wile GE, Leyendecker JR, Krehbiel KA, et al. CT and MR imaging after imaging-guided thermal ablation of renal neoplasms. Radiographics 2007 Mar–Apr; 27(2): 325–339.

Chapter 6

PRINCIPLES OF EMBOLIZATION

Jae Hyung Park

Jin Wook Chung

EMBOLOTHERAPY

General Indications

The percutaneous angiographic technique was first introduced by Seldinger (1), and modern embolotherapy was first attempted by Rösch (2) in 1972 to control duodenal bleeding. The term **embolization** refers to the induction of vascular occlusion by introducing an embolic agent into a vessel through a selectively placed catheter for therapeutic purposes.

The indications of embolotherapy are various, and include bleeding control, tumor devascularization, arteriovenous fistula and malformations, aneurysms, organ or tissue ablation, varicocele, blood flow redistribution and perigraft leakage. Tumors indicated for devascularization by embolotherapy are renal cell carcinoma (3, 4), angiomyolipoma (5), hepatic tumors (6, 7), bone and soft tissue tumors (8) and uterine fibroids (9). Liver tumor transcatheter arterial embolization (TAE) was first reported by Doyon et al. (10) and chemoembolization using Gelfoam and anticancer drugs was reported by Yamada et al. (7).

Recently, catheters with hydrophilic coatings and microcatheter systems have been developed, and currently, the precise and safe delivery of embolic materials is possible to any body location using blood vessels. The embolization process involves the precise localization of a target lesion, the selection of ideal embolic materials, complete embolization of the target lesion and preservation of non-targeted regions. For effective embolization, the selective and superselective techniques are important in terms of inducing complete embolization, and for preserving normal parenchyma and target organ function. Moreover, the recent development of the microcatheter now allows the occlusion of culprit vessels 1 mm in size without disturbing the surrounding normal parenchyma in the presence of renal bleeding.

Embolic Materials

Various embolic materials are now commercially available. Embolic materials must be designed with the following in mind: embolization level (proximal or distal), regular size and shape (constant or changing), duration of occlusion (permanent or temporary), ease of injection through the catheter (solid, elastic or liquid) and the potential risk of complication. Many embolic materials have been introduced for TAE, such as gelatin sponge particles (11), microspheres (12), autologous blood clots (13), polyvinyl alcohol particles (14), N-butyl cyanoacrylate (NBCA, glue) (15) and absolute ethanol (4).

Gelfoam

Gelatin sponge (Gelfoam, Upjohn, Kalamazoo, MI) is a porous, pliable product, which is prepared from purified pork skin, and is applied to bleeding surfaces as a hemostatic. Gelfoam is the most frequently used embolic material for the devascularization of tumors, and for vascular occlusion for bleeding control. Moreover, gelatin sponge particles of 500 to 1000 micrometers do not cause serious hepatic damage in experimental animals or humans with good hepatic

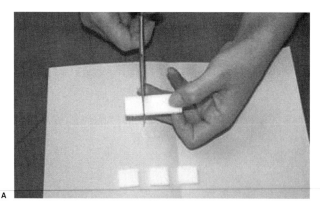
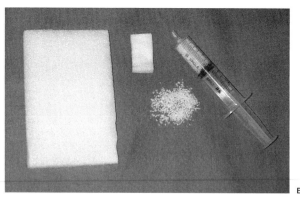

FIGURE 6.1.   Gelfoam particles. (A) A gelatin sponge sheet is easily cut into smaller size particles. (B) These particles, 2 × 2 × 2 mm cubes, can be sterilized with ethylene oxide (EO) gas in a 10 cc syringe. See Color Plate 10.

functional reserve (16). Gelfoam may be cut to the required size, usually 2- to 6-mm cubes (Figure 6.1), and can be loaded into the hub and injected using a tuberculin syringe. After passage through a micro-catheter, Gelfoam may be broken up into smaller particles, which range from 10 to 700 microns in diameter (mainly 10 to 50 μm). Gelfoam powder produces peripheral and capillary occlusion. However, its visceral use is considered dangerous as it may induce bowel infarction. Gelfoam is a useful embolic agent for the control of traumatic bleeding, gastrointestinal bleeding and solid organ bleeding and may cause effective tumor devascularization in various organs. It is usually absorbed 4 to 6 weeks after embolization.

Polyvinyl Alcohol Foam

Polyvinyl alcohol foam (PVA; Ivalon) is the product of the reaction between foamed polyvinyl alcohol and formaldehyde. It is an insoluble rigid material when dry and resilient when wet. However, it may cause a foreign body reaction in living tissue. Polyvinyl alcohol foam particles have several commercial names, for example, Ivalon Embolization Particles (Ivalon, Inc., San Diego, CA), Contour Ivalon Particles (Target Therapeutics, Fremont, CA) and PVA Foam Embolization Particles (Biodyne, Inc., Cajon, CA). Particle sizes vary from 50 μm to 1000 μm (Figure 6.2A).

It is recommended that PVA particles be prepared as a well-suspended powder in contrast medium, and it is important to prepare the contrast media such that it has the same specific gravity as the PVA particles (Figure 6.2B). Most 3F microcatheters are suitable for PVA particles of up to 500 μm. This type of suspension is commonly used for the embolization of hepatic tumors (17), renal cell carcinomas, uterine fibroids

(9), metastatic bone tumors (18), arteriovenous malformations and gastrointestinal hemorrhages.

Coils

Coils are used in an embolic manner to reduce blood flow, and level of occlusion depends on coil size. Conventional coils are of the Gianturco type and have Dacron strands attached along their entire lengths to induce thrombosis. The commonly available coil diameters are of 0.025, 0.035, and 0.038 inches, to match the diameter of guidewires. 5F to 6F angiographic catheters are suitable for 0.035-inch coils. Angiographic catheters of the same French size tapered to the diameter of 0.038-inch guidewire are necessary for 0.038-inch coils.

Microcoils are made of 0.018-inch platinum wire, and are designed for use with 3F coaxial microcatheters. They include Hilal microcoils, Tornado microcoils and Target coils with helical diameters that vary from 2 to 8 mm (Figure 6.3). Recently, these microcoils have been found to be useful for the superselective embolization of a specific branch to prevent gastrointestinal, renal and hepatic bleeding, and preserve adjacent normal parenchyma. In terms of tumor embolization, coils and microcoils are used to modify blood flow, to redirect blood flow to improve the effectiveness of intra-arterial chemotherapy or chemoembolization, and to occlude an artery of a non-targeted organ to avoid complications (Figure 6.4) (19, 20).

Absolute Ethanol

Absolute ethanol is a potent embolic agent for vascular occlusion and tissue ablation. Once infused into a vessel, it causes the denaturation of proteinaceous blood elements, which results in clot formation and

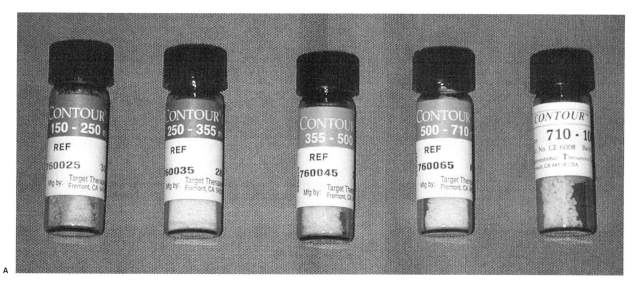

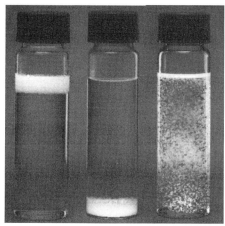

FIGURE 6.2. PVA particles. (A) PVA particles (Contour®) are available commercially in different sizes (150–1000 μm). (B) Dilution of contrast media. Particles are suspended in contrast media (*left*) and precipitated in saline (*middle*) and then freely dispersed in the bottle of specific gravity–matched contrast media (*right*). See Color Plate 11.

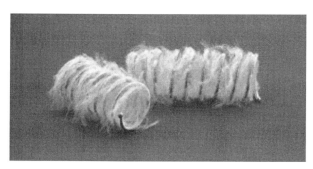

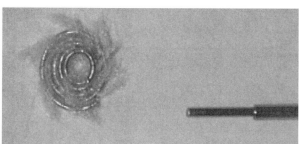

FIGURE 6.3. Microcoils. Several different types of microcoils are currently available, i.e., spiral or Tornado types, with thrombogenic Dacron fibers. See Color Plate 12.

endothelial damage and thus permanently occludes vessels. Because it is a radiolucent material, absolute ethanol may be used after mixing it with lipiodol or non-ionic contrast media to allow visualization of the agent by fluoroscopy (21). Ethanol has been used effectively to treat renal cell carcinoma (4), renal angiomyolipoma (22), hepatocellular carcinoma (23, 24), esophageal varices, and arteriovenous malformation. However, during such procedures, care should be taken to avoid reflux of the embolic material. Retrograde flow may produce inadvertent embolization of a non-target organ.

A mixture of ethanol and iodized oil has been utilized to treat tumors (Figure 6.5). In an experimental renal arterial embolization model using an ethanol-lipiodol mixture (ELM), the infusion of 50% and 75% of ELM solution resulted in embolization equal to that of absolute ethanol (21). Superselective transcatheter arterial embolization with 75% ELM was successfully applied to the treatment of a small nodular hepatocellular carcinoma with a prominent

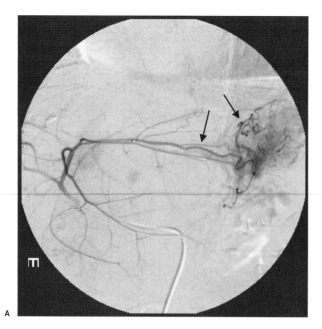

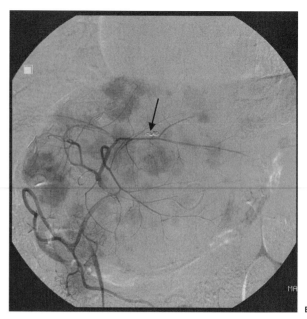

A   B

FIGURE 6.4. Redirecting blood flow by microcoil embolization for tumor treatment. (A) Selective left hepatic arteriograph revealing a prominent accessory left gastric artery (*arrows*) from the left hepatic artery supplying gastric fundus in a patient with multiple nodular type hepatoma. (B) After microcoil embolization (*arrow*), flow to the accessory left gastric artery from the left hepatic artery ceased. Chemoembolization was performed safely to control multinodular lesions via the left hepatic artery during follow-up.

feeding artery (23), and was also found to be effective and convenient for the selective or nonselective devascularization of unresectable renal cell carcinoma (25). Recently Kan et al. reported that the hepatic arterial administration of a lipiodol-ethanol mixture (LEM, ratios of 5:1, 4:1 and 3:1) creates both hepatic arterial and portal venous embolization, and it has a lobar ablation effect (26). Hepatic arterioportal shunting of these substances occurs via the peribiliary plexa (27).

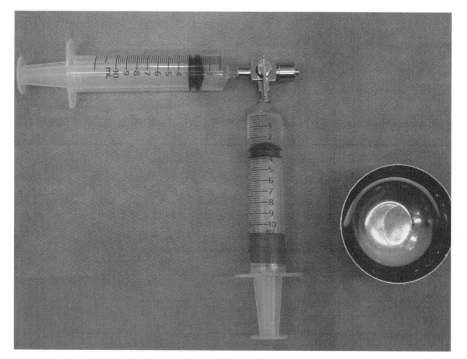

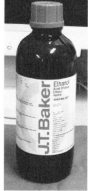

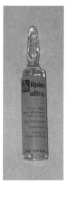

FIGURE 6.5.   A mixture of ethanol and lipiodol. Pumping method used to mix ethanol and lipiodol using two syringes connected via a three-way valve. The syringe marked with red tape contains absolute ethanol. See Color Plate 13.

Microspheres

Recently, in concert with the introduction of micro-catheter superselective embolization, TAE based on smaller microspheres has been investigated clinically. Several experimental and clinical trials using various microsphere sizes have shown that although particles smaller than 40 micrometers preferentially (6- to 12-fold) accumulate in tumor vasculatures, they may pass through sinusoids and tumor-related arteriovenous shunts into the systemic circulation, and thus, may produce serious embolic complications (28, 29).

Several different types of microspheres are used for embolization. Embospheres (Biosphere Medical, Rockland, MA), which are made of trisacryl gelatin microspheres, are being increasingly utilized because of their ease of use (Figure 6.6). They are compressible and have a hydrophilic surface, and thus, are less prone to aggregate. However, there is tendency for Embospheres to reflux proximally when flushing fluid is injected to clear a catheter or microcatheter. To pre-vent this, extreme caution should be exercised when flushing a catheter after embolization, and Embospheres should be suspended in non-ionic contrast media for about 5 minutes before injection to allow them to attain neutral buoyancy in contrast. Embospheres are flexible hydrophilic spheres, which do not aggregate in catheters and induce uniform occlusion. Moreover, Embosphere microspheres can be mixed with carboplatin, mitomycin C, 5-fluorouracil or pirarubicin without a detrimental effect on morphology, dimensions or geometric characteristics (30). Hong, et al. compared the effects of different types of embolization particles, including Embospheres and PVA particles, in a rabbit tumor model, and the concentration of the anti-cancer drug Carboplatin was found to be significantly greater within tumors in the Embosphere group (31).

Several different types of microspheres made of PVA are currently available – for example, DC Beads (Biocompatibles UK, Surrey, UK), BeadBlock (Bio-compatibles UK, Surrey, UK), Contour SE (Boston

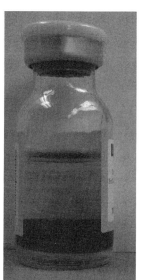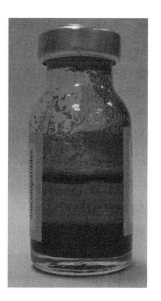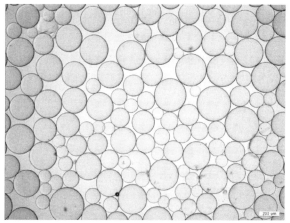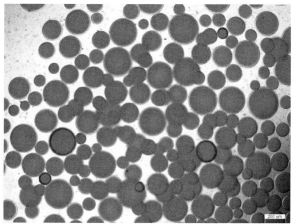

FIGURE 6.6. DC bead spheres. (A) A bottle of DC bead spheres (doxorubicin-capable beads, Biocompatible, UK) of 100–300 mm size. (B) A bottle containing DC beads after mixing with doxorubicin solution for 1 hour. (C) Microscopic view of DC beads of 100–300 mm. (D) Microscopic view of red-tinged DC beads containing doxorubicin after soaking in drug solution. See Color Plate 14.

Scientific, Natick, MA) and Surgica MaxiStat (Protein Polymer Technologies, San Diego, CA). DC bead spheres (doxorubicin-capable beads) can be loaded with doxorubicin to 25 mg/mL on hydrated beads by immersing them in a drug solution for 1 to 120 minutes (32). Moreover, when drug-eluting beads (DEB) loaded with doxorubicin were used to embolize left liver lobes in young adult Yucatan pigs, locoregional delivery of doxorubicin from DEB caused targeted tissue damage with minimal systemic impact. It is evident that this offers a promising new approach to the transarterial chemoembolization of solid tumors (33). Irinotecan drug-eluting beads (DC beads) administered as transcatheter arterial chemoembolization (TACE) have also been reported to be active and safe in patients with liver metastases from colorectal cancer (34).

Several other types of microspheres have been reported upon recently. Chitosan-coated alginate microspheres, prepared by the ionic complexation of alginate and chitosan biopolymers, were examined for embolization and chemoembolization (35). Degradable starch microspheres (DSMs) have been reported to transiently occlude small arteries and to be a potential therapy for liver metastases when mixed with anti-cancer drugs such as Irinotecan (36). Moreover, superabsorbent polymer microspheres (SAP-MS), made of sodium acrylate and vinyl alcohol copolymer, were compared with trisacryl gelatin microspheres and polyvinyl alcohol. The effect of SAP-MS was found to be similar to that of Embospheres, and they were found to be distributed homogenously in peripheral vessels and to better conform to vessel lumen (37).

Embolization: Technical Considerations

Microcatheters and Microguidewires

There are several types of microcatheters. The first generation, Tracker 18 (Target), was a stiff unbraided catheter with a tendency to flatten when passed around tight curves. Current braided microcatheters are coated with a hydrophilic material, and have better trackability and better maintain catheter lumen diameter when passed around curves. Size 18 microcatheters have an inner lumen diameter of from 0.019 to 0.021 inches and accept all microcoil sizes. Other microcatheters with larger lumens are used for administering large volumes of relatively large particles, for instance, for treating advanced hepatoma

or patients with large uterine fibroids. There are also several different types of microguidewires. Terumo microwires are easily advanced and have an excellent hydrophilic coating but may perforate small arteries more easily and thus should be used with caution.

Pre-embolization Evaluation

For efficient catheterization by superselective embolization, a pre-procedural computed tomographic (CT) evaluation is essential. Recent technical advances in CT arteriography make it possible to depict major branches of the aorta and major arterial variations before procedures. The evaluation of the relation between arterial anatomy and a tumor or a specific lesion, such as bleeding, is mandatory before embolization. A variety of arterial anatomical variations are possible for each organ. For example, there are several different anatomical variations in addition to the ten types of Michel's classification of hepatic arterial variations. Details of hepatic arterial anatomy and anatomic considerations necessary for the chemoembolization of hepatomas are described in a later chapter. Knowledge of individual anatomy is important if complete lesion embolization is to be achieved while avoiding unnecessary complications and preserving normal parenchyma as much as possible.

Roadmap and Superselective Arteriography

For accurate superselective catheterization, a roadmap function is essential during fluoroscopy for embolization. A fine feeding branch located as distally as possible may be selected for effective superselective embolization. A magnified view and oblique projections at different angles are useful when comparing real-time fluoroscopic images with roadmap images. Moreover, a proper oblique projection should be selected to separate overlapping multiple branches. For example, a right oblique projection is essential for the successful embolization of tumors of the right liver lobe to discriminate a proper feeding artery among arteries of the four Couinaud segments. Repeated angiographies are necessary to confirm the superselective position of a catheter from time to time. However, one must consider the benefit of repeated angiography versus radiation hazard.

Special shaping of the microguidewire is recommended for selective catheterization when dealing with a smaller branch of proximal origin from a relatively large artery. For example, a shepherd's hook

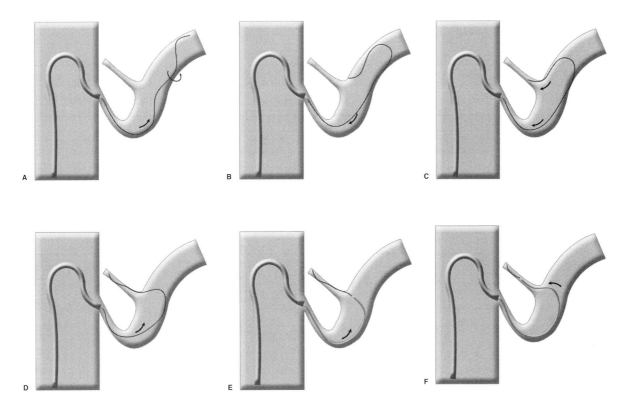

FIGURE 6.7. A useful selection technique – the shepherd's crook technique. When the origin of a small target branch forms an acute angle with the proximal portion of the major aortic branch, this technique is useful for selecting the small branch. (From Baek JH, Chung JW, Jae HJ, Lee W, Park JH. A new technique for superselective catheterization of arteries: Shepherd hook preshaping of a microguidewire. Korean J Radiol. 2007 Jun;8(3):225–230, with permission.)

technique has been described for the selection of a right inferior phrenic artery with a microcatheter and a microguidewire to control extrahepatic collaterals to a hepatoma (Figure 6.7) (38). The operator should be familiar with fine modifications of the flexible distal tip of microguidewires during superselective catheterization. A long microcatheter and a microguidewire of 150 cm are used for the superselective catheterization of a branch of the brachiocephalic arteries, such as the internal mammary artery or an omental branch of the gastroepiploic artery, as an extrahepatic supply to a peripherally located hepatoma. In cases of arterial stenosis at the arterial origin, the stenosis can be opened by angioplasty or the obstruction may be circumvented by the long catheterization of a collateral pathway.

CHEMOEMBOLIZATION

Synergistic Effects of Ischemia and Drug Therapy

During TACE, intra-arterial chemotherapy and arterial embolization are believed to act in a synergistic manner. This approach offers the potential for highly concentrated chemotherapy and a means of ischemically damaging a tumor and thus is likely to enhance tumor necrosis (39). Ischemic necrosis of a tumor due to embolization may cause failure of transmembrane pumps in tumor cells, which would result in greater absorption of chemotherapeutic agents by tumor cells (40). An increased uptake of 3H-daunomycin (an analogue of doxorubicin) by hepatoma cells was found to occur under hypoxic conditions in a cell culture experiment. So, selective hepatic arterial occlusion may facilitate increased chemotherapeutic agent uptake into liver tumors. In addition, by reducing arterial flow after embolization, chemotherapeutic agents may remain within tumor tissue for prolonged periods of time. It has been reported that the tissue concentrations of chemotherapeutic agents within tumors is 40 times higher than in surrounding normal liver parenchyma several months after TACE (41–43).

Chemotherapeutic Agents Used for Chemoembolization

When preparing a mixture of an iodized oil and chemotherapeutic agents, the chemotherapeutic

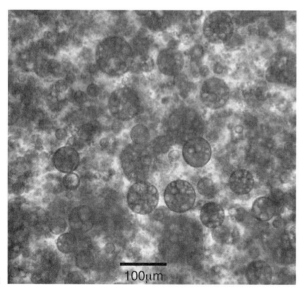

FIGURE 6.8. Doxorubicin(Adriamycin)-lipiodol emulsion formation using the pumping technique. (A) Preparation. The materials used were a single 10-mL sample of lipiodol, two bottles of doxorubicin powder and a bottle of contrast media (iopamidol). (B) Mixing of doxorubicin solution with lipiodol using the three-way stopcock. (C) Manual pumping (more than 30 times) to produce a homogenous emulsion. (D) Ready to infuse chemoembolic material with 1 cc tuberculin syringe. (E) Microscopic view of lipiodol emulsion showing variably sized droplets containing red-colored doxorubicin after pumping. See Color Plate 15.

drugs are usually pre-dissolved in a water-soluble contrast agent and then emulsified in iodized oil using a pumping method (Figure 6.8). Anti-cancer drug-iodized oil solutions or suspensions can be prepared to match the physical characteristics of the drug. Many centers use a single chemotherapeutic agent, such as doxorubicin, whereas others use combinations of different drugs (e.g., cisplatin, mitomycin or 5-fluorouracil). Japanese investigators used styrene maleic acid neocarzinostatin (SMANCS), which is highly lipophilic and is expected to be more stable when mixed with iodized oil (44, 45). Unfortunately, no data are available that clearly demonstrate the comparative merits of cytotoxic agents. Cisplatin may confer slightly better survival when administered as a cisplatin-iodized oil suspension (46, 47).

Lipiodol Chemoembolization

In the early 1980s, iodized oil (lipiodol; Andre Guerbet, Aulnay-sous-Bois, France), a lymphangiographic dye, was found to remain selectively in the neovasculature and extravascular spaces of liver tumors when injected into the hepatic artery (48, 49). Thereafter, TACE based on an iodized oil mixed with different anti-cancer agents or, more often, with an emulsion of iodized oil and anti-cancer drugs followed by Gelfoam embolization, has been increasingly used as an effective palliative treatment for unresectable tumors. Moreover, iodized oil has been used successfully not only as an embolic material but also as a carrier of chemotherapeutic agents (50). In a study on the biodistribution of doxorubicin after chemoembolization, the mixture of Lipiodol and doxorubicin was found to lower the peak concentration of doxorubicin in plasma and to increase intratumoral concentration and prolong half-life. Moreover, the combination of doxorubicin, lipiodol and gelfoam was found to produce highest intratumoral concentrations (51).

When injected into the hepatic artery, iodized oil persists selectively in the tumor for a few weeks or months because of hemodynamic differences between hypervascular hepatic tumors and liver parenchyma, and presumably because of the absence of Kupffer cells in tumors (27, 52). Nakajo et al. (53) reported that iodine-131 iodized oil accumulated in vascular tumors 7.5 to 21 times more so than in adjacent normal parenchyma. Chemotherapeutic agents can be locally delivered to a hepatocellular carcinoma (HCC) with iodized oil as a carrier, and are released slowly from the lipiodol mixture (54). In contrast, in normal liver parenchyma, iodized oil injected into the hepatic artery usually does not cause complete occlusion of the hepatic artery and accumulates in the peripheral portal vein through multiple arterioportal communications. It then subsequently passes through the sinusoids into the systemic circulation (51).

Lobar Ablation Technique with Both Arterial and Portal Embolization

The normal liver receives a dual blood supply from the hepatic artery and the portal vein. Approximately one-third of normal hepatic blood flow originates from the hepatic artery and the other two-thirds from the portal vein. About one-half of the oxygen requirement of the liver is supplied by the portal vein. Conversely, both primary and secondary liver tumors derive 90% of their blood supply from the hepatic artery with a smaller (10%) contribution from the portal vein (27, 55). Therefore, intra-arterial agents have been recommended for the targeted treatment of HCC. In an experimental study, ten times higher intratumoral concentrations of chemotherapeutic agents were observed when the chemoembolic material was administered via the hepatic artery as opposed to the portal vein (56). However, the blood supply of liver tumors is dependent on their developmental stages and growth patterns. Whereas encapsulated nodular HCCs are totally supplied by the hepatic artery, well-differentiated or early HCCs, small nodular tumors (i.e., daughter nodules) and intrahepatic metastases, and the extracapsular infiltrating edge of advanced HCC are supplied by both the portal vein and the hepatic artery (57, 58). Even in advanced-stage disease, most liver metastases have a distinct portal blood supply to the tumor periphery (59, 60). Therefore, these tumors with a portal blood supply may be resistant to intra-arterial embolotherapy, which is why it is important to simultaneously embolize hepatic arterial and portal venous supplies. When a mixture of lipiodol and an anticancer drug (i.e., doxorubicin [Adriamycin]) or lipiodol and ethanol is injected into a segmental hepatic artery, the mixture may reach the segmental portal vein via the peribiliary plexus to cause segmental or subsegmental chemoembolization (61).

REFERENCES

1. Seldinger SI. Catheter placement of the needle in percutaneous arteriography. Acta Radiol 1953; 39: 368–376.
2. Rösch J, Dotter CT, Brown MJ. Selective arterial embolization A new method for control of acute gastrointestinal bleeding. Radiology 1972; 102: 303–306.
3. Wallace S, Chuang VP, Swanson D, et al. Embolization of renal cell carcinoma. Radiology 1981; 138: 563–570.
4. Ellman BA, Parkhill BJ, Curry TS, et al. Ablation of renal tumors with absolute ethanol: A new technique. Radiology 1981; 141: 619–626.
5. Soulen MC, Faykus MH Jr., Shalnsky-Goldberg RD, et al. Elective embolization for prevention of hemorrhage from renal angiomyolipomas. J Vasc Interv Radiol 1994; 5: 587–591.
6. Chuang VP, Wallace S. Hepatic artery embolization in the treatment of hepatic neoplasms. Radiology 1981; 140: 51–58.
7. Yamada R, Sato M, Kawabata M, et al. Hepatic artery embolization in 120 patients with unresectable hepatoma. Radiology 1983; 148: 397–401.
8. Chuang VP, Soo CS, Wallace S, et al. Arterial occlusion: Management of giant cell tumor and aneurysmal bone cyst. Am J Roentgenol 1981; 136: 1127–1130.
9. Goodwin SC, Vedantham S, McLucas B, et al. Preliminary experience with uterine artery embolization for uterine fibroids. J Vasc Interv Radiol 1997; 8: 517–526.

10. Doyon D, Mouzon A, Jourde AM, et al. Hepatic arterial embolization in patients with malignant liver tumors. Ann Radiol (Paris) 1974; 17: 593–603.

11. Reuter SR, Chuang VP, Bree RL. Selective arterial embolization for control of massive upper gastrointestinal tract bleeding. Am J Roentgenol 1975; 125: 119–126.

12. Nishioka Y, Kyotani S, Okamura M, et al. A study of embolizing materials for chemo-embolization therapy of hepatocellular carcinoma: Effects of particle size and dose on chitin-containing cis-diamminedichloroplatinum (II) albumin microsphere antitumor activity in VX2 hepatic tumor model rabbits. Biol Pharm Bull 1994; 17: 1251–1255.

13. Gunji T, Kawauchi N, Akahane M, et al. Long-term outcomes of transcatheter arterial chemoembolization with autologous blood clot for unresectable hepatocellular carcinoma. Int J Oncol 2002; 21: 427–432.

14. Tadavarthy SM, Moller JH, Amplatz K. Polyvinyl alcohol (Ivalon)-a new embolic material. AJR 1975; 125: 609–616.

15. Dotter CT, Goldman ML, Rösch J. Instant selective arterial occlusion with isobutyl-2-cyanoacrylate. Radiology 1975; 114: 227–230.

16. Cho KJ, Reuter SR, Schmidt R. Effects of experimental hepatic artery embolization on hepatic function. Am J Roentgenol 1976; 127: 563–567.

17. Chuang VP, Soo CS, Wallace S. Ivalon embolization in abdominal neoplasms. Am J Roentgenol 1981; 136: 729–733.

18. Barton PP, Waneck RE, Karnel FJ, et al. Embolization of bone metastases. J Vasc Interv Radiol 1996; 7: 81–88.

19. Cho KJ, Andrews JC, Williams DM, et al. Hepatic arterial chemotherapy: Role of angiography. Radiology 1989; 173: 783–791.

20. Chuang VP, Wallace S. Hepatic arterial redistribution for intraarterial infusion of hepatic neoplasms. Radiology 1980; 135: 295–299.

21. Park JH, Jeon SC, Kang HS, et al. Transcatheter renal arterial embolization with mixture of ethanol and Lipiodol. Invest Radiol 1986; 21: 577–580.

22. Park JH, Kim WS, Han MC, et al. Renal arterial embolization with absolute ethanol. J Korean Med Sci 1987; 2: 13–18.

23. Park JH, Han JK, Chung JW, et al. Superselective transcatheter arterial embolization with ethanol and iodized oil for hepatocellular carcinoma. J Vasc Interv Radiol 1993; 4: 333–339.

24. Matsui O, Kadoya M, Yoshikawa J, et al. Small hepatocellular carcinoma: Treatment with subsegmental transcatheter arterial embolization. Radiology 1993; 188: 79–83.

25. Park JH, Kim SH, Han JK, et al. Transcatheter arterial embolization of unresectable renal cell carcinoma with a mixture of ethanol and iodized oil. Cardiovasc Intervent Radiol 1994; 17: 323–327.

26. Kan Z, Wallace S. Transcatheter liver lobar ablation: An experimental trial in an animal model. Eur Radiol 1997; 7: 1071–1075.

27. Kan Z, Ivancev K, Lunderquist A. Peribiliary plexa – an important pathways for shunting of iodized oil and silicon rubber solution from the hepatic artery to the portal vein. An experimental study in rats. Invest Radiol 1994; 29: 671–676.

28. Bastian P, Bartkowski R, Kohler H, et al. Chemoembolization of experimental liver metastases. Part I: Distribution of biodegradable microspheres of different sizes in an animal model for the locoregional therapy. Eur J Pharm Biopharm 1998; 46: 243–254.

29. Brown KT. Fatal pulmonary complications after arterial embolization with 40–120- micron tris-acryl gelatin microspheres. J Vasc Interv Radiol 2004; 15: 197–200.

30. Vallee JN, Lo D, Guillevin R, et al. In vitro study of the compatibility of tris-acryl gelatin microspheres with various chemotherapeutic agents. J Vasc Interv Radiol 2003; 14: 621–628.

31. Hong K, Kobeiter H, Georgiades CS, et al. Effects of the type of embolization particles on carboplatin concentration in liver tumors after transcatheter arterial chemoembolization in a rabbit model of liver cancer. J Vasc Interv Radiol 2005; 16: 1711–1717.

32. Lewis AL, Gonzalez MV, Lloyd AW, et al. DC bead: in vitro characterization of a drug-delivery device for transarterial chemoembolization. J Vasc Interv Radiol 2006; 17: 335–342.

33. Lewis AL, Taylor RR, Hall B, et al. Pharmacokinetic and safety study of doxorubicin-eluting beads in a porcine model of hepatic arterial embolization. J Vasc Interv Radiol 2006; 17: 1335–1343.

34. Aliberti C, Tilli M, Benea G, et al. Trans-arterial chemoembolization (TACE) of liver metastases from colorectal cancer using irinotecan-eluting beads: Preliminary results. Anticancer Res 2006; 26: 3793–3795.

35. Eroglu M, Kursaklioglu H, Misirli Y, et al. Chitosan-coated alginate microspheres for embolization and/or chemoembolization: In vivo studies. J Microencapsul 2006; 23: 367–376.

36. Morise Z, Sugioka A, Kato R, et al. Transarterial chemoembolization with degradable starch microspheres, irinotecan, and mitomycin-C in patients with liver metastases. J Gastrointest Surg 2006; 10: 249–258.

37. Khankan AA, Osuga K, Hori S, et al. Embolic effects of superabsorbent polymer microspheres in rabbit renal model: Comparison with tris-acryl gelatin microspheres and polyvinyl alcohol. Radiation Medicine 2004; 22: 384–390.

38. Baek JH, Chung JW, Jae HJ, et al. A new technique for superselective catheterization of arteries: Shepherd hook preshaping of a microguidewire. Korean J Radiol 2007; 8: 225–230.

39. Ramsey DE, Kernagis LY, Soulen MC, et al. Chemoembolization of hepatocellular carcinoma. J Vasc Interv Radiol 2002; 13: S211–S221.

40. Kruskal JB, Hlatky L, Hahnfeldt P, et al. In vivo and in vitro analysis of the effectiveness of doxorubicin combined with temporary arterial occlusion in liver tumors. J Vasc Interv Radiol 1993; 4: 741–747.

41. Sasaki Y, Imaoka S, Kasugai H, et al. A new approach to chemoembolization therapy for hepatoma using ethiodized oil, cisplatin, and gelatin sponge. Cancer 1987; 60: 1194–1203.

42. Sawada S. Transcatheter oily chemoembolization of hepatocellular carcinoma. Radiology 1989; 170: 783–786.

43. Konno T. Targeting cancer chemotherapeutic agents by use of lipiodol contrast medium. Cancer 1990; 66: 1897–1903.

44. Abe S, Okubo Y, Ejiri Y, et al. Focal therapeutic efficacy of transcatheter arterial infusion of styrene maleic acid neocarzinostatin for hepatocellular carcinoma. J Gastroenterol 2000; 35: 28–33.

45. Okusaka T, Okada S, Ueno H, et al. Transcatheter arterial embolization with zinostatin stimalamer for hepatocellular carcinoma. Oncology 2002; 62: 228–233.

46. Ueno K, Miyazono N, Inoue H, et al. Transcatheter arterial chemoembolization therapy using iodized oil for patients with unresectable hepatocellular carcinoma: Evaluation of three kinds of regimens and analysis of prognostic factors. Cancer 2000; 88: 1574–1581.

47. Kamada K, Nakanishi T, Kitamoto M, et al. Long-term prognosis of patients undergoing transcatheter arterial chemoembolization for unresectable hepatocellular carcinoma: Comparison of cisplatin lipiodol suspension and doxorubicin hydrochloride emulsion. J Vasc Interv Radiol 2001; 12: 847–854.

48. Konno T, Maeda H, Iwai K, et al. Effect of arterial administration of high-molecular-weight anticancer agent SMANCS with lipid lymphographic agent on hepatoma. Eur J Cancer Clin Oncol 1983; 19: 1053–1065.

49. Nakamura H, Tanaka T, Hori S, et al. Transcatheter embolization of hepatocellular carcinoma: Assessment of efficacy in case of resection following embolization. Radiology 1983; 147: 401–405.

50. Raoul JL, Heresbach D, Bretagne JF, et al. Chemoembolization of hepatocellular carcinomas: A study of the biodistribution and pharmacokinetics of doxorubicin. Cancer 1992; 70: 585–590.

51. Kan Z, Sato M, Ivancev K, et al. Distribution and effect of iodized poppy seed oil in the liver after hepatic artery embolization: Experimental study in several animal species. Radiology 1993; 186: 261–266.

52. Bhattacharya S, Novell JR, Winslet MC, et al. Iodized oil in the treatment of hepatocellular carcinoma. Br J Surg 1994; 81: 1563–1571.

53. Nakajo M, Kobayashi H, Shimabukuro K, et al. Biodistribution and in vivo kinetics of iodine-131 lipiodol infused via the hepatic artery of patients with hepatic cancer. J Nucl Med 1988; 29: 1066–1077.

54. Nakamura H, Hashimoto T, Oi H, et al. Transcatheter oily chemoembolization of hepatocellular carcinoma. Radiology 1989; 170: 783–786.

55. Ackerman NB. The blood supply of experimental liver metastases. IV. Changes in vascularity with increasing tumor growth. Surgery 1974; 75: 589–596.

56. Sigurdson ER, Ridge JA, Kemeny N, et al. Tumor and liver drug uptake following hepatic artery and portal vein infusion. J Clin Oncol 1987; 5: 1836–1840.

57. Wakasa K, Sakurai M, Kuroda C, et al. Effect of transcatheter arterial embolization on the boundary architecture of hepatocellular carcinoma. Cancer 1990; 65: 913–919.

58. Goseki N, Nosaka T, Endo M, et al. Nourishment of hepatocellular carcinoma cells through the portal blood flow with and without transcatheter arterial embolization. Cancer 1995; 76: 736–742.

59. Strohmeyer T, Haugeberg G, Lierse W. Angioarchitecture and blood supply of micro- and macrometastases in human livers. An anatomic-pathological investigation using injection techniques. J Hepatol 1987; 4: 181–189.

60. Taniguchi H, Daidoh T, Shioaki Y, et al. Blood supply and drug delivery to primary and secondary human liver cancers studied with in vivo bromodeoxyuridine labeling. Cancer 1993; 71: 50–55.

61. Kan Z. Dynamic study of iodized oil in the liver and blood supply to hepatic tumors. An experimental investigation in several animal species. Acta Radiol (Suppl), 1996; 408: 1–25.

Chapter 7

IMAGING IN INTERVENTIONAL ONCOLOGY: ROLE OF IMAGE GUIDANCE

Stephen B. Solomon

Advances in medical imaging have created the opportunity for minimally invasive, image-guided oncologic care. Through the 1980s and 1990s, as diagnostic scan quality improved, it became obvious to make the transition from using imaging tools simply for diagnostic use to roles that could aid in intervention. As an interventional tool, medical imaging allows visualization of anatomic targets inside the body without requiring direct, open surgical visualization. When combined with advances in medical device design and device miniaturization, medical imaging can guide devices to targets for therapy without large incisions. These less invasive, image-guided procedures offer patients an opportunity for faster, less complicated recoveries.

Interventional use of imaging equipment has different priorities compared with diagnostic uses of imaging equipment. In general, generating the highest quality image is most important for diagnosis. This means that taking more imaging time or applying more radiation are acceptable "costs" for diagnostic imaging. In contrast, patients come to interventional procedures already having undergone high-quality diagnostic imaging. For interventional procedures, in general, lower-quality imaging is an acceptable compromise for real-time imaging with lower radiation dose. Interventional procedures, therefore, prioritize imaging equipment that (1) provides real-time imaging, (2) lowers radiation dose and (3) provides greater physician access to the patient.

Although most current image-guided therapy still utilizes standard diagnostic imaging equipment, more and more imaging equipment is being customized for the particular needs of interventional procedures. These future intervention-focused improvements will help broaden the applications of image-guided therapy.

In general, medical imaging plays four key roles in image-guided therapies. These roles are (1) procedure planning, (2) device delivery, (3) intra-procedure monitoring and (4) therapy assessment. Although many of these roles are still relatively primitive, as research and development in medical imaging focus on interventional needs, it is likely that the role of medical imaging in intervention will become more integral and more widely applied.

IMAGING FOR PROCEDURE PLANNING

The first critical application of imaging in any image-guided procedure or, for that matter, any surgical procedure, is in the planning phase. In this application, the most relevant, high-quality diagnostic imaging study available must be evaluated. In many cases, the evaluation requires an assortment of imaging studies. Some may be anatomic studies such as contrast computed tomography (CT) or magnetic resonance (MR), and other studies may be physiologic studies such as positron emission tomography (PET) or single photon emission computed tomography

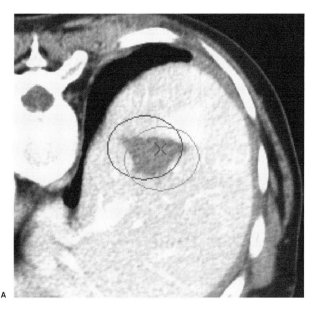

FIGURE 7.1. (A) Imaging used for planning. Planning software is used to plan overlapping thermal ablations to fully cover the tumor volume. Each circle represents the theoretical volume of necrosis from a single radiofrequency abla-tion. (B) Planning software can segment the hepatic arterial tree from a rotational angiographic study. By pointing to the tumor target, the software can identify the feeding branches as depicted in red. See Color Plate 16.

(SPECT). Older studies should be compared to newer ones to help direct the therapy.

The imaging component of the patient evaluation prior to a procedure includes answering the following basic questions: (a) Is the procedure technically feasible? (b) What is the best approach to the target? (c) Are there any anatomic variants? (d) What are the potential deleterious effects to nearby structures?

Radiation oncologists employ sophisticated planning systems to optimize their procedures. Although similar systems for interventional oncology are still in their infancy, they are being developed. One appropriate example of interventional oncology planning is mapping overlapping ablations prior to an ablation procedure (Figure 7.1). This planning can help ensure adequate tumor coverage and avoidance of critical structures. Mathematical models have been used to predict necessary ablation overlapping (1–3). In a feasibility study, robots have been used to implement an overlapping ablation plan (4). Other examples of interventional oncology planning using imaging include 3D CT hepatic arteriography prior to chemoembolization (5) and ^{99m}Tc-macroaggregated albumin (MAA) imaging prior to selective internal radiation therapy (6).

Another aspect of planning may include simulation systems that allow the physician to not just review images but also to work with instruments in a virtual procedure. Recently, many institutions have begun applying simulation software and devices to allow physicians the opportunity to "practice" prior to an actual procedure (7). Although most of these simulation systems are still nascent, it is likely that they will play an increasing role in the future (8).

IMAGING FOR DEVICE DELIVERY

To aid in device delivery, the imaging equipment used would ideally provide real-time, three-dimensional information. It also would provide physiologic information indicating areas of contrast enhancement or areas of metabolic activity. Additionally, it would provide wide access to the patient. Although current imaging tools may provide some of these features, they generally do not ideally provide all of these features. Most CT procedures, for instance, are guided without contrast and without true three-dimensionality. Research efforts are underway to improve imaging equipment to better meet these interventional imaging requirements. The following are areas of active investigation.

Advances in Real-time Imaging

CT fluoroscopy provides real-time CT images that can guide therapy. It replaces the traditional physician movement in and out of the room during each needle's incremental advance required with standard CT interventions. The downside to this technique is the increased radiation dose and the lack of three-dimensionality (9). Attempts to reduce radiation exposure by lowering imaging parameters and by providing arm extenders have been demonstrated (10).

On the other hand, MR fluoroscopy also provides real-time imaging without ionizing radiation; however, physician access to the patient in high or intermediate field systems is a major limitation (11).

Three-dimensionality

Recent advances in rotational flat panel angiography provide the real-time imaging of fluoroscopy with intermittent, snapshot "CT-like" multi-planar imaging (12, 13). Providing the CT-like image with the patient access typical of fluoroscopy will allow mainstay X-ray fluoroscopy machines to take on a more powerful role in the interventional oncology imaging armamentarium. Although visualization of dense structures such as bone and contrast-filled vessels is good, challenges still remain in soft tissue resolution. As these new machines improve, they may reduce the need for CT in many interventional procedures.

While CT, MR, and ultrasound imaging are still primarily used in 2D "slice" mode, efforts are underway to make more use of potential 3D imaging. The ability to rapidly reconstruct three-dimensional images from these two-dimensional views will aid image-guided therapy (14, 15).

Contrast Agents

Contrast agents are increasingly being applied as interactive tools during intervention. They can highlight the target that is not easily visualized on non-contrast scans. Ultrasound contrast agents can provide tissue enhancement characteristics similar to contrast CT without the nephrotoxicity of iodinated agents (16). MR agents that remain in the vascular system or those that are aimed at Kupffer cell uptake in the liver provide new tools that can be applied to specific cases.

Image Fusion

While metabolic imaging such as PET has had a major impact on oncology, its role in intervention has been limited because it lacks the anatomic detail required for guidance. Fusion of PET with CT or MR may allow utilization of both the anatomic detail of CT or MR with the physiologic information of PET (Figure 7.2; 17–19). While this is currently

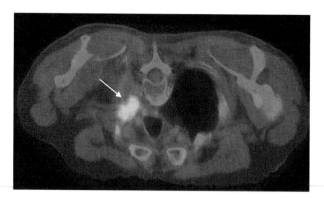

FIGURE 7.2. Imaging used for guiding therapy. Fusion of PET and CT can indicate which part of the anatomic changes still contains viable tumor. This can then guide therapy to the incompletely treated tumor. Fusion allows capitalizing on the best features of CT (anatomy) with the best features of PET (physiology). The arrow indicates the FDG-avid part of the tumor. See Color Plate 17.

actively used in diagnostic imaging, it has only been used limitedly in intervention.

Fusion has also been applied to ultrasound images fused with CT images to gain the real-time, non-ionizing radiation information of ultrasound with the exquisite anatomic detail of a diagnostic CT (20). Similar fusion of MR with ultrasound and 3D rotational fluoroscopy with 2D fluoroscopy have also been explored. These efforts toward multi-modality image fusion may really aid interventionalists, but the engineering difficulties of image registration still remain active challenges (21). Patient breathing, patient positioning and even procedure/instrument related motion present other engineering hurdles.

Navigation

Position sensors attached to medical devices can track the position of tools during a procedure. The coordinates of the tool can then be superimposed on previously acquired images or even real-time images. The real-time position information on the "old" 3D CT, for instance, may be a way to provide quasi-real-time imaging without ionizing radiation. It may also allow the physiologic images such as PET to be incorporated into an intervention. Additionally, it may allow out-of-plane trajectory imaging. However, these navigation tools, when used without a real-time imaging tool, face the same image registration engineering challenges as those of image fusion (22–26). Therefore, many navigation devices are being evaluated with a real-time imaging tool such as ultrasound.

Robotics

Robotics have been applied to several areas of medicine. Because modern imaging is digital and robots function in a digital world, it makes sense that robotics can be applied to image-guided therapy. They may have two important roles in image-guided therapy. They may act as an arm extender, thereby limiting physician radiation exposure, and they may improve procedures with their accurate tool placement (27–29). With integrated software systems, the coordinates of targets can be chosen and then the robot can deliver a tool to the prescribed location. This, however, requires that the image used for planning is registered with the patient and accounts for patient motion. These, therefore, are the same engineering challenges that are faced with navigation and fusion enhancements.

Open Access

Many of the interventional oncology tools require physician access to the patient during imaging. Physician access is important to allow real-time guidance as the physician advances a tool. Additionally, in many interventional oncology procedures, needles extend out from the patient's body. In closed gantry systems such as CT and MR, these extending needles will not fit in the gantry. In the case of MR, in particular, this can be very challenging with conventional scanners. Some open-access MR scanners provide limited access at the cost of lower field strength (30). Other solutions make use of semi-flexible needles that can bend in a closed gantry environment (31).

Radiation Exposure

Many procedures are best done utilizing CT or fluoroscopy as the guidance tool. The inherent limitation of these modalities is the radiation exposure to physician and patient. Physician exposure can be diminished with shields and arm extenders such as robots, as mentioned earlier. Modifications to the imaging equipment can also be employed to limit radiation exposure. Lowering the mA or using navigation software and fusion imaging are all approaches that can reduce radiation exposure (32, 33).

All of the aforementioned features are important areas of active research in the field of image guidance for interventional oncology procedures.

INTRA-PROCEDURAL MONITORING

An important challenge in most interventional oncologic therapies is knowing when enough therapy has been delivered. Ideally, there would be some clear endpoint for therapy completion. Imaging is one

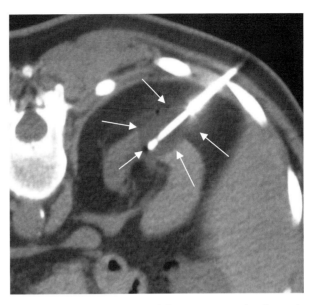

FIGURE 7.3. Imaging used for intra-procedural monitoring. Visualization of the low-density ice ball (*arrows*) around the cryoprobe during percutaneous cryotherapy allows the user to be certain that the tumor is well contained within the ice ball.

potential solution for a non-invasive measure of completeness.

A number of imaging features have been used to assess completeness of therapy. These primarily revolve around measures of blood flow. Post-embolization angiography can show a completely embolized tumor bed. Lipiodol uptake may be used to visualize progress during chemoembolization.

In ultrasound, Doppler flow and contrast imaging have been used to assess blood flow. Increased echogenicity after radiofrequency ablation (34) and acoustic shadowing associated with ice ball formation in cryotherapy (35) are two other ultrasound monitoring tools. Sonographic contrast is another method of assessing the treatment zone (36).

CT and MR also use contrast imaging to assess vascularity of the treatment zone.

Ice ball visualization on CT and MR has been used to guide cryotherapy (Figure 7.3) (37). CT low attenuation associated with percutaneous ethanol injection can guide procedure termination. Conceivably, in the future, nuclear medicine agents might be useful to measure tumor viability during a procedure.

More recently, imaging measurements of temperature have been used to determine completeness of thermal ablation. MR thermometry has been most developed for use with high-intensity focused ultrasound (38). Using proton resonance frequency changes that are associated with temperature change, one can measure tissue temperature changes in the

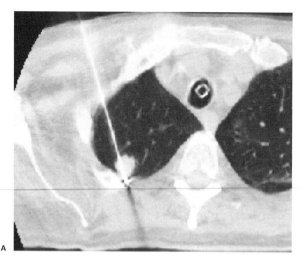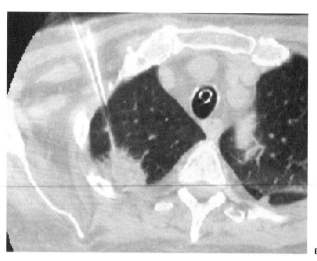

FIGURE 7.4. (A) Lung radiofrequency ablation with the probe in the tumor. (B) Immediately after the ablation, the area around the tumor looks much larger due to hemorrhage and edema. This makes using strict anatomic criteria diffi- cult to determine completeness of therapy. Post-procedure a new baseline image is necessary from which to compare future follow-up imaging.

MR to within 1°C (39). Because temperatures of ~54°C for longer than 1 second are believed to cause cell death, measuring temperature with MR can pro- vide a non-invasive tool to evaluate completeness of thermal ablation therapy. Other imaging modal- ities have been used experimentally for non-invasive thermometry. CT Hounsfield unit changes and ultrasound sound velocity changes have both been shown to correlate with temperature (40, 41).

IMAGING FOR THERAPY ASSESSMENT

Patients who receive image-guided therapy are fol- lowed with periodic diagnostic-quality imaging stud- ies. Interpretation of these images can be extremely difficult given that distinguishing expected changes after the therapy from changes associated with tumor growth can be very challenging. It is therefore crit- ical to obtain a baseline imaging study shortly after the image-guided therapy. Whichever is the choice of imaging study, it is probably best to continue to use the same modality in follow-up to allow for direct comparison.

In most cases, follow-up studies are contrast- enhanced CT or contrast-enhanced MR. PET/CT studies may be particularly helpful with fluo- rodeoxyglucose (FDG)-avid tumors but have not been rigorously proven superior. Whereas contrast- enhanced CT is the most commonly used imag- ing modality for post-therapy assessment, one study demonstrated the positive predictive value to be only 69% for evaluating completeness of therapy

(42). Subtraction imaging can be particularly useful in detecting subtle recurrence. Subtraction may be especially helpful when using contrast-enhanced MR techniques (43).

In 2000, the Response Evaluation Criteria in Solid Tumors (RECIST) were established by an international consensus group (44). These criteria became the standard for assessing response to chemo- therapy and involve measuring the diameter change of a series of up to 10 index lesions. Although these cri- teria have been useful in the systemic chemotherapy setting, they may not be useful when assessing image- guided interventions. After successful image-guided therapy, the treated lesions may in fact appear larger, not smaller than the pre-treated lesions (Figure 7.4). The increase in anatomic size on CT or MR is likely due to associated hemorrhage, edema, and inflamma- tion, as well as intentional destruction of surround- ing tissue for a safety margin (45–47). Unidimen- sional tumor measurements would suggest growth of the tumor rather than successful treatment, which is not the case. Hence, in the field of image-guided ther- apy, the RECIST criteria fail and newer methods of post-therapy assessment are mandatory.

Newer imaging techniques may provide an oppor- tunity for improved assessment of the post-therapy tumor bed. These techniques include MR diffusion, MR spectroscopy, CT/MR perfusion imaging, and PET imaging.

MR diffusion imaging assesses water molecule diffusion in the tissue. Viable tumor cells have membranes that restrict water movement, whereas necrotic cells with disrupted membranes have increased water movement. The apparent diffusion coefficient may therefore be higher in areas of necrosis than in areas of viable tumor. This technique has been particularly applied in chemoembolization cases (48). The technique is limited in areas with respiratory motion or in areas of magnetic susceptibility such as with the air in the lungs.

Assessing choline levels with ^{1}H-MR spectroscopy is another method to assess tumor viability after an image-guided therapy. Choline is an essential component of cell membrane biosynthesis. Elevated choline levels are associated with increased cell proliferation in several tumors. Post-therapy necrotic areas are believed to have low choline levels compared with areas of viable recurrent tumor (49).

A number of CT and MR enhancement and perfusion techniques have been applied to tumor imaging to provide additional information about tumor physiology. Dynamic contrast enhancement techniques measure rates of contrast enhancement in a particular area to identify viable tumor. MR imaging arterial spin labeling is another method for measuring perfusion of a particular area without administering contrast (50). All of these techniques attempt to add physiologic information to the standard anatomic information of CT and MR.

New PET imaging tracers may have increased specificity that can distinguish post-therapy inflammation from actual residual tumor. Choline and other metabolites such as thymidine can be labeled with positron-emitting isotopes for detecting tumor proliferation (51). Antibodies that specifically target cancer cells can be labeled with PET isotopes as well (52). This increased imaging specificity may be useful in assessing post-therapy tumor beds.

Other new molecular imaging techniques that provide increased tumor specificity may ultimately play a role in identifying residual disease after image-guided therapy. These tools will help improve these therapies by providing increased confidence of success and an earlier opportunity to intervene if residual viable tumor remains.

SUMMARY

Advances in imaging have enabled the field of interventional oncology. Imaging plays multiple critical roles in these new therapies. Imaging allows pre-procedure planning, tool delivery guidance, intra-procedural monitoring, and post-therapy assessment. Each of these areas is evolving. As imaging equipment becomes more customized to the task of image-guided therapy, it is likely that these procedures will become safer and more effective.

REFERENCES

1. Khajanchee YS, Streeter D, Swanstrom LL, et al. A mathematical model for preoperative planning of radiofrequency ablation of hepatic tumors. Surg Endosc 2004; 18(4): 696–701.
2. Jankun M, Kelly TJ, Zaim A, et al. Computer model for cryosurgery of the prostate. Comput Aided Surg 1999; 4(4): 193–199.
3. Villard C, Baegert C, Schreck P, et al. Optimal trajectories computation within regions of interest for hepatic RFA planning. Med Image Comput Comput Assist Interv Int Conf Med Image Comput Comput Assist Interv 2005; 8(Pt 2): 49–56.
4. Solomon SB, Patriciu A, Stoianovici DS. Tumor ablation treatment planning coupled to robotic implementation: A feasibility study. J Vasc Interv Radiol 2006; 17(5): 903–907.
5. Sze DY, Razavi MK, So SK, et al. Impact of multidetector CT hepatic arteriography on the planning of chemoembolization treatment of hepatocellular carcinoma. Am J Roentgenol 2001; 177(6): 1339–1345.
6. Ho S, Lau WY, Leung TW, et al. Clinical evaluation of the partition model for estimating radiation doses from yttrium-90 microspheres in the treatment of hepatic cancer. Eur J Nucl Med 1997 Mar; 24(3): 293–298.
7. Villard C, Soler L, Gangi A. Radiofrequency ablation of hepatic tumors: Simulation, planning, and contribution of virtual reality and haptics. Comput Methods Biomech Biomed Engin 2005; 8(4): 215–227.
8. Dawson S. Procedural simulation: A primer. J Vasc Interv Radiol 2006; 17(2 Pt 1): 205–213.
9. de Mey J, Op de Beeck B, Meysman M, et al. Real time CT-fluoroscopy: Diagnostic and therapeutic applications. Eur J Radiol 2000; 34(1): 32–40.
10. Irie T, Kajitani M, Itai Y. CT fluoroscopy-guided intervention: Marked reduction of scattered radiation dose to the physician's hand by use of a lead plate and an improved I-I device. J Vasc Interv Radiol 2001 Dec; 12(12): 1417–1421.
11. Boss A, Clasen S, Kuczyk M, et al. Magnetic resonance-guided percutaneous radiofrequency ablation of renal cell carcinomas: A pilot clinical study. Invest Radiol 2005; 40(9): 583–590.
12. Liapi E, Hong K, Georgiades CS, et al. Three-dimensional rotational angiography: Introduction of an adjunctive tool for successful transarterial chemoembolization. J Vasc Interv Radiol 2005 Sep; 16(9): 1241–1245.
13. Beldi G, Styner M, Schindera S, et al. Intraoperative three-dimensional fluoroscopic cholangiography. Hepatogastroenterology 2006; 53(68): 157–159.
14. Silverman SG, Sun MR, Tuncali K, et al. Three-dimensional assessment of MRI-guided percutaneous

cryotherapy of liver metastases. Phys Med Biol 2006; 51(12): 3251–3267.

15. Chin JL, Downey DB, Onik G, et al. Three-dimensional prostate ultrasound and its application to cryosurgery. Tech Urol 1996; 2(4): 187–193.

16. Numata K, Isozaki T, Ozawa Y, et al. Percutaneous ablation therapy guided by contrast-enhanced sonography for patients with hepatocellular carcinoma. Am J Roentgenol 2003 Jan; 180(1): 143–149.

17. Yap JT, Carney JP, Hall NC, et al. Image-guided cancer therapy using PET/CT. J Cancer 2004; 10(4): 221–233.

18. Veit P, Kuehle C, Beyer T, et al. Accuracy of combined PET/CT in image-guided interventions of liver lesions: An ex-vivo study. World J Gastroenterol 2006 Apr 21; 12(15): 2388–2393.

19. Heron DE, Smith RP, Andrade RS. Advances in image-guided radiation therapy – the role of PET-CT. Med Dosim 2006; 31(1): 3–11.

20. Wein W, Roper B, Navab N. Automatic registration and fusion of ultrasound with CT for radiotherapy. Med Image Comput Comput Assist Interv Int Conf Med Image Comput Comput Assist Interv 2005; 8(Pt 2): 303–311.

21. Solomon SB. Incorporating CT, MR imaging, and positron emission tomography into minimally invasive therapies. J Vasc Interv Radiol 2005 Apr; 16(4): 445–447.

22. Zhang H, Banovac F, Lin R, et al. Electromagnetic tracking for abdominal interventions in computer aided surgery. Comput Aided Surg 2006; 11(3): 127–136.

23. Solomon SB. Interactive images in the operating room. J Endourol 1999; 13(7): 471–475.

24. Mogami T, Dohi M, Harada J. A new image navigation system for MR-guided cryosurgery. Magn Reson Med Sci 2002; 1(4): 191–197.

25. Borgert J, Kruger S, Timinger H, et al. Respiratory motion compensation with tracked internal and external sensors during CT-guided procedures. Comput Aided Surg 2006; 11(3): 119–125.

26. Peters TM. Image-guidance for surgical procedures. Phys Med Biol 2006; 51(14): R505–540.

27. Solomon SB, Patriciu A, Bohlman ME, et al. Robotically driven interventions: A method of using CT fluoroscopy without radiation exposure to the physician. Radiology 2002; 225(1): 277–282.

28. Cleary K, Melzer A, Watson V, et al. Interventional robotic systems: Applications and technology state-of-the-art. Minim Invasive Ther Allied Technol 2006; 15(2): 101–113.

29. Hempel E, Fischer H, Gumb L, et al. An MRI-compatible surgical robot for precise radiological interventions. Comput Aided Surg 2003; 8(4): 180–191.

30. Kettenbach J, Kacher DF, Koskinen SK, et al. Interventional and intraoperative magnetic resonance imaging. Annu Rev Biomed Eng 2000; 2: 661–690.

31. Gaffke G, Gebauer B, Knollmann FD. Use of semiflexible applicators for radiofrequency ablation of liver tumors. Cardiovasc Intervent Radiol 2006 Mar-Apr; 29(2): 270–275.

32. Stoeckelhuber BM, Leibecke T, Schulz E, et al. Radiation dose to the radiologist's hand during continuous CT fluoroscopy-guided interventions. Cardiovasc Intervent Radiol 2005; 28(5): 589–594.

33. Efstathopoulos EP, Brountzos EN, Alexopoulou E, et al. Patient radiation exposure measurements during interventional procedures: A prospective study. Health Phys 2006; 91(1): 36–40.

34. Leyendecker JR, Dodd GD 3rd, Halff GA, et al. Sonographically observed echogenic response during intraoperative radiofrequency ablation of cirrhotic livers: Pathologic correlation. Am J Roentgenol 2002; 178(5): 1147–1151.

35. Mala T, Aurdal L, Frich L, et al. Liver tumor cryoablation: A commentary on the need of improved procedural monitoring. Technol Cancer Res Treat 2004; 3(1): 85–91.

36. Solbiati L, Ierace T, Tonolini M, et al. Guidance and monitoring of radiofrequency liver tumor ablation with contrast-enhanced ultrasound. Eur J Radiol 2004; 51 Suppl: S19–23.

37. Kim CK, Choi D, Lim HK, et al. Therapeutic response assessment of percutaneous radiofrequency ablation for hepatocellular carcinoma: Utility of contrast-enhanced agent detection imaging. Eur J Radiol 2005 Oct; 56(1): 66–73.

38. Permpongkosol S, Nielsen ME, Solomon SB. Percutaneous renal cryoablation. Urology 2006; 68(1 Suppl): 19–25.

39. McDannold N, Tempany CM, Fennessy FM, et al. Uterine leiomyomas: MR imaging-based thermometry and thermal dosimetry during focused ultrasound thermal ablation. Radiology 2006 Jul; 240(1): 263–272.

40. Quesson B, de Zwart JA, Moonen CT. Magnetic resonance temperature imaging for guidance of thermotherapy. J Magn Reson Imaging 2000; 12(4): 525–533.

41. Fallone BG, Moran PR, Podgorsak EB. Noninvasive thermometry with a clinical X-ray CT scanner. Med Phys 1982; 9(5): 715–721.

42. Arthur RM, Straube WL, Trobaugh JW, et al. Noninvasive estimation of hyperthermia temperatures with ultrasound. Int J Hyperthermia 2005; 21(6): 589–600.

43. Kim YS, Rhim H, Lim HK, et al. Completeness of treatment in hepatocellular carcinomas treated with image-guided tumor therapies: Evaluation of positive predictive value of contrast-enhanced CT with histopathologic correlation in the explanted liver specimen. J Comput Assist Tomogr 2006 July/August; 30(4): 578–582.

44. Boss A, Martirosian P, Schraml C, et al. Morphological, contrast-enhanced and spin labeling perfusion imaging for monitoring of relapse after RF ablation of renal cell carcinomas. Eur Radiol 2006; 16: 1226–1236.

45. Therasse P, Arbuck SG, Eisenhauer EA, et al. New guidelines to evaluate the response to treatment in solid tumors. European Organization for Research and Treatment of Cancer, National Cancer Institute of the United States, National Cancer Institute of Canada. J Natl Cancer Inst 2000; 92(3): 205–216.

46. Merkle EM, Nour SG, Lewin JS. MR imaging follow-up after percutaneous radiofrequency ablation of renal cell carcinoma: Findings in 18 patients during first 6 months. Radiology 2005; 235(3): 1065–1071.

47. Steinke K, King J, Glenn D, et al. Radiologic appearance and complications of percutaneous computed tomography-guided radiofrequency-ablated pulmonary metastases from colorectal carcinoma. J Comput Assist Tomogr 2003; 27(5): 750–757.

48. Suh RD, Wallace AB, Sheehan RE, et al. Unresectable pulmonary malignancies: CT-guided percutaneous radiofrequency ablation – preliminary results. Radiology 2003; 229(3): 821–829.

49. Kamel IR, Bluemke DA, Eng J, et al. The role of functional MR imaging in the assessment of tumor response after chemoembolization in patients with hepatocellular carcinoma. J Vasc Interv Radiol 2006; 17(3): 505–512.

50. Chen CY, Li CW, Kuo YT, et al. Early response of hepatocellular carcinoma to transcatheter arterial chemoembolization: Choline levels and MR diffusion constants – initial experience. Radiology 2006 May; 239(2): 448–456.

51. Boss A, Martirosian P, Schraml C, et al. Morphological, contrast-enhanced and spin labeling perfusion imaging for monitoring of relapse after RF ablation of renal cell carcinomas. Eur Radiol 2006 Jun; 16(6): 1226–1236.

52. van Waarde A, Jager PL, Ishiwata K, et al. Comparison of sigma-ligands and metabolic PET tracers for differentiating tumor from inflammation. J Nucl Med 2006 Jan; 47(1): 150–154.

53. Brouwers A, Mulders P, Oosterwijk E, et al. Pharmacokinetics and tumor targeting of 131I-labeled F(ab')2 fragments of the chimeric monoclonal antibody G250: Preclinical and clinical pilot studies. Cancer Biother Radiopharm 2004; 19(4): 466–477.

Chapter 8

ASSESSMENT OF TUMOR RESPONSE ON MAGNETIC RESONANCE IMAGING AFTER LOCOREGIONAL THERAPY

Manon Buijs

Josephina A. Vossen

Jean-Francois H. Geschwind

Ihab R. Kamel

Assessment of tumor response after locoregional therapy is important in determining treatment success and in guiding future therapy. Magnetic resonance (MR) imaging plays an important role in evaluating treatment response to new therapies directed toward treatment of hepatic tumors. The traditional and accepted criteria to determine tumor response in oncology, namely the Response Evaluation Criteria in Solid Tumors (RECIST), use decrease in tumor size as an indicator of successful therapy. However, because of the lack of size change early after treatment, the European Association for the Study of the Liver (EASL) criteria were introduced and are based on lack of contrast enhancement after therapy as an indicator of favorable response. A more recent evaluation method is the apparent diffusion coefficient (ADC), measured by diffusion-weighted MR imaging. Diffusion-weighted MR imaging and ADC values map the thermally induced motion of water molecules in tissues and thereby are able to provide insight into tumor microstructure. In this chapter, we discuss the role of MR imaging in assessing treatment response after various locoregional thera-

pies. We describe the role of tumor size (as recommended by RECIST) and enhancement (as suggested by EASL) as well as ADC mapping. We also discuss the MR imaging findings after radiofrequency ablation (RFA), transarterial chemoembolization (TACE) and radioembolization.

Although surgical resection and liver transplantation offer the only chance for cure in patients with hepatic malignancies, unfortunately, tumors in most patients are found to be unresectable at time of presentation, leaving palliative therapy as the only option. This has resulted in increased utilization of minimally invasive strategies as therapeutic options for both primary and metastatic hepatic malignancies (1, 2). These locoregional therapies include ablative techniques and catheter-based approaches. Ablation can be applied either chemically (percutaneous ethanol injection) or thermally (radiofrequency ablation, microwave ablation and laser ablation). Catheter-based approaches include transarterial chemoembolization and transarterial radioembolization. This method of delivery could be intraoperative, percutaneous or intra-arterial.

The aim of these treatments is to improve tumor targeting, minimize hepatotoxicity and thereby improve patients' quality of life and survival, by inducing tumor necrosis.

Assessment of tumor response after locoregional therapy is an increasingly important task in oncologic imaging. New imaging modalities play a critical role in determining treatment success and in guiding future therapy. Several monitors of tumor response have been used, including histology, tumor markers and imaging. Histological evaluation, however, is conclusive only when it shows viable tumor. Even repeated negative biopsies do not exclude the presence of viable malignancy. Although several studies have proposed the use of serological markers in diagnosing liver malignancies, the only widely used serum marker is alpha-fetoprotein. However, the sensitivity of this marker is limited. Various imaging modalities, including Doppler ultrasonography, angiography, computed tomography (CT) and MR imaging have been used to evaluate treatment response (3, 4). In this chapter, we discuss the role of MR imaging in assessing treatment response after various locoregional therapies that are commonly used at our institution.

Role of Imaging in Assessing Treatment Response

In 1981, the World Health Organization (WHO) defined criteria for objective response of a tumor to an anti-cancer agent, in an attempt to standardize the reporting of response in solid tumors (5). Even though a tumor is three dimensional, the WHO response assessment was performed on the basis of measurements from cross-sectional scans in two dimensions. However, several problems were encountered when using these WHO criteria. These include wide variations between observers in estimating the position of the lesion boundary and the number of lesions that may be used to assess for response. Furthermore, the use of relatively new imaging modalities such as CT and MR caused confusion about the use of three-dimensional measurements. These issues led to a number of modifications to the WHO criteria, resulting in a situation in which response criteria were no longer comparable among research organizations. In 2000, RECIST were introduced to rectify some of the previous issues with the WHO criteria (6). These criteria included important changes such as unidimensional tumor measurement,

selection of target lesions with a minimum size, details concerning imaging modalities and a new threshold for assignment of objective progression (7). RECIST, however, rely solely on anatomic size measurements of tumors to assess response. For this reason, the validity of RECIST has recently been questioned in view of the emergence of new locoregional anticancer therapies, because, in many cases, in spite of tumor changes, the lesion does not initially shrink (8). Shrinkage of tumor may take 6 months or more to attain the RECIST criteria for partial response (6). Occasionally, patients may not be considered to have exhibited a response in spite of the presence of tumor necrosis.

This realization, that anatomy may not change after locoregional therapies, moved the focus toward new evaluation methods. These include assessment of tumor vascular and cellular integrity, motion of water molecules and biochemical concentration. Vascular integrity is measured by the degree of extracellular contrast enhancement. The EASL has officially recommended the use of lesion enhancement on contrast-enhanced CT as the standard modality to determine treatment response of hepatocellular carcinoma (HCC) after locoregional therapy (9). This change was also reflected in the national practice guideline released by the American Association for the Study of Liver Disease on the management of HCC in 2005 (10). Areas of tumor enhancement were considered viable, whereas nonenhancing regions reflected tissue necrosis. The EASL also stated that tumor size measurements might not be accurate because these measurements would not take into account the true extent of tumor necrosis.

Diffusion-weighted MR imaging and ADC values map the thermally induced motion of water molecules in biologic tissues, known as **Brownian motion**, and are thereby able to provide insight into tumor microstructure. The motion includes not only molecular diffusion of water but also microcirculation of blood (microperfusion). The primary application of diffusion-weighted MR imaging has been in brain imaging, mainly for the evaluation of acute ischemic stroke, intracranial tumors and demyelinating disease (11–13). In the liver, diffusion-weighted imaging has been used to characterize focal hepatic lesions and to assess tumor response. Viable tumors are high in cellularity. These cells have an intact cell membrane that restricts the mobility of water molecules and causes a relatively low ADC value. Conversely, cellular necrosis causes increased membranous permeability, which allows water molecules to move freely and thus causes a relative increase in the ADC value.

Biochemical concentration can be evaluated by the use of MR spectroscopy. MR spectroscopy has been used successfully in the diagnosis of tumors in the brain (11) and breast (14) and in the evaluation of response to chemotherapy (15). In the liver, MR spectroscopy has been proven useful in evaluating diffuse hepatic disease such as hepatic steatosis, chronic hepatitis and cirrhosis (16). The role of MR spectroscopy in evaluating tumor response after locoregional therapy still has to be established. However, according to previously published in vitro and in vivo MR spectroscopy studies, the choline-containing metabolite phosphocholine is elevated in hepatic tumors as a result of increased cell turnover (17, 18). Other preliminary studies are in line with these results and show that tumor choline levels may decline after TACE, allowing the assessment of therapeutic response of HCC (19).

MR Imaging Technique

Our current MR imaging protocol uses a 1.5-T MR image scanner (CV/i, General Electric Medical Systems, Milwaukee, WI) and a phased array torso coil. The technique consists of T2-weighted fast spin-echo images (matrix size, 256 × 256; slice thickness, 8 mm; interslice gap, 2 mm; TR/TE, 5000/100; receive bandwidth, 32 kHz) and breath-hold diffusion-weighted echoplanar images (matrix, 128 × 128; slice thickness, 8 mm; interslice gap, 2 mm; b-value, 500; repetition time, 5,000–6,500 msec; echo time, 110 msec; receive bandwidth, 64 kHz).

In the initial application of diffusion-weighted MR imaging in the brain, diffusion gradients are measured multidirectional because the fiber tracks have different directionality of flow (20–23). The liver, however, has an isotropic diffusion pattern, probably due to its randomly organized structures. Therefore, the ADC is measured only in one direction (24). Higher b-values can reduce the effect of perfusion on the calculated ADC value; however, lower b-values can lead to the underestimation of ADC values (25). In prior studies performed for brain imaging, high b-values of 1000 sec/mm^2 were used. However, in our experience, a b-value of 500 sec/mm^2 had better signal-to-noise ratio compared with higher b-values. Therefore, in our institution, a b-value of 500 sec/mm^2 is used.

The final component of our imaging protocol is breath-hold unenhanced and contrast-enhanced (0.1 mmol/kg intravenous gadodiamide; Omniscan; Amersham, Princeton, NJ) T1-weighted three-dimensional fat-suppressed spoiled gradient-echo images (field of view, 320–400 mm; matrix, 192 × 160; slice thickness, 4–6 mm; repetition time, 5.1 msec; TE echo time, 1.2 msec; receive bandwidth, 64 kHz; flip angle, 15°). The contrast-enhanced images are obtained in the arterial phase (20 seconds) and portal venous phase (60 seconds).

MR Imaging after Tissue Ablation

Tissue ablation can be performed by several techniques, either chemical (e.g., ethanol ablation), thermal (e.g., radiofrequency [RF], microwave and laser ablation) or cooling effect (e.g., cryotherapy). These therapies require imaging for adequate targeting, monitoring the ablation process and follow-up. Ultrasonography (US) is most often used as the primary guidance technique, because this modality enables visualization and precise placement of the electrode. Contrast-enhanced US, CT and MR imaging are more commonly used to assess treatment response (26,27). We will discuss the role of MR imaging in evaluating therapeutic response to the most widely accepted method of tissue ablation: RFA.

RFA induces thermally mediated coagulation necrosis, resulting in cellular death, using heat and low-voltage alternating electrical current (100–500 kHz) that is delivered to the tumor by means of an electrode. This causes ionic vibrations as the ions attempt to follow the change in direction of the alternating current. Ionic vibrations result in frictional heating of the surrounding tissue. Tissue temperature above 60°C leads to changes of intra-cellular protein, lipid bilayer thawing and cell death. Temperatures above 100°C result in coagulation necrosis (28, 29). RFA can be applied percutaneously, laparoscopically or during laparotomy. Previous models of electrodes had several technological limitations that did not allow ablation in tumors larger than 3 cm. Modifications in these original designs, including hooked electrodes, internally cooled electrodes, pulsed techniques, multiple probes, multiple insertions and more powerful generators, have led to improved results (30, 31).

It is critical for physicians to select the appropriate patient population to improve therapeutic results. It is generally accepted that patient inclusion criteria for RFA are few (<5), small (<3 cm) lesions with no extrahepatic disease and near-normal liver function (32, 33). Furthermore, it has been suggested that lesions close to major structures, such as the hepatic capsule, gallbladder and major blood vessels, should not be treated with RFA. Major blood vessels may prevent adequate heating by acting as a heat sink, and proximity to the gallbladder may predispose to biliary complications.

After RFA, imaging is commonly used to assess treatment response. In our institution, MR is the modality of choice for follow-up of these lesions. Several factors influence treatment response, such as treatment approach, tumor size, tumor location, histological type and presence of confounding liver disease. Smaller lesions (<3 cm) have better necrosis and have a lower recurrence rate than larger lesions. Metastases have a higher recurrence rate, presumably because of the presence of occult disease at the time of initial ablation. Underlying cirrhosis in patients with HCC causes larger ablations than would be expected in metastatic disease, because the cirrhotic liver functions as a thermal insulator promoting better thermal coagulation, known as the oven effect (34).

Adequately treated lesions are uniformly hypo-intense on T2-weighted images, probably because of dehydration and coagulative necrosis induced by tissue heating. Occasionally, hyperintense foci may be seen on T2-weighted images corresponding to an area of tissue loss filled by fibrin or hemorrhage. A tumor that has been completely treated no longer enhances on gadolinium-enhanced MR images. However, a thin and regular (<1 mm) enhancing rim may appear immediately after treatment, most likely because of reactive hyperemia representing an inflammation reaction to the thermal injury (35, 36). Most lesions demonstrate markedly heterogeneous signal intensity on T1-weighted images caused by an uneven evolution of necrosis over time (Figure 8.1) (37). Arteriovenous shunting caused by needle puncture or thermal damage may result in wedge-shaped enhancement on the arterial phase within the liver parenchyma close to the treated lesion. However, it is expected that perfusional abnormalities vanish by 30 days after the procedure. Ideally, on MR imaging, the size of the treated lesion exceeds the size of the lesion before treatment, indicating complete ablation of the tumor margin, including a safety margin. On subsequent follow-up, the lesion shows an involution of the coagulation site. Small necrotic areas may disappear completely.

Residual or recurrent tumor manifests as a lesion with irregular and non-delineated contours and de-monstrates moderately high signal on T2-weighted images, with the same characteristics as on pre-interventional imaging. Residual or recurrent tumor is often located within or at the periphery of the ablated lesion (38). This focus may not enhance in the first 2 months after treatment; however, enhancement usually occurs on subsequent MR images. This peripheral location of treatment failure could be explained by lower energy deposition and reduced heating, remote from the needle electrode. Furthermore, tissue perfusion lowers heat accumulation due to cooling, and this phenomenon is even more marked in tissue in contact with large vessels, causing regrowth.

MR Imaging after TACE

Unlike most other organs, the liver is unique in that it has a dual blood supply via the portal vein and the hepatic artery. Normally, the portal vein is responsible for supplying most of the blood to the liver (75% to 80%), with the hepatic artery providing only a supportive role (20% to 25%) (39–41). However, in liver tumors, the hepatic artery and not the portal vein is the main supplier of blood to the tumor. This notion has been exploited in transcatheter arterial chemoembolization, in which the hepatic artery is used to deliver highly concentrated doses of chemotherapy suspended in an oily medium directly to the tumor followed by injection of embolic material to arrest blood flow within the artery (39). This technique potentiates the effects of chemotherapy by allowing the drugs to penetrate inside the cancer cells with greater ease and by preventing washout. These factors significantly reduce systemic toxicity that may result from treatment. Currently, various combinations of drugs have been reported, with most agents coming from doxorubicin or cisplatin chemotherapy families.

Assessment of tumor response by imaging after TACE is generally based on iodized oil deposition on unenhanced CT and tumor enhancement and tumor size on contrast-enhanced CT or MR imaging. Unenhanced CT can demonstrate the presence of hyperattenuating iodized oil within the tumor. Good iodized oil retention is associated with prolonged median survival but does not indicate complete necrosis (42, 43). Hyperattenuating iodized oil impairs the assessment of residual tumor enhancement on contrast-enhanced CT. In contrast to CT, the high concentration of iodized oil after chemoembolization does not affect MR signal intensity (44).

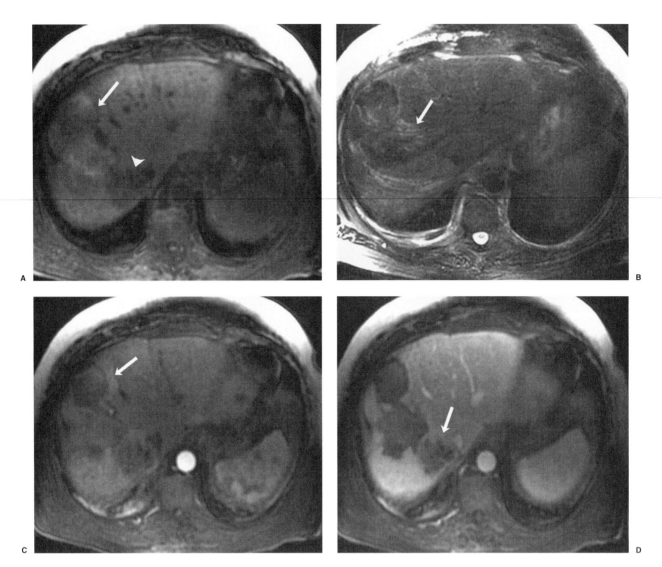

FIGURE 8.1. MR imaging after RF ablation of metastatic colorectal cancer. (A) Axial pre-gadolinium T1-weighted image shows a large region with heterogeneous high signal (*arrow*), consistent with post RFA effect and one untreated lesion with dark signal relative to liver parenchyma (*arrow-head*). (B) Axial pre-gadolinium T2-weighted image shows a rim of high signal intensity surrounding the treated lesions (*arrow*), representing reactive granulation tissue or residual tumor. (C) Gadolinium-enhanced image (repetition time/echo time, 5.1 msec/1.2 msec) again shows a rim of mild peripheral enhancement (*arrow*) in the hepatic arterial phase. (D) Gadolinium-enhanced image (repetition time/echo time, 5.1 msec/1.2 msec) shows untreated tumor with internal enhancement (*arrow*).

Contrast-enhanced MR imaging determines areas of tumor enhancement by using extracellular contrast agent. Enhancing portions of the tumor are presumed to be viable, whereas nonenhancing portions are presumed to be necrotic. The disadvantage of contrast-enhanced MR imaging is the inability to distinguish viable cells from reactive granulation tissue. Contrast enhancement in granulation tissue is believed to be caused by increased capillary permeability and marked increase in the passive distribution of gadolinium (45). After TACE, an enhancing rim can appear on contrast-enhanced MR imaging. This rim can correlate to viable tumor as well as to reactive tissue.

A recent technique for assessment of tumor response is diffusion-weighted MR imaging (46). This imaging technique is used to detect the motion of water molecules. Initially, diffusion-weighted MR imaging was limited to the brain. With the advent of the ultrafast singleshot echoplanar imaging technique, diffusion-weighted MR imaging of the abdomen has become possible.

We will discuss the MR imaging features of different tumors after TACE, including primary and metastatic liver tumors. The primary tumors we discuss are HCC and cholangiocarcinoma. The metastatic tumors we discuss are divided into

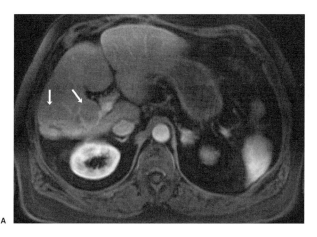

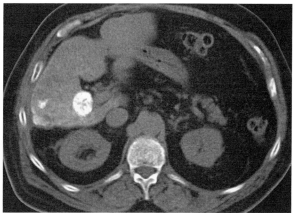

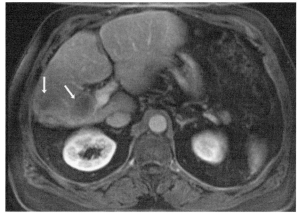

FIGURE 8.2. Changes on MR imaging after TACE of HCC. (A) Gadolinium-enhanced image (repetition time/echo time, 5.1 msec/1.2 msec) before TACE shows two enhancing liver lesions (*arrows*) in the right lobe of the liver. (B) Unenhanced CT of the abdomen following TACE of the right lobe. Notice intense deposition of iodized oil within one of the targeted masses. (C) Gadolinium-enhanced image (repetition time/echo time, 5.1 msec/1.2 msec) after TACE shows that the masses are almost completely avascular (*arrows*).

hypovascular (metastatic breast cancer) and hypervascular (metastic neuroendocrine cancer) metastases.

HCC

HCC is the fifth most common cancer in the world and represents more than 5% of all cancers (47). The majority of HCC patients (approximately 75%) are not candidates for curative treatments due to poor liver function or the presence of advanced disease. These patients may be eligible for treatment with TACE. TACE achieves partial response in 15% to 55% of patients and significantly delays tumor progression and vascular invasion (48–51). Because of its impact on survival, it has become essential to accurately determine tumor response after therapy (46).

For patients with HCC treated with TACE, signal intensity on T1- and T2-weighted images varies. Hypointensity on T2-weighted images represents necrosis. Conversely, hyperintensity on T2-weighted images corresponds to residual tumor. However, this hyperintensity can also represent hemorrhage, liquefied necrosis or inflammatory infiltration. HCC is hypervascular and enhances rapidly during the hepatic arterial phase. Enhancement declines at the portal venous phase. After TACE, on the arterial phase images, residual viable tumor is rapidly enhancing, either homogeneous or heterogeneous, whereas necrotic tumor is non-enhancing (Figure 8.2) (52, 53). On portal venous phase images, both viable tumor and inflammatory infiltration can cause persistent enhancement. After successful TACE, diffusion-weighted MR imaging shows an increase in ADC value of the targeted tumor, representing cellular necrosis. In a prior study, we demonstrated that mean tumor ADC increased after TACE by 20% (p = 0.026), whereas the ADC remained unchanged in non-tumorous liver, spleen and muscle (46).

Cholangiocarcinoma

Cholangiocarcinoma is a rare hepatic malignancy with an incidence of 1 to 2 per 100,000 persons in the United States. Only approximately 30% of patients with cholangiocarcinoma are eligible for resection because of the advanced nature of the disease at the time of diagnosis. A previous study at our institution showed that TACE provided an effective therapeutic option for patients with unresectable intrahepatic cholangiocarcinoma, with a median survival of 23 months (54).

Cholangiocarcinomas are commonly described as hypovascular tumors. They appear hypointense on T1-weighted images and hyperintense on T2-weighted images. On dynamic MR imaging, cholangiocarcinomas typically reveal minimal or moderate initial rim enhancement, followed by progressive and concentric filling with contrast material (55, 56). After TACE, necrosis is represented as dark on T1 with a central area void of contrast enhancement on gadolinium-enhanced perfusion MR imaging and increased signal on diffusion MR sequences, reflecting cell death.

Hypovascular Liver Metastases: Metastatic Breast Cancer

In the Western world, breast cancer is the most common cancer in women and, in this group, it is the second leading cause of cancer death (57). Breast cancer can spread to almost every organ of the body. The liver is the most common site of intra-abdominal metastatic disease, with metastases to the liver occurring in up to 20% of patients (58). Metastatic breast cancer is essentially incurable and TACE has become more commonly used as a treatment modality because,in many cases, metastases are confined to the liver (59).

Before TACE, most lesions are hypointense on T1, and after TACE they generally remain hypointense. According to preliminary data from our group, on gadolinium-enhanced MR imaging, overall tumor enhancement in the arterial and portal venous phases decreases significantly after TACE, by 32% and 39% respectively (p < 0.0001) (Figure 8.3). Diffusion MR imaging is also useful in monitoring response after treatment. Mean tumor ADC increases by 27% (p < 0.0001) after successful TACE, whereas the ADC remains unchanged in non-tumorous liver, spleen and muscle.

Hypervascular Liver Metastases: Metastatic Neuroendocrine Tumors

Neuroendocrine tumors (NETs) are defined as tumors that have the capacity to synthesize and secrete polypeptide products with hormonal activity (60). These tumors include both carcinoid tumors and islet tumors and represent a diverse group of rare neoplasms, with an incidence of 1 to 4 cases per 100,000 people per year (61) and unique growth pat-

terns and clinical presentation. Many primary locations of NETs are known, including the gastrointestinal and respiratory tract (62). Liver metastases occur in 46% to 93% of patients with NETs, and metastatic disease can involve large portions of the liver. Unlike most other hepatic tumors, neuroendocrine metastases rarely lead to rapid liver dysfunction and failure and are often associated with an indolent disease course. However, the presence of liver metastases influences prognosis significantly (63–65). It is generally accepted that surgical resection is the only curative treatment option for patients with hepatic neuroendocrine metasases. Unfortunately, only 10% of patients are suitable candidates for resection (66). Moreover, systemic chemotherapy in patients with diffuse and/or progressive liver metastases yields disappointing results, especially in patients with metastases from midgut origin.

Treatment of hepatic metastases with TACE seems to be an attractive palliative option, because of their slowly growing and localized hypervascular pattern. Multiple studies have demonstrated the effectiveness of TACE for hepatic metastases of NETs in achieving hormone symptoms control and reduction of tumor growth (67–70). In most previous reports, tumor response to treatment has been measured by contrast-enhanced CT or MR imaging (68, 70). In a study of 66 lesions in 26 patients with hepatic metastases from NET, we have reported the functional MR imaging findings after TACE. Mean tumor diameter before treatment was 5.5 cm and decreased to 4.5 cm after treatment. Even though the decrease in tumor size was statistically significant (p < 0.0001), the size change was small (18%), and did not fulfill the RECIST criteria for partial response. We have also reported significant decrease in tumor arterial and venous enhancement after TACE (Figure 8.4). This is particularly important because these tumors are hypervascular and TACE results in occlusion of the blood flow to the tumor vasculature. Mean pretreatment tumor enhancement in the arterial phase was 61% and decreased to 31% after treatment (p < 0.0001). Mean pretreatment tumor enhancement in the portal venous phase was 82% and decreased to 43% after treatment (p < 0.0001). We have also reported a significant increase in tumor ADC value, from 1.5 E-3 mm^2/sec before treatment to 1.8 E-3 mm^2/sec after treatment (p < 0.0001), indicating marked cellular necrosis in response to therapy.

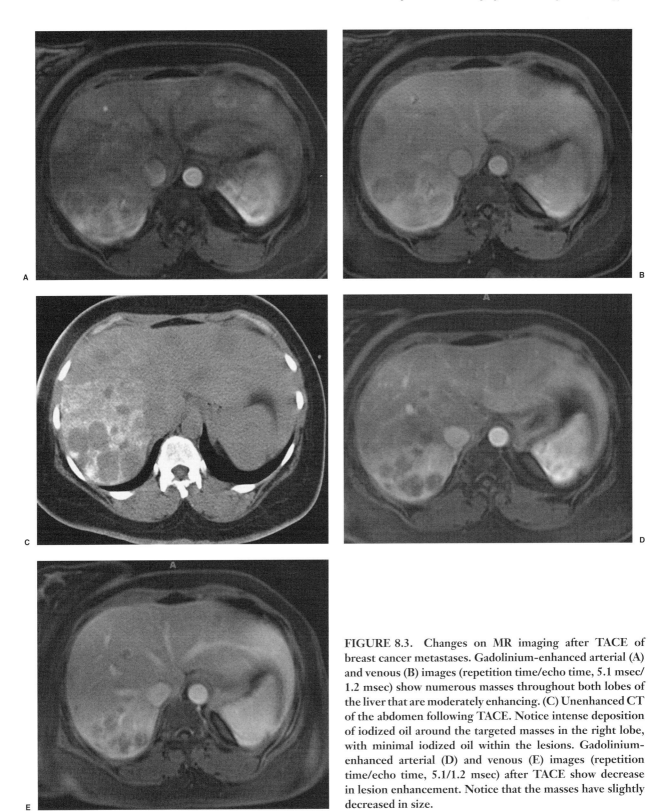

FIGURE 8.3. Changes on MR imaging after TACE of breast cancer metastases. Gadolinium-enhanced arterial (A) and venous (B) images (repetition time/echo time, 5.1 msec/ 1.2 msec) show numerous masses throughout both lobes of the liver that are moderately enhancing. (C) Unenhanced CT of the abdomen following TACE. Notice intense deposition of iodized oil around the targeted masses in the right lobe, with minimal iodized oil within the lesions. Gadolinium-enhanced arterial (D) and venous (E) images (repetition time/echo time, 5.1/1.2 msec) after TACE show decrease in lesion enhancement. Notice that the masses have slightly decreased in size.

MR Imaging after Radioembolization with Yttrium-90 Microspheres

The use of whole-liver external beam radiotherapy has limited applicability, because the liver parenchyma is radiation-sensitive and, as a result, there is a high risk of radiation-induced liver dis-ease (RILD), a clinical syndrome of anicteric hepatomegaly, ascites and increased liver enzymes occurring weeks to months after therapy. Improved results have been reported with a three-dimensional approach, thereby permitting higher levels of radiation to target regions while limiting whole liver

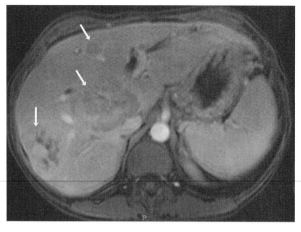

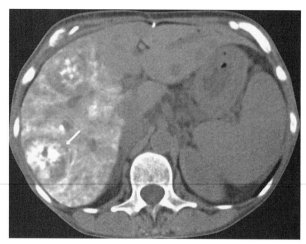

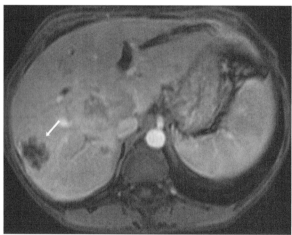

FIGURE 8.4.   Changes on MR imaging after TACE of neuroendocrine metastases. (A) Gadolinium-enhanced image (repetition time/echo time, 5.1 msec/1.2 msec) shows multiple enhancing lesions within both lobes of the liver (*arrows*). (B) Unenhanced CT of the abdomen following TACE. Notice the lipiodol deposition in and around the large right lobe lesion (*arrow*). (C) Gadolinium-enhanced image (repetition time/echo time, 5.1/1.2 msec) after TACE shows decrease in enhancement of the targeted large lesion in the right lobe (*arrow*).

exposure. However, the maximum dose that can be safely used without causing RILD is still limited by the liver parenchyma adjacent to the tumor. Radioembolization delivers internal β-radiation to liver lesions via catheter-directed intra-arterial administration of

Yttrium-90 embedded microspheres (71). The intention is to deliver a high dose of radiation selectively to the tumor, thereby causing tumor necrosis while sparing normal liver parenchyma (72,73). Lobar, segmental and subsegmental treatment can be performed.

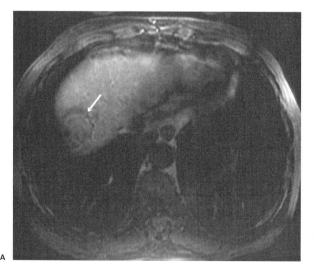

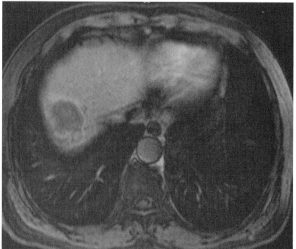

FIGURE 8.5.   Changes on MR imaging after Yttrium-90 microspheres of HCC. (A) Gadolinium-enhanced image (repetition time/echo time, 5.1 msec/1.2 msec) before TACE shows an enhancing mass (*arrow*) in the dome of the liver.

(B) Gadolinium-enhanced image (repetition time/echo time, 5.1/1.2 msec) after Yttrium-90 microspheres shows significant decrease in enhancement. Notice that the mass did not change in size.

A lung scan using technetium-99m macroaggregated albumin is performed prior to treatment, to determine the pulmonary shunting and thereby evaluate the risk of radiation pneumonitis. A shunt of 20% or less is usually acceptable (74).

Assessment of tumor response after treatment with Yttrium-90 microspheres is necessary to determine future therapeutic strategies. Some studies suggested that decrease in tumor enhancement is associated with a favorable response to therapy with Yttrium-90 microspheres (62). Preliminary data from our group showed a mean decrease in arterial enhancement of 22% (p = 0.013) and a mean decrease in venous enhancement of 25% (p = 0.012) in patients with HCC treated with Yttrium-90 microspheres (Figure 8.5).

Diffusion MR imaging has been successfully utilized to assess early tumor response after chemotherapy and radiation therapy. One report suggested diffusion-weighted MR imaging is a promising technique for evaluating early tumor response after radioembolization, with a significantly increased ADC of 65% (p = 0.004) after therapy (75). Data from our group showed an increase in ADC value of 18% (p < 0.001) (76).

CONCLUSION

MR imaging plays an important role in the follow-up of patients after locoregional therapy for hepatic neoplasms. We discussed the use of RECIST and EASL as well as functional MR imaging in the assessment of treatment response after RFA, TACE and radioembolization.

REFERENCES

1. Dodd GD, 3rd, et al. Minimally invasive treatment of malignant hepatic tumors: At the threshold of a major breakthrough. Radiographics 2000; 20(1): 9–27.
2. Goldberg SN and Ahmed M. Minimally invasive image-guided therapies for hepatocellular carcinoma. J Clin Gastroenterol 2002; 35(5 Suppl 2): S115–129.
3. Bartolozzi C, et al. Hepatocellular carcinoma: CT and MR features after transcatheter arterial embolization and percutaneous ethanol injection. Radiology 1994; 191(1): 123–128.
4. Lencioni R, Caramella D and Bartolozzi C. Hepatocellular carcinoma: Use of color Doppler US to evaluate response to treatment with percutaneous ethanol injection. Radiology 1995; 194(1): 113–118.
5. Miller AB, et al. Reporting results of cancer treatment. Cancer 1981; 47(1): 207–214.
6. Therasse P, et al. New guidelines to evaluate the response to treatment in solid tumors: European Organization for Research and Treatment of Cancer, National Cancer Institute of the United States, National Cancer Institute of Canada. J Natl Cancer Inst 2000; 92(3): 205–216.
7. Jaffe CC. Measures of response: RECIST, WHO, and new alternatives. J Clin Oncol 2006; 24(20): 3245–3251.
8. Kamel IR and Bluemke DA. Magnetic resonance imaging of the liver: assessing response to treatment. Top Magn Reson Imaging 2002; 13(3): 191–200.
9. Bruix J, et al. Clinical management of hepatocellular carcinoma. Conclusions of the Barcelona-2000 EASL conference. European Association for the Study of the Liver. J Hepatol 2001; 35(3): 421–430.
10. Bruix J and Sherman M. Management of hepatocellular carcinoma. Hepatology 2005; 42(5): 1208–1236.
11. Law M, et al. Glioma grading: Sensitivity, specificity, and predictive values of perfusion MR imaging and proton MR spectroscopic imaging compared with conventional MR imaging. Am J Neuroradiol 2003; 24(10): 1989–1998.
12. Schaefer PW, Grant PE and Gonzalez RG. Diffusion-weighted MR imaging of the brain. Radiology 2000; 217(2): 331–345.
13. Elton M. Forensic psychiatrists must be more in agreement on the evaluation of juvenile delinquents. Lakartidningen 1991; 88(34): 2668.
14. Yeung DK, Cheung HS and Tse GM. Human breast lesions: Characterization with contrast-enhanced in vivo proton MR spectroscopy – initial results. Radiology 2001; 220(1): 40–46.
15. Jagannathan NR, et al. Evaluation of total choline from in-vivo volume localized proton MR spectroscopy and its response to neoadjuvant chemotherapy in locally advanced breast cancer. Br J Cancer 2001; 84(8): 1016–1022.
16. Longo R, et al. Fatty infiltration of the liver. Quantification by 1H localized magnetic resonance spectroscopy and comparison with computed tomography. Invest Radiol 1993; 28(4): 297–302.
17. Dixon RM. NMR studies of phospholipid metabolism in hepatic lymphoma. NMR Biomed 1998; 11(7): 370–379.
18. Soper R, et al. Pathology of hepatocellular carcinoma and its precursors using proton magnetic resonance spectroscopy and a statistical classification strategy. Pathology 2002; 34(5): 417–422.
19. Chen CY, et al. Early response of hepatocellular carcinoma to transcatheter arterial chemoembolization: Choline levels and MR diffusion constants – initial experience. Radiology 2006; 239(2): 448–456.
20. Moffat BA, et al. Functional diffusion map: A noninvasive MRI biomarker for early stratification of clinical brain tumor response. Proc Natl Acad Sci USA 2005; 102(15): 5524–5529.
21. Moffat BA, et al. The functional diffusion map: An imaging biomarker for the early prediction of cancer treatment outcome. Neoplasia 2006; 8(4): 259–267.
22. Ni H, et al. Effects of number of diffusion gradient directions on derived diffusion tensor imaging indices in human brain. Am J Neuroradiol 2006;27(8):1776–1781.
23. Moseley ME, et al. Diffusion-weighted MR imaging of anisotropic water diffusion in cat central nervous system. Radiology 1990; 176(2): 439–445.

24. Taouli B, et al. Evaluation of liver diffusion isotropy and characterization of focal hepatic lesions with two single-shot echo-planar MR imaging sequences: prospective study in 66 patients. Radiology 2003; 226(1): 71–78.

25. Yamada I, et al. Diffusion coefficients in abdominal organs and hepatic lesions: Evaluation with intravoxel incoherent motion echo-planar MR imaging. Radiology 1999; 210(3): 617–623.

26. Lencioni R, Cioni D and Bartolozzi C. Percutaneous radiofrequency thermal ablation of liver malignancies: Techniques, indications, imaging findings, and clinical results. Abdom Imaging 2001; 26(4): 345–360.

27. Sironi S, et al. Small hepatocellular carcinoma treated with percutaneous RF ablation: MR imaging follow-up. Am J Roentgenol 1999; 173(5): 1225–1229.

28. Buscarini L, et al. Percutaneous radiofrequency ablation of small hepatocellular carcinoma: Long-term results. Eur Radiol 2001; 11(6): 914–921.

29. Livraghi T, et al. Percutaneous radiofrequency ablation of liver metastases in potential candidates for resection: The "test-of-time approach." Cancer 2003; 97(12): 3027–3035.

30. Goldberg SN, et al. Tissue ablation with radiofrequency using multiprobe arrays. Acad Radiol 1995; 2(8): 670–674.

31. Goldberg SN, et al. Percutaneous radiofrequency tissue ablation: Does perfusion-mediated tissue cooling limit coagulation necrosis? J Vasc Interv Radiol 1998; 9(1 Pt 1): 101–111.

32. Curley SA, et al. Early and late complications after radiofrequency ablation of malignant liver tumors in 608 patients. Ann Surg 2004; 239(4): 450–458.

33. Horkan C, et al. Radiofrequency ablation: Effect of pharmacologic modulation of hepatic and renal blood flow on coagulation diameter in a VX2 tumor model. J Vasc Interv Radiol 2004; 15(3): 269–274.

34. Livraghi T, et al. Small hepatocellular carcinoma: Treatment with radio-frequency ablation versus ethanol injection. Radiology 1999; 210(3): 655–661.

35. Bartolozzi C, et al. Assessment of therapeutic effect of liver tumor ablation procedures. Hepatogastroenterology 2001; 48(38): 352–358.

36. Rossi S, et al. Percutaneous treatment of small hepatic tumors by an expandable RF needle electrode. Am J Roentgenol 1998; 170(4): 1015–1022.

37. Shibata T, et al. Small hepatocellular carcinoma: Comparison of radio-frequency ablation and percutaneous microwave coagulation therapy. Radiology 2002; 223(2): 331–337.

38. Curley SA, et al. Radiofrequency ablation of unresectable primary and metastatic hepatic malignancies: Results in 123 patients. Ann Surg 1999; 230(1): 1–8.

39. Bergsland EK and Venook AP. Hepatocellular carcinoma. Curr Opin Oncol 2000; 12(4): 357–361.

40. Geschwind JF, et al. Novel therapy for liver cancer: Direct intraarterial injection of a potent inhibitor of ATP production. Cancer Res 2002; 62(14): 3909–3913.

41. Okuda K, et al. Natural history of hepatocellular carcinoma and prognosis in relation to treatment. Study of 850 patients. Cancer 1985; 56(4): 918–928.

42. Lee HS, et al. Therapeutic efficacy of transcatheter arterial chemoembolization as compared with hepatic resection in hepatocellular carcinoma patients with compensated liver function in a hepatitis B virus-endemic area: A prospective cohort study. J Clin Oncol 2002; 20(22): 4459–4465.

43. Stefanini GF, et al. Efficacy of transarterial targeted treatments on survival of patients with hepatocellular carcinoma: An Italian experience. Cancer 1995; 75(10): 2427–2434.

44. Yoshioka H, et al. MR imaging of the liver before and after transcatheter hepatic chemo-embolization for hepatocellular carcinoma. Acta Radiol 1990; 31(1): 63–67.

45. Lou CY, et al. Establishment and characterization of human hepatocellular carcinoma cell line FHCC-98. World J Gastroenterol 2004; 10(10): 1462–1465.

46. Kamel IR, et al. The role of functional MR imaging in the assessment of tumor response after chemoembolization in patients with hepatocellular carcinoma. J Vasc Interv Radiol 2006; 17(3): 505–512.

47. Parkin DM, et al. Estimating the world cancer burden: Globocan 2000. Int J Cancer 2001; 94(2): 153–156.

48. Lin DY, et al. Hepatic arterial embolization in patients with unresectable hepatocellular carcinoma – a randomized controlled trial. Gastroenterology 1988; 94(2): 453–456.

49. Pelletier G, et al. A randomized trial of hepatic arterial chemoembolization in patients with unresectable hepatocellular carcinoma. J Hepatol 1990; 11(2): 181–184.

50. Groupe d'Etude et de Traitement du Carcinome Hepatocellulaire. A comparison of lipiodol chemoembolization and conservative treatment for unresectable hepatocellular carcinoma. N Engl J Med 1995; 332(19): 1256–1261.

51. Bruix J, et al. Transarterial embolization versus symptomatic treatment in patients with advanced hepatocellular carcinoma: Results of a randomized, controlled trial in a single institution. Hepatology 1998; 27(6): 1578–1583.

52. De Santis M, et al. Effects of lipiodol retention on MRI signal intensity from hepatocellular carcinoma and surrounding liver treated by chemoembolization. Eur Radiol 1997; 7(1): 10–16.

53. Ito K, et al. Therapeutic efficacy of transcatheter arterial chemoembolization for hepatocellular carcinoma: MRI and pathology. J Comput Assist Tomogr 1995; 19(2): 198–203.

54. Burger I, et al. Transcatheter arterial chemoembolization in unresectable cholangiocarcinoma: Initial experience in a single institution. J Vasc Interv Radiol 2005; 16(3): 353–361.

55. Naggert JK, et al. Genomic analysis of the C57BL/Ks mouse strain. Mamm Genome 1995; 6(2): 131–133.

56. Vilgrain V, et al. Intrahepatic cholangiocarcinoma: MRI and pathologic correlation in 14 patients. J Comput Assist Tomogr 1997; 21(1): 59–65.

57. Jemal A, et al. Cancer statistics, 2006. CA Cancer J Clin 2006; 56(2): 106–130.

58. Carty NJ, et al. Patterns of clinical metastasis in breast cancer: An analysis of 100 patients. Eur J Surg Oncol 1995; 21(6): 607–608.

59. Li XP, et al. Treatment for liver metastases from breast cancer: Results and prognostic factors. World J Gastroenterol 2005; 11(24): 3782–3787.

60. Moertel CG. Karnofsky memorial lecture. An odyssey in the land of small tumors. J Clin Oncol 1987; 5(10): 1502–1522.

61. Lepage C, et al. Incidence and management of malignant digestive endocrine tumours in a well-defined French population. Gut 2004; 53(4): 549–553.

62. Modlin IM and Sandor A. An analysis of 8305 cases of carcinoid tumors. Cancer 1997; 79(4): 813–829.

63. Norton JA. S urgical treatment of neuroendocrine metastases. Best Pract Res Clin Gastroenterol 2005; 19(4): 577–583.

64. Tomassetti P, et al. Endocrine pancreatic tumors: factors correlated with survival. Ann Oncol 2005; 16(11): 1806–1810.

65. Norheim I, et al. Malignant carcinoid tumors. An analysis of 103 patients with regard to tumor localization, hormone production, and survival. Ann Surg 1987; 206(2): 115–125.

66. Schnirer II, Yao JC and Ajani JA. Carcinoid – a comprehensive review. Acta Oncol 2003; 42(7): 672–692.

67. Gupta S, et al. Hepatic artery embolization and chemoembolization for treatment of patients with metastatic carcinoid tumors: the MD. Anderson experience. Cancer J 2003; 9(4): 261–267.

68. Roche A, et al. Trans-catheter arterial chemoembolization as first-line treatment for hepatic metastases from endocrine tumors. Eur Radiol 2003; 13(1): 136–140.

69. Eriksson BK. Liver embolizations of patients with malignant neuroendocrine gastrointestinal tumors. Cancer 1998; 83(11): 2293–2301.

70. Gupta S, et al. Hepatic arterial embolization and chemoembolization for the treatment of patients with metastatic neuroendocrine tumors: Variables affecting response rates and survival. Cancer 2005; 104(8): 1590–1602.

71. Geschwind JF, et al. Yttrium-90 microspheres for the treatment of hepatocellular carcinoma. Gastroenterology 2004; 127(5 Suppl 1): S194–205.

72. Andrews JC, et al. Hepatic radioembolization with yttrium-90 containing glass microspheres: Preliminary results and clinical follow-up. J Nucl Med 1994; 35(10): 1637–1644.

73. Sarfaraz M, et al. Physical aspects of yttrium-90 microsphere therapy for nonresectable hepatic tumors. Med Phys 2003; 30(2): 199–203.

74. Buscombe JR and Padhy A. Treatment of hepatocellular carcinoma: A pivotal role for nuclear medicine? Nucl Med Commun 2001; 22(2): 119–120.

75. Deng J, et al. Diffusion-weighted MR imaging for determination of hepatocellular carcinoma response to yttrium-90 radioembolization. J Vasc Interv Radiol 2006; 17(7): 1195–1200.

76. Kamel IR, et al. Functional MR imaging assessment of tumor response after ^{90}Y microsphere treatment in patients with unresectable hepatocellular carcinoma. J Vasc Interv Radiol 2007; 18(1 Pt 1): 49–56.

PART III

ORGAN-SPECIFIC CANCERS

Primary Liver Cancer

Chapter 9

HEPATOCELLULAR CARCINOMA: EPIDEMIOLOGY, PATHOLOGY, DIAGNOSIS AND SCREENING

Philip Johnson

Hepatocellular carcinoma (HCC) is a major public health problem. Although initially thought of as a disease of the developing world, particularly sub-Saharan Africa and the Far East, it is now recognized to be of growing importance in the United States, Europe, Russia and Japan, mainly in relation to the increasing prevalence of chronic hepatitis C virus infection.

EPIDEMIOLOGY, RISK FACTORS AND PREVENTION

HCC is said to be the fifth most common cancer worldwide, and the third most common cause of cancer-related mortality (1), but these are likely to be underestimates because of underreporting in developing countries. The highest annual incidence rates, of around 100 per 100,000, occur in parts of southern Africa and the Far East (1), and as such, these areas account of at least 75% of all cases. In contrast, HCC is less common in northern Europe, the United States and Australia, although there is evidence that the frequency may be increasing, most likely in relation to

the spread of chronic hepatitis C virus infection (2). HCC usually arises in a diseased liver, usually at the stage of cirrhosis, and in this setting it is predominately a disease of men. The cirrhosis is not always symptomatic, and the development of HCC may be the first indication of the underlying cirrhosis (3, 4). HCC is now one of the leading causes of death in patients with cirrhosis. In most populations, the incidence increases with age, but the mean age tends to be lower in high-incidence areas.

The wide geographic variation in the incidence of HCC has pointed to the likely importance of environmental factors in etiology. Prime among these have been the hepatitis viruses types B and C (HBV and HCV) and exposure to aflatoxin. Beasley et al. followed up more than 22,000 Chinese males, 15% of whom were HBV carriers, for up to 9 years (5, 6). The development of HCC was almost exclusively confined to those who had serum markers of HBV infection at presentation, and the relative risk for HCC development was almost 100. The evidence is thus overwhelming that chronic HBV infection is the major etiological factor, responsible for around 75% of cases worldwide, and confers a life-time risk of HCC of around 25%. In high-incidence areas, the infection is usually acquired at birth from a carrier mother (7). There is now evidence that the annual incidence rate of HCC is starting to fall, at least among children, in countries such as Taiwan, where universal vaccination (at birth) against HBV is practiced (8). Preliminary evidence also suggests that antiviral therapy in patients with chronic hepatitis B may decrease the incidence of subsequent HCC development (9). Both these observations lend further support to the pivotal role of chronic HBV infection in the pathogenesis of HCC.

The epidemiological evidence linking chronic HCV infection and HCC is similar to that for HBV. Indeed, in Europe, Japan and the United States, the attributable risk may be even higher, although in prospective studies, only a small minority (perhaps 2% to 4%) of those infected develop HCC (10–14). It is likely that co-factors, including coexistent HBV and excessive alcohol consumption, significantly increase the risk in HCV carriers (15).

Aflatoxins, formed by the fungus _Aspergillus_ flavus (hence afla-toxin), which grows on cereals, including corn and peanuts, stored under damp conditions, are one of the most potent classes of hepatic carcinogens known. In several high HCC incidence areas of the world, a clear relation between aflatoxin intake and the incidence of HCC has been established, both by conventional dietary assessment (16) and, more recently, by the use of urinary aflatoxin biomarkers (17, 18). As well as the obvious approach of improving grain storage to overcome the problem of aflatoxin exposure, extensive studies involving chemo preventive agents are on-going (19, 20).

Excessive alcohol consumption is consistently found to be a risk factor in the West, but the risk is likely to be confined to those who have developed alcoholic cirrhosis. Cigarette consumption may also be a significant risk factor, but the relationship is confounded by the association of cigarette smoking and alcohol consumption (21).

PATHOLOGY

The key features of the pathology of the HCC are the presence and degree of underlying chronic liver disease, the gross (macroscopic features) and histological features.

Gross Pathology

Although there have been several proposals for classification of the macroscopic appearances of HCCs (21a–23), a simple descriptive classification seems to work best. This describes the tumor as "massive" (one major solitary mass with often much smaller satellite nodules in the immediate area), "multinodular" (rounded nodules spread throughout the liver) or "diffuse" (with innumerable small nodules infiltrating the liver, difficult to differentiate from cirrhotic nodules). Occasionally, "pedunculated" tumors are seen. The presence of a capsule is of prognostic significance, as is the infiltration of blood vessels, classically the portal vein (24). Fibrolamellar carcinomas are a distinct, histologically defined subgroup of HCC (discussed subsequently).

Histology

The World Health Organization classifies the histology of HCC under five headings (25):

- Trabecular (plate-like) sinusoidal

- Pseudoglandular (adenoid or acinar)

- Compact solid

- Scirrhous

- Fibrolamellar

The histological type is not of prognostic significance with the exception of the fibrolamellar variant. Furthermore, there are often areas of differing histological appearance within the same tumor and clear distinction between primary and metastatic carcinoma cannot always be made on histological grounds alone, particularly when the tumor is poorly differentiated. The presence of microvascular invasion is highly predictive of subsequent disease recurrence after surgical resection (26). The pattern of growth and the resemblance of the tumor cells to normal hepatocytes are the key observations in designating tumor as hepatocellular, and the presence of bile in tumor cells is diagnostic of HCC (27).

For patients with a liver mass and not fulfilling the conventional diagnostic criteria (discussed later), the diagnosis of HCC usually needs to be confirmed histologically. Fine-needle biopsy may be limited by sampling error/missing small lesions, and by difficulty in distinguishing well-differentiated HCC from dysplasia or from adenoma or even normal liver.

Fibrolamellar Carcinoma

These tumors are the only histological variant to have a clearly defined clinical phenotype (28, 29). Histologically, they are characterized by large eosinophilic tumor cells with granular cytoplasm and extensive fibrous lamellar strands (30). Fibrolamellar HCC typically occurs in younger patients (mean 26 years) without underlying chronic liver disease, and AFP is not elevated. In this setting, resection rates are higher and prognosis is better (median survival 5 years) (31), although this may reflect the younger age, absence of cirrhosis and low AFP, all of which are associated with a better prognosis, rather than being related directly to the histological subtype (32).

DIAGNOSIS

Establishing the diagnosis of HCC is often difficult, and controversy surrounds the role of biopsy and the criteria for histological confirmation in small tumors.

Symptoms and Presentation

HCCs seldom cause symptoms until they are more than 5 cm in diameter. The most common mode of presentation is the triad of right upper quadrant abdominal pain, weight loss and the presence of hepatomegaly, often massive. A vascular bruit can be heard in about one-quarter of cases. Symptoms have usually been present for only a few weeks or months, and delay in seeking medical investigation is not the reason for late presentation.

In addition, patients with HCC may present with signs of hepatic decompensation such as progressive ascites resistant to medical therapy, variceal hemorrhage or encephalopathy (33). Variceal hemorrhage is more common when the portal vein is occluded, but other causes of gastrointestinal hemorrhage must be borne in mind, including the direct invasion of the stomach or duodenum by tumor (34).

A particularly dramatic presentation is spontaneous rupture of the tumor. There is a sudden onset of severe abdominal pain with shock, and paracentesis reveals blood-stained ascitic fluid (35). Rarer presentations of HCC include hypoglycemia, hypercalcemia and polycythemia. As noted subsequently, HCC is increasingly diagnosed pre- or asymptomatically. This follows screening patients with cirrhosis by serial estimations of AFP and/or ultrasound examination or transplant assessment.

It is impossible to determine on clinical examination, with any confidence, whether or not cirrhosis is present. Most HCC patients have no signs of chronic liver disease and did not know, before the onset of the HCC, that they had chronic liver disease. Cirrhosis was diagnosed in only 11 of 211 patients with HCC, but at autopsy, the figure was 90% (36).

Imaging

Ultrasound examination (USS) is often the initial screen when a focal liver lesion is suspected. It is relatively cheap, sensitive, not associated with radiation disease and is especially useful for guiding percutaneous biopsy (38). Cross-sectional imaging is required to assess the extent of disease so that treatment can be planned; in particular, size, number and distribution of tumors can be established as well as the presence of macrovascular invasion and extra-hepatic disease. Both dynamic triphasic CT or gadolinium-enhanced MR imaging classically show marked enhancement in the arterial phases with relative hypovascularity (wash out) in the portal or late phases (39, 40). In a patient known to have cirrhosis and in the presence of a mass greater than 2 cm in diameter, this radiological appearance is now regarded as being diagnostic of HCC without biopsy. Between 1 and 2 cm, diagnosis is difficult and most centers still biopsy; below 1 cm further scanning at 3-month intervals is appropriate (40).

MR imaging is proving particularly useful in characterizing lesions that remain indeterminate on USS and is probably superior in this aspect to CT scanning. It is also particularly useful in correctly classifying lesions such as hemangiomas that may cause diagnostic confusion (41). Nonetheless, it must be recognized that both CT and MR imaging, even in the best hands, will miss small tumors. In addition, several studies in which MR imaging findings are correlated with findings based upon thin slicing of explanted livers found sensitivity of only 50% to 75% (39, 42, 43).

Tumor Markers

The first serologic assay for detection and clinical follow-up of patients with HCC was AFP (44, 45). The reference range varies with assays but is usually quoted as <10 ng/ml. Serum AFP is elevated above this level in 50% to 70% of HCCs and is of particular value in the diagnosis of HCC in patients with cirrhosis. However, levels of up to 400 ng/ml can occur in other, benign, liver diseases, especially chronic active hepatitis and fulminant hepatic failure (45, 46), so from a diagnostic point of view, a cut-off point is used at around 400 ng/ml.

It can also be detected in a small percentage of other, non-hepatic gastrointestinal tumors (45, 47). At a cut-off of 400 ng/ml, the sensitivity is about 50% and the specificity about 95%. However, even below the conventional cut-off point, a steadily rising AFP is strongly suggestive of HCC. AFP is also useful in monitoring the effects of all therapies (provided that the baseline level is above 400 ng/ml), for detection of disease recurrence or progression following treatment and in assessment of prognosis, with higher levels being associated with a worse prognosis. The other commonly used tumor marker is des-gamma-carboxy prothrombin protein (PIVKA-II) (48, 49). This protein is increased in up to 90% of patients with HCC, but may also be elevated in patients with vitamin K deficiency, chronic active hepatitis or metastatic carcinoma.

Histological Confirmation

The necessity for histological confirmation of HCC remains controversial. There is an increasing trend to accept characteristic imaging features in association with serum AFP according to the following rule:

In the patient with *known chronic liver disease*, if the tumor is larger than 2 cm and has been confirmed by at least two imaging procedures, *and* has the characteristic features of arterial phase hypervascularity and portal phase washout, then the diagnosis is established; only one imaging procedure is required if the serum AFP level is >400 ng/ml (40).

Nonetheless, in the area of clinical trials in HCC, both regulatory authorities and the sponsoring pharmaceutical companies often still require histological confirmation prior to recruitment. If the aforementioned selection criteria are not met, then histological confirmation is usually required, providing that it will really impact on management. For example, to undertake biopsy of an incidentally detected small tumor in a patient with advanced cirrhosis and liver failure is meddlesome.

Most surgeons prefer not to undertake percutaneous biopsy prior to surgical resection because of the risk of "seeding" in the biopsy tract and the theoretical risk of tumor dissemination. The magnitude of this risk is about 1% (50, 51). On occasion, biopsying the non-tumorous liver is carried out to aid the diagnosis of HCC. The presence of chronic liver disease may support the diagnosis of HCC rather than a secondary liver tumor.

SCREENING

In light of the limited therapeutic options for HCC once the lesion is greater than 4 to 5 cm in diameter and/or is symptomatic and the fact that high-risk groups can now be identified, screening (or, more strictly, surveillance) seems a logical approach. Many, but not all, of the appropriate criteria for a cost-effective screening program are met (52).

Furthermore, there is now no doubt that a surveillance program *does* result in the detection of tumors before they become symptomatic, typically below 3 cm in diameter (53). The major screening modality is USS, an approach that can claim sensitivity of around 70% and specificity of around 90% (52). However, it must be noted that these figures are only obtained by careful examination of the liver for small tumors by trained, experienced and diligent operators, and similar results cannot be expected outside this setting. As noted earlier, estimation of serum AFP has been widely used in a screening role but current evidence suggests that its sensitivity is insufficient.

It is also important to focus a surveillance program on appropriate patients, for example, those who are most likely to benefit from early diagnosis. Thus, the ideal candidates are those with Child's A cirrhosis; those with advanced disease who would not be suitable for resection/transplantation or radical ablative therapies should not be screened. The patient needs to be fully informed about the risks and benefits of a surveillance program. Although not formally analyzed, it is clear that whereas some patients feel reassured by surveillance, the 6-month ultrasound examinations generate extreme anxiety in others, and a balance between useful information gained and anxiety generated needs to be carefully assessed.

Short of a prospective randomized trial demonstrating a decrease in disease-specific mortality, this will not be a truly evidence-based procedure. It is now apparent that for numerous reasons such a trial will never be undertaken. Furthermore, several trials would be needed, for example, different baseline populations (stage and etiology of liver disease) and using different screening procedures (screening tools, intervals). Because antiviral therapy may reduce the risk of HCC, it is now difficult to calculate the numbers of patients who would be needed to establish efficacy, and the screening procedure seems so well established that it is unlikely that a control population could be recruited. Nevertheless, there is one trial from China (54) suggesting decreased disease-specific mortality and the preliminary results from an Italian screening program suggest that those screened are surviving longer, although the impact of lead-time bias is difficult to assess (55).

REFERENCES

1. Parkin DM, Bray F, Ferlay J, et al. Global cancer statistics, 2002. CA Cancer J Clin 2005; 55: 74–108.
2. El-Serag HB and Mason AC. Rising incidence of hepatocellular carcinoma in the United States. N Engl J Med 1999; 340: 745–750.
3. Johnson PJ and Williams R. Cirrhosis and the aetiology of hepatocellular carcinoma. J Hepatol 1987; 4(1): 140–147.
4. Zaman SN, Johnson PJ and Williams R. Silent cirrhosis in patients with hepatocellular carcinoma: Implications for screening in high-incidence and low-incidence areas. Cancer 1990; 65(7): 1607–1610.
5. Beasley RP, Hwang LY, Lin CC, et al. Hepatocellular carcinoma and hepatitis B virus: A prospective study of 22 707 men in Taiwan. Lancet 1981; 2: 1129–1133.
6. Beasley RP. Hepatitis B virus. The major etiology of hepatocellular carcinoma. Cancer 1988; 61: 1942–1956.
7. Wong VC, Lee AK and Ip HM. Transmission of hepatitis B antigens from symptom-free carrier mothers to the fetus and the infant. Br J Obstet Gynaecol 1980; 87(11): 958–965.
8. Chang MH, Chen CJ, Lai MS, et al. Universal hepatitis B vaccination in Taiwan and the incidence of hepatocellular carcinoma in children. N Engl J Med 1997; 336: 1855–1859.
9. Liaw YF, Sung JJ, Chow WC, et al. Lamivudine for patients with chronic hepatitis B and advanced liver disease. N Engl J Med 2004; 351(15): 1521–1531.
10. Colombo M. Hepatitis C virus and hepatocellular carcinoma. Semin Liver Dis 1999; 19(3): 263–269.
11. Hayashi PH and Di Bisceglie AM. The progression of hepatitis B- and C-infections to chronic liver disease and hepatocellular carcinoma: epidemiology and pathogenesis. Med Clin North Am 2005; 89(2): 371–389.
12. Davila JA, Morgan RO, Shaib Y, et al. Hepatitis C infection and the increasing incidence of hepatocellular carcinoma: A population-based study. Gastroenterology 2004; 127: 1372–1380.
13. Seeff LB and Hoofnagle JH. Epidemiology of hepatocellular carcinoma in areas of low hepatitis B and hepatitis C endemicity. Oncogene 2006; 25(27): 3771–3777.
14. Seeff LB and Hoofnagle JH. Appendix: The National Institute of Health Consensus Development Conference, Management of Hepatitis C. 2002. Clin Liver Dis 2003; 7(1): 261–287.
15. Tagger A, Gelatti U, Parrinello G, et al. Alcohol and hepatocellular carcinoma: The effect of lifetime intake and hepatitis virus infections in men and women. Am J Epidemiol 2002; 155(4): 323–331.
16. Van Rensburg SJ, Cook-Mozaffari P, Van Schalkwyk DJ, et al. Hepatocellular carcinoma and dietary aflatoxin in Mozambique and Transkei. Br J Cancer 1985; 51(5): 713–726.
17. Groopman JD, Wild CP, Hasler J, et al. Molecular epidemiology of aflatoxin exposures: Validation of aflatoxin-N7-guanine levels in urine as a biomarker in experimental rat models and humans. Environ Health Perspect 1993; 99: 107–113.
18. Ross RK, Yu MC, Henderson BE, et al. Aflatoxin biomarkers. Lancet 1992; 340(8811): 119.
19. Kensler TW, Egner PA, Wang JB, et al. Chemoprevention of hepatocellular carcinoma in aflatoxin-endemic areas. Gastroenterology 2004; 127(5 Suppl 1): S310–318.
20. Turner PC, Sylla A, Gong YY, et al. Reduction in exposure to carcinogenic aflatoxins by postharvest intervention measures in West Africa: A community-based intervention study. Lancet 2005; 365: 1950–1956.
21. Donato F, Tagger A, Gelatti U, et al. Alcohol and hepatocellular carcinoma: The effect of lifetime intake and hepatitis virus infections in men and women. Am J Epidemiol 2002; 155(4): 323–331.
21a. Kojiro M and Nakashima T. Pathology of hepatocellular carcinoma. In: Okuda K and Ishak KG (eds.), Neoplasms of the Liver, pp. 81–104. Berlin: Springer 1987.
22. Nakashima T, Kojiro M, Sakamoto K, et al. Studies of primary liver carcinoma. I. Proposal of a new gross anatomical classification of primary liver cell carcinoma. Acta Hepatologica Japanica 1974; 15: 279–291.
23. Peters RL. Pathology of hepatocellular carcinoma. In: Okuda K and Peters RL (eds.), Hepatocellular Carcinoma, pp. 107–169. New York: Wiley 1976.
24. Liver Cancer Study Group of Japan. Primary liver cancer in Japan: Clinicopathologic features and results of surgical treatment. Ann Surgery 1990; 211: 277–287.
25. Ishak KG, Anthony PP and Sobin LH. Histological Typing of Tumors of the Liver. In: WHO International Histological Classification on Tumours, 2nd edition, p. 20. Berlin: Springer 1994.
26. Chau GY, Lui WY and Wu CW. Spectrum and significance of microscopic vascular invasion in hepatocellular carcinoma. Surg Oncol Clin North Am 2003; 12(1): 25–34.
27. Kojiro M. Histopathology of liver cancers. Best Pract Res Clin Gastroenterol 2005; 19(1): 39–62.
28. Craig JR, Peters RL, Edmondson HA, et al. Fibrolamellar carcinoma of the liver: A tumor of adolescents and young adults with distinctive clinico-pathologic features. Cancer 1980; 46(2): 372–379.
29. Katzenstein HM, Krailo MD, Malogolowkin MH, et al. Fibrolamellar hepatocellular carcinoma in children and adolescents. Cancer 2003; 97(8): 2006–2012.
30. Jain M, Niveditha SR, Bharadwaj M, et al. Cytological features of fibrolamellar variant of hepatocellular carcinoma with review of literature. Cytopathology 2002; 13(3): 179–182.
31. Stipa F, Yoon SS, Liau KH, et al. Outcome of patients with fibrolamellar hepatocellular carcinoma. Cancer 2006; 106(6): 1331–1338.
32. Kakar S, Burgart LJ, Batts KP, et al. Clinicopathologic features and survival in fibrolamellar carcinoma: Comparison with conventional hepatocellular

carcinoma with and without cirrhosis. Mod Pathol 2005; 18(11): 1417–1423.

33. Melia WM, Wilkinson ML, Portmann BC, et al. Hepatocellular carcinoma in the non-cirrhotic liver: a comparison with that complicating cirrhosis. Q J Med (New Series III) 1984; 211: 391–400.

34. Yeo W, Sung JY, Ward SC, et al. A prospective study of upper gastrointestinal hemorrhage in patients with hepatocellular carcinoma. Dig Dis Sci 1995; 40(12): 2516–2521.

35. Lai EC and Lau WY. Spontaneous rupture of hepatocellular carcinoma: A systematic review. Arch Surg 2006; 141(2): 191–198.

36. Lai CL, Lam KC, Wong KP, et al. Clinical features of hepatocellular carcinoma: Review of 211 patients in Hong Kong. Cancer 1981; 47(11): 2746–2755.

37. Livraghi T, Lazzaroni S, Meloni F, et al. Risk of tumour seeding after percutaneous radiofrequency ablation for hepatocellular carcinoma. Br J Surg 2005; 92 (7): 856–858.

38. Lencioni R, Cioni C, Della Pina C, et al. Imaging diagnosis. Semin Liver Dis 2005; 25(2): 162–170. Review.

39. Rode A, Bancel B, Douek P, et al. Small nodule detection in cirrhotic livers: Evaluation with US, spiral CT, and MRI and correlation with pathologic examination of explanted liver. J Comput Assist Tomogr 2001; 25(3): 327–336.

40. Bruix J and Sherman M. Practice Guidelines Committee, American Association for the Study of Liver Diseases. Management of hepatocellular carcinoma. Hepatology 2005; 42(5): 1208–1236.

41. Lencioni R, Cioni D, Crocetti L, et al. Magnetic resonance imaging of liver tumors. J Hepatol 2004; 40(1): 162–171. Review.

42. Burrel M and Llovet JM. Barcelona Clinic Liver Cancer Group. MRI angiography is superior to helical CT for detection of HCC prior to liver transplantation: An explant correlation. Hepatology 2003; 38(4): 1034–1042.

43. Barthia B, Ward J, Guthrie JA, et al. Hepatocellular carcinoma in cirrhotic livers: Double-contrast thin-section MR imaging with pathologic correlation of explanted tissue. Am J Roentgenol 2003; 180: 577–584.

44. Abelev GI, Perova SD, Khramkova NI, et al. Production of embryonal alpha-globulin by mouse hepatomas. Transplant Bulletin 1963; 1: 174.

45. Johnson PJ. The role of serum alpha-fetoprotein estimation in the diagnosis and management of hepatocellular carcinoma. Clin Liver Dis 2001; 5(1): 145–159.

46. McIntyre R, Waldmann TA, Moertel CG, et al. Serum alpha-fetoprotein in patients with neoplasms of the GI tract. Cancer Res 1975; 35: 991–995.

47. Silver HK, Deneault J, Gold P, et al. The detection of alpha 1-fetoprotein in patients with viral hepatitis Cancer Res 1974; 34: 244–249.

48. Sakon M, Monden M, Gotoh M, et al. The effects of vitamin K on the generation of des-gamma-carboxy-prothrombin (PIVKA-II) in patients with hepatocellular carcinoma. Am J Gastroenterology 1991; 86: 339–5.

49. Nakamura S, Nouso K, Sakaguichi K, et al. Sensitivity and specificity of des-gamma-carboxy prothrombin for diagnosis of patients with hepatocellular carcinomas varies according to tumor size. Am J Gastroenterol 2006; 101(9):2038–2043.

50. Llovet JM, Vilana R, Bru C, et al. Increased risk of tumor seeding after percutaneous radiofrequency ablation for single hepatocellular carcinoma. Hepatology 2001; 22(5): 1124–1129.

51. Jaskolka JD, Asch MR, Kachura JR, et al. Needle tract seeding after radiofequency ablation of hepatic tumors. J Vasc Interv Radiol 2005; 16(4): 485–491.

52. Sherman M. Hepatocellular carcinoma: Epidemiology, risk factors, and screening. Semin Liver Dis 2005; 25(2): 143–154.

53. Mok TS, Yeo W, Yu S, et al. An intensive surveillance program detected a high incidence of hepatocellular carcinoma among Hepatitis B virus carriers with abnormal alpha-fetoprotein levels or abdominal ultrasonography results. J Clin Oncol 2005; 23(31): 8041–8047.

54. Chen JG, Parkin DM, Chen QG, et al. Screening for liver cancer: Results of a randomised controlled trial in Qidong, China. J Med Screen 2003; 10(4): 204–209.

55. Sangiovanni A, Del Ninno E, Fasani P, et al. Increased survival of cirrhotic patients with a hepatocellular carcinoma detected during surveillance. Gastroenterology 2004; 126 (4): 1005–1014.

Chapter 10

STAGING SYSTEMS FOR HEPATOCELLULAR CARCINOMA

Debashish Bose

Timothy M. Pawlik

Accurate staging of hepatocellular carcinoma (HCC) is important because it provides prognostic data as well as aids in selecting patients for appropriate clinical treatment regimens (1). Many previous studies, however, have noted differing predictors of survival following treatment of HCC (2–5). A number of staging systems have therefore been proposed, including some that rely mostly on clinical parameters [Okuda, Cancer of the Liver Italian Program (CLIP)] and others that utilize pathologic data [American Joint Committee on Cancer/International Union Against Cancer (AJCC/UICC)]. This chapter provides an overview of the major HCC staging systems and highlights the relative merits of each staging scheme.

CHILD-TURCOTTE-PUGH NOMINAL SCORE

Although not a true prognostic staging scheme for HCC, the Child-Turcotte-Pugh (CTP) score is the most basic scoring system for the assessment of liver disease. The Child-Pugh score assigns points for degree of liver dysfunction based on three biochemical markers (serum albumin, bilirubin and prothrombin time) and two clinical markers (ascites and encephalopathy) (Table 10.1). The CTP score is not an assessment of HCC stage, but it is a well-established predictor of surgical risk and prognosis in patients with liver disease. The CTP score is included here because it is used as a component of several formal HCC staging systems.

OKUDA STAGING SYSTEM

In 1985, Okuda proposed a HCC staging system based on both serum liver function tests and tumor extension (6). In the Okuda staging scheme, patients are divided into three stages of disease based on tumor extent, ascites status, bilirubin level and serum albumin level (Table 10.2). Traditionally the most widely used clinical staging system in the West, more recently the Okuda staging system has fallen out of favor. Specifically, the Okuda staging system has been criticized because it was devised based on an analysis of patients who predominantly had advanced-stage HCC. As such, the Okuda staging system does not include many of the factors that have prognostic importance in early-stage HCC, such as whether the tumor is single or multiple or whether vascular invasion is present (7). The utility of the Okuda staging system to assess the prognosis of patients with HCC is therefore limited to those with advanced, unresectable disease.

CANCER OF THE LIVER ITALIAN PROGRAM CLASSIFICATION

The CLIP staging system was proposed in 1998 as a more accurate prognostic HCC classification scheme (8). Based on a retrospective study of 435 HCC patients, the score combines data on CTP score, serum alpha-fetoprotein (AFP) level, the presence or absence of portal vein thrombosis and tumor

TABLE 10.1 Child-Turcotte-Pugh (CTP) Score

Points Assigned	1	2	3
Albumin	>3.5	2.8–3.5	<2.8
Bilirubin	<2	2–3	>3
PT (seconds prolonged)	1–3	4–6	>6
Encephalopathy	None	Controlled	Uncontrolled
Ascites	None	Controlled	Uncontrolled
Child's class	A 5–6 points		
	B 7–9 points		
	C 10–15 points		

morphology/extension (Table 10.3). Although initially derived from a retrospective analysis, the CLIP staging system has subsequently been prospectively validated (9). In fact, the prospective analysis noted that the CLIP score was more accurate and had greater predictive power than the Okuda score (9). The CLIP score stratifies HCC patients with the highest CLIP scores being associated with the poorest prognosis. Patients with CLIP scores of 0, 1, 2, 3, and 4 had median survival times of 36, 22, 9, 7, and 3 months, respectively (9). Additional studies in Canada and Japan have further validated the usefulness of the CLIP staging system. Levy et al. (10) reported that the CLIP score was a better predictor of prognosis compared with the Okuda staging system in 257 Canadian patients with HCC. Similarly, Uneo et al. (11) analyzed 663 Japanese patients with HCC and reported that the CLIP score had a better ability to stratify patients than either the Okuda staging system or the fourth edition of the Japanese tumor-node-metastasis (TNM) staging system.

Despite its ability to help predict prognosis in patients with HCC, the CLIP score does have several limitations. The CLIP system was derived from a cohort of 435 patients, almost all of whom had cirrhosis. Only 12 (2.8%) patients underwent a surgical procedure, and 182 (41.8%) had no locoregional treatment, highlighting the fact that most patients had advanced HCC (8). Tumor morphology in the CLIP score is simply designated as uni- or multi-nodular, and extent of disease is categorized as greater than or less than 50% of the liver volume. The CLIP score may therefore stratify patients with small (e.g., 2 cm) lesions and those with larger lesions similarly (e.g., if both have uni-nodular and less than 50% involvement of the liver). In addition, the CLIP staging system only allows for scoring only portal vein thrombosis that is clinically detectable; it provides no designation for microscopic vascular invasion that may be present with less advanced stages of disease. Such crude designations reflect the classification's inability to discriminate between early and advanced stage disease. This may be the reason why several studies failed to detect significant differences in the survival of patients classified as CLIP 3, 4, 5 and 6 (7, 10, 11).

BARCELONA CLINIC LIVER CANCER STAGING CLASSIFICATION

The Barcelona Clinic Liver Cancer (BCLC) staging system was designed to expand on the Okuda staging scheme so as to better incorporate patients with earlier stage tumors (12). The BCLC was developed by combining a retrospective study of patients

TABLE 10.2 The Okuda Staging System

Points	0	1
Size	<50%	>50%
Ascites	No	Yes
Albumin	=3	<3
Bilirubin	<3	=3
Okuda Stage I	0 points	
Okuda Stage II	1–2 points	
Okuda Stage III	3–4 points	

TABLE 10.3 Cancer of the Liver Italian Program System

Points	0	1	2
CTP class	A	B	C
Tumor	Uninodular <50%	Multinodular <50%	Massive >50%
AFP	<400	>400	
Portal vein thrombosis	No	Yes	

CTP, Child-Turcotte-Pugh; AFP, alpha-fetoprotein.

TABLE 10.4 Barcelona Clinic Liver Cancer System

Feature	Tumor	PH	PST	Bill	CTP
Early HCC					
Stage A1	Single	No	0	nl	
Stage A2	Single	Yes	0	nl	
Stage A3	Single	Yes	0	abn	
Stage A4	3 tumors, all <3 cm		0		A,B
Intermediate HCC					
Stage B	Large multinodular		0		A,B
Advanced HCC					
Stage C	Vascular invasion/extrahepatic spread		1–2		A,B
End-stage HCC					
Stage D	Any		3–4		C

PH, portal hypertension; PST, performance status; nl, normal; abn, abnormal.

undergoing surgical resection of HCC and a prospective study of patients with advanced HCC. The BCLC combines elements of both the Okuda scheme and Child-Pugh score into a calculus that also includes performance status and tumor characteristics (Table 10.4). The BCLC system stratifies patients into four stages: early (e.g., stage A, asymptomatic tumors amenable to resection, transplantation or percutaneous treatment); intermediate (e.g., stage B, asymptomatic multi-nodular tumors larger than 3 cm); advanced (e.g., stage C, symptomatic tumors or vascular invasion or extra-hepatic spread); and end-stage (e.g., stage D, any tumor in the setting of end-stage liver disease). BCLC stages A to C include patients who have Okuda stage 1 or 2 disease, with a performance status of 0 to 2 and a Child-Pugh classification of A or B. Groups are further stratified based on tumor number, tumor size, vascular invasion and extra-hepatic spread.

Constructed as an algorithm to direct treatment, the BCLC has been criticized on several fronts. The BCLC algorithm allocates only patients with solitary lesions and normal portal pressure for resection. Ablative techniques are also reserved for early stage patients with multi-nodular disease, while chemoembolization is proposed for intermediate and some patients with advanced disease (8). In addition, the BCLC staging system does not advocate transplantation for many patients who meet the Milan criteria – assigning many of these patients to radiofrequency ablation (RFA) or alcohol ablation. As such, the BCLC has been criticized for being overly conservative in its treatment recommendations as it potentially excludes patients from being considered for curative

treatments. For example, whereas the BCLC recommends trial-based or palliative therapy for patients with large or multi-nodular HCC, Ng et al. (13) reported a 5-year survival of 39% for this cohort of patients. Similarly, Pawlik et al. (14) reported a 5-year survival of 25% in a well-selected cohort of patients with HCC measuring greater than 10 cm. According to the BCLC treatment algorithm, these patients would have been categorically excluded from surgical consideration. The BCLC "staging" system is therefore not strictly speaking a true *staging* algorithm, but rather a *treatment* algorithm. The BCLC cannot be considered a pure prognostic staging system, nor can it be considered current with regard to its stage-based treatment recommendations.

THE CHINESE UNIVERSITY PROGNOSTIC INDEX

The Chinese University Prognostic Index (CUPI) incorporates the traditional TNM stage with certain clinical factors, including AFP level, degree of ascites and presence or absence of symptoms, as well as total bilirubin and alkaline phosphatase levels (Table 10.5) (15). Although the CUPI was successful in stratifying patients in the initial study of 926 patients used to construct the staging system, its prognostic power has not been independently corroborated.

LIVER CANCER STUDY GROUP OF JAPAN

The Liver Cancer Study Group of Japan (LCSGJ) proposed a classification of primary liver cancer based

TABLE 10.5 Chinese University Prognostic Index

		Weight		
TNM stage	I and II	−3	Low risk group = CUPI = 1	
	IIIa and IIIb	−1		
	IV	0		
Asymptomatic at presentation		−4	Intermediate risk group = CUPI 2–7	
Ascites		3		
AFP >500 ng/ml		2	High risk group = CUPI = 8	
Total bilirubin (μmol/L)	<34	0		
	34–51	3		
	>51	4		
Alkaline phosphatase = 200 IU/L		3		

TNM, tumor-node-metastasis

on the Japanese TNM system (16). In the LCSGJ classification, T stage is defined by tumor number (e.g., solitary versus multiple), tumor size (≤2 cm versus >2 cm) and the presence of portal vein, hepatic vein or bile duct invasion (present versus absent). The LCSGJ staging system has been criticized for several reasons. First, the LCSGJ scoring system considers each of the three prognostic factors (tumor number, tumor size vascular/biliary invasion) as equivalent and does not reflect how each of these factors may have a differential impact on prognosis. Second, the LCSGJ system relies solely on macroscopic pathology assessment and fails to include microscopic findings such as microvascular invasion. These shortcomings may help explain why Poon et al. (17) noted no significant difference in prognostic value comparing the more advanced stages of LCSGJ with the American Joint Committee on Cancer/International Union Against Cancer (AJCC/UICC) staging system.

The Japanese Integrated Score (JIS) scoring system has more recently been proposed as an improvement over the LCSGJ system (7). The JIS scoring system combines information on Child-Pugh class and the LCSGJ stage (Table 10.6). Whether the JIS scoring system provides any incremental improvement in discriminating the prognosis of patients with HCC remains controversial. At best, it suffers from the same shortcomings as the LCSGJ staging system and, at worst, it is simply another scoring algorithm rather than a true tumor staging system.

AMERICAN JOINT COMMITTEE ON CANCER/INTERNATIONAL UNION AGAINST CANCER

The initial AJCC/UICC TNM classification scheme for HCC was introduced in 1988. Since that time, the AJCC/UICC staging system has undergone multiple

TABLE 10.6 Japan Integrated Staging Score

Score	0	1	2	3	Stage
Japanese TNM stage	I	II	III	IV	I
CTP	A	B	C		II
					III
					IVA
					IVB
Japanese TNM (Liver Cancer Study Group of Japan)					
Factors: single tumor, >2 cm, no vessel invasion					
T1		Fulfills all 3			
T2		Fulfills 2	T1N0M0		
T3		Fulfills 1	T2N0M0		
T4		Fulfills none	T3N0M0		
N1		Regional node	T4N0M0 or any T, N1 M0		
		positivity	Any T, any N, M1		

TNM, tumor-node-metastasis

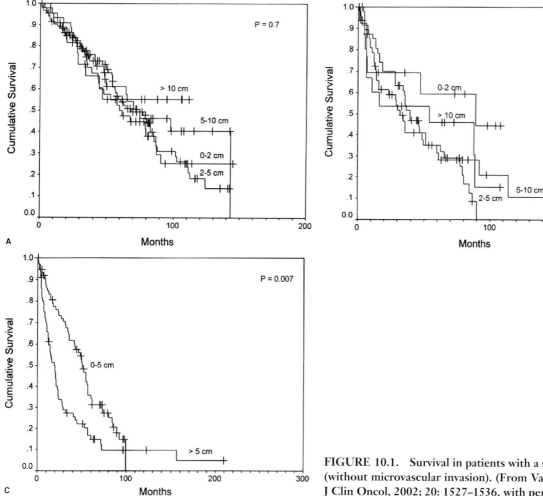

FIGURE 10.1. Survival in patients with a single T1 tumor (without microvascular invasion). (From Vauthey JN, et al., J Clin Oncol, 2002; 20: 1527–1536, with permission.)

revisions, with the most recent changes adopted in 2003. Whereas earlier versions of this staging system failed to stratify patients effectively and were criticized as being unnecessarily complex (18, 19), the most recent, sixth edition of the AJCC/UICC has not only been simplified (20, 21) but also has been independently validated (17).

The 6th edition AJCC/UICC staging system was based on an analysis of 557 patients who had undergone resection for HCC at major hepatobiliary centers in the United States, Japan and Europe (20). On multivariate analysis, factors associated with prognosis included tumor number, tumor size >5 cm, microscopic vascular invasion, invasion of a main branch of the portal or hepatic vein, and severe fibrosis/cirrhosis. In patients with a single tumor, tumor size had no effect on survival in those with no vascular invasion or microvascular invasion, regardless of how tumor size was dichotomized (Figure 10.1). The 5-year survival of patients with multiple tumors – none of which were larger than 5 cm – was the same as patients with any tumor more than 5 cm. Thus, the

influence of tumor size on prognosis is limited only to patients with multiple tumors. In the most recent AJCC/UICC staging system, T1 disease is therefore defined as any solitary tumor without vascular invasion, regardless of tumor size. In addition, the prognosis of patients with multiple tumors, none larger than 5 cm, was similar to that of patients with a single tumor with vascular invasion. Thus, these two groups of patients were combined to form the T2 classification. In contrast, T3 disease was classified as patients with multiple tumors, any of which is >5 cm, and those patients with tumors with major vascular invasion (Table 10.7). In the absence of lymph node metastasis (N0) and distant metastasis (M0), T1, T2 and T3 tumors correspond to stage I, stage II and stage IIIa disease, respectively. Patients with lymph node metastasis (N1) are designated as stage IIIb, and those patients with distant metastasis (M1) are classified as stage IV.

The AJCC/UICC staging system also includes a provision for the separate reporting of fibrosis/cirrhosis. Assessment of fibrosis/cirrhosis is performed

TABLE 10.7 AJCC-UICC TNM Staging System

T1	Single tumor, no vascular invasion
T2	Single tumor with vascular invasion or multiple none >5 cm
T3	Multiple tumors any >5 cm or involvement of major portal or hepatic vein branch
F0	Ishak grade 0–4 fibrosis (none-moderate)
F1	Ishak grade 5–6 fibrosis (severe/cirrhosis)

	T	N	M
Stage I	T1	N0	M0
Stage II	T2	N0	M0
Stage IIIa	T3	N0	M0
Stage IIIb	Any T	N1	M0
Stage IV	Any T	Any N	M1

using the fibrosis classification scheme proposed by Ishak et al. (22). The relevance of reporting hepatic fibrosis is reflected in the fact that fibrosis status affects survival within every T-stage classification (20). For example, 5-year survival is 64% for stage I patients without underlying fibrosis (F0) versus 49% for stage I patients with moderate-to-severe fibrosis (F1) (Figure 10.2).

The strengths of the AJCC/UICC system lie in the fact that the results are based on multivariate analysis of prognostic variables that are independent of any treatment algorithm and include a thorough pathologic evaluation. In addition, the staging system was derived from an analysis of a large number of patients from both the East and West. In addition, the AJCC/UICC has been prospectively validated (17). Despite this, some of the key variables in the AJCC/UICC staging system are not available prior to resection and pathologic review, making use of this staging system somewhat limited in the evaluation of patients with unresectable HCC.

HCC STAGING SYSTEMS: A SELECTIVE REVIEW OF COMPARATIVE STUDIES

Comparison of staging systems is difficult as various centers utilize different treatment algorithms and include patients with different clinicopathologic factors. Despite these limitations, several investigators have sought to compare the various HCC staging systems with regard to their ability to stratify patient prognosis.

Marrero et al. (23) retrospectively analyzed several HCC staging schemes in 239 patients from the University of Michigan. In this study, the algorithm used to direct treatment closely mirrored that proposed by the BCLC group: resection for patients without clinical portal hypertension and only a single lesion, transplantation or RFA for patients who met the Milan criteria, and transarterial chemoembolization (TACE) for patients with no portal vein thrombosis who had multi-nodular disease or a single lesion >5 cm. Although the authors stated that the treatment groups were balanced, most patients had advanced disease (cirrhosis, 98%; multiple tumors,

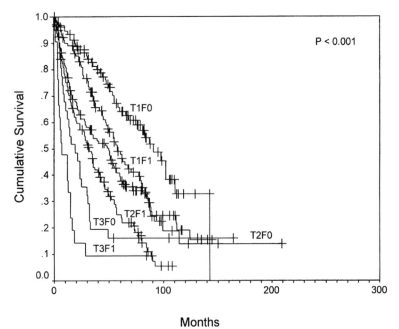

FIGURE 10.2. Survival of patients with T1, T2 and T3 tumors – effect of severe fibrosis/cirrhosis. F0 = fibrosis score 0–4, F1 = fibrosis score 5–6. (From Vauthey JN, et al., J Clin Oncol, 2002; 20: 1527–1536, with permission.)

56%) and only 4% underwent resection. The authors reported that the BCLC staging classification provided the best prognostic stratification for patients with HCC, whereas the CUPI, JIS, and AJCC/UICC TNM staging systems were significantly less useful in stratifying patients with regard to prognosis. The study, however, has been criticized for several shortcomings (24). First, it excluded patients from potentially curative therapeutic options using the same criteria as the BCLC. As such, it is not surprising that the study outcome was similar to the treatment-based "staging" system of the BCLC. Second, similar to the initial BCLC report, the Marrero data were based in large part on patients with advanced disease who did not undergo surgical resection. As such, the authors failed to prove conclusively that the BCLC is superior to other staging systems in patients with resectable HCC.

In a separate study, Cillo et al. (25) reported on 195 patients treated at the University of Padua in whom the BCLC treatment algorithm was not applied. In this study, 48% of patients underwent either resection (n = 52) or transplantation (n = 42). In general, patients were evenly divided between Childs A and B status, and more than one-half had solitary lesions; the majority of patients had cirrhosis. In this prospective study, the authors reported that the BCLC had the best independent predictive power for survival when compared with the Okuda, CLIP and JIS prognostic systems. The BCLC remained the best staging system to discriminate prognosis even when considering only surgically resected patients or when examining patients with cirrhosis.

In contrast, several studies have demonstrated the superiority of the CLIP scoring system. Tateishi et al. (26) reported that the CLIP score was superior to the BCLC. Similarly, Toyoda et al. (27) analyzed 1508 patients who were roughly equally distributed among surgical resection, percutaneous ablation and chemoembolization techniques and reported that the CLIP system was superior to the BCLC. Other studies (28, 29) have also corroborated the relative merit of the CLIP staging system as compared with the Okuda and TNM systems.

Few comparative studies have specifically investigated the relative merit of HCC staging systems in the context of interventional radiology trials. This issue is important as interventional radiologists must choose which staging system to use in planning TACE and other interventional liver-directed therapies. Tetsa

et al. (30) noted that the CLIP staging system was superior to the Okuda staging system in predicting patient survival after TACE for unresectable HCC. In a separate study, Biselli et al. (31) similarly reported that the CLIP system was better than the Okuda in correlating survival of patients treated with TACE. In contrast, Grieco et al. (32) reported better prognostic accuracy with use of the BCLC compared with either the Okuda system or the CLIP staging system for patients with unresectable HCC treated with TACE. More recently, Georgiades et al. (33) proposed that the Child-Pugh nominal liver staging system was the most accurate in predicting survival of patients with unresectable HCC treated with TACE. Given the disparate findings in the literature, no single staging system can currently be considered the standard for HCC staging in patients with unresectable HCC treated with TACE. In general, most interventional radiologists have, however, adopted the CLIP system to help predict survival following treatment with TACE.

CONCLUSION

For patients who have undergone surgical resection and for whom pathologic data therefore are available, the AJCC/UICC staging system provides the most accurate prognostic assessment. However, the majority of patients with HCC will have unresectable disease. As such, staging systems that depend on clinical and radiological factors will be more applicable. In patients treated with TACE for unresectable disease, the CLIP staging system is the most widely used and relevant staging system as it incorporates elements of underlying liver function (Child-Pugh stage) and tumor-related characteristics (e.g., tumor morphology, AFP level and presence of vascular invasion). As our understanding of HCC evolves, and as investigations into treatment options for HCC continue to expand, the prognostic staging systems for HCC will also inevitably be further refined.

REFERENCES

1. Pawlik TM, Tseng JF, Vauthey JN. Controversies in staging of hepatocellular carcinoma. Cancer Reviews: Asia-Pacific 2003; 1: 179–189.
2. Vauthey JN, Klimstra D, Franceschi D, et al. Factors affecting long-term outcome after hepatic resection for hepatocellular carcinoma. Am J Surg 1995; 169: 28–34; discussion 34–35.

3. Ikai I, Yamamoto Y, Yamamoto N, et al. Results of hepatic resection for hepatocellular carcinoma invading major portal and/or hepatic veins. Surg Oncol Clin North Am 2003; 12: 65–75, ix.

4. Fong Y, Sun RL, Jarnagin W, et al. An analysis of 412 cases of hepatocellular carcinoma at a Western center. Ann Surg 1999; 229: 790–799; discussion 799–800.

5. Kosuge T, Makuuchi M, Takayama T, et al. Long-term results after resection of hepatocellular carcinoma: Experience of 480 cases. Hepatogastroenterology 1993; 40: 328–332.

6. Okuda K, Ohtsuki T, Obata H, et al. Natural history of hepatocellular carcinoma and prognosis in relation to treatment: Study of 850 patients. Cancer 1985; 56: 918–928.

7. Kudo M, Chung H, Osaki Y. Prognostic staging system for hepatocellular carcinoma (CLIP score): Its value and limitations, and a proposal for a new staging system, the Japan Integrated Staging Score (JIS score). J Gastroenterol 2003; 38: 207–215.

8. The Cancer of the Liver Italian Program (CLIP) investigators. A new prognostic system for hepatocellular carcinoma: A retrospective study of 435 patients. Hepatology 1998; 28: 751–755.

9. The Cancer of the Liver Italian Program (CLIP) Investigators. Prospective validation of the CLIP score: A new prognostic system for patients with cirrhosis and hepatocellular carcinoma. Hepatology 2000; 31: 840–845.

10. Levy I, Sherman M. Staging of hepatocellular carcinoma: Assessment of the CLIP, Okuda, and Child-Pugh staging systems in a cohort of 257 patients in Toronto. Gut 2002; 50: 881–885.

11. Ueno S, Tanabe G, Nuruki K, et al. Prognostic performance of the new classification of primary liver cancer of Japan (4th ed) for patients with hepatocellular carcinoma: A validation analysis. Hepatol Res 2002; 24: 395–403.

12. Llovet JM, Bru C, Bruix J. Prognosis of hepatocellular carcinoma: The BCLC staging classification. Semin Liver Dis 1999; 19: 329–338.

13. Ng KK, Vauthey JN, Pawlik TM, et al. Is hepatic resection for large or multinodular hepatocellular carcinoma justified? Results from a multi-institutional database. Ann Surg Oncol 2005; 12: 364–373.

14. Pawlik TM, Poon RT, Abdalla EK, et al. Critical appraisal of the clinical and pathologic predictors of survival after resection of large hepatocellular carcinoma. Arch Surg 2005; 140: 450–457; discussion 457–458.

15. Leung TW, Tang AM, Zee B, et al. Construction of the Chinese University Prognostic Index for hepatocellular carcinoma and comparison with the TNM staging system, the Okuda staging system, and the Cancer of the Liver Italian Program staging system: A study based on 926 patients. Cancer 2002; 94: 1760–1769.

16. Makuuchi M, Belghiti J, Belli G, et al. IHPBA concordant classification of primary liver cancer: Working group report. J Hepatobiliary Pancreat Surg 2003; 10: 26–30.

17. Poon RT, Fan ST. Evaluation of the new AJCC/UICC staging system for hepatocellular carcinoma after hepatic resection in Chinese patients. Surg Oncol Clin North Am 2003; 12: 35–50, viii.

18. Staudacher C, Chiappa A, Biella F, et al. Validation of the modified TNM-Izumi classification for hepatocellular carcinoma. Tumori 2000; 86: 8–11.

19. Izumi R, Shimizu K, Ii T, et al. Prognostic factors of hepatocellular carcinoma in patients undergoing hepatic resection. Gastroenterology 1994; 106: 720–727.

20. Vauthey JN, Lauwers GY, Esnaola NF, et al. Simplified staging for hepatocellular carcinoma. J Clin Oncol 2002; 20: 1527–1536.

21. Liver (Including intrahepatic bile ducts). In: Green F, Page D, I. F, et al. (eds)., AJCC Cancer Staging Handbook, pp. 131–144. New York: Springer 2002.

22. Ishak K, Baptista A, Bianchi L, et al. Histological grading and staging of chronic hepatitis. J Hepatol 1995; 22: 696–699.

23. Marrero JA, Fontana RJ, Barrat A, et al. Prognosis of hepatocellular carcinoma: Comparison of 7 staging systems in an American cohort. Hepatology 2005; 41: 707–716.

24. Pawlik TM, Abdalla EK, Thomas M, et al. Staging of hepatocellular carcinoma. Hepatology 2005; 42: 738–739; author reply 739–740.

25. Cillo U, Vitale A, Grigoletto F, et al. Prospective validation of the Barcelona Clinic Liver Cancer staging system. J Hepatol 2006; 44: 723–731.

26. Tateishi R, Yoshida H, Shiina S, et al. Proposal of a new prognostic model for hepatocellular carcinoma: An analysis of 403 patients. Gut 2005; 54: 419–425.

27. Toyoda H, Kumada T, Kiriyama S, et al. Comparison of the usefulness of three staging systems for hepatocellular carcinoma (CLIP, BCLC, and JIS) in Japan. Am J Gastroenterol 2005; 100: 1764–1771.

28. Nanashima A, Omagari K, Tobinaga S, et al. Comparative study of survival of patients with hepatocellular carcinoma predicted by different staging systems using multivariate analysis. Eur J Surg Oncol 2005; 31: 882–890.

29. Ueno S, Tanabe G, Sako K, et al. Discrimination value of the new Western prognostic system (CLIP score) for hepatocellular carcinoma in 662 Japanese patients. Cancer of the Liver Italian Program. Hepatology 2001; 34: 529–534.

30. Testa R, Testa E, Giannini E, et al. Trans-catheter arterial chemoembolisation for hepatocellular carcinoma in patients with viral cirrhosis: Role of combined staging systems, Cancer Liver Italian Program (CLIP) and Model for End-stage Liver Disease (MELD), in predicting outcome after treatment. Aliment Pharmacol Ther 2003; 17: 1563–1569.

31. Biselli M, Andreone P, Gramenzi A, et al. Transcatheter arterial chemoembolization therapy for patients with hepatocellular carcinoma: A case-controlled study. Clin Gastroenterol Hepatol 2005; 3: 918–925.

32. Grieco A, Pompili M, Caminiti G, et al. Prognostic factors for survival in patients with early-intermediate hepatocellular carcinoma undergoing non-surgical therapy: Comparison of Okuda, CLIP, and BCLC staging systems in a single Italian centre. Gut 2005; 54: 411–418.

33. Georgiades CS, Hong K, D'Angelo M, et al. Safety and efficacy of transarterial chemoembolization in patients with unresectable hepatocellular carcinoma and portal vein thrombosis. J Vasc Interv Radiol 2005; 16: 1653–1659.

Chapter 11

HEPATOCELLULAR CARCINOMA: MEDICAL MANAGEMENT

Philip Johnson

Daniel Palmer

THE NEED FOR SYSTEMIC THERAPIES IN HEPATOCELLULAR CARCINOMA

Recent years have seen major advances in local control of hepatocellular carcinoma (HCC), and the relevant approaches are described in detail elsewhere in this volume. Thus, although surgical resection (and orthotopic liver transplantation) has long been seen as the only approach to offer cure, or at least long-term survival, other locoregional therapies including percutaneous ethanol injection and thermal ablation now appear to be rivaling surgical resection by many criteria of efficacy. However, it is clear that all these approaches (including surgical resection) are less effective as the tumor increases in size, and conventionally, most are confined to lesions smaller than 5 cm in diameter. This probably reflects the fact that as tumors increase in size, the frequency of vascular invasion increases and with it, the likelihood of metastasis. Thus, if local treatments are applied to larger lesions then the rate of recurrence increases dramatically.

Similarly, trans-catheter approaches are recognized to cause extensive tumor necrosis, but evidence of survival improvement has been more difficult to demonstrate because disease progression and tumor re-vascularization are still the rule. Thus to complement these local measures, systemic treatment is urgently required to expand the indications for local

therapies and to decrease the recurrence rate (i.e., in the adjuvant setting).

At the outset, it should be noted that, largely because of the progress in local treatment, systemic agents have moved "down the scale" so that new chemotherapeutic agents have been tried mainly in patients with advanced or even terminal disease and this necessarily limits the scope for observing effective treatments. Most, perhaps 75% to 85% of patients with HCC have underlying hepatic cirrhosis and thus patients have, in effect, two diseases with independent natural histories. Thus if clinical trials involve, as has often been the case, patients with advanced liver disease, it is difficult to know whether failure to improve survival is related to failure to halt tumor progression or progressive liver disease. For this reason, it has been suggested that, at least initially, clinical trials should be undertaken on patients with good liver function so that underlying liver disease does not complicate the situation (i.e., any improved survival can be confidently ascribed to the anti-tumor treatment).

Systemic treatments have not kept pace with advances in local treatments. However, over the past 10 years, large prospective randomized trials in patients with HCC have been forthcoming, and more attention has been focused on the optimal design of earlier-phase trials that aim to determine which new agents should progress to examination in randomized studies. This chapter starts by describing the limited progress that has been made using conventional cytotoxic agents and then progresses to look at the newer targeted agents.

CYTOTOXIC CHEMOTHERAPY

Response rates for single-agent cytotoxic chemotherapy are low, and significant durable remission is rare. The most widely used single cytotoxic agent has been doxorubicin, an anthracycline. Although an early prospective randomized trial reported a significantly increased survival (1), the absolute improvement was small, and in subsequent systematic reviews of randomized trials of doxorubicin therapy significant survival effect was not discernable (2, 3). Review of series containing more than 700 patients suggests a typical response rate of 10% to 15%, occasionally complete but usually short-lasting and partial (4). Mitoxantrone, an anthracendione, gave similar results with perhaps less toxicity, and this agent was licensed for use in HCC (5), although it was not widely regarded as "standard of care." In two recent large-scale trials of drugs that had shown promising activity in early-phase trials, Ti67, a novel tubulin-binding drug (6), and nolatrexed, a thymidylate synthase inhibitor (7), were tested with doxorubicin being used as the control arm. In the former there was no improvement in survival (6 months in both groups); in the latter, the doxorubicin patients survived significantly longer (6.9 compared to 4.7 months) (6, 7). Until very recently, no other systemic therapy has fared significantly better and systemic cytotoxic chemotherapy for HCC is now largely confined to clinical trials (4, 8–12).

Combination chemotherapy appears to give a higher response rate, although again, the duration of remission is usually short. In general, even for well-selected patients, the expected objective response is only around 20% to 30% and, as such, seems unlikely to have a significant impact on survival (4). A Phase II study of a four-drug systemic combination regimen [cisplatin, recombinant interferon alpha-2b, doxorubicin and 5-fluorouracil (PIAF)] was encouraging, showing that although the response rate was not high (25%), 9 of the 13 partial responders had their disease rendered resectable (13). However, a prospective randomized study comparing PIAF to conventional systemic doxorubicin showed that although the expected response rates for doxorubicin and PIAF were achieved (10% and 20% respectively) and survival was in line with the Phase II trial experience (8.5 months), this did not translate into a significant improvement in survival when compared to doxorubicin alone. It was suggested that any benefit in terms of the increased response rate was counteracted by increased toxicity (14). A recent Phase II trial of a similar combination – cisplatin, doxorubicin and capecitibine – showed similar results in terms of activity, with a response rate of 24% (15).

Thus, conventional cytotoxic therapy has undoubted activity but whether or not this translates into a survival advantage has not been rigorously or convincingly tested (4, 8–12).

The Systemic Component of Intra-(Hepatic)-Arterial Therapy

It is often stated that intra-arterial cytotoxic chemotherapy, either alone or in combination with arterial embolization (see Chapter 16), results in higher intra-tumor drug concentration and lower systemic exposure. The former assertion is probably true, but not the latter. There is no difference in the systemic drug levels or toxicity (e.g., in terms of neutropenia) when the same dose of drug is administered intra-arterially or intravenously (16). Whether the systemic exposure is beneficial or detrimental to the patient is unresolved.

ENDOCRINE MANIPULATION

An alternative systemic approach has been endocrine manipulation based on reports of estrogen receptor expression in some HCCs. Early small studies with anti-estrogenic and anti-androgenic agents showed some promise (17, 18). However, recent large-scale prospective controlled studies have refuted any role for hormonal agents, including tamoxifen (19–23).

OCTREOTIDE

Octreotide is a somatostatin analog that has revolutionized the treatment of symptomatic carcinoid tumors by suppressing the secretion of peptide hormones responsible for the syndrome, and that has occasionally led to shrinkage of the primary tumor and liver metastases. Because the agent may also act indirectly by suppressing tropic hormones (insulin and insulin-like growth factors) and has anti-angiogenic activity, and because somatostatin receptors have been reported, trials in HCC seem a logical choice (24, 25).

In the first study, there was a significant survival advantage and associated improvement in quality of life among those receiving octreotide, although the study was small (only 59 patients in total) and the quality-of-life instrument was not a recognized and validated tool (26). In a second study, involving 70 patients, there was no survival advantage or difference in quality of life. However, the value of this study must be questioned because the median survival of patients in both arms was less than 2 months and one-third of patients died before receiving treatment (27). However, the most recent HECTOR study was a prospective placebo-controlled randomized study in which patients with reasonable liver function were included, but there was no evidence of benefit in any subgroup of patients (28).

Somatostatin acts through five receptors, somatostatin receptors (SSTRs) 1–5, and the anti-angiogenic effect is primarily mediated through SSTR3. Somatostatin analogues are available in short-acting and long-acting preparations, and there are differences in their affinity for different SSTRs. In particular, short-acting octreotide has a higher affinity for SSTR3. Because the first trial used short-acting octreotide (26), whereas subsequent trials used long-acting preparations (27, 28), this might account for the contrasting results.

THE NEW AGE OF TARGETED THERAPIES

As noted earlier, systemic therapy has not kept pace with the rapid development of therapies that appear to give effective local control. There are several reasons. First, HCC is a relatively rare tumor in the West and has not been seen as a high priority. Facilities for clinical trials have, until recently, been limited in areas of the world where the tumor is common. For these reasons, large-scale trials, which have been widely utilized in most other areas of oncology, have not been implemented.

However, over recent years, multi-center trials have started to appear, and there is no doubt that they are feasible, but a second problem is now becoming apparent. Out of the multiplicity of agents and combinations of agents that are currently available, how should it be decided which agents should progress to randomized Phase III trials? This is further compli-cated by the fact that, in the case of several of the newer targeted agents, the conventional Phase II trials, which aim to assess the activity, are not applicable. Agents may not cause tumor shrinkage but rather disease stabilization, and this may result in the need for novel trial designs.

TARGETED THERAPIES

The term **targeted** or **targeted molecular therapies** includes recently developed drugs that target some specific part of the pathway that controls the abnormal cellular proliferation or apoptosis that characterize cancer. As has been pointed out, any drug that has an effect, such as doxorubicin or cisplatin, is in fact targeted. The distinction arises because the targets are more discrete and the drugs have, in most cases, been specifically chosen for their action upon a particular molecular target. A critical challenge in the development of these therapies is the incorporation of translational endpoints into clinical trial design in order to identify the presence of the relevant target in the tumor and to correlate this with response so that patients most likely to benefit can be selected.

This next section focuses on such novel therapies, but starts with a brief review of angiogenesis.

ANGIOGENESIS AND HEPATOCELLULAR CARCINOMA

As tumors grow to exceed the size at which oxygen enters by diffusion, a blood supply becomes essential. Thus, the process of angiogenesis (the growth of blood vessels from pre-existing vasculature) is key to both invasion and metastases. Vascular endothelial growth factor (VEGF) is the main signaling protein involved in angiogenesis and acts predominantly on cells of the vascular endothelium via VEGF receptor-2. Its production is stimulated by hypoxia via the transcription factor hypoxia inducible factor (HIF). Circulating VEGF then binds to VEGF receptors on endothelial cells, triggering a tyrosine kinase pathway, leading to angiogenesis. Normal liver cells express VEGF, and in HCC there is overexpression that appears to correlate with the degree of differentiation in established HCCs and with the degree of microvascular density in dysplastic nodules. As tumors grow, levels of VEGF increase, and in patients undergoing transarterial chemoembolization (TACE), levels are significantly higher in those who did not respond well (29–33).

For all these reasons, anti-angiogenic therapy is a logical approach to HCC treatment. To date, there are two approaches. First, the small molecules such as sorafenib or sunitinib (although, as noted subsequently, these agents have several other kinase-inhibiting properties) and secondly, monoclonal antibodies such as bevacizumab.

Sorafenib

Sorafenib is an oral multi-kinase inhibitor that targets the Ras/Raf/MAP/Erk signaling pathway, for which there is good evidence of increased activity in HCC (34–36). Of importance, it also targets receptor protein kinases for both platelet-derived growth factor (PDGF) and vascular endothelial growth factors (2 and 3). In the Phase I trial, there was a confirmed partial response in a patient with metastatic HCC (37) and in the subsequent Phase II study, although the response rate was very low, one-third (2.2%) showed stable disease with an overall median survival of 9 months (38). Despite these apparently limited efficacies, a preliminary analysis of a Phase III randomized study showed an improvement in overall survival of around 2.7 months (from 8 months in the placebo arm to 10.7 months in the treatment arm) in patients with Child-Pugh A unresectable HCC (39). A randomized Phase II study of doxorubicin plus sorafenib vs. doxorubicin alone suggests promising synergy (40).

Bevacizumab

Bevacizumab is a humanized murine anti-VEGF monoclonal antibody that, in combination with cytotoxic chemotherapy, showed significant activity in metastatic colorectal carcinoma (41). Phase II studies of bevacizumab alone and in combination with gemcitabine and oxaliplatin (GemOx) both showed moderate activity. In the latter, the response rate was 20%, and 27% had stable disease with a median survival of 9.5 months (42). The significance of these results within the context of a single-arm Phase II study is difficult to interpret. Although comparison across Phase II studies is difficult due to potential imbalances in prognostic factors in patients participating in different studies, they do not appear to be significantly better than GemOx alone (43) (RR 18%, stable disease 58%, median survival 11.5 months).

Erlotinib

Tumor angiogenesis is regulated predominantly, but by no means exclusively, through VEGF signaling.

Other key signaling pathways include epidermal growth factor (EGF), fibroblast growth factor (FGF), and transforming growth factor (TGF). These pathways also contribute directly to tumor cell growth and so represent rational targets for HCC therapy.

EGF and TGF-α play major roles in cell proliferation invasion and angiogenesis. Both are active through the EGF/human epidermal growth factor (HER) receptor that is overexpressed in HCC cell lines and in human HCC tissue (44). Erlotinib (Tarceva; Genentech, Inc., South San Francisco, CA) is an orally active inhibitor of EGFR/HER 1-related tyrosine kinase. Phillip et al. reported partial responses among 38 patients, and 12 of 38 patients (32%) were progression free at 6 months (45). Thomas et al. reported that 8 of 25 patients (32%) achieved progression-free survival (PFS) at 4 months (46).

Combining Targeted Therapies

The complexity, redundancy and cross-talk within tumor cell and endothelial cell signaling suggest that inhibition of one single pathway is unlikely to meet with dramatic success. Increased understanding of these processes does provide evidence for the rational combination of several agents, and such combinations are now entering clinical trials. This may also underpin the success of the multi-targeted kinase inhibitor sorafenib.

The promising results for bevacizumab and erlotinib used singly has inevitably led to investigation of their use in combination, with encouraging results from a Phase II study reporting a response rate of 22% in 27 patients (including one complete response) and 55% PFS at 16 weeks (47). These data are preliminary and require longer follow-up and corroboration in larger studies.

Many of the pathways inhibited by novel targeted therapies, such as Raf/Mek/Erk may also contribute to resistance to conventional chemotherapeutic agents, and combination of these agents with chemotherapy may overcome chemoresistance. A randomized Phase II study has addressed this question by combining sorafenib with systemic doxorubicin. Results are awaited.

CONCLUSION

The interventional radiologist is currently limited by tumor size in the case of thermal ablation, because above about 5 cm, recurrence failure of local control becomes increasingly common. A systemic therapy might expand the indications for this approach and decrease local recurrence rates. Similarly, although TACE is considered only palliative, it might be anticipated that antiangiogenic approaches might slow down recurrence and thereby enhance survival. With the advent of an apparently effective agent, such as sorafenib, close collaboration between interventional radiologists and medical oncologists should ensure a much brighter future for patients with this devastating disease.

REFERENCES

1. Lai CL, Wu PC, Chan GC, et al. Doxorubicin versus no antitumor therapy in inoperable hepatocellular carcinoma: A prospective randomized trial. Cancer 1988; 62(3): 479–483.

2. Simonetti RG, Leberati A, Angiolini C, et al. Treatment of hepatocellular carcinoma: A systematic review of randomized controlled trials. Ann. Oncology 1997; 8: 117–136.

3. Nerenstone SR, Ihde DC, and Friedman MA. Clinical trials in primary hepatocellular carcinoma: Current status and future directions. Cancer Treat Rev 1988; 15: 1–31.

4. Burroughs A, Hochhauser D, Meyer T. Systemic treatment and liver transplantation for hepatocellular carcinoma: Two ends of the therapeutic spectrum. Lancet Oncol 2004; 5(7): 409–418.

5. Dunk AA, Scott SC, Johnson PJ, et al. Mitozantrone as single agent therapy in hepatocellular carcinoma. J Hepatol 1985; 1(4): 395–404.

6. Posey J, Johnson P, Mok T, et al. Results of a phase 2/3 open-label, randomized trial of T138067 versus doxorubicin (DOX) in chemotherapy-naïve, unresectable hepatocellular carcinoma (HCC). Proc Am Soc Clin Oncol 2005; 23: 4035a.

7. Porta C, Ruff P, Feld R, et al. Results of a phase III, randomized controlled study, the largest ever completed in hepatocellular carcinoma (HCC), comparing the survival of patients with unresectable HCC treated with nolatrexed (NOL) or doxorubicin (DOX). American Society of Clinical Oncology Gastrointestinal Cancers Symposium San Francisco, CA, 2006; January 26–28.

8. Johnson PJ. Are there indications for chemotherapy in hepatocellular carcinoma? Surg Oncol Clin North Am 2003; 12(1): 127–134.

9. Leung TW and Johnson PJ. Systemic therapy for hepatocellular carcinoma. Semin Oncol 2001; 28(5): 514–520.

10. Palmer DH, Hussain SA, Johnson PJ. Systemic therapies for hepatocellular carcinoma. Expert Opin Investig Drugs 2004; 13(12): 1555–1568.

11. Zhu AX. Systemic therapy of advanced hepatocellular carcinoma: How hopeful should we be? The Oncologist 2006; 11(7): 790–800.

12. Abou-Alfa GK. Hepatocellular carcinoma: Molecular biology and therapy. Semin Oncol 2006; 33(6 Suppl 11): S79–83.

13. Leung TW, Patt YZ, Lau WY, et al. Complete pathological remission is possible with systemic combination chemotherapy for inoperable hepatocellular carcinoma. Clin Cancer Res 1999; 5: 1676–1681.

14. Yeo W, Mok TS, Zee B, et al. A randomized phase III study of doxorubicin versus cisplatin/interferon alpha-2b/doxorubicin/fluorouracil (PIAF) combination chemotherapy for unresectable hepatocellular carcinoma. J Natl Cancer Inst 2005; 97: 1532–1538.

15. Park SH, Lee Y, Han SH, et al. Systemic chemotherapy with doxorubicin, cisplatin and capecitabine for metastatic hepatocellular carcinoma. BMC Cancer 2006; 6: 3–8.

16. Johnson PJ, Kalayci C, Dobbs N, et al. Pharmacokinetics and toxicity of intraarterial adriamycin for hepatocellular carcinoma: Effect of coadministration of lipiodol. J Hepatol 1991; 13(1): 120–127.

17. Farinati F, Salvagnini M, de Maria N, et al. Unresectable hepatocellular carcinoma: A prospective controlled trial with tamoxifen. J Hepatol 1990; 11: 297–301.

18. Martinez Cerezo FJ, Tomas A, Donoso L, et al. Controlled trial of tamoxifen in patients with advanced hepatocellular carcinoma. J Hepatol 1994; 20: 702–706.

19. CLIP Group (Cancer of the Liver Italian Programme). Tamoxifen in treatment of hepatocellular carcinoma: A randomised controlled trial. Lancet 1998; 352: 17–20.

20. Chow PK, Tai BC, Tan CK, et al. High-dose tamoxifen in the treatment of inoperable hepatocellular carcinoma: A multicenter randomized controlled trial. Hepatology 2002; 36: 1221–1226.

21. Barbare JC, Bouche O, Bonnetain F, et al. Randomized controlled trial of tamoxifen in advanced hepatocellular carcinoma. J Clin Oncol 2005; 23: 4338–4346.

22. Grimaldi C, Bleiberg H, Gay F, et al. Evaluation of antiandrogen therapy in unresectable hepatocellular carcinoma: Results of a European Organization for Research and Treatment of Cancer multicentric double-blind trial. J Clin Oncol 1998; 16: 411–417.

23. Di Maio M, De Maio E, Morabito A, et al. Hormonal treatment of human hepatocellular carcinoma. Ann N Y Acad Sci 2006 1089: 252–261.

24. Reynaert H, Rombouts K, Vandermonde A, et al. Expression of somatostatin receptors in normal and cirrhotic human liver and in hepatocellular carcinoma. Gut 2004; 53(8): 1180–1189.

25. Blaker M, Schmitz M, Gocht A, et al. Differential expression of somatostatin receptor subtypes in hepatocellular carcinomas. J Hepatol 2004; 41(1): 112–118.

26. Kouroumalis E, Skordilis P, Thermos K, et al. Treatment of hepatocellular carcinoma with octreotide: A randomized controlled study. Gut 1998; 42: 442–447.

27. Yuen MF, Poon RT, Lai CL, et al. A randomized placebo-controlled study of long-acting octreotide for the treatment of advanced hepatocellular carcinoma. Hepatology 2002; 36: 687–691.

28. Becker G, Allgaier HP, Olschewski M, et al. Long-acting octreotide versus placebo for treatment of advanced HCC: A randomized controlled double-blind study. Hepatology 2007; 45(1): 9–15.

29. Yamane A, Seetharam L, Yamaguchi S, et al. A new communication system between hepatocytes and sinusoidal endothelial cells in liver through vascular endothelial

growth factor and Flt tyrosine kinase receptor family (Flt-1 and KDR/Flk-1). Oncogene 1994; 9: 2683–2690.

30. Yamaguchi R, Yano H, Iemura A, et al. Expression of vascular endothelial growth factor in human hepatocellular carcinoma. Hepatology 1998; 28: 68–77.

31. Chao Y, Li CP, Chau GY, et al. Prognostic significance of vascular endothelial growth factor, basic fibroblast growth factor, and angiogenin in patients with resectable hepatocellular carcinoma alter surgery. Ann Surg Oncol 2003; 10: 355–362.

32. Poon R, Lau C, Yu W, et al. High serum level of vascular endothelial growth factor predict poor response to transarterial chemoembolisation in hepatocellular carcinoma: A prospective study. Oncol Rep 2004; 11: 1077–1084.

33. von Marscall Z, Cramer T, Hocker M, et al. Dual mechanism of vascular endothelian growth factor upregulation by hypoxia in human hepatocellular carcinoma. Gut 2001; 48: 87–96.

34. Ito Y, Sasaki Y, Horimoto M, et al. Activation of mitogen-activated protein kinases/extracellular signal-regulated kinases in human hepatocellular carcinoma. Hepatology 1998; 27: 951–958.

35. McKillop IH, Schmidt CM, Cahill PA, et al. Altered expression of mitogen-activated protein kinases in a rat model of experimental hepatocellular carcinoma. Hepatology 1997; 26: 1484–1491.

36. Schmidt CM, McKillop IH, Cahilland PA, et al. Increased MAPK expression and activity in primary human hepatocellular carcinoma. Biochemical Biophysical Research Communications 1997; 236: 54–58.

37. Strumberg D, Richly H, and Hilger RA. Phase I clinical and pharmacokinetic study of the novel Raf kinase and vascular endothelial growth factor receptor inhibitor BAY 43–9006 in patients with advanced refractory solid tumors. J Clin Oncol 2005; 23: 965–972.

38. Abou-Alfa GK, Schwartz L, Ricci S, et al. Phase II study of sorafenib in patients with advanced hepatocellular carcinoma. J Clin Oncol 2006; 24(26): 4293–4300.

39. Llovet J, Ricci S, Mazzaferro V, et al. Randomized phase III trial of sorafenib versus placebo in patients with advanced hepatocellular carcinoma. Proc Am Soc Clin Oncol 2007; 25: 111s.

40. Abou-Alfa G, Johnson P, Knox J, et al. Preliminary results from a Phase II, randomized, double-blind study of sorafenib plus doxorubicin versus placebo plus doxorubicin in patients with advanced hepatocellular carcinoma. Proceedings of the 2007 meeting of the European Cancer Organization. Eur J Cancer Supp 2007; 5(259), Abstract 3500.

41. Schwartz J, Schwartz M, Lehrer D, et al. Bevacizumab in hepatocellular carcinoma (HCC) in patients without metastases and without portal vein invasion. J Clin Oncol 2005; 23: 338s suppl: abstr 4122.

42. Zhu AX, Blaszkowsky LS, Ryan DP, et al. Phase II study of gemcitabine and oxaliplatin in combination with bevacizumab in patients with advanced hepatocellular carcinoma. J Clin Oncol 2006; 24(12): 1898–1903.

43. Louafi S, Boige V, Ducreux M, et al. Gemcitabine plus oxaliplatin (GEMOX) in patients with advanced hepatocellular carcinoma (HCC): Results of a phase II study. Cancer 2007; 109(7). 1384–1390.

44. Abbruzzese JL and Thomas MB. Opportunities for targeted therapies in hepatocellular carcinoma. J Clin Oncol 2005; 23(31): 8093–8108.

45. Philip PA and Mahoney MR. Phase II study of Erlotinib (OSI-774) in patients with advanced hepatocellular cancer. J Clin Oncol 2005; 23(27): 6657–6663.

46. Thomas MB, Dutta A, Brown T, et al. A phase II open-label study of OSI-774 (NSC 718781) in unresectable hepatocellular carcinoma. Proc Am Soc Clin Oncol 2005; 23: 4083a.

47. Thomas MB, Chadha R, Iwasaki M, et al. The combination of bevacizumab and erlotinib shows significant biological activity in patients with advanced hepatocellular carcinoma. Proc Am Soc Clin Oncol 2007; 25: 214s.

Chapter 12

SURGICAL MANAGEMENT (RESECTION)

Brian D. Badgwell

Dario Ribero

Jean-Nicolas Vauthey

Hepatocellular carcinoma (HCC) is the fifth most common neoplasm worldwide, affecting more than 600,000 people annually (1). Though less prevalent in the United States, the estimated annual number of cases exceeds 16,000. Moreover, despite a decline in alcoholic liver disease and increased use of hepatitis B immunization strategies, the incidence in our country is steadily rising and has doubled between 1975 and 1998, likely due to an increase in hepatitis C virus infection (2). In the majority of patients, HCC develops in fibrotic/cirrhotic livers, and cirrhosis represents the strongest predisposing factor.

The natural history of untreated HCC varies depending on the stage at presentation and the degree of underlying liver disease. However, even in patients with early stages, the prognosis is grim if the disease is left untreated (3, 4). As primary medical therapy has failed to significantly improve survival, surgical resection and orthotopic liver transplantation (OLT) represent the only treatment options, offering a prospect for cure with 5-year survival rates of up to 50% (5–7) and 70% (8, 9), respectively.

Unfortunately, only approximately 20% to 40% (10, 11) of patients are candidates for resection due to the burden of hepatic tumor, the presence of extrahepatic spread or the extent of underlying liver disease. Despite this, liver resections are increasingly being performed due to better perioperative care,

improved imaging and advances in surgical technique.

OLT represents the only surgical option in patients with small HCC and impaired liver function. However, in view of the severe graft shortage and restricted indications for OLT, liver resection is considered the mainstay of curative therapy in patients with preserved hepatic function.

PREOPERATIVE EVALUATION

A significant aspect of the morbidity and mortality of liver resection relates to patient selection. Identification of appropriate candidates for resection is also essential to ensure optimal long-term oncologic outcome. Therefore, accurate evaluation of tumor staging, general medical fitness, underlying liver function and volume of the anticipated future liver remnant (FLR) is the key for suitable patient selection.

The assessment of tumor extent is the primary step for determining resectability and the appropriate type of surgical resection. At The University of Texas M. D. Anderson Cancer Center, each patient is staged with helical computed tomography (CT) of the thorax and the abdomen. The liver is studied using thin slices acquired during the unenhanced phase and during the arterial, portal and equilibrium phases after contrast administration. Magnetic resonance imaging (MRI) is the imaging modality of choice when contrast agents are contraindicated, better lesion characterization is needed or the anatomic relationship between tumor and major vascular or biliary structures requires further delineation.

As mortality rates after partial hepatectomy have fallen in recent years to almost zero, many centers worldwide have expanded eligibility criteria for resection. Now included are tumors once considered unresectable, such as large HCCs, multinodular and bilobar HCCs and HCCs with portal vein or hepatic vein involvement. Based on preoperative imaging, patients are considered for resection when all tumor nodules can be safely excised with negative margins and when the volume and function of the FLR is adequate. Formal contraindications for resection are the presence of extrahepatic disease, tumor thrombus in the inferior vena cava and involvement of the common hepatic artery and portal vein trunk. Extension to surrounding structures, such as the diaphragm, does not represent a contraindication if a margin negative resection can be attained.

Patient Selection

Patient age should not be considered per se a contraindication for resection, given that it has not been shown to be an independent predictor of increased operative risk. Conversely, surrogate markers of general physiologic fitness, such as the American Society of Anesthesiology (ASA) score, do significantly influence the incidence of postoperative complications. An analysis of 478 patients who had undergone liver resection demonstrated that patients with an ASA score >1 had more than three times the mortality rate and twice the morbidity of those patients with an ASA score of 1 (mortality 3% vs. 0.2% and

morbidity 16% vs. 7%, respectively) (12). These findings were confirmed in a recent study identifying the presence of comorbidities as one of the two independent factors predictive of postoperative mortality after extended hepatectomy, the other factor being perioperative blood transfusion (13). Patients with congestive heart failure, severe chronic obstructive pulmonary disease and chronic renal failure represent a prohibitive risk.

Evaluation of Liver Function

In Western countries, the Child-Pugh (CP) classification (Table 12.1), which was originally designed to estimate the risk of cirrhotic patients undergoing portocaval shunt surgery (14), has traditionally been used to evaluate hepatic function. Although no individual test accurately predicts liver function, the CP classification, combining different parameters, provides a rough estimation of the gross synthetic and detoxification capacity of the liver. In general, the risk of death after surgery increases with each CP class. Operative mortality rates for CP class A, B and C patients undergoing abdominal operations are approximately 10%, 30%, and 82%, respectively (15); therefore, liver resection is considered only in CP class A patients. Nevertheless, recent series of hepatectomy in CP class A patients have reported a wide range of perioperative mortality rates, from 0% to 16% (16–18). Critics have also pointed out that two aspects of the scoring system are ambiguous – the grading of ascites and encephalopathy. Consequently, the CP classification must be considered cautiously because it may underestimate the surgical risk.

Undiagnosed or latent portal hypertension, which is present when the portal venous pressure is greater than 10 mmHg, increases the risk for hepatic

TABLE 12.1 Child-Pugh Classification

Clinical and Biochemical Parameters	Points		
	1	2	3
Albumin (g/dL)	>3.5	2.8–3.5	<2.8
Bilirubin (mg/dL)	<2	2–3	>3
Prothrombin time			
Sec prolonged	<4	4–6	>6
%	>60	40–60	<60
INR	<1.7	1.7–2.3	>2.3
Encephalopathy	Absent	Moderate (Stage I–II)	Severe (Stage III–IV)
Ascites	Absent	Moderate	Refractory

Total points: 5–6 points: Child-Pugh A; 7–9 points: Child-Pugh B; 10–15 points: Child-Pugh C.

decompensation after hepatectomy. Portal hypertension can also lead to increased hemorrhage, coagulopathy and decreased ability to tolerate bleeding and puts the patient at risk of major complications, such as variceal bleeding and endotoxemia. In a prospective study in CP class A cirrhotic patients, Bruix et al. (19) showed that the hepatic venous pressure gradient (HVPG), a surrogate measurement of portal venous pressure, was the only predictor of hepatic decompensation following hepatic resection. Specifically, unresolved hepatic decompensation developed in 11 of 15 patients with a HVPG greater than 10 mmHg versus none of the patients with a HVPG less than 10 mmHg (p < 0.002), suggesting that the CP classification may be somewhat inaccurate in assessing risk. Thus, preoperative clinical or radiologic signs of portal hypertension, including splenomegaly, abdominal collaterals, thrombocytopenia (platelets <100,000/mm^3) and esophagogastric varices are relative contraindications for resection.

Additionally, postoperative mortality has been shown to be almost six-fold higher in a cohort of 285 patients who underwent hepatectomy for HCC when there was histologic evidence of cirrhosis and active hepatitis vs. cirrhosis alone (20). Although the presence of hepatitis does not always correlate with serum transaminase levels (21, 22), increased complication and death rates have been reported in those patients with elevated liver function tests. Patients with an aspartate aminotransferase level greater than 100 IU/L (23) or an alanine aminotransferase level at least twice normal (24) are considered to be poor candidates for major hepatic resection. Bilirubin levels greater than 2 mg/dL contraindicate hepatic resection, whereas patients with bilirubin levels between 1.1 and 2.0 mg/dL should be carefully selected and considered for only limited resection.

In Eastern countries, hepato-biliary surgeons have employed other, more sophisticated, measures to evaluate the hepatic metabolic function, such as indocyanine green (ICG) clearance, galactose elimination capacity and aminopyrine clearance. The most widely used and validated metabolic assessment is the ICG clearance test. ICG dye is given intravenously (0.5 mg/kg), whereby it binds to plasma proteins until being exclusively removed by the liver and excreted into bile. The percentage of ICG retained at 15 minutes (ICGR15) after injection is used to predict the risk of postoperative liver failure. Patient selection by ICG clearance test has reduced the mortality rate in

some centers to zero (18). Makuuchi and colleagues have incorporated the ICGR15 and two clinical features – that is, bilirubin and ascites – into a treatment-selection algorithm. In patients without ascites and bilirubin levels less than 1.0 mg/dL, ICGR15 is used to predict the number of liver segments that can be safely resected (ICGR15 <10%, extended hepatectomy and right hemihepatectomy are safe; ICGR15 10%–19%, left hemihepatectomy and bisegmentectomy are safe; ICGR15 20%–29%, only segmentectomies are safe; ICGR15 30%–39%, only wedge resections are safe; ICGR15 ≥40%, only enucleations are safe). This algorithmic approach was prospectively validated in 107 patients; the 30-day mortality rate was zero, and there were no major complications (25).

Evaluation of Future Liver Remnant Volume

Although useful, the CP classification, the ICG clearance and other hepatic reserve tests only estimate the overall hepatic function and do not provide information regarding the FLR, which may vary in size as a result of individual intrahepatic variation (26) or compensatory hypertrophy. In this context, a right or an extended right hepatectomy may result in quite variable amounts of residual parenchymal tissue. For these reasons, recent studies have emphasized an association between volume and the function of the residual liver after resection. Indeed, small FLR volumes may result in a mismatch between their functional reserve and the metabolic demands of the patient. Moreover, animal studies have suggested that small FLR sizes are associated with increases in portal pressure and flow, endothelial and Kupffer cell injury and release of proinflammatory cytokines (27, 28). Collectively, these factors result in hepatocellular injury and lack of regeneration. Therefore, in patients selected for major hepatic resection, attention has focused on the FLR volume.

The FLR volume can be accurately calculated using three-dimensional CT volumetry. Although direct measurement of the total liver volume (TLV) is feasible, it has been suggested not to be relevant for surgical planning, for several reasons (29). First, in patients with large tumors, the total volume of the liver is altered, and attempts to subtract tumor volume from TLV require additional time for calculation and lead to additive mathematical errors in volume calculation (30). These errors are greater in patients with multiple tumors or biliary dilatation in the liver to be resected. Liver volume for cirrhotic livers is often variable, so the measured TLV may not be useful as an index to which FLR volume is standardized.

An alternative, accurate method uses the estimated TLV, which is calculated using a mathematical formula that relies on the linear correlation between liver size and body surface area (BSA). The formula TLV $(\text{cm}^3) = -794.41 + 1{,}267.28 \times \text{BSA}\,(\text{m}^2)$ was recently evaluated in a meta-analysis and recommended as one of the least biased and most precise formulas for the estimation of the TLV in adults (31). The FLR/estimated TLV ratio, termed the **standardized FLR,** is then calculated to provide the percent of TLV remaining after resection.

The standardized FLR measurement has been used to establish a correlation between the anticipated liver remnant and operative outcome. In 48 patients without chronic liver disease undergoing extended hepatectomy with and without portal vein embolization, Abdalla et al. (32) showed that the postoperative complication rate was significantly increased in patients with FLR volume less than or equal to 20% of the estimated TLV. Using a different BSA-based standardized method of remnant liver calculation, a correlation between liver volume and outcome has also been demonstrated in patients with chronic liver disease. In this study, Shirabe et al. (33) reported that all deaths from liver failure occurred in patients with a remnant liver volume less than 250 ml/m² (Figure 12.1). In-hospital and intensive care unit stay, as measures of the overall postoperative course, also appear to be increased as liver remnant size decreases.

In general, a FLR of 20% is considered the minimum safe volume needed following extended hepatic resection in patients with normal underlying liver, whereas a FLR of 40% is required in patients with cirrhosis or hepatitis (33, 34). Because small FLRs are strongly correlated with increased morbidity and mortality after hepatic resection, standardized FLR measurement should be a routine part of the preoperative assessment in candidates for major hepatic resection. Liver volume analysis has revealed that the lateral left liver (segments II and III) contributes less than 20% of the TLV in more than 75% of patients in the absence of compensatory hypertrophy. Further, the right liver (segment V to VIII) contributes 70% or more of the TLV in approximately 25% of the patients; in 10% of patients, the left liver (segments II, III and IV) is expected to represent 20% or less of the TLV (26).

Portal Vein Embolization

In patients who are otherwise candidates for hepatic resection, an inadequate FLR volume – up to 20% or less than 40% of the estimated TLV in patients with normal or cirrhotic livers, respectively – may be the only obstacle to curative resection. Portal vein embolization (PVE) can be performed to prime the growth of the anticipated FLR, thereby making a major or extended hepatectomy possible. Usually, portal venous access is obtained using a percutaneous ipsilateral transhepatic technique, followed by portography and embolization of the target segments with microparticles and microcoils. The redirection of the portal flow to the FLR results in atrophy of the liver to be resected and hypertrophy of the non-embolized segments. In patients with chronic liver disease, the magnitude and rate of volume increase after PVE are less than in patients with normal liver. The FLR growth has also been shown to correlate with improved function as indicated by increased biliary excretion (35), increased technetium-99m-galactosyl human serum albumin uptake (36), and improvement in the natural history of postoperative liver function tests (37). Moreover, a recent prospective study corroborated the benefit of PVE in patients with chronic liver disease prior to right hepatectomy, showing a significant decrease in pulmonary complications, hepatic decompensation, intensive care unit stay and in-hospital stay (38). Current suggested

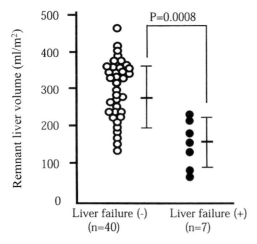

FIGURE 12.1. Small liver volume correlates with poor outcomes in patients with chronic liver disease. In this study, all deaths from liver failure occurred in patients with standardized liver remnants less than 250 ml/m² (mean: 163 ± 63 ml/m²). (From Shirabe K, et al. J Am Coll Surg 1999; 188:304–309; used with permission.)

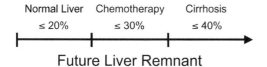

Normal Liver   Chemotherapy   Cirrhosis
≤ 20%   ≤ 30%   ≤ 40%

Future Liver Remnant

FIGURE 12.2. Proposed indications for PVE according to the extent of underlying liver disease. (From Vauthey JN, et al. In Surgery of the Liver and Biliary Tract, 4th ed, LH Blumgart, ed.; with permission.)

indications for PVE in patients with normal, injured and cirrhotic livers are presented in Figure 12.2.

SURGICAL TECHNIQUE

Advances in anesthetic and surgical techniques, as well as a thorough understanding of the liver anatomy and tumor biology, have contributed dramatically to the safety and effectiveness of liver resection for HCC. Modern surgical principles include anatomic resection, the use of vascular inflow occlusion and low central venous pressure anesthesia. New surgical approaches such as the anterior approach and liver hanging maneuver have been developed along with the use of more effective instruments for parenchymal transection.

For a safe liver resection, both the bilateral subcostal incision, with or without superior/midline extension to the xiphoid (hockey-stick incision), and the J-type incision are valid options. After mobilization of the liver, intraoperative ultrasound (IOUS) is systematically performed to confirm the extent of disease, review the intrahepatic portal and hepatic vein anatomy and define the parenchymal transection plane. IOUS identifies new nodules in 15% to 30% of patients with HCC (39, 40), although only about 25% of these new nodules are malignant. Because intraoperative liver biopsies are not useful to differentiate regenerative nodules, dysplastic nodules or early HCCs, the internal echo patterns (mosaic, hypoechoic, hyperechoic) of these new lesions can be considered to predict the histologic features. The classic description of HCC by IOUS is a mosaic pattern with posterior enhancement and lateral shadowing. In nodules that lack specific findings of HCC, malignancy is found in 24% to 30% of hypoechoic nodules and 0% to 18% of hyperechoic nodules) (39, 40). IOUS may therefore decrease recurrence through the identification of unrecognized multifocal HCC. In addition, IOUS is considered an essential aid for guidance of resection (41) and has proven useful in obtaining a margin negative resection (42).

HCC has a high propensity to invade the portal and hepatic veins. Hence, the main pathway of spread is through the bloodstream – first via the portal vein to cause intrahepatic metastasis, and later, to extrahepatic organs such as the lungs, bone and adrenal glands. On this basis, Makuuchi and colleagues introduced the concept of anatomic resection, which involves systematic removal of a hepatic segment along the path of portal blood supply that might contain portal metastases or daughter micronodules. The theoretical advantage of anatomic over non-anatomic resection has been demonstrated in two large series in which anatomic resection was found to be an independent factor for both overall and disease-free survival (43, 44). Therefore, segment-oriented anatomical resection should be proposed for any HCC, whenever technically and functionally possible. The width of a negative resection margin has also been investigated. A study predating the reports on anatomic resection showed that the rate of postoperative recurrence of HCC was not related to the width of the resection margin but rather to microvascular invasion or the presence of microsatellites (45), further supporting the superior value of the anatomic approach. As the margin size has not been found to be an independent predictor of recurrence across multiple studies, functional liver should not be sacrificed in an attempt to obtain a wide margin (45–48).

Several studies have shown that blood loss and transfusion requirements are independent predictors of major morbidity and death from surgery. Blood transfusion can add the risk of coagulopathy as well as exert immunosuppressive effects. Given this, efforts to minimize blood loss become critical. Techniques of temporary vascular occlusion such as portal triad clamping and total vascular exclusion (TVE) have been used to reduce bleeding from the cut edge of the liver. In a prospective randomized study, portal triad clamping, otherwise known as the Pringle maneuver, has been shown to significantly reduce blood loss, resulting in improved postoperative liver function (49). Further, the authors suggested that the reduction in blood loss offset the potential adverse effects of ischemia-reperfusion-induced hepatocellular injury. In a different randomized trial, Belghiti and colleagues demonstrated that intermittent Pringle maneuver – 15 minutes of inflow occlusion followed by 5 minutes of liver revascularization – is safer than continuous inflow occlusion in patients with chronic liver disease and should be considered, in this population, the technique of choice (50). Although Pringle maneuvers exceeding 4 hours have been reported, Wei and colleagues found that inflow occlusion time exceeding 80 minutes was associated with a higher mortality rate (13). TVE, a technique that involves the Pringle maneuver as well as clamping of the supra- and infra-hepatic vena cava, has not been shown to be more effective in decreasing blood loss when compared to portal triad clamping alone (51), while it is associated with increased morbidity. Indications for TVE are limited to those cases with tumor involvement of the cavo-hepatic junction (52).

When performing major or extended hepatectomies, inflow and outflow control prior to transecting the parenchyma can further reduce intraoperative blood loss. This technical conception (the extrahepatic approach), first described by Lortat-Jacob and colleagues (53), involves careful dissection of the porta hepatis to identify and selectively divide the first-order portal and hepatic artery branches. Due to the prevalence of anatomic variants of the biliary tree, we do not recommend extrahepatic hilar dissection and transection of the bile ducts. After control of the inflow, dissection of the vena cava/hepatic vein confluence allows ligation and transection of the right or the middle and/or left hepatic veins. In recent years, laparoscopic linear cutting staplers have been safely used to transect the hepatic and portal veins.

With an adequate Pringle maneuver, the hepatic vein branches represent the primary source of bleeding. In a prospective study, a direct linear correlation was found between mean caval pressure and blood loss (54). As hepatic vein pressure directly reflects the caval pressure, the maintenance of a low central venous pressure is an effective technique to reduce back bleeding from the hepatic veins (55, 56). At our institution, all patients who undergo hepatic resection have maintenance of a low central venous pressure (<5 cm H_2O), with a minimal acceptable urine output of 0.5 mL/kg per hour, until the parenchymal transection is completed. Infusions and transfusions are minimized, and transient hypotension that can occur with hepatic mobilization is treated with vasopressor support (usually phenylephrine). When the parenchymal transection is complete and hemostasis achieved, patients are rendered euvolemic with crystalloid and/or albumin infusions.

New approaches have been developed to enhance the safety of resection of large right-lobe HCCs. In these patients, the conventional technique for hepa-

tectomy – that is, mobilization of the right lobe from the retroperitoneum and anterior surface of the inferior vena cava (IVC) – may be challenging because of the tumor volume and adhesion to the diaphragm. To overcome these problems, after hilar control of the vascular inflow, the parenchyma is transected from the anterior surface of the liver down to the anterior surface of the IVC without prior mobilization of the right lobe. This anterior approach results in less intraoperative blood loss, lower transfusion requirements, a lower in-hospital death rate and significantly better overall and disease-free survival compared with the conventional approach in patients with large right-lobe HCCs. Because it may be difficult to control bleeding in the deeper parenchymal plane using this method, a technique of hanging the liver over an umbilical tape passed between the anterior surface of the IVC and the liver parenchyma (liver-hanging maneuver) has been proposed. After dissection of the space between the right and middle hepatic veins and the anterior plane of the IVC, a vascular clamp is gently pushed cranially from below to blindly complete the dissection of the middle plane along the IVC. When the clamp appears between the right and middle hepatic veins, the tape is seized and passed around the hepatic parenchyma. The parenchymal dissection is facilitated by upward traction on the tape, which allows the surgeon to follow a direct plane and facilitates exposure and hemostasis of the posterior parenchymal plane in front of the IVC.

Several different parenchymal dissection techniques have been developed to minimize blood loss and expedite hepatic resection. Advances in instrumentation, such as development of the ultrasonic aspirator, the jet cutter, the argon beam coagulator and saline-linked cautery, have all been purported to improve surgical technique. The ultrasonic dissector is a hand-held device that destroys hepatocytes by cavitation based on water content and aspirates the liquefied tissue. Vessels and biliary ducts, which contain less water, are preserved, allowing for a clear delineation of these structures within the transection plane. Saline-linked cautery (SLC) uses a metal probe to deliver radiofrequency energy conducted through a slow infusion of saline. At our institution, we recently combined these two devices in a standardized fashion (Figure 12.3): the primary surgeon dissects the hepatic parenchyma from the patient's left side, utilizing the ultrasonic dissector, while the second surgeon operates the SLC from the patient's right side.

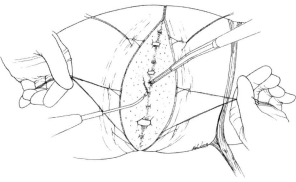

Secondary surgeon   Primary surgeon

FIGURE 12.3. Two-surgeon technique for hepatic parenchymal transection. Using the ultrasonic dissection device, the primary surgeon directs the dissection from the patient's left side. Simultaneously, the secondary surgeon operates the saline-linked cautery device from the patient's right side. Traction on 4–0 polypropylene stay sutures is used to expose the deepening transection plane. (From Aloia TA, et al. Ann Surg 2005; 242: 172–177; with permission.)

Vessels of 3 mm or smaller are coagulated and divided using the SLC device, whereas those 3 mm to 5 mm in diameter are controlled with titanium clips and divided sharply. Larger vessels and portal triads are sutured with 3–0 silk ties in continuity and divided sharply. This two-surgeon technique (57) resulted in a significant decrease in blood loss and total operative time. This is of paramount importance given that a faster parenchymal phase may reduce the time of the Pringle maneuver and therefore ischemic injury of the liver.

Drains have not been shown to be beneficial after hepatic resection for HCC. In a meta-analysis of three randomized controlled trials, the incidence of post-operative biloma was approximately 5% and either equal or even higher in drained patients compared with not drained patients (58). In one of these trials, which only included patients with chronic liver disease, drainage after resection was an independent predictor of postoperative complications (59). Drains also failed to detect significant postoperative complications such as bile leak and hemorrhage that needed surgical or radiologic interventions.

MORBIDITY AND MORTALITY

Improvements in patient selection and surgical technique have resulted in a remarkable decrease in perioperative mortality rates. A large, multi-center review from the 1970s by Foster and Berman reported a perioperative mortality rate of 21% for major hepatectomy and 58% for patients with cirrhosis (60). Currently, the mortality rate is approximately 5% with some centers approaching close to zero mortality (18, 25, 61). Refinements are multi-factorial and include surgical technique, anesthesia management, perioperative care and the establishment of high-volume referral centers specializing in hepato-biliary surgery.

Morbidity rates range from 25% to 50% in recent large series (6, 7, 11–13). In addition to complications associated with all major surgery, post-hepatectomy specific complications include right pleural effusion, subphrenic abscess, bleeding, biliary leak/fistula, ascites and hepatic insufficiency. Blood loss and the need for transfusion have clearly been shown to increase morbidity and mortality (62, 63). In a review of extended hepatectomies for HCC, multi-variate analysis identified the Pringle maneuver and blood transfusion as risk factors for morbidity with co-morbid illness and blood transfusion as independent risk factors for death (13). The risk of morbidity with Pringle maneuver was primarily for minor complications such as ascites/effusion and mainly in patients whose clamping time exceeded 80 minutes.

LONG-TERM OUTCOME

During the past two to three decades, survival after hepatic resection has markedly improved over earlier results, likely due to early diagnosis in high-risk patients screened with alpha-fetoprotein (AFP) and ultrasound, improved patient selection and surgical management. Large series have reported 30% to 50% 5-year overall survival rates following curative resection (64–66). The main cause of treatment failure is tumor recurrence. Indeed, cumulative 5-year recurrence rates of 70% to 100% have been reported after hepatic resection. Recurrence occurs in the liver remnant in about 80% to 90% (66, 67) of cases, as a result of vascular invasion leading to microsatellite tumors within the liver – that is, intrahepatic metastases (early recurrence), or second primaries in the remnant liver associated with field effect from hepatitis and cirrhosis (late recurrence).

The prognosis after potentially curative therapy depends on tumor-related factors and underlying liver disease. Thus, clinical and pathologic predictors of survival have been extensively investigated. For example, in a stepwise analysis approach on

5,800 patients, the Liver Cancer Study Group of Japan established portal involvement as the predominant prognostic factor, followed by number of tumor nodules, AFP level, tumor size, cirrhosis, age and surgical curability (as defined by resection margin, stage and absence of remaining macroscopic tumor; 68). However, different studies from Asia, Europe and North America have reported divergent predictors of survival. These studies have resulted in a number of different classification systems for HCC. In 2003, the American Hepato-Pancreato-Biliary Association (AHPBA)/American Joint Committee on Cancer (AJCC) consensus conference on staging for HCC recommended the use of the tumor-node-metastasis (TNM) staging system (69) to stratify surgical patients with respect to prognosis. Hence, outcome results will be discussed herein by presenting the basis of the current 6th edition AJCC/International Union against Cancer (UICC) staging system. Moreover, because prognosis depends essentially on whether the tumor is suitable for radical treatment, the rationale for patient selection is also discussed.

The past fifth edition of the AJCC/UICC staging system for HCC was used inconsistently, in part because of its complexity, and was believed by many clinicians to provide suboptimal prognostic information regarding patient outcome.

In 2002, in an attempt to improve the TNM staging system, the International Cooperative Study Group for HCC reviewed the clinical and pathologic data from 557 patients who had undergone resection of HCC in centers in the United States, Europe and Asia (70). Using multi-variate analysis, invasion of a main branch of the portal or hepatic vein, microvascular invasion (i.e., the presence of tumor emboli within either the central hepatic vein, the portal vein or the large capsular vessels), severe fibrosis/cirrhosis, tumor number and a tumor size greater than 5 cm were found to be independent predictors of survival. As in several other studies (71–73), vascular invasion was identified as the most important tumor-related predictor of survival (microvascular invasion, HR = 1.6, 95% CI 1.2–2.1; major vascular invasion, HR = 2.1, 95% CI 1.4–3.3). Based on this analysis, Vauthey and colleagues proposed a simplified TNM staging system, which was obtained by grouping together into three T stages subgroups of patients with similar survival after stratification according to the prognostic factors. This revised TNM staging system

was subsequently adopted in the sixth edition of the AJCC/UICC TNM staging manual (Table 12.2).

Vauthey and colleagues found that in patients with a single tumor without major or microvascular invasion, tumor size had no effect on survival, irrespective of how tumor size was dichotomized (i.e., 2, 3, 4, 5, or 10 cm). Therefore, in the current AJCC/UICC staging system, patients with solitary tumors without vascular invasion, regardless of tumor size, are classified as T1. These patients are expected to achieve a 5-year survival rate of 55%.

The prognosis of patients with multiple tumors, none larger than 5 cm, was similar to that of patients with a single tumor with microscopic vascular invasion. Thus, these two groups of patients were combined to form the new T2 class. These patients are expected to achieve a 5-year survival rate of 37%.

Patients with multiple tumors, any of which is greater than 5 cm, and those presenting with major vascular invasion were also found to have similar survival and were categorized as T3. In these patients, the 5-year survival is expected to be 15%. After its adoption, the current TNM staging system has gained wide acceptance and has been validated in both Eastern and Western populations (74, 75). Tumor size, vascular invasion and tumor number represent prognostic factors rather than selection criteria. Though associated with reduced survival, these factors cannot be used for patient selection.

In addition, conflicting data have been reported on the impact of tumor size on prognosis. Many series found tumor size to be a high-ranking and independent variable in predicting adverse outcome after resection (68), with a higher recurrence rate noted for tumors larger than 5 cm (66, 71). Conversely, other authors showed that the size of the tumor had little influence on prognosis (76–78). Pawlik and colleagues analyzed the predictors of microvascular invasion in 1073 patients, reporting that the incidence of microscopic vascular invasion increased progressively with tumor size and that high histologic grade and multiple nodules each predicted occult vascular invasion in tumors larger than 5 cm (79). The finding that tumor size and histologic grade may be markers of invasiveness can help explain why these factors failed to affect survival in studies that controlled for vascular invasion. Although some authors consider a single tumor exceeding 5 cm to be unresectable (80), patients with a single tumor of any size – that is, T1 or T2 depending on the absence or presence of microscopic

TABLE 12.2 AJCC/UICC Tumor-Node-Metastasis, Histologic Grade and Fibrosis Score Classification Scheme for Hepatocellular Carcinoma*

Primary tumor (T)	
T1	Solitary tumor without vascular invasion
T2	Solitary tumor with vascular invasion or multiple tumors, none more than 5 cm
T3	Multiple tumors more than 5 cm *or* tumor involving a major branch of the portal or hepatic vein(s)
T4	Tumor(s) with direct invasion of adjacent organs other than the gallbladder or with perforation of visceral peritoneum
Regional lymph nodes (N)	
N0	No regional lymph node metastasis
N1	Regional lymph node metastasis
Distant metastasis (M)	
M0	No distant metastasis
M1	Distant metastasis

Stage grouping			
Stage I	T1	N0	M0
Stage II	T2	N0	M0
Stage IIIA	T3	N0	M0
Stage IIIB	T4	N0	M0
Stage IIIC	Any T	N1	M0
Stage IV	Any T	Any N	M1

Histologic grade (G)	
G1	Well differentiated
G2	Moderately differentiated
G3	Poorly differentiated
G4	Undifferentiated
Fibrosis score (F)	
F0	Fibrosis score 0–4 (no fibrosis to moderate fibrosis)
F1	Fibrosis score 5–6 (severe fibrosis to cirrhosis)

*New 6th Edition.

vascular invasion – are expected to achieve 37% to 55% 5-year survival after resection.

Two contemporary studies have also specifically evaluated the outcomes after resection of HCCs larger than 10 cm (81, 82). Despite the technical problems encountered with huge tumors – such as problems with liver mobilization, access and control of the hepatic veins, Poon and colleagues demonstrated the safety of hepatic resection in this population with no significant difference in mortality when compared to resection of smaller HCCs (mortality 5.0% vs. 4.6%, p = 0.87) (81). In a separate study, we reported a 5-year survival of 27% in 300 patients who underwent partial hepatectomy for HCCs larger than 10 cm (82). Therefore, tumor size alone should not be used as exclusion criterion for resection in patients with adequate reserve who can attain a negative margin (Figure 12.4).

Unlike microscopic vascular invasion, tumor invasion of the hepatic or portal veins can be detected preoperatively. Some treatment guidelines (83, 84) allocate those individuals with major vascular invasion

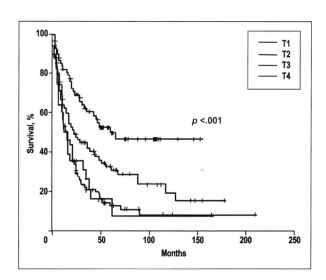

FIGURE 12.4. Survival in 300 patients resected for HCCs larger than 10 cm, according to the AJCC/UICC Staging T-classification system. Patients with T1 tumors had a significantly better outcome than did patients with T2 tumors (p < 0.001), while patients with T2 tumors had a longer median survival than did patients with T3 or T4 tumors (p < 0.001). Patients who had T3 and T4 tumors had a similar poor long-term prognosis. (From Pawlik TM, et al. Arch Surg 2005; 140: 450–458; with permission.)

into treatment algorithms consisting of only medical therapies with new anti-tumoral agents, in the setting of randomized controlled trials. Tumor involvement of the portal or hepatic veins represents a technical and oncologic challenge given that HCCs with major vascular invasion are aggressive and often multi-focal tumors. However, hepatic resection in these patients seems justified because it provides better survival rates than in their untreated counterparts. In a series of 23 patients with portal vein involvement who were treated with partial hepatectomy, Minagawa and colleagues reported a median survival of 3.4 years and 1-, 3-, and 5-year survival rates of 82%, 42%, and 42%, respectively (85). In a larger series of 102 patients with major portal or hepatic vein involvement, we reported a lower 5-year survival rate of 23% in patients without cirrhosis (86). Nonetheless, the median survival exceeded the historical survival rates in similar patients treated nonsurgically. In light of the dismal survival with ablative treatment, the contraindication for liver transplantation and the lack of effective systemic therapy, resection represents the only option for patients with HCC and major vascular invasion.

Multi-nodular HCCs lead the surgeon to face a problematic scenario. Multiple nodules may represent independent tumors derived from multiple loci of hepatocarcinogenesis or may be a manifestation of advanced disease with intrahepatic metastasis, an event associated with a poor prognosis. Further, bilobar location of the tumors contributes to the technical challenge. Indeed, surgical resection for these patients often requires major resection because of substantial tumor volume. Patients with more than three nodules, regardless the size, or those with two or three nodules, one of which exceeds 3 cm in diameter, have been considered unsuitable for resection (87). Ng and colleagues recently analyzed the outcome of 380 resected patients matching these criteria of "irresectability": the mortality rate was 2.4%, with a 5-year survival rate of 39% (88). In a series of 39 patients with bilobar tumors, Wu and colleagues reported 6-year disease-free and actuarial survival rates of 30.5% and 42.9%, respectively, after radical resection (89). Hence, when liver function permits and clearance of all tumor nodules is possible, *en-bloc* extended hepatectomy, multiple bilobar resections or hepatectomy plus local ablation of contralateral nodules should be considered for patients with bilobar HCC.

The gross appearance of the tumor (90), the presence of a capsule surrounding the tumor (66), the presence of microsatellite nodules (45) and preoperative level of AFP (66, 68, 91) have all been shown to predict the prognosis. However, the prognostic significance of these factors is highly variable among studies, and the usefulness as selection criteria for resection has never been established.

Chronic hepatitis and cirrhosis represent the strongest predisposing factors for primary HCC and critically impact both early and late survival by, first, limiting patient eligibility for hepatic resection and, second, promoting recurrence after surgery (92). In a study of 145 patients who survived more than 5 years after resection of HCC, we have reported that recurrence rates were 31% in patients with severe fibrosis or cirrhosis, compared with only 7% in patients with no fibrosis or cirrhosis, suggesting that chronic liver disease acts as a field of cancerization, contributing to new HCCs (93, 94). The effect of the underlying liver on long-term survival was also underscored in the study from the International Cooperative Study Group of HCC. The investigators found that the presence of severe fibrosis/cirrhosis was significantly associated with a worse 5-year survival, regardless of T-stage classification (Table 12.3). Therefore, the new AJCC/UICC TNM system incorporated the

TABLE 12.3 Prognosis of the Main T Categories of the New AJCC/UICC Classification

Group	Fibrosis	5-Year Survival (%)	P Value
T1 – Solitary without vascular invasion	F0	64	0.01
	F1	49	
T2 – Solitary with vascular invasion or multiple tumors ≤5 cm	F0	46	0.01
	F1	30	
T3 – Major vascular invasion or multiple tumors >5 cm	F0	17	0.005
	F1	9	

F0: fibrosis grade 0–4 and F1: fibrosis grade 5–6 according to Ishak (Iskak K; 1995 J Hepatol).
Adapted from Vauthey, et al. J Clin Oncol 2002; 20: 1527–1536, with permission.

provision of a separate report of fibrosis in every resected case of HCC using the fibrosis classification proposed by Ishak (95). (Ishak 0–2 represents no or minimal fibrosis, Ishak 3–4 incomplete bridging fibrosis, and Ishak 5–6 complete fibrosis and nodules). Patients with severe fibrosis/cirrhosis (Ishak score of 5–6) are staged as F1, whereas patients with no or moderate fibrosis (Ishak score 0–4) are staged as F0.

Although surgical resection of intrahepatic tumor recurrence is a demanding procedure because of reduced hepatic parenchyma and a more hostile environment, repeat hepatectomy has proved to be safe and worthwhile (96–101). Ten to thirty-one percent of the patients with intrahepatic recurrence can be treated with a second hepatectomy. Utilizing the same selection criteria as for primary resection, three clinicopathologic variables were found to be independent prognostic factors: absence of portal invasion at the second resection, single HCC at the primary hepatectomy and a disease-free interval of at least 1 year after the primary hepatectomy. In a series of 67 patients, the overall 5-year survival after a repeat hepatectomy was 56% – a rate comparable to those reported in many series of initial resection (101). Aggressive non-surgical treatment with ethanol injection, radiofrequency ablation and transarterial chemoembolization may yield favorable results in patients not suitable for reresection.

Hepatic resection still remains the first treatment option for most patients with HCC and is no longer limited to early stage disease. Unfavorable prognostic features at presentation cannot reliably exclude patients from surgery.

REFERENCES

1. Parkin DM, Bray F, Ferlay J, et al. Global cancer statistics, 2002. CA Cancer J Clin 2005; 55(2): 74–108.
2. El-Serag HB, Mason AC. Rising incidence of hepatocellular carcinoma in the United States. N Engl J Med 1999; 340(10): 745–750.
3. Nagasue N, Yukaya H, Hamada T, et al. The natural history of hepatocellular carcinoma. A study of 100 untreated cases. Cancer 1984; 54(7): 1461–1465.
4. Barbara L, Benzi G, Gaiani S, et al. Natural history of small untreated hepatocellular carcinoma in cirrhosis: A multivariate analysis of prognostic factors of tumor growth rate and patient survival. Hepatology 1992; 16(1): 132–137.
5. Shuto T, Hirohashi K, Kubo S, et al. Changes and results of surgical strategies for hepatocellular carcinoma: Results of a 15-year study on 452 consecutive patients. Surg Today 1998; 28(11): 1124–1129.
6. Zhou XD, Tang ZY, Yang BH, et al. Experience of 1000 patients who underwent hepatectomy for small hepatocellular carcinoma. Cancer 2001; 91(8): 1479–1486.
7. Takenaka K, Kawahara N, Yamamoto K, et al. Results of 280 liver resections for hepatocellular carcinoma. Arch Surg 1996; 131(1): 71–76.
8. Mazzaferro V, Regalia E, Doci R, et al. Liver transplantation for the treatment of small hepatocellular carcinomas in patients with cirrhosis. N Engl J Med 1996; 334(11): 693–699.
9. Llovet JM, Bruix J, Fuster J, et al. Liver transplantation for small hepatocellular carcinoma: The tumor-node-metastasis classification does not have prognostic power. Hepatology 1998; 27(6): 1572–1577.
10. Cance WG, Stewart AK, Menck HR. The National Cancer Data Base Report on treatment patterns for hepatocellular carcinomas: Improved survival of surgically resected patients, 1985–1996. Cancer 2000; 88(4): 912–920.
11. Fong Y, Sun RL, Jarnagin W, et al. An analysis of 412 cases of hepatocellular carcinoma at a Western center. Ann Surg 1999; 229(6): 790–799.
12. Belghiti J, Hiramatsu K, Benoist S, et al. Seven hundred forty-seven hepatectomies in the 1990s: An update to evaluate the actual risk of liver resection. J Am Coll Surg 2000; 191(1): 38–46.
13. Wei AC, Tung-Ping Poon R, Fan ST, et al. Risk factors for perioperative morbidity and mortality after extended hepatectomy for hepatocellular carcinoma. Br J Surg 2003; 90(1): 33–41.
14. Pugh RN, Murray-Lyon IM, Dawson JL, et al. Transection of the oesophagus for bleeding oesophageal varices. Br J Surg 1973; 60(8): 646–649.
15. Mansour A, Watson W, Shayani V, et al. Abdominal operations in patients with cirrhosis: Still a major surgical challenge. Surgery 1997; 122(4): 730–735.
16. Teh SH, Christein J, Donohue J, et al. Hepatic resection of hepatocellular carcinoma in patients with cirrhosis: Model of End-Stage Liver Disease (MELD) score predicts perioperative mortality. J Gastrointest Surg 2005; 9(9): 1207–1215.
17. Belghiti J, Regimbeau JM, Durand F, et al. Resection of hepatocellular carcinoma: A European experience on 328 cases. Hepatogastroenterology 2002; 49(43): 41–46.
18. Fan ST, Lo CM, Liu CL, et al. Hepatectomy for hepatocellular carcinoma: Toward zero hospital deaths. Ann Surg 1999; 229(3): 322–330.
19. Bruix J, Castells A, Bosch J, et al. Surgical resection of hepatocellular carcinoma in cirrhotic patients: Prognostic value of preoperative portal pressure. Gastroenterology 1996; 111(4): 1018–1022.
20. Eguchi H, Umeshita K, Sakon M, et al. Presence of active hepatitis associated with liver cirrhosis is a risk factor for mortality caused by posthepatectomy liver failure. Dig Dis Sci 2000; 45(7): 1383–1388.
21. Haber MM, West AB, Haber AD, et al. Relationship of aminotransferases to liver histological status in chronic hepatitis C. Am J Gastroenterol 1995; 90(8): 1250–1257.
22. Healey CJ, Chapman RW, Fleming KA. Liver histology in hepatitis C infection: A comparison between

patients with persistently normal or abnormal transaminases. Gut 1995; 37(2): 274–278.

23. Poon RT, Fan ST, Lo CM, et al. Long-term prognosis after resection of hepatocellular carcinoma associated with hepatitis B-related cirrhosis. J Clin Oncol 2000; 18(5): 1094–1101.

24. Noun R, Jagot P, Farges O, et al. High preoperative serum alanine transferase levels: Effect on the risk of liver resection in Child grade A cirrhotic patients. World J Surg 1997; 21(4): 390–394.

25. Torzilli G, Makuuchi M, Inoue K, et al. No-mortality liver resection for hepatocellular carcinoma in cirrhotic and noncirrhotic patients: Is there a way? A prospective analysis of our approach. Arch Surg 1999; 134(9): 984–992.

26. Abdalla EK, Denys A, Chevalier P, et al. Total and segmental liver volume variations: Implications for liver surgery. Surgery 2004; 135(4): 404–410.

27. Kawasaki T, Moriyasu F, Kimura T, et al. Changes in portal blood flow consequent to partial hepatectomy: Doppler estimation. Radiology 1991; 180(2): 373–377.

28. Panis Y, McMullan DM, Emond JC. Progressive necrosis after hepatectomy and the pathophysiology of liver failure after massive resection. Surgery 1997; 121(2): 142–149.

29. Vauthey JN, Abdalla EK, Doherty DA, et al. Body surface area and body weight predict total liver volume in Western adults. Liver Transpl 2002; 8(3): 233–240.

30. Abdalla EK, Hicks ME, Vauthey JN. Portal vein embolization: Rationale, technique and future prospects. Br J Surg 2001; 88(2): 165–175.

31. Johnson TN, Tucker GT, Tanner MS, et al. Changes in liver volume from birth to adulthood: A meta-analysis. Liver Transpl 2005; 11(12): 1481–1493.

32. Abdalla EK, Barnett CC, Doherty D, et al. Extended hepatectomy in patients with hepatobiliary malignancies with and without preoperative portal vein embolization. Arch Surg 2002; 137(6): 675–680.

33. Shirabe K, Shimada M, Gion T, et al. Postoperative liver failure after major hepatic resection for hepatocellular carcinoma in the modern era with special reference to remnant liver volume. J Am Coll Surg 1999; 188(3): 304–309.

34. Kokudo N, Makuuchi M. Current role of portal vein embolization/hepatic artery chemoembolization. Surg Clin North Am 2004; 84(2): 643–657.

35. Ijichi M, Makuuchi M, Imamura H, et al. Portal embolization relieves persistent jaundice after complete biliary drainage. Surgery 2001; 130(1): 116–118.

36. Hirai I, Kimura W, Fuse A, et al. Evaluation of preoperative portal embolization for safe hepatectomy, with special reference to assessment of nonembolized lobe function with 99mTc-GSA SPECT scintigraphy. Surgery 2003; 133(5): 495–506.

37. Vauthey JN, Chaoui A, Do KA, et al. Standardized measurement of the future liver remnant prior to extended liver resection: methodology and clinical associations. Surgery 2000; 127(5): 512–519.

38. Farges O, Belghiti J, Kianmanesh R, et al. Portal vein embolization before right hepatectomy: prospective clinical trial. Ann Surg 2003; 237(2): 208–217.

39. Kokudo N, Bandai Y, Imanishi H, et al. Management of new hepatic nodules detected by intraoperative ultrasonography during hepatic resection for hepatocellular carcinoma. Surgery 1996; 119(6): 634–640.

40. Takigawa Y, Sugawara Y, Yamamoto J, et al. New lesions detected by intraoperative ultrasound during liver resection for hepatocellular carcinoma. Ultrasound Med Biol 2001; 27(2): 151–156.

41. Torzilli G, Makuuchi M. Intraoperative ultrasonography in liver cancer. Surg Oncol Clin North Am 2003; 12(1): 91–103.

42. Lau WY, Leung KL, Lee TW, et al. Ultrasonography during liver resection for hepatocellular carcinoma. Br J Surg 1993; 80(4): 493–494.

43. Hasegawa K, Kokudo N, Imamura H, et al. Prognostic impact of anatomic resection for hepatocellular carcinoma. Ann Surg 2005; 242(2): 252–259.

44. Regimbeau JM, Kianmanesh R, Farges O, et al. Extent of liver resection influences the outcome in patients with cirrhosis and small hepatocellular carcinoma. Surgery 2002; 131(3): 311–317.

45. Poon RT, Fan ST, Ng IO, et al. Significance of resection margin in hepatectomy for hepatocellular carcinoma: A critical reappraisal. Ann Surg 2000; 231(4): 544–551.

46. Jwo SC, Chiu JH, Chau GY, et al. Risk factors linked to tumor recurrence of human hepatocellular carcinoma after hepatic resection. Hepatology 1992; 16(6): 1367–1371.

47. Yamamoto J, Kosuge T, Takayama T, et al. Recurrence of hepatocellular carcinoma after surgery. Br J Surg 1996; 83(9): 1219–1222.

48. Cha CH, Ruo L, Fong Y, et al. Resection of hepatocellular carcinoma in patients otherwise eligible for transplantation. Ann Surg 2003; 238(3): 315–321; discussion 21–23.

49. Man K, Fan ST, Ng IO, et al. Prospective evaluation of Pringle maneuver in hepatectomy for liver tumors by a randomized study. Ann Surg 1997; 226(6): 704–711.

50. Belghiti J, Noun R, Malafosse R, et al. Continuous versus intermittent portal triad clamping for liver resection: A controlled study. Ann Surg 1999; 229(3): 369–375.

51. Belghiti J, Noun R, Zante E, et al. Portal triad clamping or hepatic vascular exclusion for major liver resection: A controlled study. Ann Surg 1996; 224(2): 155–161.

52. Torzilli G, Makuuchi M, Midorikawa Y, et al. Liver resection without total vascular exclusion: Hazardous or beneficial? An analysis of our experience. Ann Surg 2001; 233(2): 167–175.

53. Lortat-Jacob JL, Robert HG, Henry C. Excision of the right lobe of the liver for a malignant secondary tumor. Arch Mal Appar Dig Mal Nutr 1952; 41(6): 662–667.

54. Johnson M, Mannar R, Wu AV. Correlation between blood loss and inferior vena caval pressure during liver resection. Br J Surg 1998; 85(2): 188–190.

55. Rees M, Plant G, Wells J, et al. One hundred and fifty hepatic resections: Evolution of technique towards bloodless surgery. Br J Surg 1996; 83(11): 1526–1529.

56. Cunningham JD, Fong Y, Shriver C, et al. One hundred consecutive hepatic resections: Blood loss, transfusion, and operative technique. Arch Surg 1994; 129(10): 1050–1056.

57. Aloia TA, Zorzi D, Abdalla EK, et al. Two-surgeon technique for hepatic parenchymal transection of the noncirrhotic liver using saline-linked cautery and ultrasonic dissection. Ann Surg 2005; 242(2): 172–177.

58. Petrowsky H, Demartines N, Rousson V, et al. Evidence-based value of prophylactic drainage in gastrointestinal surgery: A systematic review and meta-analyses. Ann Surg 2004; 240(6): 1074–1084.

59. Liu CL, Fan ST, Lo CM, et al. Abdominal drainage after hepatic resection is contraindicated in patients with chronic liver diseases. Ann Surg 2004; 239(2): 194–201.

60. Foster JH, Berman MM. Solid Liver Tumors Philadelphia: W. B. Saunders Company 1977.

61. Jaeck D, Bachellier P, Oussoultzoglou E, et al. Surgical resection of hepatocellular carcinoma. Post-operative outcome and long-term results in Europe: An overview. Liver Transpl 2004; 10(2 Suppl 1): S58–63.

62. Makuuchi M, Takayama T, Gunven P, et al. Restrictive versus liberal blood transfusion policy for hepatectomies in cirrhotic patients. World J Surg 1989; 13(5): 644–648.

63. Shimada M, Takenaka K, Fujiwara Y, et al. Risk factors linked to postoperative morbidity in patients with hepatocellular carcinoma. Br J Surg 1998; 85(2): 195–198.

64. Bismuth H, Majno P, Adam R. Hepatocellular carcinoma: From ethanol injection to liver transplantation. Acta Gastroenterologica Belgica 1999; 62(3): 330–341.

65. Capussotti L, Borgonovo G, Bouzari H, et al. Results of major hepatectomy for large primary liver cancer in patients with cirrhosis. Br J Surg 1994; 81(3): 427–431.

66. Belghiti J, Panis Y, Farges O, et al. Intrahepatic recurrence after resection of hepatocellular carcinoma complicating cirrhosis. Ann Surg 1991; 214(2): 114–117.

67. Nagasue N, Kohno H, Chang YC, et al. Liver resection for hepatocellular carcinoma: Results of 229 consecutive patients during 11 years. Ann Surg 1993; 217(4): 375–384.

68. Liver Cancer Study Group of Japan. Predictive factors for long-term prognosis after partial hepatectomy for patients with hepatocellular carcinoma in Japan. Cancer 1994; (74): 2272–2780.

69. Liver (including intrahepatic bile ducts). In Greene FL, Page DL, Fleming ID, et al., eds: American Joint Committee on Cancer Staging Manual, 6th Edition, pp. 131–144. New York, NY: Springer-Verlag 2002.

70. Vauthey JN, Lauwers GY, Esnaola NF, et al. Simplified staging for hepatocellular carcinoma. J Clin Oncol 2002; 20(6): 1527–1536.

71. Izumi R, Shimizu K, Ii T, et al. Prognostic factors of hepatocellular carcinoma in patients undergoing hepatic resection. Gastroenterology 1994; 106(3): 720–727.

72. Vauthey JN, Klimstra D, Franceschi D, et al. Factors affecting long-term outcome after hepatic resection for hepatocellular carcinoma. Am J Surg 1995; 169(1): 28–34.

73. Tsai TJ, Chau GY, Lui WY, et al. Clinical significance of microscopic tumor venous invasion in patients with resectable hepatocellular carcinoma. Surgery 2000; 127(6): 603–608.

74. Poon RT, Fan ST. Evaluation of the new AJCC/UICC staging system for hepatocellular carcinoma after hepatic resection in Chinese patients. Surg Oncol Clin North Am 2003; 12(1): 35–50, viii.

75. Ramacciato G, Mercantini P, Cautero N, et al. Prognostic evaluation of the new American Joint Committee on Cancer/International Union Against Cancer staging system for hepatocellular carcinoma: Analysis of 112

76. Lai EC, Ng IO, You KT, et al. Hepatic resection for small hepatocellular carcinoma: The Queen Mary Hospital experience. World J Surg 1991; 15(5): 654–659.

77. Kanematsu T, Takenaka K, Matsumata T, et al. Limited hepatic resection effective for selected cirrhotic patients with primary liver cancer. Ann Surg 1984; 199(1): 51–56.

78. Nagasue N, Yukaya H, Ogawa Y, et al. Clinical experience with 118 hepatic resections for hepatocellular carcinoma. Surgery 1986; 99(6): 694–701.

79. Pawlik TM, Delman KA, Vauthey JN, et al. Tumor size predicts vascular invasion and histologic grade: Implications for selection of surgical treatment for hepatocellular carcinoma. Liver Transpl 2005; 11(9): 1086–1092.

80. Llovet JM, Bustamante J, Castells A, et al. Natural history of untreated nonsurgical hepatocellular carcinoma: Rationale for the design and evaluation of therapeutic trials. Hepatology 1999; 29(1): 62–67.

81. Poon RT, Fan ST, Lo CM, et al. Extended hepatic resection for hepatocellular carcinoma in patients with cirrhosis: Is it justified? Ann Surg 2002; 236(5): 602–611.

82. Pawlik TM, Poon RT, Abdalla EK, et al. Critical appraisal of the clinical and pathologic predictors of survival after resection of large hepatocellular carcinoma. Arch Surg 2005; 140(5): 450–457.

83. Llovet JM, Bru C, Bruix J. Prognosis of hepatocellular carcinoma: The BCLC staging classification. Semin Liver Dis 1999; 19(3): 329–338.

84. Bruix J, Llovet JM. Prognostic prediction and treatment strategy in hepatocellular carcinoma. Hepatology 2002; 35(3): 519–524.

85. Minagawa M, Makuuchi M, Takayama T, et al. Selection criteria for hepatectomy in patients with hepatocellular carcinoma and portal vein tumor thrombus. Ann Surg 2001; 233(3): 379–384.

86. Pawlik TM, Poon RT, Abdalla EK, et al. Hepatectomy for hepatocellular carcinoma with major portal or hepatic vein invasion: Results of a multicenter study. Surgery 2005; 137(4): 403–410.

87. Bruix J, Sherman M. Management of hepatocellular carcinoma. Hepatology 2005; 42(5): 1208–1236.

88. Ng KK, Vauthey JN, Pawlik TM, et al. Is hepatic resection for large or multinodular hepatocellular carcinoma justified? Results from a multi-institutional database. Ann Surg Oncol 2005; 12(5): 364–373.

89. Wu CC, Ho WL, Lin MC, et al. Hepatic resection for bilobar multicentric hepatocellular carcinoma: Is it justified? Surgery 1998; 123(3): 270–277.

90. Hui AM, Takayama T, Sano K, et al. Predictive value of gross classification of hepatocellular carcinoma on recurrence and survival after hepatectomy. J Hepatol 2000; 33(6): 975–979.

91. Nagao T, Inoue S, Goto S, et al. Hepatic resection for hepatocellular carcinoma: Clinical features and long-term prognosis. Ann Surg 1987; 205(1): 33–40.

92. Matsumoto Y, Fujii H, Matsuda M, et al. Multicentric occurrence of hepatocellular carcinoma: Diagnosis and clinical significance. J Hepatobiliary Pancreat Surg 2001; 8(5): 435–440.

cirrhotic patients resected for hepatocellular carcinoma. Ann Surg Oncol 2005; 12(4): 289–297.

93. Bilimoria MM, Lauwers GY, Doherty DA, et al. Underlying liver disease, not tumor factors, predicts long-term survival after resection of hepatocellular carcinoma. Arch Surg 2001; 136(5): 528–535.

94. Vauthey JN, Walsh GL, Vlastos G, et al. Importance of field cancerisation in clinical oncology. The Lancet Oncology 2000; 1(1): 15–16.

95. Ishak K, Baptista A, Bianchi L, et al. Histological grading and staging of chronic hepatitis. J Hepatol 1995; 22(6): 696–699.

96. Suenaga M, Sugiura H, Kokuba Y, et al. Repeated hepatic resection for recurrent hepatocellular carcinoma in eighteen cases. Surgery 1994; 115(4): 452–457.

97. Kakazu T, Makuuchi M, Kawasaki S, et al. Repeat hepatic resection for recurrent hepatocellular carcinoma. Hepatogastroenterology 1993; 40(4): 337–341.

98. Matsuda Y, Ito T, Oguchi Y, et al. Rationale of surgical management for recurrent hepatocellular carcinoma. Ann Surg 1993; 217(1): 28–34.

99. Shimada M, Takenaka K, Taguchi K, et al. Prognostic factors after repeat hepatectomy for recurrent hepatocellular carcinoma. Ann Surg 1998; 227(1): 80–85.

100. Arii S, Monden K, Niwano M, et al. Results of surgical treatment for recurrent hepatocellular carcinoma: Comparison of outcome among patients with multicentric carcinogenesis, intrahepatic metastasis, and extrahepatic recurrence. J Hepatobiliary Pancreat Surg 1998; 5(1): 86–92.

101. Minagawa M, Makuuchi M, Takayama T, et al. Selection criteria for repeat hepatectomy in patients with recurrent hepatocellular carcinoma. Ann Surg 2003; 238(5): 703–710.

Chapter 13

LIVER TRANSPLANTATION FOR HEPATOCELLULAR CARCINOMA

James P. Hamilton

Paul J. Thuluvath

Liver transplantation for hepatocellular carcinoma (HCC) is an effective and potentially curative therapy for carefully selected patients. More than 80% of patients with HCC have underlying cirrhosis and HCC may be multifocal; thus, transplantation is a rational therapeutic option as it offers the potential for treatment of cancer and underlying liver disease. In the non-cirrhotic patient with HCC, surgical resection for amenable lesions is the treatment of choice. Ideal candidates for liver transplantation are those who have small tumors with no metastatic spread, underlying cirrhosis and no serious co-morbid conditions. Since the adoption of the Milan Criteria (one tumor less than 5 cm or up to three tumors, each less than 3 cm), many liver transplant centers have reported excellent recurrence-free survival and overall survival rates for HCC (1–3). The examination of United Network for Organ Sharing data confirmed a steady and significant improvement (5-year patient survival: 1987–1991, 25.3%; 1992–1996, 46.6%; 1997–2001, 61.1%) in the outcome of patients who were transplanted for HCC, indicating that the published criteria, most likely the Milan Criteria, may have contributed to better patient selection and improved survival (2, 3). In fact, in some cases, the post-transplant results for HCC are better than that for non-malignant conditions (4, 5). As the role of liver transplantation for HCC has evolved, several lines of evidence suggest that a modest expansion of the Milan Criteria may be acceptable, although this is not widely practiced. In addition, there is increasing experience with the use of neo-adjuvant therapy in order to downsize tumors to within acceptable limits, but its role is poorly defined. In this chapter, listing criteria for liver transplantation, neo-adjuvant therapy and post-surgical survival of both deceased and live-donor liver transplantation will be reviewed.

SELECTION CRITERIA

HCC is the most common tumor of the liver and carries a dismal prognosis. Worldwide, HCC ranks among the leading causes of cancer mortality, and in the United States, the frequency of HCC has doubled in the past 20 years (6). A majority of patients present with advanced cancer or liver disease such that surgical resection is contraindicated. Moreover, systemic chemotherapy has not been found to be effective for HCC. Liver transplantation has many limitations. It is not widely available, it requires multi-disciplinary expertise and moreover, it relies on organ availability, a severely limited resource. This has led to the adoption of strict selection requirements that maximize post-transplant survival and minimize tumor recurrence.

In the 1960s and 1970s, liver transplantation offered a novel therapeutic option for patients with HCC. Despite the fact that survival in many of the initial transplant patients was limited, a subset of patients with HCC did well, and these patients

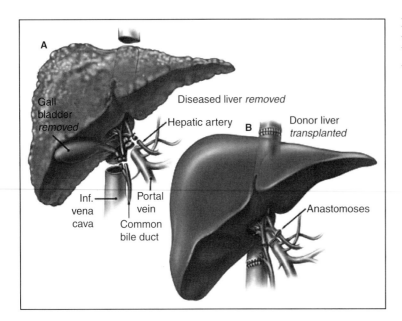

FIGURE 13.1. Schematic of orthotopic liver transplantation. (Courtesy of Johns Hopkins University School of Medicine, Division of Gastroenterology.) See Color Plate 18.

provided the basis for the selection criteria that are currently used by transplant programs to list patients. Clearly, macroscopic vascular invasion by tumor and metastatic disease are contraindications for liver transplantation. However, in patients without these findings, tumor size and number are the most important factors when determining eligibility for transplantation.

From 1963 to 1985, Starzl and colleagues transplanted 54 patients with primary tumors of the liver (HCC, hepatoblastoma, or fibrolamellar HCC) (7). In 13 of these recipients, the neoplasm was detected incidentally on pathologic examination of the explanted liver. At the time this report was published, survival in 12 of these 13 patients ranged from 4 months to 15 years. One patient died of surgical complications, and no patient had recurrence of their malignancy. By contrast, the tumor recurrence rate in the 41 patients in whom hepatic malignancy was the primary indication for transplant was 74% (7). Similarly, Bismuth et al., in a review of 60 transplanted patients, concluded that the best indication for transplantation was in patients with small (<3 cm) and solitary or binodular tumors (8). Building on the these findings, multiple European transplant centers published excellent results in transplant recipients who had solitary tumors less than 5 cm in diameter, or with up to three tumors, each less than 3 cm (9). One of these studies, conducted by Mazzaferro et al., demonstrated a greater than 70% 5-year survival in these early stage liver cancer patients. The tumor characteristics of the patients in this Italian study are

referred to as the Milan Criteria, and are currently accepted selection criteria regarding eligibility of a patient with HCC to be listed for liver transplantation. In addition, this study established early HCC as an indication for liver transplantation (11). Since the original publication, these criteria have now been validated in numerous studies totaling more than 1000 patients. A summary of some of these studies may be found in Table 13.1.

Tumor size and number are rational selection criteria because of the prognostic information that these factors relay. In the absence of metastatic disease, micro- or macroscopic vascular invasion is the best predictor of post-transplantation tumor recurrence. Vascular infiltration is considered to be a prerequisite for systemic tumor dissemination. It has been shown that the likelihood of vascular invasion is directly related to increased tumor size and number (19). Macroscopic vascular invasion of the portal or hepatic veins can usually be determined by imaging and carries a high risk of tumor recurrence and therefore portends a poor prognosis (20). The advent of high-resolution, multi-detector computed tomography (CT) scans and magnetic resonance imaging (MRI) has increased the ability to stratify patients into high- or low-risk transplant candidates. One study found that when compared to angiographic findings, multi-detector CT scans were 97% accurate at detecting vascular abnormalities (21). Microscopic tumor invasion, as defined by the presence of tumor emboli within the central hepatic vein, the portal or the large capsular vessels (20), cannot be detected with

TABLE 13.1 Survival after Liver Transplantation

Study (Ref.)	Year	No.	Selection Criteria	Survival Rate (%)
Mazzaferro, et al. (1)	1996	48	1 lesion ≤5 cm or ≤3 lesions ≤3 cm.	75*
Llovet, et al. (16)	1998	58	1 lesion ≤5 cm.	74
Bechstein, et al. (17)	1998	52	1 lesion ≤5 cm or ≤3 lesions ≤4 cm	71
Bismuth, et al. (18)	1999	45	1 lesion ≤3 cm or ≤3 lesions ≤3 cm	74
Llovet, et al. (12)	1999	79	1 lesion ≤5 cm	75
Hemming, et al. (5)	2001	112	1 lesion ≤5 cm	57
Jonas, et al. (13)	2001	120	1 lesion ≤5 cm or ≤3 lesions ≤3 cm	71
Yao, et al. (14)	2001	70	1 lesion ≤6.5 cm or ≤3 lesions ≤4.5 cm; total tumor diameter ≤8 cm	75

*4-year survival; the 5-year survival is listed for all other studies.

preoperative imaging. High serum levels of the pro-angiogenic compound, vascular endothelial growth factor (VEGF), have been shown to predict microscopic tumor invasion (22, 23), however this finding has not been fully validated and incorporated into standard clinical practice. One of the problems with VEGF is the wide range of serum values within normal subjects. Logistic regression analysis of a large cohort of transplanted tumor patients showed a correlation between microscopic vascular invasion and maximal tumor diameter. Specifically, in patients with a maximal tumor diameter of greater than 5 cm, vascular invasion was significantly more common than in than in patients with smaller tumor diameters (13). However, it is important to note that vascular invasion can be found in small HCCs as well. In an autopsy study, portal vein thrombi were found in 40% of individuals with tumors less than 5 cm (24).

Differentiation of tumors is also an important predictor of outcome (25, 26), but this information is rarely available prior to transplantation as it would require a pre-transplant core biopsy. Zavaglia et al. found that in patients with poorly differentiated HCC, the outcome was dismal, with 5-year recurrence-free survival and overall survival of 41% and 44%, respectively (20). By contrast, patients within Milan Criteria with well-differentiated tumors (and no vascular invasion) had a remarkable 97%, 5-year survival (20). In this study, only histological grade and macroscopic vascular invasion were predictors of post-transplant survival (20). There are additional reports of 50% to 60%, 3-year survival for large (>5 cm), well-differentiated HCC (27, 28). However,

pre-transplant biopsies are not routinely performed to assess tumor differentiation because the information obtained may be misleading as large tumors are known to be heterogeneous (29). In addition, biopsy of HCC may be associated with a very small risk of malignant seeding of the biopsy tract (30).

Strict selection criteria are required for liver transplantation for HCC because of limited organ availability. United Network for Organ Sharing (UNOS), which coordinates organ allocation in the United States, uses the Milan Criteria for listing and expedited transplantation of patients with HCC. Using these criteria, only patients with early HCC and, therefore, a high likelihood for prolonged post-transplant survival are candidates for transplantation (11). Regrettably, this practice results in rejecting patients with more advanced HCC, despite the suggestion that patients with slightly larger tumors may have a reasonable post-transplant outcome. It has been suggested that as many as 40% of patients with HCC that fall outside the Milan Criteria actually have low risk of recurrence (31). These circumstances have led to several proposals and much debate about expanding the indications for liver transplant as a therapy for HCC (32).

It is important to recognize that the current criteria were developed and based on studies that were performed when imaging techniques were not as sensitive as they are today. For example, when post-transplant pathologic examination is compared to preoperative imaging, tumor size is underestimated by approximately 10% to 15% (33). In addition, after a patient is listed for liver transplantation, waiting times are such that it is possible that the tumor may expand beyond acceptable limits. Accordingly, several groups have reported greater than 50%, 5-year survival in patients with tumors that are marginally larger than the current guidelines. All the tumors in these studies were negative for macroscopic or microscopic vascular invasion, without lymphatic invasion, and had no extrahepatic, metastatic foci. In one of these studies, Yao and colleagues suggested that size limits could be expanded to solitary tumors less than 6.5 cm, up to three nodules, each less than 4.5 cm, and a total tumor diameter of less than 8 cm (known as the UCSF criteria), without adversely impacting survival. However, many of these studies, which support the expansion of the criteria for HCC and transplantation, are limited by their sample size and retrospective nature (i.e., post-surgical pathologic examination of the tumor(s) was used to define the size and number) of tumor size assessment.

In summary, there is some emerging evidence, although not confirmed, that patients with tumors larger than the current guidelines (Milan Criteria) may do well after transplant. According to American Association for the Study of Liver Disease guidelines, however, the existing data cannot fully support or justify expanding the current criteria (11).

LISTING FOR TRANSPLANTATION: PRIORITIZATION FOR HCC

Patients selected for liver transplantation undergo rigorous presurgical evaluation, and patients with HCC are no exception. Prior to listing, all patients are presented at a multi-disciplinary conference, during which medical, psychiatric, social and even financial histories are reviewed. A cardiac stress test and pulmonary function test are standard. Routine imaging examinations such as a CT scan or MRI of the liver are required to evaluate tumor size and number, as well as vascular and other anatomic abnormalities. In patients with HCC, a bone scan and chest CT are also needed to evaluate for metastatic disease. A pre-listing biopsy is not required. Age-appropriate cancer screening is also mandatory, and other concurrent malignancies are a contraindication to transplant.

In response to a federal mandate, the UNOS adopted a system by which patients with the highest short-term mortality were transplanted first. In 2001, a mathematical formula known as the MELD (Model

for End-Stage Liver Disease) score was implemented for patients with chronic liver disease (35). This calculation is based on three variables: serum bilirubin, serum creatinine and prothrombin time (a MELD, or the pediatric counterpart PELD, calculator may be found at www.unos.org). Healthy patients with normal hepatic synthetic function will have a MELD score of less than 10, whereas critically ill patients can reach a maximum score of 40. Although it varies based upon region and blood type, patients at the top of the "list" typically have MELD scores greater than 20. The MELD-based allocation program provides a system by which a patient's need for transplant is defined by their risk of dying on the waiting list within 3 months. A MELD of 22 predicts a 15%, 3-month mortality. The MELD score, however, does not predict the increased risk of mortality in patients with HCC. Therefore, supplemental or bonus points are now given to patients with HCC. Patients with a solitary tumor 2 to 5 cm or three nodules each less than or equal to 3 cm (modified Milan Criteria) and no evidence of extra-hepatic spread as defined by lung imaging (CT or MRI) and bone scan, are arbitrarily granted 22 MELD points. These tumor characteristics correspond to a Stage II HCC in the modified tumor-node-metastasis (TNM) staging classification (36). An additional 10% increase (3 points) is added for every 3 months spent on the waiting list until patient is transplanted or removed from the list because of tumor progression. Patients with tumors smaller than 2 cm or larger than 5 cm are not eligible for exception points. A summary of the UNOS criteria for priority listing for transplantation is listed in Table 13.2.

TABLE 13.2 UNOS Criteria for Priority Listing for Patients with Hepatocellular Carcinoma

1. One tumor that is greater than 2 cm and less than 5 cm, or up to three lesions, the largest being less than 3 cm.
2. Evaluation must include an ultrasound and CT scan or MRI of the chest and abdomen that documents the lesion(s) and excludes metastases.
3. The diagnoses of a tumor can be made by one of the following: A vascular blush corresponding to the area of suspicion seen on the aforementioned imaging studies, AFP level of greater than 200 ng/ml, an arteriogram confirming a tumor, a biopsy confirming HCC, chemoembolization of lesion, radiofrequency, cryo- or chemical ablation of the lesion.

www.unos.org policy 3.6.4.4. 2006.

UNOS has defined the criteria for the diagnosis of HCC for the purpose of listing and to receive additional bonus points. HCC could be diagnosed on the basis of imaging, and histological confirmation is not mandatory if patients fulfill the following criteria. The patient must also have one of the following: biopsy-proven HCC, a tumor-associated vascular blush seen on imaging, alpha-fetoprotein (AFP) level greater than 200 ng/ml, angiogram confirming a tumor or chemoembolization, radiofrequency ablation or cryoablation of a suspicious hepatic lesion (35, 36). Extra-hepatic disease should be excluded by lung imaging (CT or MRI) and bone scans. Patients who have tumors that do not meet the aforementioned criteria receive no additional priority and must be listed based on MELD score.

The UNOS criteria designed to make the diagnosis of HCC are not without controversy. In a review of the UNOS database, 165 (21%) of 789 patients transplanted for HCC (and who fulfilled the UNOS criteria) between April 2003 and November 2005 did not actually have HCC on examination of the explanted liver (38). Small lesions (<2 cm) were particularly hard to differentiate from regenerating or dysplastic nodules, hemangiomas, cysts, granulomas, adenomas or other benign lesions (38). These results suggest that the specificity of preoperative imaging for the diagnosis of small HCC (<2 cm) is unacceptable, and these observations support the current UNOS policy of giving no priority to lesions less than 2 cm. In order to increase the pretransplant diagnostic accuracy, some authors advocate that all suspicious hepatic lesions should be biopsied (36), but this practice is also controversial. There is a remote (0.003%–0.009%) risk of biopsy tract seeding by tumor cells, although patient outcome is typically not affected (39–41). The risk of bleeding after a tumor biopsy exists. The diagnostic accuracy of small lesions has been questioned (42); however, an analysis of 294 hepatic lesions less than 2 cm revealed that fine-needle biopsy had a diagnostic accuracy of approximately 90% (43). Based on the current evidence, if imaging characteristics are typical (early wash out), or two separate imaging modalities are suggestive of HCC, or AFP is greater than 400 ng/ml, there is no reason to biopsy the lesion. Although not necessary for listing purposes, the authors recommend histological confirmation of suspicious lesions when a diagnosis cannot be firmly established.

TUMOR PROGRESSION WHILE ON THE WAITING LIST

A tremendous source of anxiety, not unfounded, for patients and caregivers alike is the risk of tumor progression while on the waiting list for liver transplantation. Although organ shortage varies among transplant centers and regions, wait times can range from weeks to months. As of January 2007, there were 16,993 patients awaiting liver transplant in the United States. In 2003–2004, the median wait time for a patient with a MELD score of 19 to 24 was 105 days (44). While a patient is on the waiting list, there is a risk of tumor progression beyond the limits of the Milan Criteria, decompensation of liver disease, or development of other co-morbidities that may be a contraindication for transplant. Annual dropout rates while on the waiting list are approximately 25% to 50%, depending upon geographical location (12, 45, 46). Since the implementation of the MELD exception (bonus) points for patients with HCC, the probability of being transplanted for a Stage 2 tumor within 6 months is 70% (47). From an intention-to-treat perspective, survival of patients with HCC is reduced because of dropouts from the waiting list due to death or tumor progression (48). Overall survival at 5 years is reduced from 81% to 58%, to 62% to 47% for waiting times of 6 to 12 months, with dropouts as high as 30% (49).

An analysis of the UNOS database revealed that the independent risk factors for HCC candidates dropping off the waiting list are maximum tumor size, advanced age, AFP level and MELD score at listing (50). Tumor size has been shown to predict progression and removal from transplant lists in several studies (51). Specifically, Yao and colleagues reported that tumors greater than 3 cm are nine times as likely to progress than smaller tumors (53). It is reasonable to assume that this progression risk increases linearly with increasing tumor size. This is another argument against expanding the current size criteria for liver transplantation. Tumors that increase in size rapidly may have unfavorable tumor biology and hence may not have the optimal outcome if transplanted.

AFP is used to screen for HCC in high-risk populations and has served as a diagnostic test for HCC since the 1970s (54). Other studies have confirmed that serum AFP is a marker for rapid tumor progression and dropout from the waiting list (12, 52).

Interestingly, it is not the AFP level per se; rather it is the slope by which the AFP increases that predicts rapid tumor progression (50).

There two mechanisms by which the risk of tumor progression may be reduced or eliminated. One method to abrogate tumor progression is the use of local, neo-adjuvant therapies such as transarterial chemoembolization (TACE) or radiofrequency ablation (RFA). These treatment modalities may also be used to potentially downsize tumors to within acceptable limits. Second, increasing the pool of donor organs, thereby reducing wait times, is another rational solution. This may be accomplished by the use of so-called extended criteria grafts, split-liver transplantation and living donor transplantation.

LOCALIZED THERAPY FOR HCC

Systemic chemotherapy is ineffective for HCC (11, 55). Response rates range from 10% to 20% with no survival benefit (56). Because of this, locoregional therapy has become the standard of care for the palliative treatment of patients with unresectable HCC. TACE involves the local delivery of embolic agents, iodized oil and chemotherapeutic drugs directly into tumor tissue (57). TACE is effective because the vessels feeding the tumors are embolized; therefore, the chemotherapeutic agents remain in contact with the tumor cells for a prolonged time. Numerous observational studies demonstrate the ability of TACE or RFA to induce widespread tumor necrosis and prevent tumor progression in HCC (1, 58, 59). However, it is difficult to draw meaningful conclusions from these studies due to the heterogeneity of the patient population, the variable evaluation of treatment response and differences in waiting list dropout criteria among centers. In most studies, an effective response to TACE or RFA is defined as greater that 50% tumor necrosis on pathologic examination. Tumor necrosis may also be estimated by radiological examination such as diffusion MRI; however, there is often discordance between the radiology and the histology. For example, one study using RFA found 70% necrosis by CT but only 55% tissue destruction by histology. Response rates for RFA range from 12% to 55% and 22% to 29% for TACE (12). A combination of therapies results in pathological responses up to 66%. The best results for either modality are achieved in tumors less than 3 cm. Patients with smaller tumors, however, are least likely to benefit from adjuvant therapy

as most of them are unlikely to drop out because of tumor progression.

Tumor progression on the transplant list represents a major cause of mortality for these patients. Thus, the use of neo-adjuvant therapy to delay tumor progression is a logical treatment strategy, but controlled data are lacking, and circumstantial evidence is conflicting. Some studies demonstrate that among patients who meet the Milan Criteria and are treated with neo-adjuvant therapy, there is almost no patient dropout at 6 months. However, in similar patient populations, another center reported a 15% and 25% dropout rate at 6 and 12 months, respectively. In patients who were beyond the Milan Criteria treated with TACE, Roayaie et al. (60) described a dropout rate of 46%, with nearly a third due to tumor progression. Recurrence and disease-free survival in neo-adjuvantly treated patients who received a liver transplant depend upon tumor stage rather than treatment response. Controlled studies are necessary before neo-adjuvant therapy is routinely recommended.

Another rational utilization of TACE or RFA is in an attempt to downsize tumors such that they fulfill the Milan Criteria. In the seminal study from researchers in France, 54 patients with tumors were treated with TACE prior to transplantation. TACE shrank the tumor in 19 (54%) of the 35 patients with tumors greater than 3 cm, and complete necrosis was found in 15 (28%) of the 54 patients. Five-year disease-free survival was 71% in patients who responded to TACE versus 29% in patients who had an incomplete response (p = 0.01.) Other studies have failed to demonstrate such positive survival benefit with TACE or RFA, although one study reported a 2-year survival of greater than 80% in a group of 16 patients whose tumors were successfully downsized to within acceptable limits, but the long-term disease-free survival was not reported. There is no randomized controlled trial or cohort study specifically designed to support the use of preoperative neo-adjuvant treatments in order to downsize tumors to within the Milan Criteria. The results of the existing studies, although compelling, are inconsistent and cannot justify the use of neo-adjuvant therapies in this manner.

Neo-adjuvant treatments are interventional procedures that are performed on chronically ill patients, and therefore there are considerable risks associated with these procedures. Major complications to consider are bleeding, peritonitis, biliary strictures and death from liver failure. The major complication rate for these adjuvant treatments is approximately 4% to 8%, and in one study, treatment-related death due to liver failure after TACE was 2.5%. Anecdotal reports have suggested that TACE may also increase the risk of hepatic artery thrombosis, and RFA may be associated with needle-track seeding of tumor cells.

EXTENDED CRITERIA GRAFTS

The ideal liver transplant donor is a relatively young healthy individual who is declared brain dead through some set of unfortunate circumstances. In this situation, the liver is adequately perfused by the heart until harvesting. The expansion of liver transplant lists and the concomitant lack of sufficient numbers of donor organs has led some transplant centers to experiment with so-called extended criteria grafts, such as livers from non-heart-beating donors, hepatitis B core antibody-positive donors, hepatitis C-positive donors, donors with a body mass index greater than 30, or older donors. Several centers have reported promising results – that is, equivalent survival and decreased waiting time – with the aggressive acceptance of extended criteria grafts. However, non-heart-beating donors may be troublesome because of the "warm" ischemia time – that is, the time that the liver remains in the donor after the heart has stopped. After transplantation, recipients of non-heart-beating donors have an increased risk of biliary complications due to ischemic cholangiopathy.

LIVING DONOR LIVER TRANSPLANTATION

Living donor liver transplantation has emerged as a potential treatment strategy for patients with HCC (15). In fact, live donor transplantation may be an excellent strategy to increase the donor pool and offer patients with HCC a potential cure (11). Transplant programs that have the most experience with this surgery are in Far-East Asia, where deceased organs are unavailable for social and cultural reasons. The surgery involves the resection of the right or left lobe of the donor liver and transplantation into a recipient matched by blood type and body habitus. Results from Asia and Europe indicate that the outcome after live donor transplantation for patients with HCC is similar to deceased donation. In one of the largest series, Todo et al. from Japan reported the outcomes of living donor liver transplantation in 316 patients with HCC.

Of these, 137 patients were within the Milan Criteria and others were outside the Milan Criteria. The recurrence rate was only 1.4% for those within Milan Criteria and 22.2% for those outside Milan Criteria; 3-year survival rates were 79% and 60% respectively for the groups. Complications, however, may occur in 20% to 40% of donors, and the mortality risk for the donor could be as high as 0.5% (11). Therefore, the decision to proceed with live donation must involve the risk of dropout while waiting, the length of waiting time, the 5-year recipient survival, and the risk to the donor (11). In addition, the procedure itself is more complex than deceased transplantation, and to reduce morbidity and mortality, only experienced surgeons should attempt it. Because live donation offers the chance of transplant when preoperative staging is recent, some authors propose expanding the inclusion tumor criteria. However, this issue involves a controversial interplay between the medical community and donor autonomy, and there currently are insufficient data to expand the Milan Criteria for live donation.

POST-TRANSPLANT MANAGEMENT

Other than anti-viral therapies, there is no effective intervention or management to prevent tumor recurrence after transplantation. Patients with hepatitis B can be successfully managed with nucleoside or nucleotide analogues and hepatitis B immunoglobulin. The treatment and prevention of recurrent hepatitis C remains a major problem, and cirrhosis may occur in the transplanted liver in less than 5 years.

Any patient with hepatoma found on explant requires careful surveillance with serial AFP levels and radiological examinations. Patients with large tumor size (>5 cm), vascular invasion and poorly differentiated tumors are at highest risk for tumor recurrence. Our center performs either serum AFP and CT or MRI of the chest and abdomen every 3 months post-transplant for the first year, and then every 6 months thereafter. The time of HCC recurrence is generally early, with most occurring within the first 2 years after liver transplant and the median time being approximately 1 to 1.5 years. Recurrence may occur in the liver, lungs, bone or elsewhere. Surgical resection and adjuvant therapies may be employed to help control tumor growth, but 5-year survival post liver transplant in patients with recurrence is approximately 25%. There are no data in favor of any specific immunosuppression regimen in order to diminish recurrence risk (11). Finally, careful management of post-transplant diabetes mellitus and obesity are important, as these factors are associated with an increase risk of de novo HCC.

NEW FRONTIERS

A fundamental problem with liver transplantation for HCC is that, despite our best current techniques, we are unable to predict which patient has the lowest risk of tumor recurrence after transplant. Even with the strict adherence to the Milan Criteria, up to 10% of patients will have recurrent tumors at 5 years (11). Advances in genomic research may help to develop a molecular signature that can be used to ascertain recurrence risk. For example, the Barcelona liver group found that the reduced expression of the cell cycle inhibitor $p27$ was an independent predictor of recurrence after surgical resection. In addition, another study demonstrated that the detection of the fractional allelic loss rate of a panel of nine microsatellites predicted the recurrence of HCC better than vascular invasion. With the unraveling of the human genome, we should anticipate an explosion of new molecular information to help diagnoses and management of HCC.

Chemotherapeutic agents can only be expected to improve with time as well. Recently, the U.S. Food and Drug Administration (FDA) has approved an oral drug, sorafenib, for the management of HCC. Sorafenib acts by inhibiting multiple tyrosine kinases that are involved in the signaling pathway of HCC. More biologic therapies specifically designed to attack HCC tumor cells are likely in the near future. As an example, researchers from China have developed a novel murine monoclonal antibody labeled with radioactive iodine and targeted against Hab18G/CD147, which is a common antigen seen in HCC. In this study, patients outside the Milan criteria were transplanted and randomized to treatment with this drug, Licartin or placebo. After 1 year, the treatment group enjoyed a 20% increase in survival and 30% decrease in recurrence compared with the placebo group. Clearly, these results must be validated on a larger scale, but these results are encouraging.

CONCLUSION

Liver transplantation is the optimal treatment in patients with advanced cirrhosis and small HCC, with survival rates similar to those transplanted without HCC. With adherence to strict selection criteria, 5-year survival rates are approximately 70% and tumor recurrence rates are approximately 10%. Shortage of donor organs and a long waiting period, which allow progression of both the tumor as well as the underlying liver disease, are two major limiting factors. In addition, several issues, including optimal selection criteria and the role of preoperative neoadjuvant treatment, remain unresolved. Finally, novel molecular information may lead to improved early detection of HCC or prediction of recurrence, and hence a better outcome for patients with HCC.

REFERENCES

1. Mazzaferro V, Regalia E, Doci R, et al. Liver transplantation for the treatment of small hepatocellular carcinomas in patients with cirrhosis. N Engl J Med 1996; 334: 693–699.
2. Molmenti EP, Klintmalm GB. Liver transplantation in association with hepatocellular carcinoma: An update of the International Tumor Registry. Liver Transpl 2002; 8: 736–748.
3. Figueras J, Jaurrieta E, Valls C, et al. Survival after liver transplantation in cirrhotic patients with and without hepatocellular carcinoma: A comparative study. Hepatology 1997; 25: 1485–1489.
4. Yoo HY, Patt CH, Geschwind JF, et al. The outcome of liver transplantation in patients with hepatocellular carcinoma in the United States between 1988 and 2001: 5-year survival has improved significantly with time. J Clin Oncol 2003; 21: 4329–4335.
5. Hemming AW, Cattral MS, Reed AI, et al. Liver transplantation for hepatocellular carcinoma. Ann Surg 2001; 233: 652–659.
6. El-Serag HB. Hepatocellular carcinoma: Recent trends in the United States. Gastroenterology 2004; 127: S27–34.
7. Iwatsuki S, Gordon RD, Shaw BW, Jr., et al. Role of liver transplantation in cancer therapy. Ann Surg 1985; 202: 401–407.
8. Bismuth H, Chiche L, Adam R, et al. Liver resection versus transplantation for hepatocellular carcinoma in cirrhotic patients. Ann Surg 1993; 218: 145–151.
9. Bismuth H, Chiche L, Adam R, et al. Surgical treatment of hepatocellular carcinoma in cirrhosis: Liver resection or transplantation? Transplant Proc 1993; 25: 1066–1067.
10. Jonas S, Herrmann M, Rayes N, et al. Survival after liver transplantation for hepatocellular carcinoma in cirrhosis according to the underlying liver disease. Transplant Proc 2001; 33: 3444–3445.
11. Bruix J, Sherman M. Management of hepatocellular carcinoma. Hepatology 2005; 42: 1208–1236.
12. Llovet JM, Fuster J, Bruix J. Intention-to-treat analysis of surgical treatment for early hepatocellular carcinoma: Resection versus transplantation. Hepatology 1999; 30: 1434–1440.
13. Jonas S, Bechstein WO, Steinmuller T, et al. Vascular invasion and histopathologic grading determine outcome

after liver transplantation for hepatocellular carcinoma in cirrhosis. Hepatology 2001; 33: 1080–1086.

14. Yao FY, Ferrell L, Bass NM, et al. Liver transplantation for hepatocellular carcinoma: Expansion of the tumor size limits does not adversely impact survival. Hepatology 2001; 33: 1394–1403.

15. Patt CH, Thuluvath PJ. Role of liver transplantation in the management of hepatocellular carcinoma. J Vasc Interv Radiol 2002; 13: S205–210.

16. Llovet JM, Bruix J, Fuster J, et al. Liver transplantation for small hepatocellular carcinoma: The tumor-node-metastasis classification does not have prognostic power. Hepatology 1998; 27: 1572–1577.

17. Bechstein WO, Guckelberger O, Kling N, et al. Recurrence-free survival after liver transplantation for small hepatocellular carcinoma. Transpl Int 1998; 11 Suppl 1: S189–192.

18. Bismuth H, Majno PE, Adam R. Liver transplantation for hepatocellular carcinoma. Semin Liver Dis 1999; 19: 311–322.

19. Hsu HC, Wu TT, Wu MZ, et al. Tumor invasiveness and prognosis in resected hepatocellular carcinoma: Clinical and pathogenetic implications. Cancer 1988; 61: 2095–2099.

20. Zavaglia C, De Carlis L, Alberti AB, et al. Predictors of long-term survival after liver transplantation for hepatocellular carcinoma. Am J Gastroenterol 2005; 100: 2708–2716.

21. Sahani D, Saini S, Pena C, et al. Using multidetector CT for preoperative vascular evaluation of liver neoplasms: Technique and results. AJR Am J Roentgenol 2002; 179: 53–59.

22. Poon RT, Ho JW, Tong CS, et al. Prognostic significance of serum vascular endothelial growth factor and endostatin in patients with hepatocellular carcinoma. Br J Surg 2004; 91: 1354–1360.

23. Poon RT, Ng IO, Lau C, et al. Serum vascular endothelial growth factor predicts venous invasion in hepatocellular carcinoma: A prospective study. Ann Surg 2001; 233: 227–235.

24. Yuki K, Hirohashi S, Sakamoto M, et al. Growth and spread of hepatocellular carcinoma: A review of 240 consecutive autopsy cases. Cancer 1990; 66: 2174–2179.

25. Cillo U, Vitale A, Bassanello M, et al. Liver transplantation for the treatment of moderately or well-differentiated hepatocellular carcinoma. Ann Surg 2004; 239: 150–159.

26. Wayne JD, Lauwers GY, Ikai I, et al. Preoperative predictors of survival after resection of small hepatocellular carcinomas. Ann Surg 2002; 235: 722–730; discussion 730–721.

27. Klintmalm GB. Liver transplantation for hepatocellular carcinoma: A registry report of the impact of tumor characteristics on outcome. Ann Surg 1998; 228: 479–490.

28. Tamura S, Kato T, Berho M, et al. Impact of histological grade of hepatocellular carcinoma on the outcome of liver transplantation. Arch Surg 2001; 136: 25–30; discussion 31.

29. Kojiro M. Histopathology of liver cancers. Best Pract Res Clin Gastroenterol 2005; 19: 39–62.

30. Chapoutot C, Perney P, Fabre D, et al. Needle-tract seeding after ultrasound-guided puncture of hepatocellular carcinoma. A study of 150 patients. Gastroenterol Clin Biol 1999; 23: 552–556.

31. Marsh JW, Dvorchik I. Liver organ allocation for hepatocellular carcinoma: Are we sure? Liver Transpl 2003; 9: 693–696.

32. Bruix J, Fuster J, Llovet JM. Liver transplantation for hepatocellular carcinoma: Foucault pendulum versus evidence-based decision. Liver Transpl 2003; 9: 700–702.

33. Libbrecht L, Bielen D, Verslype C, et al. Focal lesions in cirrhotic explant livers: Pathological evaluation and accuracy of pretransplantation imaging examinations. Liver Transpl 2002; 8: 749–761.

34. Burrel M, Llovet JM, Ayuso C, et al. MRI angiography is superior to helical CT for detection of HCC prior to liver transplantation: An explant correlation. Hepatology 2003; 38: 1034–1042.

35. Freeman RB, Jr., Wiesner RH, Harper A, et al. The new liver allocation system: Moving toward evidence-based transplantation policy. Liver Transpl 2002; 8: 851–858.

36. Marsh JW, Dvorchik I. Should we biopsy each liver mass suspicious for hepatocellular carcinoma before liver transplantation? –Yes. J Hepatol 2005; 43: 558–562.

37. www.unos.org policy 3.6.4.4. 2006.

38. Freeman RB, Mithoefer A, Ruthazer R, et al. Optimizing staging for hepatocellular carcinoma before liver transplantation: A retrospective analysis of the UNOS/OPTN database. Liver Transpl 2006; 12: 1504–1511.

39. Smith EH. Complications of percutaneous abdominal fine-needle biopsy [review]. Radiology 1991; 178: 253–258.

40. Schotman SN, De Man RA, Stoker J, et al. Subcutaneous seeding of hepatocellular carcinoma after percutaneous needle biopsy. Gut 1999; 45: 626–627.

41. Huang GT, Sheu JC, Yang PM, et al. Ultrasound-guided cutting biopsy for the diagnosis of hepatocellular carcinoma – a study based on 420 patients. J Hepatol 1996; 25: 334–338.

42. Bruix J, Sherman M, Llovet JM, et al. Clinical management of hepatocellular carcinoma: Conclusions of the Barcelona-2000 EASL conference, European Association for the Study of the Liver. J Hepatol 2001; 35: 421–430.

43. Caturelli E, Solmi L, Anti M, et al. Ultrasound guided fine-needle biopsy of early hepatocellular carcinoma complicating liver cirrhosis: A multicentre study. Gut 2004; 53: 1356–1362.

44. www.unos.org. 2006

45. Everhart JE, Lombardero M, Detre KM, et al. Increased waiting time for liver transplantation results in higher mortality. Transplantation 1997; 64: 1300–1306.

46. Roayaie S, Haim MB, Emre S, et al. Comparison of surgical outcomes for hepatocellular carcinoma in patients with hepatitis B versus hepatitis C: A Western experience. Ann Surg Oncol 2000; 7: 764–770.

47. Yao FY, Bass NM, Ascher NL, et al. Liver transplantation for hepatocellular carcinoma: Lessons from the first year under the Model of End-Stage Liver Disease (MELD) organ allocation policy. Liver Transpl 2004; 10: 621–630.

48. Arii S, Yamaoka Y, Futagawa S, The Liver Cancer Study Group of Japan, et al. Results of surgical and nonsurgical treatment for small-sized hepatocellular carcinomas: A retrospective and nationwide survey in Japan. Hepatology 2000; 32: 1224–1229.

49. Llovet JM, Schwartz M, Mazzaferro V. Resection and liver transplantation for hepatocellular carcinoma. Semin Liver Dis 2005; 25: 181–200.

50. Freeman RB, Edwards EB, Harper AM. Waiting list removal rates among patients with chronic and malignant liver diseases. Am J Transplant 2006; 6: 1416–1421.

51. Yao FY, Bass NM, Nikolai B, et al. Liver transplantation for hepatocellular carcinoma: Analysis of survival according to the intention-to-treat principle and dropout from the waiting list. Liver Transpl 2002; 8: 873–883.

52. Shetty K, Timmins K, Brensinger C, et al. Liver transplantation for hepatocellular carcinoma validation of present selection criteria in predicting outcome. Liver Transpl 2004; 10: 911–918.

53. Yao FY, Bass NM, Nikolai B, et al. A follow-up analysis of the pattern and predictors of dropout from the waiting list for liver transplantation in patients with hepatocellular carcinoma: Implications for the current organ allocation policy. Liver Transpl 2003; 9: 684–692.

54. Bellet DH, Wands JR, Isselbacher KJ, et al. Serum alpha-fetoprotein levels in human disease: Perspective from a highly specific monoclonal radioimmunoassay. Proc Natl Acad Sci USA 1984; 81: 3869–3873.

55. Holman M, Harrison D, Stewart A, et al. Neoadjuvant chemotherapy and orthotopic liver transplantation for hepatocellular carcinoma. NJ Med 1995; 92: 519–522.

56. Venook AP, Stagg RJ, Lewis BJ, et al. Chemoembolization for hepatocellular carcinoma. J Clin Oncol 1990; 8: 1108–1114.

57. Geschwind JF, Ramsey DE, Choti MA, et al. Chemoembolization of hepatocellular carcinoma: Results of a meta-analysis. Am J Clin Oncol 2003; 26: 344–349.

58. Geschwind JF: Interventional radiology. In: DeVita VT RS, Hellman S, (eds). Cancer, Principles and Practice of Oncology, 6th edition, pp. 32–49. Philadelphia: JB Lippincott, Williams & Wilkins 2001.

59. Stone MJ, Klintmalm GB, Polter D, et al. Neoadjuvant chemotherapy and liver transplantation for hepatocellular carcinoma: A pilot study in 20 patients. Gastroenterology 1993; 104: 196–202.

60. Roayaie S, Frischer JS, Emre SH, et al. Long-term results with multimodal adjuvant therapy and liver transplantation for the treatment of hepatocellular carcinomas larger than 5 centimeters. Ann Surg 2002; 235: 533–539.

Chapter 14

IMAGE-GUIDED ABLATION OF HEPATOCELLULAR CARCINOMA

Riccardo Lencioni

Laura Crocetti

Clotilde Della Pina

Dania Cioni

Hepatocellular carcinoma (HCC) is increasingly diagnosed at an early, asymptomatic stage owing to surveillance of high-risk patients. Patients with early stage HCC require careful diagnostic and therapeutic management. Diagnostic confirmation of small nodules detected in cirrhotic livers may be challenging. It is very difficult to distinguish well-differentiated tumors from non-malignant hepatocellular nodules on biopsy specimens. Careful assessment of lesion vascularity – through the use of state-of-the-art dynamic imaging techniques – can provide a reliable non-invasive diagnosis. Given the complexity of the disease, multidisciplinary assessment of tumor stage, liver function and physical status is required for proper therapeutic planning. Patients with early stage HCC should be considered for any of the available curative therapies, including surgical resection, liver transplantation and percutaneous image-guided ablation. Resection is currently indicated among patients with solitary HCC and extremely well-preserved liver function, who have neither clinically significant portal hypertension nor abnormal bilirubin. Liver transplantation benefits patients who have decompensated cirrhosis and one tumor smaller than 5 cm or up to three nodules smaller than 3 cm, but donor shortage greatly limits its applicability.

This difficulty might be overcome by living donation; that, however, is still at an early stage of clinical application. Image-guided percutaneous ablation is the best therapeutic choice for nonsurgical patients with early stage HCC. Although ethanol injection has been the seminal percutaneous technique, radiofrequency ablation has emerged as the most effective method for local tumor destruction and is currently used as the primary ablative modality at most institutions.

Hepatocellular carcinoma (HCC) is the fifth most common cause of cancer, and its incidence is increasing worldwide because of the dissemination of hepatitis B and C virus infection (1, 2). Patients with cirrhosis are at the highest risk of developing HCC and should be monitored every 6 months to diagnose the tumor at an asymptomatic stage (2). Lesions detected by surveillance require proper diagnostic approach. In fact, diagnostic confirmation of small nodules as true HCC may be challenging, as pathologic changes inherent in cirrhosis – such as dysplastic nodule (DN) – mimic a small tumor (3). Treatment choice is also difficult, given the complexity of the disease and the large number of potentially useful therapies, and requires careful multidisciplinary assessment of tumor stage, liver function and physical status (4–6).

PRETREATMENT EVALUATION

Imaging Assessment

In the setting of a patient with known hepatitis B or cirrhosis of other etiology, a solid nodular lesion found during surveillance has a high likelihood of being HCC. However, it has been shown by pathologic studies that many small nodules detected in cirrhotic livers do not correspond to HCC (7). The differential diagnosis between small HCC and non-malignant hepatocellular lesions may be very challenging. Percutaneous image-guided biopsy could appear as the most straightforward approach. Unfortunately, biopsy of small nodular lesions in cirrhosis is not entirely reliable. In fact, needle placement may be difficult, and a sampling error may occur. Moreover, it is very difficult to distinguish HCC from DN on small biopsy specimens, as there is no clear-cut dividing line between dysplasia and well-differentiated tumor. Therefore, a positive biopsy – as assessed by an expert pathologist – is helpful, but a negative biopsy can never be taken as a criterion to rule out malignancy (5, 6). In addition, biopsy is associated with a low – but not negligible – rate of complications, including tumor seeding along the needle track.

Current guidelines recommend further investigation of nodules detected during surveillance with dynamic imaging techniques – including contrast-enhanced ultrasound, contrast-enhanced multi-detector computed tomography (CT) and contrast-enhanced magnetic resonance imaging (MRI) (5, 6). In fact, one of the key pathologic factors for differential diagnosis that is reflected in dynamic imaging studies is the vascular supply to the lesion. Through the progression from regenerative nodule, to low-grade DN, to high-grade DN, to frank HCC, one sees loss of visualization of portal tracts and development of new arterial vessels, termed **nontriadal arteries,** which become the dominant blood supply in overt HCC lesions (3). It is this neovascularity that allows HCC to be diagnosed and is the key for imaging cirrhotic patients.

A rational diagnostic protocol should be structured according to the actual risk of malignancy and the possibility of achieving a reliable diagnosis. Because the prevalence of HCC among ultrasound-detected nodules is strongly related to the size of the lesion, the diagnostic work-up depends on the size of the lesion (6). Lesions smaller than 1 cm in diameter have a low likelihood of being HCC. However, minute hepatic nodules detected by ultrasound may become malignant over time. Therefore, these nodules need to be followed-up in order to detect growth suggestive of malignant transformation. A reasonable protocol is to repeat ultrasound every 3 months, until the lesion grows to more than 1 cm, at which point additional diagnostic techniques are applied (5). It has to be emphasized, however, that the absence of growth during the follow-up period does not rule out the malignant nature of the nodule because even an early HCC may take more than 1 year to increase in size (5). When the nodule exceeds 1 cm in size, the lesion is more likely to be HCC and diagnostic confirmation should be pursued. It is accepted that the diagnosis of HCC can be made without biopsy in a nodule larger than 1 cm that shows characteristic vascular features of HCC – i.e., arterial hypervascularization with washout in the portal venous or delayed phase – even in patients with normal alpha-fetoprotein value. Such lesions should be treated as HCC because the positive predictive value of the clinical and radiological findings exceeds 95%, provided that examinations are conducted by using state-of-the-art equipment and interpreted by radiologists with extensive expertise in liver imaging (8). For lesions ranging 1 cm to 2 cm, current guidelines recommend that typical imaging findings are confirmed by two coincident dynamic imaging modalities to allow a non-invasive diagnosis (6). If the imaging findings are not characteristic or the vascular profile is not coincidental between techniques, biopsy is recommended (6). For nodules >2 cm, a single imaging technique – out of contrast-enhanced ultrasound, contrast-enhanced multi-detector CT and contrast-enhanced MRI – showing the characteristic vascular profile of HCC mentioned earlier, may confidently establish the diagnosis (6).

It has to be pointed out that non-invasive criteria based on imaging findings can be applied only in patients with established cirrhosis (5). For nodules detected in non-cirrhotic livers, as well as for those showing atypical vascular patterns, biopsy is recommended. Although ultrasound is widely accepted for HCC surveillance, multi-detector CT or dynamic MRI is required for intrahepatic staging of the disease, as these examinations provide a comprehensive assessment of the liver parenchyma and can identify additional tumor foci.

Clinical Staging

In most solid malignancies, tumor stage at presentation determines prognosis and treatment management. Most patients with HCC, however, have two diseases – liver cirrhosis and HCC – and complex interactions between the two have major implications for prognosis and treatment choice (9). Therefore, the tumor-node-metastasis (TNM) system has limited usefulness in the clinical decision-making process because it does not take into account hepatic functional status. Several scoring systems have been developed in the past few years in attempts to stratify patients according to expected survival. However, the only system that links staging with treatment modalities is the Barcelona Clinic Liver Cancer (BCLC) staging system (4, 10).

The BCLC includes variables related to tumor stage, liver functional status, physical status and cancer-related symptoms and provides an estimation of life expectancy that is based on published response rates to the various treatments. In the BCLC system, early stage HCC includes patients with World Health Organization (WHO) performance status of 0, preserved liver function (Child-Pugh class A or B), and solitary tumor or up to three nodules smaller than 3 cm in size each, in the absence of macroscopic vascular invasion and extrahepatic spread. If the patient has Child-Pugh class A cirrhosis and a solitary tumor smaller than 2 cm in size, the stage may be defined as very early. Patients with multi-nodular HCC with neither vascular invasion nor extrahepatic spread are classified as intermediate-stage according to the BCLC staging system, provided that they have a performance status of 0 and Child-Pugh class A or B cirrhosis (3). Patients with portal vein invasion or extrahepatic disease are classified as advanced stage. The terminal stage includes patients who have either severe hepatic decompensation (Child-Pugh class C) or performance status greater than 2.

TRIAGE OF EARLY STAGE HEPATOCELLULAR CARCINOMA

Patients with early stage HCC can benefit from curative therapies, including surgical resection, liver transplantation and percutaneous ablation, and have the possibility of long-term cure, with 5-year survival figures ranging from 50% to 75% (6). However, there is no firm evidence to establish the optimal first-line treatment for early-stage HCC because of the lack of randomized controlled trials (RCTs) comparing radical therapies. Patients should be evaluated in referral centers by multi-disciplinary teams involving hepatologists, oncologists, interventional radiologists, surgeons, and pathologists to guarantee careful selection of candidates for each treatment option and to ensure the expert application of these treatments (6).

Surgical Resection

Resection is the treatment of choice for HCC in non-cirrhotic patients, who account for about 5% of the cases in Western countries. However, in patients with cirrhosis, candidates for resection have to be carefully selected to reduce the risk of postoperative liver failure. It has been shown that a normal bilirubin concentration and the absence of clinically significant portal hypertension are the best predictors of excellent outcomes after surgery (11). In experienced hands, such patients have treatment-related mortality of less than 1% to 3% and may achieve a 5-year survival higher than 70% (11–13). In contrast, survival drops to less than 50% at 5 years in patients with significant portal hypertension, and to less than 30% at 5 years in those with both adverse factors (portal hypertension and elevated bilirubin) (11). Most groups restrict the indication for resection to patients with single tumor in a suitable location. Anatomic resections – guided by intraoperative ultrasound techniques – are preferred to wedge resections as they include any microsatellite lesions possibly located in the same hepatic segment as the main tumor. In fact, it is known that neoplastic dissemination occurs at very early stages in HCC via the invasion of small peripheral portal vein branches (7). After resection, tumor recurrence rate exceeds 70% at 5 years, including recurrence due to dissemination and de novo tumors developing in the remnant cirrhotic liver. The most powerful predictors of recurrence are the presence of microvascular invasion and/or additional tumor sites besides the primary lesion (11).

Liver Transplantation

Liver transplantation is the only option that provides cure of both the tumor and the underlying chronic liver disease. It is recognized as the best treatment for patients with solitary HCC smaller than 5 cm in the setting of decompensated cirrhosis and for those with early multi-focal disease (up to three lesions, none larger than 3 cm) (1). However, for patients with a solitary small tumor in well-compensated cirrhosis, the optimal treatment strategy is still under debate (14). The reported outcomes of patients who actually underwent transplantation are better than those of patients submitted to resection, especially if the substantially lower rates of tumor recurrence – less than 10% to 20% at 5 years – are considered (14). Overall survival, however, decreases on an intention-to-treat perspective (11, 14–16). In fact, because of the lack of sufficient liver donation, there is always a waiting period between listing and transplantation, during which the tumor may grow and develop contraindications to transplantation (vascular invasion, extrahepatic spread). The rate of dropouts may be as high as 25% if the waiting list is longer than 12 months (17). Most groups perform interventional treatments – including transarterial chemoembolization (TACE) and percutaneous ablation – to achieve local control of the tumor during the waiting time. Living donor liver transplantation is a viable option to expand the number of available livers. However, it requires a highly skilled group of senior liver surgeons, increases surgery-related morbidity and carries the risk of donor mortality. In addition, the applicability of the technique is low, and only about one-fourth of potential recipients eventually undergo the procedure (14).

Image-guided Ablation

Image-guided percutaneous ablation is currently accepted as the best therapeutic choice for non-surgical patients with early stage HCC (5, 6). Over the past two decades, several methods for chemical ablation or thermal tumor destruction through localized heating or freezing have been developed and clinically tested (Table 14.1). Whereas chemical and hypertermic ablation techniques have been widely performed

TABLE 14.1 Percutaneous Methods for Ablation of Hepatocellular Carcinoma

Chemical ablation
Ethanol injection
Acetic acid injection
Thermal ablation
Radiofrequency ablation
Microwave ablation
Laser ablation
Cryoablation

via a percutaneous approach, most of the experience with cryotherapy in HCC has involved an open or laparoscopic approach. Recently, following technological advances, percutaneous ablation has also been used to treat selected patients with intermediate-stage tumors, especially in combination with TACE.

CHEMICAL ABLATION

The seminal technique used for local ablation of HCC is percutaneous ethanol injection (PEI). Ethanol induces coagulation necrosis of the lesion as a result of cellular dehydration, protein denaturation and chemical occlusion of small tumor vessels. PEI is a well-established technique for the treatment of nodular-type HCC. HCC nodules have a soft consistency and are surrounded by a firm cirrhotic liver. Consequently, injected ethanol diffuses within them easily and selectively, leading to complete necrosis of about 70% of small lesions (18). An alternate method for chemical ablation is acetic acid injection. Although acetic acid injection has been reported to increase the success rate of PEI, this technique has been used by very few investigators worldwide.

Ethanol Injection

PEI is best administered by using ultrasound guidance because ultrasound allows for continuous real-time monitoring of the injection. This is crucial to realize the pattern of tumor perfusion and to avoid excessive ethanol leakage outside the lesion. Fine non-cutting needles, with either a single end hole or multiple side holes, are commonly used for PEI. PEI is usually performed under local anesthesia and does not require patient hospitalization. The treatment schedule includes four to six sessions performed once or twice weekly. The number of treatment sessions, as well as the amount of injected ethanol per session, may vary greatly according to the size of the lesion, the pattern of tumor perfusion and the compliance of the patient. Recently, multi-pronged injection needles that allow single-session PEI treatment have been introduced in clinical practice (Figure 14.1).

Although there have not been any RCTs comparing PEI and best supportive care or PEI and surgical resection, several retrospective studies have provided indirect evidence that PEI improves the natural history of HCC: the long-term outcomes of patients with small tumors who were treated with PEI were similar to those reported in surgical series, with 5-year

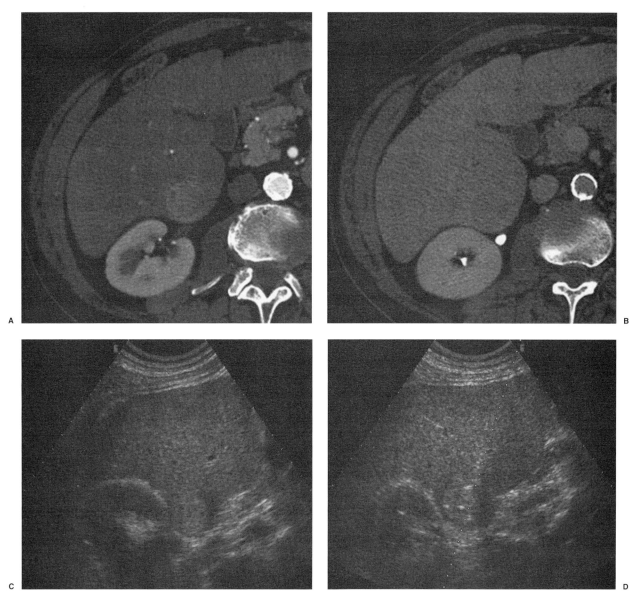

FIGURE 14.1.   Complete response of hepatocellular carcinoma after percutaneous ethanol injection. Pretreatment CT (A, B) shows a small, hypervascular tumor of segment VI. The lesion has an exophytic growth and is adjacent to the ureter and the large bowel. Placement and deployment of the multi-pronged injection needle under ultrasound guidance (C, D).

survival rates ranging 41% to 60% in Child A patients (Table 14.2) (18–23). Of importance, two cohort studies and one retrospective case-control study comparing surgical resection and PEI failed to identify any difference in survival, despite patients in PEI groups having poorer liver function (24–26).

Despite PEI's being a low-risk procedure, severe complications have been reported. In a multi-center survey including 1066 patients, one death (0.1%) and 34 complications (3.2%), including seven cases of tumor seeding (0.7%), were reported (27). The major limitation of PEI is the high local recurrence rate, which may reach 33% in lesions smaller than 3 cm and

43% in lesions exceeding 3 cm (28, 29). The injected ethanol does not always accomplish complete tumor necrosis because of its inhomogeneous distribution within the lesion – especially in presence of intratumoral septa – and the limited effect on extracapsular cancerous spread. Moreover, PEI is unable to create a safety margin of ablation in the liver parenchyma surrounding the nodule and therefore may not destroy tiny satellite lesions that – even in small tumors – may be located in close proximity of the main nodule.

Injection of large volumes of ethanol in a single session performed under general anesthesia has been reported to enable successful PEI treatment of large

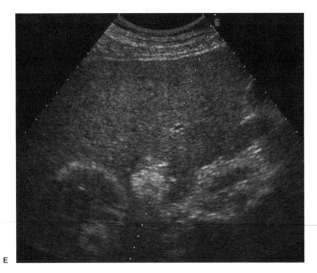

E

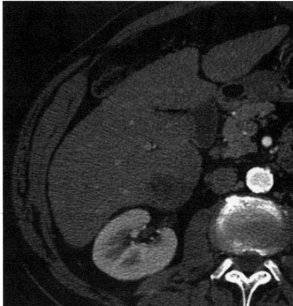

F

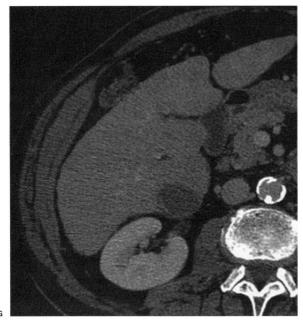

G

FIGURE 14.1. (*Continued*) Homogeneous alcohol perfusion of the whole tumor mass is accomplished (E). Posttreatment CT shows unenhancing area consistent with complete tumor ablation (F, G).

TABLE 14.2 Studies Reporting Long-term Survival Outcomes of Patients with Early-stage Hepatocellular Carcinoma Who Underwent Percutaneous Ethanol Ablation

Author and Year	Number of Patients	Survival Rates (%)		
		1-yr	3-yr	5-yr
Lencioni, et al., 1995 (18)	105	96	68	32
Livraghi, et al., 1995 (19)				
Child A, single HCC ≤5 cm	293	98	79	47
Child B, single HCC ≤5 cm	149	93	63	29
Ryu, et al., 1997 (20)				
Stage I, One to three HCC ≤3 cm*	110	98	84	54
Stage II, One to three HCC ≤3 cm*	140	91	65	45
Lencioni, et al., 1997 (21)				
Child A, One HCC ≤5 cm or three ≤3 cm	127	98	79	53
Child B, One HCC ≤5 cm or three ≤3 cm	57	88	50	28
Teratani, et al., 2002 (22)				
Age ≤70 years	516	90	65	40
Age >70 years	137	83	52	27
Ebara, et al., 2005 (23)				
One HCC ≤3 cm or three ≤3 cm	270	99	82	60

HCC, hepatocellular carcinoma.
*Clinical stage according to the Liver Cancer Study Group of Japan.

or infiltrating HCC (30). However, results of single-session PEI are based on uncontrolled investigations, and when critically compared with data about the natural history and prognosis of untreated nonsurgical HCC, the benefits of the procedure are not evident.

Acetic Acid Injection

Acetic acid injection has been proposed as a viable alternative to PEI for the treatment of HCC. Two studies compared acetic acid injection and PEI. In the first paper, 60 patients with small HCC lesions were entered into a randomized trial. The 1- and 2-year survival rates were 100% and 92%, respectively, in the acetic acid injection group, and 83% and 63%, respectively, in the PEI group. A multivariate analysis of prognostic factors showed that treatment was an independent predictor of survival (31). In contrast, in a prospective comparative study including 63 patients treated by acetic acid injection and 62 patients treated by PEI, no significant survival differences were observed between the two treatment groups (32). In summary, this alternative option for chemical ablation had limited diffusion and was not tested in large series of patients. The reported survival outcomes are not better than those obtained by several authors with PEI.

THERMAL ABLATION

Application of localized heating or freezing enables in situ destruction of malignant liver tumors, preserving normal liver parenchyma. The thermal ablative therapies involved in clinical practice can be classified as either hepatic hyperthermic treatments – including radiofrequency (RF) ablation, microwave ablation and laser ablation – or hepatic cryotherapy. Hepatic hyperthermic treatments are mainly performed via a percutaneous approach, while an open or laparoscopic approach has been widely adopted – until recently – for hepatic cryotherapy. This chapter focuses on percutaneous hyperthermic treatments, particularly RF ablation, which has been, by far, the most widely used thermal ablative modality in HCC.

The thermal damage caused by heating depends on both the tissue temperature achieved and the duration of heating. Heating of tissue at 50° to 55°C for 4 to 6 minutes produces irreversible cellular damage. At temperatures between 60°C and 100°C, near-immediate coagulation of tissue is induced, with irreversible damage to mitochondrial and cytosolic enzymes of the cells. At more than 100° to 110°C, tissue vaporizes and carbonizes (33). For adequate destruction of tumor tissue, the entire target volume must be subjected to cytotoxic temperatures. Different physical mechanisms are involved in the hepatic hyperthermic treatments in order to generate a lethal temperature. A common important factor that affects the success of thermal ablation is the ability to ablate all viable tumor tissue and possibly an adequate tumor-free margin. Ideally, a 360°, 0.5- to 1-cm thick ablative margin should be produced around the tumor (33). This cuff would ensure that microscopic invasions around the periphery of a tumor have been eradicated. Thus, the target diameter of an ablation – or of overlapping ablations – must be larger than the diameter of the tumor that undergoes treatment (34).

Thermal ablation is usually performed with the patient under intravenous sedation, with standard cardiac, pressure and oxygen monitoring. Targeting of the lesion can be performed with ultrasound, CT or MR imaging. The guidance system is chosen largely on the basis of operator preference and local availability of dedicated equipment such as CT fluoroscopy or open MR systems. Real-time ultrasound/CT (or ultrasound/MRI) fusion imaging substantially improves the ability to guide and monitor liver tumor ablation procedures. Current virtual navigation systems allow the definition of the extent of the liver tumor burden, planning and simulatation of the insertion of the needle and prediction of the amount of the induced necrosis (Figure 14.2). During the procedure, important aspects to be monitored include how well the tumor is being covered and whether any adjacent normal structures are being affected at the same time. Although the transient hyperechoic zone that is seen at ultrasound within and surrounding a tumor during and immediately after RF ablation can be used as a rough guide to the extent of tumor destruction, MR is currently the only imaging modality with validated techniques for real-time temperature monitoring. To control an image-guided ablation procedure, the operator can utilize the image-based information obtained during monitoring or automated systems that terminate the ablation at a critical point in the procedure. At the end of the procedure, most systems allow the clinician to ablate the needle track, which is aimed at preventing any tumor cell dissemination.

Contrast-enhanced ultrasound performed after the end of the procedure may allow an initial

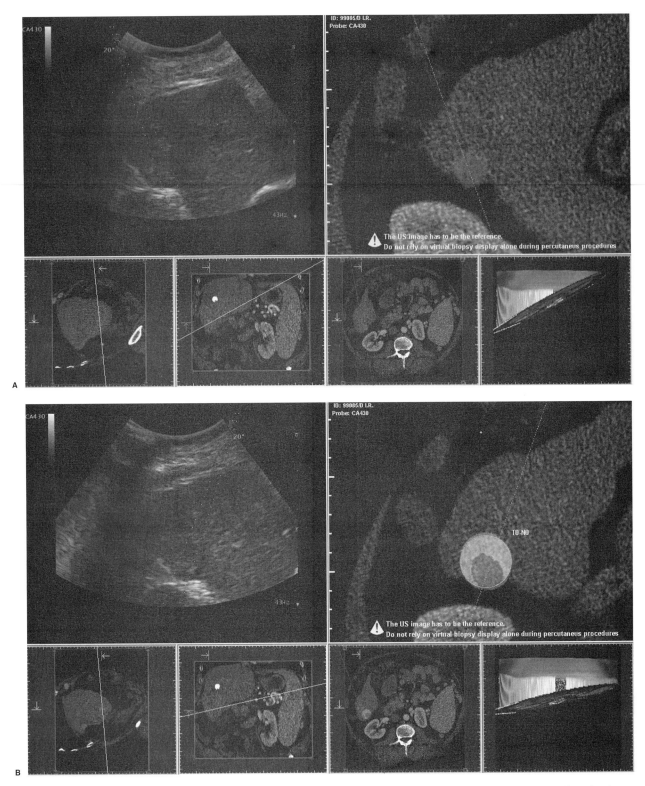

FIGURE 14.2. RF ablation performed with the assistance of a virtual navigation system. Tumor is depicted at real-time ultrasound/CT fusion imaging. The tumor volume is high-lighted (A). Ablation track is selected and predicted volume of ablation is shown by the system (B).

evaluation of treatment effects. However, contrast-enhanced CT or MR imaging are recognized as the standard modalities to assess treatment outcome. CT and MR images obtained after treatment show successful ablation as a non-enhancing area with or without peripheral enhancing rim. The enhancing rim that may be observed along the periphery of the ablation zone appears a relatively concentric, symmetric and uniform process in an area with smooth inner margins. This is a transient finding that

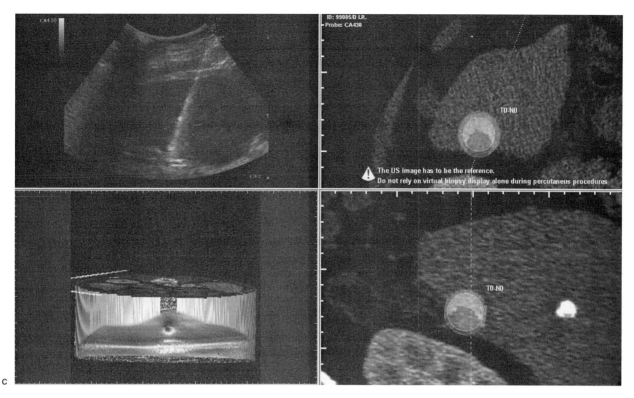

FIGURE 14.2.   (Continued) Actual electrode placement following the planned path (C). Computer confirms proper coverage of the tumor.

represents a benign physiologic response to thermal injury (initially, reactive hyperemia; subsequently, fibrosis and giant cell reaction; Figure 14.3). Benign periablational enhancement needs to be differentiated from irregular peripheral enhancement due to residual tumor that occurs at the treatment margin. In contrast to benign periablational enhancement, residual unablated tumor often grows in scattered, nodular or eccentric patterns (35). Later follow-up imaging studies should be aimed at detecting the recurrence of the treated lesion (i.e., local tumor progression), the development of new hepatic lesions or the emergence of extrahepatic disease.

Radiofrequency Ablation

The goal of RF ablation is to induce thermal injury to the tissue through electromagnetic energy deposition. The patient is part of a closed-loop circuit that includes a RF generator, an electrode needle and a large dispersive electrode (ground pads). An alternating electric field is created within the tissue of the patient. Because of the relatively high electrical resistance of tissue in comparison with the metal electrodes, there is marked agitation of the ions present in the target tissue that surrounds the electrode, since the tissue ions attempt to follow the changes in direction of alternating electric current. The agitation results in frictional heat around the electrode. The discrepancy between the small surface area of the needle electrode and the large area of the ground pads causes the generated heat to be focused and concentrated around the needle electrode. Several electrode types are available for clinical RF ablation, including internally cooled electrodes and multi-tined expandable electrodes with or without perfusion (35).

RF ablation has been the most widely assessed alternative to PEI for local ablation of HCC (36). Histologic data from explanted liver specimens in patients who underwent RF ablation showed that tumor size and presence of large (3 mm or more) abutting vessels significantly affect local treatment effect. Complete tumor necrosis was pathologically shown in 83% of tumors less than 3 cm and 88% of tumors in nonperivascular location (37). Three RCTs compared RF ablation versus PEI for the treatment of early-stage HCC (Table 14.3) (38–40). The first trial, performed in European centers, failed to show a statistically significant difference in overall survival between patients who received RF ablation and those treated with PEI (38). However, survival advantages were identified in a subgroup analysis of a trial coming from Taiwan (39) and in a Japanese study, although

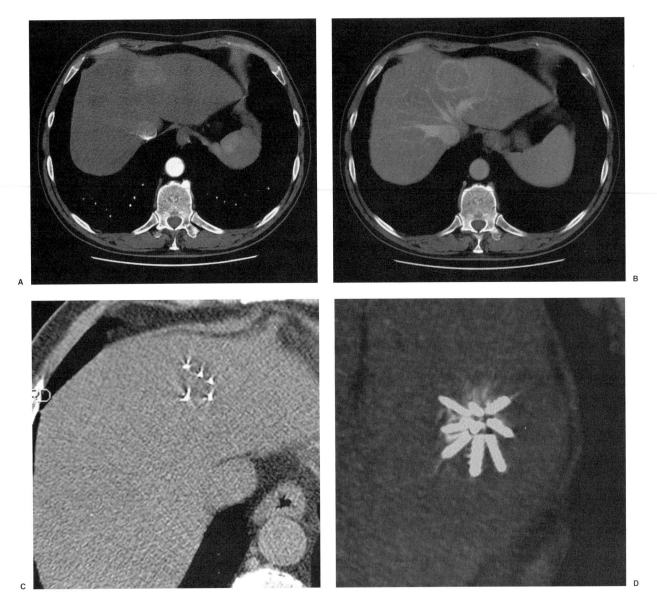

FIGURE 14.3. Complete response of hepatocellular carcinoma treated with RF ablation. Pre-treatment CT shows hypervascular tumor (A, B). Expandable multi-tined electrode is placed into the lesion (C, D).

in the latter the survival benefit was not confirmed in the subgroup analysis of patients with solitary tumors (40). All three investigations showed that RF ablation had higher local anti-cancer effect than PEI, leading to a better local control of the disease. Therefore, RF ablation appears to be the preferred percutaneous treatment for patients with early stage HCC on the basis of more consistent local tumor control.

Recently, the long-term survival outcomes of RF ablation-treated patients were reported (Table 14.4). In the first published report, 206 patients with early stage HCC who were not candidates for resection or transplantation were enrolled in a prospective, intention-to-treat clinical trial (41). RF ablation was considered as the first-line non-surgical treatment and was actually performed in 187 (91%) of 206 patients. Nineteen (9%) of 206 patients had to be excluded from RF treatment because of the unfavorable location of the tumor. In patients who underwent RF ablation, survival depended on the severity of the underlying cirrhosis and the tumor multiplicity. Patients in Child class A with solitary HCC had a 5-year survival rate of 61%. Three other studies confirmed that survival of chemonaive patients with well-compensated cirrhosis bearing early-stage HCC ranges from 43% to 64% (42–44). Of interest, in a randomized trial of RF ablation versus surgical resection in patients with solitary HCC less than 5 cm

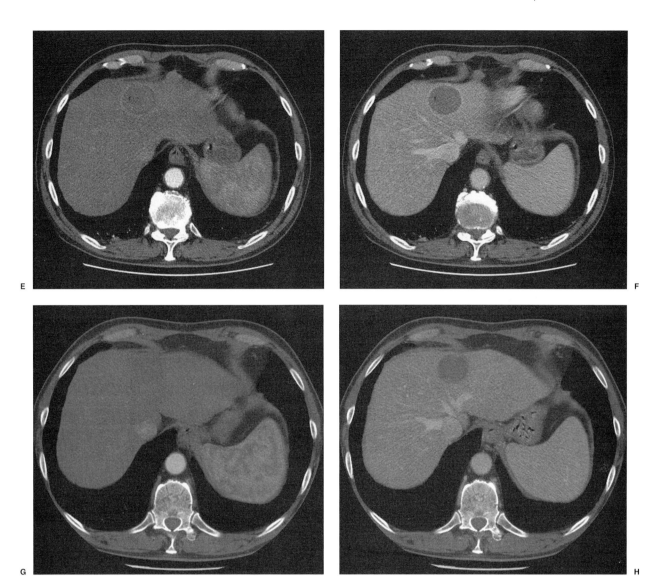

FIGURE 14.3. (Continued) Post-treatment CT shows non-enhancing tumor with peripheral enhancing rim, suggesting complete ablation with perilesional reaction (E, F). Follow-up CT at 3 months confirms complete response with disappearance of perilesional enhancement (G, H).

TABLE 14.3 Randomized Studies Comparing RF Ablation and Percutaneous Ethanol Injection in the Treatment of Early-stage Hepatocellular Carcinoma

Author and Year	Complete Response (%)	2-year Local Progression (%)	Survival Rates 2-yr	3-yr	P
Lencioni, et al., 2003 (38)					
PEI (n = 50)	82	38*	88	NA	
RF ablation (n = 52)	95	4*	96	NA	NS
Lin, et al., 2004 (39)					
PEI – low dose (n = 52)	88	45	61	50	
PEI – high dose (n = 53)	92	33	63	55	
RF ablation (n = 52)	96	18	82	74	≤.05
Shiina, et al., 2005 (40)					
PEI (n = 114)	100	11	82	63	
RF ablation (n = 118)	100	2	90	80	≤.05

PEI, percutaneous ethanol injection; RF, radiofrequency; NA, not available; NS, not significant.
*2-year local recurrence-free survival: PEI 62%, RF ablation 96%.

TABLE 14.4 Studies Reporting Long-term Survival Outcomes of Patients with Early-stage Hepatocellular Carcinoma Who Underwent Percutaneous RF Ablation

Author and Year	Number of Patients	Survival Rates (%)		
		1-yr	3-yr	5-yr
Lencioni, et al., 2005 (41)				
Child A, one HCC ≤5 cm or three ≤3 cm	144	100	76	51
One HCC ≤5 cm	116	100	89	61
Child B, one HCC ≤5 cm or three ≤3 cm	43	89	46	31
Tateishi, et al., 2005 (42)				
Naive patients*	319	95	78	54
Non-naive patients†	345	92	62	38
Cabassa, et al., 2006 (43)	59	94	65	43
Choi, et al., 2007 (44)				
Child A, one HCC ≤5 cm or three ≤3 cm	359	NA	78	64
Child B, one HCC ≤5 cm or three ≤3 cm	160	NA	49	38

HCC, hepatocellular carcinoma.
*Patients who received RF ablation as primary treatment.
†Patients who received RF ablation for recurrent tumor after previous treatment including resection, ethanol injection, microwave ablation and transarterial embolization.

in diameter, no differences in overall survival rates and cumulative recurrence-free survival rates were observed (45).

RF ablation of HCC is associated with very low mortality rates and acceptable morbidity. Recently, three separate multi-center surveys have reported mortality rates ranging from 0.1% to 0.5%, major complication rates ranging from 2.2% to 3.1% and minor complication rates ranging from 5% to 8.9% (46). The most common causes of death were sepsis, hepatic failure, colon perforation and portal vein thrombosis, whereas the most common complications were intraperitoneal bleeding, hepatic abscess, bile duct injury, hepatic decompensation and grounding pad burns (47–49). Minor complications and side effects were usually transient and self-limiting. An uncommon late complication of RF ablation is tumor seeding along the needle track. In patients with HCC, tumor seeding occurred in 8 (0.5%) of 1,610 cases in a multi-center survey (47) and in 1 (0.5%) of 187 cases in a single-institution series (41). Lesions with subcapsular location and an invasive tumoral pattern, as shown by a poor differentiation degree, seem to be at higher risk for such a complication (50). Although these data indicate that RF ablation is a relatively safe procedure, a careful assessment of the risks and benefits associated with the treatment has to be made in each individual patient by a multi-disciplinary team.

Despite the many published reports, some questions concerning image-guided RF ablation in HCC treatment are still unanswered. Some authors have reported that RF ablation may be a safe and effective bridge to liver transplantation (51–54). However, randomized studies would be needed to determine advantages and disadvantages of RF ablation with respect to TACE for HCC patients awaiting transplantation. Recent studies have reported encouraging initial results in the treatment of intermediate-size HCC lesions with a combination of RF ablation and balloon catheter occlusion of the tumor arterial supply or prior TACE (55–59). However, further clinical trials are warranted to determine the survival benefit associated with this approach.

Microwave Ablation

Microwave ablation is the term used for all electromagnetic methods of inducing tumor destruction by using devices with frequencies greater than or equal to 900 kHz. The passage of microwaves into cells or other materials containing water results in the rotation of individual molecules. This rapid molecular rotation generates and uniformly distributes heat, which is instantaneous and continuous until the radiation is stopped. Microwave irradiation creates an ablation area around the needle in a column or round shape, depending on the type of needle used and the generating power (60).

The local effect of treatment in HCC was assessed by examining the histological changes of the tumor after microwave ablation (61, 62). In one study, 89% of 18 small tumors were ablated completely (61). Coagulative necrosis with faded nuclei and eosinophilic cytoplasm were the predominant findings in the ablated areas. There were also areas in which the tumors maintained their native morphological features as if the area was fixed, but their cellular activity was destroyed as demonstrated by succinic dehydrogenase stain. One study compared microwave ablation and PEI in a retrospective evaluation of 90 patients with small HCC (63). The overall 5-year survival rates for patients with well-differentiated HCC treated with microwave ablation and PEI were not significantly different. However, among the patients with moderately or poorly differentiated HCC, overall survival with microwave ablation was significantly better than with PEI. In a large series including 234 patients, the 3- and 5-year survival rates were 73% and 57%, respectively (64). At a multivariate analysis, tumor size, number of nodules and Child-Pugh classification had a significant effect on survival (65). Only one randomized trial compared the effectiveness of microwave ablation with that of RF ablation (66). Seventy-two patients with 94 HCC nodules were randomly assigned to RF ablation and microwave ablation groups. Unfortunately, in this study, the data were analyzed with respect to lesions and not to patients. Although no statistically significant differences were observed with respect to the efficacy of the two procedures, a tendency favoring RF ablation was recognized with respect to local recurrences and complications rates.

Laser Ablation

The term **laser ablation** should be used for ablation with light energy applied via fibers directly inserted into the tissue. A great variety in laser sources and wavelength is available. In addition, different types of laser fibers, modified tips and single or multiple laser applicators can be used. From a single, bare 400-μm laser fiber, a spherical volume of coagulative necrosis up to 2 cm in diameter can be produced. Use of higher power results in charring and vaporization around the fiber tip. Two methods have been developed for producing larger volumes of necrosis. The first consists of firing multiple bare fibers arrayed at 2-cm spacing throughout a target lesion, whereas the second uses cooled-tip diffuser fibers that can deposit up to 30 W

over a large surface area, thus diminishing local overheating (67).

To date, few data are available concerning the clinical efficacy of laser ablation. No randomized trial to compare laser ablation with any other treatment has been published thus far. In one study including 74 patients with early-stage HCC, overall survival rates were 68% at 3 years and 15% at 5 years, respectively (68). Laser ablation appears to be relatively safe, with a major complication rate less than 2% (69). The major drawback of current laser technology appears to be the small volume of ablation that can be created with a single-probe insertion. Insertion of multiple fibers is technically cumbersome and may not be feasible in lesions that are not conveniently located. New devices could overcome this limitation.

CONCLUSION

Several image-guided ablation techniques have been developed to treat non-surgical patients with HCC. These minimally invasive procedures can achieve effective and reproducible tumor destruction with low morbidity. Percutaneous ablation is accepted as the best therapeutic choice for patients with early stage HCC when resection or transplantation are precluded. On the basis of the current evidence, RF ablation seems to offer higher cumulative survival and recurrence-free survival rates compared with other image-guided treatments and is accepted as the primary ablative modality at most institutions. Further trials are needed to establish the clinical value of image-guided ablation in combination with intra-arterial treatments (70).

REFERENCES

1. Llovet JM, Burroughs A, Bruix J. Hepatocellular carcinoma. Lancet 2003; 362: 1907–1917.
2. Sherman M. Hepatocellular carcinoma: Epidemiology, risk factors, and screening. Semin Liver Dis 2005; 25: 143–154.
3. Lencioni R, Cioni D, Della Pina C, et al. Imaging diagnosis. Semin Liver Dis 2005; 25: 162–170.
4. Bruix J, Boix L, Sala M, et al. Focus on hepatocellular carcinoma. Cancer Cell 2004; 5: 215–219.
5. Bruix J, Sherman M, Llovet JM, et al.; EASL Panel of Experts on HCC. Clinical management of hepatocellular carcinoma: Conclusions of the Barcelona-2000 EASL conference. European Association for the Study of the Liver. J Hepatol 2001; 35: 421–430.
6. Bruix J, Sherman M. Management of hepatocellular carcinoma. Hepatology 2005; 42: 1208–1236.

7. Kojiro M, Roskams T. Early hepatocellular carcinoma and dysplastic nodules. Semin Liver Dis 2005; 25: 133–142.

8. Levy I, Greig PD, Gallinger S, et al. Resection of hepatocellular carcinoma without preoperative tumor biopsy. Ann Surg 2001; 234: 206–209.

9. Johnson PJ. Hepatocellular carcinoma: Is current therapy really altering outcome? Gut 2002; 51: 459–462.

10. Llovet JM, Bru C, Bruix J. Prognosis of hepatocellular carcinoma: The BCLC staging classification. Semin Liver Dis 1999; 19: 329–338.

11. Llovet JM, Fuster J, Bruix J. Intention-to-treat analysis of surgical treatment for early hepatocellular carcinoma: Resection versus transplantation. Hepatology 1999; 30: 1434–1440.

12. Fong Y, Sun RL, Jarnagin W, et al. An analysis of 412 cases of hepatocellular carcinoma at a Western center. Ann Surg 1999; 229: 790–800.

13. Wayne JD, Lauwers GY, Ikai I, et al. Preoperative predictors of survival after resection of small hepatocellular carcinomas. Ann Surg 2002; 235: 722–731.

14. Llovet JM, Schwartz M, Mazzaferro V. Resection and liver transplantation for hepatocellular carcinoma. Semin Liver Dis 2005; 25: 181–200.

15. Jonas S, Beckstein WO, Steinmuller T, et al. Vascular invasion and histopathologic grading determine outcome after liver transplantion for hepatocellular carcinoma in cirrhosis. Hepatology 2001; 33: 1080–1086.

16. Yao FY, Ferrel L, Bass NM, et al. Liver transplantation for hepatocellular carcinoma: Expansion of tumor size limits does not adversely impact survival. Hepatology 2001; 33: 1394–1403.

17. Yao FY, Bass NM, Nikolai B, et al. Liver transplantation for hepatocellular carcinoma: Analysis of survival according to the intention-to-treat principle and dropout from the waiting list. Liver Transpl 2002; 8: 873–883.

18. Lencioni R, Bartolozzi C, Caramella D, et al. Treatment of small hepatocellular carcinoma with percutaneous ethanol injection: Analysis of prognostic factors in 105 Western patients. Cancer 1995; 76: 1737–1746.

19. Livraghi T, Giorgio A, Marin G, et al. Hepatocellular carcinoma and cirrhosis in 746 patients: Long-term results of percutaneous ethanol injection. Radiology 1995; 197: 101–108.

20. Ryu M, Shimamura Y, Kinoshita T, et al. Therapeutic results of resection, transcatheter arterial embolization and percutaneous transhepatic ethanol injection in 3225 patients with hepatocellular carcinoma: A retrospective multicenter study. Jpn J Clin Oncol 1997; 27: 251–257.

21. Lencioni R, Pinto F, Armillotta N, et al. Long-term results of percutaneous ethanol injection therapy for hepatocellular carcinoma in cirrhosis: A European experience. Eur Radiol 1997; 7: 514–519.

22. Teratani T, Ishikawa T, Shiratori Y, et al. Hepatocellular carcinoma in elderly patients: Beneficial therapeutic efficacy using percutaneous ethanol injection therapy. Cancer 2002; 95: 816–823.

23. Ebara M, Okabe S, Kita K, et al. Percutaneous ethanol injection for small hepatocellular carcinoma: Therapeutic efficacy based on 20-year observation. J Hepatol 2005; 43: 458–464.

24. Castells A, Bruix J, Bru C, et al. Treatment of small hepatocellular carcinoma in cirrhotic patients: A cohort study comparing surgical resection and percutaneous ethanol injection. Hepatology 1993; 18: 1121–1126.

25. Yamamoto J, Okada S, Shimada K, et al. Treatment strategy for small hepatocellular carcinoma: Comparison of long-term results after percutaneous ethanol injection therapy and surgical resection. Hepatology 2001; 34: 707–713.

26. Daniele B, De Sio I, Izzo F, et al., CLIP Investigators. Hepatic resection and percutaneous ethanol injection as treatments of small hepatocellular carcinoma: A Cancer of the Liver Italian Program (CLIP 08) retrospective case-control study. J Clin Gastroenterol 2003; 36: 63–67.

27. Di Stasi M, Buscarini L, Livraghi T, et al. Percutaneous ethanol injection in the treatment of hepatocellular carcinoma: A multicenter survey of evaluation practices and complication rates. Scand J Gastroenterol 1997; 32: 1168–1173.

28. Khan KN, Yatsuhashi H, Yamasaki K, et al. Prospective analysis of risk factors for early intrahepatic recurrence of hepatocellular carcinoma following ethanol injection. J Hepatol 2000; 32: 269–278.

29. Koda M, Murawaki Y, Mitsuda A, et al. Predictive factors for intrahepatic recurrence after percutaneous ethanol injection therapy for small hepatocellular carcinoma. Cancer 2000; 88: 529–537.

30. Livraghi T, Benedini V, Lazzaroni S, et al. Long-term results of single-session percutaneous ethanol injection in patients with large hepatocellular carcinoma. Cancer 1998; 83: 48–57.

31. Ohnishi K, Yoshioka H, Ito S, et al. Prospective randomized controlled trial comparing percutaneous acetic acid injection and percutaneous ethanol injection for small hepatocellular carcinoma. Hepatology 1998; 27: 67–72.

32. Huo TI, Huang YH, Wu JC, et al. Comparison of percutaneous acetic acid injection and percutaneous ethanol injection for hepatocellular carcinoma in cirrhotic patients: A prospective study. Scand J Gastroenterol 2003; 38: 770–778.

33. Goldberg SN, Gazelle GS, Mueller PR. Thermal ablation therapy for focal malignancies: A unified approach to underlying principles, techniques, and diagnostic imaging guidance. AJR Am J Roentgenol 2000; 174: 323–331.

34. Dodd GD 3rd, Frank MS, Aribandi M, et al. Radiofrequency thermal ablation: Computer analysis of the size of the thermal injury created by overlapping ablations. AJR Am J Roentgenol 2001; 177: 777–782.

35. Goldberg SN, Charboneau JW, Dodd GD 3rd, et al; International Working Group on Image-guided Tumor Ablation. Image-guided tumor ablation: Proposal for standardization of terms and reporting criteria. Radiology 2003; 228: 335–345.

36. Lencioni R, Crocetti L. A critical appraisal of the literature on local ablative therapies for hepatocellular carcinoma. Clin Liver Dis 2005; 9: 301–314.

37. Lu DS, Yu NC, Raman SS, et al. Radiofrequency ablation of hepatocellular carcinoma: Treatment success as defined by histologic examination of the explanted liver. Radiology 2005; 234: 954–960.

38. Lencioni R, Allgaier HP, Cioni D, et al. Small hepatocellular carcinoma in cirrhosis: Randomized comparison of radiofrequency thermal ablation versus percutaneous ethanol injection. Radiology 2003; 228: 235–240.

39. Lin SM, Lin CJ, Lin CC, et al. Radiofrequency ablation improves prognosis compared with ethanol injection for hepatocellular carcinoma ≤4 cm. Gastroenterology 2004; 127: 1714–1723.

40. Shiina S, Teratani T, Obi S, et al. A randomized controlled trial of radiofrequency ablation versus ethanol injection for small hepatocellular carcinoma. Gastroenterology 2005; 129: 122–130.

41. Lencioni R, Cioni D, Crocetti L, et al. Early-stage hepatocellular carcinoma in cirrhosis: Long-term results of percutaneous image-guided radiofrequency ablation. Radiology 2005; 234: 961–967.

42. Tateishi R, Shiina S, Teratani T, et al. Percutaneous radiofrequency ablation for hepatocellular carcinoma. Cancer 2005; 103: 1201–1209.

43. Cabassa P, Donato F, Simeone F, et al. Radiofrequency ablation of hepatocellular carcinoma: Long-term experience with expandable needle electrodes. Am J Roentgenol 2006; 185: S316–321.

44. Choi D, Lim HK, Rhim H, et al. Percutaneous radiofrequency ablation for early-stage hepatocellular carcinoma as a first-line treatment: Long-term results and prognostic factors in a large single-institution series. Eur Radiol 2007; 17: 684–692.

45. Chen MS, Li JQ, Zheng Y, et al. A prospective randomized trial comparing percutaneous local ablative therapy and partial hepatectomy for small hepatocellular carcinoma. Ann Surg 2006; 243: 321–328.

46. Rhim H. Complications of radiofrequency ablation in hepatocellular carcinoma. Abdom Imaging 2005; 30: 409–418.

47. Livraghi T, Solbiati L, Meloni MF, et al. Treatment of focal liver tumors with percutaneous radio-frequency ablation: Complications encountered in a multicenter study. Radiology 2003; 26: 441–451.

48. De Baere T, Risse O, Kuoch V, et al. Adverse events during radiofrequency treatment of 582 hepatic tumors. AJR Am J Roentgenol 2003; 181: 695–700.

49. Bleicher RJ, Allegra DP, Nora DT, et al. Radiofrequency ablation in 447 complex unresectable liver tumors: Lessons learned. Ann Surg Oncol 2003; 10: 52–58.

50. Llovet JM, Vilana R, Bru C, et al; Barcelona Clinic Liver Cancer (BCLC) Group. Increased risk of tumor seeding after percutaneous radiofrequency ablation for single hepatocellular carcinoma. Hepatology 2001; 33: 1124–1129.

51. Fontana RJ, Hamidullah H, Nghiem H, et al. Percutaneous radiofrequency thermal ablation of hepatocellular carcinoma: A safe and effective bridge to liver transplantation. Liver Transpl 2002; 8: 1165–1174.

52. Wong LL, Tanaka K, Lau L, et al. Pre-transplant treatment of hepatocellular carcinoma: Assessment of tumor necrosis in explanted livers. Clin Transplant 2004; 18: 227–234.

53. Lencioni R, Cioni D, Crocetti L, et al. Percutaneous ablation of hepatocellular carcinoma: State-of-the-art. Liver Transpl 2004; 10: S91–97.

54. Lu DS, Yu NC, Raman SS, et al. Percutaneous radiofrequency ablation of hepatocellular carcinoma as a bridge to liver transplantation. Hepatology 2005; 41: 1130–1137.

55. Rossi S, Garbagnati F, Lencioni R, et al. Percutaneous radio-frequency thermal ablation of nonresectable hepatocellular carcinoma after occlusion of tumor blood supply. Radiology 2000; 217: 119–126.

56. Yamasaki T, Kurokawa F, Shirahashi H, et al. Percutaneous radiofrequency ablation therapy for patients with hepatocellular carcinoma during occlusion of hepatic blood flow: Comparison with standard percutaneous radiofrequency ablation therapy. Cancer 2002; 95: 2353–2360.

57. Kitamoto M, Imagawa M, Yamada H, et al. Radiofrequency ablation in the treatment of small hepatocellular carcinomas: Comparison of the radiofrequency effect with and without chemoembolization. Am J Roentgenol 2003; 181: 997–1003.

58. Lencioni R, Della Pina C, Bartolozzi C. Percutaneous image-guided radiofrequency ablation in the therapeutic management of hepatocellular carcinoma. Abdom Imaging 2005; 30: 401–408.

59. Veltri A, Moretto P, Doriguzzi A, et al. Radiofrequency thermal ablation (RFA) after transarterial chemoembolization (TACE) as a combined therapy for unresectable non-early hepatocellular carcinoma (HCC). Eur Radiol 2006; 16: 661–669.

60. Lu MD, Chen JW, Xie XY, et al. Hepatocellular carcinoma: US-guided percutaneous microwave coagulation therapy. Radiology 2001; 221: 167–172.

61. Yamashiki N, Kato T, Bejarano PA, et al. Histopathological changes after microwave coagulation therapy for patients with hepatocellular carcinoma: Review of 15 explanted livers. Am J Gastroenterol 2003; 98: 2052–2059.

62. Yu NC, Lu DS, Raman SS, et al. Hepatocellular carcinoma: Microwave ablation with multiple straight and loop antenna clusters – pilot comparison with pathologic findings. Radiology 2006; 239: 269–275.

63. Seki T, Wakabayashi M, Nakagawa T, et al. Percutaneous microwave coagulation therapy for patients with small hepatocellular carcinoma: Comparison with percutaneous ethanol injection therapy. Cancer 1999; 85: 1694–1702.

64. Dong B, Liang P, Yu X, et al. Percutaneous sonographically guided microwave coagulation therapy for hepatocellular carcinoma: Results in 234 patients. Am J Roentgenol 2003; 180: 1547–1541.

65. Liang P, Dong B, Yu X, et al. Prognostic factors for survival in patients with hepatocellular carcinoma after percutaneous microwave ablation. Radiology 2005; 235: 299–307.

66. Shibata T, Iimuro Y, Yamamoto Y, et al. Small hepatocellular carcinoma: Comparison of radio-frequency ablation and percutaneous microwave coagulation therapy. Radiology 2002; 223: 331–337.

67. Vogl TJ, Muller PK, Hammerstingl R, et al. Malignant liver tumors treated with MR imaging-guided laser-induced thermotherapy: Technique and prospective results. Radiology 1995; 196: 257–265.

68. Pacella CM, Bizzarri G, Magnolfi F, et al. Laser thermal ablation in the treatment of small hepatocellular carcinoma: Results in 74 patients. Radiology 2001; 221: 712–720.

69. Vogl TJ, Straub R, Eichler K, et al. Malignant liver tumors treated with MR imaging-guided laser-induced thermotherapy: Experience with complications in 899 patients (2,520 lesions). Radiology 2002; 225: 367–377.

70. Lencioni R, Della Pina C, Crocetti L, et al. Percutaneous ablation of hepatocellular carcinoma. Recent Results Cancer Res 2006; 167: 91–105.

Chapter 15

EMBOLIZATION OF LIVER TUMORS: ANATOMY

Jin Wook Chung

Jae Hyung Park

In transcatheter management of hepatic tumors, it is essential to understand hepatic vascular anatomy in detail to enhance therapeutic results and prevent complications due to non-target treatment.

The purpose of this chapter is to review celiac trunk and hepatic artery variations, non-hepatic arteries arising from hepatic arteries and extra-hepatic collateral supply to hepatic tumors.

Celiac Trunk Anatomy

Normal Celiac Trunk Anatomy and Variations

The celiac trunk is a wide branch from the front of the aorta just below the aortic hiatus of the diaphragm. It passes nearly horizontally forward and slightly to the right above the pancreas and the splenic vein, and divides into three major branches of the left gastric artery (LGA), common hepatic artery (CHA) and splenic artery. It may give off one or both inferior phrenic arteries, dorsal pancreatic artery and rarely, colic or jejunal branches (Figure 15.1) (1). The superior mesenteric artery (SMA) separately arises from the aorta inferior to the origin of the celiac axis. Usually, the LGA is the first major branch of the celiac trunk. However, in about 4% of the population, the LGA directly arises from the supraceliac or juxtaceliac aorta, which represents the most common form of celiac trunk variation. If inferior phrenic arteries arise from the celiac trunk, their origin is almost always located proximal to the LGA (Figure 15.1).

Celiac trunk variation is found in approximately 10% of the general population (2). Celiac trunk variations can be considered as the result of the origin of the CHA, LGA, splenic artery and SMA from the aorta in different combinations. Among 15 possible combinations of their origin (Figure 15.2), we could find 13 types in clinical practice and the literature. In describing celiac trunk and hepatic artery variations, it is extremely important to define the terminology used. The CHA should be defined as the common trunk of a hepatic artery (regardless of its size or anatomical distribution) and the gastroduodenal artery (GDA). According to our experience, the most common type of celiac trunk variation was the common trunk of the CHA and splenic artery and the separate origins of the LGA and the SMA from the aorta, which was followed by two separate trunks from the aorta in combination of the CHA and SMA (hepatomesenteric trunk) and that of the LGA and splenic artery (gastrosplenic trunk) (Figure 15.3). The CHA can also arise from the hepatogastric trunk, hepatosplenomesenteric trunk and celiacomesenteric trunk, or directly from the aorta. Rarely, the CHA can arise from the LGA in normal celiac trunk anatomy.

Occasionally, there are situations in which it is difficult to define the celiac trunk anatomy because of embryological communicating channels (Figure 15.4) and absent CHA (Figure 15.5). In the situations of separate origin of the proper hepatic artery (PHA) and GDA or the separate origin of the right hepatic

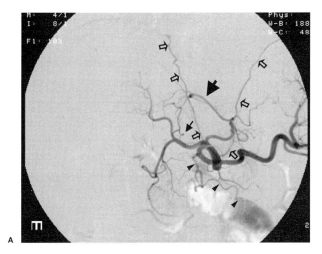 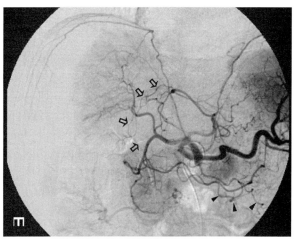

FIGURE 15.1. Normal celiac trunk with an aberrant left hepatic artery, a jejunal branch and a long hepatic falciform artery. (A) The first branches of the celiac trunk are the inferior phrenic arteries (*open arrows*). The left gastric artery gives off the aberrant left hepatic artery (*thick arrow*) sup-plying liver segments 2 and 3. Arrowheads indicate a jejunal branch from the proximal splenic artery and the thin arrow indicates the right gastric artery from the segment 4 hepatic artery. (B) Open arrows indicate the hepatic falciform artery arising from the aberrant left gastric artery.

artery (RHA) and left hepatic artery (LHA) and GDA, the CHA does not exist according to the aforementioned definition of the CHA (Figure 15.5).

Adequate celiac trunk angiography includes proper opacification of the LGA and inferior phrenic arter-ies off the celiac trunk, considering the possibility of extra-hepatic collateral supply from inferior phrenic arteries and aberrant LHA from the LGA. Otherwise, selective catheterization of the LGA or inferior phrenic arteries may be necessary.

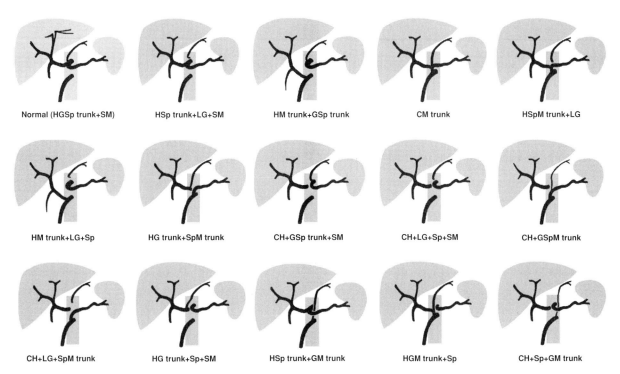

FIGURE 15.2. Schematic diagrams of possible 15 types of celiac trunk variations. The last two types have not been observed. CH, common hepatic artery; CM, celiacomesenteric; GM, gastromesenteric; GSp, gastro-splenic; GSpM, gastrosplenomesenteric; HG, hepatogas-tric; HGM, hepatogastromesenteric; HGSp, hepatogastro-splenic; HM, hepatomesenteric; HSp, hepatosplenic; HSpM, hepatosplenomesenteric; LG, left gastric artery; SM, supe-rior mesenteric artery; Sp, splenic artery; SpM, splenomes-enteric.

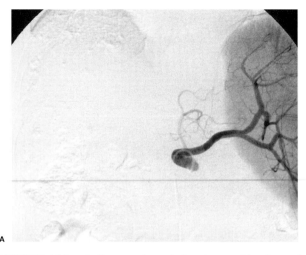

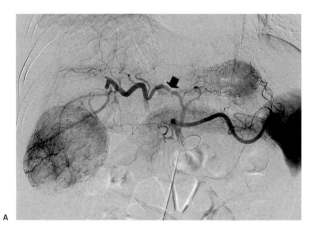

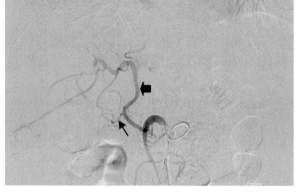

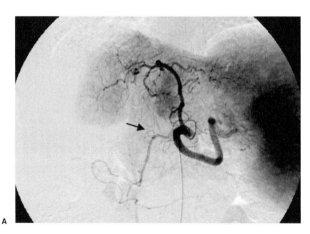

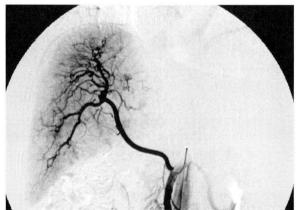

FIGURE 15.3. Celiac trunk variation in combination of gastrosplenic trunk (A) and hepatomesenteric trunk (B). Because of the associated celiac stenosis, superior mesenteric arteriogram shows hypertrophied collateral circulation via the dorsal pancreatic artery from the superior mesenteric artery (*thick arrow*) and an anastomotic channel (*thin arrows*) between the ascending part of the segment 2 hepatic artery and the fundic branch of the left gastric artery (*arrowheads*). When there is an accessory left gastric artery from the left hepatic artery, the fundic branch from the left gastric artery is usually replaced by it. Note the early branching of the right hepatic artery from the common hepatic artery (*open arrow*).

FIGURE 15.4. Ambiguous celiac trunk anatomy due to persistent embryological communicating channels (*thick arrows*). Because they are widely patent and almost equal in diameter, it is impossible to determine the celiac trunk anatomy, whether the common hepatic artery is replaced from the left gastric artery or replaced from the superior mesenteric artery. The thin arrow indicates the origin of the right gastroepiploic artery.

FIGURE 15.5. Ambiguous celiac trunk anatomy due to absent common hepatic artery. (A) The entire left hepatic artery is replaced from the left gastric artery. The gastroduodenal artery arises from the celiac trunk as usual with the right gastric artery (*arrow*). (B) The entire right hepatic artery is replaced from the superior mesenteric artery.

Celiac Stenosis or Occlusion

Celiac stenosis or occlusion is the initial obstacle in transcatheter management of hepatic tumors. For successful and uneventful placement of a catheter in the target hepatic arteries, it is important to recognize celiac stenosis early and to understand the anatomy and hemodynamic alteration related to celiac stenosis. If the celiac trunk is severely stenotic or occluded, particular skill is required to pass a catheter through it or along alternative collateral pathways without causing arterial injury (3).

Reported causes of celiac trunk stenosis or occlusion are atherosclerosis, dissection, injury from previous catheter manipulation, surgical trauma, Takayasu arteritis and extrinsic compression by the median arcuate ligament (4). Among them, the two major causes are atherosclerosis and extrinsic compression by the median arcuate ligament of the diaphragm. The extrinsic compression is a kind of congenital abnormality, and the onset of atherosclerosis is an age-dependent event. Thus, the incidence of celiac stenosis and the proportion of the two etiologies in the group with celiac stenosis vary according to the age and gender of the study population. Derrick et al. (5) found that in 110 unselected autopsy cases, its incidence was 21%, whereas Bron and Redman (4) noted an incidence of 12.5% among 713 patients referred for abdominal aortography. They found that the most important etiology of celiac stenosis was atherosclerosis. In contrast to the general belief that atherosclerosis is the major cause of the celiac stenosis, there are studies that report extrinsic compression by the median arcuate ligament of the diaphragm as the major cause of celiac stenosis in asymptomatic individuals and the Asian population (6, 7). According to a series of David and Harold (6), 12 of 50 asymptomatic individuals had celiac stenosis of 50% or more. On lateral aortography, the proximal celiac trunk showed a U-shaped configuration with compression along the superior aspect, a characteristic of impingement by the median arcuate ligament of the diaphragm (Figure 15.6). Thus, most cases of celiac stenosis in that series resulted from median arcuate ligament compression. In an Asian study using spiral CT scan and direct pressure measurement, the incidence of hemodynamically significant celiac stenosis in an asymptomatic population was 7.3%, and the most important etiology was extrinsic compression by the median arcuate ligament of the diaphragm (7). In that study,

atherosclerosis was only a minor cause of celiac stenosis. Deep expiration accentuates the compression of the celiac axis by the median arcuate ligament of the diaphragm (Figure 15.7) (8).

Although celiac stenosis is frequently encountered, clinically significant ischemia is rarely reported due to rich collateral circulation. The collateral circulation associated with celiac stenosis develops via pathways of the pancreaticoduodenal arcades, dorsal pancreatic arteries, replaced or accessory RHAs, interlobar collaterals, or gastric anastomosis (Figures 15.6 and 15.8; 9). Celiac trunk or hepatic artery variations greatly affect the pattern of collateralization (9). According to the severity of celiac stenosis, the flow direction of the GDA or CHA is reversed by retrograde flow from the SMA. In severe celiac stenosis, celiac arteriography poorly visualizes hepatic arterial territory due to competitive unopacified flow from the SMA, and superior mesenteric arteriography better opacifies hepatic arterial territory through hypertrophied pancreaticoduodenal arcade or dorsal pancreatic artery pathways (Figure 15.6). Severe celiac stenosis, especially associated with concomitant SMA stenosis, and unusual extra-hepatic collateral pathways may develop. We have to remember that the hepatic segment unusually supplied by extra-hepatic arterial collaterals (i.e., from the internal mammary artery) cannot be opacified either by celiac arteriography or by superior mesenteric arteriography. It is important to identify each segmental hepatic artery to avoid incomplete angiography and treatment. Interlobar collaterals in celiac stenosis may cause untoward embolization of non-target organ due to reversed flow of hepatic arteries. In that occasion, it is necessary to embolize interlobar collaterals for safe and effective treatment (Figure 15.8).

For safe and successful catheterization of the occluded celiac trunk, it is important to understand its etiology and the corresponding anatomy and to adjust catheterization techniques to suit them. In transcatheter management of hepatic tumors with an occluded celiac trunk, the access route to the hepatic arteries determines the success and completeness of the procedure. If possible, access through the occluded celiac trunk is superior to that through the pancreaticoduodenal arcades in microcatheter manipulation and superselective catheterization of tumor-feeding arteries. In our experience, catheterization through the pancreaticoduodenal

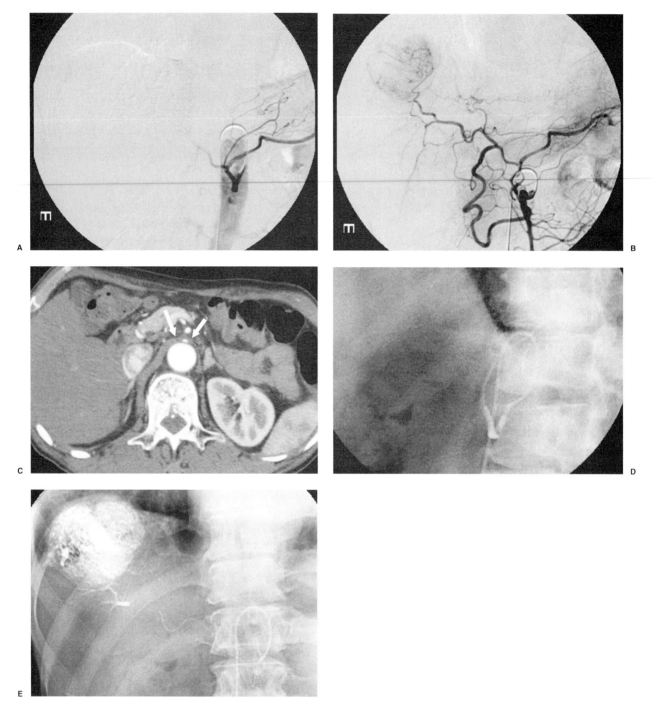

FIGURE 15.6. Severe celiac stenosis and segmental chemoembolization via the stenotic celiac trunk. (A) Celiac arteriogram shows acute downward angulation of the celiac trunk with poor opacification of the common hepatic artery due to reversed competitive flow from the gastroduodenal artery. (B) Superior mesenteric arteriography demonstrates excellent opacification of hepatic arteries and the splenic artery via hypertrophied pancreaticoduodenal arcade and dorsal pancreatic artery. The common hepatic artery is atrophic due to chronic celiac stenosis. (C) Thin-section arterial phase CT scan reveals severe compression of the proximal celiac trunk by the median arcuate ligament of the diaphragm (*arrows*). (D) Test injection of the celiac axis in left anterior oblique projection shows characteristic appearance of the celiac stenosis due to median arcuate ligament compression. (E) It was possible to advance a microcatheter through the severely stenotic celiac axis and select the right anterior segment hepatic artery. Segmental chemoembolization was successfully performed.

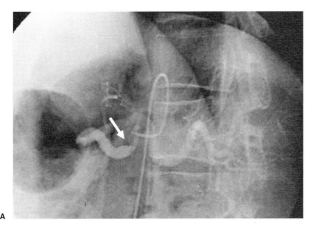

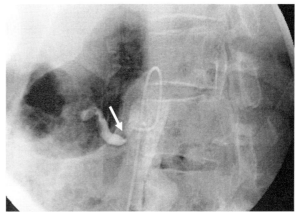

FIGURE 15.7.   Accentuation of celiac compression by the median arcuate ligament of the diaphragm during expiration. (A) Celiac arteriogram during inspiration shows mild focal stenosis at the superior aspect of the proximal celiac trunk *(arrow).* **(B) Deep expiration accentuates celiac trunk compression and almost stops the blood flow through the celiac trunk.**

arcade required more procedure time and, sometimes, additional devices. Therefore, we suggest that catheterization through the occluded celiac trunk should be the initial approach with an occluded celiac trunk. For the inexperienced angiographer, there is increased risk of arterial dissection as a result of repeated attempts at catheterization of the celiac trunk when the trunk is significantly stenotic or occluded. According to the cause of celiac occlusion, it is recommended to use appropriate catheterization techniques to minimize arterial injury. The pancreaticoduodenal arcade is the most common collateral pathway in cases of common hepatic or celiac arterial occlusion. It can be an alternative route for hepatic chemoembolization in patients with celiac occlu-

sion. The techniques to catheterize the target hepatic arteries in celiac occlusion were described in detail by Kwon et al. (10). Even the LHA arising from the LGA can be catheterized in the retrograde fashion through the pancreaticoduodenal arcade. The gastric anastomosis between the RGA and LGA can be a route for successful catheterization of the LHA arising from the occluded or severely stenotic LGA in patients with celiac trunk variation.

With the recent advances in helical CT technology, it became possible to detect celiac stenosis and predict its etiologies. Thin-section helical CT successfully demonstrates the median arcuate ligament of the diaphragm obstructing the celiac axis. The CT findings of celiac compression by the median

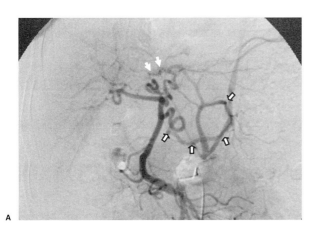

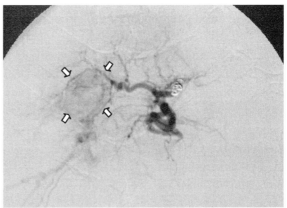

FIGURE 15.8.   Celiac stenosis and embolization of intrahepatic collateral channels in a patient with celiac trunk variation of hepatomesenteric trunk and aberrant left hepatic artery from the left gastric artery. (A) Superior mesenteric arteriogram demonstrates hypertrophied anastomotic channels between the right gastric artery and the left gastric artery *(open arrows),* **and between the segment 4 hepatic artery and aberrant left hepatic artery from the left gastric artery** *(arrows).* **The flow of the left gastric artery is also reversed. (B) After coil embolization of the intrahepatic collateral channel, selective segment 4 hepatic arteriography reveals tumor stain** *(open arrows).* **The tumor was successfully treated with chemoembolization.**

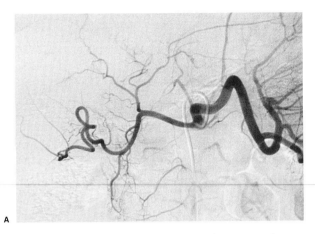
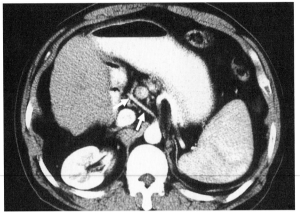

A   B

FIGURE 15.9. Unusual anatomical course of the common hepatic artery, which arises from the celiac trunk and runs through the portocaval space (*arrows*).

arcuate ligament are effacement or narrowing of the celiac axis by an anterior soft tissue band (Figure 15.6), dilated peripancreatic collateral vessels and poststenotic dilation of the distal celiac axis (7, 11). In most patients with celiac occlusion due to median arcuate ligament compression, it is possible to pass a microcatheter through the compressed potential lumen (Figure 15.6). Therefore, in selective catheterization of the occluded celiac axis, it is quite useful to carefully review helical CT scans. Thin-section helical CT in arterial phase may also demonstrate major collateral vessels, including unusual ones, and enable preprocedural evaluation of their anatomy for successful catheterization.

Hepatic Artery Anatomy

Normal Hepatic Artery Anatomy and Variations in Its Origin and Anatomic Course

In normal celiac trunk anatomy, the CHA typically bifurcates into the GDA and PHA, and the PHA bifurcates into the RHA and LHA. The classic CHA lies in the hepatoduodenal ligament to the left of the common bile duct and anterior to the portal vein. Therefore, the hepatic artery runs across the portal vein anteriorly. This standard hepatic arterial anatomy has been reported in 50% to 65% of patients on cadaveric and angiographic investigations (2, 12).

There is a wide spectrum of hepatic artery variations encompassing the territory of variant hepatic arteries (from the CHA to subsegmental hepatic arteries), their aberrant origin and their abnormal anatomical course.

As CHA variations, the CHA arises from the SMA in the hepatomesenteric trunk as a celiac trunk variation. In the hepatomesenteric trunk, the CHA could take various anatomical pathways in relation to the pancreas and the portal vein. Most times, it runs through the portocaval space or across the portal vein anteriorly. Occasionally, it may pass through or below the pancreas head. Rarely, the CHA arising from the celiac trunk passes through the portocaval space, when it looks normal on celiac arteriography (Figure 15.9). The CHA rarely arises from the LGA through the fissure for the ligamentum venosum (Figure 15.10). When the CHA arises from the LGA, it sequentially gives off the LHA, RHA and GDA.

As PHA variation, the PHA may arise from the LGA, celiac trunk, GDA, SMA or directly from the aorta, with the GDA separately arising from the celiac trunk or SMA.

In hepatic artery variations, the vascular territory of variant hepatic arteries can vary from subsegmental to lobar distribution. In addition, hepatic artery variations can coexist (Figure 15.11). The aberrant RHA can arise from the SMA, celiac trunk or directly from the aorta, with an incidence of 15% to 20%. The aberrant LHA arises from the LGA with a similar incidence. The most common variants of the hepatic artery are the aberrant LHA from the LGA and the aberrant RHA from the SMA. The aberrant RHA from the SMA is usually the first major artery arising from the SMA. This vessel almost always possesses the origin of the main cystic or accessory cystic artery (13). Occasionally, it may arise from the pancreaticoduodenal trunk. The aberrant LHA from the LGA runs within the ligamentum venosum with a characteristic appearance and frequently sends

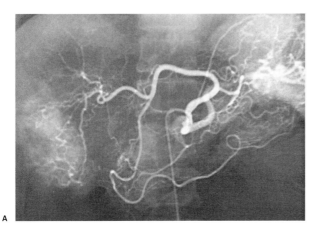 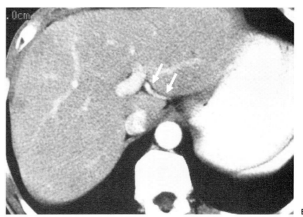

FIGURE 15.10.   The anomalous origin of the common hepatic artery from the left gastric artery. It passes through the fissue for the ligamentum venosum on CT scan (*arrows*).

smaller branches to the stomach and esophagus (Figure 15.11; 14). In aberrant LHA from the LGA, all of the side branches before reaching the umbilical point are esophageal or gastric branches.

Variant arteries running through the fissure for the ligamentum venosum include the CHA, PHA and LHA from the LGA. The accessory LGA from the LHA or PHA, the left inferior phrenic artery from LHA and aberrant left gastric venous drainage also can pass through the fissure for ligamentum venosum. Variant arteries running through the portocaval space include the RHA from the CHA, the RHA and CHA from the celiac trunk, the RHA and PHA and CHA from the SMA and RHA from the aorta.

Aberrant origin of subsegmental or segmental hepatic arteries may not be easily recognized on celiac arteriography. Careful interpretation of dynamic CT, tracing of individual segmental hepatic arteries on celiac arteriography, adequate opacification of the LGA on celiac angiography and routine SMA arteriography can avoid missing them. Most of these variant hepatic arteries can be accurately predicted with thin-section helical dynamic CT (Figures 15.10 and 15.11).

There are also hepatic artery variations within the CHA in about 10% of patients. Multiple hepatic arteries arise from the CHA as separate trunks, as trifurcation, two or three hepatic arterial trunks sequentially off the CHA or aberrant origin of the RHA or LHA from the GDA or pancreaticoduodenal artery.

All of these hepatic artery variations can coexist with celiac trunk variations.

If competitive flow from a dual arterial supply is noted due to hepatic artery variations, embolization or fractionation of the therapeutic agent may be con-

sidered. If tortuosity of the vessel prevents safe administration of the therapeutic agent, embolization of the artery may be required (13).

Intrahepatic Variations in Branching Segmental Hepatic Arteries

There are also diverse variations in intrahepatic branching of segmental hepatic arteries. The RHA is one of the most constant vessels of the liver. The right hepatic lobe can be partly supplied by an accessory RHA from SMA or celiac trunk in fewer than 5% of the population (15, 16). Rarely, a segmental RHA arises from the LHA (Figure 15.12). The anterior and posterior section of the right hepatic lobe is commonly supplied by multiple arteries. Segment 5 and 7 were predominantly supplied by one artery, and segments 6 and 8, by two arteries (16).

The left hepatic lobe is supplied by the one LHA (from the PHA or LGA) only in less than half of the population (15, 17). The aberrant LHA from the LGA can supply the whole left hepatic lobe, segment 2 and 3 and a part of segment 4, segment 2 and 3, segment 2 and 4, or segment 2 alone. Segment 4 was usually supplied by two or three hepatic arteries. Left medial arterial branches arise from the LHA on the umbilical portion of the portal vein, arise from the LHA before reaching the umbilical portion of the portal vein or arise from the RHA (18).

The caudate lobe is usually supplied by multiple arteries (2). According to our experience, almost all caudate arteries arise from the proximal segment of hepatic arteries, including the PHA, the ascending part of the main LHA or middle hepatic artery, the main RHA and the proximal segment of the right anterior and posterior segmental artery

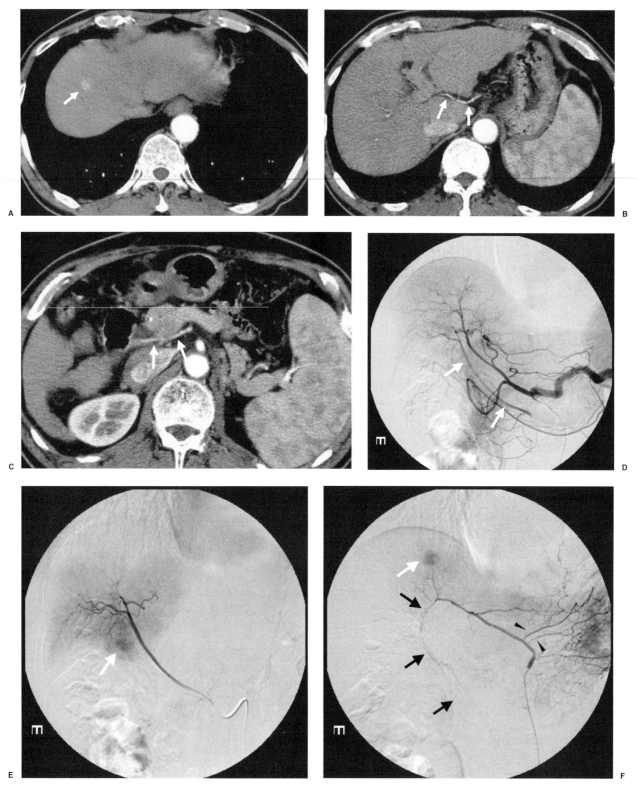

FIGURE 15.11. Recognition of multiple variant hepatic arteries in a patient. (A) Arterial-phase CT scan shows a small enhancing nodule in hepatic segment 4. (BC) CT scan also demonstrates the presence of aberrant left hepatic artery in the fissure for the ligamentum venosum (*arrows* in B) and aberrant right hepatic artery in the portocaval space (*arrows* in C). (D) There is no tumor stain on common hepatic arteriography. The missing right posterior segmental artery (faintly opacified by the reflux of the contrast material via the pancreaticoduodenal arcade) and the left hepatic artery supplying hepatic segment 2 and 4 should be recognized. (E) Selective angiogram of the right posterior segmental artery from the superior mesenteric artery shows another tumor stain (*arrow*). (F) Selective left hepatic arteriogram shows the aberrant left hepatic artery supplying hepatic segment 2 and 4 and tumor stain in segment 4 (*white arrow*). All of the side branches before reaching the umbilical point (*arrowheads*) are gastric or esophageal branches. Note the hepatic falciform artery arising from the segment 4 hepatic artery (*black arrows*).

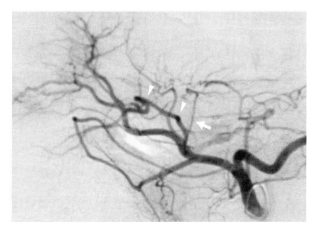

FIGURE 15.12. Intrahepatic variation. The right posterior segmental artery (*arrowheads*) **arises from the proper hepatic artery as the first branch with the segment 3 hepatic artery** (*arrow*).

(Figure 15.13). The caudate lobe is divided into three subsegments of the Spiegel lobe, paracaval portion and caudate process. The paracaval portion and caudate process almost always are supplied by feeders

from the main RHA or the proximal segment of its branches. In contrast, the hepatic artery supplying the Spiegel lobe is evenly distributed to the proximal segment of hepatic arteries. Because the caudate lobe is supplied by multiple feeders from the RHA and LHA, wedged injection of a caudate hepatic artery frequently demonstrates anastomotic channels between multiple feeders and between the RHA and LHA.

Segmental Localization of Liver Tumors

Accurate segmental localization is important for effective segmental transcatheter management of hepatic tumors and inaccurate segmentation in CT interpretation can lead to prolonged procedure time and erroneous treatment of innocent hepatic segment. The conventional method dividing hepatic segments according to Couinaud's classification is based on the concept of three vertical planes that divide the liver into four segments and a transverse scissura

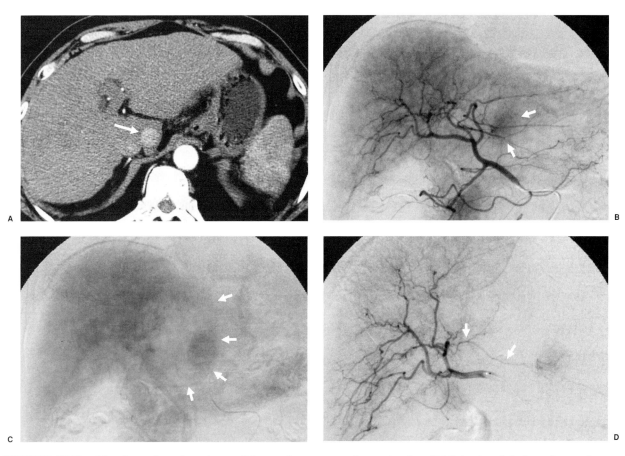

FIGURE 15.13. Blood supply and territory of the caudate lobe. (A) Arterial-phase CT scan shows nodular enhancing tumor (arrow) at the Spiegel lobe of the caudate lobe. (B) Common hepatic arteriogram shows an ill-defined tumor stain (*arrows*). **(C) Delayed parenchymal phase image shows the typical outline of the caudate lobe** (*arrows*) **on antero-** posterior projection. **(D) Selective right hepatic arteriogram shows a feeding artery from the proximal segment of the right anterior segmental artery** (*arrows*). **Iodized-oil CT scan was obtained immediately after segmental lipiodol chemoembolization.**

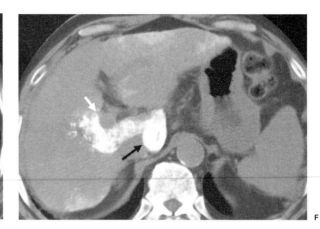

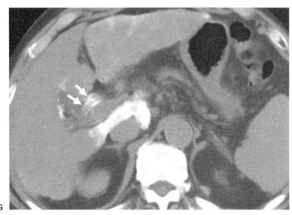

FIGURE 15.13. (Continued) (E) Iodized-oil CT scan at the level of the middle hepatic vein (*black arrow*) shows the cross-sectional anatomical location of the paracaval portion (*white arrows*). (F) Iodized-oil CT scan at the level of the tumor (*black arrow* with compact iodized-oil uptake) shows the territory of the caudate lobe. The caudate hepatic artery supplies a far posterior aspect of the hepatic segment 4 (*white arrow*). (G) Iodized-oil CT scan at the level of the central bile duct (the bifurcation area). There is iodized-oil uptake in the wall of the bile duct (*arrows*), which implies the caudate hepatic artery can supply the bile duct or anastomose with a bile duct artery.

that further subdivides the segments into two subsegments each (19–21). Although convenient for daily radiologic practice, clinical and extraclinical studies have demonstrated that the shape and localization of the hepatic segments based on this conventional method do not always match real situations (22–24). As an example, the segment 8 extends posterior to the right hepatic vein (23,24). In addition, in contrast to the vague conventional concept of posterosuperior-anteroinferior relationship of segment 2 and segment 3, the average orientation of the intersegmental plane between segment 2 and segment 3 is slightly slanted anteriorly from the vertical plane (Figure 15.14) (25). The scissurae may curve, undulate or even interdigitate within the liver (22). Radiological determination of the segmental and subsegmental portal venous anatomy can be done by evaluation of the overlapping transverse slices in an interactive cine mode or by performing three-dimensional rendering (22).

Non-hepatic Arteries Arising from Hepatic Arteries

A **non-hepatic artery** is defined as an artery that arises from the PHA or its distal branches and supplies organs and areas other than hepatic parenchyma.

Non-hepatic arteries include the cystic artery, RGA, hepatic falciform artery, accessory LGA, pancreaticoduodenal artery and left inferior phrenic artery, in descending order of frequency. Some of these non-hepatic arteries can be detected only on superselective angiography with use of a microcatheter, especially hepatic falciform arteries and small accessory LGA and RGA. Therefore, to identify these arteries, careful analysis of celiac axis arteriograms and superselective angiograms is required. According to a recent investigation using a microcatheter and superselective angiography (26), the most frequent site of origin of non-hepatic arteries except the cystic artery was the LHA. More than two-thirds of the patients had one or more non-hepatic arteries from the LHA and one-third of patients had gastric arteries from the LHA. In contrast, only 3% of the non-hepatic arteries except the cystic artery arose from the RHA. More than 40% of patients had multiple non-hepatic arteries.

In describing the origin sites of non-hepatic arteries, it is necessary to define the terminology of the PHA. In general, the PHA is defined as the common trunk of the RHA and LHA. According to the definition of the PHA, when the RHA or LHA has aberrant

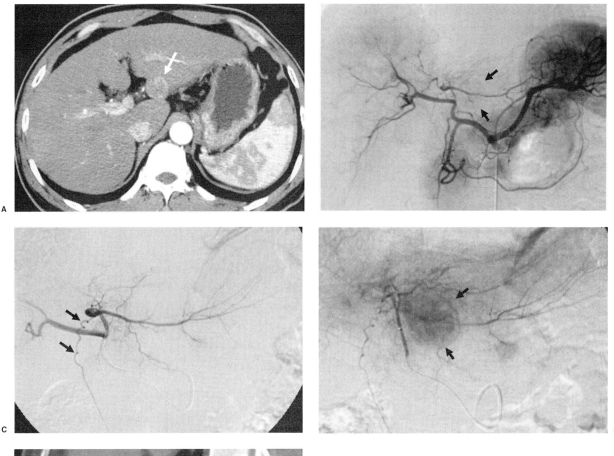

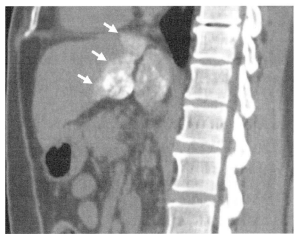

FIGURE 15.14.   Segmental localization of a tumor in the left lateral segment of the liver. (A) Small nodular enhancing tumor (*arrow*) is located at the posterior aspect of the left lateral segment below the level of the left portal vein. (B) On celiac arteriography, the tumor (*arrows*) overlaps with the segment 3 hepatic artery. (C) Selective angiogram of the segment 3 hepatic artery shows no tumor stain. Note the hepatic falciform artery arising from the segment 3 hepatic artery (*arrows*). (D) Segment 2 hepatic arteriogram shows nodular tumor stain (*arrows*). Lipiodol chemoembolization was performed exclusively at the segment 2 hepatic artery. (E) Sagittal reformatted image of the immediate iodized-oil CT demonstrates the orientation of the intersegmental plane between segment 2 and 3, which is slanted posteriorly at the superior aspect and undulating in its contour.

origins, there is no PHA. We adopted the term **PHA equivalent** to describe the hepatic arterial trunk arising from the CHA in the situation of aberrant origin of the RHA or LHA from the CHA or other sites. For example, an LHA arising from the PHA differs from one arising directly from the CHA when the RHA aberrantly originates from the SMA, celiac trunk or aorta. We assumed that when the PHA was absent as a result of an aberrant hepatic artery origin (or when two separate hepatic arterial trunks arose from the CHA), the (first) arterial trunk arising from the CHA is equivalent to the PHA.

Inadvertent infusion of therapeutic materials at a hepatic artery proximal to the origin of a non-hepatic artery may unavoidably induce diverse complications after transcatheter liver-directed therapies. They include cholecystitis or gallbladder infarction, gastroduodenal mucosal lesions, pulmonary oil embolism and supraumbilical skin rash. Therefore, the preprocedural identification of non-hepatic arteries arising from the hepatic arteries is important to reduce complications related to various transcatheter therapies such as chemoembolization, intra-arterial infusion chemotherapy, and brachytherapy

(13). Advances in microcatheters and digital subtraction angiography systems enable identification of small tumor-feeding vessels and permit selective insertion of microcatheters into small segmental or subsegmental arteries distal to the non-hepatic arteries. This superselective procedure can reduce not only hepatic parenchymal injury but also unintentional infusion of chemoembolic agent into the non-hepatic arteries. If superselective catheterization of tumor-feeding arteries is not possible, it is essential to use appropriate preventive measures: embolization of a non-hepatic artery with adequate embolic materials before the therapeutic infusion or infusion through an occlusion balloon catheter to redirect blood flow in non-hepatic arteries toward the liver (27, 28). Flow to the non-target organ is maintained by distal collateral vessels. If the non-hepatic artery acts as the tumor-feeding vessel, it should be treated superselectively by advancing a microcatheter to a tumor feeder from the nonhepatic artery. If superselective catheterization is not possible, other alternative therapeutic methods, including surgery, ablation therapy and injection therapy, should be considered (13).

Right Gastric Artery

The RGA usually arises from the hepatic artery, descends to the pyloric end of the stomach, and passes from right to left along the lesser curvature, supplying it with branches, and anastomosing with the LGA (Figure 15.15) (1). Usually, the RGA is the minor contributor to the gastric perfusion when compared with the LGA. Occasionally, the RGA is larger than the LGA or too small to identify on celiac or common hepatic arteriography as the RGA. In cases of aberrant anatomy and small RGA, the LGA may be used to identify the origin of the RGA (13). When cannulation of the RGA is difficult as a result of tortuosity or orientation of the origin, retrograde catheterization through the anastomotic arcade between the LGA and RGA can be a good alternative and has proved to be effective for RGA embolization (29, 30).

Regardless of the presence or absence of anatomic variations, the most common origin site of the RGA is the PHA (40% to 59%) or its equivalent followed by the LHA (17% to 45%) (Figure 15.1). In about three-fourths of the patients, the RGA arises from the PHA or its distal branches. In the remaining patients, the RGA arises from the bifurcation point of the CHA or GDA (Figure 15.15). The RGA rarely arises from the CHA or RHA (2, 14, 26, 30).

Identification of the RGA is crucial for transcatheter management of hepatic tumors, as gastroduodenal necrosis, ulceration and perforation have all been identified as complications of inadvertent delivery of chemotherapeutic agent (29, 30). In hepatic arterial infusion chemotherapy, successful embolization of the RGA was accomplished in more than 90% of patients and sufficient embolization of the RGA significantly reduced the incidence of endoscopically confirmed acute mucosal lesions (31). Depending on the regional therapy being considered, the need for prophylactic embolization of the gastric variants must be taken into account (13).

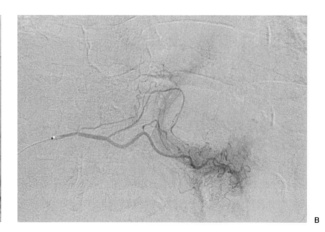

A B

FIGURE 15.15. Recognition of gastric arteries. **(A)** Celiac arteriogram shows trifurcation of the common hepatic artery into the left hepatic artery, right hepatic artery and gastroduodenal artery. The right gastric artery arises from the trifurcation of the common hepatic artery and anastomoses with the left gastric artery (*black arrows*). The artery indicated by white arrows arises from the ascending segment of the left hepatic artery before reaching the umbilical point, which strongly suggests the possibility of the accessory left gastric artery. **(B)** On selective angiography, it supplies the distal esophagus and the cardia of the stomach.

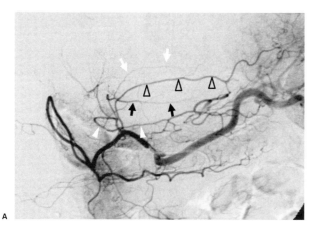
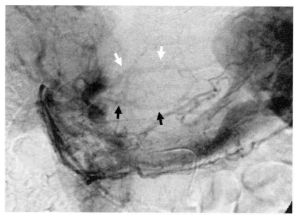

FIGURE 15.16.   Recognition of the accessory left gastric artery. (A) The accessory left gastric artery (*open arrowheads*) arises from the segment 4 hepatic artery and the right gastric artery (*white arrowheads*) arises from the left lateral hepatic artery. (B) On portal phase, the segment 3 (*black arrows*) and segment 2 hepatic arteries (*white arrows*) have their accompanying portal vein. In contrast, the accessory left gastric artery does not have the accompanying portal vein.

Accessory Left Gastric Artery

The accessory LGA runs from the liver to the stomach and supplies the esophagus and the cardia and fundus of the stomach (2, 32). In 1928, Adachi reported that accessory LGA was seen in 47 of 252 autopsies (17.9%). In contrast, Michels (2) reported an accessory LGA prevalence of only 3% among 200 anatomic dissections, which indicates a lower incidence in the Western population than in Asian populations (26, 32).

Considering the results of previous cadaveric and angiographic studies, the variant LHA and accessory LGA may be remnants of the embryologic communicating channel between the liver and stomach through the lesser omentum (26, 32). Therefore, it may not be surprising that the accessory LGA is not found in patients with a variant LHA from the LGA.

Because esophageal and gastric mucosa might be adversely affected by the infusion of therapeutic agents into the hepatic artery (28, 32–34), it is important to recognize the accessory LGA and differentiate gastric wall stain of the accessory LGA from a hepatic tumor of the left hepatic lobe (32).

The most common origin of the accessory LGA is the LHA. Occasionally, the accessory LGA can arise from the PHA and rarely from the RHA or CHA. It is possible to identify an accessory LGA by visualizing the point of branching, the course of the artery and the characteristic tortuosity of the peripheral branches. Branching occurs at the ascending segment of the LHA before the LHA reaches the umbilical point, at which the LHA kinks and divides into segmental branches. In the portal phase, the accessory LGA does not have an accompanying portal vein (Figure 15.16). Peripheral arterial branches around and in the gastric wall have a characteristic coiled appearance. In patients with the accessory LGA, the LGA from the celiac trunk do not have a fundic branch on celiac arteriography (Figure 15.15). When the accessory LGA is small, it is necessary to perform selective left hepatic arteriography or selective angiography of the suspected accessory LGA (Figure 15.17). Rarely, the accessory LGA arises from the LHA as a common trunk with the left inferior phrenic artery, mediastinal branch or bronchial artery.

Hepatic Falciform Artery

The hepatic falciform artery (HFA) arises as a terminal branch from the middle hepatic artery or LHA, which runs within the hepatic falciform ligament with the umbilical vein. The falciform ligament consists of a double fold of peritoneum located anterior to the liver, dividing the medial and lateral segments of the left lobe of the liver. With progression of liver cirrhosis, the falciform ligament in front of the liver is shifted to the right depending on the degree of atrophy of the right hepatic lobe. Therefore, the classic orientation of HFA is the initial short rightward segment before escaping the left intersegmental fissure (sometimes in coiled appearance in anteroposterior projection) and long leftward and downward segment before reaching the anterior abdominal wall (Figures 15.1, 15.11 and 15.14); (35, 36). The HFA provides partial blood supply around the umbilicus and communicates with branches of the internal mammary and superior epigastric arteries (Figure 15.18)

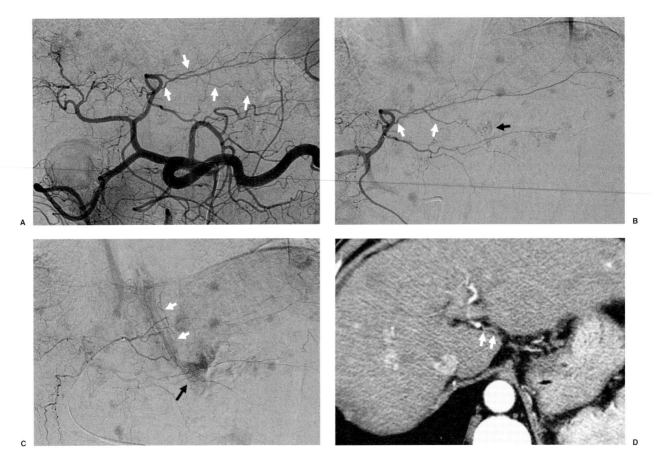

FIGURE 15.17. Recognition of the accessory left gastric artery. **(A)** Celiac arteriogram shows an artery arising from the left hepatic artery just before the umbilical point (*arrows*). It has a rather undulating course and terminal tortuosity. The right gastric artery arises from the bifurcation point of the proper hepatic artery. **(B)** Selective left hepatic arteriogram shows ill-defined stain at the end of the artery (*black arrow*) in the background of small multiple nodular tumor stain in the left hepatic lobe. **(C)** Selective angiogram obtained using a microcatheter shows esophageal (*white arrows*) and gastric stain (*black arrow*). **(D)** Arterial-phase scan in 2.5-mm collimation demonstrates this small accessory left gastric artery in the fissure for the ligamentum venosum (*arrows*).

(2, 27, 35). The HFA may function as a collateral pathway to the liver in cases of celiac trunk or hepatic artery occlusion.

In a detailed anatomic study, Michels (2) found the HFA in 70% of 200 cadaveric dissections. Angiographic studies reported a dramatically wide range of its frequency, from 2% to 52%, depending on the quality of angiography [screen-film angiography vs digital subtraction angiography (DSA)], celiac angiography versus selective left hepatic arteriography using a microcatheter and study design (prospective versus retrospective) (26, 27, 36, 37). It may be necessary to prolong DSA runs to allow for opacification of the vessel as a result of sluggish and competitive flow from the internal mammary and superior epigastric arteries (37). In a prospective study (26), only 62% of the HFA were recognized by celiac arteriography, which was the lowest detection rate on celiac arteriography among the non-hepatic arteries. The remaining cases were identified on superselec-

tive left hepatic arteriography. The HFA showed wide ranges of sizes and lengths. Most HFAs detected only by superselective angiography were much shorter in length than the others. The most common origin of the HFA is segment 4 hepatic artery regardless of the presence of hepatic arterial variation. In no cases did the HFA arise from the segment 2 hepatic artery (26).

The clinical significance of an angiographically patent HFA is that supraumbilical skin rash may be caused by exposure of the skin to toxic chemicals during chemoembolization or infusion chemotherapy through this artery (35, 37). There is a controversy over whether prophylactic embolization of the HFA is necessary. The HFA is clearly associated with supraumbilical skin rash, epigastric pain and skin necrosis after chemoembolization (27, 37, 39). However, it is also true that delivery of chemoembolic agents into the HFA does not always induce skin complications. Usually, the long HFA has a greater chance of reaching supraumbilical skin area. However, not

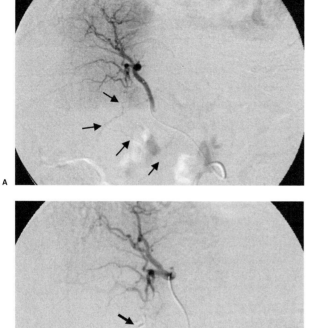

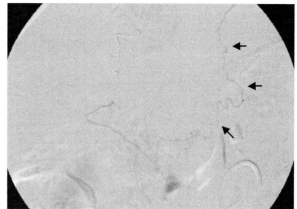

FIGURE 15.18. The hepatic falciform artery anastomosing with superior epigastric artery of the internal mammary artery. (A) Left hepatic arteriogram shows the falciform artery in its characteristic appearance (*arrows*). (B) Its selective angiogram using a microcatheter reveals the anastomosis with a superior epigastric vessel (*arrows*). (C) Embolization was successfully performed by casting the artery with glue (*arrows*).

every long HFA causes supraumbilical skin rash when chemoembolic materials is infused. On the contrary, even small HFAs occasionally induce skin lesions. Therefore, depending on the therapeutic materials used in transcatheter management and technical feasibility, the strategy for embolization of the HFA (optional or prophylactic embolization) can be determined. If the skin reaction to the therapeutic material is immediate in action and short-term in duration, optional embolization can be chosen. If preventive embolization is not feasible, it is recommended to perform therapeutic infusion with careful observation of the supraumbilical skin and symptoms. With intra-arterial brachytherapy, prophylactic embolization is necessary because non-target administration of yttrium-90 microspheres into the HFA will result in a highly localized midabdominal burning sensation for a period of days or weeks (13). Microcoils or glue can be used for embolization of the HFA (Figure 15.18).

Left Inferior Phrenic Artery

The two most common origins of the inferior phrenic arteries (IPAs) are the aorta immediately above or adjacent to the celiac trunk or the celiac trunk as a common trunk. The left IPA occasionally arises from the LHA. It is well-known that chemoembolization

through the IPA can induce shoulder pain, atelectasis of the basal lung and pleural effusion (40, 41). In case of a systemic-pulmonary shunt through the IPA, chemoembolization through the IPA may cause pulmonary embolism (42). The left IPAs from the LHA frequently form a common trunk with the accessory LGA (Figure 15.19). We have experienced a case of hemoptysis after chemoembolization in a patient with hepatocellular carcinoma, in whom the left IPA originated from the LHA.

Pancreaticoduodenal Arteries

The vascular anatomy of the pancreas head and the duodenum is very complex. Several named arteries, including pancreaticoduodenal arcade, dorsal pancreatic artery, supraduodenal or retroduodenal artery, contribute to complex flow dynamics in this region. Each of these vessels warrants consideration when regional therapy is to be considered (13). Adequate bolus injection and proper identification of these vessels may prevent therapy-induced pancreatitis (43), duodenal ulceration or perforation (44).

The pancreaticoduodenal arcades supply the head of the pancreas and the C loop of the duodenum, at least one being anterior and at least one posterior to the head of the pancreas (2). The anterior

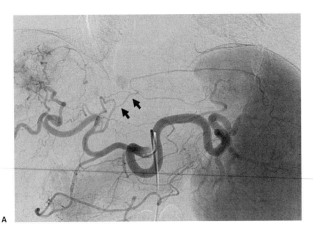

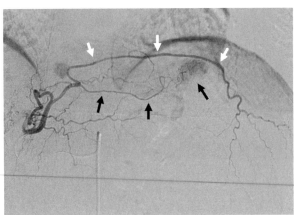

FIGURE 15.19. The left inferior phrenic artery arising from the accessory left gastric artery as a common trunk. (A) Celiac angiogram shows the origin of a nonhepatic artery from the left hepatic artery (*arrows*). (B) On selective angiog-raphy, it consists of the left inferior phrenic artery (*white arrows*) and the accessory left gastric artery producing the gastric fundus stain (*black arrows*).

pancreaticoduodenal arcade is formed by the anterior superior pancreaticoduodenal artery (PDA), the smaller of the two end branches of the GDA. The posterior pancreaticoduodenal arcade is formed by the retroduodenal artery (posterior superior PDA), usually the first branch of the GDA before or immediately after it passes behind the duodenum. The two arcades either unite with the SMA via separate inferior PDA given off by the SMA, one for each arcade, or end in a common inferior PDA. The posterior arcades are more cephalad than the anterior arcades.

The pancreaticoduodenal arcades are the most common collateral pathways from the SMA to the celiac branches. Although in most cases both the anterior and posterior arcades developed as collateral pathways between the SMA and the CHA, occasion-ally one arcade developed as a single channel (Figure 15.6) (9).

Michels (2) reported that the posterior PDA arose from the first branch of the GDA in 90% of 200 dissections, from the RHA in 5%, from the PHA in 4% and from the artery being replaced by a branch from the dorsal pancreatic artery in 1%. In a prospective study (26), the incidence of the posterior superior PDA arising from the PHA or its distal branches was 7%. This condition was particularly prevalent in patients with a variant hepatic artery originating from the GDA. Of 13 patients with a variant hepatic artery arising from the GDA, the prevalence of the postero-superior PDA was 54% (7 of 13). In other words, the posterior pancreaticoduodenal arcade is an important route of hepatic artery variation (Figure 15.20).

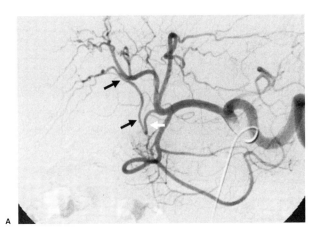

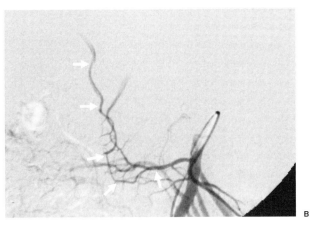

FIGURE 15.20. Accessory right hepatic artery arising from the posterior superior pancreaticoduodenal arcade formed between the proper hepatic artery and the superior mesenteric artery. (A) Celiac angiogram shows aberrant origin of the segment 6 hepatic artery from the proper hepatic artery in unusual configuration (*arrows*). (B) Superior mesen-teric arteriogram clearly shows the communicating arcade (*arrows*) between the aberrant segment 6 hepatic artery and the posterior inferior pancreaticoduodenal artery. Therefore, it can be said the segment 6 hepatic artery originates from the posterior superior pancreaticoduodenal artery.

The dorsal pancreatic artery is the first large pancreatic branch of the splenic artery. In an anatomic study of 200 cadavers by Michels (13), the dorsal pancreatic artery was seen to arise from the splenic artery in 39% of cases. However, in 61% of cases it arose from other sources, such as the CHA (12%), SMA (14%) or celiac artery (22%). A dorsal pancreatic artery of SMA origin has numerous anastomotic connections with the celiac and SMA branches and therefore has an important role in the collateral circulation in patients with celiac axis stenosis. The dorsal pancreatic artery typically divides into two right branches and one left branch (2). One of the right branches joins the pancreaticoduodenal arcade, whereas the other becomes the artery to the uncinate process of the pancreas. The left branch becomes the transverse pancreatic artery. The pancreatica magna or caudal pancreatic arteries of the splenic artery anastomose with the transverse pancreatic artery. The fourth branch of the dorsal pancreatic artery often descends below the inferior border of the pancreas behind the splenic vein to communicate with the SMA or one of its branches (the jejunal, middle colic or accessory middle colic artery), thereby constituting an important longitudinal collateral pathway between the celiac artery and the SMA (9).

The supraduodenal artery has been described as a distinctive artery that may arise from the GDA (27%), CHA (20%), LHA (20%), RHA (13%) and cystic arteries (10%) (13, 45). Anastomoses with the extra-hepatic biliary ductal arterial supply have been described in gross dissection (46).

Cystic Artery and Biliary Plexus

Based on the cadaveric dissection of 500 specimens, Daseler et al. (46) reported an incidence of cystic artery arising from a classic location (RHA arising from the PHA) of 72%, with an incidence of accessory or duplicated cystic arteries of 3%. Other origins of the cystic artery include replaced/accessory RHA (18%), LHA (7%), CHA (3%), GDA (1%) and several other unusual origins (13). The cystic artery usually has two branches, a superficial (peritoneal) branch and a deep (non-peritoneal) branch (Figure 15.21) (13). It may contribute blood supply to extra-hepatic bile ducts.

The cystic artery must be identified before transcatheter management of hepatic tumors to prevent or minimize the risks of chemical cholecystitis or ischemic or radiation necrosis. Therefore, catheterization distal to the cystic artery is recommended. Occasionally, the cystic artery may feed the tumor. The superselective catheterization of tumor-feeding arteries from the cystic artery with lack of gallbladder wall staining allows safe delivery of therapeutic agents (Figure 15.21) (13).

The blood supply to the biliary tree is via a microscopic peribiliary plexus that is seldom visualized angiographically. It may enlarge when it supplies the tumor invading the bile ducts or major portal vein (Figures 15.22 and 15.23). The extra-hepatic bile duct system is supplied by multiple arteries from the cystic artery, PDA and RHA (47, 48). The right and left intrahepatic bile ducts are surrounded by a vascular plexus supplied from the main right and left hepatic arteries, segmental arteries, GDA and accessory hepatic arteries. This plexus is closely associated with the arteries supplying the caudate lobe. The caudate lobe and biliary plexus provide collateral connections between the right and left livers (49). Biliary necrosis is a relatively rare occurrence because there lies a rich extra-hepatic arterial supply for the biliary system.

Extra-hepatic Collateral Arteries

Extra-hepatic collateral arteries (EHCs) commonly supply hepatic tumors if the tumors are large or peripherally located, irrespective of the hepatic artery patency (Figures 15.24 and 15.25) (50, 51). Exophytic growth and extracapsular infiltration of hepatic tumors can cause adhesion or direct invasion into adjacent organs, including the diaphragm, omentum, abdominal wall, gallbladder, stomach, colon, adrenal gland and kidney, which creates blood supply to the tumors from these organs. Hepatic artery occlusion or attenuation of peripheral hepatic arteries due to repeated transcatheter managements may initiate or exaggerate extra-hepatic collateral supply to the tumors (Figures 15.26 and 15.27) (52–55).

EHCs include IPAs (Figures 15.24, 15.26 and 15.27), omental branches (Figure 15.27), cystic artery (Figure 15.21), internal mammary arteries (IMAs) (Figures 15.25 and 15.27), intercostal (Figure 15.26) or lumbar arteries, adrenal arteries, gastric arteries, renal or renal capsular artery (Figure 15.26), colic branches from the SMA and collateral vessels from the GDA or PDAs (Figure 15.23) (3, 40, 41, 50–61). The IPAs, IMAs, and intercostal arteries communicate with each other and with peripheral hepatic arterial branches through the diaphragm

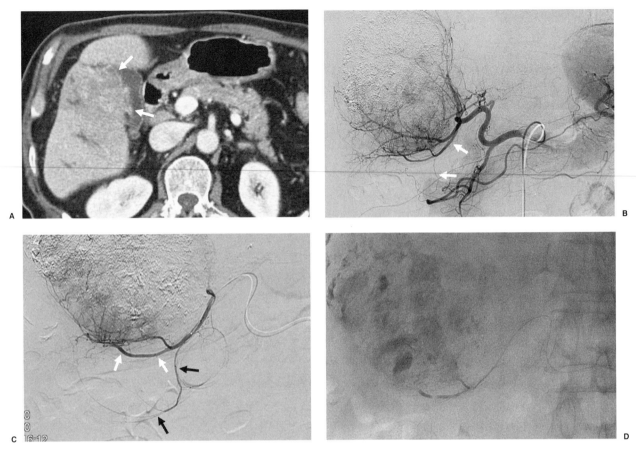

FIGURE 15.21. Hepatocellular carcinoma supplied by deep cystic artery and its selective embolization. (A) CT scan shows compression or direct invasion of the gallbladder by a tumor (*arrows*). (B) The common hepatic arteriogram shows hypervascular tumor suspected to be supplied by the hypertrophied cystic artery (*arrows*). (C) Selective angiogra-phy of the cystic artery demonstrates tumor stain exclusively supplied by the deep branch (*white arrows*). The superficial branch (*black arrows*) did not contribute to the tumor. (D) Chemoembolization was performed at the deep branch of the cystic artery.

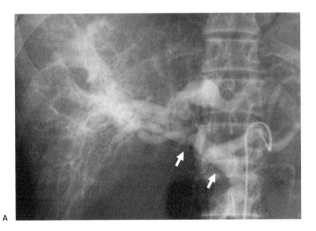
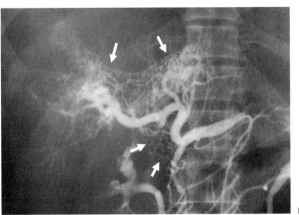

FIGURE 15.22. Dilated periportal, and peribiliary collat-eral network in a patient with hepatocellular carcinoma invading the main portal vein and severe arterioportal shunt. (A) Common hepatic arteriography demonstrates a diffuse tumor in the right hepatic lobe invading the main portal vein and severe arterioportal shunt. Note the hepatofugal opaci-fication of the main portal vein (*arrows*) and its tributaries. (B) After Gelfoam embolization of the arterioportal shunt, numerous fine arterial networks appeared along the central portal vein and bile ducts including the hepatoduodenal lig-ament (*arrows*). The tributaries of the gastroduodenal artery also contribute to these anastomotic networks.

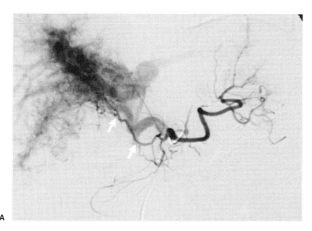

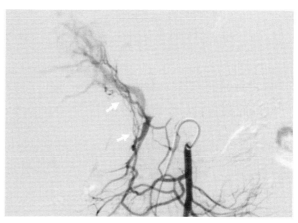

FIGURE 15.23. Dilated periportal and peribiliary collateral vessels along the hepatoduodenal ligament in a patient with hepatocellular carcinoma invading the right portal vein and severe arterioportal shunt. **(A)** Celiac arteriogram demonstrates a diffuse tumor in the right hepatic lobe invading the right portal vein and severe arterioportal shunt. Note the hypertrophied collateral vessel in the hepatoduodenal ligament (*arrows*) supplied by the dorsal pancreatic artery from the splenic artery. **(B)** Superior mesenteric arteriogram reveals additional multiple collateral channels supplied by the pancreaticoduodenal artery (*arrows*).

(Figures 15.24–15.27) (41, 50–58). The right renal capsular artery, middle adrenal artery and inferior adrenal artery run through the hepatorenal ligament and enter the liver (55). The branches of the right and middle colic arteries may enter the liver through adhesion between the liver and colon at the paracolic gutter (53). The RGA and LGA anastomose with each other and enter the liver via the lesser omentum. The bile duct artery or collaterals from the GDA or PDA run through the hepatoduodenal ligament and enter the liver. The cystic artery may give off a small hepatic artery branch (62) or communicate with the branch of a hepatic artery through the deep branch of the cystic artery at the gallbladder fossa (63). The omental

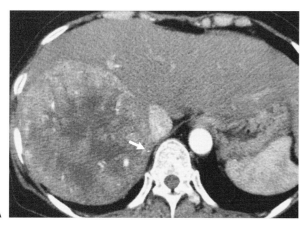

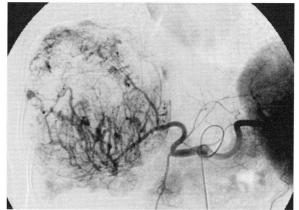

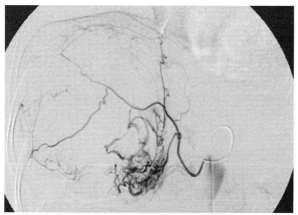

FIGURE 15.24. Large hepatocellular carcinoma supplied by the right inferior phrenic artery at its initial presentation. **(A)** Helical CT scan in the arterial phase shows a large hypervascular tumor at the right hepatic lobe abutting the posterior diaphragm. The arrow indicates the right inferior phrenic artery. Its hypertrophy is not remarkable. **(B)** On celiac arteriography, the celiac trunk and hepatic arteries are widely patent. **(C)** Right inferior phrenic arteriogram shows its aortic origin and tumor vascularity.

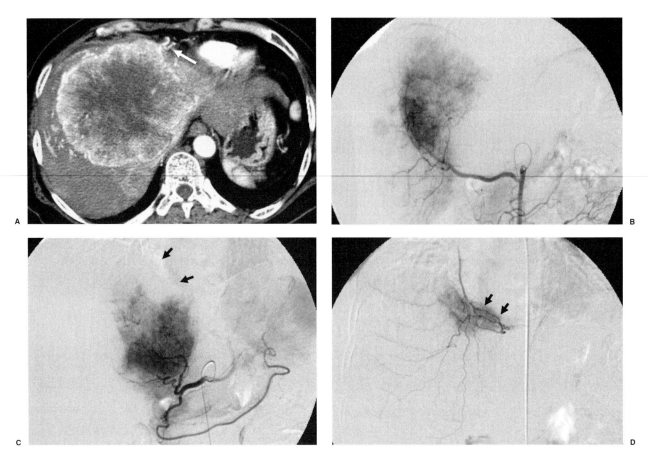

FIGURE 15.25. Large hepatocellular carcinoma abutting the anterosuperior diaphragm supplied by the right internal mammary artery at its initial presentation. **(A)** Helical CT scan in the arterial phase shows a large hypervascular tumor replacing the segment 4 and 8 abutting the anterosuperior diaphragm. The arrow indicates hypertrophied tumor feeding artery. **(B)** The right hepatic artery is replaced from the superior mesenteric artery. **(C)** Common hepatic arteriogram demonstrates a defect of the tumor stain at the superior diaphragmatic aspect (*arrows*). **(D)** The defect area is supplied by a phrenic branch (*arrows*) from the right internal mammary artery.

arteries may enter the liver by adhesion of the omentum to the liver (59–60).

Multiple EHCs can supply a tumor (Figure 15.27). Once extra-hepatic collateral supply develops, the effective control of the tumors with transcatheter managements can be made possible by the proper management of not only the hepatic arterial supply but also extra-hepatic collateral supply (Figure 15.26) (41, 50, 55, 56, 59–61). It is known to be possible to perform chemoembolization through EHCs at high success rates and safety (50, 55). Therefore, radiologists should become familiar with the spectrum of EHCs that supply hepatic tumors, the factors that lead to their formation and their characteristic imaging appearance at CT and conventional angiography to detect them at an early stage. Delivery of therapeutic materials into EHCs should be performed with a thorough knowledge of the vascular anatomy and should be performed superselectively with coax-

ial microcatheters to avoid complications due to nontarget delivery (50).

Prevalence and Causes

Basically, the hepatic tumors at subcapsular locations or exophytic growth carry the risk of extra-hepatic collateral supply. According to our prospective investigation using 479 patients with hepatocellular carcinomas (51), 23% of the tumors in the subcapsular location or that demonstrated exophytic growth had extra-hepatic collateral supply at the initial presentation. In the past literature, most EHCs were discovered after the hepatic arterial blood supply had been interrupted by surgical ligation, temporary balloon occlusion, repeated embolization or mechanical injury to the hepatic artery (52–54). However, we found that almost all the patients with extra-hepatic collateral supply had widely patent hepatic arteries (Figures 15.24 and 15.25).

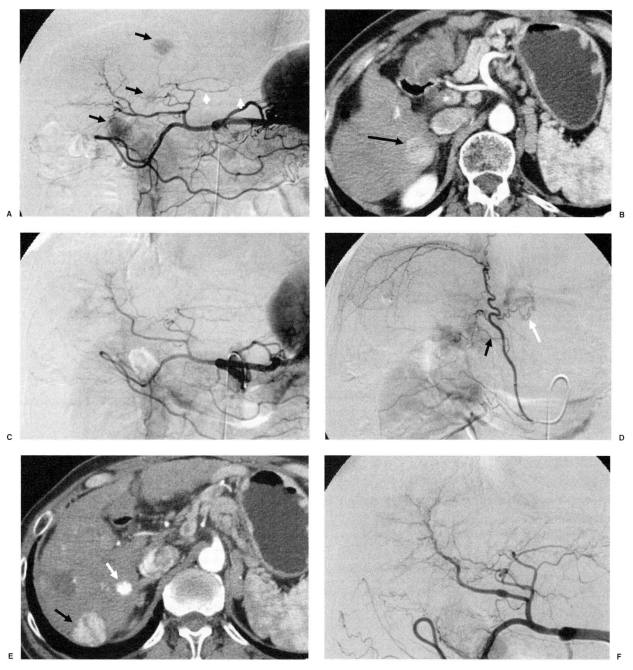

FIGURE 15.26. Hepatocellular carcinoma exclusively supplied by extrahepatic collateral arteries after repeated sessions of chemoembolization. (A) The patient had multiple nodular tumors (*black arrows*) at the initial presentation. Note the accessory left gastric artery (*white arrows*). (B) Five repeated sessions of chemoembolization were performed and all the tumors at the intial presentation showed complete response. During follow-up, a recurrent tumor (*arrow*) developed at the segment 7 abutting the adrenal gland. (C) Celiac arteriogram showed no tumor stain; however, the peripheral hepatic arteries were attenuated. (D) With a suspicion of extrahepatic arterial supply, right inferior phrenic arteriography was performed. The tumor was exclusively supplied by a feeder (black arrow) from the right inferior phrenic artery. The white arrow indicates a feeder for inferior phrenic-pulmonary shunt. (E) On follow-up CT scan, the treated tumor showed complete response (*white arrow*). But, another recurrent tumor (*black arrow*) developed at segment 7 abutting the posterior diaphragm. (F) The tumor was not supplied by the hepatic arteries at all.

The prevalence of extra-hepatic collateral supply to hepatocellular carcinoma at initial presentation was determined by tumor size (51). There was an abrupt increase in the prevalence of an extra-hepatic collateral supply to hepatocellular carcinoma with a tumor size in the range of 4 to 6 cm. When the tumor was smaller than 4 cm, the prevalence of extra-hepatic collateral supply at the initial chemoembolization session was less than 3% (6 of 253 tumors). Instead, when the tumor was bigger than 6 cm, the prevalence of

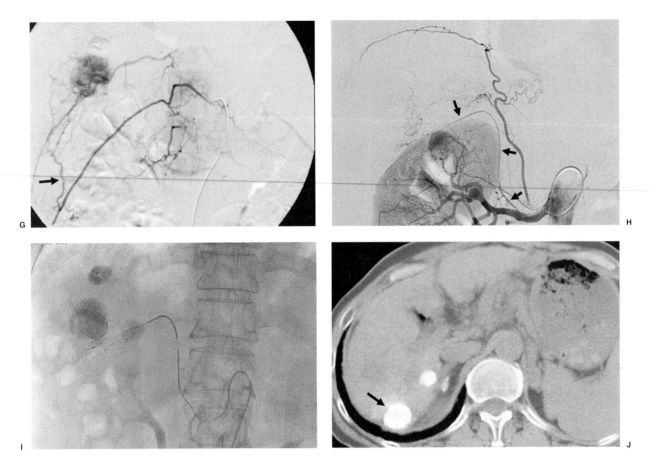

FIGURE 15.26. (Continued) **(G)** It was totally supplied by the 11th intercostal artery. Note the hypertrophied feeding artery (*arrow*) which arises from the intercostal artery at the diaphragmatic attachment site and ascends along the diaphragm to reach the tumor. **(H)** There was a local progression of the treated tumor at the follow-up CT (*not shown*) and the residual viable tumor was supplied by the renal capsular artery (*arrows*) from the right renal artery. **(I)** The renal capsular artery was selectively catheterized using a microcatheter and chemoembolization was performed. **(J)** Iodized-oil CT scan taken 2 weeks after the procedure shows compact accumulation of iodized-oil in the tumor.

extra-hepatic collateral supply was 63% (65 of 107 tumors).

Hepatic artery occlusion or attenuation of peripheral hepatic arteries due to repeated transcatheter managements (Figures 15.26 and 15.27), iatrogenic dissection, surgical ligation or celiac stenosis or occlusion may initiate or exaggerate extra-hepatic collateral supply to the tumors. According to our prospective investigation (51), as the number of chemoembolization sessions increased, the cumulative probability of EHCs also increased, and particularly for those EHCs supplying recurrent tumors (Figure 15.26). Whereas patients who initially had a large primary tumor usually had EHCs supplying the primary tumor (Figures 15.24 and 15.25), patients with a small tumor usually had EHCs supplying a recurrent tumor after several chemoembolization sessions (Figure 15.26). The increasing probability of finding EHCs for large tumors during repeated chemoembolization procedures can be explained by

the growth of invisible tiny tumor foci that were initially supplied by EHCs or local tumor progression to seek EHCs (i.e., the primary tumor grows to reach a subcapsular location; it grows exophytically; or it invades an adjacent organ, resulting in the creation of EHCs). In contrast, for patients with small primary tumors (<5 cm), most of the EHCs supplied the recurrent tumors that developed after multiple chemoembolization sessions. Peripheral hepatic artery attenuation or occlusion was frequently associated with these circumstances (Figure 15.26). Therefore, the increasing probability of EHCs for small tumors during repeated chemoembolization procedures can be explained by a sequence of events: peripheral hepatic artery occlusion due to repeated chemoembolization procedure, the development of EHCs supplying the peripheral zone of the liver parenchyma, and then subsequent remote-site tumor recurrence at the peripheral zone supplied by the EHCs.

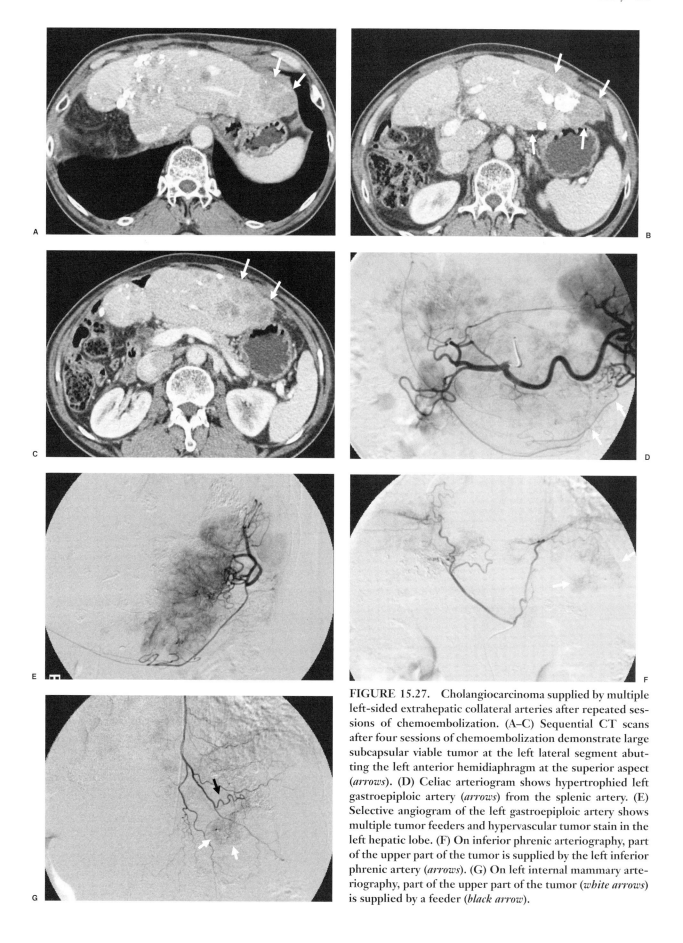

FIGURE 15.27. Cholangiocarcinoma supplied by multiple left-sided extrahepatic collateral arteries after repeated sessions of chemoembolization. (A–C) Sequential CT scans after four sessions of chemoembolization demonstrate large subcapsular viable tumor at the left lateral segment abutting the left anterior hemidiaphragm at the superior aspect (*arrows*). (D) Celiac arteriogram shows hypertrophied left gastroepiploic artery (*arrows*) from the splenic artery. (E) Selective angiogram of the left gastroepiploic artery shows multiple tumor feeders and hypervascular tumor stain in the left hepatic lobe. (F) On inferior phrenic arteriography, part of the upper part of the tumor is supplied by the left inferior phrenic artery (*arrows*). (G) On left internal mammary arteriography, part of the upper part of the tumor (*white arrows*) is supplied by a feeder (*black arrow*).

A previous abdominal operation may predispose a patient to early formation of collateral vessels to a tumor due to postoperative omental or peritoneal adhesion. In cases of recurrent tumor at the resection margin, collateral supply from omental arteries should be considered. Peripheral hepatic infarction after chemoembolization sometimes induces omental or peritoneal adhesion, and EHCs can develop through the adhesion.

How to Predict: Suggestive Findings

Because selective angiography of individual collateral vessels is tedious and time-consuming, it is essential to try to determine first whether parasitic or collateral blood supply is present (50). The initial CT scan provides useful information, and CT signs of direct invasion into adjacent organs or extracapsular infiltration indicate the presence of EHCs. Tumors with an exophytic growth pattern are prone to collateral vessel development. It is sometimes possible to observe hypertrophied EHCs (Figure 15.25). Follow-up CT scans are also useful. A peripheral iodized oil retention defect within the tumor or delayed development of viable tumor at the peripheral portion of the treated tumor at follow-up CT indicates the presence of EHCs (Figure 15.26). In a tumor that recurs after surgery at the resection margin, the presence of omental collateral vessels should be suspected and investigated. Peripheral local recurrence in a patient with attenuated peripheral hepatic arteries after repeated chemoembolization is frequently supplied by EHC. The correlation of CT and angiographic findings is essential. If a tumor observed at CT or CT arterial portography is not demonstrated at hepatic angiography, collateral vessels must be investigated (55). When tumor staining on hepatic angiograms has a focal defect or a focal iodized oil retention defect is noted during hepatic arteriography or iodized oil infusion, alternative feeder vessels are a possibility (Figure 15.25). A hypertrophied omental branch or right IPA may be noted on celiac angiograms (Figure 15.27). If the serum alpha-fetoprotein level is persistently elevated even after successful devascularization of the hepatic artery, we recommend an investigation of EHCs to the liver.

There is a close relationship between the tumor location and possible EHCs (50,55). Tumors located at the posterior surface of the right lobe and abutting the diaphragm are most likely to be fed by the right IPA (Figure 15.24). The right intercostal and lumbar arteries usually supply tumor in the lateral and posteroinferior aspect of the right lobe and, when the IPA is attenuated by repeated chemoembolization procedures, reach the territory of the IPA (Figure 15.26). Blood supply from the right IMA is seen when the tumor is located beneath the anterior part of the diaphragm or abutting the anterior abdominal wall (Figures 15.25 and 15.27). Tumors located near the right renal fossa are fed by the right renal capsular artery or adrenal arteries. Tumors located at the anterior surface of the right lobe of the liver or at the lower edge of the right lobe or medial segment of the left liver are fed by the omental or colic arteries. Potential feeders for the tumors in the lateral segment of the liver are the left or right gastric arteries, omental arteries from the right or left gastroepiploic arteries, short gastric arteries and left inferior phrenic or internal mammary arteries (Figure 15.27). The cystic artery mainly feeds tumors located near the gallbladder fossa (see Figure 15.21), but it infrequently supplies the tumor in the right lobe or medial segment of the liver at a distance from the gallbladder fossa when the hepatic artery is attenuated. Tumors arising in the caudate lobe tend to be fed by the right IPA, LGA and pancreatic arteries. Adjacent EHCs are connected to each other, and their distribution shows individual variation. Transcatheter management of an EHC induces redistribution of blood supply in adjacent collateral arteries.

Anatomy of Extra-hepatic Collateral Arteries
Inferior Phrenic Arteries

There is a close contact between the liver and the diaphragm, and the blood supply to the diaphragm can reach the liver by direct adherence. The IPA supplies most of the diaphragm, including the area in contact with the bare area of the liver. Thus, the right IPA is the most common collateral pathway and accounts for almost half of all EHCs. It anastomoses with the adjacent arteries, including the internal mammary, intercostal, and adrenal arteries.

The right and the left IPAs usually originate from the celiac trunk or directly from the aorta as a common trunk or independent origins (see Figures 15.1, 15.24 and 15.27). Less frequently, they arise from the renal arteries (Figure 15.26) or, rarely, from the left gastric or hepatic arteries (see Figure 15.19). On arterial phase CT scans, we can frequently identify the vertical segment of the hypertrophied IPA (see

Figure 15.24) and guess its origin. With thin-section multi-detector CT, its origin and branching pattern can be directly viewed in most cases. When the IPA originates, from the celiac axis with median arcuate ligament compression, selective catheterization of the IPA is frequently difficult. In that case, special techniques using a catheter with a large side hole (64) or microguide wire loop technique (65) is quite useful. Occasionally, the IPA is occluded or severely stenotic and reconstructed via retroperitoneal anastomosis from the adrenal artery, pancreatic arteries from SMA or dorsal pancreatic artery, LGA or contralateral IPA (66). These anastomotic pathways can be used to continue transcatheter treatments of the tumors.

The tumors supplied by IPA were almost always located in the posterior segment, the dome of the right hepatic lobe, and the caudate lobe of the liver. Especially when the tumor is located in liver segment 7 and is in contact with the right hemidiaphragm, selective angiography of the right IPA is mandatory (55). When the tumor is located in liver segments 2 or 3 and abuts the left hemidiaphragm, the possibility of a collateral blood supply from the left IPA should be kept in mind.

Patients commonly complain of shoulder pain or chest tightness during embolization of the IPA. Transient pleural effusion, basal atelectasis, pulmonary oil embolism or hemoptysis and diaphragmatic weakness may develop after the procedure (41, 67). Because the IPA is also a potential source for collateralization to the pulmonary circulation, the presence or absence of IPA-pulmonary shunt should be determined before delivery of therapeutic material into the IPA (Figure 15.26d).

Internal Mammary Arteries

Angiographic anatomy of the IMA supplying hepatic tumors has been recently investigated in detail (Figure 15.28) (68). The IMA usually arises from the proximal part of the subclavian artery, opposite the origin of the vertebral artery. The lateral costal branch, which seldom supplies the diaphragm, arises above the first rib and courses laterally and downward into the lateral chest wall. The pericardiacophrenic artery usually arises above the second intercostal space and gives branches to the pleura, pericardium and diaphragm. At the level of the sixth intercostal space, the IMA divides into two end arteries, the musculophrenic and superior epigastric arteries. The musculophrenic artery passes

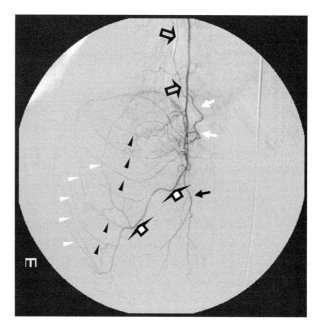

FIGURE 15.28. Angiographic anatomy of the right internal mammary artery in a patient whose right inferior phrenic artery was previously embolized. At the level of the sixth intercostal space, the internal mammary artery divides into the musculophrenic (*short thick white arrows*) and superior epigastric arteries (*black arrow*). The long descending branch indicated by an open arrow is the pericardiacophrenic artery which is rarely demonstrated. The phrenic branch (*white arrows*) arises from the main trunk of the internal mammary artery just above the diaphragm. Among multiple branches of the internal mammary artery, this phrenic branch most commonly supplies hepatic tumors. The musculophrenic artery gives off the paired anterior intercostal arteries (*black arrowheads*) and the ascending phrenic branches (*white arrowheads*).

obliquely downward and laterally, behind the seventh, eighth, and ninth costal cartilages. It perforates the diaphragm near the ninth costal cartilage and terminates opposite the last intercostal space. It gives off two anterior intercostal branches to each of the seventh, eighth, and ninth intercostal spaces and vertical diaphragmatic branches, which anastomose with the branches of the IPA. The anterior intercostal arteries and the hypertrophied vertical diaphragmatic branches from the musculophrenic artery create a lattice appearance (Figure 15.28). The superior epigastric artery passes vertically downward and anastomoses with the inferior epigastric artery. It gives off some branches to the diaphragm, which extend into the falciform ligament of the liver and anastomose with the LHA (55).

In anatomy textbooks, a pericardiacophrenic artery is described that accompanies the phrenic nerve between the pleura and the pericardium. However, according to our experience, it rarely reaches the diaphragm and supplies hepatic tumors. We found that the phrenic branch is the most common side branch of the IMA supplying hepatic tumors (Figures 15.25d and 15.28) (68). It usually arises between the fourth and sixth intercostal spaces and passes through anterior pericardial fat. Although anatomy textbooks offer no information about this branch, Singh stated that "muscular branches to the diaphragm" arose between the third and sixth intercostal cartilages and were found in 20 of 100 patients (69).

Regardless of the patency of the hepatic artery, when a hepatic tumor is located in ventral hepatic areas, abutting the diaphragm and anterior abdominal wall, the IMAs may serve as feeding arteries. Tumors located in liver segment 4 were most commonly supplied by the phrenic branch of the right IMA. On the other hand, tumors located in liver segment 8 were most commonly supplied by the right musculophrenic artery. Tumors located in liver segment 2 or 3 were fed by the right or left IMA in even distribution. Occasionally both IMAs can supply the tumor (68).

In patients who underwent chemoembolization through the right IPA, a tumor in the posterior location can be supplied by the right IMA because previous chemoembolization through the IPA causes the right IMA to take over the territory of the right IPA through anastomotic channels (68).

Cutaneous complications may occur after chemoembolization of the IMA. Understanding vascular anatomy of the IMA and selective catheterization of tumor-feeding arteries are prerequisites to prevent skin necrosis after the procedure (70).

Intercostal and Lumbar Arteries

Nine pairs of posterior intercostal arteries originate from the dorsal aspect of the thoracic aorta. They anastomose with the anterior intercostal branches of IMA after giving off the dorsal branch, the collateral intercostal branch and the muscular branch. Lower posterior intercostal arteries anastomose with the IPA at the insertion site of the diaphragm. A hypertrophied intercostal artery may be observed as a dot-like or linear structure just inferior to the ribs on arterial phase CT scans (58). Tumors abutting the inferolateral aspect of the diaphragm are frequently supplied by the posterior intercostal arteries. Tumors invading the abdominal wall are also found to be supplied by the lower intercostal, subcostal or lumbar arteries. The intercostal artery always passes the

diaphragm insertion site to supply the hepatic tumors, abutting the diaphragm and making a sharp upward turn near the costochondral junction (Figure 15.26G) (58). A microcatheter should be advanced beyond the diaphragmatic insertion to the thoracic cage, where a sharp upward turn is seen, to avoid possible complications such as skin necrosis and spinal infarction (58). The common levels of the intercostal arteries that supply hepatic tumors are T10, T9 and T11, in order of frequency (58). Occasionally, hepatic tumors that abut the posteroinferior diaphragm can be supplied by the subcostal or lumbar arteries.

When the right IPA is obliterated by the previous treatment, the ICAs can supply a tumor at the dome of the liver.

Cystic Artery

The cystic artery is the first branch of the RHA and usually supplies the liver parenchyma near the gallbladder bed. When the tumor protrudes to the gallbladder fossa, it may be supplied by the cystic artery (see Figure 15.21), despite an intact hepatic artery. When hepatic arteries are attenuated because of repeated chemoembolization, a tumor located at a distance from the gallbladder fossa may be fed by the cystic artery. Embolization of the cystic artery may cause cholecystitis or gallbladder infarction, but chemoembolization after selective catheterization into the tumor-feeding branch is usually safe (see Figure 15.21) (61).

Omental Arteries

The omental branch (Figure 15.27) from the gastroepiploic artery (or, in rare cases, from the dorsal pancreatic artery) is the second most common collateral vessel. Omental branches usually are small and branch at an acute angle from the gastroepiploic artery. Several omental branches exist in healthy patients, but they are hardly recognized on angiograms. Whereas most of the other EHCs enter the liver via the suspensory ligament or bare area of the liver, the omental branch supplies the tumor by direct adhesion to the omentum. When an omental branch supplies a tumor, it becomes sufficiently dilated to be recognizable at celiac angiography (59, 60). Therefore, a careful review of celiac angiograms is a first step toward detecting the omental branch that supplies a hepatic tumor. Because the greater omentum is remarkably mobile, the omental branch can supply a tumor in any intraperitoneal portion of the liver. In patients with severe liver cirrhosis, the liver shrinks so markedly that an exophytic tumor in the liver dome surrounded by the omentum can be supplied by an omental branch with a very long path (50). These omental branches arise from the right and left gastroepiploic arteries (Figure 15.27). The left gastroepiploic artery arises from the distal splenic artery. Omental branches from the left gastroepiploic artery frequently supply an exophytic tumor at the dome of the right hepatic lobe.

Adrenal Arteries

If a tumor extends inferomedially, adrenal arteries can supply the tumor. The adrenal gland has three sources of arterial supply: a superior adrenal artery that arises from the IPA, a middle adrenal artery that arises from the lateral aspect of the aorta at a level between the celiac and renal arteries and an inferior adrenal artery that arises from the superior aspect of the ipsilateral renal artery. Normal adrenal gland staining is triangular. On inferior phrenic angiograms, superior adrenal artery and normal adrenal gland staining are usually observed. Therefore, normal adrenal gland staining must not be confused with tumor staining on inferior phrenic angiograms.

Renal and Renal Capsular Arteries

If a tumor extends posteroinferiorly, it may be fed by the renal and renal capsular arteries (Figure 15.26). The superior capsular artery usually arises together with the inferior adrenal artery from the renal artery and follows a characteristic tortuous path over the superior pole of the kidney. Perforating capsular arteries arise from arcuate and interlobular arteries, which may supply the tumor in contact with the kidney. In advanced cases of hepatic tumors, multiple arteries supply the tumor, and it may be difficult to differentiate the renal capsular artery, renal artery and inferior adrenal artery.

Gastric Arteries

When a hepatic tumor has broad contact with the stomach, gastric arteries can supply the tumor. The LGA usually arises from the celiac trunk and infrequently from the supraceliac aorta. The RGA commonly arises from the proper hepatic and left hepatic arteries and infrequently arises from the gastroduodenal and common hepatic arteries. Short gastric arteries arise from the splenic artery and supply the gastric fundus. Normal stomach stain can often mimic tumor stain. To prevent inadvertent embolization of the stomach, selective catheterization should be attempted, but this technique cannot be accomplished in many cases (55).

Colic Branches

Because of exophytic growth and extracapsular infiltration, hepatic tumors may have direct contact with the intra-abdominal organs, such as the colon and stomach. When an exophytic tumor is located in the inferior tip of the right hepatic lobe, the hepatic flexure of the colon can be in close contact with the tumor. A branch of the SMA, particularly the right or middle colic branch, may supply the tumor under these conditions (50).

Gonadal Artery

The gonadal arteries (the testicular artery in men and the ovarian artery in women) supply the perirenal fat and ureter in the abdomen as well as the gonads (1). They usually originate from the anterolateral aspect of the abdominal aorta at the level of the second lumbar vertebra, 2.5 to 5 cm below the renal artery, and passes inferolaterally under the peritoneum on the psoas major (Figure 15.29) (1). However, the origin of the gonadal artery varies from L1 to L4 because of the migration of the gonad along the gubernaculums (71). At the proximal segment of the gonadal artery, small variable twigs branch off to the adjacent retroperitoneal area: some extend to the renal hilum to supply the renal pelvis and the adjacent ureter, whereas others communicate with the superior renal capsular and adrenal vessels (72). Therefore, if a tumor in liver segment 6 invades the kidney or perirenal fat, a branch from the gonadal artery can theoretically supply the tumor (Figure 15.29).

Interestingly, the gonadal arteries supplying hepatic tumors usually show anatomic variation of a high origin and a common trunk with the adrenal artery. Moreover, they run laterally and slightly upward and then descend at right angles, whereas usually the gonadal artery runs obliquely downward (73). These anatomic variations could cause the gonadal artery to course near the kidney, thus better enabling a branch of the gonadal artery to supply the tumor.

Transcatheter Management of Extrahepatic Collateral Arteries

When EHCs are chemoembolized, there is a risk of embolizing non-target branches, which can lead

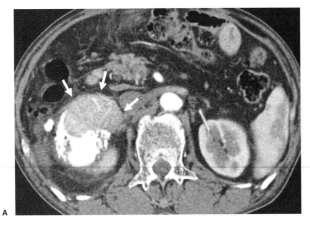

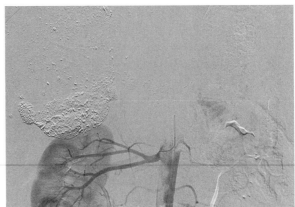

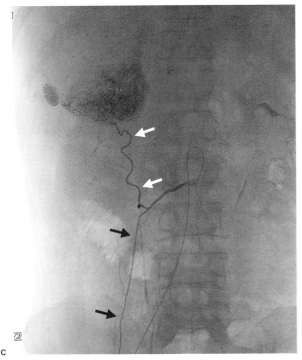

FIGURE 15.29. Hepatocellular carcinoma supplied by the right testicular artery. (A) Helical CT scan in the arterial phase shows an exophytic tumor with a peripheral viable portion (*arrows*). (B) The right renal and adrenal arteries do not supply the tumor. (C) The right testicular artery (*black arrows*) arises from the aorta at the lower margin of the second lumbar vertebra and gives off single large tumor feeder (*white arrows*).

to a variety of complications, depending on location (74). Cutaneous problems, such as itching, erythema and necrosis, may arise when the internal mammary, intercostal or lumbar artery is embolized (70). Gastrointestinal erosion, ulceration or perforation can be caused by gastric, omental and colic branch artery embolization (34). Paraplegia may result from the inadvertent embolization of spinal branches arising from intercostal or lumbar collateral vessels, and embolization of the cystic artery may cause cholecystitis or gallbladder infarction (74). Chemoembolization of the IPA may result in shoulder pain, pleural effusion, basal atelectasis, pulmonary embolization or diaphragmatic weakness (41, 67).

To avoid these complications, selective catheterization should be achieved by first placing the catheter tip as close as possible to the specific branch or branches supplying a neoplasm. Second, embolic materials should be infused incrementally to prevent them from refluxing into a non-target branch. Third, coils and gelatin-sponge particles may be used to occlude and protect the territory of the normal distal branches before chemoembolization. Fourth, to reduce pain, it is recommended that a small amount of 1% lidocaine be injected intra-arterially during embolization (50).

Because terminal branches of adjacent EHCs are anastomosed to each other, multiple EHCs can supply one tumor. If an EHC is proximally embolized or is complicated by an arterial spasm during catheterization or if there is a local recurrence after chemoembolization of an EHC, adjacent vessels can take over its territory. For example, a recurrent tumor previously supplied via the IPA may be supplied by the intercostal or IMA at a subsequent chemoembolization session. It is important to catheterize EHCs by using a meticulous technique with microcatheters to prevent spasm or arterial injury and to investigate the presence or absence of collateral circulation from adjacent vessels. In advanced stages of hepatic tumors, chemoembolization through EHCs may not improve tumor control, because it is extremely difficult to embolize multiple feeder vessels from hepatic arteries and EHCs effectively (50).

REFERENCES

1. Williams PL, Warwick R. Gray's Anatomy, 36th edition Philadelphia: Saunders 1980.
2. Michels NA. Blood Supply and Anatomy of the Upper Abdominal Organs. pp.152–154, 256–259, 374–375. Philadelphia, JB Lippincott 1955.
3. Soo CS, Chuang VP, Wallace S, et al. Treatment of hepatic neoplasm through extrahepatic collaterals. Radiology 1983; 144: 485–494.
4. Bron KM, Redman HC. Splanchnic artery stenosis and occlusion: Incidence, arteriographic and clinical manifestations. Radiology 1969; 92: 323–328.
5. Derrick JR, Pollard HS, Moore RM. The pattern of arteriosclerotic narrowing of the celiac and superior mesenteric arteries. Ann Surg 1959; 149: 684–689.
6. David CL, Harold AB. High incidence of celiac axis narrowing in asymptomatic individuals. AJR Am J Roentgenol 1972; 116: 426–429.
7. Park CM, Chung JW, Kim HB, et al. Celiac axis stenosis: Incidence and etiologies in asymptomatic individuals. Korean J Radiol 2001; 2: 8–13.
8. Reuter S. Accentuation of celiac compression by the median arcuate ligament of the diaphragm during deep expiration. Radiology 1971; 98: 561.
9. Song SY, Chung JW, Kwon JW, et al. Collateral pathways in patients with celiac axis stenosis: angiographic-spiral CT correlation. Radiographics 2002; 22: 881–893.
10. Kwon JW, Chung JW, Song SY, et al. Transcatheter arterial chemoembolization for hepatocellular carcinomas in patients with celiac axis occlusion. J Vasc Interv Radiol 2002; 13: 689–694.
11. Patten RM, Coldwell DM, Ben-Menachem Y. Ligamentous compression of the celiac axis: CT findings in five patients. AJR Am J Roentgenol 1991; 156: 1101–1103.
12. Covey AM, Brody LA, Maluccio MA, et al. Variant hepatic arterial anatomy revisited: Digital subtraction angiography performed in 600 patients. Radiology 2002; 224: 542–547.
13. Lie DM, Salem R, Bui JT, et al. Angiographic considerations in patients undergoing liver-directed therapy. J Vasc Interv Radiol 2005; 16: 911–935.
14. VanDamme JP, Bonte J. Vascular Anatomy in Abdominal Surgery New York: Thieme 1990.
15. Couinaud C. Liver anatomy: Portal (and suprahepatic) or biliary segmentation. Dig Surg 1999; 16: 459–467.
16. Mlakar B, Gadijev EM, Ravnik D, et al. Anatomical variations of the arterial pattern in the right hemiliver. Eur J Morphology 2002; 40: 267–273.
17. Mlakar B, Gadzijev E, Ravnik D, et al. Anatomical variations of the arterial pattern in the left hemiliver. Eur J Morphology 2002 Apr; 40(2): 115–120.
18. Yoshimura H, Uchida H, Ohishi H, et al. Evaluation of "M-point" in hepatic artery to identify left medial segment of liver: angiographic study. Eur J Radiol 1986 Aug; 6(3): 195–198
19. Soyer P, Bluemke DA, Bliss DF, et al. Surgical segmental anatomy of the liver: Demonstration with spiral CT during arterial portography and multiplanar reconstruction. AJR Am J Roentgenol 1994; 163: 99–103.
20. Lafortune M, Madore E, Patriquin H, et al. Segmental anatomy of the liver: A sonographic approach to the Couinaud nomenclature. Radiology 1991; 181: 443–448.
21. Couinaud C. Le foie: Études anatomiques et chirurgicales Paris, France: Masson 1957; pp. 9–12.
22. Fasel J, Selle D, Evertsz C, et al. Segmental anatomy of the liver: Poor correlation with CT. Radiology 1998; 206: 151–156.
23. Cho A, Okazumi S, Takayama W, et al. Anatomy of the right anterosuperior area (segment 8) of the liver: Evaluation with helical CT during arterial portography. Radiology 2000; 214: 491–495.
24. Ohashi I, Ina H, Okada Y, et al. Segmental anatomy of the liver under the right diaphragmatic dome: Evaluation with axial CT. Radiology 1996; 200: 779–783.
25. Lee HY, Chung JW, Park JH, et al. A new and simple practical plane dividing hepatic segment 2 and 3 of the liver: Evaluation of its validity. Korean J Radiol 2007; 8: 302–310.
26. Song SY, Chung JW, Lim HG, et al. Nonhepatic arteries originating from the hepatic arteries: Angiographic analysis in 250 patients. J Vasc Interv Radiol 2006; 17: 461–469.
27. Ueno K, Miyazono N, Inoue H, et al. Embolization of the hepatic falciform artery to prevent supraumbilical skin rash during transcatheter arterial chemoembolization for hepatocellular carcinoma. Cardiovasc Intervent Radiol 1995; 18: 183–185.
28. Nakamura H, Hashimoto H, Sawada S, et al. Prevention of gastric complications in hepatic arterial chemoembolization: Balloon catheter occlusion technique. Acta Radiol 1991; 32: 81–82.
29. Hashimoto M, Heianna J, Tate E, et al. The feasibility of retrograde catheterization of the right gastric artery via the left gastric artery. J Vasc Interv Radiol 2001; 12: 1103–1106.
30. Yamagami T, Nakamura T, Iida S, et al. Embolization of the right gastric artery before hepatic arterial infusion chemotherapy to prevent gastric mucosal lesions: Approach through the hepatic artery versus the left gastric artery. AJR Am J Roentgenol 2002; 179: 1605–1610.
31. Inaba Y, Arai Y, Matsueda K, et al. Right gastric artery embolization to prevent acute gastric mucosal lesions in patients undergoing repeat hepatic arterial infusion chemotherapy. J Vasc Interv Radiol 2001; 12: 957–963.
32. Nakamura H, Uchida H, Kuroda C, et al. Accessory left gastric artery arising from left hepatic artery: angiographic study. AJR Am J Roentgenol 1980; 134: 529–532.

33. Chuang PV, Wallace S, Stroehlein J, et al. Hepatic artery infusion chemotherapy: Gastroduodenal complications. Am J Roentgenol 1982; 137: 347–350.

34. Hirakawa M, Iida M, Aoyagi K, et al. Gastroduodenal lesions after transcatheter arterial chemo-embolization in patients with hepatocellular carcinoma. Am J Gastroenterol 1988; 83: 837–840.

35. Williams DM, Cho KJ, Ensminger WD, et al. Hepatic falciform artery: Anatomy, angiographic appearance, and clinical significance. Radiology 1985; 156: 339–340.

36. Baba Y, Miyazono N, Ueno K, et al. Hepatic falciform artery: Angiographic findings in 25 patients. Acta Radiol 2000; 41: 329–333.

37. Gibo M, Hasuo K, Inoue A, et al. Hepatic falciform artery: Angiographic observations and significance. Abdom Imaging 2001; 26: 515–519.

38. Kim DE, Yoon HK, Ko GY, et al. Hepatic falciform artery: Is prophylactic embolization needed before short-term hepatic arterial chemoinfusion? Am J Roentgenol 1999; 172: 1597–1599.

39. Ibukuro K, Tsukiyama T, Mori K, et al. Hepatic falciform ligament artery: Angiographic anatomy and clinical importance. Surg Radiol Anat 1998; 20: 367–371.

40. Dupart G, Charnsangvej C, Wallace S, et al. Inferior phrenic artery embolization in the treatment of hepatic neoplasm. Acta Radiol 1988; 29: 427–429.

41. Chung JW, Park JH, Han JK, et al. Transcatheter oily chemoembolization of the inferior phrenic artery in hepatocellular carcinoma: The safety and potential therapeutic role. J Vasc Interv Radiol 1998; 9: 495–500.

42. Sakamoto I, Aso N, Nagaoki K. Complications associated with transcatheter arterial embolization for hepatic tumors. Radiographics 1998; 18: 605–619.

43. Sammon J, Baron R. Phase II study of Spherex (degradable starch microspheres) injected into the hepatic artery in conjunction with doxorubicin and cisplatin in the treatment of advanced-stage hepatocellular carcinoma: Interim analysis. Semin Oncol 1997; 24(Suppl 6): S6–S97.

44. Choplin RH, Gelfand DW, Hunt TH. Gastric perforation from hepatic artery infusion chemotherapy. Gastrointest Radiol 1983; 8: 133–134.

45. Bianchi HF, Albanese EF. The supraduodenal artery. Surg Radiol Anat 1989; 11: 37–40.

46. Daseler EH, Anson BJ, Hambley WC, et al. The cystic artery and constituents of the hepatic pedicle: A study of 500 specimens. Surg Gynecol Obstet 1947; 85:47–63.

47. Chen WJ, Ying DJ, Liu ZJ, et al. Analysis of the arterial supply of the extrahepatic bile ducts and its clinical significance. Clin Anat 1999; 12(4): 245–249.

48. Tohma T, Cho A, Okazumi S, et al. Communicating arcade between the right and left hepatic arteries: Evaluation with CT and angiography during temporary balloon occlusion of the right or left hepatic artery. Radiology 2005; 237: 361–365.

49. Stapleton GN, Hickman R, Terblanche J. Blood supply of the right and left hepatic ducts. Br J Surg 1998 Feb; 85(2): 202–207.

50. Kim HC, Chung JW, Lee W, et al. Recognizing extrahepatic collateral vessels that supply hepatocellular carcinoma to avoid complications of transcatheter arterial chemoembolization. Radiographics 2005; 25: S25–39.

51. Chung JW, Kim HC, Jae HJ, et al. Transcatheter arterial chemoembolization of hepatocellular carcinoma: Prevalence and causative factors of extrahepatic collateral arteries in 479 patients. Korean J Radiol 2006; 7: 257–266.

52. Michels NA. Collateral arterial pathways to the liver after ligation of the hepatic artery and removal of the celiac axis. Cancer 1953; 6: 708–724.

53. Charnsangavej C, Chuang VP, Wallace S, et al. Angiographic classification of hepatic arterial collaterals. Radiology 1982; 144: 485–494.

54. Takeuchi Y, Arai Y, Inaba Y, et al. Extrahepatic arterial supply to the liver: Observation with a unified CT and angiography system during temporary balloon occlusion of the proper hepatic artery. Radiology 1998; 209: 121–128.

55. Miyayama S, Matsui O, Taki K, et al. Extrahepatic blood supply to hepatocellular carcinoma: Angiographic demonstration and transcatheter chemoembolization. Cardiovasc Intervent Radiol 2006; 29: 39–48.

56. Kim JH, Chung JW, Han JK, et al. Transcatheter arterial embolization of the internal mammary artery in hepatocellular carcinoma. J Vasc Interv Radiol 1995; 6: 71–74.

57. Nakai M, Sato M, Kawai N, et al. Hepatocellular carcinoma: Involvement of the internal mammary artery. Radiology 2001; 219: 147–152.

58. Park SI, Lee DY, Won JY, et al. Extrahepatic collateral supply of hepatocellular carcinoma by the intercostal arteries. J Vasc Interv Radiol 2003; 14: 461–468.

59. Miyayama S, Matsui O, Akakura Y, et al. Hepatocellular carcinoma with blood supply from omental branches: Treatment with transcatheter arterial embolization. J Vasc Interv Radiol 2001; 12: 1285–1290.

60. Won JY, Lee DY, Lee JT, et al. Supplemental transcatheter arterial chemoembolization through a collateral omental artery: treatment for hepatocellular carcinoma. Cardiovasc Intervent Radiol 2003; 26: 136–140.

61. Miyayama S, Matsui O, Nishida H, et al. Transcatheter arterial chemoembolization for unresectable hepatocellular carcinoma fed by the cystic artery. J Vasc Interv Radiol 2003; 14: 1155–1161.

62. Komatsu T, Matsui O, Kadoya M, et al. Cystic artery origin of the segment V hepatic artery. Cardiovasc Intervent Radiol 1999; 22: 165–167.

63. Tanigawa N, Sawada S, Okuda Y, et al. A case of small hepatocellular carcinoma supplied by the cystic artery. Am J Roentgenol 1998; 170: 675–676.

64. Miyayama S, Matsui O, Akakura Y, et al. Use of a catheter with a large side hole for selective catheterization of the inferior phrenic artery. J Vasc Interv Radiol 2001; 12: 497–499.

65. Baek JH, Chung JW, Jae HJ, et al. A new technique for superselective catheterization of arteries originating from a large artery at an acute angle: Shepherd-hook preshaping of a micro-guide wire. Korean J Radiol 2007; 8: 225–230.

66. Miyayama S, Matsui O, Taki K, et al. Transcatheter arterial chemoembolization for hepatocellular carcinoma fed by the reconstructed inferior phrenic artery: Anatomical and technical analysis. J Vasc Interv Radiol 2004; 15: 815–823.

67. Shin SW, Do YS, Choo SW, et al. Diaphragmatic weakness after transcatheter arterial chemoembolization of interior phrenic artery for treatment of hepatocellular carcinoma. Radiology 2006; 241: 581–588.

68. Kim HC, Chung JW, Choi SH, et al. Hepatocellular

carcinoma supplied by the internal mammary artery: Angiographic anatomy in 97 patients. Radiology 2007; 242: 925–932.

69. Singh RN. Radiographic anatomy of the internal mammary arteries. Cathet Cardiovasc Diagn 1981; 7: 373–386.

70. Arora R, Soulen MC, Haskal ZJ. Cutaneous complications of hepatic chemoembolization via extrahepatic collaterals. J Vasc Interv Radiol 1999; 10: 1351–1356.

71. Machnicki A, Grzybiak M. Variations in testicular arteries in fetuses and adults. Folia Morphol (Warsz) 1997; 56: 277–285.

72. Khademi M, Seebode JJ, Falla A. Selective spermatic arteriography for localization of an impalpable undescended testis. Radiology 1980; 136: 627–634.

73. Kim HC, Chung JW, Jae HJ, et al. Hepatocellular carcinoma: Transcatheter arterial chemoembolization of the gonadal artery. J Vasc Interv Radiol 2006; 17: 703–709.

74. Chung JW, Park JH, Han JK, et al. Hepatic tumors: Predisposing factors for complications of transcatheter oily chemoembolization. Radiology 1996; 198: 33–40.

Chapter 16

TRANSCATHETER ARTERIAL CHEMOEMBOLIZATION: TECHNIQUE AND FUTURE POTENTIAL

Eleni Liapi

Christos S. Georgiades

Kelvin Hong

Jean-Francois H. Geschwind

Transcatheter arterial chemoembolization (TACE) is one of the most commonly performed procedures in interventional radiology and over the past 20 years, has significantly contributed to the evolution of this subspecialty (1, 2). TACE exploits the initial observation that most hepatic malignancies receive their blood supply largely by the hepatic artery, and selectively delivers intra-arterially high doses of chemotherapy to the tumor bed, while sparing the surrounding hepatic parenchyma (3, 4). Despite its promising design, TACE has not proved yet to be as effective as in theory. Several variations in the application of the technique, as well as the heterogeneity of chemotherapeutic regimens, are some of the most important challenges toward a thorough investigation of its clinical benefits (5). It is therefore essential for interventional radiologists to standardize the technique in order to maximize its effectiveness and help future advancements. In this chapter, we review the technical and clinical part of the procedure, as well as current results and future potential of TACE.

DEFINITION OF TACE, HISTORICAL BACKGROUND AND UNDERLYING PRINCIPLES OF TUMOR DAMAGE

TACE is defined as the infusion of a mixture of chemotherapeutic agents with or without iodized oil followed by embolization with particles (6). The technique was introduced in 1977 by Yamada, who intra-arterially delivered gelatin-sponge pieces permeated with 10 mg of mitomycin C or 20 mg of doxorubicin (Adriamycin), after super-selecting the tumor feeding artery of unresectable hepatomas (3, 4). A decade later, the observation that the injection of lipiodol, an iodinated ester derived from poppy seed oil, can be selectively up-taken and retained by primary HCC and hepatic metastases of colonic and neuroendocrine tumors, led to the establishment of this compound as an important part of the injected chemotherapeutic mixture (7–9). Moreover, lipiodol was found to effectively engage the chemotherapeutic agents, while leading to dual embolization and tumor necrosis.

Theoretically, embolization of the feeding vessel should cause ischemia of the tumor and, when combined with chemotherapy, should result in tumor necrosis; however, several reports suggest that TACE may actually accelerate the rate of intrahepatic recurrence or extrahepatic metastases (10). The mechanisms involved in chemoembolization-induced metastases are not well understood. Animal studies have shown that tumor ischemia and hypoxia up-regulate several molecular factors, such as vascular endothelial growth factor (VEGF) and hypoxia inducible factor-1 (HIF-1), thereby preventing cell apoptosis and stimulating tumor growth (10, 11). In clinical studies assessing embolization and angiogenesis, elevated levels of hypoxia-induced VEGF were reported 7 days after chemoembolization and, when obtained before chemoembolization, helped predict worse survival in patients with hepatocellular carcinoma (HCC) undergoing chemoembolization (12). These observations need to be further tested in the clinical setting to demonstrate the role of possible interactions between hypoxia and the effect of embolization during a chemoembolization procedure.

PATIENT SELECTION AND INDICATIONS FOR TACE

Nowadays, chemoembolization is the preferred treatment for palliation of unresectable HCC (13–15). TACE is also employed as an adjunctive therapy to liver resection or as a bridge to liver transplantation, as well as prior to or after radiofrequency ablation (16–20). Other palliative applications of TACE include unresectable cholangiocarcinomas (21), carcinoid and pancreatic islet tumors and sarcomas metastatic to the liver (22, 23). The efficacy of TACE in patients with colorectal metastases is less established (24).

Not all patients with unresectable primary or metastatic liver tumor will benefit from chemoembolization. One important aspect in the selection of patients is the presence of adequate liver function. In patients with advanced liver disease, treatment-induced liver failure may offset the anti-tumoral effect or survival benefit of the intervention. Predictors of outcome are related to tumor burden (tumor size, vascular invasion, and alpha-fetoprotein [AFP] levels), liver functional impairment (Child-Pugh [CP], bilirubin, ascites), performance status (Karnofsky index, Eastern Cooperative Oncology

Group [ECOG] scale), and response to treatment. Interestingly, in a comparison of 12 liver staging systems, the CP nominal liver staging system was the most accurate in predicting survival of patients with unresectable HCC treated with TACE (25). Overall, the best candidates are patients with preserved liver function and asymptomatic lesions without vascular invasion or extrahepatic spread.

CONTRAINDICATIONS FOR TACE

Historically, contraindications to TACE have included increased serum bilirubin level, low serum albumin level, severe liver dysfunction as indicated by CP score, impaired hepatopetal flow (i.e., portal vein obstruction) and biliary obstruction. Several recent studies have challenged these traditional contraindications, favoring a super-selective approach as well as an adjustment of the chemotherapeutic dosage that may minimize liver damage. Absolute contraindications for TACE such as absence of hepatopedal blood flow and presence of encephalopathy and biliary obstruction are now considered relative ones. Several articles have demonstrated little negative impact on hepatic function in cases of portal vein tumoral thrombosis and chemoembolization can be safely performed if hepatopetal collateral flow is present (26, 27).

Current absolute contraindications for TACE now include tumor resectability, intractable systemic infection and the synergistic effect of poor synthetic function (Child-Pugh C) and compromised hepatopetal flow. Relative contraindications include a variety of other factors including, but not limited to, serum bilirubin greater than 2 mg/dL, lactate dehydrogenase greater than 425 U/L, aspartate aminotransferase greater than 100 U/L, tumor burden involving more than 50% of the liver, presence of extrahepatic metastases, poor performance status, cardiac or renal insufficiency, ascites, recent variceal bleeding or significant thrombocytopenia, intractable arteriovenous fistula, surgical portocaval anastomosis, severe portal vein thrombosis, and tumor invasion to the inferior vena cava (IVC) and right atrium. Table 16.1 summarizes the list of absolute and relative contraindications for TACE.

PATIENT PREPARATION

In our institution, all patients undergo a baseline gadolinium-enhanced magnetic resonance imaging

TABLE 16.1 Contraindications for TACE

ABSOLUTE
1. Tumor resectability
2. Extensive intractable infection
3. Extensive liver disease combined with compromised hepatopetal flow

RELATIVE
1. Borderline liver function
2. Total bilirubin >4 mg/dl
3. Portal vein thrombosis
4. Uncorrectable coagulopathy
5. Poor general health
6. Significant arteriovenous shunting through the tumor
7. Encephalopathy

(MRI) study of the liver with perfusion/diffusion sequences, in order to assess the extent and viability of tumor and plan future treatment. A dual-phase MRI or computed tomogram (CT) is also acceptable, but the addition of the diffusion sequences may reliably demonstrate and quantify tumor necrosis (28). In addition to information regarding tumor viability, cross-sectional imaging may add valuable information regarding its vascular supply. For instance, the presence of portal vein thrombosis and/or variant vascular anatomy may alter the embolization part of the procedure or reduce the procedure time and contrast load.

Patients are premedicated depending on the tumor histology, renal function and prior surgical and medical history. Patients whose sphincter of Oddi function has been eliminated – that is, hepatojejunostomy, sphincterotomy patients or patients with percutaneous or internal biliary stents – are at high risk for developing a hepatic abscess following TACE. Stringent 24-hour bowel preparation and intravenous administration of broad-spectrum antibiotics prior to the procedure all but eliminate this possibility. Because the procedure is performed with the patient under conscious sedation, an 8-hour fasting status is required.

TECHNICAL CONSIDERATIONS

Although many different chemoembolization protocols have been used in the past, the combination of some chemotherapeutic agents and a vehicle such as lipiodol constitutes the basis of most procedures. Single-drug therapies or a combination of agents may be used. The most widely used single chemotherapeutic agent is doxorubicin, and the combination of

cisplatin, doxorubicin and mitomycin C is the most common drug combination infused. The latest trends in the employment of the technique favor a more selective (segmental or subsegmental arterial catheter placement) approach (29). Non-occlusive and occlusive techniques have been described (30). Improved tumor response has been shown when chemoembolization can be repeated multiple times with maintenance of long-term arterial patency (31, 32). Several types of embolic agents have been utilized in conjunction with lipiodol for chemoembolization, including gelfoam powder and pledgets, polyvinyl alcohol, starch and glass or tris-acryl gelatin microspheres (30). The gelatin sponges cause only temporary thrombosis lasting about 2 weeks, whereas polyvinyl alcohol and tris-acryl gelatin microspheres create a more permanent effect.

Following, we describe the Johns Hopkins Hospital protocol, which consists of segmental or subsegmental chemoembolization with use of the triple chemotherapeutic cocktail of doxorubicin, mytomicin and cisplatin with lipiodol, followed by the injection of embospheres (33).

TECHNIQUE

After informed consent is obtained, the patient is brought to the interventional radiology suite, placed on the fluoroscopy table supine and both groins are prepared in a sterile fashion. Following volume loading with normal saline and administration of conscious sedation, the single-wall Seldinger technique with an 18-gauge needle is used to access the right common femoral artery. A 5-French vascular sheath is then placed into the artery over a 0.035 guidewire Under fluoroscopic guidance, a 5-French catheter (Simmons-1 or Cobra) is then used to select the superior mesenteric artery (SMA) and the celiac axis.

The angiogram of the SMA is carried well into the portal venous phase, in order to assess possible variant vascular anatomy (accessory or replaced hepatic artery) and retrograde flow through the gastroduodenal artery (GDA), as well as visualize and identify the patency of the portal vein (Figures 16.1A–C and 16.2A–B). A celiac angiogram may adequately demonstrate hepatic branch anatomy, possible presence of replaced left hepatic artery, or other variant arteries. If possible, the right inferior phrenic artery should be interrogated to exclude malignant parasitization of blood flow. It is necessary that the injection

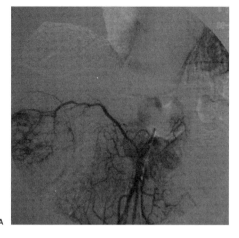
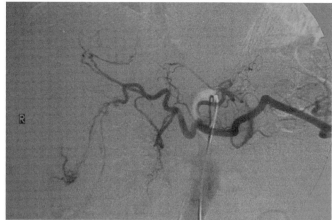
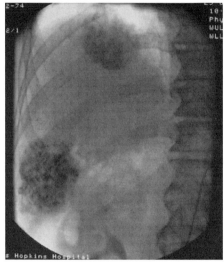

FIGURE 16.1.   Digital subtraction angiography (DSA). Anteroposterior views of the superior mesenteric artery, celiac axis and selective accessory right hepatic artery in a 55-year-old male patient with unresectable multifocal HCC treated with TACE. (A) Accessory right hepatic artery arising off the superior mesenteric artery, supplying multiple lesions. (B) DSA of the celiac axis demonstrates the presence of a right hepatic artery. (C) Selective angiogram of the accessory right hepatic artery, showing two hypervascular lesions.

rates used should balance adequate opacification of the targeted vessels without unnecessary reflux of contrast material into the aorta or other vessels proximal to the injection site. Over the guidewire, the 5-Fr catheter is next advanced into the desired hepatic artery branch. Depending on tumor location, a selective hepatic arteriogram demonstrates the tumor "blush" (Figure 16.3A–D). Special attention should be paid to the falciform, phrenic, right or accessory gastric arteries, supraduodenal, retroduodenal,

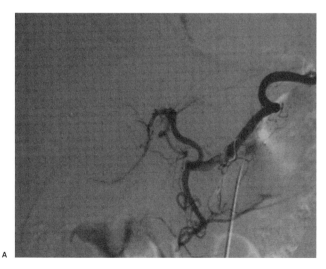
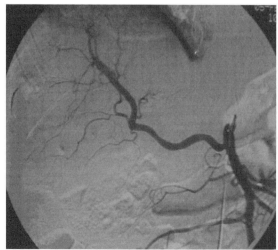

FIGURE 16.2.   DSA Anteroposterior views of the celiac axis, SMA and right hepatic artery of 71-year-old male patient with HCC. (A) DSA view of the celiac axis, showing little hepatic perfusion. (B) DSA view of the SMA showing a replaced right hepatic artery.

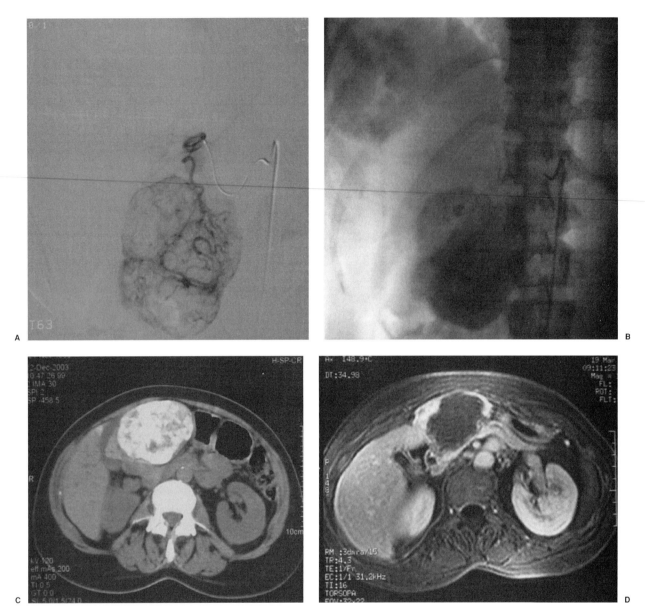

FIGURE 16.3. (A) DSA Anteroposterior view of a segmental right branch in a female patient with metastatic leiomyosarcoma, showing a hypervascular lesion. (B) Spot image after TACE demonstrates lipiodol deposition in the treated lesion. (C) Non-contrast CT scan within 24 hours following the procedure shows good lipiodol deposition. (D) T1-weighted gadolinium-enhanced MR image 6 weeks after TACE, showing significant tumor necrosis.

retroportal and cystic arteries, so as to avoid non-target embolization. The catheter should be advanced beyond the GDA. In difficult cases with complex vascular anatomy, the utilization of three-dimensional rotational angiography may help in minimizing procedure risks or complications and lead a more effective lesion targeting (34).

Reversal of flow can be demonstrated by a microcatheter injection with relatively high injection rates. It is also important to identify any arteriovenous shunting patterns, which have been reported to occur in 31% to 63% of cases between second-order branches (35). In such cases, direct embolization of recognized shunts, even in the setting of portal vein thrombosis, followed by chemoembolization may prove effective.

After this initial visceral vascular evaluation has been performed, the vessel of interest targeting the specific tumor bed is subsequently accessed. A solution containing cisplatin 100 mg, doxorubicin 50 mg and mitomycin C 10 mg in a 1:1 to 2:1 mixture with ethiodol is subsequently injected, until stasis is achieved. Then, 5 to 10 mL of intra-arterial lidocaine is injected for immediate analgesia and to diminish post-procedural symptoms. This is followed by injection of 1 to 2 ml of mixture containing embosphere particles (100 to 500 μm in size), suspended in 1:1 ratio in contrast medium. The embolization endpoint is not artery occlusion, but reduction in arterial inflow, for prevention of quick chemotherapy washout. Closure of femoral artery access can be achieved with use of a closure device when no standard contraindication prevails after the performance of common femoral arteriography. A recent study on patients treated with TACE showed that repetitive use of a collagen-plug closure device after each procedure does not impose patients to further risks (27).

RECOVERY

After proper hemostasis is achieved, the patient is placed on a patient-controlled analgesia (PCA) pump with intravenous hydration and sent to the floor. Frequent vital signs monitoring is required for only the 4-hour post-procedure period, after which routine nursing checks are adequate. When needed, medication should include (in addition to the morphine or fentanyl PCA) anti-nausea and additional pain medication for breakthrough pain. After the initial observation period, the patient is encouraged to ambulate under supervision. The use of a closure device can reduce the observation period to 2 hours (36). As soon as the patient ambulates, the Foley catheter (if one was placed) is removed and oral intake is advanced as tolerated. Within 24 hours following the procedure, a non-contrast CT of the abdomen is obtained to document the distribution of lipiodol and the degree of lipiodol uptake by the tumor.

FOLLOW-UP AND EVALUATION OF RESPONSE TO TREATMENT

For maximal benefit, patients should be advised to return for a follow-up clinical visit 4 to 6 weeks after treatment. During this visit, liver function tests, as well as a perfusion-diffusion MRI scan of the liver, are performed. Decision to retreat is based upon the combination of imaging and laboratory findings as well as the patient's clinical performance status.

According to the World Health Organization (WHO) and the Response Evaluation Criteria in Solid Tumors (RECIST), reduction in tumor size is the optimal outcome of every non-surgical treatment (37, 38). Additionally, tumor enhancement on CT or

MRI delineate viability, as enhancing portions of the tumor are presumed to be viable whereas the non-enhancing ones are presumed necrotic (39–41). Following chemoembolization, the presence of lipiodol on CT scans may remain for more than 2 months and therefore may obscure true tumor enhancement. Perfusion-diffusion MRI can successfully overcome this obstacle, as lipiodol does not obscure gadolinium enhancement, and measurement of increased free water content within the tumor translates into cancerous cell death (Figure 16.3A–D) (28) . Furthermore, diffusion MRI may prove more useful in the early post-treatment period after TACE, when tumors are not expected to change in size despite the fact that they may be nonviable (42, 43).

Lack of satisfactory response after one session of TACE does not predict eventual response, and repeated treatments targeting the same lesion are sometimes necessary. The emergence of any contraindications to TACE between consecutive procedures precludes re-treatment; thus, prior to each procedure, the relevant laboratory values should be obtained and the patient re-evaluated.

COMPLICATIONS AND SIDE EFFECTS

TACE has been reported to be frequently complicated by pain, fever, nausea, fatigue and elevated transaminases, commonly referred to as the **post-embolization syndrome.** These symptoms are usually self-limited and are more common in cases in which large tumors are treated. In selected cases, careful post-operative monitoring is required to differentiate post-embolization syndrome from other, more serious, complications, such as liver abscess, gallbladder infarction and septicemia.

Complications due to non-target embolization include necrosis in undesirable arterial beds, such as the cystic artery and gastrointestinal, cutaneous and phrenic capillary beds. Hepatic arterial pseudoaneurysm formation or arterial stenosis may occur following difficult or inelegant catheter manipulations. Liver failure and hepatorenal syndrome are more likely to occur in debilitated patients with advanced disease and those with impaired liver function or compromised portal flow; in such individuals, it is important to weigh the possible complications of the procedure against its potential benefits. Other uncommon problems following TACE include ischemic cholecystitis, pulmonary or cerebral embolization,

TABLE 16.2 Complications of TACE

Post-embolization syndrome (pain, fever, nausea, fatigue and leukocytosis)
Liver abscess
Gallbladder infarction
Septicemia
Irreversible liver failure
Hepatorenal syndrome
Pulmonary oil embolization
Cerebral embolization

hypothyroidism, or the development of a pleural effusion. Table 16.2 summarizes a list of most commonly encountered side effects and complications of TACE.

SURVIVAL BENEFIT

The median survival of patients with inoperable HCC is 4 to 7 months (which can be extended with maximal supportive care to approximately 10 months). Despite that chemoembolization had early in its course proved to reduce tumor growth, initial large randomized trials failed to demonstrate a survival advantage (44–46). In 2002, two published randomized controlled published showed a survival advantage for TACE in selected patients with preserved liver function and supportive maintenance (14, 15). A meta-analysis that included seven randomized trials of arterial embolization for unresectable HCC provided further support of the efficacy of TACE (17). Compared with control (either conservative treatment or less favorable therapy, such as intravenous 5-fluorouracil), there was a statistically significant improvement in 2-year survival with arterial chemoembolization (17). TACE showed a median survival of more than 2 years and, although rarely, converted some patients into operable candidates. In the future, it is highly unlikely that more randomized controlled studies with conservative or less favorable treatments will be initiated, since serious ethical considerations may rise.

There is less experience with TACE in the treatment of hepatic metastases (23). Several studies have excellent symptomatic and biologic complete response rates of 70% to 73% of patients with metastatic carcinoid treated with chemoembolization (47). The efficacy of TACE in other groups, such as patients with colorectal metastasis, is less established (48).

CURRENT RESEARCH ON TACE

Drug-loaded (doxorubicin or irinotecan loaded) microspheres have recently been developed for intra-arterial injection (49). Doxorubicin-eluting beads (DC Bead for loading by the physician and PRECISION Bead preloaded with doxorubicin, Biocompatibles UK Ltd, Surrey, UK) were initially tested on the rabbit Vx-2 tumor model and demonstrated consistent drug release over time, with excellent tumor control (49). The results of Phase I/II studies have been recently published, and initial results seem rather encouraging (50–52). Irinotecan-eluting beads for metastatic colon cancer are also under development (53, 54).

HCC is one of the most vascular solid cancers, associated with a high propensity for vascular invasion. One of the most critical and specific factors for blood vessel formation is VEGF (55). Today, a variety of strategies are available for targeting VEGF, although VEGF blockade with monoclonal antibodies is the most studied approach (56,57). Bevacizumab (Avastin, Genentech Inc, San Francisco, CA) is the first U.S. commercially available anti-VEGF, humanized monoclonal antibody that binds VEGF and prevents the interaction of VEGF with its receptors on the surface of endothelial cells (58). When unblocked, this interaction may lead to endothelial cell proliferation and new blood vessel formation (59). This antibody has shown both cytostatic and cytotoxic effects in clinical trials (60,61). VEGF expression is known to play an important role in the development of HCC and the degree of its expression is reported to be associated with tumor size and histologic grade (62, 63). Currently, there are three National Cancer Institute NCI Phase II trials evaluating the safety and efficacy of bevacizumab in patients with primary unresectable liver cancer. In our institution, a Phase II trial of bevacizumab with TACE for HCC has just completed patient enrollment with initial promising results. TACE is performed on day 1 of a 42-day therapy cycle and bevacizumab (10 mg/kg) is administered intravenously on days 7, 8, and 22. Data from this trial may guide to the development of novel antiangiogenic liver cancer regimens.

CONCLUSION

Chemoembolization is routinely performed in many institutions throughout the world. Standardization of the technique is essential to conduct large prospective randomized trials and meta-analyses, and this may prove difficult to achieve, as there is no consensus regarding the chemotherapeutic agents, embolic materials, technique and treatment planning. Although the standardization of the technique is necessary to boost the effectiveness of the procedure and subsequently improve patient survival, it is also imperative to promote research in other areas, such as the application of combination therapies or further employment of gene and molecular therapies, in order to give new dimensions to this locoregional therapy.

REFERENCES

1. Stuart K. Chemoembolization in the management of liver tumors. Oncologist, 2003 October 1; 8(5): 425–437.

2. Roche A, Girish B, de Baere T, et al. Trans-catheter arterial chemoembolization as first-line treatment for hepatic metastases from endocrine tumors. Eur Radiol, 2003; 13(1): 136.

3. Yamada R, Nakatsuka H, Nakamura K, et al. Hepatic artery embolization in 32 patients with unresectable hepatoma. Osaka City Med J, 1980; 26(2): 81–96.

4. Yamada R, Sato M, Kawabata M, et al. Hepatic artery embolization in 120 patients with unresectable hepatoma. Radiology, 1983 Aug; 148(2): 397–401.

5. Geschwind JF. Chemoembolization for hepatocellular carcinoma: Where does the truth lie? J Vasc Interv Radiol, 2002 Oct; 13(10): 991–994.

6. Brown DB, Gould JE, Gervais DA, et al. Transcatheter therapy for hepatic malignancy: Standardization of terminology and reporting criteria. J Vasc Interv Radiol, 2007; 18(12): 1469–1478.

7. Nakakuma K, Tashiro S, Hiraoka T, et al. Studies on anticancer treatment with an oily anticancer drug injected into the ligated feeding hepatic artery for liver cancer. Cancer, 1983 Dec 15; 52(12): 2193–2200.

8. Konno T, Maeda H, Iwai K, et al. Effect of arterial administration of high-molecular-weight anticancer agent SMANCS with lipid lymphographic agent on hepatoma: A preliminary report. Eur J Cancer Clin Oncol, 1983 Aug;19; (8): 1053–1065.

9. Clouse ME, Perry L, Stuart K, et al. Hepatic arterial chemoembolization for metastatic neuroendocrine tumors. Digestion, 1994; 55 Suppl 3: 92–97.

10. Xiong ZP, Yang SR, Liang ZY, et al. Association between vascular endothelial growth factor and metastasis after transcatheter arterial chemoembolization in patients with hepatocellular carcinoma. Hepatobiliary Pancreat Dis Int, 2004 Aug; 3(3): 386–390.

11. Kobayashi N, Ishii M, Ueno Y, et al. Co-expression of Bcl-2 protein and vascular endothelial growth factor in hepatocellular carcinomas treated by chemoembolization. Liver, 1999 Feb; 19(1): 25–31.

12. Sergio A, Cristofori C, Cardin R, et al. Transcatheter arterial chemoembolization (TACE) in hepatocellular carcinoma (HCC): The role of angiogenesis and invasiveness. Am J Gastroenterol, 2008 Jan 2 [Epub ahead of print].

13. Groupe d'Etude et de Traitement du Carcinome Hepatocellulaire. A comparison of lipiodol chemoembolization and conservative treatment for unresectable hepatocellular carcinoma. N Engl J Med, 1995 May 11; 332(19): 1256–1261.

14. Lo CM, Ngan H, Tso WK, et al. Randomized controlled trial of transarterial lipiodol chemoembolization for unresectable hepatocellular carcinoma. Hepatology, 2002 May; 35(5): 1164–1171.

15. Llovet JM, Real MI, Montana X, et al. Arterial embolisation or chemoembolisation versus symptomatic treatment in patients with unresectable hepatocellular carcinoma: A randomised controlled trial. Lancet, 2002 May 18; 359(9319): 1734–1739.

16. Aoki T, Imamura H, Hasegawa K, et al. Sequential preoperative arterial and portal venous embolizations in patients with hepatocellular carcinoma. Arch Surg, 2004; 139(7): 766–774.

17. Llovet JM, Burroughs A, and Bruix J. Hepatocellular carcinoma. Lancet, 2003 Dec 6; 362(9399): 1907–1917.

18. Llovet JM. Treatment of hepatocellular carcinoma. Curr Treat Options Gastroenterol, 2004 Dec; 7(6): 431–441.

19. Arii S, Yamaoka Y, Futagawa S, The Liver Cancer Study Group of Japan. et al. Results of surgical and nonsurgical treatment for small-sized hepatocellular carcinomas: A retrospective and nationwide survey in Japan. Hepatology, 2000 Dec; 32(6): 1224–1229.

20. Livraghi T, Meloni F, Morabito A, et al. Multimodal image-guided tailored therapy of early and intermediate hepatocellular carcinoma: Long-term survival in the experience of a single radiologic referral center. Liver Transpl, 2004 Feb; 10(2 Suppl 1): S98–106.

21. Burger I, Hong K, Schulick R, et al. Transcatheter arterial chemoembolization in unresectable cholangiocarcinoma: Initial experience in a single institution. J Vasc Interv Radiol, 2005 Mar; 16(3): 353–361.

22. Liapi E, Geschwind JF, Vossen JA, et al. Functional MRI evaluation of tumor response in patients with neuroendocrine hepatic metastasis treated with transcatheter arterial chemoembolization. AJR Am J Roentgenol, 2008 Jan; 190(1): 67–73.

23. Sullivan KL. Hepatic artery chemoembolization. Semin Oncol, 2002 Apr; 29(2): 145–151.

24. Vogl TJ, Zangos S, Eichler K, et al. Colorectal liver metastases: Regional chemotherapy via transarterial chemoembolization (TACE) and hepatic chemoperfusion: An update. Eur Radiol, 2007 Apr; 17(4): 1025–1034.

25. Georgiades CS, Liapi E, Frangakis C, et al. Prognostic accuracy of 12 liver staging systems in patients with unresectable hepatocellular carcinoma treated with transarterial chemoembolization. J Vasc Interv Radiol, 2006 October 1; 17(10): 1619–1624.

26. Chung JW, Park JH, Han JK, et al. Hepatocellular carcinoma and portal vein invasion: Results of treatment with transcatheter oily chemoembolization. Am J Roentgenol, 1995 August 1; 165(2): 315–321.

27. Georgiades CS, Hong K, D'Angelo M, et al. Safety and efficacy of transarterial chemoembolization in patients with unresectable hepatocellular carcinoma and portal vein thrombosis. J Vasc Interv Radiol, 2005 December 1; 16(12): 1653–1659.

28. Kamel IR, Bluemke DA, Ramsey D, et al. Role of diffusion-weighted imaging in estimating tumor necrosis after chemoembolization of hepatocellular carcinoma. Am J Roentgenol, 2003, Sept; 181(3): 708–710.

29. Kothary N, Weintraub JL, Susman J, et al. Transarterial chemoembolization for primary hepatocellular carcinoma in patients at high risk. J Vasc Interv Radiol, 2007; 18(12): 1517–1526.

30. Bruix J, Sala M, and Llovet JM. Chemoembolization for hepatocellular carcinoma. Gastroenterology, 2004 Nov; 127(5 Suppl 1): S179–188.

31. Jaeger HJ, Mehring UM, Castaneda F, et al. Sequential transarterial chemoembolization for unresectable advanced hepatocellular carcinoma. Cardiovasc Intervent Radiol, 1996 Nov–Dec; 19(6): 388–396.

32. Geschwind JF, Ramsey DE, van der Wal BC, et al. Transcatheter arterial chemoembolization of liver tumors: Effects of embolization protocol on injectable volume of chemotherapy and subsequent arterial patency. Cardiovasc Intervent Radiol, 2003 Mar–Apr; 26(2): 111–117.

33. Liapi E, Georgiades CC, Hong K, et al. Transcatheter arterial chemoembolization: current technique and future promise. Tech Vasc Interv Radiol, 2007 Mar; 10(1): 2–11.

34. Liapi E, Hong K, Georgiades CS, et al. Three-dimensional rotational angiography: Introduction of an adjunctive tool for successful transarterial chemoembolization. J Vasc Interv Radiol, 2005 Sept; 16(9): 1241–1245.

35. Okuda K, Musha H, Yamasaki T, et al. Angiographic demonstration of intrahepatic arterio-portal anastomoses in hepatocellular carcinoma. Radiology, 1977 Jan 1; 122(1): 53–58.

36. Hong K, Liapi E, Georgiades CS, et al. Case-controlled comparison of a percutaneous collagen arteriotomy closure device versus manual compression after liver chemoembolization. J Vasc Interv Radiol, 2005 March 1; 16(3): 339–345.

37. Therasse P, Arbuck SG, Eisenhauer EA, et al. New guidelines to evaluate the response to treatment in solid tumors: European Organization for Research and Treatment of Cancer, National Cancer Institute of the United States, National Cancer Institute of Canada. J Natl Cancer Inst, 2000 Feb 2; 92(3): 205–216.

38. Tsuchida Y and Therasse P. Response evaluation criteria in solid tumors (RECIST): New guidelines. Med Pediatr Oncol, 2001 Jul; 37(1): 1–3.

39. Murakami R, Yoshimatsu S, Yamashita Y, et al. Treatment of hepatocellular carcinoma: Value of percutaneous microwave coagulation. AJR Am J Roentgenol, 1995 May; 164(5): 1159–1164.

40. Castrucci M, Sironi S, De Cobelli F, et al. Plain and gadolinium-DTPA-enhanced MR imaging of hepatocellular carcinoma treated with transarterial chemoembolization. Abdom Imaging, 1996 Nov–Dec; 21(6): 488–494.

41. Bartolozzi C, Lencioni R, Caramella D, et al. Treatment of hepatocellular carcinoma with percutaneous ethanol injection: Evaluation with contrast-enhanced MR imaging. AJR Am J Roentgenol, 1994 Apr; 162(4): 827–831.

42. Lim HK and Han JK. Hepatocellular carcinoma: Evaluation of therapeutic response to interventional procedures. Abdom Imaging, 2002 Mar–Apr; 27(2): 168–179.

43. Takayasu K, Arii S, Matsuo N, et al. Comparison of CT findings with resected specimens after chemoembolization with iodized oil for hepatocellular carcinoma. AJR Am J Roentgenol, 2000 Sep; 175(3): 699–704.

44. Bruix J, Llovet JM, Castells A, et al. Transarterial embolization versus symptomatic treatment in patients with advanced hepatocellular carcinoma: Results of a randomized, controlled trial in a single institution. Hepatology, 1998 Jun; 27(6): 1578–1583.

45. Livraghi T, Giorgio A, Marin G, et al. Hepatocellular carcinoma and cirrhosis in 746 patients: Long-term results of percutaneous ethanol injection. Radiology, 1995 Oct; 197(1): 101–108.

46. Simonetti RG, Liberati A, Angiolini C, et al. Treatment of hepatocellular carcinoma: A systematic review of randomized controlled trials. Ann Oncol, 1997 Feb; 8(2): 117–136.

47. Gupta S, Johnson MM, Murphy R, et al. Hepatic arterial embolization and chemoembolization for the treatment of patients with metastatic neuroendocrine tumors. Cancer, 2005; 104(8): 1590–1602.

48. Lang EK and Brown CL, Jr. Colorectal metastases to the liver: Selective chemoembolization. Radiology, 1993 November 1; 189(2): 417–422.

49. Geschwind JF, Khwaja A, and Hong K. New intraarterial drug delivery system: Pharmacokinetics and tumor response in an animal model of liver cancer. ASCO Annual Meeting, 2005, Orlando, Florida.

50. Varela M, Real MI, Burrel M, et al. Chemoembolization of hepatocellular carcinoma with drug eluting beads: Efficacy and doxorubicin pharmacokinetics. J Hepatol, 2007; 46(3): 474–481.

51. Reyes D, Geschwind J-FH, et al. Intraarterial doxorubicin-eluting microspheres for patients with unresectable hepatocellular carcinoma: A pilot study. CIRSE, 2007; Athens, Greece: European Society of Cardiovascular Interventional Radiology, 2007, p. 16.

52. Poon RT, Tso WK, Pang RW, et al. A phase I/II trial of chemoembolization for hepatocellular carcinoma using a novel intra-arterial drug-eluting bead. Clin Gastroenterol Hepatol, 2007 Sep; 5(9): 1100–1108.

53. Yoshizawa H, Nishino S, Shiomori K, et al. Surface morphology control of polylactide microspheres enclosing irinotecan hydrochloride. Int J Pharm, 2005; 296(1–2): 112–116.

54. Aliberti C, Tilli M, Benea G, et al. Trans-arterial chemoembolization (TACE) of liver metastases from colorectal cancer using irinotecan-eluting beads: Preliminary results. Anticancer Res, 2006 Sep–Oct; 26(5B): 3793–3795.

55. Ferrara N and Henzel WJ. Pituitary follicular cells secrete a novel heparin-binding growth factor specific for vascular endothelial cells. Biochem Biophys Res Commun, 1989 Jun 15; 161(2): 851–858.

56. Wang Y, Fei D, Vanderlaan M, et al. Biological activity of bevacizumab, a humanized anti-VEGF antibody in vitro. Angiogenesis, 2004; 7(4): 335.

57. Motl S. Bevacizumab in combination chemotherapy for colorectal and other cancers. Am J Health Syst Pharm, 2005 May; 62(10): 1021–1032.

58. Food and Drug Administration. Bevacizumab FDA approval letter, 2004.

59. Kim KJ, Li B, Winer J, Armanini M, et al. Inhibition of

vascular endothelial growth factor-induced angiogenesis suppresses tumour growth in vivo. Nature, 1993 Apr 29; 362(6423): 841–844.

60. Cobleigh MA, Langmuir VK, Sledge GW, et al. A phase I/II dose-escalation trial of bevacizumab in previously treated metastatic breast cancer. Semin Oncol, 2003 Oct; 30(5Suppl 16): 117–124.

61. Yang JC, Haworth L, Sherry RM, et al. A randomized trial of bevacizumab, an anti-vascular endothelial growth factor antibody, for metastatic renal cancer. N Engl J Med, 2003 July 31; 349(5): 427–434.

62. Imaeda T, Kanematsu M, Mochizuki R, et al. Extracapsular invasion of small hepatocellular carcinoma: MR and CT findings. J Comput Assist Tomogr, 1994 Sept–Oct; 18(5): 755–760.

63. Yamaguchi R, Yano H, Iemura A, et al. Expression of vascular endothelial growth factor in human hepatocellular carcinoma. Hepatology, 1998 Jul; 28(1): 68–77.

Chapter 17

NEW CONCEPTS IN TARGETING AND IMAGING LIVER CANCER

Eleni Liapi

Christos S. Georgiades

Kelvin Hong

Jean-Francois H. Geschwind

Ongoing research in the discipline of image-guided interventional oncology for hepatic malignancies seeks to discover and implement novel and effective therapeutic approaches in order to benefit patients with unresectable liver cancer. Research in this area incorporates advancements in the knowledge of liver cancer biology, new concepts in targeting liver cancer, development of novel drugs, improvement of intra-arterial drug delivery and technological advances of imaging systems.

This chapter is an overview of the most recent knowledge in liver cancer biology, new locoregional therapies for liver cancer and new imaging concepts for monitoring locoregional treatment response.

NEW CONCEPTS IN TARGETING LIVER CANCER

Targeting Angiogenesis

The fundamental role of angiogenesis in tumor progression was first suggested by Folkman et al. in a classic study describing that tumors cannot grow beyond 1 mm or 2 mm without the formation of new blood vessels (1). This complex process facilitates tumor progression and, eventually, tumor metastatic spread (1, 2). Several factors, including tumor hypoxia, growth factors, cytokines, oncogene activation and other mutations interact to stimulate angiogenesis (2, 3). Therefore, targeted inhibition of angiogenesis can be achieved at any of the aforementioned different levels, with treatments including the neutralization of growth factors with monoclonal antibodies (mAbs), the inhibition of downstream signaling from tyrosine kinase receptors and interference with the interaction between proliferating endothelial cells and matrix components.

Hepatocellular carcinoma (HCC) is one of the most vascular solid cancers, associated with a high propensity for vascular invasion. One of the most critical and specific factors for blood vessel formation is vascular endothelial growth factor (VEGF) (4). VEGF is an endothelial cell mitogen that regulates proliferation, permeability and survival of endothelial cells through inhibition of apoptosis (4–7). Its expression has been shown to be prognostic for a number of solid tumors, including colorectal hepatic metastases and HCC (8–10). Up-regulation of VEGF has been correlated with increased tumor invasion, intratumoral microvessel density, disease recurrence and poor prognosis (11–13). Over the past decade, intense research activity has succeeded in demonstrating the role of VEGF as a valid target for cancer therapy and has led to the development and clinical testing of numerous novel angiogenesis inhibitors (5, 14, 15).

Today, a variety of strategies are available for targeting VEGF, although VEGF blockade with mAbs is the most studied approach (16, 17). Bevacizumab (Avastin, Genentech Inc, San Francisco, CA) is the first commercially available anti-VEGF in the United States, humanized monoclonal antibody that binds VEGF and prevents the interaction of VEGF and its receptors on the surface of endothelial cells (18). When unblocked, this interaction may lead to endothelial cell proliferation and new blood vessel formation (14). This antibody has shown both cytostatic and cytotoxic effects in clinical trials (19, 20). Objective responses, such as reduction in tumor growth and increase in time to tumor progression, have been documented for various types of solid tumors (17, 19–23). VEGF expression is known to play an important role in the development of HCC, and the degree of its expression is reported to be associated with tumor size and histologic grade (24, 25). However, there are a limited number of studies suggesting a potential therapeutic role for bevacizumab (26). A recent pilot study

suggested that bevacizumab can be given safely at both 5 mg/kg and 10 mg/kg in HCC patients with localized unresectable HCC, preserved liver function and no significant esophageal varices (27). In another pilot study, selected HCC patients undergoing transcatheter arterial chemoembolization (TACE) additionally received intravenous bevacizumab, which was well tolerated and prolonged disease control (28). Currently, there are three National Cancer Institute (NCI) Phase II trials evaluating the safety and efficacy of bevacizumab in patients with primary unresectable liver cancer (29–31). In our institution, a Phase II trial of bevacizumab with TACE for HCC has just started enrolling patients. TACE is designed to be performed on day 1 of a 42-day therapy cycle, and intravenous bevacizumab (10 mg/kg) will be administered on days 7, 8 and 22 (Figure 17.1A, B). These data may guide to the development of novel antiangiogenic liver cancer regimens and/or enhanced anti-tumoral activity with combinations of traditional local chemotherapeutic treatments with angiogenesis inhibitors. The integration of bevacizumab to the transcatheter arterial delivery formulas of chemotherapy for liver cancer seems challenging, as the formation of new blood vessels may effectively be reduced while maintaining high intratumoral cytotoxic chemotherapeutic concentrations.

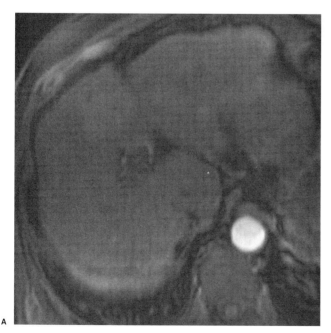 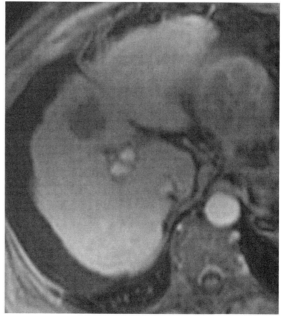

A

B

FIGURE 17.1. Contrast-enhanced T1-weighted MR images before (A) and after (B) one cycle of TACE combined with intravenous infusion of bevacizumab (10 mg/kg) in an 84-year-old man with unresectable HCC. Note that the tumor decreased in size and vascularity (Courtesy of Diane Reyes, RN, BS, Johns Hopkins Hospital, Baltimore, MD).

Targeting Glucose Tumor Metabolism

It long has been known that cancer cells frequently exhibit increased glycolysis and depend largely on this metabolic pathway for generation of adenosine triphosphatase (ATP) to meet their energy needs (32). Molecular studies have shown that HCC cells have an increased expression of the type II isoform of hexokinase, a key enzyme in the glycolytic pathway for maintaining high glycolytic performance (33). Moreover, when exposed to hypoxic conditions, hepatoma cells activate the type II hexokinase promoter up to seven-fold (34). In a recent clinical study, metastatic liver cancer displayed significantly high hexokinase II mRNA expression, and hexokinase II protein expression was localized in the cancer cells near necrotic regions, suggesting that glycolysis increases in tumors that have an insufficient oxygen supply from the vessels (35). Another clinical study has recently demonstrated that hypoxia stimulates HCC cellular growth through hexokinase II induction, and its inhibition induces apoptotic cell death (36).

3-Bromopyruvate (3-BrPa) is a potent ATP inhibitor, potentially via the hexokinase II pathway, with concurrent glycolysis inhibition (Figure 17.2) (37).

Preliminary experiments on the rabbit VX2 tumor model for liver cancer with direct intraarterial infusion of 3-BrPa showed very specific necrosis of the implanted lesions (37, 38). Additionally, intraarterial injection did not affect the viability of surrounding normal liver tissues, nor damage the animals' major tissues during systemic infusion (37). The mechanism of innate resistance of normal cells against 3-BrPa treatment has not yet been clarified, although it might be related to the difference of hexokinase II expression levels between normal and cancer cells (39).

In a study conducted on human hepatoma cell lines, 3-BrPa induced HCC cell apoptosis, besides inhibiting ATP production (36). This apoptotic cell type of death was likely responsible for the full effect of 3-BrPa on growth suppression, as induced apoptosis reached more than 90% within 6 hours of treatment (36). It should be noted that previous studies have suggested that apoptosis is an ATP-dependent process (40). In another study, cell death induced by 3-BrPa was shown to contain both apoptotic and necrotic components, in a ratio depending on the 3-BrPa concentration (41). The aforementioned study also demonstrated the ability of 3-BrPa to preferentially kill cancer cells with mitochondrial defects

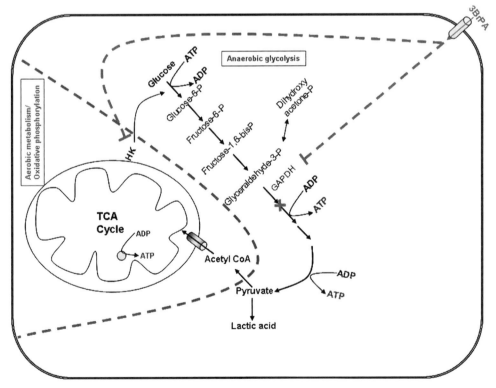

FIGURE 17.2. Proposed mechanism of action of 3-bromopyruvate. (*Adapted from* Geschwind JF, et al. Novel therapy for liver cancer: Direct intraarterial injection of a potent inhibitor of ATP production. Cancer Res 62, 3909–3913, July 15, 2002; with permission.) See Color Plate 19.

and tumor cells in a hypoxic environment (41). In the same study, depletion of ATP by glycolytic inhibition induced apoptosis in multi-drug resistant cells, suggesting that deprivation of cellular energy supply may be an effective way to overcome multi-drug resistance (41).

Further development and studies of this glycolytic inhibitor are necessary to establish its clinical therapeutic safety and efficacy. The direct intra-arterial infusion of 3-BrPa may serve as an effective approach for targeting liver cancer. Moreover, the use of 3-BrPa may have broad applications in cancer treatment, considering the glycolytic inhibitory effect observed in a wide spectrum of human cancers.

Targeting Hypoxia

Traditional interventional oncologic approaches for the treatment of HCC support the induction of tumor hypoxia by embolizing the feeding artery, as oxygen depletion is claimed to arrest tumor cell proliferation and lead to apoptosis and necrosis (42). However, tumor response rate is not always satisfactory, and only a small population of patients may benefit from this treatment (43). Recent data suggest that HCC cells likely have a compensatory mechanism, rendering cells in a hypoxic microenvironment the ability to survive or even proliferate more efficiently than cells in a normoxic condition (44). Several factors, such as hypoxia-inducible factor 1 (HIF-1), are involved in tumor progression/metastasis and activated in various cancers. HIF-1 is a transcription factor that enhances many types of gene expression including those involved in angiogenesis, cell proliferation, glucose metabolism, erythropoiesis and cell survival.

HIF-1α, which plays a major role in HIF-1 activation, has been shown to be overexpressed in preneoplastic hepatocytic lesions from a very early stage during hepatocarcinogenesis in mice and humans (45). HIF-1α stabilization occurring as a consequence of intermittent hypoxia may also be an important cause for radiotherapy (and possibly chemotherapy) treatment resistance. Fortunately, there is considerable interest in the development of drugs that can inhibit HIF-1 promoter activity. As such, HIF-1 is an important target to be considered in combination with cytotoxic locoregional therapies.

Targeting Malignant Stem Cells

Gene therapy, first introduced in 1990, is considered a promising new therapeutic modality against cancer, and currently about 60% of the clinical trial protocols for gene therapy have addressed the treatment of cancer. The main concept of gene therapies lies on the existence of a tumor stem cell compartment within a solid tumor. The identification of the specific pathways involved in malignant stem cell survival and proliferation has recently provided new opportunities for targeted therapies.

The transfer of therapeutic genes to liver tumors or to the peritumoral tissue seems particularly attractive for the potential treatment of liver cancer and metastasis, given that local delivery may increase the direct uptake of the DNA carrier complex into the target tissue compared with systemic delivery. Furthermore, though the intravenously infused genes enter the liver efficiently, it has been shown that most of them are completely trapped by Kupffer cells, thereby making it impossible to direct a gene to hepatocytes or tumor cells. One recent study demonstrated that it is feasible to use an iodized oil emulsion for gene delivery (46). Another recent study evaluated the therapeutic potential of hepatotropic nanoparticles for gene therapy of liver tumor in a rat model (47). These nanoparticles do not contain a viral genome and display the hepatitis B virus L antigen, which is essential to confer hepatic specificity.

Hepatic arterial infusion (HAI) has been examined as a means of regional delivery of gene therapy for liver metastases. Based on the fact that the *p53* gene is frequently defective or deleted in colorectal and other cancers, two approaches using recombinant adenoviruses have been investigated. The first uses a replication-incompetent virus encoding wild-type *p53* to infect cancer cells and replace the deficient gene product. HAI of one such adenoviral vector (Adp53 or SCH58500) was well tolerated in a Phase I study and achieved significant transgene expression at higher doses; this vector is currently being studied further, both alone and in combination with HAI of floxuridine (FUDR) (48). A second approach uses replication-selective viruses lacking the *E1B 55-kDa* gene as a means of targeted oncolysis. This gene product binds to *p53* and inhibits it, allowing for viral replication and cytotoxicity. A virus lacking the *E1B 55-kDa* gene is unable to inhibit wild-type *p53* and, therefore, selectively replicates in *p53*-deficient cancer cells while sparing normal cells. One such virus, Onyx-15 (aka *dl*1520) was administered via HAI to 11 patients with refractory metastatic gastrointestinal cancers to the liver, with no dose-limiting toxicity and

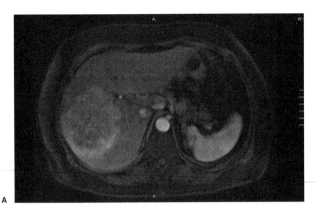
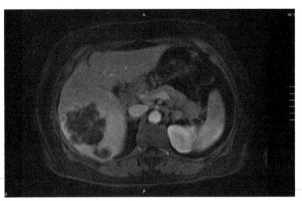

FIGURE 17.3. Contrast-enhanced T1-weighted axial MR images before (A) and after (B) one session of hepatic arterial chemoembolization with doxorubicin-eluting beads in a 65- year-old woman with unresectable HCC. Note the remarkable tumor shrinkage and devascularization.

documented replication in vivo (49). Further studies of these approaches are warranted.

DRUG-ELUTING MICROSPHERES: THE NEW CONCEPT IN TACE

Currently, there is intense research activity in the area of nanotechnology and drug-delivery systems. The ideal drug-loaded carriers should deliver the agent precisely, release it in a controlled and sustained manner and achieve high intra-tumor drug concentration for a sufficient period, without damaging the surrounding hepatic parenchyma. Several drug-delivery systems for intra-arterial treatment of hepatic lesions, such as polyvinyl alcohol microspheres and plcg-microspheres, have been recently tested (50–53). Polyvinyl alcohol (PVA) hydrogel microspheres can be loaded with a single chemotherapeutic agent, such as doxorubicin or irinotecan, and infused intra-arterially for selective tumor targeting (54–56). Doxorubicin-eluting beads (DC Bead for loading by the physician and PRECISION Bead preloaded with doxorubicin, Biocompatibles UK Ltd., Surrey, UK) were initially tested on the rabbit Vx-2 tumor model and demonstrated consistent drug release over time with excellent tumor control. These preliminary animal data showed that the concentration of doxorubicin within the tumor remains high up to 7 days post-transcatheter infusion, suggesting continuous release of doxorubicin from the microspheres, whereas systemic drug concentration is kept at minimal levels (57). Phase I and II clinical trials in Europe, the United States and Hong Kong for treatment of unresectable primary liver cancer with doxorubicin-eluting beads have recently completed enrollment.

The results in patients with unresectable HCC have been extremely promising, with an advantageous pharmacokinetic profile, reduced side effects and improved tumor response by imaging when compared with conventional TACE (Figure 17.3A,B) (51, 54).

Smaller-size drug-eluting beads (100–300 μm) seem to lodge distally in the tumor vasculature, possibly at the level of pathologic arterioportal microshunts, thereby allowing slow elution of the doxorubicin out of the beads, in turn leading to a more pronounced initial tumor response. However, a higher complication rate has been reported, presumably related to smaller-size beads. Irinotecan-eluting beads are also being currently investigated in the treatment of patients with colorectal cancer metastases to the liver (56, 58, 59).

NEW PERCUTANEUOUS APPROACHES FOR TREATMENT OF LIVER CANCER

Intrahepatic Delivery of α-Galactosylceramide-Pulsed Dendritic Cells

Dendritic cells (DCs) effectively elicit immune responses to self and foreign antigens. These specialized antigen-presenting cells can induce the generation of both antigen-specific cytotoxic T lymphocytes and T helper cells. In this regard, conventional DCs pulsed with tumor-associated antigens in various forms, including peptide or tumor cell lysates, have been applied to human cancer treatment. Recent research in DC biology has revealed that they also contribute to innate immune responses by activating natural killer (NK) cells and natural killer T (NKT) cells via interleukin-12 (IL-12) secretion and direct cellular interaction. As the liver contains both a large compartment of innate immune cells (NK cells and NKT cells) and acquired immune cells (T cells), DC-based vaccine trials against liver cancer have been initiated (60). Although tumor-specific T cells were promoted by vaccination in most patients, clinical benefits have thus far only been observed in only a minority of treated individuals.

The glycolipid antigen α-galactosylceramide (α-GalCer) induces activation of NKT cells. α-GalCer presented by DCs efficiently stimulates NKT cells implicated in innate immunity and has been recently tested as a novel anti-tumor therapy. In vivo animal studies have shown that systemic administration of α-GalCer can lead to anti-tumor effects against various tumors (including melanoma, sarcoma, colon carcinoma and lymphoma) in hepatic and lung metastasis models. Intravenous administration of α-GalCer pulsed DCs leads to more potent anti-tumor activities than direct administration of α-GalCer alone in mouse metastatic tumor models. Based on the promising results of preclinical studies demonstrating the anti-tumor potential of α-GalCer, several Phase I clinical studies have been done in cancer immunotherapy using intravenous administration of α-GalCer or α-GalCer-loaded DCs, but with limited clinical responses. This might partly be because intravenously administered α-GalCer or α-GalCer-loaded DCs may not be delivered efficiently to the tumor site.

Although the anti-tumor effect of α-GalCer has been demonstrated in murine metastatic liver tumor, no clinical trial against liver cancer has been reported to date. For further development of liver cancer treatment, intrahepatic (IH) injection of α-GalCer-loaded DCs, expected to be the most efficient delivery system for tumor lesions, should be tested with respect to inducing effective anti-tumor therapy.

Percutaneous Injection with [166]Holmium Chitosan Complex (Milican) for the Treatment of Small Hepatocellular Carcinoma

Holmium-166 ([166]Ho) is a product of the neutron activation of holmium-165 and is predominantly a high-energy β-emitter ($E_{max} = 1.84$ MeV) with radiotherapeutic properties appropriate for ablation therapy. It also emits γ-ray photons (81 keV, 6.2%) detectable by scintillation imaging. Its relatively short half-life (26.8 hours) and proper mean penetration depth (2.2 mm) permit effective treatment without

isolation, and with a low risk of radiation hazard. Microspheres loaded with radioactive [166]Ho have been investigated in several preclinical studies and have been shown to be potentially useful agents for internal radiation therapy for hepatic tumors (61, 62).

A recent Phase IIb clinical trial of the percutaneous [166]Ho/chitosan complex ([166]Ho/CHICO, Milican, Dong Wha Pharmaceutical Co., Seoul, Korea) injection (PHI) evaluated the long-term therapeutic efficacy and safety of PHI in patients with tumors up to 3 cm (63). Two months after PHI, complete tumor necrosis was achieved in 31 of 40 patients (77.5%) with HCC lesions 3 cm or less and in 11 of 12 patients (91.7%) with HCC up to 2 cm. Tumors recurred in 28 patients during the long-term follow-up period, of which 24 recurred at another intrahepatic site. The 1-year and 2-year cumulative local recurrence rates were 18.5% and 34.9%, respectively. The survival rates at 1, 2 and 3 years were 87.2%, 71.8% and 65.3%, respectively. Transient bone marrow depression was a serious adverse event requiring hospitalization in two patients. A Phase III randomized active control trial is clearly warranted for further testing of the safety and efficacy of PHI among a larger study population.

NEW APPROACHES IN IMAGING TUMOR RESPONSE AFTER TREATMENT: IMAGING BIOMARKERS

Part of the successful and expanding use of locoregional therapies may be attributed to advances in radiological imaging, which has altered patients' management by offering not only early tumor detection but also effective monitoring of tumor response to therapy and, more recently, individual early tailoring of therapy. The goal of any locoregional therapy is the complete ablation of any given tumor with minimal damage to the surrounding liver parenchyma. While cure is the ultimate clinical endpoint for any form of medical treatment, valid endpoints of measuring response to therapy with locoregional therapies or increased patient survival are also considered favorable endpoints for any locoregional therapy.

Anatomic imaging using one- or two-dimensional measurements to characterize cancers has been used traditionally to make these measurements in all aspects of cancer patient management, from diagnosis and staging to monitoring response to therapy and disease progression. However, these measurements made by using standard anatomic imaging techniques are often inadequate for monitoring the effects of drugs or locoregional therapies that do not cause tumor shrinkage or for cancers that progress slowly or metastasize diffusely. Newer imaging modalities including volumetric and functional imaging show high promise as the basis for characterizing better biomarkers of cancer. Unlike anatomic imaging, functional imaging methods display biochemical and physiologic underlying cancer abnormalities rather than the structural consequences of these abnormalities.

Diffusion-weighted MR Imaging

Diffusion magnetic resonance (MR) imaging is based on motion of water molecules across cell membranes. Viable tumors are highly cellular, with intact cell membranes, which restrict the motion of water molecules, therefore producing low apparent diffusion coefficient (ADC) values. Diffusion-weighted MR imaging has been lately successfully used to assess response to radiation or systemic chemotherapy in patients with brain and breast cancers (64, 65).

A recent study showed that diffusion-weighted imaging may provide functional information on a molecular level regarding the viability of tumor cells after TACE, allowing therefore a cellular-based assessment of treatment response after TACE (66). Viable tumor cells have intact cellular membrane, which restricts the movement of water molecules, resulting in low ADC values. With cellular death, cellular membranes eventually are disrupted, and diffusion of water molecules is no longer restricted, leading to an increase of the ADC values within the necrotic tumor tissue, therefore confirming the presence and invasion of extracellular water inside the cancerous cells. In this study, there was a statistically significant decrease in the ADC value of treated HCC after TACE, compared to values before treatment (p = 0.026). In this way, the ADC value measurements allow for the accurate quantification of the degree of cellular damage, and this may prove especially valuable after TACE because of the wide spectrum of histopathologic findings, ranging between complete necrosis and the absence of necrosis (Figure 17.4A–C) (67–69).

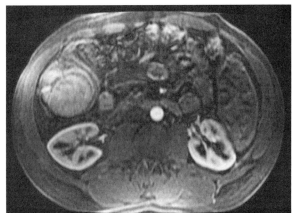

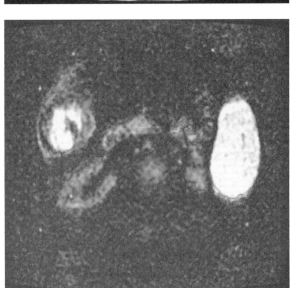

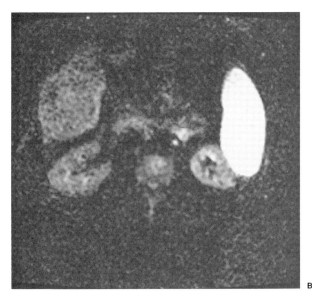

FIGURE 17.4.   Contrast-enhanced T1-weighted axial MR image (A) and diffusion-weighted MR image (B) before treatment with TACE in a 65-year-old man with unresectable HCC. Diffusion-weighted MR image (C) after treatment with TACE. Note the increased hyperintensity inside the tumor, representing increased water mobility across the destroyed cancer cell membranes.

Dynamic Contrast-enhanced MR Imaging

Dynamic contrast-enhanced magnetic resonance imaging (DCE-MRI) is a noninvasive imaging technique that can be used to measure properties of tissue microvasculature. DCE-MRI is sensitive to differences in blood volume and vascular permeability that can be associated with tumor angiogenesis and is a promising method as well as a potential biomarker for characterizing tumor response to antiangiogenic treatment. Tumor microvascular measurements by DCE-MRI have been found to correlate with prognostic factors such as tumor grade, microvessel density (MVD) and VEGF expression and with recurrence and survival outcomes. Moreover, DCE-MRI changes measured during treatment have been shown to correlate with outcome, suggesting a role for DCE-MRI as a predictive marker (70, 71).

The accuracy of DCE-MRI relies on the ability to model the pharmacokinetics of an injected tracer, or contrast agent, using the signal intensity changes on sequential MRIs. Signal intensity changes can be rapid immediately after (small molecular weight) contrast injection, and thus the temporal sampling rate is important. However, increasing the temporal sampling rate of MRI has direct consequences on critical image characteristics such as spatial resolution, signal-to-noise ratio and the volume of anatomy covered. The trade-offs between temporal resolution and spatial resolution for DCE-MRI are not clear, and cannot easily be tested. MVD measured histopathologically gives a partial picture of the tissue microvasculature but does not reflect its functional properties, including permeability, that contribute to the DCE-MRI measurement.

Prospective clinical trials are needed with primary aims designed to test standardized DCE-MRI methods for both data acquisition and marker quantification. A prospective evaluation of DCE-MRI will require a change in the way imaging is performed as part of clinical trials. Like those for tissue- and serum-based biomarkers, the assay methods used to measure the imaging biomarker are critical. The technical specification for measuring an imaging biomarker must be well defined, and adherence to these specifications must be monitored. Changes will be required to the clinical practice culture to emphasize the importance of maintaining technical standards for quantitative imaging. Consistent methodologies for contrast administration are also needed to ensure the reproducibility of DCE-MRI measurements.

^{18}Fluoro-deoxy-glucose Positron-emission Tomography

Formal recognition by the NCI of the potential importance of positron-emission tomography [^{18}Fluoro-deoxy-glucose (FDG) PET] in monitoring treatment response has been motivated by the search for biomarkers as endpoints of clinical trials to help reduce the growing cost of obtaining new drug approvals (72). The hope is that ^{18}F-FDG PET may be a true surrogate that can be used in place of classic endpoints in evaluating treatment response. A second motivation has been dissatisfaction with the classic anatomy-based imaging methods for assessing treatment response, such as the World Health Organization (WHO) criteria or the Response Evaluation Criteria in Solid Tumors (RECIST) (73). A third motivation has been the growing evidence in major cancers that ^{18}F-FDG uptake represents important underlying cancer biology and is a predictor of aggressive tumor behavior and treatment response (72).

Recently available combined PET/CT systems provide accurately fused functional and morphologic datasets in a single session. The potential advantage of PET/CT compared with PET alone is based on lesion detection and localization as demonstrated in initial evaluations. PET/CT imaging possibly proved more accurate when evaluating the ablative zone for residual tumor than image analysis based on morphologic data alone. The advantages of fused PET/CT datasets over PET alone and CT alone are related to accurate localization of focally increased glucose metabolism in terms of therapeutic planning in an area of residual tumor, offering guidance of subsequent interventional procedures to these areas of viable tumor cells. PET/CT therefore may be expected to play a distinctive role in follow-up of patients undergoing RFA of liver lesions for the detection of residual tumor and local tumor recurrence (74).

There are significant challenges to developing robust imaging biomarkers. It requires both establishing that one or more functional measurements sensitively capture the biology of interest, and defining a measurement method that can be applied in a reliable and standardized fashion. Specification of the measurement method can be complex, as in the case of MRI, in which many experimental variables influence the signal. Thus, optimizing and subsequently standardizing functional imaging measurement methods present a significant task.

CONCLUSION

Current research continues to unravel the mechanisms of hepatocarcinogenesis and identify key relevant molecular targets for therapeutic intervention. Because of the heterogeneity and aggressive nature of the disease, we should at first focus on testing the promising agents and regimens in patients with relatively preserved hepatic function and good performance status. However, because underlying cirrhosis with impaired hepatic function is a common finding in patients with HCC, we should consequently assess the safety and toxicity profiles of the newer agents and regimens in such populations. Furthermore, because most hepatic tumors show extensive heterogeneity and display different sensitivities toward therapy, it is important to tailor our medical treatment to the biology of the tumor. To reach this level of sophistication in the therapeutic approach to liver cancer, we need mechanistic information regarding the underlying oncogenic processes and highly specific inhibitors. While searching for these oncogenic processes and testing new targeted agents for liver cancer, it is also imperative to incorporate imaging studies and surrogate markers in an attempt to understand the potential mechanisms of action of these new agents.

REFERENCES

1. Folkman J. Tumor angiogenesis: Therapeutic implications. N Engl J Med, 1971; 285(21): 1182–1186.
2. Yancopoulos GD, Davis S, Gale NW, et al. Vascular-specific growth factors and blood vessel formation. Nature, 2000; 407(6801): 242.
3. Bergers G and Benjamin LE. Tumorigenesis and the angiogenic switch. Nat Rev Cancer, 2003 Jun; 3(6): 401–410.
4. Ferrara N and Henzel WJ. Pituitary follicular cells secrete a novel heparin-binding growth factor specific for vascular endothelial cells. Biochem Biophys Res Commun, 1989; 161(2): 851–858.
5. Hicklin DJ and Ellis LM. Role of the vascular endothelial growth factor pathway in tumor growth and angiogenesis. J Clin Oncol, 2005; 23(5): 1011–1027.
6. Dvorak HF, Brown LF, Detmar M, et al. Vascular permeability factor/vascular endothelial growth factor, microvascular hyperpermeability, and angiogenesis. Am J Pathol, 1995; 146(5): 1029–1039.
7. Ferrara N. Vascular endothelial growth factor: Molecular and biological aspects. Curr Top Microbiol Immunol, 1999; 237: 1–30.
8. Schneider BP and Miller KD. Angiogenesis of breast cancer. J Clin Oncol, 2005 Mar 10; 23(8): 1782–90.
9. Fan F, Wey JS, McCarty MF, et al. Expression and function of vascular endothelial growth factor receptor-1 on human colorectal cancer cells. Oncogene, 2005; 24(16): 2647–2653.
10. Jeng KS, Sheen IS, Wang YC, et al. Prognostic significance of preoperative circulating vascular endothelial growth factor messenger RNA expression in resectable hepatocellular carcinoma: A prospective study. World J Gastroenterol, 2004; 10(5): 643–648.
11. Ng IO, Poon RT, Lee JM, et al. Microvessel density, vascular endothelial growth factor and its receptors Flt-1 and Flk-1/KDR in hepatocellular carcinoma. Am J Clin Pathol, 2001; 116(6): 838–845.
12. Yao DF, Wu XH, Zhu Y, et al. Quantitative analysis of vascular endothelial growth factor, microvascular density and their clinicopathologic features in human hepatocellular carcinoma. Hepatobiliary Pancreat Dis Int, 2005; 4(2): 220–6.
13. Takahashi Y, Kitadai Y, Bucana CD, et al. Expression of vascular endothelial growth factor and its receptor, KDR, correlates with vascularity, metastasis, and proliferation of human colon cancer. Cancer Res, 1995; 55(18): 3964–3968.
14. Kim KJ, Li B, Winer J, et al. Inhibition of vascular endothelial growth factor-induced angiogenesis suppresses tumour growth in vivo. Nature, 1993; 362(6423): 841–844.
15. Levene AP, Singh G, Palmieri C. Therapeutic monoclonal antibodies in oncology. J R Soc Med, 2005 Apr 1; 98(4): 146–152.
16. Wang Y, Fei D, Vanderlaan M, et al. Biological activity of bevacizumab, a humanized anti-VEGF antibody in vitro. Angiogenesis, 2004; 7(4): 335.
17. Motl S. Bevacizumab in combination chemotherapy for colorectal and other cancers. Am J Health Syst Pharm, 2005; 62(10): 1021–1032.
18. Food and Drug Administration. Bevacizumab FDA approval letter, 2004.
19. Cobleigh MA, Langmuir VK, Sledge GW, et al. A phase I/II dose-escalation trial of bevacizumab in previously treated metastatic breast cancer. Semin Oncol, 2003; 30(5 Suppl 16): 117–124.
20. Yang JC, Haworth L, Sherry RM, et al. A randomized trial of bevacizumab, an anti-vascular endothelial growth factor antibody, for metastatic renal cancer. N Engl J Med, 2003; 349(5): 427–434.
21. Kerr C. Bevacizumab and chemotherapy improves survival in NSCLC. The Lancet Oncology, 2005; 6(5): 266.
22. Petrylak DP. The current role of chemotherapy in metastatic hormone-refractory prostate cancer. Urology, 2005; 65(5, Supplement 1): 3.
23. Rini BI. VEGF-targeted therapy in metastatic renal cell carcinoma. Oncologist, 2005; 10(3): 191–197.
24. Imaeda T, Kanematsu M, Mochizuki R, et al. Extracapsular invasion of small hepatocellular carcinoma: MR and CT findings. J Comput Assist Tomogr, 1994; 18(5): 755–760.
25. Yamaguchi R, Yano H, Iemura A, et al. Expression of vascular endothelial growth factor in human hepatocellular carcinoma. Hepatology, 1998; 28(1): 68–77.
26. Graepler F, Gregor M, and Lauer UM. [Anti-angiogenic therapy for gastrointestinal tumours]. Z Gastroenterol, 2005; 43(3): 317–329.
27. Schwartz JD SM, Lehrer D, Coll D, et al. Bevacizumab in hepatocellular carcinoma (HCC) in patients without

metastasis and without invasion of the portal vein. Orlando, Florida: American Society of Clinical Oncology, Gastrointestinal Cancers Symposium; 2005.

28. Britten C, Finn RS, Gomes AS, et al. A pilot study of IV bevacizumab in hepatocellular carcinoma patients undergoing chemoembolization. ASCO Annual Meeting; Orlando, Florida, 2005.

29. Geschwind JF. Bevacizumab and Chemoembolization in Treating Patients with Liver Cancer that Cannot Be Removed by Surgery. National Cancer Institute Clinical Trials Database, accessed 30/12/2007.

30. Britten C. A Phase II Study of rhuMAb VEGF (Bevacizumab) in Patients with Hepatocellular Carcinoma Receiving Chemoembolization. National Cancer Institute (NCI) Database, accessed 30/12/2007.

31. Peck-Radosavljevic M. Transarterial Chemoembolisation Plus Bevacizumab for Treatment of Hepatocellular Carcinoma. National Cancer Institute (NCI), 2007.

32. Warburg O. On the origin of cancer cells. Science, 1956; 123(3191): 309–314.

33. Rempel A, Mathupala SP, Griffin CA, et al. Glucose catabolism in cancer cells: Amplification of the gene encoding type II hexokinase. Cancer Res, 1996; 56(11): 2468–2471.

34. Shinohara Y, Ichihara J, Terada H. Remarkably enhanced expression of the type II hexokinase in rat hepatoma cell line AH130. FEBS Letters, 1991; 291(1): 55.

35. Yasuda S, Arii S, Mori A, et al. Hexokinase II and VEGF expression in liver tumors: correlation with hypoxia-inducible factor-1[alpha] and its significance. J Hepatol, 2004; 40(1): 117.

36. Gwak G-Y, Yoon J-H, Kim KM, et al. Hypoxia stimulates proliferation of human hepatoma cells through the induction of hexokinase II expression. J Hepatol, 2005; 42(3): 358.

37. Geschwind J-FH, Ko YH, Torbenson MS, et al. Novel therapy for lver cancer: Direct intraarterial injection of a potent inhibitor of ATP production. Cancer Res, 2002; 62(14): 3909–3913.

38. Geschwind JF, Georgiades CS, Ko YH, et al. Recently elucidated energy catabolism pathways provide opportunities for novel treatments in hepatocellular carcinoma. Expert Rev Anticancer Ther, 2004; 449–457.

39. Foubister V. Energy blocker to treat liver cancer. Drug Discovery Today, 2002; 7(18): 934.

40. Leist M, Single B, Castoldi AF, et al. Intracellular adenosine triphosphate (ATP) concentration: A switch in the decision between apoptosis and necrosis. J Exp Med, 1997; 185(8): 1481–1486.

41. Xu R-H, Pelicano H, Zhou Y, et al. Inhibition of glycolysis in cancer cells: A novel strategy to overcome drug resistance associated with mitochondrial respiratory defect and hypoxia. Cancer Res, 2005; 65(2): 613–621.

42. Llovet JM, Bruix J. Systematic review of randomized trials for unresectable hepatocellular carcinoma: Chemoembolization improves survival. Hepatology, 2003; 37(2): 429–442.

43. Lo CM, Ngan H, Tso WK, et al. Randomized controlled trial of transarterial lipiodol chemoembolization for unresectable hepatocellular carcinoma. Hepatology, 2002; 35(5): 1164–1171.

44. Yang ZF, Poon RT, To J, et al. The potential role of hypoxia inducible factor-1{alpha} in tumor progression after hypoxia and chemotherapy in hepatocellular carcinoma. Cancer Res, 2004; 64(15): 5496–5503.

45. Tanaka H, Yamamoto M, Hashimoto N, et al. hypoxia-independent overexpression of hypoxia-inducible factor-{alpha} as an early change in mouse hepatocarcinogenesis. Cancer Res, 2006; 66(23): 11263–11270.

46. Kim YI, Chung JW, Park JH, et al. Intraarterial gene delivery in rabbit hepatic tumors: Transfection with non-viral vector by using iodized oil emulsion. Radiology, 2006; 240(3): 771–777.

47. Iwasaki Y, Ueda M, Yamada T, et al. Gene therapy of liver tumors with human liver-specific nanoparticles. Cancer Gene Ther, 2006; 14(1): 74–81.

48. Reid T, Warren R, Kirn D. Intravascular adenoviral agents in cancer patients: Lessons from clinical trials. Cancer Gene Ther, 2002; 9(12): 979–986.

49. Reid T, Galanis E, Abbruzzese J, et al. Intra-arterial administration of a replication-selective adenovirus (dl1520) in patients with colorectal carcinoma metastatic to the liver: A phase I trial. Gene Ther, 2001; 8(21): 1618–1626.

50. Qian J, Truebenbach J, Graepler F, et al. Application of poly-lactide-co-glycolide-microspheres in the transarterial chemoembolization in an animal model of hepatocellular carcinoma. World J Gastroenterol, 2003; 9(1): 94–98.

51. Constantin M, Fundueanu G, Bortolotti F, et al. Preparation and characterisation of poly(vinyl alcohol)/cyclodextrin microspheres as matrix for inclusion and separation of drugs. Int J Pharm, 2004; 285(1–2): 87–96.

52. Vallee JN, Lo D, Guillevin R, et al. In vitro study of the compatibility of tris-acryl gelatin microspheres with various chemotherapeutic agents. J Vasc Interv Radiol, 2003; 14(5): 621–628.

53. Fujiwara K, Hayakawa K, Nagata Y, et al. Experimental embolization of rabbit renal arteries to compare the effects of poly L-lactic acid microspheres with and without epirubicin release against intraarterial injection of epirubicin. Cardiovasc Intervent Radiol, 2000; 23(3): 218–223.

54. Varela M, Real MI, Burrel M, et al. Chemoembolization of hepatocellular carcinoma with drug eluting beads: Efficacy and doxorubicin pharmacokinetics. J Hepatol, 2007; 46(3): 474–481.

55. Lewis AL, Gonzalez MV, Lloyd AW, et al. DC bead: In vitro characterization of a drug-delivery device for transarterial chemoembolization. J Vasc Interv Radiol, 2006; 17(2): 335–342.

56. Taylor RR, Tang Y, Gonzalez MV, et al. Irinotecan drug eluting beads for use in chemoembolization: In vitro and in vivo evaluation of drug release properties. Eur J Pharma Sci, 2007; 30(1): 7–14.

57. Hong K, Khwaja A, Liapi E, et al. New intra-arterial drug delivery system for the treatment of liver cancer: Preclinical assessment in a rabbit model of liver cancer. Clin Cancer Res, 2006; 12(8): 2563–2567.

58. Taylor RR, Tang Y, Gonzalez MV, et al. Irinotecan drug eluting beads for use in chemoembolization: In vitro and in vivo evaluation of drug release properties. Eur J Pharma Sci, 2007; 30(1): 7–14.

59. Aliberti C, Tilli M, Benea G, et al. Trans-arterial chemoembolization (TACE) of liver metastases from

colorectal cancer using irinotecan-eluting beads: Preliminary results. Anticancer Res, 2006; 26(5B): 3793–3795.

60. Yukio I, Kouichirou T, Shigeru G, et al. A phase I study of autologous dendritic cell-based immunotherapy for patients with unresectable primary liver cancer. Cancer Immunology, Immunotherapy, 2003; 52(3): 155–161.

61. Nijsen JF, Zonnenberg BA, Woittiez JR, et al. Holmium-166 poly lactic acid microspheres applicable for intra-arterial radionuclide therapy of hepatic malignancies: effects of preparation and neutron activation techniques. Eur J Nucl Med, 1999; 26(7): 699–704.

62. Mumper RJ, Yun Ryo U, Jay M. Neutron-activated holmium-166-poly (L-lactic acid) microspheres: A potential agent for the internal radiation therapy of hepatic tumors. J Nucl Med, 1991; 32(11): 2139–2143.

63. Kim JK, Han K-H, Lee JT, et al. Long-term clinical outcome of Phase IIb clinical trial of percutaneous injection with holmium-166/chitosan complex (Milican) for the treatment of small hepatocellular carcinoma. Clin Cancer Res, 2006; 12(2): 543–548.

64. Hamstra DA, Chenevert TL, Moffat BA, et al. Evaluation of the functional diffusion map as an early biomarker of time-to-progression and overall survival in high-grade glioma. PNAS, 2005; 102(46): 16759–16764.

65. Hall DE, Moffat BA, Stojanovska J, et al. Therapeutic efficacy of DTI-015 using diffusion magnetic resonance imaging as an early surrogate marker. Clin Cancer Res, 2004; 10(23): 7852–7859.

66. Kamel IR, Bluemke DA, Eng J, et al. The role of functional MR imaging in the assessment of tumor response after chemoembolization in patients with hepatocellular carcinoma. J Vasc Interv Radiol, 2006; 17(3): 505–512.

67. Sakurai M, Okamura J, Kuroda C. Transcatheter chemoembolization effective for treating hepatocellular carcinoma. A histopathologic study. Cancer, 1984; 54(3): 387–392.

68. Di Carlo V, Ferrari G, Castoldi R, et al. Pre-operative chemoembolization of hepatocellular carcinoma in cirrhotic patients. Hepatogastroenterology, 1998; 45(24): 1950–1954.

69. Paye F, Jagot P, Vilgrain V, et al. Preoperative chemoembolization of hepatocellular carcinoma: A comparative study. Arch Surg, 1998; 133(7): 767–772.

70. Miller JC, Pien HH, Sahani D, et al. Imaging angiogenesis: Applications and potential for drug development. J Natl Cancer Inst, 2005; 97(3): 172–187.

71. Padhani AR, Leach MO. Antivascular cancer treatments: Functional assessments by dynamic contrast-enhanced magnetic resonance imaging. Abdominal Imaging, 2005; 30(3): 325–342.

72. Juweid ME, Cheson BD. Positron-emission tomography and assessment of cancer therapy. N Engl J Med, 2006; 354(5): 496–507.

73. Jaffe CC. Measures of response: RECIST, WHO, and new alternatives. J Clin Oncol, 2006; 24(20): 3245–3251.

74. Patrick V, Gerald A, Hrvoje S, et al. Detection of residual tumor after radiofrequency ablation of liver metastasis with dual-modality PET/CT: Initial results. Eur Radiol, 2006; 16(1): 80–87.

Chapter 18

INTRAHEPATIC CHOLANGIOCARCINOMA

Christos S. Georgiades

Kelvin Hong

Jean-Francois H. Geschwind

EPIDEMIOLOGY

Intrahepatic cholangiocarcinoma (ICC) is primary liver cancer with cholangiocytic molecular and histopathologic characteristics located peripheral to the biliary ductal confluence. Cholangiocarcinomas, in general, represent only 15% of primary liver cancers (1), with ICC composing only about 15% of those. These numbers have contributed to the pervasive perception that ICC is a rare cancer, and compared with cancers that globally impact health care (i.e., colon, breast, lung cancers), indeed it is. However, an accelerated increase in incidence has recently been demonstrated, which, coupled with the very poor prognosis imparted by this cancer, has raised concerns. From 1975 to 2000, the age-adjusted incidence of ICC in the United States has increased from 0.32 per 100,000 to 0.85 per 100,000, or roughly an increase from 800 to 2800 newly diagnosed cases per year (2). More concerning is that this 165% increase in age-adjusted incidence (2, 3) is accelerating, with current estimates showing an annual percentage increase in incidence of 9.11% (2). Prognosis is almost universally poor, with little change in demonstrated survival over the past 25 years despite novel and more aggressive treatments. In 1975, the 1- and 5-year survival rates were 15.8% and 2.6% respectively. Twenty-five years later (2000) and despite sig-

nificant medical advances in cancer treatment 1-, 2- and 5-year survival rates have essentially remained stable, at 25%, 13% and 3.5% respectively (2, 3). Even for the few patients who are initially deemed resectable, post-operative 1-, 3- and 5-year survival is 58%, 33% and 33%, respectively (4, 5). Mortality from ICC is increasing slightly faster than the incidence, with an annual percentage change of +9.44%. This suggests that ICC is not only increasing in incidence but in virulence as well.

Advances in pathophysiology have been able to identify different subtypes of ICC. This is crucial as respective patient survival appears to be different. For example, mean survival for the regular type ICC is 16 months, whereas that of the intra-ductal papillary neoplasm of the liver (IPNL) ICC subtype is 47 months (6). As we better understand the behavior of ICC, we must try to define as best we can its subtype, location, physiologic and imaging behavior and, along with the patient's clinical status, explore all avenues of treatment.

The advent of non-surgical techniques in the treatment of ICC offers new hope in the form of percutaneous ablation (i.e., radiofrequency ablation [RFA]) or transarterial chemoembolization (TACE). Although mainly offered to patients with unresectable hepatocellular carcinoma (HCC) or certain secondary hepatic malignancies, TACE has recently been shown to extend the median survival of patients with mass-forming ICC. Reported median survival was 23 months in 17 TACE-treated patients in the series, with 2 of 17 becoming resectable after TACE (7). RFA has been shown effective in the treatment of HCC (and other small neoplasms such as lung cancers and renal cell cancers, provided they are sufficiently small and percutaneously accessible). For HCCs 3 cm or less, RFA is similar to resection in terms of recurrence or disease-free progression. Data on ICC are scarce due to the low incidence of disease; however, initial reports are encouraging, with reported 100% necrosis in accessible ICC that are 3 cm or less (8, 9). Whatever the subtype of ICC, most patients are unresectable at presentation, thus eliminating the only curative options, which are resection or transplantation. Chemotherapy and external radiation therapy have been ineffective (10), which highlights the importance of new treatment techniques such as TACE.

PATHOPHYSIOLOGY

The majority (approximately 70%) of cholangiocarcinomas occur at or, by the time of diagnosis, involve the biliary confluence and are thus termed **Klatskin-type neoplasms.** Another 10% to 15% involve the common hepatic/bile duct (CH/BD) alone, whereas the remaining 15% to 20% are of the intrahepatic type. Risk factors for cholangiocarcinoma are mainly conditions that result in chronic inflammation or chronic cholestasis (1, 11, 12). Table 18.1 tabulates these identified risk factors. Though initially the distinction between ICC and extrahepatic cholangiocarcinomas seemed arbitrary and based on anatomic location, recent evidence suggests that the ICC type is pathophysiologically and possibly genotypically different from the rest of cholangiocarcinomas. Phenotypically, primary non-stromal hepatic neoplasms can be hepatic, cholangitic or the rare mixed hepatic-cholangitic type. Genotypic aberrations (such as the *p53* mutation) have been documented in patients with ICC-complicated cirrhosis, suggesting ICC and HCC may arise from the same hepatic precursor cells (13). Mechanisms of multi-sep carcinogenesis implicate chronic infectious or inflammatory conditions (parasitosis or cirrhosis) that, via formation of carcinogens, result in DNA damage and biliary ductal epithelial prolifera-

TABLE 18.1 Risk Factors for Cholangiocarcinoma

	Risk Factor	Adjusted Odds Ratio	Reference
1	Cirrhosis	27.2	2, 11
2	Alcoholic liver disease	7.4	11
3	Hepatitis C infection	6.1	2, 11
4	HIV	5.9	11
5	Inflammatory bowel disease	2.3	1, 11
6	Diabetes mellitus	2.0	11
7	Primary sclerosing cholangitis		2
8	Hepatolithiasis		1, 2, 12
9	Thorotrast		1, 2
	Choledochal cysts		2
	Hepatitis B infection		2
	Liver fluke infestation (*Clonorchis sinensis* and *Opisthorchis viverrini*)		1, 11, 12

tion (1, 14–16). Non-inflammatory conditions, especially familial cholestatic diseases, have also been implicated in mutagenesis. These conditions are collectively termed **progressive familial intrahepatic cholestasis** (PFIC) and include primary biliary cirrhosis (PBC), primary sclerosis cholangitis (PSC) and autoimmune cholangitis/hepatitis (AICH) (17). Notwithstanding the above, the majority of patients have no risk factors at presentation. Recent studies have also indicated that ICCs are different from HCCs not only in the specific mutations necessary to cause neoplasia but also in their energy metabolism. Whereas HCCs appear to up-regulate hexokinase II (HKII) as a means to increase their energy production, ICCs show no such increase in HKII; rather they show preference in generating energy via the pentose phosphate pathway (18). Despite such recent advances in the genetics and energy metabolism pathways of ICCs, treatment options are still limited to surgery for the few surgical candidates or palliative biliary stenting or radiation therapy. The failure of these discoveries to yield effective chemical therapies has propelled minimally invasive techniques such as RFA or TACE to the forefront of treatment options.

DIAGNOSIS

Patients with ICC usually present with upper abdominal pain, weight loss and fatigue. Clinical investigation commonly uncovers elevated liver function tests

(LFTs). Alanine amino transferase (ALT) and aspartate aminotransferase (AST) are frequently abnormal at presentation. Hyperbilirubinemia is rarer because the peripheral nature of ICC causes only focal and minimal to no biliary ductal dilatation (19). Computed tomography (CT), magnetic resonance imaging (MRI) and ultrasonography (US) are equally sensitive in detecting the primary tumor; however, contrast-enhanced CT or MRI is required to determine resectability, treatment planning and response to treatment. Despite the fact that on gross pathology the tumor appears dense, fibrous and minimally necrotic, it tends to encircle vessels and other structures with minimal distortion (19). This is shown on Figure 18.1, in which vessels are noted crossing a large, solid ICC apparently uncompressed.

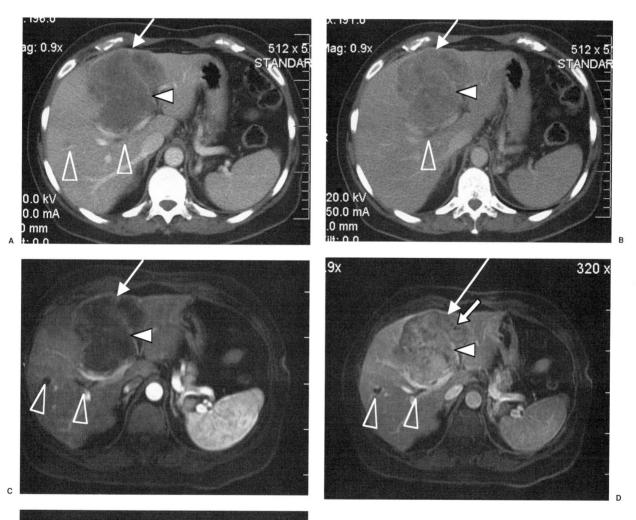

FIGURE 18.1.   Fifty-five-year-old woman presenting with 3-month duration of right upper quadrant dull pain moderately responsive to NSAIDs. Pain persistence led to a CT of the abdomen. CT findings led to a contrast-enhanced MRI. Arterial (A) and venous (B) phase CT of the liver show a 7 × 6 cm solid, well-defined, hypervascular mass distorting the capsule of the liver anteriorly (*arrow*). Similar findings are noted on the arterial (C) and venous (D) phases of the contrast-enhanced MRI of the liver. Even though this is a solid lesion, vessels (*arrowhead*) and bile ducts (*block arrow*, best discernible on late-phase contrast-enhanced MRI) are seen traversing it, not an uncommon finding in ICCs. Mild biliary ductal dilatation, a common finding in ICCs, is also noted (*open arrowheads*). T2-weighted MRI image of the same patient (E) shows increased signal throughout the tumor but low enough to exclude a hemangioma.

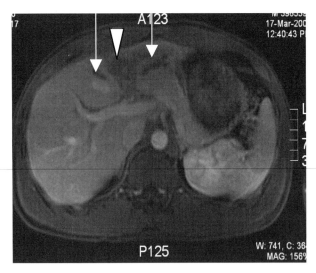

FIGURE 18.2. Fifty-eight-year-old man presenting with incidentally noted elevated total bilirubin. Axial, venous phase, contrast-enhanced MRI of liver shows a 4 × 2 cm, ill-defined, mildly enhancing mass in the left lobe of the liver (*arrowhead*). Biliary ductal dilatation is also noted peripheral to the mass (*arrows*). If bilirubin is greater than 4 mg/dl (as was the case here) and before TACE can be performed, a percutaneously placed biliary drain catheter is required in order to lower the bilirubin to below that level.

Fine-needle aspiration or core-needle biopsy is adequate for diagnosis. Surgical resection may reveal small intrabiliary stones or small bile abscesses, which explain the leukocytosis that patients frequently have on presentation. On imaging, there are two types of ICC, which correspond to two distinct pathologic subtypes. The first is a peripheral, mass-forming lesion as noted on Figures 18.1 and 18.4. This sub

type presents earlier due to volume-related symptoms. The second is the peripheral but infiltrating type, which spreads along Glisson's sheath. This subtype has a propensity to spread and metastasize earlier than the first but present symptomatically later. There is controversy on the usefulness of cancer markers for the diagnosis of ICC. One-third of patients will have a mildly elevated carcinoembryonic antigen (CEA) at time of presentation (19). Also, AFP may be elevated, especially in poorly differentiated cholangiocarcinomas, because both hepatocytes and cholangiocytes differentiate from the same progenitor cells. However, the incidence of elevated CEA and AFP in patients with ICC is too low to be of diagnostic significance or to be used for surveillance in a reliable manner.

TREATMENT

Liver transplantation or resection are the only accepted curative options for patients with ICC. However, most patients are not surgical candidates at time of presentation. For these, the only options are intra-arterial or percutaneous techniques, with the most popular (but still limited in numbers of patients receiving them) being RFA or TACE.

Radiofrequency Ablation

The use of RFA to treat inoperable ICC is a natural extension from the interventional radiologists' experience in treating HCC with percutaneous

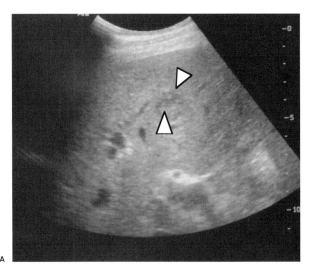

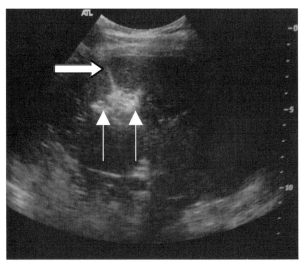

FIGURE 18.3. Sixty-five-year-old man with a small (2 × 1.5 cm) incidentally noted mass-forming cholangiocarcinoma (*arrowheads*, A). The shaft (*block arrow*) and open tines (*arrows*) of a 3-cm Boston Scientific RFA probe placed under US guidance are seen (B). The echogenic shadows around

the tines represent gas bubbles forming during ablation as temperatures reach up to 100°C. Because of these changes, the lesion is no longer visible, thus initial probe positioning is crucial for optimal ablation.

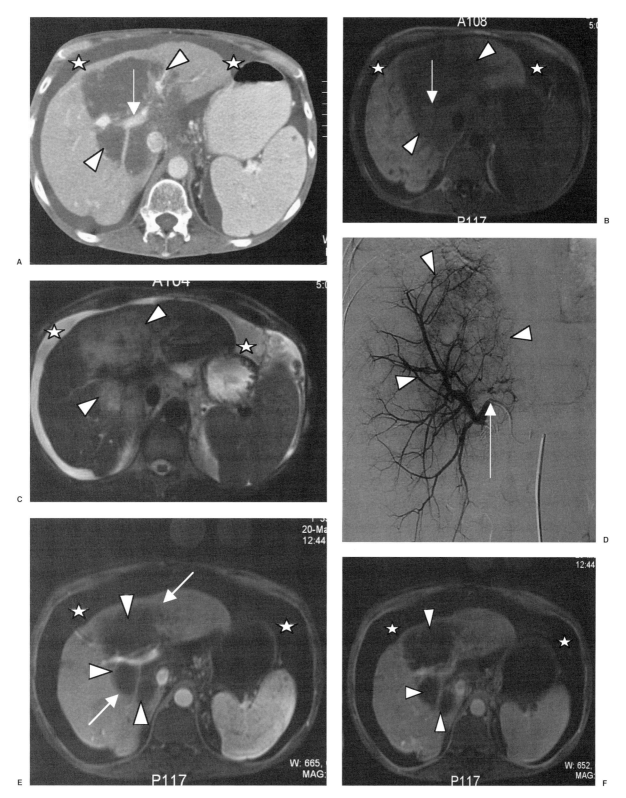

FIGURE 18.4. Sixty-eight-year-old man with history of liver cirrhosis presented with a large (9 × 8 cm) mass on his first surveillance CT. Patient admitted to many-month history of vague abdominal pain, but attributed it to his known ascites (*asterisk*). Axial contrast-enhanced, venous-phase CT of the liver (A) and a non-contrast-enhanced, T1-weighted MRI (B), show a solid, hypovascular mass (*arrowheads*) that, as is the case in the patient in Figure 18.1, allows vessels (*arrows*) to traverse it with minimal distortion. Again as in Figure 18.1, T2-weighted MRI shows increased signal throughout the tumor but again low enough to exclude a hemangioma (C). Digital subtraction, right hepatic arte-riogram using a microcatheter (*arrow*) reveal the hypervascular nature of this ICC (*arrowheads*) (D). Repeat contrast-enhanced MRI of the liver was obtained 3 weeks after TACE. Arterial (E) and venous (F) phase images reveal near-complete necrosis and cystic transformation (*arrowheads*) of the tumor with minimal shrinkage. A thin rim of enhancement (*arrows*) is seen, representing either residual tumor or a hypervascular fibrotic, inflammatory capsule commonly seen after TACE. When response to TACE is above 75% necrosis, as in this case, a repeat MRI is planned in 6 weeks. Additional TACE is offered only if an enlarging tumor is again noted. See Color Plate 20.

techniques. For HCC, tumor-free survival and over-all survival after RFA are strongly related to tumor size at time of treatment. In patients with tumor size of up to 2 cm, there was an 85% complete response rate defined as no enhancement on follow-up CT and no recurrence during the following 6 months (20). For lesions larger than 2 cm, the rate of treatment failure increases, with tumors up to 3 cm showing a 75% complete response rate (20). Tumor-free survival for HCC 3 cm or less is nearly identical for RFA vs. surgically treated patients. The 1-, 2-, 3- and 5-year survival rates for HCC lesions, 3 cm or less in diameter and Child-Pugh class A or B, were 94%, 86%, 68% and 40%, respectively (21). Although the response rate for larger HCC lesions (>3 cm in diameter) is expectedly lower than for those less than 3 cm, encouraging results were reported by Livraghi et al. (22). Complete or near-complete response (>90% necrosis) was reported in 79% of the treated lesions with a diameter of 4 cm. A vessel proximal to the lesion may act as a heat sink, as the blood carries away useful energy. This phenomenon may necessitate prolonged treatment or even limit treatment efficacy and it can be seen in all local ablative techniques that depend on heat to cause tissue necrosis (23). These results may not necessarily be extended to ICC; however, if RFA is technically feasible – that is, the ICC is mass-forming and not the infiltrating type, smaller than 4 cm and accessible percutaneously – in which case the efficacy of RFA for ICC should be comparable to that for HCC. Overall efficacy and survival may even be better as most patients with ICC do not suffer from advanced cirrhosis like their HCC counterparts.

Technique

RFA can be performed in most cases under conscious sedation and using any imaging modality that suits the operator best. Most commonly, US is used as it is faster and provides real-time probe-positioning feedback. CT fluoro- or even regular CT guidance can be used, and, occasionally MRI, assuming the probe is MRI compatible. The caveat is that whatever imaging modality is used for guidance, the lesion is visible. When a lesion is not visible under one of the aforementioned modalities, another should be used as there is no relationship between lesion detectability among modalities. Probe selection should be such that the ablated volume would cover the lesion plus an additional radius beyond it (up to 1 cm) to minimize chances of local recurrence. For example, a 2-cm lesion should be treated with at least a 3 cm probe. Larger or irregular lesions may require overlapping treatments for complete ablation. The actual ablation protocol depends on (1) the ablation technique (RFA, microwave coagulation, cryoablation); (2) the type of probe (Boston Scientific, RITA or Valleylab); and (3) the organ being ablated (lung vs. liver vs. bone vs. kidney). Manufacturers include specific protocols for each case with the generator. Patient preparation is uncomplicated and includes informed consent, 8-hour fasting status and antibiotics in some cases. Post-procedure care is directed toward patient comfort with adequate analgesia.

Follow-up

The most specific imaging modality for follow up is a positron emission tomography (PET)/CT, which becomes even more valuable if a positive baseline PET/CT exists. Care should be exercised not to obtain a PET scan too early as inflammatory changes may be confused with residual cancer. A 3-month delay after RFA is recommended, at which time any activity is likely residual cancer. For liver and kidney tumors that have been ablated, a dual-phase MRI or CT may be adequate in showing any residual tumor, and a 1-month wait period is usually adequate. Even if there is residual tumor, retreatment with the same ablative method should be attempted, assuming the residual tumor is accessible. No scientific study conclusively shows the maximal number or size of lesions that can be effectively treated with RFA in the liver; however, a consensus exists in the literature of a maximum of six lesions of 3 cm or less each. Each patient should have his or her own specific planning treatment, however, as these are only guidelines.

TACE

TACE has been found to prolong the life expectancy of patients with unresectable HCC and has become the mainstay of treatment for such patients (24–26). Experience with treating cholangiocarcinoma with TACE has been very limited because most cholangiocarcinomas are infiltrating, centrally located and without clearly defined blood supply on angiograms. As experience with HCC grew and it became clear that well-defined, mass-forming, vascular lesions respond well to TACE, attention was turned to treating ICC, which happen to be, by and large, mass forming and well defined. Initial results with TACE for ICC are encouraging. Burger et al. (7) have shown that TACE-treated patients with mass-forming ICC have a median survival of 23 months, which is longer than the published survival of historical controls of 6 to 8 months. Additionally, 2 of 17 of their patients have become surgical candidates and underwent resection after TACE-related shrinkage of the ICC. The basic principles that make TACE possible and effective are the same irrespective of the type of neoplasm. Normal liver is supplied both by the portal vein (70%) and hepatic artery (30%), whereas hepatic neoplasms receive their blood supply nearly exclusively from the hepatic artery. This limits injury to liver parenchyma while tumors "see" a chemotherapy concentration of up to 100-fold compared with systemic chemotherapy. This increase in chemotherapy concentration, coupled with the prolongation of the chemotherapy residence time within the tumor (as a result of the embolization part of TACE) results in the greater tumoricidal effect and lesser systemic toxicity than experienced with systemic chemotherapy.

Technique

The technique is identical to that of TACE for HCC; however, ICC patients tend to have biliary obstruction, which, if total bilirubin is above 4 mg/dl, may necessitate insertion of a percutaneous biliary drain catheter to reduce bilirubin to below that level. This, however, compromises the sphincter of Oddi and results in colonization of the biliary epithelium with gut flora. The resulting TACE-related (and RFA) injury to the biliary epithelium, which is supplied by the hepatic arterial system, carries a high risk (30%–70%) of abscess formation. Bowel preparation and periprocedural broad-spectrum intravenous antibiotics mitigate but do not eliminate this risk. In cases in which the patient has a biliary tube or has had a hepatojejunostomy, informed consent should include the risk of liver abscess formation. Patients are brought in as outpatients 2 hours prior to procedure and premedicated with diphenylhydramine (50 mg, IV), dexamethasone (10 mg, IV), cefazolin (1 g, IV), metronidazole (500 mg, IV) and ondansetron (24 mg, IV). Access to the common femoral artery is obtained, after which diagnostic visceral and selective hepatic arteriography is performed to better delineate the

blood supply to the tumor and document portal vein patency. After hypervascular tumor blush is identified, the branch vessels feeding the tumor are selectively catheterized. These branches represent either the left or right hepatic artery, or both.

Chemotherapy mixture used at our institution is a cocktail of 100 mg cisplatin (Bristol Myers Squibb, Princeton, NJ), 50 mg doxorubicin hydrocloride (Adriamycin; Pharmacia-Upjohn/Kalamazoo, MI) and 10 mg mitomycin C (Bedford Laboratories, Bedford, OH). These chemotherapeutic agents are emulsified in a 1:1 to 2:1 ratio with ethiodol (Savage Laboratories, Melville, NY) and injected under fluoroscopy, ensuring no reflux. Then, 5 to 10 ml of intra-arterial lidocaine is injected for immediate analgesia and to diminish post-procedural symptoms. This is followed by 1 to 4 ml of 150- to 250-μm embosphere particles (Biosphere Medical, Boston, MA) in order to reduce the arterial inflow to the tumor without however, effecting, complete embolization of the artery. The decision to use embospheres is made based on evidence obtained in animals that a higher concentration of chemotherapy could be achieved within the tumor (abstract SIR 2003). After each procedure, the patient is admitted for overnight observation, placed on patient-controlled analgesia, cefazolin (500 mg, IV q8hr × 3d), metronidazole (500 mg, IV q8 × 3), ondansetron (8 mg, IC q12hr prn) and dexamethasone (8 mg, IV q8). A non-contrast-enhanced CT scan of the liver is obtained immediately prior to discharge. Evidence of the technical success of the procedure was demonstrated by focal deposition of the mixture of lipiodol (and therefore chemotherapeutic agent) in the tumor and relative sparing of the non-tumorous liver parenchyma.

Patient Follow-up

Patients are followed on a routine basis at 6-week intervals with contrast-enhanced dual-phase MRI, LFTs and a clinic visit. Indication for subsequent TACE treatment depends on overall clinical status/ Eastern Cooperative Oncology Group (ECOG) performance status, liver function reserve and tumor viability. Twenty-five percent to seventy-five percent necrosis after TACE prompts additional TACE treatment and the 6-week follow-up cycle restarts. Conversely, treatment was terminated when tumor necrosis was estimated to be greater than 75% on MRI, or there was a decline in clinical status or a score of

TABLE 18.2 Contraindications to TACE

1.	ECOG 3	
2	Child-Pugh C	
3	Significant encephalopathy	
4	Significant extrahepatic disease	
5	Total bilirubin >4 mg/dl	Relative contraindication (can be treated with biliary drainage)
6	Compromised sphincter of Oddi (HJ or biliary tube)	Relative contraindication

Child-Pugh C. Contraindications to TACE are shown on Table 18.2.

CONCLUSION

ICCs, for a multitude of reasons, are receiving more attention from the medical community than they have in the past. First, new understanding regarding the pathophysiology of these neoplasms has shown that ICCs are, indeed, different types of neoplasms from their more common central infiltrating counterparts. They have been shown to have different risk factors, genotype and phenotype as well as different clinical course. Second, the incidence of ICC has been on the rise and this increase is expected to continue (2). Third, the advent of still-palliative but effective treatment methods such as RFA and TACE has provided viable treatment alternatives to patients who, thus far, if unresectable, were offered no effective treatment options. In order to ensure these patients receive the maximum benefit from these novel treatments, careful patient selection, preparation and stringent follow-up and treatment protocols are required. A multidisciplinary team (oncology, gastrointestinal surgery, transplant surgery, diagnostic and interventional radiology) should review the patient's status and come to a consensus on the optimum course of treatment. Once RFA or TACE is decided upon, patient counseling, proper informed consent and preparation (premedication, hydration, etc.) are crucial in maximizing the chances of effective treatment and minimizing potential complications. Treatment technique should be followed stringently, and immediate post-operative care should aim to minimize complications and maximize patient comfort. Follow-up with LFTs and contrast-enhanced MRI is required to determine the patient's response to treatment and need for retreatment. It is also crucial for the multidisciplinary team to remain engaged in the patient's care, as a small minority of these patients will become resectable after TACE, thus offering an opportunity for cure for an otherwise uniformly fatal disease.

REFERENCES

1. Parkin DM, Ohshima H, Srivatanakul P, et al. Cholangiocarcinoma: Epidemiology, mechanisms of carcinogenesis and prevention. Cancer Epidemiol Biomarkers Prev, 1993 Nov–Dec; 2(6): 537–544.
2. Shaib Y and El-Serag HB. The epidemiology of cholangiocarcinoma. Semin Liver Dis, 2004 May; 24(2): 115–125.
3. Shaib YH, Davila JA, McGlynn K, et al. Rising incidence of intrahepatic cholangiocarcinoma in the United States: A true increase? J Hepatol, 2004 Mar; 40(3): 472–477.
4. Patel T. Increasing incidence and mortality of primary intrahepatic cholangiocarcinoma in the United States. Hepatology, 2001 Jun; 33(6): 1353–1357.
5. Uenishi T, Hirohashi K, Kubo S, et al. Clinicopathological factors predicting outcome after resection of mass-forming intrahepatic cholangiocarcinoma. Br J Surg, 2001 Jul; 88(7): 969–974.
6. Yeh TS, Tseng JH, Chen TC, et al. Characterization of intrahepatic cholangiocarcinoma of the intraductal growth-type and its precursor lesions. Hepatology, 2005 Sep; 42(3): 657–664.
7. Burger I, Hong K, Schulick R, et al. Transcatheter arterial chemoembolization in unresectable cholangiocarcinoma – initial experience in a single institution. J Vasc Interv Radiol, 2005; 16: 353–361
8. Zgodzinski W and Espat NJ. Radiofrequency ablation for incidentally identified primary intrahepatic cholangiocarcinoma. World J Gastroenterol, 2005 Sep 7; 11(33): 5239–5240.
9. Chiou YY, Hwang JI, Chou YH, et al. Percutaneous ultrasound-guided radiofrequency ablation of intrahepatic cholangiocarcinoma. Kaohsiung J Med Sci, 2005 Jul; 21(7): 304–309.
10. Khan SA, Thomas HC, Davidson BR, et al. Cholangiocarcinoma. Lancet, 2005 Oct 8; 366(9493): 1303–1314.
11. Shaib YH, El-Serag HB, Davila JA, et al. Risk factors of intrahepatic cholangiocarcinoma in the United States: A case-control study. Gastroenterology, 2005 Mar; 128(3): 620–626.
12. Okuda K, Nakanuma Y, and Miyazaki M. Cholangiocarcinoma: Recent progress. Part 1: Epidemiology and etiology. J Gastroenterol Hepatol, 2002 Oct; 17(10): 1049–1055.
13. Nomoto K, Tsuneyama K, Cheng C, et al. Intrahepatic cholangiocarcinoma arising in cirrhotic liver frequently expressed p63-positive basal/stem-cell phenotype. Pathol Res Pract, 2006; 202(2): 71–76.
14. Kuroki T, Tajima Y, and Kanematsu T. Hepatolithiasis and intrahepatic cholangiocarcinoma: Carcinogenesis based on molecular mechanisms. J Hepatobiliary Pancreat Surg, 2005; 12(6): 463–466.
15. Kassahun WT, Gunl B, Tannapfel A, et al. Alpha(1)- and

beta(2)-adrenoceptors in the human liver with mass-forming intrahepatic cholangiocarcinoma: Density and coupling to adenylate cyclase and phospholipase C. Naunyn Schmiedebergs Arch Pharmacol, 2005 Nov; 372(3): 171–181. Epub 2005 Nov 15.

16. Obama K, Ura K, Satoh S, et al. Up-regulation of PSF2, a member of the GINS multiprotein complex, in intrahepatic cholangiocarcinoma. Oncol Rep, 2005 Sep; 14(3): 701–706.

17. Poupon R, Chazouilleres O, and Poupon RE. Chronic cholestatic diseases. J Hepatol, 2000; 32(1 Suppl): 129–140.

18. Lee JD, Yang WI, Park YN, et al. Different glucose uptake and glycolytic mechanisms between hepatocellular carcinoma and intrahepatic mass-forming cholangiocarcinoma with increased (18)F-FDG uptake. J Nucl Med, 2005 Oct; 46(10): 1753–1759.

19. Miin-Fu Chen. Peripheral cholangiocarcinoma (cholangiocellular carcinoma): Clinical features, diagnosis and treatment. J Gastroenterol Hepatol, 1999; 14: 1144–1148.

20. Sironi S, Livraghi T, Meloni F, et al. Small hepatocellular carcinoma treated with percutaneous RF ablation: MR imaging follow-up. AJR Am J Roentgenol, 1999; 173: 1225–1229.

21. Rossi S, Di Stassi M, Buscarini E, et al. Percutaneous RF interstitial thermal ablation in the treatment of hepatic cancer. AJR Am J Roentgenol, 1996; 167: 759–768.

22. Livraghi T, Goldberg SN, Lazzaroni S, et al. Hepatocellular carcinoma: Radio frequency ablation of medium and large lesions. Radiology, 2000; 214: 761–768.

23. Shuichi O. Local ablation therapy for hepatocellular carcinoma. Semin Liver Dis, 1999; 19: 323–327.

24. Llovet JM, Real MI, Montana X, et al. Arterial embolization or chemoembolization versus symptomatic treatment in patients with unresectable hepatocellular carcinoma: A randomized controlled trial. Lancet, 2002; 359: 1734–1739.

25. Camma C, Schepis F, Orlando A, et al. Transarterial chemoembolization for unresectable hepatocellular carcinoma: Meta-analysis of randomized controlled trials. Radiology, 2002; 224: 47–54.

26. Lo CM, Ngan H, Tso WK, et al. Randomized control trial of transarterial lipiodol chemoembolization for unresectable hepatocellular carcinoma. Hepatology, 2002; 35(5): 1164–1171.

Liver Metastases

Chapter 19

MEDICAL MANAGEMENT OF COLORECTAL LIVER METASTASIS

Wen W. Ma

Wells A. Messersmith

Colorectal cancer is the third most common cancer in the United States, and about 145,000 new cases are expected each year (1). Approximately 15% to 30% of all colorectal cancer patients have synchronous liver metastases at initial diagnosis, and up to 60% will develop hepatic metastases at some point during their disease course (2–4). Therefore, liver metastases from colorectal cancer are a common oncologic problem. Because management of patients with colorectal liver metastases frequently involves medical oncologists, surgical oncologists, interventional radiologists and other specialists, a multidisciplinary setting is optimal.

Palliative chemotherapy remains the mainstay of treatment for patients with widely metastatic colorectal cancer, and survival has increased significantly with the introduction of novel agents. However, 5-year survival of such patients remains anecdotal. Advances in surgical and interventional techniques, however, have made cure a possibility for some colorectal cancer patients with liver-only metastases. Patients with initially resectable colorectal liver metastases have achieved impressive 5-year survival rates of 30% to 70% following metastatectomy (4–6). Unfortunately, only 20% to 30% of patients with colorectal liver metastases are candidates for resection at initial presentation (7, 8).

Preoperative or neoadjuvant chemotherapy may improve the rate of successful metastatectomy, limit the extent of hepatectomy and improve postoperative recovery in this group of patients. In patients with unresectable liver metastases, neoadjuvant chemotherapy can potentially render previously unresectable liver metastases amenable to surgery. The 5-year survival rate of those who subsequently undergo hepatic metastatectomy has been reported to be 20% to 40% (9). Unfortunately, 70% to 80% of these patients develop recurrence, with more than one-half in the liver.

Chemotherapy remains an important treatment modality in the management of colorectal liver-only metastases. Whether post-metastatectomy adjuvant chemotherapy can reduce the risk of liver recurrence remains unproven. Chemotherapy can be administered systemically or regionally to the liver through the hepatic artery. To fully understand the role of chemotherapy in these settings, this chapter will discuss the active systemic chemotherapeutic agents in metastatic colorectal cancer.

SYSTEMIC CHEMOTHERAPY IN ADVANCED COLORECTAL CANCER

According to a meta-analysis of 13 randomized trials, systemic chemotherapy prolongs survival and improves quality of life for patients with advanced colorectal cancers when compared to best supportive care alone (10). Fluorouracil forms the core of systemic therapy for advanced colorectal cancers, and the survival of these patients roughly doubled around the turn of the century with the advent of new chemotherapeutic agents such as oxaliplatin, irinotecan, cetuximab and bevacizumab (Figure 19.1) (11). The regimens that combine these active agents proved to be superior to single-agent fluorouracil regimens (Table 19.1).

CYTOTOXIC AGENTS

Fluoropyrimidines

Fluorouracil is a fluorinated pyrimidine that is metabolized to fluorodeoxyuridine monophosphate (FdUMP), which inhibits thymidylate synthase and interferes with pyrimidine nucleotide synthesis. Fluorouracil is usually co-administered with leucovorin, a reduced folate that stabilizes the binding of FdUMP to thymidylate synthase and enhances the inhibition of DNA synthesis.

Fluorouracil and leucovorin are administered intravenously in a variety of dosing schedules. In the loading bolus schedules, fluorouracil and leucovorin are administered in bolus daily for 5 consecutive days and repeated every 28 days (Mayo regimen) (13); in the weekly bolus schedule, fluorouracil and leucovorin are given weekly for 6 of every 8 weeks (Roswell Park regimen) (14). For the infusional regimen, leucovorin and fluorouracil are administered in bolus followed by 22 hours of fluorouracil infusion through a central venous catheter on days 1 and 2 and repeated every 2 weeks (15).

These regimens differ in their toxicities, which may partly guide their use clinically. The bolus regimens tend to be associated with bone marrow suppression, mucostomatitis and diarrhea, whereas palmar-plantar erythrodysesthesia ("hand-foot syndrome") is more common in the infusional regimen. Central venous access is required for the infusional regimen. The difference in quality of life and cost between the infusional and bolus regimens is marginal, and the infusional method seems to be

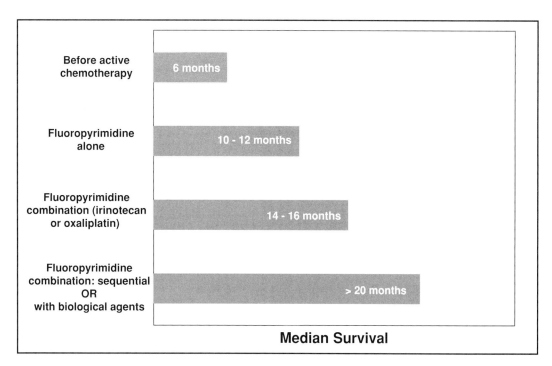

FIGURE 19.1.   Median survival of patients with advanced colorectal cancer.

TABLE 19.1 Systemic Chemotherapeutic Agents for Metastatic Colorectal Cancer

Active Agents	
Cytotoxic Agents	**Biological Agents**
Fluorouracil	Bevacizumab
Capecitabine	Cetuximab
Oxaliplatin	
Irinotecan	
Commonly Used Regimens	
5-FU/LV	bolus (Mayo)
	– bolus fluorouracil daily for 5 days; repeat every 28 days weekly bolus (Roswell Park)
	– bolus weekly fluorouracil for 6 out of 8 weeks infusional (de Gramont)
	– bolus fluorouracil followed by continuous infusion over 22 hours for 2 days; repeat every 2 weeks
IFL (Saltz)	Irinotecan on day 1 and bolus fluorouracil followed by continuous infusion for 2 days; repeat every 2 weeks
FOLFOX	Oxaliplatin and infusional fluorouracil; repeat every 2 weeks
FOLFIRI	Irinotecan and infusional fluorouracil; repeat every 2 weeks
CAPOX	Oxaliplatin and capecitabine for 14 days; repeat every 3 weeks
Bevacizumab with fluorouracil-containing regimen	Bevacizumab with 5-FU/LV, IFL, FOLFIRI or FOLFOX
Cetuximab and irinotecan	Cetuximab weekly and irinotecan

marginally more effective than the bolus approach (16–20).

Oral Fluoropyrimidines

Oral fluoropyrimidines offer an attractive alternative to intravenous fluorouracil without the inconvenience of intravenous access and associated complications. However, intestinal absorption of oral fluorouracil is erratic due to variable concentration of dihydropyrimidine dehydrogenase, a major catabolic enzyme of the fluoropyrimidine, in the gastrointestinal mucosa (21). Oral fluorouracil prodrugs and coadministration of oral fluorouracil with dihydropyrimidine dehydrogenase inhibitors were developed to overcome this problem.

Capecitabine, a fluoropyrimidine carbamate, is an oral prodrug that undergoes enzymatic conversion in the liver to fluorouracil (22). The side-effect profile is similar to that of the infusional fluorouracil regimen, with hand-foot syndrome as the predominant toxicity. However, stomatitis, nausea, vomiting, bone marrow suppression and diarrhea are observed as well. Capecitabine was superior to the daily bolus "Mayo" regimen in terms of objective response rate (about 25% vs. 16% respectively) in two randomized control trials but did not confer significant survival advantage (median survival: about 12.9 vs. 12.8 months respectively) (23–25).

Another oral fluoropyrimidine with response and survival rates similar to intravenous fluorouracil was tegafur, another prodrug of fluorouracil, plus uracil, an inhibitor of dihydropyrimidine dehydrogenase (26, 27). The combination is usually administered together with oral leucovorin and is approved by regulatory agencies outside of the United States. S-1 is another fluorouracil-based oral combination drug that has mainly been developed in Asia (28–33).

Hence, oral fluoropyrimidines seem to be a safe and convenient alternative for patients with advanced or metastatic colorectal cancer (34). However, the benefit of oral fluoropyrimidines over the less toxic fluorouracil schedules, such as the weekly Roswell-Park and the infusional regimens, has not been demonstrated. The possibility of replacing intravenous fluorouracil in combination regimens with oral fluoropyrimidines is being explored in various clinical trials (35, 36). The cost-effectiveness of capecitabine monotherapy over the Mayo regimen remains controversial and is primarily attributed to the savings in hospital-related costs (37–40).

Irinotecan

Irinotecan (also known as CPT-11) is a semisynthetic derivative of the natural alkaloid camptotecin and exerts its cytotoxic effects by inhibiting topoisomerase I, which is necessary for the proper uncoiling of DNA for replication and transcription. The drug is hydrolyzed to its more potent active metabolite, SN38 or 7-ethy-10-hydroxycampthotecin, by carboxylesterase (41). Irinotecan and its metabolites interact with the DNA replication forks, leading to DNA fragmentation by stabilizing single-chain DNA breaks and subsequent cell death.

When compared to infusional fluorouracil or best supportive care, irinotecan showed single-agent activity in patients with advanced colorectal cancer who had previously received bolus fluorouracil, with improvement in median survival and quality of life (42, 43).

In first-line advanced colorectal cancer therapy, irinotecan improved median survival by about 2 months and almost doubled the response rate when combined with fluorouracil and leucovorin in two randomized trials (44, 45). In the North American trial, irinotecan added to weekly bolus-schedule fluorouracil (IFL) was compared to the bolus fluorouracil Mayo regimen and patients who received IFL had a longer median survival (14.8 vs. 12.6 mo., p = 0.04) and higher response rate (39% vs. 21%, p < 0.001; Figure 19.2). In the European trial, irinotecan combined with infusional fluorouracil (FOLFIRI) was compared to infusional fluorouracil regimens.

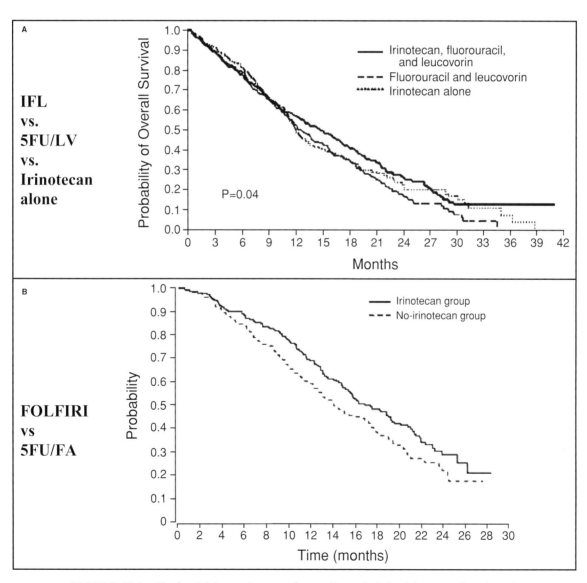

FIGURE 19.2. Kaplan-Meier estimates of overall survival for irinotecan-based regimens. [(A) *From* Saltz LB, Cox JV, Blanke C, et al. Irinotecan plus fluorouracil and leucovorin for metastatic colorectal cancer. Irinotecan Study Group. N Engl J Med 2000; 343(13): 905–914; (B) *from* Douillard JY, Cunningham D, Roth AD, et al. Irinotecan combined with fluorouracil compared with fluorouracil alone as first-line treatment for metastatic colorectal cancer: a multicentre randomised trial. Lancet 2000; 355(9209): 1041–1047; with permission.]

TABLE 19.2 Important Toxicities of Systemic Chemotherapy Agents Used in Colorectal Cancers

Fluorouracil	Mucostomatitis
Capecitabine	Diarrhea
	Bone marrow suppression
	Hand-foot syndrome
Irinotecan	Diarrhea
	Bone marrow suppression
	Nausea
	Vomiting
Oxaliplatin	Sensory neuropathy
	Cold-induced dysesthesias
	Electrolytes disturbance
	Bone marrow suppression
Cetuximab	Anaphylaxis (less common)
	Rash
	Diarrhea
Bevacizumab	Anaphylaxis (less common)
	Hypertension
	Proteinuria
	Wound dehiscence*
	Gastrointestinal perforation*
	Thromboembolic disease*
	Bleeding*

*Not statistically significant.

Similar efficacy was found in patients who received the FOLFIRI, with improvement of median survival from 4.4 to 6.7 months (p < 0.001) and response rate from 35% to 22% (p < 0.01).

The toxicity of irinotecan includes diarrhea, bone marrow suppression, nausea and vomiting, and correlates retrospectively with a polymorphism of uridine diphosphate glucuronosylytransferase isoform 1A1 (UGT1A1). SN38, the active metabolite, is cleared by UGT1A1 during glucuronidation in the liver. Reduced UGT1A1 activity increases SN38 level and is especially correlated with bone marrow suppression and gastrointestinal toxicities (46, 47). A FDA-approved clinical test for UGT1A1 poylmorphism is available, and individualizing irinotecan dosage based on patients' pharmacogenomic profile may eventually be clinically feasible (48) (Table 19.2).

Oxaliplatin

Oxaliplatin is a third-generation diaminocyclo-hexane-containing platinum compound that forms bulky DNA adducts and induces cellular apoptosis (49). Unlike previous generations of platinum compounds, oxaliplatin showed promising activity against human colorectal cell lines in preclinical studies. In clinical studies, oxaliplatin had limited single-agent efficacy but was highly synergistic with fluo-

ropyrimidines in first- and second-line therapy for metastatic colorectal cancers (50–52). One possible mechanism was down-regulation of thymidylate synthase by oxaliplatin (53–55).

In metastatic colorectal cancers, oxaliplatin can be administered with fluorouracil and leucovorin in different ways, with different dosages and method of administration, but it is generally referred to as the FOLFOX regimen. For example, oxaliplatin was combined with bolus fluorouracil followed by 46 hours of continuous infusion fluorouracil together with leucovorin in FOLFOX6; and with bolus followed by 22 hours of infusional fluorouracil and leucovorin for 2 consecutive days in FOLFOX4.

In second-line setting, patients with metastatic colorectal cancer who received FOLFOX following IFL failure had a better outcome in median time to progression and response rate compared with those who received bolus and infusional fluorouracil and leucovorin (56). In three first-line randomized trials, the oxaliplatin-containing regimens showed consistently better time to progression, response rate and overall survival than fluorouracil and leucovorin alone (57,58). In one study comparing FOLFOX4 with infusional fluorouracil, median progression-free survival was 9.0 vs. 6.2 months (p = 0.0003); response rate was 50.7% vs. 22.3% (p = 0.0001); and median survival was 16.2 vs. 14.7 months (p = 0.12) (59).

Oxaliplatin also has been administered with oral capecitabine. The combination proved to be safe in previously untreated metastatic colorectal cancer patients in various Phase II trials (35, 60–62). Two European trials demonstrated reasonable efficacy and acceptable toxicity in patients older than 70 years old, with response rate and median survival about 40% and 14 months respectively. However, the role of this convenient regimen in the first-line therapy of metastatic colorectal cancer has yet to be validated in randomized trials.

Side effects from oxaliplatin are quite distinct from cisplatin and carboplatin. Nephrotoxicity, ototoxicity and alopecia are less common than with first- and second-generation platinums (63–65). Approximately 15% of patients who receive oxaliplatin-based regimens, however, develop a unique neuropathy of grade 3 or 4 (indicating that activities of daily living are affected). There is an acute, reversible, transient and cold-induced paresthesia of hands, feet, oral or pharyngeal regions during or for a short time following infusion, and a cumulative, dose-dependent, longer-lasting peripheral dysesthesia following months of treatment that is usually reversible when the medication is stopped. There is also higher frequency of grade 3 and 4 neutropenia and diarrhea in oxaliplatin-containing regimens. Fortunately, the neuropathy reverses in more than 99% of patients to a level not interfering with activities of daily living within 18 months after oxaliplatin is discontinued (66).

Irinotecan and Oxaliplatin in First-line Therapy

When administered with infusional fluorouracil and leucovorin, both irinotecan (FOLFIRI) and oxaliplatin (FOLFOX) appear to be equally efficacious in patients with previously untreated metastatic colorectal cancer (67, 68). The choice for first-line therapy was then often guided by the regimens' side effects and institutional practice.

Oxaliplatin and irinotecan were compared in a multicenter trial (N9741) conducted in North America. Seven hundred and ninety-five patients with previously untreated metastatic colorectal cancer were randomized to receive the infusional fluorouracil regimen with oxaliplatin (FOLFOX), bolus fluorouracil with irinotecan (IFL) or irinotecan plus oxaliplatin (IROX) (69). Note that the irinotecan was administered with bolus 5-FU, which likely accounts for some of the study findings. Patients who received

FOLFOX had a superior outcome (median time to progression of 8.7 months, response rate of 45% and median survival time of 19.5 months) than those who received IFL (median time to progression of 6.9 months, response rate of 31% and median survival time of 15.0 months) and IROX. In this trial, most patients proceeded to second-line treatment after failure of the initial first-line therapy. It is important to note that some of these patients received the other active agent during second-line therapy, and oxaliplatin was not widely available in North America for the duration of the trial, which may explain in part the inferior outcome of patients who received IFL. The study further supports the superiority of infusional fluorouracil.

A European randomized trial provided direct evidence of comparable efficacy between irinotecan and oxaliplatin when administered with infusional fluorouracil as first-line therapy for patients with metastatic colorectal cancers (68). Overall response rate (31% vs. 34%), median time to progression (7 vs. 7 months) and overall survival (14 vs. 15 months) were not statistically different between the both groups (FOLFIRI vs. FOLFOX respectively) (Figure 19.3). Patients in the FOLFIRI arm reported more alopecia and gastrointestinal disturbances, whereas those in the FOLFOX arm experienced more neuropathy and thrombocytopenia.

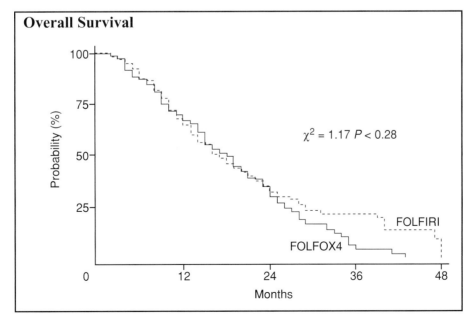

FIGURE 19.3. Kaplan-Meier estimates of overall survival and time to progression for FOLFIRI vs. FOLFOX4. (*From* Colucci G, Gebbia V, Paoletti G, et al: Phase III randomized trial of FOLFIRI versus FOLFOX4 in the treatment of advanced colorectal cancer: A multicenter study of the Gruppo Oncologico dell'Italia Meridionale. J Clin Oncol 2005; 23(22):4866–4875; with permission.)

TABLE 19.3 Efficacy of Systemic Chemotherapy for Metastatic Colorectal Cancer (First-line)

Regimens	Study	Design	N	ORR (%)	PFS (mo.)	Median Survival (mo.)	Reference
5-FU/Leucovorin (LV)		Meta-analysis	1219				(19)
	Bolus		612	14	**4-yr. OS:** 1%	11.3	
	Infusional		607	22	**4-yr. OS:** 2.6%	12.1	
IFL							
	Saltz, 2000	Phase III	231	39	7.0	14.8	(44)
	Goldberg, 2004		264	31	6.9	15.0	(69)
FOLFIRI							
	Tournigand, 2004*	Phase III	109	54	8.0	21.5[†]	(67)
	Colucci, 2005		164	31	7	14	(68)
	Souglakos, 2006		147	33.6	6.9	19.5	(71)
FOLFOX							
	de Gramont, 2000	Phase III	210	50.7	9.0	16.2	(59)
	Tournigand, 2004*		111	56	8.5	20.6[‡]	(67)
	Goldberg, 2004		267	45	8.7	19.5	(69)
	Colucci, 2005		172	34	7	15	(68)
FOLFOXIRI							
	Souglakos, 2006	Phase III	138	43	8.4	21.5	(71)
Capecitabine							
	Van Cutsem, 2004	Phase III		18.9	5.2	13.2	(25)
CAPOX							
	Cassidy	Phase II	96	55	7.7	19.5	(35)
	Feliu, 2006[§]		50	36	5.8	13.2	(62)

*Data from patients treated with first-line therapy.
[†]OS for patients treated with FOLFIRI initially.
[‡]OS for patients treated with FOLFOX initially.
[§]Study population ≥70 years of age.
ORR, Overall response rate (CR+PR); PFS, progression-free survival; OS, overall survival.

When administered with oral capecitabine, oxaliplatin (CapOx) and irinotecan (CapIri) seem to have comparable efficacy in patients with previously untreated colorectal cancers in small studies (70).

Efficacy of adding both oxaliplatin and irinotecan to first-line therapy in patients with previously untreated colorectal cancers was studied in a European trial randomizing patients to receive oxaliplatin, irinotecan, leucovorin and infusional fluorouracil (FOLFOXIRI) and FOLFIRI (71). No significant differences in overall survival, time to progression or response rate were observed. However, patients in the FOLFOXIRI arm were more likely to have resection of lung and liver metastases than the FOLFIRI arm (10% vs. 4%; p = 0.08), suggesting a potential role in managing patients with colorectal liver metastases. It is important to note that metastatectomy was not a primary endpoint in the trial. The FOLFOXIRI regimen was also more toxic than FOLFIRI, with higher frequency of alopecia, diarrhea and neuropathy.

The sequence in which patients with metastatic colorectal cancers are treated with FOLFOX and FOLFIRI does not seem to affect survival significantly (67). In fact, survival seemed to be maximized as long as these three active agents were available to all eligible patients with metastatic colorectal cancer during the course of treatment (Tables 19.3 and 19.4) (72).

BIOLOGICAL AGENTS

With advances in knowledge of the cellular and molecular events underlying oncogenesis, a new class of chemotherapeutic agents is impacting clinical management. Unlike conventional cytotoxic agents that frequently affect nonspecific processes such as cellular metabolism and DNA synthesis, these novel "biologic" agents disrupt cellular signaling pathways important for tumor growth, survival, differentiation, metastasis and angiogenesis. As such, they have distinct side-effect profiles that tend to be more

TABLE 19.4 Efficacy of Biologic-based Regimen Therapy for Metastatic Colorectal Cancer

Regimens	Study	Design	N	ORR (%)	PFS (mo.)	Median Survival (mo.)	Reference
First-line *First-line*							
Bevacizumab + IFL							
	Hurwitz, 2004	Phase III	402	44.8	10.6	20.3	73
Second-line *Second-line*							
Bevacizumab + FOLFOX4							
	Giantonio, 2005	Phase III	290	–	7.4	12.5	74
Cetuximab							
	Saltz, 2004	Phase II	57	9	1.4	6.4	75
	Cunningham, 2004	Phase III	111	10.8	1.5	6.9	76
Cetuximab + irinotecan							
	Saltz, 2001	Phase II	121	17	2.8		77
	Cunningham, 2004	Phase III	218	22.9	4.1	8.6	76

ORR, Overall response rate (CR+PR); PFS, progression-free survival.

tolerable. Thus far, targeting epidermal growth factor receptor (EGFR) and angiogenesis pathways have yielded promising results in the treatment of patients with metastatic colorectal cancer.

Cetuximab and Epidermal Growth Factor Receptor

EGFR, or Her-1, is a transmembrane receptor tyrosine kinase that belongs to the erbB, or Her, receptor family. Upon binding with a ligand such as epidermal growth factor (EGF) or transforming growth factor (TGF-α), EGFR pairs with another EGFR receptor (homodimerization) or another member of the erbB family (heterodimerization). Dimerization leads to receptor autophosphorylation and activation of intracellular signaling pathways that regulate cellular growth, survival, migration, adhesion and differentiation (Figure 19.4). The receptor was found to be abnormally activated in many epithelial malignancies, including colorectal cancer (78, 79).

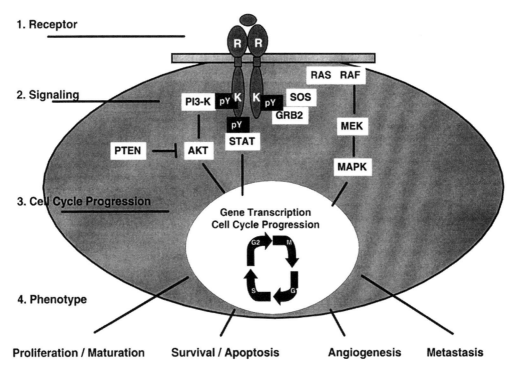

FIGURE 19.4.   EGF signaling pathway. (*From* Baselga J: Targeting the epidermal growth factor receptor: A clinical reality. J Clin Oncol 2001; 19(18 Suppl):41S–44S; with permission.)

EGFR became a target of interest in colorectal cancer therapy when expression or up-regulation of the EGFR gene was found in 60% to 80% of cases (81–84). Overexpression of EGFR in colorectal cancer was also associated with poorer prognosis (85, 86). Inhibition of EGFR can be achieved by targeting the extracellular domain with monoclonal antibodies or the intracellular tyrosine kinase with small molecule inhibitors (87).

Cetuximab is a chimeric murine/human immunoglobulin G1 (IgG1) monoclonal antibody highly specific for EGFR and has a higher affinity than EGF and TGF-α, thereby blocking the ligand-dependent autophosphorylation of the receptor. Although preclinical studies showed primarily cytostatic single-agent activity, cetuximab plus irinotecan was highly synergistic in irinotecan-refractory colorectal cancer xenografts when tumor growth would have continued with respective agents alone (88–90).

Cetuximab was the first of its class to be approved by the Food and Drug Administration in the United States (FDA) for treatment of colorectal cancer in patients who had failed previous chemotherapy. The response rates for cetuximab alone and cetuximab plus irinotecan were 9% and 17% respectively in two nonrandomized trials involving colorectal cancer patients previously treated with an irinotecan-based regimen (75, 77). In a multi-institutional randomized study, 329 patients with metastatic colorectal cancer who progressed on irinotecan-based regimen were randomized to receive either cetuximab plus irinotecan or cetuximab monotherapy (76). The patients receiving cetuximab plus irinotecan had a better response rate (22.9% vs. 10.8%; p = 0.007) and median time to progression (4.1 vs. 1.5 months; p < 0.001) than cetuximab monotherapy, although median survival rates were not significantly different (8.6 vs. 6.9 months; p = 0.48). The combination of cetuximab plus oxaliplatin-based regimen (FOLFOX) in irinotecan-refractory metastatic colorectal cancer appeared to be safe when examined in a multi-institutional randomized trial. The efficacy of this combination is actively being explored (91).

The side effects of cetuximab were fairly well tolerated. In the trials, about 75% of patients developed a mild acneiform-like rash, of which 12% was grade 3. About 3% of patients developed hypersensitivity infusional reactions when receiving therapy. The development of rash to anti-EGFR therapy seemed to correlate with objective response, but this relationship needs to be better defined in a properly designed clinical study (92).

In previous cetuximab trials, only patients with EGFR expression by immunohistochemical stain were eligible due to preclinical evidence suggesting predictive value of EGFR expression for cetuximab efficacy. This led to the initial approval of cetuximab therapy for patients with EGFR-expressing colorectal cancer by the FDA. However, the degree of EGFR expression seems to be unrelated to response, and patients with EGFR-negative colorectal cancers have responded to cetuximab as well (93,94). Hence, EGFR expression by the contemporary immunohistochemical analysis techniques does not seem to predict cetuximab response, and patients with EGFR-negative colorectal cancer should not be excluded from cetuximab-based therapy.

On the horizon, panitumumab, a fully humanized monoclonal antibody targeting EGFR, is undergoing evaluation in clinical trials and theoretically decreases the problem of hypersensitivity to murine proteins. In a multicenter Phase III randomized trial in patients with previously treated metastatic colorectal cancer, patients who received panitumumab and best supportive care reported a partial response rate of 8%. About 90% of the patients experienced the acneiform rash. Hypersensitivity infusion reaction to panitumumab was also lower that that reported for the chimeric cetuximab (95). Panitumumab has the advantage of bi-weekly administration, which correlates nicely with infusional 5-FU regimens. A decision regarding FDA approval is expected shortly.

Bevacizumab and Angiogenesis

Angiogenesis delivers essential nutrients and oxygen for sustained growth and metastasis in tumors and presents a rational target in cancer therapy (96). These tumor-induced blood vessels are often structurally and functionally abnormal, impairing the effective delivery of chemotherapeutic agents to the cancer (97). The abnormal process is thought to be driven by an imbalance of pro- and antiangiogenic factors, and disrupting the process by neutralizing vascular endothelial growth factor (VEGF), a key ligand for angiogenesis, has been a focus in colorectal cancer therapy (98).

Bevacizumab is a humanized recombinant monoclonal antibody that binds VEGF and inhibits ligand-dependent angiogenesis. The drug's efficacy was demonstrated in two randomized controlled trials,

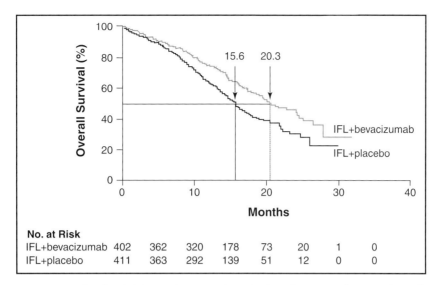

FIGURE 19.5. Kaplan-Meier estimates of survival with IFL with or without beva-cizumab. (*From* Hurwitz H, Fehrenbacher L, Novotny W, et al. Bevacizumab plus irinote-can, fluorouracil, and leucovorin for metastatic colorectal cancer. N Engl J Med. 2004; 350(23): 2335–2342; with permission.)

which led to approval by the FDA for use with any intravenous fluorouracil-containing regimen in first-line metastatic colorectal cancer therapy (99). Several mechanisms have been speculated to explain the activity of bevacizumab and other antiangiogenic agents, including starving the tumor of essential nutrients and oxygen by inhibition of formation of tumor vasculature, and improving the delivery of chemotherapeutic agents by normalizing the tumor vasculature and decreasing interstitial pressures in tumors.

In a small randomized Phase II trial, 104 patients were randomized to receive weekly bolus fluorouracil and leucovorin (5-FU/LV; control arm), bevacizumab 5 mg/kg or 10 mg/kg plus 5-FU/LV ("low-dose" and "high-dose" bevacizumab arms respectively; 100). Compared with the control arm, patients in both bevacizumab arms had better response rate (control: 17%; low dose: 40%; high dose: 24%), longer median time to progression (5.2, 9.0 and 7.2 months respectively) and longer median survival (13.8, 21.5 and 16.1 months respectively). Interestingly, the low-dose bevacizumab arm seemed to be superior to the high-dose arm, which was partly attributed to some imbalance in randomization resulting in more patients with poor prognostic factors in the latter group. The dose of 5 mg/kg for bevacizumab was thus chosen for the subsequent Phase III trial. Bleeding (gastrointestinal and epistaxis), hypertension, thrombosis and protein-uria were more frequent in the bevacizumab arms.

In the interim, IFL became the standard first-line therapy for metastatic colorectal cancer in United States (see earlier discussion). As such, the subsequent Phase III trial used IFL as the control regimen and 813 patients with previously untreated metastatic colorectal cancer were randomized to IFL plus placebo, IFL plus bevacizumab 5 mg/kg and 5-FU/LV plus bevacizumab 5 mg/kg (73). The 5-FU/LV/bevacizumab arm was discontinued during a planned interim analysis when the data monitoring committee found the addition of bevacizumab to IFL had an acceptable safety profile. The intention-to-treat analysis showed a superior median survival for the IFL plus bevacizumab arm compared to control (20.3 vs. 15.6 months, p < 0.001) (Figure 19.5). The study arm also had a better response rate (44.8% vs. 34.8%, p = 0.004) and median duration of response (10.4 vs. 7.1 months, p = 0.001). Reversible hypertension and proteinuria were more frequent in the study arm. Other rare but serious adverse events included thrombotic events, gastrointestinal perforation (1.5% of the patients in the bevacizumab arm) and wound dehiscence.

The role of bevacizumab with oxaliplatin-based regimen for second-line therapy for patients with metastatic colorectal cancer was studied in a randomized Phase III study (E3200). (74, 101) In the study, patients were randomly assigned to FOLFOX4 alone or FOLFOX4 plus high dose bevacizumab (10 mg/kg). Preliminary analysis of 829 patients showed superior median survival in the bevacizumab plus FOLFOX4 arm. Dose reduction of bevacizumab to 5 mg/kg was allowed in the study for hypertension, bleeding, thrombosis, proteinuria and abnormal liver tests. About 56% of 240 patients in the FOLFOX4 plus bevacizumab arm had bevacizumab dose reduction and the overall survival was not statistically different from the group without dose reduction (102).

Despite the clear role of bevacizumab with intravenous fluorouracil-based regimens in first- and second-line therapy for patients with metastatic colorectal cancer, more clinical questions still need to be clarified, such as efficacy of continuing bevacizumab into second-line therapy and synergism with oral fluoropyrimidines. Studies addressing the combination of bevacizumab and cetuximab are ongoing.

NEOADJUVANT CHEMOTHERAPY FOR COLORECTAL LIVER METASTASIS

Modern chemotherapy has not only improved the survival of patients with metastatic colorectal cancer, but also the associated tumor shrinkage has rendered some metastatic disease patients as surgically resectable. As described in previous sections, response rate has tripled with the introduction of new systemic chemotherapeutic agents. When administered appropriately in a multi-disciplinary setting, contemporary systemic chemotherapy offers the potential for cure in selected patients with metastatic disease when combined with surgery and interventional techniques.

Neoadjuvant or preoperative chemotherapy also offers the opportunity to evaluate the biology of the colorectal cancer and facilitate the choice of the most appropriate postoperative chemotherapy regimen. In addition, micro-metastatic disease can be treated earlier with a neoadjuvant approach instead of delaying systemic chemotherapy therapy until after recovery from metastatectomy (9). The use of hepatic arterial chemotherapy in unresectable colorectal liver metastases is discussed in other chapters.

Choice of Neoadjuvant Chemotherapy Regimen

The potential of systemic chemotherapy in improving the surgical management of colorectal liver metastases was reported in a number of case series and prompted many investigators to examine the benefit of neoadjuvant chemotherapy more systematically (115). A large percentage of the studies employed oxaliplatin-containing regimens (Table 19.5).

Bismuth et al. have reported their experience with neoadjuvant therapy (103, 105). This retrospective study reviewed the management of 701 patients with unresectable colorectal liver metastases treated with preoperative chronomodulated intravenous fluorouracil, folinic acid and oxaliplatin. The criteria for resectability were not predefined, and the general considerations were tumor size, location, multinodularity and extrahepatic disease. About 13.6% of these patients responded and underwent curative-intent resection. The patients received a mean of 10.6 months of neoadjuvant chemotherapy. The 5-year survival rate from the start of neoadjuvant chemotherapy in patients who underwent resection was about 39%, and 46% developed recurrence.

In a series of 151 patients presented with unresectable colorectal liver metastases treated with the combination of fluorouracil, leucovorin and oxaliplatin, 59% of patients had more than 50% shrinkage in their metastases, 51% underwent curative intent surgery and 38% achieved complete resection of live metastases (104). The 5-year survival rate for the patients who underwent curative-intent resection was 28%. The criteria for unresectability were defined as more than four liver metastases, greater than 5 cm diameter, tumor location, percentage of liver involvement and invasion of intrahepatic vasculature. Seventy-two percent of patients who had complete resection relapsed within a median time of 12 months, with most recurrences in the liver. Relapse rate of those who underwent curative-intent resection was 79%.

The benefit of irinotecan and oxaliplatin regimens in patients with initially unresectable colorectal metastases was examined in a secondary analysis of the Phase III Intergroup trial N9741 involving 795 patients with metastatic colorectal cancer (69, 106). It is important to note that N9741 was not originally designed to study the benefit of systemic chemotherapy on the survival of patients with unresectable colorectal liver metastases after secondary metastatectomy. The authors reviewed 450 patients who could potentially benefit from surgical metastatectomy, and 24 patients (5%) underwent curative resection of metastatic disease. Twenty of the twenty-four (92%) resected patients received an oxaliplatin-based regimen. About 70% of the resected patients relapsed and most recurred in the resected organ. The median survival for resected patients was about 42.4 months.

A prospective Phase II trial examined the efficacy of neoadjuvant high-dose fluorouracil and folinic acid in 53 initially unresectable colorectal metastases

TABLE 19.5 Evidence for Neoadjuvant Systemic Chemotherapy in Unresectable Colorectal Liver Metastases

Design	Study	No.	Regimens	ORR (%)	% Curative-intent Metastatectomy	OS (5-yr.)/ Median Survival	RecurR (%)	Reference
Retrospective	Bismuth, 1996	330	**5FU/Lv/oxaliplatin (Chrono)**	–	16	40%/–	46	103
	Giacchetti, 1999	151	**5FU/LV/oxaliplatin**	59	51	50%/48 mo.	79	104
	Adam, 2001	701	**5FU/Lv/oxaliplatin (Chrono)**	–	14	39%/–	–	105
Retrospective analysis of phase III trial	Goldberg, 2004 Delaunoit, 2005	450	IFL FOLFOX4 IROX	67	5	4-yr.: 37%/42 mo.	–	69, 106
Secondary analysis of 2 phase II trials	Masi, 2006	74	**FOLFOXIRI**	72	26	–/37 mo.	42	107
Phase II	Wein, 2001	53	**Infusional 5FU**	41	17	–/17 mo.	–	108
	Gaspar, 2003 (abstract)	22	**FOLFOX4**	50	45	–/–	–	109
	Alberts, 2005	42	**FOLFOX4**	60	40	–/26 mo.	73	110
	Pozzo, 2004	40	**Irinotecan/5FU/FA**	48	33	–/–	–	111
	Quenet, 2004 (abstract)	25	**FOLFIRINOX**	72	56	–/–	–	112
	De La Camara, 2004 (abstract)	22	**FOLFOXIRI**	–	50	–/–	–	113
Pilot data	Gruenberger, 2006	9	**CAPOX + bevacizumab**	–	88	–/–	–	114

ORR, overall response rate (CR+PR) in patients who received neoadjuvant chemotherapy; OS, overall survival of patients who underwent curative-intent metastatectomy; RecurR, recurrence rate (% of resected patients); Chrono, chronomodulated; FOLFOIRINOX, irinotecan/oxaliplatin/5FU/LV.

233

(108). Response rate with the regimen was 41%, and 17% of the patients receiving the chemotherapy underwent curative intent resection. The median survival of the patients who had secondary metastatectomy was 17 months, with a median follow-up of 41 months. Criteria for unresectability included distant metastases involving more than one organ, distant diffuse bilateral involvement in a single organ and close vicinity of metastases or local recurrence to central vessels, bile ducts or other structures making curative resection impossible. Each patient was evaluated by two experienced liver surgeons.

The efficacy of neoadjuvant oxaliplatin-based regimen (FOLFOX4) was evaluated in a North Central Cancer Treatment Group (NCCTG) Phase II study involving 42 assessable patients with unresectable liver-only colorectal metastases (110). Resectability of the hepatic metastases was evaluated by a liver surgeon and was based on the distribution of multiple lesions or the proximity of large lesions adjacent to major vessels that would preclude a tumor-free margin resection. Response occurred in 60% of patients receiving neoadjuvant therapy, and 40% underwent curative-intent resection. A median of 10 cycles, or 5 months, of treatment was administered and the median survival was 26 months.

A European Phase II trial evaluated the efficacy of neoadjuvant IFL on the resection rate and survival of patients with initially unresectable colorectal liver metastases (111). Resectability of the metastases was determined by a team consisting of a hepatobiliary surgeon, an oncologist and a radiologist based on the tumor location, number of metastases, size of lesion, liver reserve after resection and presence of extra-hepatic disease. Response rate to the regimen was 48% and 32.5% of the patients underwent curative-intent hepatic resection following the chemotherapy. All patients were alive at a median follow-up of 19 months and the median time to progression was 14.3 months.

The high response rates of oxaliplatin- and irinotecan-containing regimens prompted investigators to examine the efficacy of chemotherapy containing both highly active agents. FOLFOXIRI was evaluated in a Phase I/II and subsequent Phase II trials involving 74 patients with initially unresectable metastases (116, 117). The primary sites of metastatic disease were liver (81%), lung (26%) and abdomen (36%). The regimen achieved an impressive response rate of 72% and a median survival of 26 months. However, surgical metastatectomy was not part of these two prospective studies, and a secondary analysis examined the outcome of patients with initially unresectable metastases who receive FOLFOX-FIRI followed by metastatectomy with curative intent (107). Thirty patients (41%) of the 53 patients who responded to the chemotherapy were considered for surgical resection. Eventually, 26% (of 74) underwent metastatectomy, and median survival was 36.8 months, compared with 22.2 months among the other 34 chemotherapy-responsive patients who did not undergo resection.

The efficacy of chemotherapy containing both oxaliplatin and irinotecan was evaluated in other two smaller prospective studies (112, 113). Preliminary data showed a response rate of about 72%, and more than 50% of patients receiving the regimen underwent potentially curative resection. Survival of these patients was still unknown at the time of this writing.

The biological agents bevacizumab and cetuximab have improved the outcome of patients with metastatic colorectal cancer when combined with cytotoxic agents. There is an interest in integrating these biologic agents into neoadjuvant therapy, given the significant tumor response rate associated with such regimens. In a pilot study, eight of nine patients (88%) treated with bevacizumab, capecitabine and oxaliplatin achieved tumor response (114). However, caution is required when considering bevacizumab as neoadjuvant therapy due to the potential adverse effects of bevacizumab on liver regeneration and wound healing, and prospective studies are needed (118, 119).

Effects of Neoadjuvant Chemotherapy on Surgical Outcome

A positive correlation between response rate to systemic chemotherapy and the rate of secondary liver metastatectomy was reported in retrospective analyses and underlined the effort to develop more active regimens for neoadjuvant therapy (120). However, systemic chemotherapy also has the potential to degrade surgical outcome.

Steatohepatitis occurred in about a third of patients who received cytotoxic chemotherapy in a retrospective series. Patients receiving oxaliplatin were at a high risk for sinusoidal injury in the liver (121, 122). In a series of 248 patients with metastatic colorectal hepatic metastases receiving preoperative fluoropyrimidine-based chemotherapy, 8.9% developed steatosis, 8.4% had steatohepatitis and 5.4% had sinusoidal dilation that was primarily associated with oxaliplatin (123). Patients receiving irinotecan were also at a higher risk of steatohepatitis. The study concluded that patients with steatohepatitis had an increased 90-day postoperative mortality than those without.

Bevacizumab use was associated with a higher frequency of postoperative complications, such as bleeding and wound dehiscence, in a retrospective analysis of a pivotal Phase III trial evaluating IFL with and without bevacizumab in patients with metastatic colorectal cancer (73, 124). In addition, VEGF was found to be critical for liver regeneration following resection or injury in preclinical studies. An 8-week wait period free from bevacizumab before hepatic resection has been recommended to allow systemic VEGF levels to normalize (118).

Neoadjuvant chemotherapy should be administered with caution in patients who may become candidates for liver metastatectomy. A balance has to be achieved between improved resectability with optimal tumor shrinkage and avoiding complications that can compromise patient outcome following hepatic metastatectomy.

Future Directions

Evidence for neoadjuvant chemotherapy in patients with colorectal liver metastases is limited by the lack of well-designed randomized trials. Patient selection had been an important confounding problem because the definition of resectability had been inconsistent between studies, rendering it difficult to compare results. Future trials should examine clinically relevant endpoints, such as the rate of successful metastatectomy and survival following successful neoadjuvant chemotherapy and surgery. The optimal dose and timing of neoadjuvant chemotherapy in relation to surgery also need to be defined.

ADJUVANT CHEMOTHERAPY FOLLOWING HEPATIC METASTATECTOMY

Approximately 70% of patients relapse following surgical resection of colorectal cancer liver metastases and up to one-half of recurrences are in the liver

(8, 125, 126). Postoperative chemotherapy seems logical to reduce the risk of recurrence and improve survival after metastatectomy, but its use has been based on extrapolation of experience from adjuvant therapy for resected primary tumors.

Adjuvant Chemotherapy after Resection of Primary Tumor

The improvement in overall survival and disease-free survival supports the use of adjuvant chemotherapy as standard treatment in patients with stage III, or node-positive, colon cancer following surgery.

As in metastatic colorectal cancers, fluorouracil-based regimens form the backbone of colorectal cancer adjuvant therapy (127–129). Both bolus and infusional single-agent fluorouracil are comparable in efficacy in resected patients, although the latter has more hematological toxicity. Capecitabine, an oral prodrug of fluorouracil, has been shown to be an effective alternative to intravenous bolus fluorouracil in stage III disease (130).

Oxaliplatin-based regimens are currently accepted as the standard following resection of the primary tumor. In the Multi-center International Study of Oxaliplatin/5-Fluorouracil/Leucovorin in the Adjuvant Treatment of Colon Cancer (MOSAIC) trial, 6 months of oxaliplatin plus FOLFOX4 following surgery reduced the relative relapse risk by 24% and improved disease-free survival compared to infusional fluorouracil and leucovorin at 4-year follow-up (66, 131). Similar risk reduction was reported by the multi-center Phase III trial (NSABP C-07) in patients who received 6 months of oxaliplatin plus bolus fluorouracil and leucovorin (FLOX) at 3-year follow-up (132).

In contrast to the metastatic disease setting, the addition of irinotecan to adjuvant therapy failed to improve disease-free survival in patients with resected primary colorectal cancer (133–135). The role of biological agents, such as bevacizumab and cetuximab, in adjuvant therapy is being evaluated.

Postoperative Chemotherapy after Hepatic Metastatectomy

Definitive data supporting the use of adjuvant chemotherapy for resected colorectal liver metastases are lacking. In the multi-center randomized Fondation Francaise de Cancérologie Digestive (FFCD) 9002 trial, 162 patients were randomized over

10 years to either 6 months of bolus intravenous fluorouracil and folinic acid or observation (136). Adjuvant therapy improved 5-year disease-free (33% vs. 24%) and overall survival (51% vs. 44%) compared with observation only. The low accrual rate indicated the challenge of such trials.

The benefit of perioperative chemotherapy in patients with potentially resectable colorectal liver metastases is being evaluated in an ongoing European Organisation for Research and Treatment of Cancer (EORTC) Intergroup 40983 trial (137). Three hundred and sixty-four patients were randomized to observation or receiving 3 months of preoperative and 3 months of postoperative FOLFOX4. Interim analysis indicated that perioperative chemotherapy could be administered safely.

Many experts recommend 4 to 6 months of chemotherapy following resection of liver metastases, extrapolating experience in using adjuvant chemotherapy. Which regimens to use and the optimal duration of therapy remain unanswered questions, and may depend on previous treatment individual patients have received. Multi-disciplinary management in specialized centers in generally recommended. Patients with resected colorectal cancer liver metastases should be encouraged to enroll in clinical trials.

SYSTEMIC CHEMOTHERAPY IN CHEMOEMBOLIZATION

Transarterial chemoembolization (TACE) is widely used in the management of primary and secondary liver cancers (138–141). TACE offers an appropriate option with impressive response rate in selected hepatic metastases, such as sarcomas and carcinoid tumors, which otherwise are unresponsive to systemic chemotherapy (142); however, the role of TACE in colorectal hepatic metastases is less established (143). Survival of patients with colorectal liver metastases treated with TACE with or without systemic fluorouracil therapy is comparable to systemic chemotherapy alone (144–148). With newer chemotherapeutic agents and interventional strategies now available, however, the role of TACE for colorectal liver metastases is being re-examined, and impressive initial results have been reported.

The role of the newer biological agents with chemoembolization in colorectal hepatic metastases is yet unknown. Angiogenesis is implicated in the pathogenesis of many cancers, including colorectal carcinomas. High pretreatment VEGF levels were found to be associated with progressive disease following TACE in unresectable hepatocellular carcinoma (149). In addition, preclinical and human studies suggested that hypoxia resulting from insults, such as TACE and radiation, can lead to an adaptive increase in VEGF level, neovascularization and potentially recurrence (150–153). The combination of bevacizumab with TACE is being studied, and initial results from a pilot study of 30 patients with hepatocellular carcinoma has been presented (154). Serial angiograms were performed to assess neovascularization. Preliminary results on seven patients reported hypertension, proteinuria and variceal bleed as the main bevacizumab-related toxicities. The approach appeared to be feasible and relatively well-tolerated, but efficacy data and analysis of pre- and post-treatment angiogenic factors are not yet available.

REFERENCES

1. American Cancer Society. Cancers Facts & Figures 2005, ed. 1 Atlanta: American Cancer Society, 2005.
2. Gilbert JM. Distribution of metastases at necropsy in colorectal cancer. Clin Exp Metastasis, 1983; 1(2): 97–101.
3. Tong D, Russell AH, Dawson LE, et al. Second laparotomy for proximal colon cancer. sites of recurrence and implications for adjuvant therapy. Am J Surg, 1983; 145(3): 382–386.
4. Fong Y, Cohen AM, Fortner JG, et al. Liver resection for colorectal metastases. J Clin Oncol, 1997 15(3): 938–946.
5. Adam R. Chemotherapy and surgery: New perspectives on the treatment of unresectable liver metastases. Ann Oncol, 2003; 14 Suppl 2: ii13–16.
6. Adam R, Delvart V, Pascal G, et al. Rescue surgery for unresectable colorectal liver metastases downstaged by chemotherapy: A model to predict long-term survival. Ann Surg, 2004; 240(4): 644–657; discussion 657–658.
7. Stangl R, Altendorf-Hofmann A, Charnley RM, et al. Factors influencing the natural history of colorectal liver metastases. Lancet, 1994; 343(8910): 1405–1410.
8. Scheele J, Stang R, Altendorf-Hofmann A, et al. Resection of colorectal liver metastases. World J Surg, 1995; 19(1): 59–71.
9. Leonard GD, Brenner B, and Kemeny NE. Neoadjuvant chemotherapy before liver resection for patients with unresectable liver metastases from colorectal carcinoma. J Clin Oncol, 2005; 23(9): 2038–2048.
10. Palliative chemotherapy for advanced or metastatic colorectal cancer. Colorectal meta-analysis collaboration. Cochrane Database Syst Rev (2) (2): CD001545, 2000.
11. Meyerhardt JA and Mayer RJ. Systemic therapy for colorectal cancer. N Engl J Med, 2005; 352(5): 476 487.

12. Rustum YM. Thymidylate synthase: A critical target in cancer therapy? Front Biosci, 2004; 9: 2467–2473.

13. Poon MA, O'Connell MJ, Wieand HS, et al. Biochemical modulation of fluorouracil with leucovorin: Confirmatory evidence of improved therapeutic efficacy in advanced colorectal cancer. J Clin Oncol, 1991; 9(11): 1967–1972.

14. Petrelli N, Herrera L, Rustum Y, et al. A prospective randomized trial of 5-fluorouracil versus 5-fluorouracil and high-dose leucovorin versus 5-fluorouracil and methotrexate in previously untreated patients with advanced colorectal carcinoma. J Clin Oncol, 1987; 5(10): 1559–1565.

15. de Gramont A, Bosset JF, Milan C, et al. Randomized trial comparing monthly low-dose leucovorin and fluorouracil bolus with bimonthly high-dose leucovorin and fluorouracil bolus plus continuous infusion for advanced colorectal cancer: A French intergroup study. J Clin Oncol, 1997; 15(2): 808–815.

16. Lokich JJ, Moore CL, and Anderson NR. Comparison of costs for infusion versus bolus chemotherapy administration: Analysis of five standard chemotherapy regimens in three common tumors. Part one. Model projections for cost based on charges. Cancer, 1996; 78(2): 294–299.

17. Lokich JJ, Moore CL, Anderson NR. Comparison of costs for infusion versus bolus chemotherapy administration. Part two. Use of charges versus reimbursement for cost basis. Cancer, 1996; 78(2): 300–303.

18. Kohne CH, Wils J, Lorenz M, et al. Randomized phase III study of high-dose fluorouracil given as a weekly 24-hour infusion with or without leucovorin versus bolus fluorouracil plus leucovorin in advanced colorectal cancer: European Organization of Research and Treatment of Cancer Gastrointestinal Group study 40952. J Clin Oncol, 2003; 21(20): 3721–3728.

19. Meta-analysis Group in Cancer. Efficacy of intravenous continuous infusion of fluorouracil compared with bolus administration in advanced colorectal cancer. J Clin Oncol 1998; 16(1): 301–308.

20. Meropol NJ. Turning point for colorectal cancer clinical trials. J Clin Oncol, 2006; 24(21): 3322–3324.

21. Milano G, Ferrero JM, and Francois E. Comparative pharmacology of oral fluoropyrimidines: A focus on pharmacokinetics, pharmacodynamics and pharmaco-modulation. Br J Cancer, 2004; 91(4): 613–617.

22. Pentheroudakis G and Twelves C. The rational development of capecitabine from the laboratory to the clinic. Anticancer Res, 2002; 22(6B): 3589–3596.

23. Van Cutsem E, Twelves C, Cassidy J, et al. Oral capecitabine compared with intravenous fluorouracil plus leucovorin in patients with metastatic colorectal cancer: Results of a large phase III study. J Clin Oncol, 2001; 19(21): 4097–4106.

24. Hoff PM, Ansari R, Batist G, et al. Comparison of oral capecitabine versus intravenous fluorouracil plus leucovorin as first-line treatment in 605 patients with metastatic colorectal cancer: Results of a randomized phase III study. J Clin Oncol, 2001; 19(8): 2282–2292.

25. Van Cutsem E, Hoff PM, Harper P, et al. Oral capecitabine vs intravenous 5-fluorouracil and leucovorin: Integrated efficacy data and novel analyses from two large, randomised, Phase III trials. Br J Cancer, 2004; 90(6): 1190–1197.

26. Douillard JY, Hoff PM, Skillings JR, et al. Multicenter phase III study of uracil/tegafur and oral leucovorin versus fluorouracil and leucovorin in patients with previously untreated metastatic colorectal cancer. J Clin Oncol, 2002; 20(17): 3605–3616.

27. Carmichael J, Popiela T, Radstone D, et al. Randomized comparative study of tegafur/uracil and oral leucovorin versus parenteral fluorouracil and leucovorin in patients with previously untreated metastatic colorectal cancer. J Clin Oncol, 2002; 20(17): 3617–3627.

28. Tsunoda A, Shibusawa M, Tsunoda Y, et al. Antitumor effect of S-1 on DMH induced colon cancer in rats. Anticancer Res, 1998; 18(2A): 1137–1141.

29. Konno H, Tanaka T, Baba M, et al. Therapeutic effect of 1 M tegafur-0.4 M 5-chloro-2,4-dihydroxypyridine-1 M potassium oxonate (S-1) on liver metastasis of xeno-transplanted human colon carcinoma. Jpn J Cancer Res, 1999; 90(4): 448–453.

30. Maehara Y, Sugimachi K, Kurihara M, et al. Clinical evaluation of S-1, a new anticancer agent, in patients with advanced gastrointestinal cancer. S-1 Cooperative Gastrointestinal Study Group. Gan To Kagaku Ryoho, 1999; 26(4): 476–485.

31. Takemoto H, Fukunaga M, Ooshiro R, et al. A case of peritoneal dissemination disappeared by CPT-11 + TS-1 combination chemotherapy. Gan To Kagaku Ryoho, 2005; 32(11): 1768–1770.

32. Nakao K, Tsunoda A, Amagasa H, et al. A case report of poorly-differentiated adenocarcinoma in sigmoid colon cancer with liver and pulmonary metastasis responding to TS-1 and CPT-11. Gan To Kagaku Ryoho, 2006; 33(1): 109–112.

33. Kanazawa S, Seo A, Tokura N, et al. Liver metastasis from sigmoid colon cancer with peritoneal dissemination showed a complete response to TS-1. Gan To Kagaku Ryoho, 2006; 33(1): 113–117.

34. Ward S, Kaltenthaler E, Cowan J, et al. Clinical and cost-effectiveness of capecitabine and tegafur with uracil for the treatment of metastatic colorectal cancer: Systematic review and economic evaluation. Health Technol Assess, 2003; 7(32): 1–93.

35. Cassidy J, Tabernero J, Twelves C, et al. XELOX (capecitabine plus oxaliplatin): Active first-line therapy for patients with metastatic colorectal cancer. J Clin Oncol, 2004; 22(11): 2084–2091.

36. Bennouna J, Perrier H, Paillot B, et al. A phase II study of oral uracil/ftorafur (UFT) plus leucovorin combined with oxaliplatin (TEGAFOX) as first-line treatment in patients with metastatic colorectal cancer. Br J Cancer, 2006; 94(1): 69–73.

37. Ward S, Kaltenthaler E, Cowan J, et al. Clinical and cost-effectiveness of capecitabine and tegafur with uracil for the treatment of metastatic colorectal cancer: Systematic review and economic evaluation. Health Technol Assess, 2003; 7(32): 1–93.

38. Jansman FG, Postma MJ, van Hartskamp D, et al. Cost-benefit analysis of capecitabine versus 5-fluorouracil/leucovorin in the treatment of colorectal cancer in the Netherlands. Clin Ther, 2004; 26(4): 579–589.

39. Hieke K, Kleeberg UR, Stauch M, et al. Costs of treatment of colorectal cancer in different settings in Germany. Eur J Health Econ, 2004; 5(3): 270–273.

40. Faithfull S and Deery P. Implementation of capecitabine (Xeloda) into a cancer centre: UK experience. Eur J Oncol Nurs, 2004; 8 Suppl 1: S54–62.

41. Pizzolato JF and Saltz LB. The camptothecins. Lancet, 2003; 361(9376): 2235–2242.

42. Cunningham D, Pyrhonen S, James RD, et al. Randomised trial of irinotecan plus supportive care versus supportive care alone after fluorouracil failure for patients with metastatic colorectal cancer. Lancet, 1998; 352(9138): 1413–1418.

43. Rougier P, Van Cutsem E, Bajetta E, et al. Randomised trial of irinotecan versus fluorouracil by continuous infusion after fluorouracil failure in patients with metastatic colorectal cancer. Lancet, 1998; 352(9138): 1407–1412.

44. Saltz LB, Cox JV, Blanke C, et al. Irinotecan plus fluorouracil and leucovorin for metastatic colorectal cancer. Irinotecan Study Group. N Engl J Med, 2000; 343(13): 905–914.

45. Douillard JY, Cunningham D, Roth AD, et al. Irinotecan combined with fluorouracil compared with fluorouracil alone as first-line treatment for metastatic colorectal cancer: A multicentre randomised trial. Lancet, 2000; 355(9209): 1041–1047.

46. Gupta E, Lestingi TM, Mick R, et al: Metabolic fate of irinotecan in humans: Correlation of glucuronidation with diarrhea. Cancer Res, 1994; 54(14): 3723–3725.

47. Gupta E, Wang X, Ramirez J, et al. Modulation of glucuronidation of SN-38, the active metabolite of irinotecan, by valproic acid and phenobarbital. Cancer Chemother Pharmacol, 1997; 39(5): 440–444.

48. Innocenti F, Undevia SD, Iyer L, et al. Genetic variants in the UDP-glucuronosyltransferase 1A1 gene predict the risk of severe neutropenia of irinotecan. J Clin Oncol, 2004; 22(8): 1382–1388.

49. Raymond E, Faivre S, Chaney S, et al. Cellular and molecular pharmacology of oxaliplatin. Mol Cancer Ther, 2002; 1(3): 227–235.

50. Becouarn Y, Ychou M, Ducreux M, et al. Phase II trial of oxaliplatin as first-line chemotherapy in metastatic colorectal cancer patients. Digestive Group of French Federation of Cancer Centers. J Clin Oncol, 1998; 16(8): 2739–2744.

51. Diaz-Rubio E, Sastre J, Zaniboni A, et al. Oxaliplatin as single agent in previously untreated colorectal carcinoma patients: A phase II multicentric study. Ann Oncol, 1998; 9(1): 105–108.

52. Levi F, Perpoint B, Garufi C, et al. Oxaliplatin activity against metastatic colorectal cancer. A phase II study of 5-day continuous venous infusion at circadian rhythm modulated rate. Eur J Cancer, 1993; 29A(9): 1280–1284.

53. Plasencia C, Taron M, Martinez E, et al. Down-regulation of thymidylate synthase gene expression after oxaliplatin administration: Implications for the synergistic activity of sequential oxaliplatin/5FU in sensitive and 5FU-resistant cell lines. Proc Am Assoc Cancer Res, 2001; 42: 508, (abstr).

54. Fischel JL, Formento P, Ciccolini J, et al. Impact of the oxaliplatin-5 fluorouracil-folinic acid combination on respective intracellular determinants of drug activity. Br J Cancer, 2002; 86(7): 1162–1168.

55. Yeh KH, Cheng AL, Wan JP, et al. Down-regulation of thymidylate synthase expression and its steady-state mRNA by oxaliplatin in colon cancer cells. Anticancer Drugs, 2004; 15(4): 371–376.

56. Rothenberg ML, Oza AM, Bigelow RH, et al. Superiority of oxaliplatin and fluorouracil-leucovorin compared with either therapy alone in patients with progressive colorectal cancer after irinotecan and fluorouracil-leucovorin: Interim results of a phase III trial. J Clin Oncol, 2003; 21(11): 2059–2069.

57. Giacchetti S, Perpoint B, Zidani R, et al. Phase III multicenter randomized trial of oxaliplatin added to chronomodulated fluorouracil-leucovorin as first-line treatment of metastatic colorectal cancer. J Clin Oncol, 2000; 18(1): 136–147.

58. Grothey A, Deschler B, Kroening H, et al. Phase III study of bolus 5-fluorouracil (5-FU)/ folinic acid (FA) (Mayo) vs weekly high-dose 24h 5-FU infusion/ FA + oxaliplatin (OXA) (FUFOX) in advanced colorectal cancer (ACRC). Proc Am Soc Clin Oncol, 2002; 21: (abstr 512).

59. de Gramont A, Figer A, Seymour M, et al. Leucovorin and fluorouracil with or without oxaliplatin as first-line treatment in advanced colorectal cancer. J Clin Oncol, 2000; 18(16): 2938–2947.

60. Shields AF, Zalupski MM, Marshall JL, et al. Treatment of advanced colorectal carcinoma with oxaliplatin and capecitabine: A phase II trial. Cancer, 2004; 100(3): 531–537.

61. Comella P, Natale D, Farris A, et al. Capecitabine plus oxaliplatin for the first-line treatment of elderly patients with metastatic colorectal carcinoma: Final results of the southern Italy Cooperative Oncology Group trial 0108. Cancer, 2005; 104(2): 282–289.

62. Feliu J, Salud A, Escudero P, et al. XELOX (capecitabine plus oxaliplatin) as first-line treatment for elderly patients over 70 years of age with advanced colorectal cancer. Br J Cancer, 2006; 94(7): 969–975.

63. Raymond E, Faivre S, Woynarowski JM, et al. Oxaliplatin: Mechanism of action and antineoplastic activity. Semin Oncol, 1998; 25(2 Suppl 5): 4–12.

64. Raymond E, Chaney SG, Taamma A, et al. Oxaliplatin: A review of preclinical and clinical studies. Ann Oncol, 1998; 9(10): 1053–1071.

65. Grothey A: Oxaliplatin-safety profile: Neurotoxicity. Semin Oncol, 2003; 30(4 Suppl 15): 5–13.

66. de Gramont A, Boni C, Navarro M, et al. Oxaliplatin/ 5FU/LV in the adjuvant treatment of stage II and stage III colon cancer: Efficacy results with a median follow-up of 4 years. Journal of Clinical Oncology, ASCO Annual Meeting Proceedings, 2005; Vol 23, No 16S, Part I of II (June 1 Supplement): 3501 (abstr).

67. Tournigand C, Andre T, Achille E, et al. FOLFIRI followed by FOLFOX6 or the reverse sequence in advanced colorectal cancer: A randomized GERCOR study. J Clin Oncol, 2004; 22(2): 229–237.

68. Colucci G, Gebbia V, Paoletti G, et al. Phase III randomized trial of FOLFIRI versus FOLFOX4 in the treatment of advanced colorectal cancer: A multicenter study of the Gruppo Oncologico dell'Italia Meridionale. J Clin Oncol, 2005; 23(22): 4866–4875.

69. Goldberg RM, Sargent DJ, Morton RF, et al. A randomized controlled trial of fluorouracil plus leucovorin, irinotecan, and oxaliplatin combinations in patients with

previously untreated metastatic colorectal cancer. J Clin Oncol 2004; 22(1): 23–30.

70. Grothey A, Jordan K, Kellner O, et al. Randomized phase II trial of capecitabine plus irinotecan (CapIri) vs capecitabine plus oxaliplatin (CapOx) as first-line therapy of advanced colorectal cancer (ACRC). Proc Am Soc Clin Oncol, 2003; 22: (Abstr 1022).

71. Souglakos J, Androulakis N, Syrigos K, et al. FOL-FOXIRI (folinic acid, 5-fluorouracil, oxaliplatin and irinotecan) vs. FOLFIRI (folinic acid, 5-fluorouracil and irinotecan) as first-line treatment in metastatic colorectal cancer (MCC): A multicentre randomised phase III trial from the Hellenic Oncology Research Group (HORG). Br J Cancer, 2006; 94(6): 798–805.

72. Grothey A, Sargent D, Goldberg RM, et al. Survival of patients with advanced colorectal cancer improves with the availability of fluorouracil-leucovorin, irinotecan, and oxaliplatin in the course of treatment. J Clin Oncol, 2004; 22(7): 1209–1214.

73. Hurwitz H, Fehrenbacher L, Novotny W, et al. Bevacizumab plus irinotecan, fluorouracil, and leucovorin for metastatic colorectal cancer. N Engl J Med, 2004; 350(23): 2335–2342.

74. Giantonio BJ, Catalano PJ, Meropol NJ, et al. High-dose bevacizumab improves survival when combined with FOLFOX4 in previously treated advanced colorectal cancer: Results from the Eastern Cooperative Oncology Group (ECOG) study E3200. Journal of Clinical Oncology, ASCO Annual Meeting Proceedings, Vol 23, No 16S, Part I of II (June 1 Supplement), 2005, 2 (abstr).

75. Saltz LB, Meropol NJ, Loehrer PJ S, et al. Phase II trial of cetuximab in patients with refractory colorectal cancer that expresses the epidermal growth factor receptor. J Clin Oncol, 2004; 22(7): 1201–1208.

76. Cunningham D, Humblet Y, Siena S, et al. Cetuximab monotherapy and cetuximab plus irinotecan in irinotecan-refractory metastatic colorectal cancer. N Engl J Med, 2004; 351(4): 337–345.

77. Saltz L, Rubin MS, and Hochster HS. Cetuximab (IMC-C225) plus irinotecan (CPT-11) is active in CPT-11-refractory colorectal cancer (CRC) that expresses epidermal growth factor receptor (EGFR). Proc Am Soc Clin Oncol, 2001; 20: (abstr 7).

78. Carpenter G and Cohen S: Epidermal growth factor. J Biol Chem, 1990; 265(14): 7709–7712.

79. Real FX, Rettig WJ, Chesa PG, et al. Expression of epidermal growth factor receptor in human cultured cells and tissues: Relationship to cell lineage and stage of differentiation. Cancer Res, 1986; 46(9): 4726–4731.

80. Baselga J: Targeting the epidermal growth factor receptor: A clinical reality. J Clin Oncol, 2001; 19(18 Suppl): 41S–44S.

81. Yasui W, Sumiyoshi H, Hata J, et al. Expression of epidermal growth factor receptor in human gastric and colonic carcinomas. Cancer Res, 1988; 48(1): 137–141.

82. Messa C, Russo F, Caruso MG, et al. EGF, TGF-alpha, and EGF-R in human colorectal adenocarcinoma. Acta Oncol, 1998; 37(3): 285–289.

83. Porebska I, Harlozinska A, and Bojarowski T. Expression of the tyrosine kinase activity growth factor receptors (EGFR, ERB B2, ERB B3) in colorectal adenocarcinomas and adenomas. Tumour Biol, 2000; 21(2): 105–115.

84. Salomon DS, Brandt R, Ciardiello F, et al. Epidermal growth factor-related peptides and their receptors in human malignancies. Crit Rev Oncol Hematol, 1995; 19(3): 183–232.

85. Mayer A, Takimoto M, Fritz E, et al. The prognostic significance of proliferating cell nuclear antigen, epidermal growth factor receptor, and mdr gene expression in colorectal cancer. Cancer, 1993; 71(8): 2454–2460.

86. Hemming AW, Davis NL, Kluftinger A, et al. Prognostic markers of colorectal cancer: An evaluation of DNA content, epidermal growth factor receptor, and ki-67. J Surg Oncol, 1992; 51(3): 147–152.

87. Baselga J: Why the epidermal growth factor receptor? The rationale for cancer therapy. Oncologist, 2002; 7 Suppl 4: 2–8.

88. Fan Z, Baselga J, Masui H, et al. Antitumor effect of anti-epidermal growth factor receptor monoclonal antibodies plus cis-diamminedichloroplatinum on well established A431 cell xenografts. Cancer Res, 1993; 53(19): 4637–4642.

89. Goldstein NI, Prewett M, Zuklys K, et al. Biological efficacy of a chimeric antibody to the epidermal growth factor receptor in a human tumor xenograft model. Clin Cancer Res, 1995; 1(11): 1311–1318.

90. Prewett MC, Hooper AT, Bassi R, et al. Enhanced anti-tumor activity of anti-epidermal growth factor receptor monoclonal antibody IMC-C225 in combination with irinotecan (CPT-11) against human colorectal tumor xenografts. Clin Cancer Res, 2002; 8(5): 994–1003.

91. Badarinath S, Mitchell EO, Hennis CD, et al. Cetuximab plus FOLFOX for colorectal cancer (EXPLORE): Preliminary safety analysis of a randomized phase III trial. Journal of Clinical Oncology, ASCO Annual Meeting Proceedings (Post-Meeting Edition), 2004; Vol 22, No 14S (July 15 Supplement): 3531 (abstr).

92. Perez-Soler R and Saltz L. Cutaneous adverse effects with HER1/EGFR-targeted agents: Is there a silver lining? J Clin Oncol, 2005; 23(22): 5235–5246.

93. Lenz H, Mayer RJ, and Gold PJ. Activity of cetuximab in patients with colorectal cancer refractory to both irinotecan and oxaliplatin. Journal of Clinical Oncology, ASCO Annual Meeting Proceedings (Post-Meeting Edition), 2004; Vol 22, No 14S (July 15 Supplement): 3510 (abstr).

94. Chung KY, Shia J, Kemeny NE, et al. Cetuximab shows activity in colorectal cancer patients with tumors that do not express the epidermal growth factor receptor by immunohistochemistry. J Clin Oncol, 2005; 23(9): 1803–1810.

95. Gibson TB, Ranganathan A, and Grothey A. Randomized phase III trial results of panitumumab, a fully human anti-epidermal growth factor receptor monoclonal antibody, in metastatic colorectal cancer. Clin Colorectal Cancer, 2006; 6(1): 29–31.

96. Folkman J. Seminars in medicine of the Beth Israel Hospital, Boston: Clinical applications of research on angiogenesis. N Engl J Med, 1995; 333(26): 1757–1763.

97. Jain RK. Normalizing tumor vasculature with anti-angiogenic therapy: A new paradigm for combination therapy. Nat Med, 2001; 7(9): 987–989.

98. Ferrara N, Gerber HP, LeCouter J. The biology of VEGF and its receptors. Nat Med, 2003; 9(6): 669–676.

99. Ferrara N, Hillan KJ, and Novotny W. Bevacizumab (Avastin), a humanized anti-VEGF monoclonal antibody for cancer therapy. Biochem Biophys Res Commun, 2005; 333(2): 328–335.

100. Kabbinavar F, Hurwitz HI, Fehrenbacher L, et al. Phase II, randomized trial comparing bevacizumab plus fluorouracil (FU)/leucovorin (LV) with FU/LV alone in patients with metastatic colorectal cancer. J Clin Oncol, 2003; 21(1): 60–65.

101. Giantonio BJ, Catalano PJ, Meropol EP, et al. High-dose bevacizumab in combination with FOLFOX4 improves survival in patients with previously treated advanced colorectal cancer: Results from the Eastern Cooperative Oncology Group (ECOG) study E3200. 2005 ASCO Gastrointestinal Cancers Symposium; Abstract 169a (abstr).

102. Giantonio BJ, Catalno PJ, O'Dwyer PJ, et al. Impact of bevacizumab dose reduction on clinical outcomes for patients treated on the Eastern Cooperative Oncology Group's study E3200. Journal of Clinical Oncology, ASCO Annual Meeting Proceedings, Part I Vol 2006; 24, No 18S (June 20 Supplement): 3538 (abstr).

103. Bismuth H, Adam R, Levi F, et al. Resection of non-resectable liver metastases from colorectal cancer after neoadjuvant chemotherapy. Ann Surg, 1996; 224(4): 509–520; discussion 520–522.

104. Giacchetti S, Itzhaki M, Gruia G, et al. Long-term survival of patients with unresectable colorectal cancer liver metastases following infusional chemotherapy with 5-fluorouracil, leucovorin, oxaliplatin and surgery. Ann Oncol, 1999; 10(6): 663–669.

105. Adam R, Avisar E, Ariche A, et al. Five-year survival following hepatic resection after neoadjuvant therapy for nonresectable colorectal. Ann Surg Oncol, 2001; 8(4): 347–353.

106. Delaunoit T, Alberts SR, Sargent DJ, et al. Chemotherapy permits resection of metastatic colorectal cancer: Experience from Intergroup N9741. Ann Oncol, 2005; 16(3): 425–429.

107. Masi G, Cupini S, Marcucci L, et al. Treatment with 5-fluorouracil/folinic acid, oxaliplatin, and irinotecan enables surgical resection of metastases in patients with initially unresectable metastatic colorectal cancer. Ann Surg Oncol, 2006; 13(1): 58–65.

108. Wein A, Riedel C, Kockerling F, et al. Impact of surgery on survival in palliative patients with metastatic colorectal cancer after first line treatment with weekly 24-hour infusion of high-dose 5-fluorouracil and folinic acid. Ann Oncol, 2001; 12(12): 1721–1727.

109. Gaspar EM, Artigas V, Montserrat E, et al. Single centre study of L-OHP/5-FU/LV before liver surgery in patients with NOT optimally resectable colorectal cancer isolated liver metastases. Proc Am Soc Clin Oncol, 2003; 22: (abstr 1416).

110. Alberts SR, Horvath WL, Sternfeld WC, et al. Oxaliplatin, fluorouracil, and leucovorin for patients with unresectable liver-only metastases from colorectal cancer: A North Central Cancer Treatment Group phase II study. J Clin Oncol, 2005; 23(36): 9243–9249.

111. Pozzo C, Basso M, Cassano A, et al. Neoadjuvant treatment of unresectable liver disease with irinotecan and 5-fluorouracil plus folinic acid in colorectal cancer patients. Ann Oncol, 2004; 15(6): 933–939.

112. Quenet F, Nordlinger B, Rivoire M, et al. Resection of previously unresectable liver metastases from colorectal cancer (LMCRC) after chemotherapy (CT) with CPT-11/L-OHP/LV5FU (FOLFIRINOX): A prospective phase II trial. Journal of Clinical Oncology, ASCO Annual Meeting Proceedings (Post-Meeting Edition), 2004; Vol 22, No 14S (July 15 Supplement): 3613 (abstr).

113. De La Camara J, Rodriguez J, Rotellar F, et al. Triplet therapy with oxaliplatin, irinotecan, 5-fluorouracil and folinic acid within a combined modality approach in patients with liver metastases from colorectal cancer. Journal of Clinical Oncology, ASCO Annual Meeting Proceedings (Post-Meeting Edition), 2004; Vol 22, No 14S (July 15 Supplement): 3593.

114. Gruenberger T, Gruenberger B, and Scheithauer W. Neoadjuvant therapy with bevacizumab. J Clin Oncol, 2006; 24(16): 2592–2593; author reply, 2593–2594.

115. Fowler WC, Eisenberg BL, and Hoffman JP. Hepatic resection following systemic chemotherapy for metastatic colorectal carcinoma. J Surg Oncol, 1992; 51(2): 122–125.

116. Falcone A, Masi G, Allegrini G, et al. Biweekly chemotherapy with oxaliplatin, irinotecan, infusional fluorouracil, and leucovorin: A pilot study in patients with metastatic colorectal cancer. J Clin Oncol, 2002; 20(19): 4006–4014.

117. Masi G, Allegrini G, Cupini S, et al: First-line treatment of metastatic colorectal cancer with irinotecan, oxaliplatin and 5-fluorouracil/leucovorin (FOLFOXFIRI): Results of a phase II study with a simplified biweekly schedule. Ann Oncol, 2004; 15(12): 1766–1772.

118. Ellis LM, Curley SA, and Grothey A. Surgical resection after downsizing of colorectal liver metastasis in the era of bevacizumab. J Clin Oncol, 2005; 23(22): 4853–4855.

119. Chong G, Cunningham D. Improving long-term outcomes for patients with liver metastases from colorectal cancer. J Clin Oncol, 2005; 23(36): 9063–9066.

120. Folprecht G, Grothey A, Alberts S, et al. Neoadjuvant treatment of unresectable colorectal liver metastases: Correlation between tumour response and resection rates. Ann Oncol, 2005; 16(8): 1311–1319.

121. Kooby DA, Fong Y, Suriawinata A, et al. Impact of steatosis on perioperative outcome following hepatic resection. J Gastrointest Surg, 2003; 7(8): 1034–1044.

122. Rubbia-Brandt L, Audard V, Sartoretti P, et al. Severe hepatic sinusoidal obstruction associated with oxaliplatin-based chemotherapy in patients with metastatic colorectal cancer. Ann Oncol, 2004; 15(3): 460–466.

123. Vauthey JN, Pawlik TM, Ribero D, et al. Chemotherapy regimen predicts steatohepatitis and an increase in 90-day mortality after surgery for hepatic colorectal metastases. J Clin Oncol, 2006; 24(13): 2065–2072.

124. Hurwitz H, Fehrenbacjer T, Cartwright T, et al. Wound healing/bleeding in metastatic colorectal cancer patients who undergo surgery during treatment with bevacizumab. Journal of Clinical Oncology, ASCO Annual Meeting Proceedings (Post-Meeting Edition), 2004; Vol 22, No 14S (July 15 Supplement): 3702 (abstr).

125. Fong Y, Fortner J, Sun RL, et al. Clinical score for predicting recurrence after hepatic resection for metastatic

colorectal cancer: Analysis of 1001 consecutive cases. Ann Surg, 1999; 230(3): 309–318; discussion 318–321.

126. Figueras J, Valls C, Rafecas A, et al. Resection rate and effect of postoperative chemotherapy on survival after surgery for colorectal liver metastases. Br J Surg, 2001; 88(7): 980–985.

127. Andre T, Colin P, Louvet C, et al. Semimonthly versus monthly regimen of fluorouracil and leucovorin administered for 24 or 36 weeks as adjuvant therapy in stage II and III colon cancer: Results of a randomized trial. J Clin Oncol, 2003; 21(15): 2896–2903.

128. Chau I, Norman AR, Cunningham D, et al. A randomised comparison between 6 months of bolus fluorouracil/leucovorin and 12 weeks of protracted venous infusion fluorouracil as adjuvant treatment in colorectal cancer. Ann Oncol, 2005; 16(4): 549–557.

129. Poplin EA, Benedetti JK, Estes NC, et al. Phase III Southwest Oncology Group 9415/Intergroup 0153 randomized trial of fluorouracil, leucovorin, and levamisole versus fluorouracil continuous infusion and levamisole for adjuvant treatment of stage III and high-risk stage II colon cancer. J Clin Oncol, 2005; 23(9): 1819–1825.

130. Twelves C, Wong A, Nowacki MP, et al. Capecitabine as adjuvant treatment for stage III colon cancer. N Engl J Med, 2005; 352(26): 2696–2704.

131. Andre T, Boni C, Mounedji-Boudiaf L, et al. Oxaliplatin, fluorouracil, and leucovorin as adjuvant treatment for colon cancer. N Engl J Med, 2004; 350(23): 2343–2351.

132. Wolmark N, Wieand HS, Kuebler JP, et al. A phase III trial comparing FULV to FULV + oxaliplatin in stage II or III carcinoma of the colon: Results of NSABP protocol C-07. Journal of Clinical Oncology, ASCO Annual Meeting Proceedings, 2005; Vol 23, No 16S, Part I of II (June 1 Supplement): 3500 (abstr).

133. Van Cutsem E, Labianca R, Hossfeld D, et al. Randomized phase III trial comparing infused irinotecan / 5-fluorouracil (5-FU)/folinic acid (IF) versus 5-FU/FA (F) in stage III colon cancer patients (pts). (PETACC 3). Journal of Clinical Oncology, ASCO Annual Meeting Proceedings, 2005; Vol 23, No 16S, Part I of II (June 1 Supplement): 8 (abstr).

134. Ychou M, Raoul JL, Douillard JY, et al: A phase III randomized trial of LV5FU2+CPT-11 vs. LV5FU2 alone in adjuvant high risk colon cancer (FNCLCC Accord02/FFCD9802). Journal of Clinical Oncology, ASCO Annual Meeting Proceedings, 2005; Vol 23, No 16S, Part I of II (June 1 Supplement): 3502 (abstr).

135. Saltz LB, Niedzwiecki D, Hollis D, et al. Irinotecan plus fluorouracil/leucovorin (IFL) versus fluorouracil/leucovorin alone (FL) in stage III colon cancer (intergroup trial CALGB C89803). Journal of Clinical Oncology, ASCO Annual Meeting Proceedings (Post-Meeting Edition), 2004; Vol 22, No 14S (July 15 Supplement): 3500 (abstr).

136. Portier G, Rougier P, Milan C, et al. Adjuvant systemic chemotherapy (CT) using 5-fluorouracil (FU) and folinic acid (FA) after resection of liver metastases (LM) from colorectal (CRC) origin. Results of an intergroup phase III study (trial FFCD-ACHBTH-AURC 9002). Proc Am Soc Clin Oncol, 2002; 21: (abstr 528) (abstr).

137. Nordlinger B, Sorbye H, Debois M, et al. Feasibility and risks of pre-operative chemotherapy (CT) with FOL-FOX 4 and surgery for resectable colorectal cancer liver metastases (LM). Interim results of the EORTC intergroup randomized phase III study 40983. Journal of Clinical Oncology, ASCO Annual Meeting Proceedings, Vol 2005; 23, No 16S, Part I of II (June 1 Supplement): 3528 (abstr).

138. Llovet JM, Burroughs A, and Bruix J. Hepatocellular carcinoma. Lancet, 2003; 362(9399): 1907–1917.

139. Bruix J, Sala M, and Llovet JM. Chemoembolization for hepatocellular carcinoma. Gastroenterology, 2004; 127(5 Suppl 1): S179–88.

140. Diculescu M, Atanasiu C, Arbanas T, et al. Chemoembolization in the treatment of metastatic ileocolic carcinoid. Rom J Gastroenterol, 2002; 11(2): 141–147.

141. Salman HS, Cynamon J, Jagust M, et al. Randomized phase II trial of embolization therapy versus chemoembolization therapy in previously treated patients with colorectal carcinoma metastatic to the liver. Clin Colorectal Cancer, 2002; 2(3): 173–179.

142. Gupta S, Yao JC, Ahrar K, et al. Hepatic artery embolization and chemoembolization for treatment of patients with metastatic carcinoid tumors: The M.D. Anderson experience. Cancer J, 2003; 9(4): 261–267.

143. Sullivan KL. Hepatic artery chemoembolization. Semin Oncol, 2002; 29(2): 145–151.

144. Sanz-Altamira PM, Spence LD, Huberman MS, et al. Selective chemoembolization in the management of hepatic metastases in refractory colorectal carcinoma: A phase II trial. Dis Colon Rectum, 1997; 40(7): 770–775.

145. Tellez C, Benson AB, 3rd, Lyster MT, et al. Phase II trial of chemoembolization for the treatment of metastatic colorectal carcinoma to the liver and review of the literature. Cancer, 1998; 82(7): 1250–1259.

146. Leichman CG, Jacobson JR, Modiano M, et al. Hepatic chemoembolization combined with systemic infusion of 5-fluorouracil and bolus leucovorin for patients with metastatic colorectal carcinoma: A Southwest Oncology Group pilot trial. Cancer, 1999; 86(5): 775–781.

147. Bavisotto LM, Patel NH, Althaus SJ, et al. Hepatic transcatheter arterial chemoembolization alternating with systemic protracted continuous infusion 5-fluorouracil for gastrointestinal malignancies metastatic to liver: A phase II trial of the Puget Sound Oncology Consortium (PSOC 1104). Clin Cancer Res, 1999; 5(1): 95–109.

148. You YT, Changchien CR, Huang JS, et al. Combining systemic chemotherapy with chemoembolization in the treatment of unresectable hepatic metastases from colorectal cancer. Int J Colorectal Dis, 2006; 21(1): 33–37.

149. Poon RT, Lau C, Yu WC, et al. High serum levels of vascular endothelial growth factor predict poor response to transarterial chemoembolization in hepatocellular carcinoma: A prospective study. Oncol Rep, 2004; 11(5): 1077–1084.

150. Li X, Feng GS, Zheng CS, et al. Influence of transarterial chemoembolization on angiogenesis and expression of vascular endothelial growth factor and basic fibroblast growth factor in rat with Walker-256 transplanted hepatoma: An experimental study. World J Gastroenterol, 2003; 9(11): 2445–2449.

151. Chung YL, Jian JJ, Cheng SH, et al. Sublethal irradiation induces vascular endothelial growth factor and promotes growth of hepatoma cells: Implications for radiotherapy of hepatocellular carcinoma. Clin Cancer Res, 2006; 12(9): 2706–2715.

152. Roy-Chowdhury S, Peng Y, Wei D, et al. Evaluation of serum vascular endothelial growth factor (VEGF) levels following trans-arterial chemoembolization (TACE) of hepatic malignancies of gastrointestinal (GI) origin. Journal of Clinical Oncology, ASCO Annual Meeting Proceedings, 2005; Vol 23, No 16S, Part I of II (June 1 Supplement): 3087 (abstr).

153. Schwartz JD, Zuo Q, Lehrer D, et al. Serum vascular endothelial growth gactor (VEGF) and hepatocyte growth factor (HGF) are increased following transarterial chemoembolization (TACE) in unresectable hepatocellular carcinoma (HCC). 2006 ASCO Gastrointestinal Cancers Symposium; abstract No. 218 (abstr).

154. Britten CD, Finn RS, Gomes AS, et al. A pilot study of IV bevacizumab in hepatocellular cancer patients undergoing chemoembolization. Journal of Clinical Oncology, ASCO Annual Meeting Proceedings, 2005; Vol 23, No 16S, Part I of II (June 1 Supplement): 4138.

Chapter 20

SURGICAL RESECTION OF HEPATIC METASTASES

Michael A. Choti

PRIMARY LIVER CANCER

Hepatocellular carcinoma (HCC) is the most common type of common primary liver cancer and is associated with more than one million cases diagnosed worldwide each year. Other histologic types, including intrahepatic cholangiocarcinoma, while less common than HCC, are also experiencing a rise in incidence in the United States in recent years (1, 2). Complex management options confront those treating patients with primary liver cancer, making a multi-disciplinary team comprising hepatologists, diagnostic and interventional radiologists, medical oncologists, radiation oncologists, transplant surgeons and surgical oncologists important for optimal care. In patients without cirrhosis, surgical resection of primary liver cancer with partial hepatectomy is the treatment of choice; however, no more than 30% of patients have resectable disease, and when cirrhosis is present, fewer than 10% are resectable (3, 4). The presence of extrahepatic disease, lack of sufficient hepatic function reserve, multi-focal disease within the liver and suboptimal tumor location are all common reasons for unresectability in these patients.

HEPATIC METASTASES

Metastatic disease is the most common malignancy of the liver in the United States. The liver is the most common site for developing metastases, accounting for more than one-half of cases of advanced cancer. Although primary tumors originating from gastrointestinal sites are more likely than others to develop hepatic metastases, many tumors arising in other locations, including those of the breast and lung, also commonly develop hepatic metastases. Cancer of the colon and rectum account for the majority of primary tumors that develop isolated liver metastases and are candidates for surgical resection. This malignancy is the third most commonly diagnosed cancer in the United States and second overall in cancer mortality (5). Approximately 20% of patients have clinically recognizable liver metastases at the time of their primary diagnosis. After resection of a primary colorectal cancer in the absence of apparent metastatic disease, approximately 50% of patients will subsequently manifest metastatic liver disease (6). Given these figures, one can expect that at least 30,000 patients in the United States will develop metastatic colorectal cancer confined to the liver, each year.

The potential for developing liver metastases from neuroendocrine tumors depends upon the tumor type. Appendiceal carcinoid tumors and insulinomas rarely develop liver metastases, whereas small bowel carcinoid tumors and other islet cell tumors, including gastrinoma and glucagonoma, develop hepatic metastatic disease in up to 40% of cases. Other less common malignancies can also demonstrate a pattern of liver-predominant metastases. These include gastrointestinal stromal tumors (GIST), retroperitoneal sarcoma and ocular melanomas. Other tumor types, including renal cell carcinoma, Wilms' tumor and breast cancer, although they do not metastasize principally to the liver, can occasionally develop isolated liver metastases.

SELECTING PATIENTS FOR SURGICAL RESECTION

Perioperative mortality associated with liver resection has decreased from 20% in several decades ago to close to 1% in patients undergoing liver resection in more recent years (7, 8). In deciding which patients will tolerate a major liver resection, a number of factors need to be considered, including patient comorbidities. Patients with an American Society of Anesthesiology (ASA) score of greater than 1 have been shown to have more than three times the mortality rate and twice the morbidity of patients with an ASA of 1 (9). These patients with higher ASA scores reflect a group of patients with more underlying coronary artery disease, congestive heart failure or renal insufficiency, as well as other debilitating states that place this patient population at greater risk for postoperative complications. A major goal of the preoperative evaluation, therefore, is to identify patients who are at a high operative risk so that those who represent a prohibitive risk can be excluded, whereas patients with manageable comorbidities can have these conditions addressed preoperatively in an attempt to reduce their risk.

The health and function of the non-tumor-bearing liver is clearly one of the most important factors impacting resectability and outcomes following liver resection. In patients undergoing surgery for hepatic metastases, cirrhosis is rarely present. However, increasing use of prolonged preoperative combination chemotherapy can result in significant steatosis, steatohepatitis and sinusoidal dilatation. These changes can, in some cases, be associated with increased postoperative morbidity. In patients with cirrhosis, the postoperative morbidity following partial hepatectomy remains significant, primarily related to liver dysfunction. Assessment of hepatic functional reserve is important when deciding whether resection should be pursued. Prognostically useful data for both surgical and medical patients may be obtained from staging using the functional Child-Pugh classification system. Thrombocytopenia can be useful to estimate the extent of portal hypertension. Another method, the indocyanine green retention rate, can also provide an estimate of underlying liver function (10). Although this test is used in some centers, it is not employed with great frequency in most cases. Imaging techniques may shed light on the extent of cirrhosis in some cases. Specifically, computed tomography (CT) scan or magnetic resonance imaging (MRI) can identify loss of liver volume or hepatic contour changes indicative of more extensive cirrhosis; visualization of portal vein collaterals, splenomegaly or ascites can indicate more advanced disease.

DEFINING RESECTABILITY IN PATIENTS WITH HEPATIC METASTASES

In the past, resection of hepatic colorectal metastases was not attempted in patients who had more than three or four metastases, hilar adenopathy, metastases within 1 cm of major vessels such as the vena cava or main hepatic veins or extrahepatic disease. More recent studies, however, demonstrate that patients with these clinicopathologic factors can achieve long-term survival following hepatic resection and therefore should not be excluded from surgical consideration. Specifically, the number of metastases is no longer considered a contraindication to surgery (11, 12). Similarly, contiguous extension to adjacent anatomical structures and local or regional recurrence at the site of the primary colorectal cancer are not contraindications to resection. An increasing number of studies also indicates that although survival may be reduced in patients with extrahepatic colorectal metastases (13), complete resection of limited extrahepatic disease in conjunction with resection of hepatic metastases can result in long-term survival.

Taken together, these data have led to a shift in the definition of resectability from criteria based on the characteristics of the metastatic disease to new criteria based on whether a macroscopic and microscopic complete (R0) resection of the liver disease can be achieved. Currently, hepatic colorectal metastases should be defined as resectable when it is anticipated that disease can be completely resected, two adjacent liver segments can be spared, adequate vascular inflow, outflow and biliary drainage can be preserved and the volume of the liver remaining after resection is sufficient (Table 20.1). Instead of resectability being defined by what is removed, decisions regarding resectability should now focus on what will remain following resection.

The size of the remnant volume considered safe varies with the condition of the hepatic parenchyma. In healthy livers, a remnant liver volume greater than 20% to 30% of the estimated total liver volume is

TABLE 20.1 Criteria Defining Resectability for Surgical Resection

1. Macroscopic and microscopic (R0) treatment of the disease is feasible with either resection alone or resection combined with radiofrequency ablation.
2. At least two adjacent liver segments can be spared.
3. Adequate vascular inflow, outflow and biliary drainage can be preserved.
4. Sufficient remnant liver volume (>20% of the total estimated liver volume in normal liver, >40% of total estimated liver volume in cirrhotic liver).

considered sufficient (14, 15). In contrast, patients with cirrhosis need at least 40% remnant liver volume in order to avoid postoperative liver failure. CT or MRI can now provide an accurate, reproducible method for preoperatively measuring the volume of the future liver remnant (14). In cases in which major hepatectomy is planned and there is concern regarding insufficient liver volume, these patients should be considered for preoperative portal vein embolization (PVE) to induce hypertrophy of the contralateral hemiliver (16). PVE has been shown to increase the size of the future liver remnant; however, no evidence to date has clearly demonstrated improved outcomes following PVE compared with no PVE. Likely, the selective use of PVE may enable the performance of an extended hepatectomy in a subset of patients who otherwise would not have been candidates for safe resection.

TECHNIQUES FOR LIVER RESECTION

The main goal of the liver resection is to precisely remove the involved portion of liver with an adequate surgical margin and preserve sufficient hepatic reserve. Major hepatic resections can be divided into right and left hepatectomy (or hemi-hepatectomy) or extended hepatectomy, depending on the number of liver segments removed. All or part of the caudate lobe can be included as part of a major liver resection or can be resected separately. When performing major hepatic resection, the vascular structures supplying the liver being removed are typically isolated extrahepatically prior to parenchymal dissection. The relevant portal pedicle can be secured at the hilum, either as a group within the intrahepatic hilum or by individual isolation of the portal vein and hepatic artery (17). Selective extrahepatic ligation of inflow allows for the demarcation of the portion of the liver to be removed.

Minor resections can be either segmental resections or non-anatomic wedge resections. Wedge resections typically make no attempt to isolate vascular structures supplying the area being removed and are generally reserved for small peripheral lesions. When such resections are being performed for cancer and with curative intent, care must be taken to maintain an adequate margin around the tumor as wedge resections are more often associated with positive or close margins. Hepatic segmentectomy can be considered an anatomic minor resection, intermediate between major hepatic resection and that of a wedge resection. Such resections can be of a single segment or multiple adjacent segments in one or both hemi-livers. Provided adequate tumor margins are achieved, segmental resections have the advantage of preserving hepatic parenchyma compared with major liver resections. Intrahepatic anatomic landmarks visualized with intraoperative ultrasonography can be used to plan segmental resections, and vascular pedicles are typically controlled within the liver substance. Temporary total inflow occlusion is often helpful during these types of resections.

A variety of techniques has been described for the division of the liver substance itself. The traditional method utilizes blunt parenchymal dissection either manually, or with a crushing clamp or suction device. Vascular and biliary structures are identified within the liver and ligated or clipped. Other parenchymal dividing techniques utilize devices such as the ultrasonic cavitron or a saline jet irrigator to divide the liver by disrupting the parenchyma. Newer devices use saline-enhanced radiofrequency energy or a plane of thermal ablation to achieve coagulative necrosis of the liver substance to achieve hemostasis during or before the dissection. Surgical stapling devices have also greatly improved the ease in which liver resection can be performed. In addition to facilitating division of the extrahepatic vascular pedicles, staplers can be used to divide larger pedicles within the liver parenchyma. The superiority of any one single method has not been established, and which technique to use should depend on the individual surgeon's experience.

LIVER RESECTION FOR PRIMARY LIVER CANCER

In non-cirrhotic patients, operative mortality following liver resection is typically less than 2%. The

TABLE 20.2 Reported 5-Year Survival Following Resection of Colorectal Liver Metastasis with Curative Intent

Investigator (Ref.)	Year of Publication	Years Included in Study	5-year Survival (%)
Scheele et al. (24)	1995	1960–1992	39
Fong et al. (25)	1999	1985–1998	37
Choti et al. (26)	2002	1993–1999	58
Abdalla et al. (29)	2004	1992–2002	58
Fernandez et al. (30)	2004	1992–2002	58
Pawlik et al. (28)	2005	1990–2004	58

presence of cirrhosis is associated with lower resectability rate and higher mortality. While earlier reports demonstrated substantially increased operative mortality rates following resection for patients with cirrhosis, more current studies from both Western and Eastern investigators showed similar postoperative mortality rates (<5%) for patients with and without cirrhosis (18–21). As has been demonstrated with other complex operative procedures, centers with increased experience and greater number of liver resections performed are associated with decreased perioperative mortality (22).

Following partial hepatectomy, the overall 5-year survival rates are reported between 40% and 68% (19, 20, 23). Clinical and pathologic features have prognostic implications following partial hepatectomy. Similar to results following liver transplantation, important factors associated with poor prognosis include large tumor size, multi-focal disease and presence of vascular invasion. Other variables that have been associated with prognosis include alphafetoprotein level, presence of cirrhosis and histologic grade (19, 23).

LIVER RESECTION FOR HEPATIC COLORECTAL METASTASES

Overall, the perioperative mortality of liver resection for colorectal metastases is approximately 1% in most current reported series (26–29). In experienced hands, even major hepatic resections (hemihepatectomy or extended hepatectomy), which are performed in about one-half of the cases, result in perioperative mortality rates of less than 5% (26–29). The potential for adverse outcome and the complexity of these operations justifies the recommendation that major liver resection be performed at centers and by surgeons having experience with such procedures.

Complication rates for liver resection of metastatic disease are approximately 15%. The major morbidity associated specifically with liver resection includes hemorrhage, perihepatic abscess, bile leak or fistula, pleural effusion and hepatic failure.

With regard to survival, large series from the 1960s through the mid-1990s reported 5-year survival rates in the range of 33% to 36% for patients with colorectal liver metastases resected with curative intent (24, 25). However, more recent data have shown an improved 5-year survival rate of 58% following complete resection of colorectal liver metastases (Table 20.2) (26, 28–30). This improvement in overall survival likely reflects improvement in patient selection and surgical technique, and more effective adjuvant therapy.

Several clinicopathologic factors predictive of patient survival after hepatic resection have been identified (24–26). These include stage, grade and nodal status of the primary colorectal tumor; disease-free interval from diagnosis of primary tumor to diagnosis of liver metastases; number and distribution of liver metastases; level of preoperative carcinoembryonic antigen (CEA); and presence of extrahepatic disease. Although preoperative factors may be generally instructive, these factors should not be used to exclude patients from surgical consideration. Patients with one or multiple negative prognostic factors can still derive a significant survival advantage from hepatic resection of their colorectal metastases (32).

LIVER RESECTION FOR NON-COLORECTAL METASTASES

The role of liver resection for hepatic metastases from non-colorectal tumors has not been studied as well as that for metastases from colorectal primaries. Selected patients with neuroendocrine metastases may benefit from aggressive surgical resection because of the slow tumor growth and often significant symptoms related to hormone production and tumor bulk (33, 34). Even when all disease cannot be resected, uncontrolled reports suggest that when symptomatic or when greater than 90% of disease can be resected, palliative or cytoreductive surgery may be also of benefit in patients with hepatic metastases from neuroendocrine primaries.

The role of liver resection in non-colorectal non-neuroendocrine metastases is even less clear. Several small retrospective series have reported 5-year survival rates of 0% to 37% (34–36). Recently, a large retrospective registry series from France reported 5-year overall and disease-free survival rates of 36% and 21% respectively (37). In particular, in patients with metastases from GIST/sarcoma, renal, adrenal and breast cancer in whom isolated liver metastases are found, liver resection may be considered. Because in these diseases metastases confined to the liver are uncommon, careful imaging of the lung, brain and bone should be performed before hepatic resection is considered. More importantly, any decision to consider locoregional therapy on these diseases, including resection, should be highly individualized and based on specific favorable biology rather than any strict guidelines based on primary site or histology.

CONCLUSION

Liver resection currently represents one of the most effective therapeutic options for patients with primary and secondary liver cancer. Recent improvements in whole-body and hepatic imaging have allowed for more accurate selection of patients who may benefit most from resection. In addition, assessment for the presence of underlying liver disease can reduce postoperative complications related to hepatic dysfunction. Traditional clinicopathologic factors, although helpful in stratifying patients with regard to prognosis, should not be used to exclude otherwise resectable patients from surgery, particularly those with hepatic colorectal metastases. The use of modern surgical techniques is reducing perioperative morbidity and mortality, while PVE, preoperative therapy and combining resection with other approaches such as ablation can expand the population of patients who are candidates for surgical treatment. Perhaps the most important strategy when considering the multitude of therapeutic options for patients with either primary

or secondary liver cancer is the development of an individual treatment plan based on discussion among a multi-disciplinary team of specialists, including the surgeons, hepatologists, oncologists and radiologists.

REFERENCES

1. El-Serag HB and Mason AC. Rising incidence of hepatocellular carcinoma in the United States. N Engl J Med, 1999 Mar 11; 340(10): 745–750.
2. DeOliveira ML, Cunningham SC, Cameron JL, et al. Cholangiocarcinoma: Thirty-one-year experience with 564 patients at a single institution. Ann Surg, 2007 May; 245(5): 755–762.
3. Mor E, Kaspa RT, Sheiner P, et al. Treatment of hepatocellular carcinoma associated with cirrhosis in the era of liver transplantation. Ann Intern Med, 1998 Oct 15; 129(8): 643–653.
4. Farmer DG, Rosove MH, Shaked A, et al. Current treatment modalities for hepatocellular carcinoma. Ann Surg, 1994 Mar; 219(3): 236–247.
5. Jemal A, Murray T, Ward E, et al. Cancer Statistics, 2005. CA Cancer J Clin, 2005; 55: 10–30.
6. Steele G, Jr and Ravikumar TS. Resection of hepatic metastases from colorectal cancer: Biologic perspective. Ann Surg, 1989; 210: 127–138.
7. Capussotti L and Polastri R. Operative risks of major hepatic resections. Hepatogastroenterology, 1998; 45: 184–190.
8. Sitzmann JV and Greene PS. Perioperative predictors of morbidity following hepatic resection for neoplasm: A multivariate analysis of a single surgeon's experience with 105 patients. Ann Surg, 1994; 219: 13–17.
9. Belghiti J, Hiramatsu K, Benoist S, et al. Seven hundred forty-seven hepatectomies in the 1990s: An update to evaluate the actual risk of liver resection. J Am Coll Surg, 2000; 191: 38–46.
10. Farges O, Malassagne B, Flejou JF, et al. Risk of major liver resection in patients with underlying chronic liver disease: A reappraisal. Ann Surg, 1999; 229(2): 210–215.
11. Kokudo N, Imamura H, Sugawara Y, et al. Surgery for multiple hepatic colorectal metastases. J Hepatobiliary Pancreat Surg, 2004;11: 84–91.
12. Weber SM, Jarnagin WR, DeMatteo RP, et al. Survival after resection of multiple hepatic colorectal metastases. Ann Surg Oncol, 2000; 7: 643–650.
13. Iwatsuki S, Dvorchik I, Madariaga JR, et al. Hepatic resection for metastatic colorectal adenocarcinoma: A proposal of a prognostic scoring system. J Am Coll Surg, 1999; 189: 291–299.
14. Abdalla EK, Denys A, Chevalier P, et al. Total and segmental liver volume variations: Implications for liver surgery. Surgery, 2004 Apr; 135(4): 404–410.
15. Yigitler C, Farges O, Kianmanesh R, et al. The small remnant liver after major liver resection: How common and how relevant? Liver Transpl, 2003 Sep; 9(9): S18–25.
16. Abdalla EK, Hicks ME, and Vauthey JN. Portal vein embolization: Rationale, technique and future prospects. Br J Surg, 2001; 88: 165–175.
17. Khatri VP, Petrelli NJ, and Belghiti J. Extending the frontiers of surgical therapy for hepatic colorectal metastases:

Is there a limit? J Clin Oncol, 2005 Nov 20; 23(33): 8490–8499.

18. Farges O, Malassagne B, Flejou JF, et al. Risk of major liver resection in patients with underlying chronic liver disease: A reappraisal. Ann Surg, 1999; 229(2): 210–215.

19. Lee CS, Sheu JC, Wang M, et al. Long-term outcome after surgery for asymptomatic small hepatocellular carcinoma. Br J Surg, 1996; 83(3): 330–333.

20. Vauthey JN, Klimstra D, Franceschi D, et al. Factors affecting long-term outcome after hepatic resection for hepatocellular carcinoma. Am J Surg, 1995; 169.

21. Poon RT, Fan ST, Lo CM, et al. Long-term survival and pattern of recurrence after resection of small hepatocellular carcinoma in patients with preserved liver function: Implications for a strategy of salvage transplantation. Ann Surg, 2002 Mar; 235(3): 373–382.

22. Choti MA, Bowman HM, Pitt HA, et al. Should hepatic resections be performed at high-volume referral centers? J Gastrointest Surg, 1998; 2:11–20.

23. Poon RT, Fan ST, Lo CM, et al. Difference in tumor invasiveness in cirrhotic patients with hepatocellular carcinoma fulfilling the Milan criteria treated by resection and transplantation: Impact on long-term survival. Ann Surg, 2007 Jan; 245(1): 51–58.

24. Scheele J, Stang R, Altendorf-Hofmann A, et al. Resection of colorectal liver metastases. World J Surg, 1995; 19: 59–71.

25. Fong Y, Fortner J, Sun RL, et al. Clinical score for predicting recurrence after hepatic resection for metastatic colorectal cancer: Analysis of 1001 consecutive cases. Ann Surg, 1999; 230: 309–318; discussion 318–321.

26. Choti MA, Sitzmann JV, Tiburi MF, et al. Trends in long-term survival following liver resection for hepatic colorectal metastases. Ann Surg, 2002; 235: 759–766.

27. Fong Y, Cohen AM, Fortner JG, et al. Liver resection for colorectal metastases. J Clin Oncol, 1997; 15: 938–946.

28. Pawlik TM, Scoggins CR, Zorzi D, et al. Effect of surgical margin status on survival and site of recurrence after hepatic resection for colorectal metastases. Ann Surg, 2005; 241: 715–722, discussion 722–714.

29. Abdalla EK, Vauthey JN, Ellis LM, et al. Recurrence and outcomes following hepatic resection, radiofrequency ablation, and combined resection/ablation for colorectal liver metastases. Ann Surg, 2004; 239: 818–825.

30. Fernandez FG, Drebin JA, Linehan DC, et al. Five-year survival after resection of hepatic metastases from colorectal cancer in patients screened by positron emission tomography with F-18 fluorodeoxyglucose (FDG-PET). Ann Surg, 2004; 240: 438–447.

31. Nordlinger B, Guiguet M, Vaillant JC, et al. Surgical resection of colorectal carcinoma metastases to the liver. A prognostic scoring system to improve case selection, based on 1568 patients. Association Française de Chirurgie. Cancer, 1996; 77: 1254–1262.

32. Pawlik TM, Abdalla EK, Ellis LM, et al. Debunking dogma: Surgery for four or more colorectal liver metastases is justified. J Gastrointest Surg, 2006 Feb; 10(2): 240–248.

33. Chen H, Hardacre JM, Uzar A, et al. Isolated liver metastases from neuroendocrine tumors: Does resection prolong survival? J Am Coll Surg, 1998 Jul; 187(1): 88–92.

34. Harrison LE, Brennan MF, Newman E, et al. Hepatic resection for noncolorectal, nonneuroendocrine metastases: A fifteen-year experience with ninety-six patients. Surgery, 1997; 121: 625–632.

35. Benevento A, Boni L, Frediani L, et al. Result of liver resection as treatment for metastases from noncolorectal cancer. J Surg Oncol, 2000 May; 74(1): 24–29.

36. Chen H, Pruitt A, Nichol TL, et al. Complete hepatic resection of metastases from leiomyosarcoma prolongs survival. J Gastrointest Surg, 1998; 2(2): 151–155.

37. Adam R, Chiche L, Aloia T, et al. Hepatic resection for noncolorectal nonendocrine liver metastases: Analysis of 1,452 patients and development of a prognostic model. Ann Surg, 2006 Oct; 244(4): 524–535.

Chapter 21

CLINICAL MANAGEMENT OF PATIENTS WITH COLORECTAL LIVER METASTASES USING HEPATIC ARTERIAL INFUSION

Fidel David Huitzil Melendez

Nancy Kemeny

Liver metastases from colorectal cancer is a suitable clinical model for regional drug delivery for several reasons: as a result of portal venous drainage, the liver can be the first and only site of metastatic disease in patients with colorectal cancer (1). This is in contrast with other gastrointestinal malignancies, in which liver metastases are frequently a marker of widespread disease, as is the case of gastric cancer and pancreatic cancer (2). In addition, colon cancer has favorable tumor biology compared with other gastrointestinal or non-gastrointestinal malignancies. When liver resections were performed under the same criteria for liver metastases from colon cancer and from gastric cancer, 5-year overall survival was 30% for colon cancer patients and 0% for gastric cancer patients (3). Furthermore, the hepatic artery (HA) is the main blood supply of liver metastases (4). Totally implantable infusion systems have been developed (5), and the surgical techniques have improved (5), allowing a higher percentage of patients to receive regional treatment for longer periods of time.

Identification of ideal candidates is critical for optimal clinical results. Selection criteria focus on identifying patients with liver-only metastatic disease, with suitable hepatic arterial anatomy for pump placement. For this purpose, work-up should include computed tomography scan of the chest, abdomen and pelvis with liver angiography. Positron emission tomographic scans are not routinely performed, but they can be helpful in determining the nature of enlarged periportal lymph nodes or other indeterminate lesions (6). Surgery is considered a potentially curative treatment for patients with colorectal cancer metastatic to the liver, even for patients who require a two-stage hepatectomy (7) or repeated resections after local recurrence (8). Unfortunately, only a minority of patients presents with liver lesions amenable to resection. Even after successful resection, recurrence rates are high, and approximately 50% of recurrences occur in the liver (9). Accordingly, the clinical applications of HAI for patients with metastatic colorectal cancer to the liver fall into three different categories:

1. Unresectable disease
2. Borderline resectability
3. Adjuvant treatment after resection of liver metastases

TABLE 21.1 Randomized Trials of versus Systemic Chemotherapy for Unresectable Liver Metastases

Study (Ref.)	Arms[a]	No.	Primary Endpoint	% Receiving Tx in HAI Arm	Crossover to HAI	Response (CR + PR)	Median Survival (mo.)
MSKCC (12)	HAI	48	Response	94	Yes	50%*	17
	SYS	51				20%	12
NCI (13)	HAI	32	Survival	66	No	62%*	17[†]
	SYS	32				17%	12[†]
NCOG (14)	HAI	67	TTF liver	75	Yes	42%*	16.5
	SYS	76				10%	15.8
City of Hope (15)	HAI	31	TTF/Survival	100	Yes	55%*	13.8
	SYS	10				20%	11.6
NCCTG (16)	HAI	39	Survival	85	No	48%	12.6
	SYS	35				12%	10.5
French (17)	HAI	81	Survival	87	No	44%*	15*
	SYS	82				9%	11
English (18)	HAI	51	Survival	96	No	NR	13.5*
	SYS	49				NR	7.5
MRC/EORTC (19)	HAI[b]	145	Survival	63	No	22%[‡]	14.7
	SYS	145				19%	14.8
German (10)	HAI[c]	54	TTP	69	No	43%*	12.7
	SYS	57				20%	17.6
CALGB (54)	HAI	68	Survival	87	No	48%*	24*
	SYS	67				25%	20

*$p < 0.05$. [†]based on published Kaplan-Meier curves. [‡]responses were calculated at a single time point (12 weeks). Notes: [a]HAI, hepatic arterial infusion; SYS, systemic. [b]All trials used HAI-FUDR except this study, which used HAI-FU. [c]This study had two groups of HAI therapy. The group using HAI-FU is not listed on this table.

UNRESECTABLE DISEASE

The clinical utility of hepatic arterial infusion (HAI) was initially tested in the setting of unresectable disease. Clinical trials were directed toward confirming the hypothesis that direct perfusion of chemotherapy through the HA could improve outcomes compared with systemic administration of chemotherapy in patients with liver metastases from colorectal cancer. It should be noted that when initial studies were done, fluoropyrimidines were the only active agents in colon cancer. Ten randomized studies compared HAI to systemic chemotherapy (Table 21.1) (10–19). All studies used floxuridine (FUDR) or fluorouracil (FU) alone via HAI therapy. Some studies used ports and not pumps. We now know that:

1. FUDR + dexamethasone combination is better than FUDR alone or FU alone (20).

2. HAI is better than portal vein infusion (4).

3. Totally implantable pumps are superior to catheters or ports (21).

4. Aggressive dose adjustment algorithms based on liver function tests are necessary to minimize biliary toxicity and enhance treatment duration.

5. Improvement in imaging studies helps avoid inclusion of patients with extrahepatic disease (6, 22).

6. Surgical experience in pump placement is needed to minimize complications (5).

Heterogeneity in these key elements observed among clinical trials may explain different results in terms of efficacy and toxicity. Furthermore, these trials also differed in primary endpoint, and not all trials were powered or designed to demonstrate improved survival. Results from these randomized studies can be summarized as follows:

1. Almost all the studies showed an increase in response rate.

2. Two earlier European studies demonstrated an increase in survival with HAI, but appropriate systemic therapy was not always used (18, 23).

3. Two recent European trials did not show an increase in survival, the first being the Medical

Research Council (MRC) and European Organization for the Research and Treatment of Cancer (EORTC) study [19], which randomized patients to HAI – FU/leucovorin (LV) via a port (using a port rather than a pump) and (using FU rather than FUDR) vs. systemic FU/LV. In this study, 37% of the patients assigned to the HAI arm did not receive treatment, and 29% had to stop treatment. No differences were seen in response rate at 12 weeks (22% versus 19%, for HAI and systemic, respectively) and no differences were seen in toxicity, progression-free survival (PFS) or survival. The study was not analyzed to look at the patients who actually received treatment. The second negative trial in terms of survival was conducted by the German Cooperative Group (10) and randomized patients to HAI-FUDR, HAI-FU/LV, or systemic FU/LV. Tumor response rates were 43.2% and 45%, versus 19.7%, and development of extrahepatic disease was 40.5%, 12.5%, versus 18.3% for the HAI-FUDR, HAI-FU/LV, and systemic FU/LV groups, respectively. Toxicity data indicated that FU/LV therapy was much more toxic than FUDR. A port was used, rather than a pump, and dosing for FUDR was different from the American studies in that FUDR was reduced from 0.2 to 0.15 mg/kg/day after three cycles rather than adjusting for patient toxicity. The median survival was 12.7, 18.7 and 17.6 months for the HAI – FUDR, HAI-FU/LV and systemic FU/LV groups, respectively. Only 66% of patients randomized to HAI of FUDR were treated, but all were included in the survival analysis. Eight patients in the HAI-FUDR group died before ever receiving treatment, perhaps explaining the very low survival with HAI-FUDR.

4. The Cancer and Leukemia Group B (CALGB) (11) trial differs from the other HAI studies in that it included the use of dexamethasone (Dex) in the HAI arm (24). HAI-FUDR+Dex+LV was compared with systemic bolus FU/LV. No crossover was allowed. The time to hepatic progression was better in the HAI arm (9.8 months vs. 7.3 months, p = 0.034), but the time to extrahepatic progression was better in the systemic arm (14.8 months vs. 7.7 months in the HAI group, p <0.029). Despite these striking differences in the pattern of progression of disease, the HAI group had a significant increase in survival, 24.4 months versus 20 months in the systemic group (p = 0.0034), suggesting that control of hepatic disease may be more important than control of extrahepatic disease in terms of survival. There was a quality-of-life (QoL) assessment performed as part of the study, and the HAI group experienced improved QoL measured at 3 and 6 months.

5. There are differences between the CALGB study (11) and the European studies, which could possibly explain differences in the outcomes. The CALGB study used pumps instead of ports, and HAI therapy included FUDR with Dex to decrease toxicity (24). Survival was based on intent to treat in all three studies, and the actual number of patients treated was much lower in the European studies – 66% in the German study and 63% in the English study – whereas it was 86% in the CALGB study. The CALGB study did demonstrate that regional therapy alone can improve survival over systemic FU/LV, and the HAI alone therapy produced a survival similar to that which is seen utilizing the new agents.

A fair conclusion from these trials is that HAI of FUDR provides better locoregional control than systemic administration of fluoropyrimidines, and despite poor extrahepatic control, has the potential to demonstrate improvement in survival over systemic 5-FU if optimally delivered in well-selected patients treated and evaluated in well-designed controlled trials. However, systemic fluoropyrimidines no longer constitute the only active agents in colon cancer. Availability of new active drugs including irinotecan, oxaliplatin, cetuximab and bevacizumab has translated into increased survival for patients with colorectal cancer treated with systemic therapy. Accordingly, the objectives of current studies of HAI therapy have changed. The new hypothesis is that HAI chemotherapy can be safely administered concomitantly with new systemic therapies, and that this combination is able to further improve outcomes over both HAI – FUDR alone or systemic therapy with new agents alone.

In this regard, a Phase I study of HAI – FUDR combined with systemic irinotecan (CPT-11) (25) in 46 previously treated patients (45% had previous CPT-11) reported a response rate of 74%, a time to progression of 8.1 months, and a median survival of 20 months. Thirteen of the sixteen patients with prior

CPT-11 exposure responded to this regimen. The maximum tolerated dose (MTD) for patients who did not undergo cryosurgery was 100 mg/m² of irinotecan weekly for 3 of 4 weeks with concurrent HAI – FUDR (0.16 mg/kg/d × pump volume/flow rate) plus Dex for 14 days of a 28-day cycle.

A second Phase I study examined concurrent systemic oxaliplatin (Oxali) plus FU/LV or Oxali plus CPT-11 along with HAI – FUDR/Dex in 36 previously treated patients (74% had received prior CPT-11). The observed response rate in 21 patients treated with Oxali/CPT-11/HAI-FUDR was 90%, with a median survival of 36 months, and a 1-year survival of 90% (26). The MTD for the Oxali/irinotecan/HAI – FUDR combination was Oxali 100 mg/m² every 2 weeks, irinotecan 150 mg/m² every 2 weeks, and FUDR 0.12 mg/kg × 30 ml divided by pump flow rate administered over 14 days with Dex 25 mg, followed by 2-week infusion of heparinized saline. For the group of 15 patients treated with Oxali/FU/LV/HAI-FUDR, the observed response rate was 87%. The MTD for the Oxali/FU/LV combination was Oxali 100 mg/m², LV 400 mg/m², and FU 1400 mg/m² by continuous infusion over 48 hours (700 mg/m²/day). FUDR was administered as described for the Oxali/irinotecan combination group.

Response rates from these Phase I trials of combination therapy with HAI – FUDR and new systemic agents are encouraging and compare favorably to results in the second-line setting obtained with systemic chemotherapy alone or HAI-FUDR alone (Table 21.2). These results compare favorably, even in the first-line setting (Table 21.3).

In the future, randomized studies comparing HAI or HAI plus new agents versus the new agents alone would be appropriate, both in the first- and in the second-line setting.

BORDERLINE RESECTABILITY

Further evidence of the clinical utility of HAI-FUDR comes from trials evaluating resectability rates in patients with colon cancer and liver only metastases initially considered unresectable or not optimally resectable.

For appropriate interpretation of these results, one should remember that resection is only possible in about 85% of patients with clinically resectable liver metastases (27). Even in patients who undergo neoadjuvant chemotherapy despite harboring clinically resectable liver metastases, resection rates are 80%. This has been shown in a prospective study of neoadjuvant chemotherapy with FU/LV and oxaliplatin in 20 patients with primarily resectable liver metastases of colorectal cancer in whom resectability was only 80% (28).

With this background, prospective uncontrolled trials evaluating neoadjuvant systemic chemotherapy with new active drugs in the first-line setting for unresectable liver metastases from colorectal cancer have shown resectability rates of 10% to 37.5% (Table 21.3). These studies share methodological concerns about whether the same criteria of resectability were applied before and after neoadjuvant chemotherapy. For example, the study by Alberts (29) showed 33% resectability rate after intravenous infusional 5FU and oxaliplatin (FOLFOX); however, on independent review, 10% of these patients were considered to be resectable prior to chemotherapy. Prospective randomized trials of systemic chemotherapy for patients with metastatic colorectal cancer in the first-line setting have also reported retrospectively determined resectability rates. For example, Tournigand (30) reported 22% resectability rate for FOLFOX and 9% resectability rate for intravenous infusional 5FU and irinotecan (FOLFIRI), and Hurwitz (31) reported 2% resectability rate for IFL. Of note, these trials do include patients with liver-only metastatic disease plus patients with extrahepatic disease, perhaps explaining the low resectability rates. An interesting retrospective study was reported by Masi (32) on 74 patients with unresectable metastatic colorectal cancer. These patients were treated with FOLFOXIRI in the first-line setting, and a secondary operation could be performed in 26% of the patients.

In the second-line setting, FOLFOX has shown resectability rates of 0%, despite response rate of 33% as shown by a retrospective study (33).

On the other hand, HAI-FUDR as a single agent (0.2 mg/kg/day for 14 days) with Dex 20 mg for patients with liver-only unresectable disease from colorectal cancer has shown a response rate of 39% and resectability rate of 26% in 23 patients evaluated in the second-line setting (Table 21.4) (34). Metastases were believed to be unresectable on the basis of multifocality alone (more than five metastases) in 15 cases and the need for an extensive resection associated with a high risk of postoperative liver failure in eight cases. Patients received a median of three cycles of

TABLE 21.2 Efficacy of Hepatic Arterial Infusion (HAI) of FUDR, Systemic Therapy or Both in Previously Treated Patients with Isolated Hepatic Metastases from CRC: Second-line Therapy

Regimen (Ref.)	N	Response Rate (CR + PR) (%)	TTP (mo.)	Comments
HAI alone				
FUDR alone (55)	49	33	–	RR 62% (after first-line adjuvant) RR 23% (after first-line metastatic)
FUDR + Mit + BCNU (55)	45	47	–	RR 50% (after first-line adjuvant) RR 47% (after first-line metastatic)
FUDR + LV + Dex (56)	29	52	–	72% doubled alkaline phosphatase at 6 mo.
Mit + FUDR + Dex (57)	37	70	–	Biliary sclerosis 9.5%
SYS alone				
CPT-11 (58) (75% liver mets)	166	11	3.9	Prior treatment for mets: 70% Prior treatment adjuvant: 28%
Erbitux (78)	111	11	1.5	100% had received CPT-11 and
CPT-11 + Erbitux (78)	218	23	4.1	63% had received oxaliplatin
Oxaliplatin (59) (59% liver mets)	156	1.3	1.6	100% had received IFL RECIST criteria (independent review)
FOLFOX (59) (81% liver mets)	152	10	4.6	
FOLFOX (59) (75.9% liver mets)	271	8.6	4.7 (PFS)	Prior treatment with fluoropyrimidine and CPT11 required.
Bev (60) (70.8% liver mets)	230	3.3	2.7 (PFS)	
FOLFOX + Bev (60) (73.4% liver mets)	271	22.7	7.3 (PFS)	RECIST criteria (no independent review)
Erbitux + Bev (61)	40	20	4	Progression on irinotecan containing regimen.
CPT-11 + Erbitux + Bev (61)	41	37	5.8	
SYS alone (liver-only mets)				
FOLFOX 4	15	33	6.2	
HAI + SYS				
FUDR + Dex + SYS – CPT-11 (25)	38	74	8.1	45% had prior CPT-11. Response by WHO criteria.
FUDR + Dex + SYS Oxali/CPT-11 (26)	21	90	16.4 (hepatic) 16.9 (extrahepatic)	74% had prior CPT-11. Response by WHO criteria.
FUDR + Dex + SYS – Oxali/FU/LV (26)	15	87	9.4 (hepatic) 10.8 (eh)	

HAI, Hepatic arterial infusion; SYS, systemic; FUDR, floxuridine; CRC, colorectal cancer; RR, response rate; CR, complete response; PR, partial response; Mit, Mitomycin C; LV, leucovorin; Dex, dexamethasone; Oxali, oxaliplatin; FU, 5-fluorouracil; Bev, bevacizumab; RECIST, response evaluation criteria in solid tumors; WHO, World Health Organization; PFS, progression-free survival; N, number of patients.

TABLE 21.3 Prospective Trials Evaluating Neoadjuvant Systemic Chemotherapy for Unresectable Disease: Resectability Rate in First-line Setting

Investigator (Ref.)	Treatment	N	Resectability Rate (%)	Comments
Pozzo (62)	FOLFIRI	40	32.5	Number and size of metastases were criteria for unresectability
Alberts (63)	FOLFOX	42	33	10% patients resectable by independent surgical review prior to chemotherapy
Quenet (64)	Oxali/CPT-11/FU/LV	24	37.5	Patients with uncertain resectability included
Abad (65)	Oxali/CPT-11/FU	47	26	Surgery possible in 40% of patients with liver-only mets
Ho (66)	FOLFIRI	40	10	87% unresectable because of bilobar disease
Wein (67)	FU/LV	53	11	Only 41% of the patients had liver-only disease

TABLE 21.4 Initially Unresectable Disease: Resectability Rate after HAI ± Systemic Therapy

	HAI ± SYS	N	Previous Chemo (%)	Response	Resection Rate
FUDR Based					
Clavien (68)	HAI-FUDR+ Dex + LV	23	100 (86% CPT-11)	39%	26%
Kemeny (69)	HAI-FUDR + Dex SYS-CPT-11 + Oxali	47	55	81%	43%
Non-FUDR Based					
Noda (36)	HAI-FU SYS-UFT	51	–	78%	47%
Carnaghi (77)	HAI-FU SYS-Oxali/LV	39	50	41%	21%
Zelek (70)	HAI pirarubin SYS-FU + LV + CPT-11	31	0	48%	29%
Bouchahda (39)	HAI-Oxali/CPT-11/FU*	28	100	32%	7%

FUDR. Among the six resected patients, one died at 18 months and five remained alive with follow-up ranging from 20 months to 5 years. Only one patient experienced a recurrence in the liver that was treated with RFA, remaining disease-free after 2-year follow-up.

Combination of HAI-FUDR+Dex with systemic irinotecan and Oxali has shown 86% response rate and 30% resection rate in 44 patients initially considered unresectable, 78% of them treated in the second-line setting (35). No systemic therapy has reported such response rates or resectability rates in the second-line setting.

Resection rates after HAI of drugs other than FUDR in combination with systemic chemotherapy have also been reported (Table 21.4). Noda (36) reported on 51 patients treated with HAI of FU for two consecutive days per week and oral uracil/tegafur (UFT) for 5 days per week for 6 months. At completion of treatment, 61% of patients were considered clinically resectable, but only 24 patients agreed on hepatectomy. Resected patients had a 5-year survival rate of 42%. Garassino (37) tested concomitant systemic Oxali (85 mg/m^2 day 1), folinic acid (FA) (75 mg/m^2 day 1, 2) followed by HAI of FU (300 mg/m^2 bolus day 1, 2 and 22-hour HAI of FU 1200 mg/m^2) in an every 2-week cycle in 39 patients with colorectal liver metastases (49% chemonaive). A catheter was used for HAI, with 28% rate of early discontinuation. In 34 assessable patients, response rate was 41% (53% for chemonaive and 29% in pre-treated patients). Resectability rate was 15%. Median overall survival was 22 months. Zelek (38) treated 31 patients with non-resectable hepatic metastases from colorectal cancer with systemic FOLFIRI and

HAI of pirarubicin. HAI was administered via a per-cutaneous catheter. A partial response was observed in 48% of the patients. The authors questioned the additive effect of HAI pirarubicin. A curative resection (R0) was possible in nine patients. In patients with R0, median progression-free survival was 20.2 months, whereas it was 4.2 months in the other patients. Bouchahda (39) used a combination regimen of irinotecan, Oxali and 5-FU, all administered by HAI, using a multi-channel pump. Irinotecan 160 mg/m^2 was administered day 1, oxaliplatin 20 mg/m^2 day 2 through 5 and 5-FU 600 mg/m^2/d day 2– through 5 in four 21-day courses. All 28 patients had received at least one prior chemotherapy regimen. Response rate was 32% in 25 assessable patients. A curative resection was possible in two patients. Main toxicities include grade 3 to 4 diarrhea in 21% of patients and grade 3 to 4 vomiting in 14% of patients. Treatment was discontinued for thrombosis in six patients and grade 3 abdominal pain in three patients.

This evidence suggests that the combination of systemic chemotherapy with new agents and HAI chemotherapy can result in high response rates and resectability in patients with initially unresectable liver-only metastases. More importantly, it has been shown that long-term survival is possible for patients who are down-staged with systemic chemotherapy to a point where curative resection is feasible (40). Therefore, although in metastatic disease not amenable to surgical resection, increased response rates do not necessarily imply survival benefit, the scenario of liver-only metastases should be considered independently, and response rates and, more specifically, resectability rates may be considered reasonable endpoints. Definite proof of this concept should come from clinical trials. Well-designed trials for patients with initially unresectable metastatic disease to the liver comparing treatment with optimal systemic chemotherapy versus the combination of optimal systemic chemotherapy and HAI – FUDR are needed. Optimal clinical trial design to appropriately evaluate response rates, resectability rates and survival in this scenario should consider the following: (1) overall survival as the primary end-point; (2) inclusion of patients with liver-only metastatic disease; (3) predefined setting, either first-line treatment or second-line treatment; (4) predefined criteria for unresectability to be applied both before neoadjuvant chemotherapy and after neoadjuvant chemotherapy; (4) prospective determination of resectability done by an experienced liver surgeon, blind to chemotherapy status, ideally with independent surgical review of resectability; (5) predefined studies and timing for re-evaluation of resectability status, considering median time to response; (6) testing of the most active chemotherapy combinations in terms of response in a randomized fashion.

ADJUVANT TREATMENT AFTER RESECTION OF LIVER METASTASES

Predictors of recurrence and survival after resection of liver metastases have been analyzed and a clinical risk score has been developed (9). Adverse prognostic factors include a node-positive primary, disease-free interval from primary to metastases less than 12 months, more than one hepatic tumor, largest tumor greater than 5 cm and carcinoembryonic antigen (CEA) level greater than 200 ng/ml. Five-year survival rates for resected patients are approximately 30%. Patients with zero risk factors have a 60% 5-year survival versus 18% with five risk factors. Only the minority of patients will achieve cure with resection alone, and the need of adjuvant treatment is evident. Patterns of recurrence after liver resection of colorectal cancer metastases have been reported: the liver is involved in 43% of the resected cases, while extra-hepatic recurrence is observed in 60% of resected patients (41). Patterns of recurrence appear to vary depending on number of liver lesions and other primary tumor characteristics. For patients with a single lesion treated with a wedge resection, the site of first disease progression is the liver in 30% of the patients, whereas liver and extrahepatic recurrences are observed in 13% of patients and extrahepatic recurrences only are observed in 17% of patients (42).

For patients with multiple liver tumors, the most frequent site of initial recurrence was the lung in 32% of the patients, followed by the liver in 28% of the patients and by multiple recurrence sites in 17% of the patients (43). No randomized trial of adjuvant systemic chemotherapy vs. surgery alone after curative resection of liver metastases from colorectal origin has demonstrated statistically significant overall survival benefit. Improved disease-free survival (DFS) has been shown in a recently reported multicenter randomized trial comparing adjuvant chemotherapy to surgery alone (44). Patients randomized to chemotherapy received FA (200 mg/m^2) and bolus FU (400 mg/m^2) each day for 5 consecutive days every 28 days for six cycles. Follow-up was performed every 3 months for 2 years and then once per year until death or until the end of the study. Follow-up included clinical examination, abdominal ultrasonography, chest x-rays, and CEA. Computed tomography was reserved only for cases with abnormal findings in previously mentioned studies. Intention to treat analysis was based on 171 patients. The 5-year DFS rate, after adjustment for major prognostic factors, was 33.5% for patients in the chemotherapy group and 26.7% in the control group (odds ratio for recurrence or death = 0.66, 95% CI 0.46—0.96, p = 0.028). A trend toward increased overall survival did not reach statistical significance: 5-year overall survival was 51.1% in the chemotherapy group and 41.1% in the control group (odds ratio for death = 0.73, 95% CI, 0.48 – 1.10; p = 0.13. The authors discussed reasons for a failed impact in overall survival: (1) Sample size was not calculated to demonstrate an overall survival benefit, as it was a secondary endpoint. (2) The study was further underpowered as it closed prematurely due to low accrual. (3) A suboptimal regimen, which was standard when the trial initiated, was used. (4) Treatment of recurrences with second-line chemotherapy or repeat liver resections, made it difficult to identify the effect of adjuvant chemotherapy on overall survival.

Of note, a pooled analysis of individual patient data from 18 randomized phase III colon cancer adjuvant trials including 20,898 patients has demonstrated that DFS and overall survival are highly correlated, and DFS may be an appropriate endpoint for adjuvant colon cancer clinical trials (45). However, whether this applies to trials of adjuvant chemotherapy after liver resection of metastases is not known. A second randomized trial could not demonstrate any survival advantage in DFS or in overall survival. The study by Langer (46) randomized 129 patients to be treated by adjuvant chemotherapy after metastasectomy or chemotherapy in the event of recurrent disease after resection of metastatic disease. Chemotherapy consisted of LV and bolus 5-FU daily for 5 days, every 4 weeks for 6 months. This trial was also closed prematurely due to slow accrual. The group randomized to adjuvant chemotherapy experienced median DFS of 39 months and median overall survival of 53 months, compared with median DFS of 20 months and median overall survival of 43 months in the control group. Hazard ratio (adjuvant chemotherapy vs. control) for DFS was 1.28 (95% CI 0.76–2.14, p = 0.35); and hazard ratio for overall survival was 1.3 (0.71–2.36, p = 0.39). Lack of statistical significance in observed survival differences may be attributed to incomplete accrual, resulting in an underpowered study.

Randomized adjuvant studies with HAI after liver resection for liver metastases from colorectal cancer have also been conducted with variable results. As in the setting of unresectable disease, these trials have important differences in terms of the primary endpoint, power to detect statistically significant differences in the selected endpoint, drug used for HAI, device used for HAI, actual duration of treatment, whether or not combination with systemic chemotherapy was allowed in the experimental and control arms, time of randomization (preoperative vs. intraoperative) and actual proportion of patients treated. Results of these studies are summarized in Table 21.5.

The first reported trial was that of Lorenz et al (47). Patients were treated with HAI of 5-FU plus FA for 5 days, every 28 days for 6 months. The control arm was assigned to observation alone. A port was used. In the treatment group, the average number of cycles received was four. Randomization was preoperative: 108 to adjuvant therapy and 111 to resection only. Twenty-four patients in the HAI group and 13 patients in the control group did not receive the assigned treatment. Of the 84 patients that initiated treatment as randomized, only 73 of them had chemotherapy data for analysis. A curative resection was possible in 88.7% of 226 randomized patients. Survival was the primary endpoint. Median survival was 34.5 months for the HAI group vs. 40.8 months for the control group (p = 0.1519). The trial was stopped early because it was considered that the chances to detect a survival benefit were low. Treated patients actually had an increase in DFS versus those receiving no therapy.

Kemeny et al. conducted a second randomized trial (48), with significant differences in clinical trial design and results. The study was performed in a single center and was powered to demonstrate a 2-year overall survival benefit for patients treated with the combination of systemic chemotherapy (bolus 5-FU 325 mg/m^2/d for 5 days, preceded daily by LV 200 mg/m^2, every 4 weeks for six cycles) and HAI of FUDR (0.25 mg/kg/day + 20 mg of Dex + 50,000 UI of heparin for 14 days, pump emptied at day 14, and 1-week rest before next cycle, for a total of six cycles) over patients treated with systemic chemotherapy alone (5-FU 370 mg/m^2/d for 5 days every 4 weeks for six cycles). Pretreated patients with 5-FU and LV received 5-FU alone at a higher dose through a continuous infusion in both arms (850 mg/m^2 for 5 days every 5 weeks in the combined treatment arm and

TABLE 21.5 Adjuvant Therapy after Liver Resection: Randomized Trials of HAI versus SYS or Control

Ref.	No.	3-Year Survival (%)		5-Year Survival (%)	
		HAI	SYS or Control	HAI	SYS or Control
Lorenz (47)	201*	50	50	50	30
Kemeny (48)	156	70	60	59	46
Tono (72)	19	78	50	78	50
Kemeny (73)	75[†]	70	70	60	35[¶]
Lygidakis (74)	122	80	71	73	60
Asahara (75)	38	100	60	100	47[‡]
Kusonoki (76)[§]	58	78	30	60	30

HAI, Hepatic arterial infusion; SYS, systemic; N, number of patients
*Treated patients, not everyone randomized.
[†]Patients entered in study, not everyone randomized.
[‡]4-Year survival.
[¶]Updated figures (116).
[§]Non-randomized.

1000 mg/m^2 for 5 days in the monotherapy arm). Randomization was done intraoperatively, after successful liver resection, and stratification was done by number of liver metastases and treatment history. A pump was used for delivery of HAI of FUDR. The 156 patients who underwent complete resection of hepatic metastases from colorectal cancer were randomized to combination treatment (74 patients) or to systemic chemotherapy alone (82 patients). Of note, 514 patients were initially considered for liver resection, but 128 patients were found ineligible as unresectable metastases, extrahepatic disease or both were detected. Additional, 230 patients did not participate for other reasons: 105 patients declined, 28 had previously received fluorouracil and LV (an initial exclusion criteria), 13 lived far away from the treatment center, 11 had poor arterial supply to the liver, 16 were not considered appropriate for the protocol, 5 had had prior hepatic resection, 3 had no tumor, 35 were excluded as result of the surgeon's decision and 14 were excluded for miscellaneous reasons. The study was positive for its primary endpoint. The actuarial 2-year overall survival rate was 86% in the combination arm and 72% in the monotherapy arm (p = 0.03). Median survival was 72.2 months in the combined-therapy arm and 59.3 months in the monotherapy arm.

Of note, the impact on survival free of hepatic progression was more pronounced than the impact on overall progression-free survival. Median survival free of hepatic progression had not been reached in the combination treatment arm and was 42.7 months in the monotherapy arm, after a median follow-up of 62.7 months. Median overall progression-free survival was 37.4 months in the combined therapy group and 17.2 months in the monotherapy group (p = 0.07). These results have been updated after a median follow-up of 10.3 years (49). Secondary endpoints have been re-evaluated. Overall progression-free survival is now significantly greater in the combined-therapy group than in the monotherapy group (31.3 vs. 17.2 months, p = 0.02). The median survival free of hepatic progression has not yet been reached in the combined therapy group and is 32.5 months in the monotherapy group (p < 0.01). Median overall survival is now 68.4 months in the combination group and 58.8 months in the monotherapy group (p = 0.10). Ten-year survival was 41% in the HAI + systemic treatment group and 27% in the systemic alone group. Of note, patients with highest risk of recur-

rence appeared to derive the greatest benefit from combination treatment. Patients with a high clinical risk score (35) had a median survival of 60 months if assigned to combination treatment and 38.3 months if assigned to monotherapy (p = 0.13) and a 10-year survival rate of 38.7% in the combined-therapy group and 16.3% in the monotherapy group. Overall, this trial demonstrated that improvement in survival with combination of systemic chemotherapy and HAI of FUDR over systemic chemotherapy alone was possible, basically through decreasing the rate of hepatic recurrence.

A third trial conducted in Japan randomized 19 patients intraoperatively to receive adjuvant treatment with HAI of 5-FU for 4 days, 3 days rest to complete 6 weeks of treatment (50). A port was used. Primary endpoint was not specified, and observed median DFS was 62.6 months after hepatectomy in the HAI group and 13.8 months in the control group. Median survival was 62.6 months in the HAI group and 39.9 months in the control group. The 1-, 3- and 5-year cumulative survival rates in the HAI group were 88.9%, 77.8% and 77.8%, respectively and 100%, 50% and 50%, respectively, in the control groups (p = 0.2686).

The Eastern Cooperative Oncology Group conducted a multicenter randomized trial limited to patients with one to three resectable liver metastases from colorectal cancer (51). The study was powered to evaluate improvement in time to recurrence and hepatic disease-free survival. The control arm received no further therapy. The experimental arm received postoperative HAI of FUDR, 14 days on and 14 days off, for a maximum of four cycles (starting at 0.1 mg/kg/d or 0.05 mg/kg/d if the patient had had a lobectomy, and doubling the dose in subsequent cycles to a maximum of 0.2 mg/kg/d if no significant toxicity was observed) and systemic chemotherapy with 5-FU at 200 mg/m^2/d as a 14-day continuous infusion during the days of rest of HAI and for additional eight cycles after completion of HAI infusion at 300 mg/m^2/d, 14 days on, 14 days off. Randomization was done preoperatively, and patients found ineligible after randomization were excluded from the analysis (non-intention-to-treat analysis). A pump was used for HAI. Of 109 patients randomized, 75 patients were considered assessable: 45 in the control group and 30 in the chemotherapy group. After a median follow-up of 51 months, the 4-year recurrence-free rate was 25.2% in the control arm and 45.7% in the chemotherapy arm (p = 0.04) and the liver-recurrence-free rate was 43% in the control arm and 66.9% in the chemotherapy arm (p = 0.03). Median survival of assessable patients was 49.4 months in the control arm and 63.7 months in the chemotherapy arm (p = 0.6). Lack of survival benefit was explained in terms of insufficient sample size and possible subsequent treatment including re-resection and pump placement in the control arm.

Other authors have compared systemic immunotherapy with mitomycin-C, 5-FU, folinic acid and interleukin-2 (IL-2) versus the same regimen administered half dose through the HA and half dose systemically in 122 patients in a randomized study (52). Median survival for the systemic therapy arm was 66 months whereas median survival for the combined locoregional and systemic arm was 79 months (log rank, p = 0.04). The combination of oral uracil/tegafur (UFT) vs. oral UFT with HAI of 5-FU has also been tested in a non-randomized study conducted in Japan, where UFT is a popular adjuvant treatment after liver resection. An improvement in cumulative 5-year survival rate was reported for the combination arm: 59% for the combination arm and 27% for UFT alone (p = 0.00001) (53).

In conclusion, adjuvant therapy after liver resection is useful. HAI – FUDR/Dex and systemic chemotherapy can improve overall survival over systemic chemotherapy alone. Improvements in systemic 5-FU chemotherapy for metastatic disease have resulted in clinical trials testing the addition of irinotecan or Oxali to adjuvant 5-FU-based chemotherapy after resection. The addition of Oxali has resulted in an improvement of disease-free survival after primary colon resection. It needs to be seen whether this combination will improve results after liver resection. Trials with HAI – FUDR/Dex plus new systemic agents are ongoing. The National Surgical Adjuvant Breast and Bowel Project (NSABP) is testing HAI – FUDR plus systemic Oxali and capecitabine vs. systemic alone.

DOSING AND ADJUSTMENT ALGORITHMS

Here, we summarize our recommendations regarding dose adjustment for HAI of FUDR to minimize biliary toxicity. Clinical trials have traditionally used a 14-day HAI of FUDR followed by a 2-week or 3-

week period of rest. For calculating FUDR dosing, it is important to remember that a pump has a fixed volume and a fixed flow rate. At the authors' institution, 30-ml pumps are used. The flow rate is variable from pump to pump and is determined at time of laparotomy when priming the pump. The average pump has a flow rate of 1.2 ml/day. On day 14, when the pump must be emptied of the drug, a residual volume of 16 ml to 17 ml will be obtained. During the rest period, the pump is filled with heparinized saline to ensure pump patency. If the pump is not to be used for longer periods of time, filling it with glycerol can ensure patency for up to 6 weeks. Liver function tests must be obtained every 2 weeks, when the pump is filled and when the pump is emptied. Results on both dates are considered to make the decision whether the patient needs dose reductions or even dose interruptions, following the schema shown in Table 21.6. The algorithm to recommence treatment after hold is shown in Table 21.7 Of note, the alkaline phosphatase is considered the most sensible indicator of biliary toxicity. If patient develops a total bilirubin ≥3.0 mg/dl, the pump should be emptied and Dex 20 mg plus heparin 30,000 U and saline 30 ml placed in the pump q 14 days. Once there is no longer evidence of toxicity, Dex dose should be tapered in increments of 5 mg every 14 days. Tapering will continue unless enzymes increase. FUDR should be permanently discontinued unless there is evidence of disease progression (increasing CEA, worsening CT scan, worsening clinical status) AND bilirubin has returned to ≤1.5 mg/dl. In this case, FUDR can be restarted as follows: Use 25% of the last FUDR dose given with Dex, heparin and saline in the pump for 7 days. Pump should be emptied after 7 days, and patients given a 3-week rest period. This treatment and treatment schedule should continue as long as bilirubin remains ≤1.5 mg/dl and liver enzyme values do not increase.

There are two forms in which the FUDR dose can be calculated and expressed in literature. The reader must be aware to avoid misinterpretations. We recommend the second formula, which considers pump flow rate.

First formula (pump flow rate is not considered)

FUDR mg × kg × 14

Example: 70-kg patient. Dosing 0.2 mg/kg/d

0.2 mg × 70 kg × 14 days = 196 mg

TABLE 21.6 FUDR Dose-modification Schema

	Reference Value*	% FUDR Dose
SGOT (at pump emptying or day of planned retreatment, whichever is higher)	0 to <2 × reference value	100
	2 to <3 × reference value	80
	3 to <4 × reference value	50
	>4 × reference value	Hold[a]
ALK PHOS (at pump emptying or day of planned retreatment, whichever is higher)	0 to <1.2 × reference value	100
	1.2 to <1.5 × reference value	50
	>1.5 × reference value	Hold[b]
TOT BILI (at pump emptying or day of planned retreatment, whichever is higher)	0 to <1.2 × reference value	100
	1.2 to <1.5 × reference value	50
	>1.5 × reference value	Hold[c]

If SGOT >4 × reference value, alkaline phosphatase >1.5 × reference value, total bilirubin >1.5 × reference value, then treatment will be held and will not be reinstituted until values come down to more normal levels, as indicated in section "Recommencing FUDR Treatment After Hold."

[a]SGOT elevation, [b]alkaline phosphatase elevation, [c]total bilirubin elevation.

*Reference value is the value obtained on the day the patient received last FUDR dose. To determine if an FUDR dose modification is necessary, compare reference value to either the value obtained on the day the pump was emptied or on day of planned pump filling, whichever is higher.

NOTE: If alkaline phosphatase or total bilirubin shows a continual rise from day 1 of treatment, then the day 1 value will be used as the reference value for that patient when determining whether to hold treatment, and time of re-treatment after hold.

Second formula (the pump flow rate is taken into consideration)

FUDR mg × kg × pump volume (30 ml)/pump flow rate (ml/d)

Example: 70-kg patient. Dosing 0.12 mg × 70 × 30 = 252/1.2 (pump flow rate) = 210 mg

CONCLUSION

Colon cancer metastatic to the liver has become one of the best examples of how a multi-modality approach can improve patients' outcomes. Input from surgeons, medical oncologists, radiologists, interventional radiologists, radiation oncologists and gastroenterologists is necessary for making the best treatment decisions regarding patients with colorectal cancer metastatic to the liver. We have presented evidence that specialists in liver-directed chemotherapy need to join the multi-disciplinary team in order to improve treatment results. The state of the art is dynamic and improvements in surgical techniques, ablation techniques, systemic chemotherapy and regional therapy are continuous and demand constant re-evaluation of the relative benefit of each of these treatments in relation to the others. Regional chemotherapy is not the exception. However, we have presented evidence that improvements in systemic chemotherapy do not mitigate benefits of regional therapy. Rather, these two forms of treatment can be safely combined, and the combination effectively improves the results of each individual treatment. Randomized controlled trials with updated treatment strategies for patients with unresectable disease, borderline resectability or in the adjuvant setting after liver resection of metastases from colorectal cancer are encouraged.

Finally, the identification of new drugs suitable for HAI may be another way of improving regional therapy. A clear understanding of ideal pharmacokinetic characteristics is necessary for better selection of

TABLE 21.7 Recommencing Treatment after Hold

Reason for Treatment Delay	Chemotherapy Resumed When Value Has Returned to:	% FUDR Dose
SGOT elevation	2 × reference value	25% of last dose
Alkaline phosphatase elevation	1.2 × reference value	25% of last dose
Total bilirubin elevation	1.2 × reference value	25% of last dose

drugs to be tested in the HAI model. Systematic determination of clearance and hepatic extraction rates for candidate drugs is mandatory. Only in this way may the spectrum of drugs useful through HAI increase and ultimately improve treatment results in terms of efficacy and toxicity.

REFERENCES

1. Weiss L, Grundmann E, Torhorst J, et al. Haematogenous metastatic patterns in colonic carcinoma: An analysis of 1541 necropsies. J Pathol, 1986 Nov; 150(3): 195–203.

2. Kemeny N, Kemeny M, and Lawrence TS. Liver Metastases. In: Abeloff AJ, Niederhuber JE, and Kastan MB et al. (eds) Clinical Oncology, pp. 1141–1178. Philadelphia: Elsevier, 2004.

3. Imamura H, Matsuyama Y, Shimada R, et al. A study of factors influencing prognosis after resection of hepatic metastases from colorectal and gastric carcinoma. Am J Gastroenterol, 2001 Nov; 96(11): 3178–3184.

4. Sigurdson ER, Ridge JA, Kemeny N, et al. Tumor and liver drug uptake following hepatic artery and portal vein infusion. J Clin Oncol, 1987; 5(11): 1836–1840.

5. Allen PJ, Nissan A, Picon AI, et al. Technical complications and durability of hepatic artery infusion pumps for unresectable colorectal liver metastases: An institutional experience of 544 consecutive cases. J Am Coll Surg, 2005; 201(1): 57–65.

6. Ruers TJ, Langenhoff BS, Neeleman N, et al. Value of positron emission tomography with [F-18]fluoro-deoxyglucose in patients with colorectal liver metastases: A prospective study. J Clin Oncol, 2002; 20(2): 388–395.

7. Adam R, Laurent A, Azoulay D, et al. Two-stage hepatectomy: A planned strategy to treat irresectable liver tumors. Ann Surg, 2000; 232(6): 777–785.

8. Nordlinger B, Vaillant JC, Guiguet M, et al. Survival benefit of repeat liver resections for recurrent colorectal metastases: 143 cases. Association Francaise de Chirurgie. J Clin Oncol, 1994; 12(7): 1491–1496.

9. Fong Y, Fortner J, Sun RL, et al. Clinical score for predicting recurrence after hepatic resection for metastatic colorectal cancer: Analysis of 1001 consecutive cases. Ann Surg, 1999; 230(3): 309–318; discussion 318–321.

10. Lorenz M and Muller HH. Randomized, multicenter trial of fluorouracil plus leucovorin administered either via hepatic arterial or intravenous infusion versus fluorodeoxyuridine administered via hepatic arterial infusion in patients with nonresectable liver metastases from colorectal carcinoma. J Clin Oncol, 2000; 18(2): 243–254.

11. Kemeny NE, Niedzwiecki D, Hollis DR, et al. Hepatic arterial infusion versus systemic therapy for hepatic metastases from colorectal cancer: A randomized trial of efficacy, quality of life, and molecular markers (CALGB 9481). J Clin Oncol, 2006; 24(9): 1395–1403.

12. Kemeny N, Daly J, Reichman B, et al. Intrahepatic or systemic infusion of fluorodeoxyuridine in patients with liver metastases from colorectal carcinoma: A randomized trial. Ann Intern Med, 1987; 107(4): 459–465.

13. Chang AE, Schneider PD, Sugarbaker PH, et al. A prospective randomized trial of regional versus systemic continuous 5-fluorodeoxyuridine chemotherapy in the treatment of colorectal liver metastases. Ann Surg, 1987; 206(6): 685–693.

14. Hohn DC, Stagg RJ, Friedman MA, et al. A randomized trial of continuous intravenous versus hepatic intraarterial floxuridine in patients with colorectal cancer metastatic to the liver: The Northern California Oncology Group trial. J Clin Oncol, 1989; 7(11): 1646–1654.

15. Wagman LD, Kemeny MM, Leong L, et al. A prospective, randomized evaluation of the treatment of colorectal cancer metastatic to the liver. J Clin Oncol, 1990; 8(11): 1885–1893.

16. Martin JK Jr, O'Connell MJ, Wieand HS, et al. Intra-arterial floxuridine vs. systemic fluorouracil for hepatic metastases from colorectal cancer: A randomized trial. Arch Surg, 1990; 125(8): 1022–1027.

17. Rougier P, Laplanche A, Huguier M, et al. Hepatic arterial infusion of floxuridine in patients with liver metastases from colorectal carcinoma: Long-term results of a prospective randomized trial. J Clin Oncol, 1992; 10(7): 1112–1118.

18. Allen-Mersh TG, Earlam S, Fordy C, et al. Quality of life and survival with continuous hepatic-artery floxuridine infusion for colorectal liver metastases. Lancet, 1994; 344(8932): 1255–1260.

19. Kerr DJ, McArdle CS, Ledermann J, et al. Medical Research Council's Colorectal Cancer Study Group; European Organisation for Research and Treatment of Cancer Colorectal Cancer Study Group. Intrahepatic arterial versus intravenous fluorouracil and folinic acid for colorectal cancer liver metastases: A multicentre randomised trial. Lancet, 2003; 361(9355): 368–373.

20. Kemeny N, Steiter K, Niedzweiecki D, et al. A randomized trial of intrahepatic infusion of fluorouridine (FUDR) with dexamethasone versus FUDR alone in the treatment of metastatic colorectal cancer. Cancer, 1992; 69: 327–334.

21. Civalleri D, DeCian F, Pellicci R, et al. Differential device performances for hepatic arterial chemotherapy: A technical report on totally implantable pumps and ports for both continuous and bolus infusion. Eur Surg Res, 1998; 30(1): 26–33.

22. Strasberg SM, Dehdashti F, Siegel BA, et al. Survival of patients evaluated by FDG-PET before hepatic resection for metastatic colorectal carcinoma: A prospective database study. Ann Surg, 2001; 233(3): 293–299.

23. Rougier P, Laplanche A, Huguier M, et al. Hepatic arterial infusion of floxuridine in patients with liver metastases from colorectal carcinoma: Long-term results of a prospective randomized trial. J Clin Oncol, 1992; 10(7): 1112–1118.

24. Kemeny N, Seiter K, Niedzwiecki D, et al. A randomized trial of intrahepatic infusion of fluorodeoxyuridine with dexamethasone versus fluorodeoxyuridine alone in the treatment of metastatic colorectal cancer. Cancer, 1992; 69(2): 327–334.

25. Kemeny N, Gonen M, Sullivan D, et al. Phase I study of hepatic arterial infusion of floxuridine and dexamethasone with systemic irinotecan for unresectable hepatic metastases from colorectal cancer. J Clin Oncol, 2001; 19(10): 2687–2695.

26. Kemeny N, Jarnagin W, Paty P, et al. Phase I trial of systemic oxaliplatin combination chemotherapy with hepatic
arterial infusion in patients with unresectable liver metastases from colorectal cancer. J Clin Oncol, 2005; 23(22):
4888–4896.

27. Allen PJ, Kemeny N, Jarnagin W, et al. Importance of
response to neoadjuvant chemotherapy in patients undergoing resection of synchronous colorectal liver metastases. J Gastrointest Surg, 2003; 7(1): 109–115; discussion
116–117.

28. Wein A, Riedel C, Brückl W, et al. Neoadjuvant treatment
with weekly high-dose 5-fluorouracil as 24-hour infusion, folinic acid and oxaliplatin in patients with primary
resectable liver metastases of colorectal cancer. Oncology,
2003; 64(2): 131–138.

29. Alberts SR, Horvath WL, Sternfeld WC, et al. Oxaliplatin, fluorouracil, and leucovorin for patients with unresectable liver-only metastases from colorectal cancer: A
North Central Cancer Treatment Group phase II study.
J Clin Oncol, 2005; 23(36): 9243–9249.

30. Tournigand C, André T, Achille E, et al. FOLFIRI followed by FOLFOX6 or the reverse sequence in advanced
colorectal cancer: A randomized GERCOR study. J Clin
Oncol, 2004; 22(2): 229–237.

31. Hurwitz H, Fehrenbacher L, Novotny W, et al. Bevacizumab plus irinotecan, fluorouracil, and leucovorin for
metastatic colorectal cancer. N Engl J Med, 2004; 350(23):
2335–2342.

32. Masi G, Cupini S, Marcucci L, et al. Treatment with
5-fluorouracil/folinic acid, oxaliplatin, and irinotecan
enables surgical resection of metastases in patients with
initially unresectable metastatic colorectal cancer. Ann
Surg Oncol, 2006; 13(1): 58–65.

33. Gaspar EM, Artigas V, Montserrat E, et al. Single-centre
study of L-OHP/5-FU/LV before liver surgery in patients
with NOT optimally resectable colorectal cancer isolated
liver metastases. ASCO Annual Meeting, 2003, American
Society of Clinical Oncology, Chicago, Illinois.

34. Clavien PA, Selzner N, Morse M, et al. Downstaging of
hepatocellular carcinoma and liver metastases from colorectal cancer by selective intra-arterial chemotherapy.
Surgery, 2002; 131(4): 433–442.

35. Kemeny N, Jarnagin W, Paty P, et al. Phase I trial of systemic oxaliplatin combination chemotherapy with hepatic
arterial infusion in patients with unresectable liver metastases from colorectal cancer. J Clin Oncol, 2005; 23(22):
4888–4896.

36. Noda M, Yanagi H, Yoshikawa R, et al. Second-look hepatectomy after pharmacokinetic modulating chemotherapy (PMC) combination with hepatic arterial 5FU
infusion and oral UFT in patients with unresectable hepatic colorectal metastases. ASCO Annual Meeting, 2004,
American Society of Clinical Oncology, New Orleans,
Louisiana.

37. Garassino IC, Rimassa L, Zuradelli M, et al. Definitive results of hybrid chemotherapy with intravenous (iv)
oxaliplatin (OXA) and folinic acid (FA), and intra-hepatic
infusion (HAI) of 5-fluorouracil (5-FU) in patients with
colorectal liver metastases. ASCO Annual Meeting, 2005,
American Society of Clinical Oncology, Atlanta, Georgia.

38. Zelek L, Bugat R, Cherqui D, et al. Multimodal therapy
with intravenous biweekly leucovorin, 5-fluorouracil and

irinotecan combined with hepatic arterial infusion pirarubicin in non-resectable hepatic metastases from colorectal
cancer (a European Association for Research in Oncology
trial). Ann Oncol, 2003; 14(10): 1537–1542.

39. Bouchahda M, Adam R, Giacchetti S, et al. Effective
salvage therapy of liver-only colorectal cancer metastases with chronomodulated irinotecan-fluorouracil-
oxaliplatin via hepatic artery infusion. ASCO Annual
Meeting, 2006, American Society of Clinical Oncology,
Atlanta, Georgia.

40. Adam R, Delvart V, Pascal G, et al. Rescue surgery for
unresectable colorectal liver metastases downstaged by
chemotherapy: A model to predict long-term survival.
Ann Surg, 2004; 240(4): 644–657; discussion 657–658.

41. Topal B, Kaufman L, Aerts R, et al. Patterns of failure
following curative resection of colorectal liver metastases.
Eur J Surg Oncol, 2003 Apr;29(3):248–53.

42. White RR, Avital I, Sofocleous CT, et al. Rates and patterns of recurrence for percutaneous radiofrequency ablation and open wedge resection for solitary colorectal liver
metastasis. J Gastrointestinal Surg, 2007; 11(3): 256–263.

43. Kornprat P, Jarnagin WR, Gonen M, et al. Outcome
after hepatectomy for multiple (four or more) colorectal metastases in the era of effective chemotherapy. Ann
Surg Oncol, 2007; 14(3): 1151–1160.

44. Portier G, Elias D, Bouche O, et al. Adjuvant systemic
chemotherapy using 5-fluorouracil and folinic acid after
resection of liver metastases from colorectal origin. Proc
Am Soc Clin Oncol, 21: 2002; (abstr 528).

45. Sargent DJ, Wieand HS, Haller DG, et al. Disease-free
survival versus overall survival as a primary end point for
adjuvant colon cancer studies: individual patient data from
20,898 patients on 18 randomized trials. J Clin Oncol,
2005; 23(34): 8664–8670.

46. Langer B, Bleiberg H, Labianca R, et al. Fluorouracil
(FU) plus l-leucovorin (l-LV) versus observation after
potentially curative resection of liver or lung metas-
tases from colorectal cancer (CRC): Results of the ENG
(EORTC/NCIC CTG/GIVIO) randomized trial. ASCO
Annual Meeting, 2002, American Society of Clinical
Oncology, Orlando, Florida.

47. Lorenz M, Müller HH, Schramm H, et al. Randomized
trial of surgery versus surgery followed by adjuvant hepatic arterial infusion with 5-fluorouracil and folinic acid
for liver metastases of colorectal cancer. German Cooperative on Liver Metastases (Arbeitsgruppe Lebermetastasen). Ann Surg, 1998; 228(6): 756–762.

48. Kemeny N, Huang Y, Cohen AM, et al. Hepatic arterial infusion of chemotherapy after resection of hepatic
metastases from colorectal cancer. N Engl J Med, 1999;
341(27): 2039–2048.

49. Kemeny NE and Gonen M. Hepatic arterial infusion after
liver resection. N Engl J Med, 2005; 352(7): 734–735.

50. Tono T, Hasuike Y, Ohzato H, et al. Limited but definite efficacy of prophylactic hepatic arterial infusion
chemotherapy after curative resection of colorectal liver
metastases: A randomized study. Cancer, 2000; 88(7):
1549–1556.

51. Kemeny MM, Adak S, Gray B, et al. Combined-modality
treatment for resectable metastatic colorectal carcinoma
to the liver: Surgical resection of hepatic metastases in combination with continuous infusion of chemotherapy – an

intergroup study. J Clin Oncol, 2002; 20(6): 1499–1505.

52. Lygidakis NJ, Sgourakis G, Vlachos L, et al. Metastatic liver disease of colorectal origin: The value of locoregional immunochemotherapy combined with systemic chemotherapy following liver resection. Results of a prospective randomized study. Hepatogastroenterology, 2001; 48(42): 1685–1691.

53. Kusunoki M, Yanagi H, Noda M, et al. Results of pharmacokinetic modulating chemotherapy in combination with hepatic arterial 5-fluorouracil infusion and oral UFT after resection of hepatic colorectal metastases. Cancer, 2000; 89(6): 1228–1235.

54. Kemeny NE, Niedzwiecki D, Hollis DR, et al. Hepatic arterial infusion (HAI) versus systemic therapy for hepatic metastases from colorectal cancer; a CALGB randomized trial of efficacy, quality of life (QOL), cost effectiveness, and molecular markers. ASCO Annual Meeting, 2003, American Society of Clinical Oncology, Chicago, Illinois.

55. Kemeny N, Cohen A, Seiter K, et al. Randomized trial of hepatic arterial floxuridine, mitomycin, and carmustine versus floxuridine alone in previously treated patients with liver metastases from colorectal cancer. J Clin Oncol, 1993; 11(2): 330–335.

56. Kemeny N, Conti JA, Cohen A, et al. Phase II study of hepatic arterial floxuridine, leucovorin, and dexamethasone for unresectable liver metastases from colorectal carcinoma. J Clin Oncol, 1994; 12(11): 2288–2295.

57. Kemeny N, Eid A, Stockman J, et al. Hepatic arterial infusion of floxuridine and dexamethasone plus high-dose mitomycin C for patients with unresectable hepatic metastases from colorectal carcinoma. J Surg Oncol, 2005; 91(2): 97–101.

58. Rothenberg ML, Cox JV, DeVore RF, et al. A multicenter, phase II trial of weekly irinotecan (CPT-11) in patients with previously treated colorectal carcinoma. Cancer, 1999; 85(4): 786–795.

59. Rothenberg ML, Oza AM, Bigelow RH, et al. Superiority of oxaliplatin and fluorouracil-leucovorin compared with either therapy alone in patients with progressive colorectal cancer after irinotecan and fluorouracil-leucovorin: interim results of a phase III trial. J Clin Oncol, 2003; 21(11): 2059–2069.

60. Giantonio BJ, Catalano PJ, Meropol NJ, et al. High-dose bevacizumab improves survival when combined with FOLFOX4 in previously treated advanced colorectal cancer: Results from the Eastern Cooperative Oncology Group (ECOG) study E3200. ASCO Annual Meeting, 2005, American Society of Clinical Oncology, Orlando, Florida.

61. Saltz LB, Lenz H, Hochster H, et al. Randomized Phase II trial of cetuximab/bevacizumab/irinotecan (CBI) versus cetuximab/bevacizumab (CB) in irinotecan-refractory colorectal cancer. ASCO Annual Meeting, 2005, American Society of Clinical Oncology, Orlando, Florida.

62. Pozzo C, Basso M, Quirino M, et al. Long-term follow-up of colorectal cancer (CRC) patients treated with neoadjuvant chemotherapy with irinotecan and fluorouracil plus folinic acid (5-FU/FA) for unresectable liver metastases. ASCO Annual Meeting, 2006, American Society of Clinical Oncology, Atlanta, Georgia.

63. Alberts SR, Horvath WL, Sternfeld WC, et al. Oxaliplatin, fluorouracil, and leucovorin for patients with unresectable liver-only metastases from colorectal cancer: A North Central Cancer Treatment Group phase II study. J Clin Oncol, 2005; 23(36): 9243–9249.

64. Quenet F, Nordlinger B, Rivoire M, et al. Resection of previously unresectable liver metastases from colorectal cancer (LMCRC) after chemotherapy (CT) with CPT-11/L-OHP/LV5FU (FOLFIRINOX): A prospective phase II trial. ASCO Annual Meeting, 2004, American Society of Clinical Oncology, New Orleans, Louisiana.

65. Abad A, Anton A, Massuti B, et al. Resectability of liver metastases (LM) in patients with advanced colorectal cancer (ACRC) after treatment with the combination of oxaliplatin (OXA), irinotecan (IRI) and 5FU: Final results of a phase II study. ASCO Annual Meeting, 2005, American Society of Clinical Oncology, Orlando, Florida.

66. Ho WM, Ma B, Mok T, et al. Liver resection after irinotecan, 5-fluorouracil, and folinic acid for patients with unresectable colorectal liver metastases: A multicenter phase II study by the Cancer Therapeutic Research Group. Med Oncol, 2005; 22(3): 303–312.

67. Wein A, Riedel C, Köckerling F, et al. Impact of surgery on survival in palliative patients with metastatic colorectal cancer after first line treatment with weekly 24-hour infusion of high-dose 5-fluorouracil and folinic acid. Ann Oncol, 2001; 12(12): 1721–1727.

68. Clavien PA, Selzner N, Morse M, et al. Downstaging of hepatocellular carcinoma and liver metastases from colorectal cancer by selective intra-arterial chemotherapy. Surgery, 2002; 131(4): 433–442.

69. Huitzil FD, Capanu M, Paty P, et al. Predictive factors for resection of unresectable metastases from colorectal cancer in patients treated with hepatic arterial infusion (HAI) with floxuridine (FUDR) and dexamethasone (DEX) plus IV oxaliplatin (Oxali) and irinotecan (CPT). 2008 Gastrointestinal Cancers Symposium 2008. Orlando, Florida.

70. Zelek L, Bugat R, Cherqui D, et al. Multimodal therapy with intravenous biweekly leucovorin, 5-fluorouracil and irinotecan combined with hepatic arterial infusion pirarubicin in non-resectable hepatic metastases from colorectal cancer (a European Association for Research in Oncology trial). Ann Oncol, 2003; 14(10): 1537–1542.

71. Lorenz M, Müller HH, Schramm H, et al. Randomized trial of surgery versus surgery followed by adjuvant hepatic arterial infusion with 5-fluorouracil and folinic acid for liver metastases of colorectal cancer. German Cooperative on Liver Metastases (Arbeitsgruppe Lebermetastasen). Ann Surg, 1998; 228(6): 756–762.

72. Tono T, Hasuike Y, Ohzato H, et al. Limited but definite efficacy of prophylactic hepatic arterial infusion chemotherapy after curative resection of colorectal liver metastases: A randomized study. Cancer, 2000; 88(7): 1549–1556.

73. Kemeny MM, Adak S, Gray B, Macdonald JS, et al. Combined-modality treatment for resectable metastatic colorectal carcinoma to the liver: Surgical resection of hepatic metastases in combination with continuous infusion of chemotherapy – an intergroup study. J Clin Oncol, 2002; 20(6): 1499–1505.

74. Lygidakis NJ, Sgourakis G, Vlachos L, et al. Metastatic liver disease of colorectal origin: The value of locoregional immunochemotherapy combined with systemic chemotherapy following liver resection. Results of a prospective randomized study. Hepatogastroenterology, 2001; 48(42): 1685–1691.

75. Asahara T, Kikkawa M, Okajima M, et al. Studies of postoperative transarterial infusion chemotherapy for liver metastasis of colorectal carcinoma after hepatectomy. Hepatogastroenterology, 1998; 45(21): 805–811.

76. Kusunoki M, Yanagi H, Noda M, et al. Results of pharmacokinetic modulating chemotherapy in combination with hepatic arterial 5-fluorouracil infusion and oral UFT after resection of hepatic colorectal metastases. Cancer, 2000; 89(6): 1228–1235.

77. Carnaghi C, Santoro A, Rimassa L, et al. The efficacy of hybrid chemotherapy with intravenous oxaliplatin and folinic acid and intra-hepatic infusion of 5-fluorouracil in patients with colorectal liver metastases: A phase II study. Invest New Drugs, 2007; 25(5): 479–485.

78. Cunningham D, Humblet Y, Siena S, et al. Cetuximab monotherapy and cetuximab plus irinotecan in irinotecan-refractory metastatic colorectal cancer. NEJM, 2004; 351(4): 337–345.

Chapter 22

COLORECTAL METASTASES: ABLATION

Luigi Solbiati

The liver is the first, most common and often unique site of metastasis of colorectal cancer. Approximately 50% of colorectal cancer patients develop recurrent disease involving the liver during the course of their diseases.

Nowadays, multiple treatment options for colorectal metastases are available, including hepatic resection, chemoembolization, intra-arterial and systemic chemotherapy and thermal ablative therapies (cryoablation, laser-therapy and radiofrequency ablation [RFA]) (1, 2).

Over the past few years, advances in diagnostic imaging modalities such as contrast-enhanced ultrasound, multi-detector helical computed tomography (CT) and magnetic resonance imaging (MRI) with liver-specific contrast agents allow early detection and accurate quantification of liver metastatic involvement (3–6). As a result, correct selection of patients for different treatment options is usually possible.

If cure is the therapeutic goal, hepatic resection remains the most effective treatment option for liver metastases of colorectal origin (1–2, 7–10). However, patients eligible for resection are only a minority (30% to 35%, according to surgical literature) (11) because of many different occurrences: patients with metastases in difficult anatomical locations (e.g., adjacent to large blood vessels) or with new metastases or local recurrences after previous hepatic resection, patients with multiple bilobar liver metastases,

patients refusing or not eligible for surgery for general health reasons or associated pathological conditions that increase anesthesiologic risk cannot undergo resection and are all potential candidates for local ablation therapy. In fact, there are several potential advantages of local ablation over surgical resection:

1. Feasibility of treatment in previously resected patients and nonsurgical candidates due to number and/or intrahepatic location of metastatic deposits, age and co-morbidity;

2. Repeatability of treatment when incomplete and when local recurrence or development of new metachronous lesions occur;

3. Applicability in combination with systemic or regional chemotherapy;

4. Minimal invasiveness with limited complications rate and preservation of liver function;

5. Limited hospital stays and procedure costs.

Ablations can be performed by a percutaneous, laparoscopical or laparotomic approach: In this chapter, I address technical aspects and results only of percutaneously performed ablations.

TECHNICAL NOTES

Thermal ablations of liver metastases are performed in most centers with radiofrequency (using both cool-tip and multi-hooked needles), but laser and cryoprobes also are employed (1, 12–19). Microwaves are under investigation as an ablative modality and will soon become commercially available.

Cool-tip and multi-hooked electrodes can achieve comparable volumes of necrosis. In general, ablations with cool-tip electrodes are faster and technically easier, whereas multi-hooked electrodes allow accurate real-time monitoring of temperatures at the periphery of treated targets. Because it is not feasible to monitor in real-time the exact location of each hook, particularly in relation to "risky" anatomical structures, the use of multi-hooked electrodes is technically more challenging than that of cool-tip needles.

Temporary occlusion of portal vein, intra-tumoral injection of saline solution during radiofrequency energy deposition and pre-treatment liposomal chemotherapy administration can be used to increase the volume of necrosis achieved by thermal energy (20–22).

Several reasons account for the greater complexity of ablation of liver metastases in comparison with that of hepatocellular carcinomas: metastases do not have a peripheral capsule, generally develop in non-cirrhotic (i.e., regularly vascularized) liver parenchyma and have infiltrative growth, which requires achieving a 0.5- to 1-cm "safety halo" of ablated normal liver tissue at the periphery to decrease the occurrence of post-treatment local regrowth. The "heat sink effect" due to the presence of large venous vessels adjacent to metastatic tissue is also a limiting factor for the achievement of complete ablation of hepatic metastases. Considering all these problems, it is generally accepted that ablation of colorectal metastases is applicable to patients with one to five metachronous liver metastases measuring up to 3.5 to 4 cm in largest diameter (but preferably not exceeding 3 cm) from previous radically treated colorectal cancer, in whom surgery is not performable, contraindicated or simply refused (23–27). Some patients with large lesions or more than five nodules may undergo ablation after successful tumor debulking by means of chemotherapy (neoadjuvant).

Patient enrollment in the treatment process requires an anesthesiologist's evaluation. Laboratory tests include full blood count, coagulation screen, urea, electrolytes, liver function test and tumor markers.

Percutaneous ablation of colorectal metastases is mostly performed under conscious sedation. General anesthesia using endotracheal intubation and mechanical ventilation may be applied only for treatments of lesions adjacent to the Glisson's capsule (usually painful) or to risky anatomical structures, or when extended breath holds are necessary during the procedure, depending on the position of the lesion within the liver. As a result, international guidelines recommend performing percutaneous ablations in a dedicated operating room, where general anesthesia, endotracheal intubation and mechanical ventilation can be optimally performed if needed. Standard surgical asepsis rules must be strictly observed by the operating team. Patients receive antibiotic prophylaxis (i.e., ceftriaxone) prior to the treatment; antihemetic and analgesic drugs as needed postoperatively.

Percutaneous ablation is a minimally invasive procedure, so there are few absolute contraindications to its use. Exclusion criteria include the presence of severe coagulopathy, renal or liver failure, portal vein neoplastic thrombosis and obstructive jaundice. Active extrahepatic disease is a contraindication to ablation, with the exception of coexisting small lung metastases, which generally have very slow growth (compared with the fast development of hepatic metastases) and do not interfere with the oncologic goal of ablation of liver lesions.

Caution has to be taken not to damage adjacent structures. Liver lesions adjacent to the hepatic hilum, gallbladder, stomach and colon are potential candidates for ablation procedure yet require precise and careful planning. Adjacent vascular structures do not represent an obstacle alone: High blood flow in major hepatic vessels allows prompt dissipation of the warming effect secondary to the source of energy employed (heat sink effect) while the biliary system is vulnerable, especially if harboring bacteria. Gastric wall or bowel loop proximity to the area of treatment, considering the safety margin, may be a critical issue for treatment indications when selecting candidates. Perforations of bowel loops by heating may occur many hours after ablation and may be clinically misleading, being usually less painful than perforations due to inflammatory diseases. Relatively simple practical measures such as positioning of the patient and selection of a safe path to the target or intraperitoneal injection of 500 ml of dextrose (to create "artificial ascites") can provide adequate distance to avoid injury of critical structures.

Percutaneous ablations can be guided by sonography, CT or MRI. Sonography is employed in most centers because of some favorable aspects: real-time control, low cost, no use of ionizing radiations (28). CT or MRI guidance is mandatory when sonographic targeting is not possible, with significantly increased procedure time.

When sonography is used as the modality of guidance, contrast-enhanced ultrasound (CEUS) is particularly useful for pretreatment planning, targeting of lesions undetectable in basal studies and immediate control of early results of treatment.

B-mode and color/power Doppler ultrasound are not reliable to assess the size and completeness of induced coagulation necrosis at the end of the energy application; furthermore, additional repositioning of the electrode is usually made difficult by the hyperechogenic "cloud" appearing around the distal probe. Therefore, CEUS is performed at the presumed end of the treatment to enable rapid assessment of the extent of achieved tissue ablation and to discover viable tumor requiring additional immediate treatment (29).

Real-time US/CT fusion imaging technology allows targeting lesions visible only with CT, to calculate in real-time the volume to treat prior to the treatment and to guide further electrode insertions into the same target, often completely "obscured" for sonography by the gas formation created by RFA (Figures 22.1 and 22.2) (30).

Ablation is considered successful when complete coagulative necrosis of the lesion and a safety margin are obtained. Initial cross-sectional examinations are crucial to assess completeness of treatment, exclude complications and provide a baseline image for follow-up purposes. Spiral contrast-enhanced CT (or MR) scan at 24 hours (or at 1 month) after ablation is the most widely used early follow-up study.

Patients continue to undergo contrast-enhanced multi-detector CT or MR scans on a routine basis in the long-term assessment of therapeutic response, allowing prompt identification of new lesions (Figures 22.1 and 22.2). Cross-sectional imaging studies obtained at 3- to 4-month intervals need to be integrated with liver function tests and serum carcinoembryonic antigen (CEA) levels to detect local or distant recurrences.

Nevertheless, although continuous efforts are being implemented to increase the resolution and accuracy of imaging techniques, residual peripheral microscopic foci of malignancy or within the treated lesion may go undetected (particularly when contrast-enhanced CT is the imaging modality employed) and give rise to local recurrence in the short-term.

Consequently, new imaging modalities are being taken into account in order to provide more reliable assessment of thoroughness of treatment and higher sensitivity for the detection of local recurrences.

Fluorodeoxyglucose (FDG)-labeled positron emission tomography (PET) is a complementary imaging modality in case of uncertain treatment response when applied after a reasonable time interval from the treatment. Areas of abnormal FDG uptake following ablative procedures have been reported to represent disease relapse or residual viable tumor following ablation with a high degree of sensitivity (31). In some institutions, it has been proposed as a whole-body surveillance technique in treated patients.

CEUS can be helpful for the differentiation between necrosis and viable metastatic tissue, given that necrotic areas do not enhance in any vascular phase, whereas viable neoplastic nodules clearly enhance in arterial and early portal phase, becoming markedly hypovascular (thus undistinguishable from necrotic areas) in late portal phase (Figure 22.3).

Currently, MRI is more accurate than contrast-enhanced CT for the detection of viable tumoral areas and local recurrences (Figure 22.4) (32), but especially diffusion-weighted MRI combined with contrast-enhanced MRI will become, in the near future, the most reliable imaging modality for the differentiation between viable tumor tissue and necrosis, as demonstrated in recent studies (33, 34).

RESULTS

The 5-year overall survival rate following surgical resection of colorectal metastases has been reported to range between 25% and 40%, but many successfully resected patients develop recurrence in the liver or extrahepatic sites and repeated resection can be performed in only a minority of them (1, 7–11, 35–37). Prognostic factors include stage of primary tumor, biologic factors (CEA level, differentiation, cellular ploidy), number of hepatic lesions and size of dominant lesion and infiltration of resection margins. It has been demonstrated that RFA increases the possibilities of curative treatment in patients with liver recurrence after hepatectomy from 17% to 26%, and is preferred over repeated surgery because it is less invasive (38).

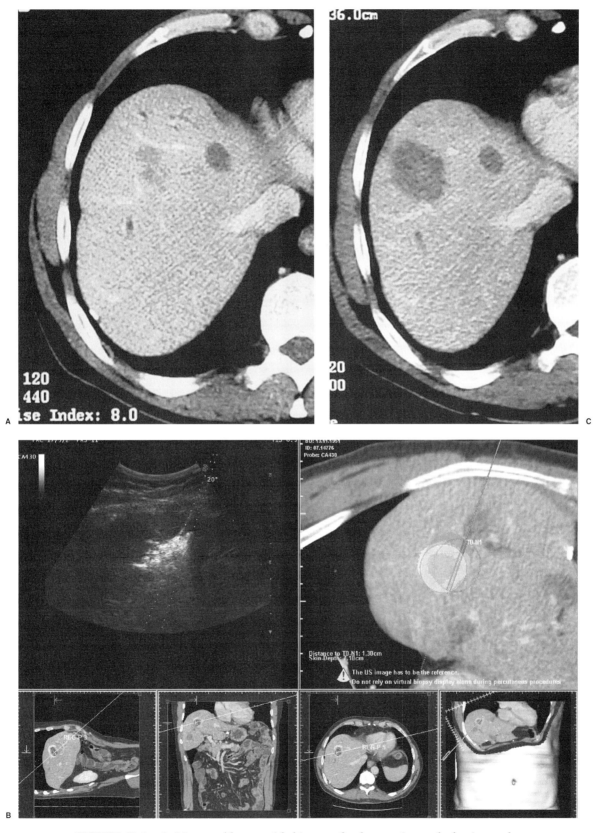

FIGURE 22.1.   A 56-year-old man with history of colon carcinoma had prior wedge resection of one metastasis in the left lobe and RFA of a second lesion in segment IV. (A) Two years later, a new metastasis in segment VIII is seen adjacent to the small and markedly hypodense area in segment IV, representing complete necrosis of the previous ablation. (B) Using real-time CT-US fusion imaging, the new metastasis is clearly identified and targeted with cool-tip radiofrequency probe. (C) 24-hour post-treatment CT scan shows complete ablation with sufficiently large "safety halo."

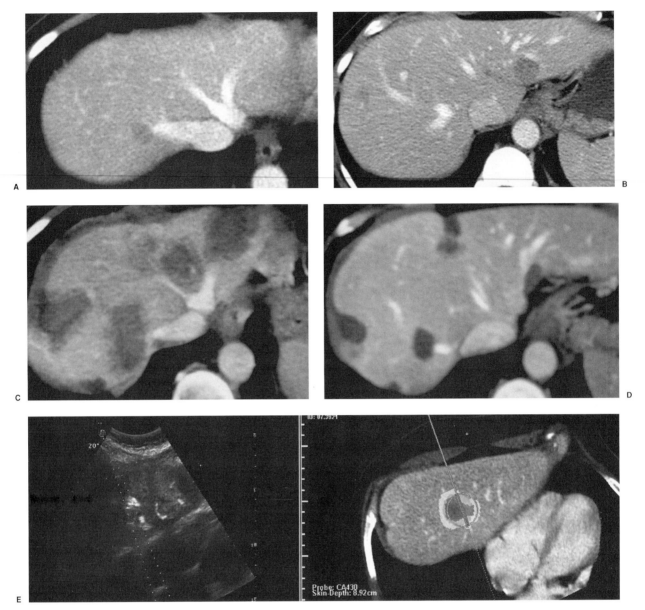

FIGURE 22.2. A 43-year-old patient with history of colon carcinoma surgically resected and systemic chemotherapy. Follow-up CT scans show the presence of six small liver metastases (one is visible in A, two in B). (C) All the lesions were treated with cool-tip RFA in a single session and large necrotic areas were achieved. (D) Three years after ablation, all the necrotic areas show marked shrinkage, but a new metastasis appears in segment IV, adjacent to one of the areas of necrosis. (E) This new metastasis was precisely treated with real-time CT-US fusion imaging. See Color Plate 21.

Although literature data of results achieved with cryoablation or microwave ablation of colorectal metastases are very limited, several published series reported significant results with laser and, mostly, RF ablation, concerning local control rate, complications, long-term follow-up and survival.

Two studies on laser ablation of colorectal metastases recently were published. In the first study (15), in 44 patients 61% of the tumors (46 of 75) were completely ablated. The likelihood of complete ablation was significantly higher for metastases smaller than 3 cm, and overall survival was 30 ± 12.7 months

in patients with complete ablation and 20.2 ± 10.2 months in patients with partial ablation. In the second study (19) in 603 patients, local recurrence rates ranged from 1.9% for metastases up to 2 cm in diameter to 4.4% for metastases larger than 4 cm; 3- and 5- year survival rates were 56% and 37% respectively, with a median survival of 3.5 years. No major complications were reported in either study.

As for RFA of colorectal metastases, several studies performed by different groups have been published in the last years, with significant data concerning long-term survival rates of treated patients that are mostly

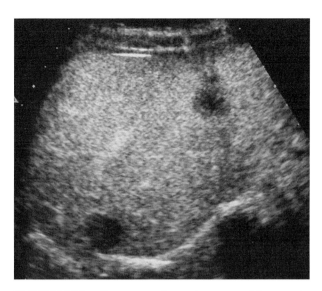

FIGURE 22.3. Contrast-enhanced sonographic scan in early portal phase in a patient with history of colorectal metastasis in segment VII, treated with RFA. The completely necrotic area in segment VII appears avascular and well demarcated. A new metastasis is visible in segment IV and shows moderate peripheral enhancement and ill-defined margins. See Color Plate 22.

comparable with those reported in surgical literature. These results are reported in Table 22.1.

In the largest multi-center Italian study (41) of 423 patients, 3- and 5-year survival rates of 47%

and 24% were reported. In a study from the Cleveland Clinic (24), 135 patients underwent RFA because they were not good candidates for resection and 80% of these patients had already received chemotherapy. The median overall survival was 28.9 months. Predictors of survival included size of the lesion and baseline CEA values. A median survival of 38 months was found for lesions 3 cm or less, 34 months for lesions 3 to 5 cm and 21 months for lesions greater than 5 cm.

On the other hand, in another series (43) of 348 patients treated with intention to cure, 190 had resection only, 101 had RFA and 57 had RFA alone. Recurrences were lowest with resection (52%) vs. 64% for RFA and resection, and 84% for RFA alone. Liver-only recurrence after RFA was 44%. The 4-year survival rate was 65% for resection, 36% for resection and RFA and 22% for RFA alone. Of course, RFA was usually a component of therapy when resection was not possible. Therefore, this is not a true comparison of RFA vs. resection.

Literature reports have also demonstrated that RFA is a safe procedure, with low rates of complications and mortality. Major complications such as hemorrhage, cholecystitis or gastric or bowel wall involvement have been reported in a small percentage

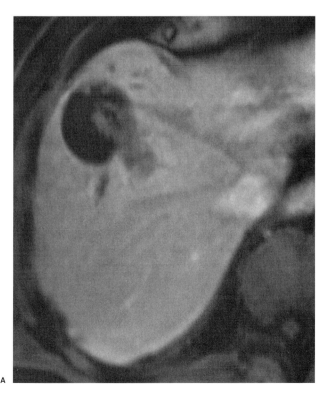

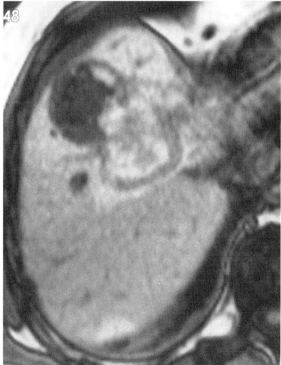

A   B

FIGURE 22.4. **(A)** T1-weighted MRI scan showing local medial-posterior recurrence of colorectal metastasis in segment VIII treated 1 year earlier. The treated area unusu-ally shows liquid changes. **(B)** After local retreatment, complete necrosis of the neoplastic recurrence is shown by T1-weighted MRI.

TABLE 22.1 Local Control and Long-Term Survival after RFA for Colorectal Cancer Liver Metastases: Literature Review

Author (Ref.)	N	No. Mets	Size (cm)	Technique	F/up (mo.)	Local Control (%)	Survival (%)
Solbiati L, 2006 (unpublished data)	128	261	0.5–6.6 mean 2.0	percutaneous	3–126	83.1	3-year: 62 5-year: 39.5
Berber E, 2005 (24)	135	432	1.2–10.2	laparoscopic	12–52		3-year: 28 median: 28.9
Gillams AR, 2004 (39)	167	354	1–12 mean 3.9	percutaneous	0–89 Mean: 17	74.9	5-year: 26
Veltri A, 2005 (21)	98	163	0.5–8.0 mean: 2.7	percutaneous intraop	12–108	59	3-year: 48 5-year: 30
Jakobs TF, 2006 (40)	68	183	0.5–5.0 mean: 2.2	percutaneous	8–38 Mean: 21	82	3-year: 68
Tumor RFA Italian Network (Lencioni R) 2005 (41)	423	543	0.5–5.0 mean: 2.7	percutaneous	1–78 Mean: 19	85.4 R0: 88.2	3-yr: 47 5-year: 24
Sorensen, et al, 2007 (42)	102	332		percutaneous	1–92 mean: 23.6		3-year: 64 5-year: 44

of cases, ranging from 0.7% to 5.7%. Mortality rates reported ranged from 0.5% to 1.4% (44, 45).

In the most recent and still unpublished long-term follow-up study at our institution, 128 patients have been treated with RFA over a period of 7 years. Twelve percent of them had previous surgery for liver neoplastic involvement, and repeated resection was considered unfeasible or too invasive. One to five metastases (mean 2.28) were ablated in each patient for a total of 261 treated lesions. Of the treated lesions, 87.5% were 3 cm or less in size; the remaining 12.5% were larger than 3 cm. Local tumor control was achieved in 83.1% of lesions, whereas local recurrence occurred in the remaining 16.9% (77.2% of these recurring metastases were larger than 3 cm). In our experience, the time interval from treatment to recurrence was related to the size of the lesion: local relapse occurred virtually in all cases during the first 12-month-period. The median time to local recurrence was 9.3 months. Repeated RFA was carried out in 37.6% of metastases with progressive local tumor growth. Distant, metachronous metastases developed at follow-up in 36% of our patients. The estimated median time until detection of new metastases was 12.3 months in our experience. The Kaplan-Meier survival analyses of the overall survival rates at 1, 3 and 5 years in our series are 96.2%, 62.0% and 39.5% respectively; resulting in estimated median survival of 51 months. No major complication was recorded in our experience. Fever was seldom observed following the treatment and receded with antipyretic drugs. No impairment in liver function tests was observed. Minimal pleural effusion was documented in a few cases by CT performed at 24 hours and usually resolved within a week.

RFA proposed after previous chemotherapy regimens is still associated with worse survival as it applies to extensive liver disease stage, chemotherapy-refractory tumor or diffuse extrahepatic disease. The comparison between RFA used as first-line or second-line regimen, or in the salvage setting investigated by Machi et al. (46) showed the greater survival benefit of its use as a first-line therapeutic option. Randomized control trials assessing the value of combined adjuvant systemic chemotherapy are urgently required in the short term.

Not so long ago, the "test of time" approach was proposed by surgeons to delay the resection of liver metastases in order to allow additional, still undetected lesions to develop and become identifiable, thus limiting the number of resections carried out in patients who may ultimately develop more metastases. On the one hand, RFA applied in this setting can significantly decrease the number of potential resections, hence resulting in complete tumor control in some of these patients, avoiding major surgery. Furthermore, offering a treatment option such as RFA to cancer patients rather than a "wait-and-see" behavior is favorable for the patient. In a recent study, using RFA as "test of time" before resection in a group of

88 potentially operable patients with 134 metastases from colorectal carcinoma followed for a period of 18 to 75 months, RFA was successful in 60.2% of patients and 43.4% of these were disease-free at the period of the study, whereas the remaining patients (56.6%) developed new untreatable intra- or extra-hepatic metastases. RFA was unsuccessful in 39.8% of patients: 57.1% of these underwent resection, the remaining 42.9% developed new untreatable metastases. No patient became untreatable because of the growth of incompletely ablated lesions. In summary, 50% of patients were spared surgery that would have been non-curative, while 26.1% additional patients avoided resection because of the curative result of RFA (47).

CONCLUSIONS

Percutaneous ablation is an established therapeutic option for liver colorectal metastases, which may obviate the need for a major surgery and result in prolonged survival and chance for cure.

Accurate selection of patients and lesions to be treated and use of state-of-the-art technology for guiding and performing ablations are of crucial importance for achieving good results.

Extensive operators' experience and technical advances provide larger coagulation volumes and therefore allow safe and effective treatment of medium and occasionally even large metastases. In experienced hands, thermal ablation can achieve local control in up to 85% to 90% of treated lesions. Repeated thermal ablations for either local recurrences or new metastases are technically feasible and very often performed.

Results of RFA in terms of global and disease-free survival currently approach those reported for surgical metastasectomy. Adverse effects rates, costs and hospitalization associated with thermal ablation are usually lower than those of surgical resection.

Recently increased awareness among referring oncologists, satisfactory results in long-term survival reported in scientific literature and minimal invasiveness of RFA vs. surgery contributed to the widely accepted status of a valid therapeutic option for local treatment of patients with limited metastatic liver disease. The overlapping long-term outcome of both surgical resection and RFA will allow, in the future, randomized studies comparing RFA versus resection for resectable metastatic liver tumors, enabling

a proper evaluation of RFA impact. However, RFA should not replace hepatic resection, whenever applicable, especially for large metastases, because of the higher risk of local recurrence due to residual viable tumor tissue within the necrotic area.

REFERENCES

1. Fahy BN, Jarnagin WR. Evolving techniques in the treatment of liver colorectal metastases: Role of laparoscopy, radiofrequency ablation, microwave coagulation, hepatic arterial chemotherapy, indications and contraindications for resection, role of transplantation, and timing of chemotherapy. Surg Clin North Am, 2006; 86: 1005–1022.
2. Nordlinger B and Rougier P. Nonsurgical methods for liver metastases including cryotherapy, radiofrequency ablation and infusional treatment: What's new in 2001? Curr Opin Oncol, 2002; 14: 420–423.
3. Sica GT, Ji H, and Ros PR. CT and MR imaging of hepatic metastases. Am J Roentgenol, 2000; 174: 691–698.
4. Valls C, Andia E, Sanchez A, et al. Hepatic metastases from colorectal cancer: Preoperative detection and assessment of resectability with helical CT. Radiology, 2001; 218: 55–60.
5. Quaia E, Bertolotto M, Forgacs B, et al. Detection of liver metastases by pulse inversion harmonic imaging during Levovist late phase: Comparison with conventional ultrasound and helical CT in 160 patients. Eur Radiol, 2003; 13: 475–483.
6. Albrecht T, Blomley MJ, Burns PN, et al. Improved detection of hepatic metastases with pulse-inversion US during the liver-specific phase of SHU 508A: Multicenter Study. Radiology, 2003; 227: 361–370.
7. Fong Y, Salo J. Surgical therapy of hepatic colorectal metastasis. Semin Oncol, 1999; 26: 514–523.
8. Hugh TJ, Kinsella AR, and Poston GJ. Management strategies for colorectal liver metastases – Part I. Surg Oncol, 1997; 6: 19–30.
9. Liu LX, Zhang WH, and Jiang HC. Current treatment for liver metastases from colorectal cancer. World J Gastroenterol, 2003; 9: 193–200.
10. Yoon SS and Tanabe KK. Surgical treatment and other regional treatments for colorectal cancer liver metastases. Oncologist, 1999; 4: 197–208.
11. McKay A, Dixon E, and Taylor M. Current role of radiofrequency ablation for the treatment of colorectal liver metastases. Br J Surg, 2006; 93: 1192–1201.
12. Goldberg SN, Gazelle GS, and Mueller PR. Thermal ablation therapy for focal malignancy: A unified approach to underlying principles, techniques, and diagnostic imaging guidance. Am J Roentgenol, 2000; 174: 323–331.
13. Goldberg SN, Solbiati L, Hahn PF, et al. Large-volume tissue ablation with radiofrequency by using a clustered, internally cooled electrode technique: Laboratory and clinical experience in liver metastases. Radiology, 1998; 209: 371–379.
14. Lencioni R, Goletti O, Armillotta N, et al. Radiofrequency thermal ablation of liver metastasis with cooled-tip electrode needle: Results of a pilot clinical trial. Eur Radiol, 1998; 8: 1205–1211.

15. Pacella CM, Valle D, Bizzarri G, et al. Percutaneous laser ablation in patients with isolated unresectable liver metastases from colorectal cancer: Results of a phase II study. Acta Oncologica, 2006; 45: 77–83.

16. Rossi S, Buscarini E, Garbagnati F, et al. Percutaneous treatment of small hepatic tumors by an expandable RF needle electrode. Am J Roentgenol, 1998; 170: 1015–1022.

17. Solbiati L, Goldberg SN, Ierace T, et al. Hepatic metastases: Percutaneous radio-frequency ablation with cooled-tip electrodes. Radiology, 1997; 205: 367–373.

18. Solbiati L, Ierace T, Goldberg SN, et al. Percutaneous US-guided radio-frequency tissue ablation of liver metastases: Treatment and follow-up in 16 patients. Radiology, 1997; 202: 195–203.

19. Vogl TJ, Straub R, Eichler K, et al. Colorectal carcinoma metastases in liver: Laser-induced interstitial thermotherapy – local tumor control rate and survival data. Radiology, 2004; 230: 450–458.

20. DeBaere T, Bessoud B, Dromain C, et al. Percutaneous radiofrequency ablation of hepatic tumors during temporary venous occlusion. Am J Roentgenol, 2002; 178: 53–59.

21. Rhim H, Goldberg SN, Dodd GD 3rd, et al. Essential techniques for successful radio-frequency thermal ablation of malignant hepatic tumors. Radiographics, 2001; 21: S17–35.

22. Goldberg SN, Kamel IR, Kruskal JB, et al. Radiofrequency ablation of hepatic tumors: Increased tumor destruction with adjuvant liposomal doxorubicin therapy. Am J Roentgenol, 2002; 179: 93–101.

23. Abitabile P, Hartl U, Lange J, et al. Radiofrequency ablation permits an effective treatment for colorectal liver metastasis. Eur J Surg Oncol, 2007; 33: 67–71.

24. Berber E, Pelley R, and Siperstein AE. Predictors of survival after radiofrequency thermal ablation of colorectal cancer metastases to the liver: A prospective study. J Clin Oncol, 2005; 23: 1358–1364.

25. Leen E and Horgan PG. Radiofrequency ablation of colorectal liver metastases. Surg Oncol, 2007; 16: 47–51.

26. Pereira PL. Actual role of radiofrequency ablation of liver metastases. Eur Radiol, 2007; 17: 2062–2070.

27. Solbiati L, Livraghi T, Goldberg SN, et al. Percutaneous radiofrequency ablation of hepatic metastases from colorectal cancer: Long-term results in 117 patients. Radiology, 2001; 221: 159–166.

28. Tonolini M and Solbiati L. Ultrasound imaging in tumor ablation. In: vanSonnenberg E, McMullen W, Solbiati L, (eds), Tumor Ablation: Principles and Practice pp. 135–147. New York: Springer, 2005.

29. Solbiati L, Tonolini M and Ierace T. Guidance of percutaneous tumor ablation. In: Lencioni R, (ed), Enhancing the Role of Ultrasound with Contrast Agents pp. 69–76. Heidelberg: Springer, 2006.

30. Solbiati L, Cova L, and Ierace T. US-CT fusion for performing radiofrequency ablation of small or poorly visualized liver tumors. Eur Radiol, 2005; 15 (Suppl 3): C45.

31. Anderson GS, Brinkmann F, Soulen MC, et al. FDG positron emission tomography in the surveillance of hepatic tumors treated with radiofrequency ablation. Clin Nucl Med, 2003; 28: 192–197.

32. Vossen JA, Buijs M, and Kamel IR. Assessment of tumor response on MR imaging after locoregional therapy. Tech Vasc Interv Radiol, 2006; 9: 125–132.

33. Koh DM, Scurr E, Collins DJ, et al. Colorectal hepatic metastases: Quantitative measurements using single-shot echo-planar diffusion-weighted MR imaging. Eur Radiol, 2006; 16: 1898–1905.

34. Taouli B, Vilgrain V, Dumont E, et al. Evaluation of liver diffusion isotropy and characterization of focal hepatic lesions with two single-shot echo-planar MR imaging sequences: Prospective study in 66 patients. Radiology, 2003; 226: 71–78.

35. Fong Y, Fortner J, Sun RL, et al. Clinical score for predicting recurrence after hepatic resection for metastatic colorectal cancer: Analysis of 1001 consecutive cases. Ann Surg, 1999; 230: 309–321.

36. Registry of Hepatic Metastases: Resection of the liver for colorectal carcinoma metastases: A multi-institutional study of indications for resection. Surgery, 1998; 103: 278–288.

37. Scheele J, Stang R, Altendorf-Hofmann A, et al. Resection of colorectal carcinoma metastases to the liver: A prognostic scoring system to improve case selection, based on 156 patients. Cancer, 1996; 77:1254–1262.

38. Elias D, DeBaere T, Smayra T, et al. Percutaneous radiofrequency thermoablation as an alternative to surgery for treatment of liver tumour recurrence after hepatectomy. Br J Surg, 2002; 89: 752–756.

39. Gillams AR and Lees WR. Radio-frequency ablation of colorectal liver metastases in 167 patients. Eur Radiol, 2004; 14: 2261–2267.

40. Jakobs TF, Hoffmann RT, Trumm C, et al. Radiofrequency ablation of colorectal liver metastases: Mid-term results in 68 patients. Anticancer Res, 2006; 26: 671–680.

41. Lencioni R, Crocetti L, Cioni D, et al. Percutaneous radiofrequency ablation of hepatic colorectal metastases: Technique, indications, results and new promises. Invest Radiol, 2004; 39: 689–697.

42. Sorensen SM, Mortensen FV, and Nielsen DT. Radiofrequency ablation of colorectal liver metastases: Long-term survival. Acta Radiol, 2007; 48: 253–258.

43. Abdalla EK, Vauthey JN, Ellis LM, et al. Recurrence and outcomes following hepatic resection, radiofrequency ablation and combined resection/ablation for colorectal liver metastases. Ann Surg, 2004; 239: 818–827.

44. DeBaere T, Risse O, Kuoch V, et al. Adverse events during radiofrequency treatment of 582 hepatic tumors. Am J Roentgenol, 2003; 181: 695–700.

45. Livraghi T, Solbiati L, Meloni MF, et al. Treatment of focal liver tumors with percutaneous radiofrequency ablation: Complications encountered in a multicenter study. Radiology, 2003; 226: 441–451.

46. Machi J, Oishi AJ, Sumida K, et al. Long-term outcome of radiofrequency ablation for unresectable liver metastases from colorectal cancer: Evaluation of prognostic factors and effectiveness in first- and second-line management. Cancer J, 2006; 12: 318–326.

47. Livraghi T, Solbiati L, Meloni F, et al. Percutaneous radiofrequency ablation of liver metastases in potential candidates for resection: The "test of time" approach. Cancer, 2003; 97: 3027–3035.

Chapter 23

COLORECTAL METASTASES: CHEMOEMBOLIZATION

Catherine M. Tuite

The prognosis of patients with colorectal carcinoma is related to the degree of penetration of the primary tumor through the bowel wall, the presence or absence of nodal involvement and the presence or absence of distant metastases (1–3). In 2005, there were an estimated 104,950 new cases of colon cancer in the United States and 56,290 deaths from the disease (4). Autopsy series have shown up to 38% of patients who die from colorectal cancer may have the liver as the sole site of metastases (6). Even for patients with other sites of involvement, more than 50% die from metastatic liver disease (7). Several studies establish that resection of colorectal liver metastases improves long-term survival (7–9); however, for the 75% of patients with colorectal liver metastases found to be unresectable, palliative treatments remain an option. Since the late 1990s, systemic chemotherapy regimens have changed significantly, and there are now five active agents used to treat advanced disease, including those that target angiogenesis and epidermal growth factor receptor (10). Despite the improved response rates and progression-free survival obtained by these agents, especially when given in combination (11–14), most patients eventually develop disease progression. Chemoembolization may be offered to these patients, particularly those with liver-dominant metastases.

Chemoembolization is one of several regional therapies for colorectal liver metastases. It is the only one that provides a two-fold line of attack, since it involves the simultaneous infusion of chemotherapeutic and embolic agents. Because the embolic particles slow the passage of chemotherapy through the hepatic circulation, drug concentrations in the tumor reach levels up to 25 times greater than with infusion alone, and remain within tumor cells for as much as 1 month after infusion (15–18). Embolic agents also render the treated tissue ischemic, resulting in tumor hypoxia. Hypoxia potentiates the effects of cytotoxic drugs by increasing their uptake and retention by tumor cells (19). Recent studies suggest that ischemia increases angiogenesis in tumor cells, possibly triggering tumor growth (20–22). One might interpret this to indicate that hepatic arterial embolization alone would be a less effective treatment than chemoembolization; however, no study thus far shows a difference in survival between the two (20, 23).

PATIENT SELECTION

Patient selection is critically important when considering treatment with chemoembolization. In order to select good candidates for chemoembolization, all patients require a thorough pre-procedure assessment. This evaluation includes a tissue diagnosis, cross-sectional imaging of the liver and, if not previously performed, of other regions such as the lungs to exclude significant extrahepatic disease. Laboratory studies, including complete blood count (CBC), parathyroid/International Normalized Ratio (PT/INR), creatinine, liver function tests and carcinoembryonic antigen (CEA) level, should be obtained before each chemoembolization session.

Patients should have multiple, non-resectable liver lesions that have been refractory to other treatments. Ideal patients have liver metastases only; however, those with minimal or indolent extra-hepatic disease may also benefit when the degree of liver involvement drives survival. Candidates should have an adequate performance status (Eastern Cooperative Oncology Group 0–2) and no active comorbid conditions. Although less common in patients with colorectal liver metastases than primary liver cancer until very late in the disease, patients with underlying liver dysfunction should be treated with caution. To that end, a subgroup of patients has been defined who have a constellation of findings that preclude safe treatment with chemoembolization due to the high risk of liver failure. This constellation includes all of the following: more than 50% of the liver volume replaced by tumor, lactate dehydrogenase greater than 425 IU/L, aspartate aminotransferase greater than 100 IU/L and total bilirubin greater than 2.0 IU/L (24). Bland embolization, leaving out the chemotherapy, does not decrease the risk for patients with contraindications to hepatic embolization.

Patients with even main portal vein thrombosis can be treated safely as long as sufficient collaterals exist with hepatopetal flow (25). Patients with untreatable biliary obstruction, even with normal serum bilirubin level, are at high risk of biliary necrosis. Patients whose obstruction is treated with a biliary stent or who have a biloenteric anastamosis are at very high risk of gram-negative bacteremia and liver abscess formation (26, 27), which can be mitigated somewhat with an aggressive peri-procedural antibiotic regimen (28). Any patient with contraindications to angiography such as anaphylactoid reactions to intravascular radiographic contrast, uncorrectable coagulopathy, severe renal insufficiency or contraindications to chemotherapy such as severe cytopenias or severe cardiac dysfunction cannot receive chemoembolization.

CHEMOEMBOLIZATION REGIMENS

There is no standard protocol for chemoembolization, and the agents used vary widely among centers. No clinical trial has compared the different techniques. In the United States, the most commonly used drugs include a combination of cisplatin doxorubicin (Adriamycin) and mitomycin C, all of which exhibit preferential extraction when delivered intrahepatically and can achieve favorable liver/systemic drug concentration ratios, thereby minimizing systemic toxicity (29). Agents used to achieve embolization also vary widely, including polyvinyl alcohol, gelatin sponge, starch microspheres and collagen particles. Most protocols include lipiodol, or ethiodized oil (ethiodol), a naturally iodinated fatty acid ethyl ester of poppyseed oil. An effective strategy causes occlusion of both the distal hepatic arterioles and the portal venules, thus trapping the chemotherapeutic drugs between the two, as occurs with an oily and particulate-based combination of embolics (17,30,31). Hepatocellular carcinoma selectively takes up ethiodol, perhaps resulting in more selective toxicity to the tumor cells (31,32); however, no such data have been shown to apply to adenocarcinomas (33). Some regimens call for the delivery of the chemotherapeutic drug(s) and oil emulsion followed by particulate embolization, or may involve a "sandwich" technique in which embolization with particles is done first, followed by injection of the liquid phase, then further embolization with additional particles (31). One commonly used protocol combines the liquid and particulate agents together. Pharmacokinetic data suggest that the chemotherapeutic drugs in the aqueous phase of the solution will wash out unless efflux is simultaneously arrested by the particles (34).

TREATMENT

Most often, patients are admitted to the interventional radiology service on the morning of the procedure, after having fasted overnight. A Foley catheter may be inserted, and vigorous hydration is initiated. Prophylactic antibiotics and antiemetics are administered intravenously, both typically continued until discharge. Usually, the procedure is performed while the patient receives moderate (conscious) sedation.

Diagnostic arteriography is always performed before injection of the chemoembolic solution. A superior mesenteric angiogram identifies variant vascular supply to the liver, including an accessory or replaced right hepatic artery, retrograde flow through the gastroduodenal artery and patency and flow direction of the portal vein. A celiac arteriogram should be performed to assess the hepatic branch anatomy, including the presence of variant supply to the left hepatic lobe. Replaced and accessory hepatic arteries are quite common and must be catheterized beyond gastric or mesenteric branches for safe chemoembolization (Figure 23.1). Next, selective hepatic arteriograms should be performed. Careful evaluation of the left hepatic artery will identify the location of

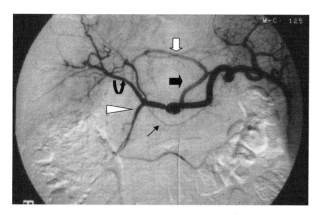

FIGURE 23.1. Celiac arteriogram demonstrates an accessory left hepatic artery (*white arrow*) arising from the left gastric artery (*thick black arrow*). A faint tumor blush supplied by branches of the right hepatic artery (*curved arrow*) is also seen. In order to safely treat this tumor, the catheter must be advanced beyond both the gastroduodenal artery (*white arrowhead*) and the right gastric artery (*thin black arrow*).

the right or accessory gastric arteries and, often, the phrenic and falciform supply. A selective right hepatic arteriogram will identify the location of the cystic artery and any supraduodenal or retroduodenal vessels, as well. Basic mesenteric arteriography need be performed only prior to the first session. Subsequent chemoembolizations usually only require evaluation of the specific vessel(s) supplying the tumor(s) to be treated. For an exhaustive review of the angiographic considerations in hepatic arterial therapy, interested readers are directed to an excellent review article by Liu et al. (35).

Once the arterial anatomy and tumor supply are clearly identified, the catheter is advanced superselectively into the right or left hepatic arterial supply, often with the aid of coaxially introduced microcatheters and wires. Whole-liver chemoembolization is not recommended due to an unwarranted high rate of toxicity (36), and some practitioners advocate segmental or subsegmental delivery of chemoembolics, particularly when liver function is marginal. It is important not to induce spasm and pseudostasis by using a standard angiographic catheter in a small vessel (less than twice the diameter of the catheter). When the catheter is removed and spasm relieved, flow to the tumor will return. Once the catheter is positioned for treatment, a final arteriogram is performed to confirm the anatomy before chemotherapy is injected. This can be accomplished even through a microcatheter. Those specifically designed for intrahepatic arterial therapy can tolerate injection rates of up to 8 to 12 ml at 2 to 3 ml/sec.

The chemoembolic mixture is injected in 1-ml increments until near-complete stasis of blood flow is identified. Excessive embolization must be avoided, particularly for patients in whom repeated chemoembolizations are anticipated. Most microcatheters contain about 1.0 to 1.5 ml emulsion, and if this additional volume is injected during a final flush of the catheter after an acceptable endpoint has been reached, overembolization can easily occur. With the ideal endpoint, the treated arteries appear as a "tree in winter," with no tumor blush seen, but preservation of flow in the segmental and lobar branches.

After the procedure, intravenous hydration, antiemetics and intravenous antibiotics are continued. Narcotics, perchlorpromazine and acetaminophen are supplied for symptoms of pain, nausea and fever. The patient may be discharged when oral intake of at least fluids is adequate and parenteral narcotics are no longer required for adequate pain relief. A 1- to 2-day hospital stay post procedure is typical. Upon discharge, the patient is given prescriptions for oral antibiotics for 5 days, as well as antiemetics and oral narcotics as necessary. The patient returns to the interventional radiology outpatient office for follow-up with repeated imaging and laboratory evaluation in 1 month or to the interventional suite in 3 to 4 weeks for additional chemoembolization. It is not necessary to re-image the liver until all tumor has been treated. For bilobar disease, patients will require two to four treatments, depending on the arterial supply. Patients who respond to treatment are followed approximately every 3 months, and retreatment is considered for responders who develop intrahepatic recurrence.

Side effects after chemoembolization are common. Post-embolization syndrome, consisting of pain, fever, nausea and sometimes vomiting, is seen to some degree in nearly all patients and is due to hepatocyte and tumor necrosis. Fatigue and anorexia lasting 4 to 6 weeks are quite common as well. Patients whose right hepatic artery is chemoembolized proximal to the cystic artery (as may be unavoidable due to anatomic restrictions) will experience a prolonged post-embolization syndrome (37) and may develop sterile ischemic chemical cholecystitis that resolves with conservative treatment (Figure 23.2A,B). The incidence of major complications after chemoembolization is 2% to 7% (38–40). Major complications of hepatic embolization include hepatic insufficiency or infarction, abscess, biliary necrosis and non-target embolization of the gut. Other complications occur less than 1% of the time, including periprocedural

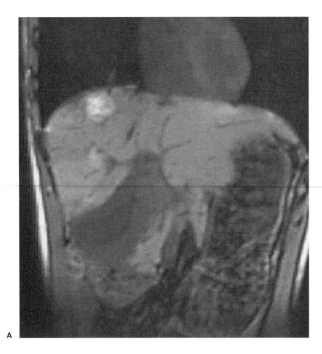

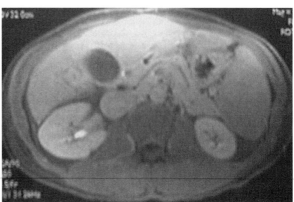

FIGURE 23.2. (A) Coronal T1-weighted magnetic resonance image of post-embolization ischemic chemical cholecystitis in a patient who was readmitted for prolonged post-embolization syndrome. (B) Axial T1-weighted magnetic resonance image 3 months later.

cardiac events, renal insufficiency, anemia requiring transfusion and complications related to angiography (41, 42). Thirty-day mortality rates have been reported to be 1% to 4% (33).

OUTCOMES IN COLORECTAL CARCINOMA

Since the 1980s, numerous studies for the treatment of metastatic colorectal cancer to the liver have been reported by centers in both the United States and elsewhere (Table 23.1). These studies used a variety of anticancer drugs and embolic agents; many include an oily embolic. Most of these patients had failed systemic therapy. Overall responses vary from 14% to 87%, and median survivals range from 7 to 29 months. It is important to realize that these survivals are longer than what would be expected in studies of systemic chemotherapy in patients who have failed standard therapy (29). In two more recent reports of

TABLE 23.1 Chemoembolization of Colorectal Liver Metastases

Reference	N	Anticancer Drug	Embolic	% Response	Median Survival (mo.)
Aronsen, 1979 (49)	7	Fluorouracil	DSM	57	7
Wollner, 1986 (51)	15	Mitomycin	DSM	20	7
Starkhammer, 1987 (50)	11	Mitomycin	DSM	63	N/A
Kobayashi, 1987 (43)	7	Adriamycin, Mitomycin	Lipiodol	78	N/A
Lorenz, 1989 (48)	11	Mitomycin	DSM	35	7
Kameyama, 1992 (44)	11	Cisplatin	Lipiodol	41	N/A
Daniels, 1992 (52)	52	CAM	Collagen	34	11
Meakem, 1992 (53)	11	CAM	Collagen	71	N/A
Lang, 1993 (45)	46	Adriamycin	Lipiodol	87	23
Feun, 1994 (46)	6	Cisplatin	Lipiodol	33	N/A
Martinelli, 1994 (42)	13	Fluorouracil, Interferon	PVA	25	9.3
Stuart, 1995 (47)	20	Fluorouracil, Mitomycin,	Lipiodol, gelfoam	59	7
Sanz-Altimira, 1997 (54)	40	Fluorouracil, Mitomycin	Lipiodol, gelfoam	63	24
Tellez, 1998 (33)	30	CAM	Collagen	63	29
Bavisotto, 1999 (55)	20	Cisplatin	PVA	70	14
Salman, 2002 (56)	24	Fluorouracil, Interferon	PVA	20.8	15
Popov, 2002 (58)	11	Mitomycin	Gelfoam	N/A	9
Voigt, 2002 (59)	10	Mitomycin, Interferon	DSM	50	Not reached
Muller, 2003 (57)	66	Melphalan	Lipiodol, gelfoam	76.6	Not reached

N, Number of patients; N/A, not available; DSM, degradable starch microspheres; CAM, cisplatin, Adriamycin, mitomycin; PVA, polyvinyl alcohol.

chemoembolization, median survival was not reached after an observation period of 28 months (57, 59). These results compare favorably with systemic chemotherapy regimens containing irinotecan or oxaliplatin in combination with fluorouracil; median overall survival durations consistently approach 20 months and, in some studies, are as high as 24 months (12, 60, 61).

Chemoembolization also shows promise as an adjuvant/neoadjuvant treatment when combined with local ablative techniques. Vogl et al. (62) report that in patients with tumors measuring up to 8 cm in diameter, tumor regression after chemoemboliza-tion allowed for additional treatment with image-guided laser-induced thermotherapy. When the two modalities were combined, mean survival time was 26.2 months, a significant improvement over a survival of 12.8 months achieved in patients who received chemoembolization alone.

For the treatment of patients with colorectal liver metastases, chemoembolization has been shown to be safe option among the many treatments with a palliative role in this difficult disease. Unfortu-nately, without a Phase III trial, we will not know if chemoembolization offers an absolute survival bene-fit for patients with colorectal liver metastases.

REFERENCES

1. Steinberg SM, Barkin JS, Kaplan RS, et al. Prognostic indicators of colon tumors: The Gastrointestinal Tumor Study Group experience. Cancer, 1986 May 1; 57(9): 1866–1870.
2. Chafai N, Chan CL, Bokey El, et al. What factors influ-ence survival in patients with unresected synchronous liver metastases after resection of colorectal cancer? Col-orectal Dis, 2005 Mar; 7(2): 176–181.
3. Stangl R, Altendorf-Hofmann A, Charnley RM, et al. Factors influencing the natural history of colorectal liver metastases. Lancet, 1994; 343: 1405–1410.
4. American Cancer Society: Cancer Facts and Figures 2005 Atlanta, GA: American Cancer Society, 2005.
5. Gilbert HA, Kagan AR. Metastases: Incidence, detection and evaluation without histologic confirmation. In: Weiss L (ed.), Fundamental Aspects of Metastasis, pp. 385–405. Amsterdam: North Holland, 1976.
6. Liu L, Shang W, and Jiang H. Current treatment for liver metastases from colorectal cancer. World J Gastroenterol, 2003; 9(2): 193–200.
7. Wagner JS, Adson MA, Van Heerden JA, et al. The nat-ural history of hepatic metastases from colorectal can-cer: A comparison with resective treatment. Ann Surg, 1984;199: 502–508.
8. Wanebo HJ, Semoglou C, Attiyeh F, et al. Surgical man-agement of patients with primary operable colorectal can-

cer and synchronous liver metastases. Am J Surg, 1978; 135: 81–85.
9. Bramhall SR, Gur U, Coldham C, et al. Liver resection for colorectal metastases. Ann R Coll Surg Engl, 2003; 85: 334–339.
10. Bartlett DL, Berlin J, Lauwers GY, et al. Chemother-apy and regional therapy of hepatic colorectal metastases: Expert consensus statement. Ann Surg Oncol, 2006; 13(10): 1284–1292.
11. Douillard JY, Cunningham D, Roth AD, et al. Irinotecan combined with fluorouracil compared with fluorouracil alone as first-line treatment for metastatic colorectal cancer: A multicentre randomised trial. Lancet, 200; 355: 1041–1047.
12. Goldberg RM, Sargent DJ, Morton RF, et al. A ran-domized controlled trial of fluorouracil plus leucovorin, irinotecan, and oxaliplatin combinations in patients with previously untreated metastatic colorectal cancer. J Clin Oncol, 2004 Jan 1; 22(1): 23–30.
13. Rothenberg ML, Oza Am, Bigelow RH, et al. Superiority of oxaliplatin and fluorouracil-leucovorin compared with either therapy alone in patients with progressive colorec-tal cancer after inrinotecan and fluorouracil-leucovorin: Interim results of a phase III trial. J Clin Oncol, 2003; 21: 2059–2069.
14. Rothenberg ML, LaFleur B, Levy DE, et al. Randomized phase II trial of the clinical and biological effects of two dose levels of gefitinib in patients with recurrent colorec-tal adenocarcinoma. J Clin Oncol, 2005; 23: 9265–9274.
15. Nakamura H, Hashimoto T, Oi H, et al. Transcatheter oily chemoembolization of hepatocellular carcinoma. Radiology, 1989; 170: 783–786.
16. Sasaki Y, Imaoka S, Kasugai H, et al. A new approach to chemoembolization therapy for hepatoma using ethiodized oil, cisplatin, and gelatin sponge. Cancer, 1987; 60: 1194–1203.
17. Konno T. Targeting cancer chemotherapeutic agents by use of lipiodol contrast medium. Cancer, 1990; 66: 1897–1903.
18. Egawa H, Maki A, Mori K, et al. Effects of intra-arterial chemotherapy with a new lipophilic anticancer agent, estradiol-chlorambucil (KM2210), dissolved in lipiodol on experimental liver tumor in rats. J Surg Oncol, 1990; 44(2): 109–114.
19. Kruskal JB, Hlatky L, Hahnfeldt P, et al. In vivo and in vitro analysis of the effectiveness of doxorubicin combined with temporary arterial occlusion in liver tumors. J Vasc Interv Radiol, 1993; 4(6): 741–747.
20. Ramsey DE, Kernagis LY, Soulen MC, et al. Chemoem-bolization of hepatocellular carcinoma. J Vasc Interv Radiol, 2002; 13(9 Pt 2): S211–221.
21. Li X, Feng GS, Zheng CS, et al. Expression of plasma vascular endothelial growth factor in patients with hep-atocellular carcinoma and effect of transcatheter arterial chemoembolization therapy on plasma vascular endothe-lial growth factor level. World J Gastroenterol, 2004; 10(19): 2878–2882.
22. Liao X, Yi J, Li X, et al. Expression of angiogenic fac-tors in hepatocellular carcinoma after transcatheter arte-rial chemoembolization. J Huazhong Univ Sci Technol Med Sci, 2003; 23(3): 280–282.
23. Camma C, Shepis F, Orlando A, et al. Transarte-rial chemoembolization for unresectable hepatocellular

carcinoma: Meta-analysis of randomized controlled trials. Radiology, 2002; 224(1): 47–54.

24. Charnsangavej C, Carrasco CH, Wallace S, et al. Hepatic arterial flow distribution with hepatic neoplasms: Significance in infusion chemotherapy. Radiology, 1987 Oct; 165(1): 71–73.

25. Pentecost MJ, Daniels JR, Teitelbaum GP, et al. Hepatic chemoembolization: Safety with portal vein thrombosis. J Vasc Interv Radiol, 1993 May–Jun; 4(3): 347–351.

26. Song SY, Chung JW, Han JK, et al. Liver abscess after transcatheter oily chemoembolization for hepatic tumors: Incidence, predisposing factors and clinical outcome. J Vasc Interv Radiol, 2001; 12: 313–320.

27. Kim W, Clark TWI, Baum RA, et al. Risk factors for liver abscess formation after hepatic chemoembolization. J Vasc Interv Radiol, 2001; 12: 965–968.

28. Geschwind JF, Kaushik S, Ramsey DE, et al. Influence of a new prophylactic antibiotic therapy on the incidence of liver abscesses after chemoembolization treatment of liver tumors. J Vasc Interv Radiol, 2002; 13: 1163–1166.

29. Stuart K. Chemoembolization in the management of liver tumors. The Oncologist, 2003; 8: 425–437.

30. Kan Z, Ivancev K, Hagerstrand I, et al. In vivo microscopy of the liver after injection of lipiodol into the hepatic artery and portal vein in the rat. Acta Radiol, 1989; 30(4): 419–425.

31. Kan Z, Sato M, Ivancev I, et al. Distribution and effect of iodized poppyseed oil in the liver after hepatic artery embolization: Experimental study in several animal species. Radiology, 1993; 186(3): 861–866.

32. Kobayashi H, Hidaka H, Kajiya Y, et al. Treatment of hepatocellular carcinoma by transarterial injection of anticancer agents in iodized oil suspension or of radioactive iodized oil solution. Acta Radiol Diagn, 1986; 27(2): 139–147.

33. Tellez C, Benson AB 3rd, Lyster MT, et al. Phase II trial of chemoembolization for the treatment of metastatic colorectal carcinoma to the liver and review of the literature. Cancer, 1998; 82(7): 1250–1259.

34. Solomon B, Soulen MC, Baum RA, et al. Chemoembolization of hepatocellular carcinoma with cisplatin, doxorubicin, mitomycin-c, ethiodol and polyvinyl alcohol: Prospective evaluation of response and survival in U.S. population. J Vasc Inter Radiol, 1999; 10: 793–798.

35. Liu DM, Salem R, Bui JT, et al. Angiographic considerations in patients undergoing liver directed therapy. J Vasc Interv Radiol, 2005; 16: 911–935.

36. Borner M, Castiglione M, Triller J, et al. Considerable side effects of chemoembolization for colorectal carcinoma metastatic to the liver. Ann Oncol, 1992; 3(2): 113–115.

37. Leung DA, Goin JE, Sickles C, et al. Determinants of postembolization syndrome after hepatic chemoembolization. J Vasc Interv Radiol, 2001; 12: 321–326.

38. Berger DH, Carrasco CH, Hohn DC, et al. Hepatic artery chemoembolization or embolization for primary and metastatic liver tumors: Post-treatment management and complications. J Surg Oncol, 1995; 60: 116–121.

39. Sakamoto I, Aso N, Nagaoki K, et al. Complications associated with transcatheter arterial embolization for hepatic tumors. Radiographics, 1998; 18: 605.

40. Chung JW, Park JH, Han JK, et al. Hepatic tumors: Predisposing factors for complications of transcatheter oily chemoembolization. Radiology, 1996; 198(1): 33–40.

41. Soulen MC. Chemoembolization of hepatic malignancies. Oncology, 1994; 8(4): 77–89.

42. Martinelli DJ, Wadler S, Bakal CW, et al. Utility of embolization or chemoembolization as second-line treatment in patients with advanced or recurrent colorectal carcinoma. Cancer, 1994; 74(6): 1706–1712.

43. Kobayashi H, Inoue H, Shimada J, et al. Infra-arterial injection of doxorubicin/mitomycin-C lipiodol suspension in liver metastases. Acta Radiol, 1987; 28(3): 275–280.

44. Kameyama M, Imaoka S, Fukuda I, et al. Delayed washout of intratumor blood flow is associated with good response to intra-arterial chemoembolization for liver metastasis of colorectal cancer. Surgery, 1992; 114(1): 97–101.

45. Lang EK and Brown CL. Colorectal metastasis to the liver: Selective chemoembolization. Radiology, 1993; 189:417–422.

46. Feun LG, Reddy KR, Yrizarry JM, et al. A phase II study of chemoembolization with cisplatin and lipiodol for primary and metastatic liver cancer. Am J Clin Oncol, 1994; 17(5): 405–410.

47. Stuart K, Huberman M, Posner M, et al. Chemoembolization for colorectal liver metastases [abstract]. Proc Am Soc Clin Oncol, 1995; 14(439): 190.

48. Lorenz M, Hermann G, Kirkowa-Reimann M, et al. Temporary chemoembolization of colorectal liver metastases with degradable starch microspheres. Eur J Surg Oncol, 1989; 15: 453–462.

49. Aronsen KF, Hellkant C, Holmberg J, et al. Controlled blocking of hepatic artery flow with enzymatically degradable microspheres combined with oncolytic drugs. Eur Surg Res, 1979; 11: 99–106.

50. Starkhammar H, Hakansson L, Morales O, et al. Intraarterial mitomycin-C treatment of unresectable liver tumors: Preliminary results on the effect of degradable starch microspheres. Acta Oncol, 1987; 26: 295–300.

51. Wollner IS, Walker-Andrews SC, Smith JE, et al. Phase II study of hepatic arterial degradable starch microspheres and mitomycin. Cancer Drug Deliv, 1986; 4: 279–284.

52. Daniels S, Pentecost M, Teitelbaum G, et al. Hepatic artery chemoembolization for carcinoma of colon using angiostat collagen and cisplatin, mitomycin and doxorubicin: Response, survival and serum drug levels. Proc Am Soc Clin Oncol, 1992; 11: 171.

53. Meakem TJ III, Unger EC, Pond GD, et al. CT findings after hepatic chemoembolization. J Comput Assist Tomogr, 1992; 16(6): 916–920.

54. Sanz-Altimira PM, Spence LD, Huberman MS, et al. Selective chemoembolization in the management of hepatic metastases in refractory colorectal carcinoma: A phase II trial. Dis Colon Rectum, 1997; 40(7): 770–775.

55. Bavisotto LM, Patel NH, Althaus SJ, et al. Hepatic transcatheter arterial chemoembolization alternating with systemic protracted continuous infusion 5-fluorouracil for gastrointestinal malignancies metastatic to the liver: A phase II trial of the Puget Sound Oncology Consortium (PSOC 1104). Clin Cancer Res, 1999; 5(1): 95–109.

56. Salman HS, Cynamon J, Jagust M, et al. Randomized phase II trial of embolization versus chemoembolization therapy in previously treated patients with colorectal

carcinoma metastatic to the liver. Clin Colorectal Cancer, 2002; 2(3): 173–179.

57. Muller H, Nakchbandi V, Chatzisavvidis I, et al. Repetitive chemoembolization with melphalan plus intraarterial immunochemotherapy with 5-fluorouracil and granulocyte-macrophage colony stimulating factor (GM-CSF) as effective first- and second-line treatment of disseminated colorectal liver metastases. Hepatogastroenterology, 2003; 50(54): 1919–1926.

58. Popov I, Lavrnic S, Jelic S, et al. Chemoembolization for liver metastases from colorectal carcinoma: Risk or benefit. Neoplasma, 2002; 49(1): 43–48.

59. Voigt W, Behrmann C, Schlueter A, et al. A new chemoembolization protocol in refractory liver metastases of colorectal cancer: A feasibility study. Onkologie, 2002; 25(2): 158–164.

60. Santini D, Vincenzi B, Schiavon G, et al. Chronomodulated administration of oxaliplatin plus capecitabine (XELOX) as first-line chemotherapy in advanced colorectal cancer patients: Phase II study. Cancer Chemother Pharmacol, 2006 Aug 31 [Epub ahead of print].

61. Goldberg RM, Sargent DJ, Morton RF, et al. Randomized controlled trial of reduced-dose bolus fluorouracil plus leucovorin and irinotecan or infused fluorouracil plus leucovorin and oxaliplatin in patients with previously untreated metastatic colorectal cancer: A North American intergroup trial. J Clin Oncol, 2006; 24(21): 3347–3353.

62. Vogl TJ, Mack MG, Balzer JO, et al. Liver metastases: Neoadjuvant downsizing with transarterial chemoembolization before laser-induced thermotherapy. Radiology, 2003; 229: 457–464.

RADIOEMBOLIZATION WITH ^{90}YTTRIUM MICROSPHERES FOR COLORECTAL LIVER METASTASES

Bassel Atassi

Saad Ibrahim

Pankit Parikh

Robert K. Ryu

Kent T. Sato

Robert J. Lewandowski

Riad Salem

^{90}Yttrium (^{90}Y) microspheres are 20- to 40-μ particles that emit beta radiation. Because the microspheres are delivered via the hepatic arterial route, the process can be considered "internal" rather than external radiation. The treatment algorithm is analogous to that followed with transarterial chemoembolization (TACE). Clinical history, physical examination, laboratory values and performance status are obtained. Patients are initially evaluated and staged using cross-sectional imaging techniques (computerized tomography [CT], magnetic resonance imaging [MRI], positron emission tomography [PET]). Once a patient is considered a possible candidate for therapy, evaluation using mesenteric angiography followed by treatment on a lobar basis is undertaken. Patients are followed clinically to assess toxicities and response prior to proceed-

ing with treatment to the other lobe. A comprehensive review of the technical and methodological considerations in ^{90}Y has been previously published (1–3).

Two devices are commercially available. TheraSphere (glass) was approved in 1999 by the Food and Drug Administration (FDA) under a Humanitarian Device Exemption (HDE) for the treatment of unresectable hepatocellular carcinoma (HCC) in patients with or without portal vein thrombosis who can have appropriately positioned hepatic arterial catheters (4). SIR-Spheres (resin) were granted full pre-marketing approval in 2002 by the FDA for the treatment of colorectal metastases in conjunction with intrahepatic floxuridine (FUDR) (5). Both devices have European approval for liver neoplasia and approvals in various Asian countries.

OVERVIEW

Patients with metastatic cancer to the liver from a colorectal primary tumor may be treated using surgical resection alone, providing a chance for long-term cure. In patients with surgically unresectable liver disease with or without extrahepatic disease, systemic chemotherapy has become the standard of care for first- and second-line treatment (6, 7). Combination therapy of angiogenesis inhibitors with surgical resection has now become an integral part of first- and second-line therapies (8). Patients with liver-dominant disease who have failed standard first- and second-line therapies may be considered for treatment using ^{90}Y.

The liver is the most common site of metastases, primarily due to the spread of cancer cells through the portal circulation. In fact, approximately 60% of patients diagnosed with colorectal carcinoma eventually experience liver disease as the predominant site (9). If possible, surgical resection of metastatic hepatic disease is the treatment of choice. However, surgical resection is feasible in fewer than 20% of patients (9). Novel approaches such as ^{90}Y have a particular application in such settings.

PATIENT SCREENING AND SELECTION

Patient Presentation

Factors to consider in patients with colorectal metastases to the liver include Eastern Cooperative Oncology Group (ECOG) performance status, history of chemotherapy, surgical resection, infusion pump placement with surgically altered vascularity and imaging findings of liver-dominant disease. Of particular interest is the growing pool of patients undergoing liver-directed therapy after failure of growth-factor inhibitors, such as bevacizumab and cetuximab. Findings on cross-sectional imaging in patients with liver metastases are relatively consistent and often demonstrate bilobar disease. PET should play an integral role in the staging and clinical follow-up of patients receiving ^{90}Y therapy (10–13). The use of PET in this setting is analogous to its clinical use in patients with lymphoma (14).

Patients with metastatic disease to the liver should be staged appropriately prior to radioembolization. They should have liver-only or liver-dominant disease. Some may present with painful bulky tumors that require palliation. Unless contraindi-cated, patients should have completed standard-of-care chemotherapy. In such cases, palliative options such as TACE, bland embolization and ^{90}Y may be considered (10, 15).

As described in the oncologic literature, the best indicators of overall liver function include prothrombin time (PT), albumin and total bilirubin (16). Just as patients with these three parameters in the normal range have better outcomes following systemic chemotherapy, ^{90}Y patients will also have better long-term outcomes if these three biochemical factors are within normal range (16). Ideally, prior to treatment with ^{90}Y, patients should have recent laboratory values, including liver function and complete blood count with differential. Carcinoembryonic antigen (CEA) is the most commonly utilized tumor marker for screening, initial staging and assessment of response to treatment in colorectal cancer.

Vascular Anatomy, Gastrointestinal Flow and Pulmonary Shunt

Given the propensity for arterial variants and hepatic tumors to exhibit arterio-venous shunting, all patients being evaluated for ^{90}Y must undergo pretreatment mesenteric angiography (17–20) and assessment of lung shunting. Meticulous, detailed, power-injected digital subtraction angiography of the hepatic and visceral vasculature should be performed in all patients prior to treatment. Vessels that must be interrogated include the celiac, common and proper hepatic, gastroduodenal artery (GDA) and right and left hepatic arteries. Knowledge of the arterial anatomy allows for the administration of ^{90}Y, with one treatment to each target vascular bed (usually the hepatic lobe or segment) at 30- to 60-day intervals. This topic has been addressed in detail by previous investigators (17, 20).

During each step of the visceral angiogram, potential gastric or small bowel flow must be assessed. The celiac arteriogram is used to detect the presence of arterial variants, such as the replaced left hepatic artery or double hepatic arteries, as well as parasitization of blood flow to the liver tumors (17, 21, 22). Depending on the proximity of the left gastric branch to the other hepatic branches (such as with a gastro-hepatic trunk), coil embolization of this vessel may be warranted, as this will minimize the risk of reflux during ^{90}Y infusion. The GDA should be identified and prophylactically embolized. The right gastric artery should also be identified during angiography. Although this vessel is often seen to arise from the left hepatic artery, it can also arise from the common, proper or right hepatic artery, as well as the GDA (17, 22, 23). Depending on the anatomic location of this vessel and the relative ease with which distal catheterization may be achieved for infusion, prophylactic coil embolization may be undertaken in order to minimize inadvertent deposition of ^{90}Y into the gastrointestinal bed. Other vessels that should be identified include the cystic, supraduodenal, retroduodenal, falciform, accessory left gastric, and right and left inferior phrenic arteries (17, 20, 22).

One of the concerns with administration of 20- to 40-μ ^{90}Y microspheres is direct shunting to the lungs, possibly resulting in radiation pneumonitis (24). Once the catheter is placed in the proper hepatic artery, 4 to 5 mCi ^{99m}Tc-macroaggregated albumin (MAA) is administered intra-arterially. Because the size of ^{99m}Tc-MAA closely mimics that of ^{90}Y microspheres, it is assumed that the distribution of the microspheres will be identical to ^{99m}Tc-MAA, and this distribution is used in the planning process. Lung shunting is assessed using planar or single photon emission computed tomography (SPECT) gamma cameras. In patients with metastatic disease, significant shunting is rare unless the tumor burden is very high. Hence, lung shunting can be assessed once with catheter placement and ^{99m}Tc-MAA injection within the proper hepatic artery at the time of the planning visceral arteriogram.

The lungs can tolerate 30 Gy per treatment session and 50 Gy cumulatively (25). Therefore, when treatment planning is undertaken and lung shunting is identified, the total cumulative pulmonary dose must be calculated. Patients may be treated if their cumulative pulmonary dose does not exceed 50 Gy for all planned infusions of ^{90}Y.

TREATMENT PROCESS

Dosimetry

TheraSphere

The recommended activity of TheraSphere that should be delivered to a lobe of the liver containing tumor is between 80 Gy and 150 Gy. This wide range exists to give the treating physician clinical flexibility. The most commonly used dose range is 120 to 130 Gy, a range that balances safety and efficacy. Assuming

TheraSphere ^{90}Y microspheres distribute in a uniform manner throughout the liver and ^{90}Y undergoes complete decay in situ, radioactivity required to deliver the desired dose to the liver can be calculated using the following formula:

$$\text{Activity required (GBq)} = \frac{[\text{Desired dose (Gy)}] \times [\text{target liver mass (kg)}]}{50}$$

Given that a fraction of the microspheres will flow into the pulmonary circulation without lodging in the arterioles, when lung shunt fraction (LSF) and vial residual (R) are taken into account, the actual dose delivered to the target volume after the vial is infused becomes (18):

$$\text{Dose (Gy)} = \frac{50 [\text{Injected activity (GBq)}] \times (1\text{-LSF}) \times (1\text{-R})}{\text{target liver mass (kg)}}$$

Liver volume (cc) is estimated with CT, and then converted to mass using a conversion factor of 1.03 mg/ml.

SIR-Spheres

Assuming SIR-Spheres ^{90}Y microspheres distribute in a uniform manner throughout the liver and undergo complete decay in situ, radioactivity delivered to the liver can be calculated using one of two available methods.

The first method incorporates body surface area and estimate of tumor burden as follows (5, 26):

SIR-Spheres: Activity required (GBq) =
BSA (m^2) $-$ 0.2 + (% tumor involvement/100)

where BSA is body surface area.

The second method is based on a broad estimate of tumor burden. The larger the tumor burden, the higher the recommended activity in increments of 0.5 GBq per 25% tumor burden. For either SIR-Spheres dosimetry model, activity (GBq) is decreased depending on the extent of LSF ($\leq$10% LSF: no reduction, 10% to 15% LSF: 20% reduction, 15% to 20% LSF: 40% reduction, >20% LSF: no treatment).

Calculation of Lung Dose

Radiation pneumonitis is a theoretical concern with ^{90}Y treatment. Previous preclinical and clinical studies with ^{90}Y microspheres demonstrated that up to 30 Gy to the lungs could be tolerated with a single injection, and up to 50 Gy for multiple injections (25).

For this reason, patients with ^{99m}Tc-MAA evidence of potential pulmonary shunting resulting in lung doses greater than 50 Gy should not be treated.

The absorbed lung radiation dose is the total cumulative dose of all treatments (27):

Cumulative absorbed lung radiation dose =

$$50 \times \text{lung mass} \sum_{i=1}^{n} A_i \times LSF_i$$

where A_i = activity infused (correcting for R in vial), LSF_i = lung shunt fraction during infusion, n = number of infusions, approximate vascular lung mass (for both lungs, including blood) = 1 kg (28).

POST PROCEDURAL CARE AND FOLLOW-UP

Post Procedure Considerations

Because ^{90}Y therapy has a low toxicity profile, the treatment can be performed on an outpatient basis. Given the possibility of small unrecognized arterial vessels coursing to the gastrointestinal system, most treatment approaches recommend the routine use of prophylactic anti-ulcer medications in all patients at the time of discharge in order to minimize the risks of gastrointestinal irritation (29). Gastric coating agents may also be used. In some cases, unless contraindicated (e.g., diabetes), a tapering 5-day steroid dose pack is also given to counteract fatigue.

Because ^{90}Y is a beta emitter, most patients will have less than 1 mrem per hour surface readings following implantation. Hence, standard biohazard precautions are sufficient to protect others from exposure once they have been discharged. With resin microspheres, trace amounts (25–50 kBq/l/GBq) of urinary excretion are a possibility in the first 24 hours after implantation (30). Investigators should refer to the product inserts, institutional radiation safety committees, as well as state and federal regulatory agencies for guidance on ^{90}Y use and patient discharge instructions.

Side Effects and Toxicities

The most common side effect of treatment is fatigue (50%). The majority of patients experience transient fatigue, with vague flu-like symptoms. This may be likely related to the short-lived and low-dose radiation effects on the normal hepatic parenchyma (10, 22, 31). It is also not unusual for symptoms of shaking, chills and fever to occur several days following treatment, likely as a response to tumor lysis (1%). Other possible side effects include abdominal pain, nausea, vomiting and radiation cholecystitis. Radiation-induced liver disease is a possibility, particularly in patients with compromised liver function at initial treatment.

1. **Post-embolization Syndrome (20%–30%):** It is not uncommon for patients to experience abdominal pain in the target organ during infusion (resin microspheres). This often resolves within 30 to 60 minutes with the use of narcotics (22, 32). Post-embolization syndrome may occur in up to one-half of patients. This syndrome is not as severe as that observed with chemoembolization and is dominated by fatigue and constitutional symptoms (31–33).

2. **Radiation gastritis/GI ulcer/pancreatitis ($\leq$5%):** Attenuated radiation to adjacent structures is another clinical concern. Treatment to the left lobe of the liver may cause radiation gastritis secondary to its proximity to the stomach. Another example of attenuated radiation effect is that of a right pleural effusion, a finding occasionally seen following right-lobe treatment. Gastrointestinal ulceration and non-target administration of microspheres should be minimized using angiographic techniques previously described (17, 22, 23, 29). Non-target administration of microspheres can result in pancreatitis (5, 30).

3. **Radiation pneumonitis ($\leq$1%):** Proper lung shunting studies and incorporation of this information in dosimetry models should be practiced universally. The risk of radiation pneumonitis is mitigated if cumulative lung dose is limited to 50 Gy (25).

4. **Radiation hepatitis ($\leq$1%):** Another possible complication of radioembolization is radiation hepatitis. This mechanism involves the irradiation of normal parenchyma beyond that which is tolerated. The classical findings of anicteric ascites, elevated alkaline phosphatase, thrombocytopenia and veno-occlusive disease occurred in those patients receiving greater than 30 Gy to the liver. More recently, investigators have reported that HCC were able to tolerate 39.8 Gy, whereas patients with liver metastases could tolerate 45.8 Gy without inducing radiation hepatitis (34).

5. **Lymphopenia (40%):** Lymphopenia is another possible clinical sequela of ^{90}Y infusion, usually as a result of the sensitivity of lymphocytes to radiation.

6. **Biliary injury (≤10%):** Theoretically, given the microsphere size of 20 to 60 μ being quite similar to the vascular diameter of the peribiliary plexus, microspheres may lodge in these vessels and cause microscopic injury (17). Possibilities include abscess formation, biliary necrosis, bilomas and radiation cholecystitis (35).

7. **Radiation cholecystitis (≤2%):** Radioembolization may cause radiation cholecystitis. Although clinically relevant radiation cholecystitis requiring cholecystectomy is not common, imaging findings of gallbladder injury (enhancing wall, mural rent) are quite common (22, 35). Patients who do not develop acute cholecystitis may experience symptoms of chronic right upper quadrant pain and biliary dyskinesia.

Treatment of the Second Lobe

Thirty days following the first treatment, response to the first infusion and overall clinical status of the patient must be assessed. Liver function tests, complete blood count with differential and tumor markers, as well as cross-sectional imaging, are obtained. Depending on the presence or absence of extra-hepatic disease, tumor markers may increase, remain unchanged or decrease from baseline, making interpretation difficult. If they are increased, tumor lysis or tumor progression in the liver or extra-hepatic sites may be implicated. If they are unchanged, an argument could be made that there has been interval stabilization or improvement in tumor burden. Due to the uncertainty in interpretation of tumor markers at 30 days, their use in the assessment of clinical response should be reserved for long-term follow-up. The follow-up imaging modality used to assess tumor response should be consistent with that employed for baseline imaging. If MRI is utilized, diffusion-weighted imaging permits the documentation of necrosis and cell death (36). CT may limit the ability to definitively document tumor necrosis. However, other indirect criteria can be used, such as size of the lesion and relative alterations in vascularity and enhancement. Follow-up functional imaging such as MRI or PET may be helpful (11–13, 36).

CT/PET Evaluation of Tumor Response

Imaging evaluation of the metastatic cancer patient involves CT, MRI and PET. PET scanning has emerged as an integral imaging modality in the assessment of treatment response to ^{90}Y. Whereas CT provides anatomic information of tumor burden, PET is better at characterizing the functional status of the tumor, both prior to and following treatment. In several studies published by Wong, metastatic colorectal liver lesions were evaluated using CT and PET before and after successful ^{90}Y treatment. PET was found to be consistently superior at assessing tumor response to therapy compared with CT (11–13). Moreover, reduction in metabolic activity measured by PET was correlated with a reduction in CEA.

LITERATURE REVIEW

SIR-Spheres

Gray published a Phase III randomized clinical trial of 74 patients conducted to assess whether a single injection of SIR-Spheres in combination with intra-hepatic floxuridine (FUDR) could increase the tumor response rate, time to disease progression in the liver and increase survival compared with FUDR alone (37). Treatment-related toxicities or change in quality of life were also examined. The mean SIR-Spheres dose administered was 2.156 ± 0.32 GBq. Six of 34 patients (18%) in the hepatic artery chemotherapy (HAC) arm had at least a partial response (PR), whereas 16 of 36 patients (44%) in the HAC + ^{90}Y arm had at least a PR. The partial and complete response rate (PR + CR) was significantly greater for patients receiving SIR-Spheres when measured by tumor area (44% vs. 17.6%, p = 0.01) tumor volumes (50% vs. 24%, p = 0.03) and CEA (72% vs. 47%, p = 0.004). The median time to disease progression in the liver was significantly longer for patients receiving SIR-Spheres in comparison with patients receiving HAC alone when measured by either tumor area (9.7 vs. 15.9 months, p = 0.001), tumor volume (7.6 vs. 12.0 months, p = 0.04) or CEA (5.7 vs. 6.7 months, p = 0.06). The 1-, 2-, 3- and 5-year survival rates for patients receiving SIR-Spheres were 72%, 39%, 17% and 3.5%, compared with 68%, 29%, 6.5% and 0% for HAC alone. Cox regression analysis suggests an improvement in survival for patients treated with SIR-Spheres who survive more than 15 months (p = 0.06). There was no increase in grade 3 or 4 treatment-related toxicity and no loss of quality of life for patients receiving SIR-Spheres in comparison with patients receiving HAC alone.

Investigators reported on a 50-patient cohort with extensive colorectal liver metastases not suitable for either resection or cryotherapy (38). The study compared experience with ⁹⁰Y alone (n = 7) and in combination (n = 43) with fluorouracil (5-FU). For all patients, ⁹⁰Y microspheres were administered as a single treatment within 10 days of hepatic artery port placement. The dose was titrated to the estimated extent of disease ($\leq$25% liver replacement: 2 GBq, 25% to 50% liver replacement: 2.5 GBq, and >50% liver replacement: 3 GBq. Median CEA levels were reduced to 25% of baseline values at 1 month post treatment with ⁹⁰Y, and remained at or below 30% of baseline when followed for 6 months. Median survival for all liver metastases patients from the time of diagnosis was 14.5 months (range 1.9 to 91.4) and from the time of treatment was 9.8 months (range 1.0 to 30.3). The same group published on 38 patients with extensive colorectal liver metastases who received SIR-Spheres (39). The treatments were well tolerated, and no treatment-related mortality was observed. Response to SIR-Spheres therapy, as indicated by decreasing tumor markers and serial 3-monthly CT scans, were seen in more than 90% of patients. Estimated survival at 6, 12 and 18 months was 70%, 46% and 46%, respectively, and was principally driven by the development of extra-hepatic metastases.

Van Hazel et al. reported a randomized study of 21 patients (11 patients received SIR-Spheres + 5-FU/leucovorin (LV); 10 patients received the 5-FU/LV alone). The mean administered radiation dose in those receiving SIR-Spheres was 2.25 GBq. The authors concluded that the administration of SIR-Spheres along with a standard chemotherapeutic regimen significantly increased treatment-related response (10 vs. 0 patients demonstrated a PR on follow-up CT), time to disease progression (18.6 vs. 3.6 months) and survival (29.4 vs. 12.8 months) compared with chemotherapy alone. Despite the fact that there were more toxicities associated with the combination therapy, there was no difference in quality of life over a 3-month period (26).

The series discussed subsequently lack detail on SIR-Spheres treatment dose and method (lobar, pump, etc.).

Van Hazel presented results on a Phase I/II dose-escalation study combining SIR-Spheres with systemic chemotherapy. Seventeen chemonaive patients with liver metastases from colorectal cancer were entered into the study. Chemotherapy consisted of the 5-FU/LV/oxaliplatin (FOLFOX4) regimen, modified with an oxaliplatin dose escalated from 30 mg/m² to 85 mg/m² in order to assess safety and tolerability. SIR-Spheres were implanted by injection into the hepatic arterial system using transcatheter techniques on days 3 or 4 of the first chemotherapy cycle. Most patients experienced nausea or abdominal pain within 48 hours of ⁹⁰Y. Mild peripheral neuropathy was evident in 6 of the first 11 patients, appearing between cycles 10 and 12. Grade 3 or 4 transient neutropenia was seen in 5 of 11 patients. Three grade 3 events were documented in 2 of 3 patients at the 30 mg/m² tier (diarrhea, nausea/vomiting, fever). Six grade 3 events were seen in 4 of 8 patients in the 60 mg/m² tier (diarrhea, nausea/vomiting, abdominal pain, fever, leukopenia, anemia). At the time of presentation, only one grade 3 had been exhibited in 1 of 6 patients in the 85 mg/m² tier (nausea/vomiting). PR [based on Response Evaluation Criteria in Solid Tumors (RECIST)] were seen in all (100%) of the first 11 patients. The median time to liver progression, at the time of presentation, was 11 months. The authors concluded that SIR-Spheres in combination with oxaliplatin appear to possess an acceptable toxicity profile (40).

Goldstein presented on a Phase I dose-escalation study with irinotecan. Twenty-five patients who had failed previous chemotherapy but were irinotecan naive were entered into the study. PR were seen in 9 of 17 patients, median time to liver progression was 7.5 months and median survival was 12 months (41).

Lim reported on a 30-patient cohort comprising patients with liver metastases from colorectal origin that had failed 5-FU-based therapies (42). There was a 33% response rate, with median response duration of 8.3 months, and a time to progression of 5.3 months. Response rate and progression-free survival were lower in patients who had failed prior chemotherapy (21% and 3.9 months, respectively).

Kennedy recently reported on a seven-center multi-institutional study. Two-hundred-eight patients who had failed irinotecan and/or oxaliplatin-based chemotherapy were treated with SIR-Spheres on a lobar and whole-liver basis. Imaging response was 35%, whereas PET response was 91%. Survival was 10.5 months and 4.5 months for responders and non-responders respectively (43).

Investigators recently reported on the use of resin microspheres as first-line therapy in combination with systemic chemotherapy. A Phase I study of SIR-Spheres therapy with modified FOLFOX4 systemic chemotherapy was conducted in patients with inoperable liver metastases from colorectal cancer who had not previously received chemotherapy for metastatic disease. Oxaliplatin (30 to 85 mg/m^2) was administered for the first three cycles with full FOLFOX4 doses from cycle 4 until cycle 12. The primary endpoint was toxicity. Twenty patients were enrolled in the study. Five patients experienced National Cancer Institute (NCI; Bethesda, MD) grade 3 abdominal pain, two of whom had microsphere-induced gastric ulcers. The dose-limiting toxicity was grade 3 or 4 neutropenia, which was recorded in 12 patients. One episode of transient grade 3 hepatotoxicity was recorded. Mean splenic volume increased by 92% following 6 months of protocol therapy. PRs were demonstrated in 18 patients and stable disease in two patients. Two patients underwent partial hepatic resection following protocol therapy. Median progression-free survival was 9.3 months, and median time to progression in the liver was 12.3 months. The maximum-tolerated dose was 60 mg/m^2 of oxaliplatin for the first three cycles, with full FOLFOX4 doses thereafter (44).

In an independent series, investigators reported on 35 patients with colorectal metastases to the liver having failed two lines of chemotherapy. The aim of the study was to evaluate toxicity, clinical response and quality of life in patients with unresectable colorectal liver metastases submitted to selective internal radiotherapy with ^{90}Y microspheres. Pre-treatment evaluation included a CT scan, blood tests, a PET scan and arteriography of celiac trunk, hepatic and superior mesenteric artery; extrahepatic uptakes and pulmonary shunts more than 10% were excluded by a Scinti-scan. Other exclusion criteria were liver dysfunction and anatomical vascular anomalies. The clinical response was evaluated by CT-scan following the RECIST criteria. Median follow-up was 4 months. Median number of metastases was four (range, 1 to 15); 38% of cases presented hepatic involvement up to 25%. The median SIRT dose delivered was 1.7 GBq. Median pulmonary shunt was 6%. No operative mortality occurred; early toxicity (within 48 hours) was 20.6%, shown as fever, acute pain and leukocytosis. The late toxicity was 24.1% with chronic pain, jaundice and nausea being

the most frequent. All the toxic events were graded 2 or 3 according to the World Health Organization scale. Preliminary results were available in terms of clinical response after 6 weeks: 12.5% had a PR; 75%, a stable disease; whereas progression of disease, was observed in 12.5% of the patients (45).

TheraSphere

Goin performed a dose-escalation study in 43 colorectal metastases patients (46). The study assessed dose-related effects on survival, tumor response and toxicity. There were no life-threatening or fatal toxicities. The median survival was 408 days (95% confidence interval: 316–565 days). Two patients had a complete response, 8 had a PR and 35 (81%) were at least stable. Higher doses were associated with greater tumor response and increased survival (p = 0.05). In addition, tumor hypervascularity (p = 0.01), higher baseline performance status (p = 0.002) and less liver involvement (p = 0.004) were associated with enhanced response or survival.

Wong presented data on TheraSphere treatment of eight patients with unresectable colorectal liver metastases (13). Tumor response was evaluated using imaging (CT/MRI) and metabolic evaluation via ^{18}fluorodeoxyglucose (^{18}FDG)-PET and serum carcinoembryonic antigen (CEA). Five of the eight patients had an improvement in their tumor activity, as assessed by a decrease in ^{18}FDG-PET metabolic activity and confirmed by parallel changes in serum CEA. However, as observed in other studies, the use of imaging by CT/MRI illustrated that only some of the tumors that responded by metabolic criteria revealed a corresponding decrease in size. The authors concluded that there was a significant metabolic response to TheraSphere treatment in patients with unresectable colorectal liver metastases. The same group presented data on 27 patients with metastatic colorectal cancer to the liver (12). Tumor response was evaluated via ^{18}FDG-PET and serum CEA. The study evaluated the use of ^{18}FDG-PET to quantify the metabolic response to treatment, comparing visual estimates to standardized hepatic uptake values. Visual estimates indicated 20 patients responded to treatment, whereas 7 patients experienced progression or no change in their disease. There was a significant correlation (r = 0.75, p ≤ 0.0001) between the response group identified through visual estimation and that determined by hepatic standardized uptake values. There was no statistically significant correlation observed with CEA values (p = 0.13), which was attributed to the effect of extra-hepatic lesions.

Lewandowski reported on 27 patients with unresectable colorectal cancer treated with TheraSphere using a targeted dose of 135 to 150 Gy. Tumor response measured by PET imaging exceeded that of CT imaging for first- (88% vs. 35%) and second-treated (73% vs. 36%) lobes, respectively. Tumor replacement of 25% or less (compared with over 25%) was associated with a statistically significant increase in median survival (339 days vs. 162 days).

Atassi presented a 71-patient cohort with metastatic colorectal cancer treated using a targeted dose of 120 Gy on a lobar basis. Partial tumor response by RECIST was 35%. Survival from first treatment at 1 and 2 years was 39.1% and 22.1% respectively. Factors associated with prolonged survival included baseline ECOG performance status, number of tumors, and presence or absence of extra-hepatic disease. ECOG scores of 0 or 1 were associated with median survival of 566 and 219 days, respectively (p ≤ 0.0001). Tumor nodules of four or fewer or greater than four were associated with median survival of 566 and 216 days, respectively (p ≤ 0.0001). The presence or absence of extra-hepatic disease was related to median survival of 187 and 407 days, respectively (p ≤ 0.003) (47).

CONCLUSION

The unique aspects of ^{90}Y therapy are its minimal toxicity profile and effective local therapeutic effect, combined with minimal exposure to normal liver tissue in properly selected patients. Diligent vascular mapping during the treatment planning angiogram with embolization of the gastroduodenal and right gastric arteries, as well as other perforating vessels, will minimize the likelihood of inadvertent deposition to gastric structures. Other than mild-to-moderate constitutional symptoms, the theoretical or potential side effects of radioembolization include non-target radiation, radiation pneumonitis and radiation hepatitis. Post-procedural follow-up of the patient to assess any treatment-emergent side effects and tumor response is conducted at 30 days and then at 2- to 3-month intervals thereafter. The unique characteristics of radioembolization using ^{90}Y coupled with the minimally invasive nature provide an attractive therapeutic option for patients for whom

there are few alternatives. The technical and clinical demands of patient selection, treatment planning, ^{90}Y administration and clinical follow-up require a dedicated interdisciplinary team willing to work cooperatively to achieve the best result for the patient. Although to date clinical results with radioembolization are promising, they have yet to be subjected to large-scale, controlled trials. Efforts are under way to complete these studies.

REFERENCES

1. Salem R and Thurston KG. Radioembolization with 90yttrium microspheres: A state-of-the-art brachytherapy treatment for primary and secondary liver malignancies: Part 1: Technical and methodologic considerations. J Vasc Interv Radiol, 2006; 17(8): 1251–1278.
2. Salem R and Thurston KG. Radioembolization with 90Yttrium microspheres: A state-of-the-art brachytherapy treatment for primary and secondary liver malignancies: Part 2: Special topics. J Vasc Interv Radiol, 2006; 17(9): 1425–1439.
3. Salem R and Thurston KG. Radioembolization with yttrium-90 microspheres: A state-of-the-art brachytherapy treatment for primary and secondary liver malignancies: Part 3: Comprehensive literature review and future direction. J Vasc Interv Radiol, 2006; 17(10): 1571–1593.
4. TheraSphere Yttrium-90 microspheres package insert, MDS Nordion, Kanata, Canada. 2004.
5. SIR-Spheres Yttrium-90 microspheres package insert, SIRTeX Medical, Lane Cove, Australia. 2004.
6. Messersmith W, Laheru D, and Hidalgo M. Recent advances in the pharmacological treatment of colorectal cancer. Expert Opin Investig Drugs, 2003; 12(3): 423–434.
7. Mulcahy MF and Benson AB, 3rd. Bevacizumab in the treatment of colorectal cancer. Expert Opin Biol Ther, 2005; 5(7): 997–1005.
8. Hoff PM. Future directions in the use of antiangiogenic agents in patients with colorectal cancer. Semin Oncol, 2004; 31(6 Suppl 17): 17–21.
9. Sasson AR and Sigurdson ER. Surgical treatment of liver metastases. Semin Oncol, 2002; 29(2): 107–118.
10. Lewandowski RJ, Thurston KG, Goin JE, et al. 90Y Microsphere (TheraSphere) treatment for unresectable colorectal cancer metastases of the liver: Response to treatment at targeted doses of 135–150 Gy as measured by (18f) fluorodeoxyglucose positron emission tomography and computed tomographic imaging. J Vasc Interv Radiol, 2005; 16(12): 1641–1651.
11. Wong CY, Qing F, Savin M, et al. Reduction of metastatic load to liver after intraarterial hepatic Yttrium-90 radioembolization as evaluated by (18F) fluorodeoxyglucose positron emission tomographic imaging. J Vasc Interv Radiol, 2005; 16(8): 1101–1106.
12. Wong CY, Salem R, Qing F, et al. Metabolic response after intraarterial 90Y-glass microsphere treatment for colorectal liver metastases: comparison of quantitative

and visual analyses by 18F-FDG PET. J Nucl Med, 2004; 45(11): 1892–1897.

13. Wong CY, Salem R, Raman S, et al. Evaluating ^{90}Y-glass microsphere treatment response of unresectable colorectal liver metastases by (18F) FDG PET: A comparison with CT or MRI. Eur J Nucl Med Mol Imaging, 2002; 29(6): 815–820.

14. Jerusalem G, Hustinx R, Beguin Y, et al. Evaluation of therapy for lymphoma. Semin Nucl Med, 2005; 35(3): 186–196.

15. Tellez C, Benson AB 3rd, Lyster MT, et al. Phase II trial of chemoembolization for the treatment of metastatic colorectal carcinoma to the liver and review of the literature. Cancer, 1998; 82(7): 1250–1259.

16. Yu AS and Keeffe EB. Management of hepatocellular carcinoma. Rev Gastroenterol Disord, 2003; 3(1): 8–24.

17. Liu DM, Salem R, Bui JT, et al. Angiographic considerations in patients undergoing liver-directed therapy. J Vasc Interv Radiol, 2005; 16(7): 911–935.

18. Salem R, Thurston KG, Carr BI, et al. Yttrium-90 microspheres: Radiation therapy for unresectable liver cancer. J Vasc Interv Radiol, 2002; 13(9 Pt 2): S223–229.

19. Rhee TK, Omary RA, Gates V, et al. The effect of catheter-directed CT angiography on Yttrium-90 radioembolization treatment of hepatocellular carcinoma. J Vasc Interv Radiol, 2005; 16(8): 1085–1091.

20. Lewandowski RJ, Sato KT, Atassi B, et al. Radioembolization with ^{90}Y microspheres: Angiographic and technical considerations. Cardiovasc Intervent Radiol, 2007; 30(4): 571–592.

21. Kim HC, Chung JW, Lee W, et al. Recognizing extrahepatic collateral vessels that supply hepatocellular carcinoma to avoid complications of transcatheter arterial chemoembolization. Radiographics, 2005; 25 Suppl 1: S25–39.

22. Murthy R, Nunez R, Szklaruk J, et al. Yttrium-90 microsphere therapy for hepatic malignancy: Devices, indications, technical considerations, and potential complications. Radiographics, 2005; 25 Suppl 1: S41–55.

23. Salem R, Lewandowski RJ, Sato KT, et al. Technical aspects of radioembolization with ^{90}Y microspheres. Tech Vasc Interv Radiol, 2007 Mar;10(1):12–29.

24. Ho S, Lau WY, Leung TW, et al. Partition model for estimating radiation doses from yttrium-90 microspheres in treating hepatic tumours. Eur J Nucl Med, 1996; 23(8): 947–952.

25. Ho S, Lau WY, Leung TW, et al. Clinical evaluation of the partition model for estimating radiation doses from yttrium-90 microspheres in the treatment of hepatic cancer. Eur J Nucl Med, 1997; 24(3): 293–298.

26. Van Hazel G, Blackwell A, Anderson J, et al. Randomised phase 2 trial of SIR-Spheres plus fluorouracil/leucovorin chemotherapy versus fluorouracil/leucovorin chemotherapy alone in advanced colorectal cancer. J Surg Oncol, 2004; 88(2): 78–85.

27. Berger MJ. Distribution of absorbed dose around point sources of electrons and beta particles in water and other media. J Nucl Med, 1971; Suppl 5: 5–23.

28. Snyder W, Ford M, Warner G, et al. S Absorbed Dose Per Unit Cumulated Activity for Selected Radionuclides and Organs. New York: Society of Nuclear Medicine, 1975–1976.

29. Yip D, Allen R, Ashton C, et al. Radiation-induced ulceration of the stomach secondary to hepatic embolization with radioactive yttrium microspheres in the treatment of metastatic colon cancer. J Gastroenterol Hepatol, 2004; 19(3): 347–349.

30. SIRTeX Medical Training Manual, SIRTeX Medical, Lane Cove, Australia, 2005.

31. Salem R, Lewandowski RJ, Atassi B, et al. Treatment of unresectable hepatocellular carcinoma with use of ^{90}Y microspheres (TheraSphere): Safety, tumor response, and survival. J Vasc Interv Radiol, 2005; 16(12): 1627–1639.

32. Murthy R, Xiong H, Nunez R, et al. Yttrium 90 resin microspheres for the treatment of unresectable colorectal hepatic metastases after failure of multiple chemotherapy regimens: Preliminary results. J Vasc Interv Radiol, 2005; 16(7): 937–945.

33. Kennedy AS, Coldwell D, Nutting C, et al. Resin ^{90}Y-microsphere brachytherapy for unresectable colorectal liver metastases: Modern USA experience. Int J Radiat Oncol Biol Phys, 2006; 65(2): 412–425.

34. Dawson LA, Normolle D, Balter JM, et al. Analysis of radiation-induced liver disease using the Lyman NTCP model. Int J Radiat Oncol Biol Phys, 2002; 53(4): 810–821.

35. Lewandowski R and Salem R. Incidence of radiation cholecystitis in patients receiving Y-90 treatment for unresectable liver malignancies. J Vasc Interv Radiol, 2004; 15(2 pt 2): S162.

36. Geschwind JF, Artemov D, Abraham S, et al. Chemoembolization of liver tumor in a rabbit model: Assessment of tumor cell death with diffusion-weighted MR imaging and histologic analysis. J Vasc Interv Radiol, 2000; 11(10): 1245–1255.

37. Gray B, Van Hazel G, Hope M, et al. Randomised trial of SIR-Spheres plus chemotherapy vs. chemotherapy alone for treating patients with liver metastases from primary large bowel cancer. Ann Oncol, 2001; 12(12): 1711–1720.

38. Stubbs RS, Cannan RJ, and Mitchell AW. Selective internal radiation therapy with [90]yttrium microspheres for extensive colorectal liver metastases. J Gastrointest Surg, 2001; 5(3): 294–302.

39. Stubbs RS, Cannan RJ, and Mitchell AW. Selective internal radiation therapy (SIRT) with [90]yttrium microspheres for extensive colorectal liver metastases. Hepatogastroenterology, 2001; 48(38): 333–337.

40. Van Hazel G, Price D, Bower G, et al. Selective internal radiation therapy (SIRT) for liver metastases with concomitant systemic oxaliplatin, 5-fluorouracil and folinic acid: A phase I/II dose escalation study. ASCO GI Symposium 2005, Miami, Florida.

41. Goldstein D, Van Hazel G, Pavlakis N, et al. Selective internal radiation therapy (SIRT) plus systemic chemotherapy with irinotecan: A phase I dose escalation study. American Society of Clinical Oncology, 2005, Orlando, Florida.

42. Lim LC, Gibbs P, Yip D, Shapiro J, et al. A prospective evaluation of treatment with selective internal radiation therapy (SIR-Spheres) in patients with unresectable liver metastases from colorectal cancer previously treated with 5-FU based chemotherapy. BMC Cancer, 2005; 5(1): 132.

43. Kennedy AS, Coldwell D, Nutting C, et al. Resin ^{90}Y-microsphere brachytherapy for unresectable colorectal

liver metastases: Modern USA experience. Int J Radiat Oncol Biol Phys, 2006; 65(2): 412–425.

44. Sharma RA, Van Hazel GA, Morgan B, et al. Radioembolization of liver metastases from colorectal cancer using yttrium-90 microspheres with concomitant systemic oxaliplatin, fluorouracil, and leucovorin chemotherapy. J Clin Oncol, 2007; 25(9): 1099–1106.

45. Mancini R, Carpanese L, Sciuto R, et al. A multicentric phase II clinical trial on intra-arterial hepatic radiotherapy with ^{90}yttrium SIR-Spheres in unresectable, colorectal liver metastases refractory to i.v. chemotherapy: Preliminary results on toxicity and response rates. In Vivo, 2006; 20(6A): 711–714.

46. Goin JE, Dancey JE, Hermann GA, et al. Treatment of unresectable metastatic colorectal carcinoma to the liver with intrahepatic Y-90 microspheres: A dose-ranging study. World J Nucl Med, 2003; 2: 216–225.

47. Atassi B, Lewandowski R, Mulachy M, et al. Treatment with Yttrium-90 microspheres of unresectable metastatic colorectal cancer to the liver: Safety, treatment response and survival. ASCO GI Symposium 2006, San Francisco, California.

Chapter 25

CARCINOID AND RELATED NEUROENDOCRINE TUMORS

Richard R. P. Warner

Michelle Kang Kim

A convincing and large body of evidence for the benefit of much more aggressive treatment of neuroendocrine tumors (NETs) has accumulated in recent years (1–6). The interventional radiologist is frequently involved by this trend and hence must have a general knowledge of the many aspects of these tumors. In general, NETs are much slower growing than are the more commonly encountered malignancies. Furthermore, they are rare. Hence, they are usually diagnosed later in their course. Distant metastases are found in 12.9% of all carcinoids at the time of their diagnosis, and the majority of metastases are from small intestinal primary tumors, with the most frequent site of distant metastasis being the liver (7, 8). However, even when far advanced, these tumors usually are amenable to aggressive treatment that would not be undertaken for other, more common malignancies at an equally advanced stage.

NOMENCLATURE AND DESCRIPTION

NETs represent a heterogeneous group of lesions with widely varying natural histories. The term *carcinoid* was initially coined to describe a carcinoma-like tumor that was believed to be less aggressive than adenocarcinoma (9). It is now known, however, that although they tend to grow more slowly than most other malignancies, these lesions actually represent a wide array of biologic and clinical behavior.

There has been considerable confusion in the literature regarding the classification and nomenclature of NETs and carcinoids. Pathologists have historically referred to all NETs as carcinoids because of their similar histologic appearance. In contrast, clinicians have generally used *carcinoid* to mean a serotonin-producing tumor. Another source of confusion has been the description of pathologic behavior. Whereas the term *typical* has generally referred to tumors with little pleomorphism and rare mitotic figures, *atypical* has referred to poorly differentiated lesions with increased mitotic activity. In keeping with the varying degrees of differentiation, typical lesions have generally been associated with a more indolent clinical course, whereas atypical lesions have implied a more aggressive clinical course.

Because of these inconsistencies, the World Health Organization adopted the terms *neuroendocrine tumor* and *neuroendocrine carcinoma*. This distinction draws attention to the differences among the well-differentiated NETs, well-differentiated neuroendocrine carcinomas and poorly differentiated NETs (10).

In recent years, development and increased availability of sensitive diagnostic imaging modalities, such as computed tomography (CT) and magnetic resonance imaging (MRI), somatostatin receptor scintigraphy, positron emission tomography (PET) scanning and endoscopy, as well as the availability of blood and urinary marker assays, have improved the understanding of the wide spectrum of clinical behavior and courses manifested by these lesions. There have been recent improvements in survival (7, 11); this may be related to our improved understanding and more aggressive approach in management of these lesions.

ORIGIN

Initially, neuroendocrine tumors were thought to arise embryologically from the neural crest. They are known, however, to arise mainly from neuroendocrine stem cells of the gastrointestinal tract and pancreatic islets of Langerhans; other sites of neuroendocrine cells include the lung, bronchus, thymus and thyroid (12, 13). The term *neuroendocrine* arose from similarities of these cells with neural cells, as well as the endocrine functions served by the substances they secrete. Like neural cells, they produce biologically active hormones, contain secretory granules, and have markers such as chromogranin-A, synaptophysin and neuron-specific enolase. However, unlike neural cells, they lack axons and synapses. In addition, they secrete bioactive hormones that function as transmitters. Because these cells stain positively for chromaffin, with chromium salts and similar stains, neuroendocrine cells are also known as enterochromaffin cells.

NETs are frequently defined by the hormones they produce and the resulting clinical syndrome. For instance, the gastrinomas are associated with excessive gastrin and insulinomas are associated with excessive insulin production. The clinical syndrome results from the excessive production of the tumor's bioactive substances. In contrast, NETs that do not produce an excessive amount of hormone are termed *non-functioning neuroendocrine tumors*. As one might expect, these tumors produce no clinical syndrome.

DISTRIBUTION

Carcinoids comprise more than three fourths of all NETs. Two-thirds are of gastroenteropancreatic origin and one-quarter arise in the lung and thymus. Fewer than 8% arise in unusual sites such as ovaries, testes, prostate, bladder, kidney and breast (7).

NETs have also been classified based upon their embryologic origin. Foregut tumors include those originating from the bronchi, stomach, pancreas, gallbladder and duodenum. Midgut tumors include those of the small intestine, appendix and proximal colon. Finally, the hindgut includes tumors of the distal colon, rectum and genitourinary tract. This classification is meaningful because tumors arising from these different sites entail different treatments and prognoses.

INCIDENCE

Earlier studies have demonstrated a rate of fewer than two newly diagnosed carcinoids per 100,000 of the general population reported per year in the United States (14–17). However, more recent studies estimate an increasing incidence, with approximately three to four newly diagnosed cases reported per year per 100,000 of the population (7, 18–20). This increased incidence most likely reflects increased detection and awareness rather than increased disease prevalence.

Although NETs represent only 2% of all gastrointestinal malignancies, autopsy studies have demonstrated a much higher incidence. In one study, when the entire pancreas was examined, 10% of patients had diminutive asymptomatic NETs (21).

Within the gastrointestinal tract, the majority of carcinoids originate from the small intestine, usually the ileum. The next most common sites of gastrointestinal carcinoids are the rectum and appendix.

Of the functioning pancreatic NETs, insulinomas and gastrinomas are the most common entities, but non-functioning pancreatic NETs are even more frequent. Although the latter had initially been thought to release no hormonal products, they are now known to frequently produce chromogranin-A and pancreatic polypeptide. These peptide neurohumoral products, however, cause no symptoms.

Carcinoid syndrome occurs in 40% to 60% of midgut carcinoids with liver metastases, in a smaller percent of metastatic foregut carcinoids and almost never with metastatic hindgut carcinoids (22, 23). Only a minority of all metastatic carcinoids, 20% to 40%, manifest carcinoid syndrome. With the passage of time, the majority of progressive unresectable carcinoids of the gastrointestinal tract and pancreatic NETs eventually metastasize to the liver (7). A similar spread to the liver can be predicted in a smaller percentage of progressing unresected foregut and hindgut carcinoids. In a small number of metastatic foregut carcinoids, the carcinoid syndrome can sometimes occur even without liver metastases. Carcinoid

TABLE 25.1 Neuroendocrine Tumor Syndromes

Tumor	Syndrome	Hormone	Clinical Features	Site	% Malignant	Standard Treatment*
Carcinoid	Carcinoid syndrome	Serotonin, bradykinin, tachykinins, prostaglandin and others	Facial flushing, diarrhea, bronchospasm, right-heart failure, hypotension	GI tract, lung, pancreas, ovary	12.9 overall, >25 midgut carcinoids	Surgery, octreotide, chemotherapy
Insulinoma	Insulinoma	Insulin, C-peptide	Hypoglycemia, weight gain	Pancreas	10	Surgery, diet, IV dextrose, chemotherapy, diazoxide
Gastrinoma	Zollinger-Ellison syndrome	Gastrin	Severe peptic ulcer, gastric hypersecretion, diarrhea	70% duodenum, 25% pancreas	60–90	PPI drugs, surgery, octreotide
VIPoma	Verner-Morrison syndrome, pancreatic cholera, WDHA syndrome	Vasoactive intestinal peptide (VIP)	Diarrhea, hypokalemia, achlorhydria, flushing, weight loss	90% pancreas	>50	IV fluids, K^+, surgery, octreotide, chemotherapy
Glucagonoma	Glucagonoma syndrome	Glucagon	Diabetes, skin rash, DVT, depression	Pancreas	>50	Surgery, diet, insulin, octreotide, anticoagulant, chemotherapy
Somatostatinoma	Somatostatinoma syndrome	Somatostatin	Diabetes, gallstones, weight loss, steatorrhea	56% pancreas, 44% upper intestine	70–80	Surgery, insulin, pancreatic digestive enzymes
Extremely Rare Tumors						
ACTHoma	Ectopic Cushing's syndrome	Adrenocorticotropic hormone	Hypertension, diabetes, weakness	Lung, pancreas, thymus	>99	Surgery, chemotherapy, octreotide
PTHrPoma	Hyperparathyroidism	Parathyroid hormone-related peptide	Hypercalcemia, nephrolithiasis	Pancreas, lung, thymus	>99	Surgery, chemotherapy
GRFoma	Acromegaly	Growth hormone releasing factor	Acromegaly	Pancreas, lung, thymus	>30	Surgery, chemotherapy, octreotide
Others						
Pheochromocytoma	Pheochromocytoma syndrome	Vasopressors, catecholamines	Hypertension, flushing, palpitations, headache, diaphoresis	Adrenal, sympathetic ganglia	3–13	Anti-hypertension drugs, surgery, chemotherapy, I^{131} MIBG

*Cytoreduction for all tumor syndromes when metastases are not totally resectable.
PPI, Proton pump inhibitor; WDHA, Watery diarrhea, hypokalemia, achlorhydria; DVT, Deep venous thrombosis.

292

TABLE 25.2 Interventional Radiology Procedures for Carcinoid/NETs

Biopsy
Hepatic artery catheterization, angiogram and embolus injection with or without chemotherapy or radioisotope (^{90}Y)
Radiofrequency ablation (RFA)
Cryoablation
Relief of jaundice (stent/catheter)
Percutaneous drainage of abscess or effusion
Intratumoral injection of alcohol or other medication (rarely performed)

TABLE 25.3 Clinical Features of Carcinoid Syndrome

Major	Minor
Flushing	Peptic ulcer
Diarrhea	Hypoalbuminemia
Pellagra	Muscle wasting
Venous telangiectasia	Arthralgias
Bronchospasm	Myopathy
Cardiac manifestations	Fibrosis
Hepatomegaly	Hyperglycemia
Brawny edema	

syndrome produced by liver metastases infrequently results from metastatic primary carcinoids of islet cell origin in the pancreas. Fifteen percent to thirty percent of pancreatic NETs (islet cell tumors) do not cause clinical endocrine syndromes (non-functioning tumors). The remainder are of varying types, each with its own rare syndrome and related specific medical treatment (Table 25.1).

ROLE OF THE INTERVENTIONAL RADIOLOGIST

The management of carcinoid/NETs may involve the interventional radiologist to perform biopsy as well as a variety of therapeutic procedures, some for cytoreduction of tumors, others for relief of obstructive processes, and for drainage of abscesses and effusions (Table 25.2). Various aspects of these procedures will be discussed in relation to carcinoid but apply to all NETs. In patients with NETs and liver metastases with or without endocrine syndrome, liver failure is the most common cause of death. Cytoreduction of liver tumors has been demonstrated to prolong survival and is indicated if significant liver metastases are present and especially if there is evidence of progression of liver tumors. Excision, ablation or embolotherapy are indicated for the palliation of poorly controlled endocrine syndrome and also can be used to reduce extensive and inoperable liver metastases in the sometimes successful effort to convert a large burden of tumor disease to a resectable state (4, 5).

CARCINOID SYNDROME

Carcinoid syndrome is composed of one or more prominent symptoms resulting from release of increased amounts of potent vasoactive substances produced by the tumor into the systemic circulation (Table 25.3). This usually requires liver metastases, but tumors with venous drainage into the caval system rather than the portal system can produce carcinoid syndrome without liver metastases. The major manifestations of carcinoid syndrome are facial flushing, diarrhea and bronchospasm. Initially these occur as intermittent, widely spaced, fleeting episodes but eventually can become more prolonged or even chronic. Additional major features are right-sided heart failure with tricuspid regurgitation and pulmonic valve stenosis and hepatomegaly. Arrhythmias also may occur. Other cardiac manifestations are very common but usually occur late in the course of the disease. Minor features of the syndrome are non-specific but often present. An outline of the many modalities used in treating carcinoid syndrome is presented in Table 25.4.

TABLE 25.4 Treatment of Carcinoid Syndrome

I. Supportive Measures
　Somatostatin analogs (octreotide, lanreotide)
　Standard antidiarrheal medications
　Nutritional factors (niacin, multivitamins, hematinics, food supplements, electrolytes)
　Anti-ulcer medications
II. Surgery
　Resection for cure
　Debulking (RFA, cryoablation and other procedures for palliation)
　Embolotherapy with or without chemotherapy
III. Anti-proliferative Treatment
　Biotherapy (somatostatin analog/α-interferon)
　Radiotherapy (external beam, intrahepatic artery ^{90}Y microspheres, systemic PRRT,* ^{131}I MIBG)
　Chemotherapy (systemic)
　Hepatic artery embolus therapy with chemotherapy[†]
　Hepatic artery bland embolus therapy[‡]

*Peptide receptor radiotherapy (^{90}Y, ^{177}LU, ^{68}GA).
[†]HACE.
[‡]HAE.

CARCINOID CRISIS

One of the most important and serious concerns for the interventional radiologist undertaking an invasive procedure in a carcinoid patient is the avoidance of a carcinoid crisis and how to manage it if it occurs. **Carcinoid crisis** is an abrupt change in the hemodynamics of a carcinoid tumor patient and is characterized by red flushing of the face, hypotension or even shock, tachycardia, and sometimes dyspnea, with or without bronchospasm. In a small minority of cases, the episode may be accompanied by hypertension (24). These attacks can be provoked by anesthesia, adrenergic stimuli (both endogenous and exogenous) such as anxiety or epinephrine, adrenergic vasopressors or, the injection of irritating chemicals into the tumor or suddenly rendering tumors ischemic (embolus injection). These episodes result from the abrupt release of the tumor's potent vasoactive products into the systemic circulation. Octreotide can be life saving in reversing a carcinoid crisis attack and is also usually effective in preventing these episodes when given preoperatively (25, 26).

Even patients with apparently non-functioning carcinoids who have never exhibited any clinical features of the carcinoid syndrome are at risk, especially if they have been found to have any increase in blood or urine carcinoid markers (serotonin, chromogranin-A, 5-hydroxyindole acetic acid [5-HIAA]). These markers should have been assayed in all cases previously or as part of the evaluation for the treatment (27). In the patient who has never had octreotide, it is prudent to administer a small 50-μg subcutaneous dose several days or more prior to the procedure to check for tolerance and for the very infrequent idiosyncratic reaction to the drug. In the somatostatin analog therapy-naïve patient without carcinoid syndrome 100 to 250 μg of octreotide should be given by subcutaneous injection 1 or 2 hours before the invasive procedure, and additional drug should be immediately available for intravenous use if needed during the procedure. For the patient with carcinoid syndrome, preoperative prophylaxis should be 250 to 500 μg subcutaneously depending on the patient's dose of maintenance octreotide that was previously required for controlling their symptoms. A continuous intravenous infusion of 100 μg/hour should be administered during the procedure and for 24 hours thereafter. However, if a carcinoid crisis occurs during the procedure, an intravenous bolus of 100 to 500 μg of octreotide should be given and thereafter the continuous intravenous infusion should be maintained at 100 μg/hour. Pulmonary carcinoids sometimes produce histamine and other products, and therefore, in addition to octreotide, control of this crisis may also require intravenous H-1 and H-2 blockers and corticosteroids.

In patients with shock not rapidly responding to octreotide and intravenous fluids, general measures in treating shock, such as airway intubation, should be rapidly applied and vasopressors may also be necessary. Because of the provocative effect of adrenergic agonists on carcinoid syndrome, this type of drug must be used with great caution. Dopamine appears to be the safest and is usually effective in this situation if large doses of octreotide are simultaneously administered. Nevertheless, dopamine should be tapered and discontinued as soon as possible.

Patients with hypertensive carcinoid crisis should be managed with octreotide in the same way as those patients with classic carcinoid crisis but may also require intravenous anti-hypertensive medications if they do not promptly respond to octreotide (24). In such cases, we employ the following drugs in the sequence listed: labetalol, hydralazine, nitroglycerine, sodium nitroprusside.

BIOPSY

Histologic diagnosis by biopsy of tumor tissue is essential for the diagnosis and determination of the type of NET. This is accomplished by standard and appropriate immunohistochemical stains – that is, gastrin, serotonin, vasoactive intestinal polypeptide (VIP), glucagon, insulin, adrenocorticotropic hormone (ACTH) and so on. Furthermore, in addition to establishing the diagnosis, biopsy can facilitate predicting the degree of aggressiveness or indolence of the tumor by determining its proliferation index. This is done by counting the percent of cells staining positively for Ki-67 (MIB-1). This is also determined by counting the percentage of tumor cells exhibiting mitosis and judging the extent of differentiation of the cells along with the presence or absence of foci of necrosis. Some immunohistochemical stains can help determine the site of origin of metastatic NETs. TTF-1 points to an origin from an organ derived from the embryologic foregut such as the lung. CDX-2 staining strongly positive implicates a midgut (intestinal) origin. Because foregut and midgut carcinoids as well as other NETs respond differently to various chemotherapy regimens and also have somewhat different natural courses, these special histologic studies of biopsied NETs can aid the clinician in management of the patient. With the burgeoning development of new cancer drugs targeted to specific membrane or intracellular enzymes or other essential molecular signaling and controlling substances, it is becoming important to do special stains for specific tissue markers (VEGFR, EGFR, C-KIT, etc.) which may indicate the likelihood of response to specific new target-oriented drugs. Furthermore, it is now recognized that carcinoids and all NETs in general are very heterogeneous tumors that, though looking alike on standard histologic examination, can each, with special stains, be distinguished as quite different in their biological behavior and response to treatment. Fine-needle aspiration (FNA) biopsy, though helping to establish that a tumor is a neuroendocrine neoplasm, usually provides too scanty a sampling of cells to permit all of the various studies noted earlier. Therefore, a core needle biopsy is much preferred over FNA whenever possible.

EMBOLOTHERAPY WITH AND WITHOUT CHEMOTHERAPY (HACE/HAE)

The rationale of this treatment is the proven observation that metastatic tumors in the liver derive almost all of their blood supply from the hepatic artery, whereas most of the blood to the normal hepatic parenchyma is from the portal vein. Hence, metastatic tumors can be made ischemic by interrupting their arterial supply. Concurrent hepatic artery injection of chemotherapy can produce greater concentrations of the drugs in the tumor and longer dwelling time than can be obtained with systemic or portal vein injection. Furthermore, ischemia appears to enhance the tumor's response to chemotherapy. Hypervascular tumors, such as carcinoid/NETs, appear to receive a larger proportion of the drugs and particles injected into the hepatic artery, and perhaps that accounts for their greater response to embolotherapy in comparison to that of less vascular tumors such as colorectal metastases (29–30). The general indications for these and other interventional cytoreductive treatments for carcinoid/NETs are indicated in Table 25.5.

Embolotherapy consists of injection of therapeutic agents through a percutaneously introduced catheter

TABLE 25.5 Indications for HACE, HAE, and RFA in Carcinoid/NETs

Palliation of poorly controlled endocrine syndrome
Progressing metastatic tumor in liver
Attempt to convert unresectable liver metastases to resectable status

positioned in the proper hepatic arteries or their branches. Angiography of the celiac and superior mesenteric artery (SMA) is performed with imaging carried out through the portal venous phase in order to determine the patency of the portal vein and the presence of collaterals or anatomical variants. Then, following appropriate positioning of the catheter, an injection is made consisting of contrast or iodinated oil (lipiodol), chemotherapy and embolic particles. Unfortunately, there is no general uniformity as to the chemotherapy agents used, their dosage, the size and type of particles and the sequence in which these are administered – if not injected simultaneously as a mixture. Because arteries to extra-hepatic structures usually arise from the common hepatic artery or its branches, the therapeutic injection should not be given proximal to the gastroduodenal artery (GDA). It must be emphasized that even if no branches to sites outside of the liver are seen arising from the left or right hepatic artery, it is still prudent not to attempt treating the entire liver at one session because treatment of the entire liver at one time is associated with increased mortality (30). In addition, if the patient has a functioning tumor causing the carcinoid syndrome, there is a greater risk of precipitating carcinoid crisis. Therefore, treatment should be selectively given to one lobe at a time or even to a smaller portion of the liver. Avoidance of injecting the cystic artery is desirable, but when not possible, the procedure is not precluded.

When native hepatic arteries were previously occluded, various collateral vessels have been treated successfully with bland emboli only, because of the potential communication of cutaneous vessels and hence the risk of cutaneous ischemic ulceration. The usual communicating vessels are the inferior phrenic, internal mammary and intercostal arteries (32, 33).

Particles used for embolization are: gelatin sponge (Gelfoam), polyvinyl alcohol (PVA-Contour), Embospheres, Bead Block and lipiodol (Ethiodol). Because of the wide variation in HACE/HAE protocols, no one regimen has been determined to be superior. The size of particles used ranges from 20 μg to 500 μg or even larger. From one to three chemotherapy drugs are used, injected individually or (doxorubicin) mixed with lipiodol and injected, then followed by embolus injection. Very often, three drugs (mitomycin-C, doxorubicin and cisplatin) are mixed in contrast dye and embolus suspension and all injected together. The dosages of these drugs vary. A popular schedule is 20 mg mitomycin-C, 30 mg doxorubicin and 50 mg lyophilized cisplatin. The total volume makes an injection of 18 to 20 ml. This is injected until stasis is seen, with care to stop the injection prior to reflux, even if the entire dosage has not been administered. Many other drugs also used for intravenous chemotherapy have been tried or are still being evaluated for hepatic artery injection (28).

No study of transarterial treatment of metastatic cancer of the liver has yet demonstrated a difference in survival between HACE and HAE (34, 35), although advocates of each type of treatment have presented data in support of their viewpoints. However, there is evidence that these therapies do prolong survival. The proponents for chemoembolotherapy appear to outnumber those in favor of bland embolotherapy. Most of the studies bearing on these two modalities have been carried out in patients with hepatocellular carcinoma. However, a recent study comparing chemoembolization with bland embolization of NET metastases to the liver reported a clear trend favoring chemoembolization for greater improvement in TTP, symptom control and survival (36).

Another emerging transarterial therapy for NET metastases in the liver (and also for colorectal metastases and HCC) is selective hepatic artery injection of yttrium-90 (^{90}Y) microspheres. Early results of this radioembolization appear to equal or even better those of chemoembolization (37).

PORTAL VEIN OCCLUSION

Portal vein occlusion has been considered a contraindication for hepatic artery chemoembolus injection. However, it has been observed in hepatocellular carcinoma patients with portal vein occlusion that chemoembolus injected selectively into secondary or tertiary tumor vessels can be done with benefit and without serious side effects (38, 39). Though there are no similar studies in NETs, it seems likely that the same observation would also pertain in these hypervascular tumors. There are many other rela-

TABLE 25.6 Contraindications for HACE/HAE

Uncontrollable carcinoid syndrome
Liver failure (jaundice, bilirubin >2.0 mg/dl, encephalopathy)
Ascites
>50%–80% of liver replaced by tumor
Incorrectable coagulation defect
Extensive extrahepatic metastatic tumor
Congestive heart failure
Severe malnutrition
Severe hyperuricemia
Portal vein obstruction
Impaired renal function (creatinine >2.0 mg/dl)

tive and absolute contraindications to HACE/HAE (Table 25.6).

LIVER FAILURE

In patients with severe hepatic functional impairment, hepatic artery infusion of chemotherapy alone can be considered and is likely to be tolerated if given in reduced dosage (40). The benefits, however, are questionable. HACE/HAE for a patient with bilirubin of 20 mg/dl or higher or serum albumin under 2.8 μg/dl carries an increased risk of liver failure and should be restricted to a very limited segment of the liver at any one session, if done at all (32, 41, 42).

REPEAT TREATMENT

Repeat treatment for an untreated segment of the liver may be done as soon as 2 to 4 weeks after prior treatment but should not be undertaken until manifestations of the post-embolization syndrome have subsided. If a second or third embolotherapy is planned to complete treatment of the entire liver, imaging between treatments is not essential unless the intervals are very prolonged or there is a question regarding a complication (35, 43).

EVALUATING RESPONSE

Response to treatment by imaging after HACE/HAE should not be evaluated until 4 to 6 weeks after all tumor-bearing areas have been treated. The main changes on CT are signs of tumor necrosis, decrease in tumor size and absence of arterial phase enhancement if it was present prior to treatment. Decrease in tumor size need not occur as an indication of decrease in tumor cell mass. Sometimes the tumor may even

TABLE 25.7 Evaluation of Response to Cytoreductive Treatment

Subjective (change in symptoms)
Objective
- change in size, shape, and texture of tumors (physical exam, imaging)
- change in level of chemical markers (5-HIAA, CGA, serotonin, gastrin, glucagon, etc.)

increase in size after effective HACE/HAE. On MRI, disappearance of arterial enhancement is an indicator of tumor necrosis (29, 31). Follow-up imaging with MRI should not be done sooner than 2 months after HACE/HAE (Table 25.7).

DURATION OF RESPONSE

HACE/HAE palliates hormone symptoms in more than 90% of carcinoid/NET patients with clinical endocrine symptoms resulting from liver metastases (31). The mean duration of response in such patients may be nearly 2 years in some instances. The benefit of these therapies when administered for the relief of pain is of shorter duration, with a mean of approximately 6 months.

PRE-PROCEDURAL PREPARATION (35, 43)

- Intravenous hydration with normal saline starting the night before the procedure.

- Octreotide for carcinoids (see treatment of carcinoid crisis).

- Immediately prior to the procedure, anti-emetic medication and octreotide should be administered.

- Corticosteroids (hydrocortisone 100 mg intravenously every 8 hours) for carcinoid syndrome patients.

- Broad-spectrum antibiotics (particularly to cover gram-negative enteric organisms) starting the night before the procedure.

- Bowel prep – discretionary.

POST-PROCEDURAL MANAGEMENT

Besides standard immobilization for arterial puncture, the patient should be continued on intraveous fluids and antibiotics (35). Steroids should be rapidly tapered over a 2- to 3-day period and anti-emetics and analgesics administered as necessary. Octreotide should be continued in dosage commensurate with the severity of the carcinoid syndrome. Parenteral proton-pump inhibitors (PPI) or H_2-blocking drugs should be administered. Oral feedings and medications can be resumed as soon as the patient's condition permits. Antibiotics should be continued orally for approximately 5 days after the procedure.

Following HACE/HAE, most patients will have at least some of the features of the post-embolization syndrome, consisting of nausea, vomiting, anorexia, right upper quadrant or epigastric pain, fever, weakness, leukocytosis and transient worsening of liver chemistries – particularly transaminases (42). The last usually recedes within a week, as do the pain and vomiting. Anorexia and weakness may last longer, wholly subsiding over a period as long as 1 month. Treatment is symptomatic in addition to hydration with electrolytes and parenteral analgesia. Parenteral PPI or H_2-blocking medication for protection against peptic ulceration is often used. The absence of any post-embolization symptoms may predict a minimal beneficial response to the hepatic artery treatment. Patients with carcinoid syndrome may experience transient worsening of the syndrome for several days to several weeks following the procedure.

The intermittent infusion of 1% lidocaine between aliquots of chemotherapy with or without lipiodol has been suggested as a means of decreasing post-embolization pain (44). This practice has not been widely used. The risks and complications of embolotherapy for carcinoid/NETs are listed in Table 25.8.

TABLE 25.8 Risks and Complications of Embolotherapy for Carcinoid/NETs

Severe postembolization syndrome
Extrahepatic perfusion of injected agents
Infarction of gallbladder or liver
Tumor lysis syndrome
Carcinoid crisis (causing acute renal failure, acute myocardial infarction, acute ischemic cerebrovascular incident)
Liver failure
Infection
Gastrointestinal tract bleeding/ulcer
Disseminated intravascular coagulation (DIC) syndrome
Biloma requiring drainage
Pulmonary arterial oil embolus
Arterial puncture site complications (hemorrhage, thrombosis, embolus, aneurysm)

^{90}YTTRIUM HEPATIC BRACHYTHERAPY

In the past few years, hepatic brachytherapy utilizing intrahepatic artery injection of ^{90}Y-bearing microspheres has emerged as a therapy at least equally effective as HACE/HAE for treating hepatic metastases of carcinoid and other NETs. This treatment appears to be gentler and of longer effectiveness. The Food and Drug Administration has approved ^{90}Y-bearing resin microspheres (SirSpheres) along with chemotherapy for treatment of colorectal hepatic metastases. However, it has been rather widely used off label for carcinoids/NETs (43). A second microsphere ^{90}Y agent (Theraspheres) approved for HCC has also been administered to carcinoid/NETs with equally good tolerance and response. This type of therapy with radioisotope-bearing microspheres is somewhat more demanding technically and requires specific training, regulatory agency approval and participation of a radiation oncologist or nuclear medicine specialist. Indications and contraindications for ^{90}Y microsphere hepatic artery treatment are similar to those of HACE/HAE. The risks and sequelae of this treatment are also similar to those of standard embolotherapy plus the risks associated with the injection of radiotherapeutic isotope. Tumor response to intrahepatic brachytherapy with a beta-emitting isotope is very gradual, and hence follow-up imaging should not be done sooner than 3 to 4 months after the procedure. Changes indicating regression of metastatic tumors in the liver in response to this treatment occasionally may not reach their maximum degree until as long as 1 year following the treatment (46).

RADIOFREQUENCY ABLATION

Radiofrequency ablation (RFA) performed by the interventional radiologist is usually done percutaneously and can be performed on multiple metastatic liver tumors if accessible and between 1 and 5 cm in diameter. It can also be done by the surgeon at laparoscopy or open surgery. The number, size and location of NET lesions in the liver will determine the choice of cytoablation either by surgical excision, RFA, cryoablation, HACE/HAE or radioembolization. In some instances, some or all four of these modalities will be utilized sequentially. It is our general impression that the outcome of HACE embolotherapy is better if it is done before RFA.

In addition to the customary risks of RFA, there is the additional risk in a patient with carcinoid syndrome of provoking a transient worsening of the syndrome due to release of vasoactive substances by necrosing tumor for several days after the procedure, or of triggering a carcinoid crisis during or immediately after the procedure (47).

PHEOCHROMOCYTOMA (48)

We include this functioning endocrine tumor in our discussion because some of the similarities of its syndrome are sometimes confused with carcinoid syndrome, resulting in incorrect treatment. Recognition of the correct syndrome and its prompt, adequate, specific treatment is imperative given that each of these two syndromes has a lethal potential. Pheochromocytoma is not a neoplasm arising from the neuroendocrine system but derives from cells of neuroectodermal origin from the adrenal medulla or, less often, from sympathetic ganglia elsewhere in the body. Paroxysmal or sustained hypertension are the outstanding most common features of this syndrome and are most often accompanied by one or more of the following: headache, diaphoresis, facial and even body flushing, palpitations, syncope and chest pain. The hypertensive crises that characterize pheochromocytoma can be precipitated by surgery, anesthesia, angiography and a fairly wide variety of drugs, including various antidepressants, droperidol, glucagon, metoclopramide, phenothiazines and naloxone. Physical exertion, trauma and anxiety may also precipitate these crises. Carcinoid crisis can look quite the same because of extreme flushing, palpitations and tachycardia but is usually associated with hypotension or even shock. However, infrequently, carcinoid crisis is associated with hypertension and in such instances can be very easily confused with a paroxysmal pheochromocytoma attack.

Malignant pheochromocytoma with metastasis to lungs, bone, liver or lymph nodes or just local extension is quite rare, occurring in only 3% to 13% of all cases. The interventional radiologist may be called upon in such cases for biopsying suspected lesions or for RFA or transarterial bland or chemoembolization of liver lesions. Because of the functional lability of these tumors and the risk of their provocation by either procedure or drugs associated with the procedure, it is essential that the patient has been pretreated for a number of days with a combination of alpha and beta blockers such as phenoxybenzamine or doxazosin, labetalol or other beta blockers. Calcium channel blockers such as nicardipine are also sometimes used, as is metyrosine, a catecholamine-synthesis blocker. Appropriate preoperative preparation usually takes 10 to 14 days and should be supervised by a knowledgeable cardiologist or endocrinologist.

In particularly labile cases, the attendance of an anesthesiologist throughout the procedure is recommended for intraoperative hemodynamic monitoring and possible administration of fast-acting intravenous vasodilators and beta blockers such as sodium nitroprusside and esmolol, or the use of intravenous vasoconstrictors, as necessary.

Following the ablation of lesions, typical monitoring is necessary for hyper- or hypotensive reactions for at least several days and can include postoperative hypoglycemia due to reactive hyperinsulinemia.

Following surgical resection of non-metastasizing but functioning pheochromocytomas, the catecholamine levels usually return to normal in approximately 2 weeks and chromogranin-A levels also become normal. The blood pressure normalizes also. Reports of response to RFA or transhepatic cytoreduction of metastatic lesions have been relatively scarce and no standard has been established to predict a timetable for anticipated response. Treatment with ^{131}I metaiodobenzylguanidine has been in use in Europe for several decades with fairly good response reported. However, in the United States, though in use for many years for imaging, it is available for therapy only on an experimental basis in a few centers.

REFERENCES

1. Öberg K. Diagnosis and treatment of carcinoid tumors. Expert Rev Anticancer Ther, 2003; 3: 863–877.
2. Yao KA, Talamonti MS, Nemcek A, et al. Indications and results of liver resection and hepatic chemoembolization for metastatic gastrointestinal neuroendocrine tumors. Surgery, 2001; 130: 677–685.
3. Chung MH, Pisegna J, Spirt M, et al. Hepatic cytoreduction followed by a novel long-acting somatostatin analog: A paradigm for intractable neuroendocrine tumors metastatic to the liver. Surgery, 2001; 130: 954–962.
4. Que FG, Sarmiento JM, and Nagorney DM. Hepatic surgery for metastatic gastrointestinal neuroendocrine tumors. Cancer Control, 2002; 9: 67–79.
5. Sarmiento JM, Heywood G, Rubin J, et al. Surgical treatment of neuroendocrine metastases to the liver: A plea for resection to increase survival. J Am Coll Surg, 2003; 197: 29–37.
6. de Herder WW, Krenning EP, van Eijck CH, et al. Considerations concerning a tailored, individualized therapeutic management of patients with (neuro)endocrine tumours of the gastrointestinal tract and pancreas. Endocr Relat Cancer, 2004; 11: 19–34.
7. Modlin IM, Lye KD, Kidd M. A 5-decade analysis of 13,715 carcinoid tumors. Cancer 2003;97:934–959.
8. Berge T and Linell F. Carcinoid tumors: Frequency in a defined population during a 12-year period. ACTA Pathol Microbiol Scan, 1976; 84: 322–330.
9. Oberndorfer S. Karzinoide Tumoren des Dunndarms. Frank Z Pathol, 1907; 1: 426–429.
10. Solcia E, Kloppel G, Sobin LH, et al. Histological typing of endocrine tumors, 2nd edition. WHO International Histological Classification of Tumors. Berlin: Springer, 2000.
11. Quaedvlieg PF, Visser O, Lamers CB, et al. Epidemiology and survival in patients with carcinoid disease in The Netherlands. An epidemiological study with 2,391 patients. Ann Oncol, 2001; 12: 295–300.
12. Rindi G, Leiter AB, Kopin AS, et al. The "normal" endocrine cell of the gut: Changing concepts and new evidences. Ann NY Acad Sci, 2004; 1014: 1–12.
13. Pictet RL, Rall LB, Phelps P, et al. The neural crest and the origin of the insulin-producing and other gastrointestinal hormone-producing cells. Science, 1976; 191: 191–192.
14. Eriksson B and Öberg K. Neuroendocrine tumours of the pancreas. Br J Surg, 2000; 87: 129–131.
15. Delcore R, Friesen SR. Gastrointestinal neuroendocrine tumors. J Am Coll Surg, 1994; 178: 187–211.
16. Lam KY and Lo CY. Pancreatic endocrine tumors: A 22-year clinicopathological experience with morphological, immunohistochemical observation and a review of the literature. Eur J Surg Oncol, 1997; 23: 36–42.
17. Buchanan KD, Johnston CF, O'Hare MM, et al. Neuroendocrine tumors: A European review. Am J Med, 1986; 81(Suppl 6B): 14–22.
18. Modlin IM, Sandor A. An analysis of 8,305 cases of carcinoid tumors. Cancer, 1997; 79: 813–829.
19. Hemminki K and Li X. Incidence trends and risk factors of carcinoid tumors: A nationwide epidemiologic study from Sweden. Cancer, 2001; 92: 2204–2210.
20. Hemminki K and Li X. Familial carcinoid tumors and subsequent cancers: A nationwide epidemiologic study from Sweden. Int J Cancer, 2001; 94: 444–448.
21. Kimura W, Kuroda A, and Morioka Y. Clinical pathology of endocrine tumors of the pancreas: Analysis of autopsy cases. Dig Dis Sci, 1991; 36: 933–942.
22. Öberg K. Carcinoid tumors, carcinoid syndrome and related disorders. In: Larsen, Kronenberg, Melmed and Polonsky, eds. Williams' Textbook of Endocrinology, 10th edition, pp. 1857–1876. Philadelphia, PA: WB Saunders, 2003.
23. Mani S, Modlin IM, Ballantyne G, et al. Carcinoids of the rectum. J Am Coll Surg, 1994; 179: 231–248.
24. Warner RR, Mani S, Profeta J, et al. Octreotide treatment of carcinoid hypertensive crisis. Mt Sinai J Med, 1994; 61: 349–355.
25. Kvols LK, Martin JK, Marsh HM, et al. Rapid reversal of carcinoid crisis with a somatostatin analog. N Engl J Med, 1985; 313: 1229–1230.

26. Kinney MA, Warner ME, Nagorney DM, et al. Perianesthetic risks and outcomes of abdominal surgery for metastatic carcinoid tumours. Br J Anaesth, 2001; 87: 447–452.

27. Ardill JES and Erikkson B. The importance of the measurement of circulating markers in patients with neuroendocrine tumours of the pancreas and gut. Endocr Relat Cancer, 2003; 10: 459–462.

28. De Baere T. Hepatic malignancies: Rationale for local and regional therapies. J Vasc Interv Radiol, Suppl (s1–s132) 2005; 16: 4–8.

29. Brown DB, Geschwind JF, Soulen MC, et al. Society of interventional radiology position statement on chemoembolization of hepatic malignancies. J Vasc Interv Radiol, 2006; 17: 217–223.

30. Ramage JK, Davies AH, Ardill J, et al. Guidelines for the management of gastroenteropancreatic neuroendocrine (including carcinoid) tumours. Gut, Suppl 4, 2005; 54: iv1–16.

31. Brown KT, Koh BY, Brody LA, et al. Particle embolization of hepatic neuroendocrine metastases for control of pain and hormonal symptoms. J Vasc Interv Radiol, 1999; 10: 397–403.

32. Tajima T, Honda H, Kuroiwa T, et al. Pulmonary complications after hepatic artery chemoembolization or infusion via the inferior phrenic artery for primary liver cancer. J Vasc Interv Radiol, 2002; 13: 893–900.

33. Arora R, Soulen M, and Haskol Z. Cutaneous complications of hepatic chemoembolization via extra hepatic collaterals. J Vasc Interv Radiol, 1999; 10: 1351–1356.

34. Strosberg JR, Choi J, Cantor AD, et al. Selective hepatic artery embolization for treatment of patients with metastatic carcinoid and pancreatic endocrine tumors. Cancer Control, 2006; 13: 72–78.

35. Brown DB, Cardella JF, Sacks D, et al. Quality improvement guidelines for transhepatic arterial chemoembolization, embolization, and chemotherapeutic infusion for hepatic malignancy. J Vasc Interv Radiol, 2006; 17: 225–232.

36. Ruutiainen AT, Soulen MC, Tuite CM, et al. Chemoembolization and bland embolization of neuroendocrine tumor metastases to the liver. J Vasc Interv Radiol, 2007; 18: 847–855.

37. Kennedy AS, Dezarn WA, McNeillie P, et al. Radioembolization for unresectable neuroendocrine hepatic metastases using resin ^{90}Y-microspheres: Early results in 148 patients. Am J Clin Oncol, 2008; 31: 271–279.

38. Walser EM, Champion SE, Montoya M, et al. Chemoembolization improves survival in patients with hepatocellular carcinoma and severely reduced portal perfusion. (Abstract 80). J Vasc Interv Radiol, 2005; Suppl (s1–s32); 16: 530.

39. Pentecost MJ, Daniels JR, Teitelbaum GP, et al. Hepatic chemoembolization: Safety with portal vein thrombosis. J Vasc Interv Radiol, 1993; 4: 347–351.

40. Ikeda M, Maeda S, Shibata J, et al. Transcatheter arterial chemotherapy with and without embolization in patients with hepatocellular carcinoma. Oncology, 2004; 66: 24–31.

41. Berger DH, Carrasco CH, Hohn DC, et al. Hepatic artery chemoembolization or embolization for primary and metabolic liver tumors. Post treatment management and complications. J Surg Oncol, 1995; 60: 116–121.

42. Stuart K. Chemoembolization in the management of liver tumors. The Oncologist, 2003; 8: 425–437.

43. Geschwind JF, Kaushik S, Ramsey DE, et al. Influence of a new prophylactic antibiotic therapy on the incidence of liver abscess after chemoembolization of liver tumors. J Vasc Interv Radiol, 2002; 13: 1163–1666.

44. Hartnell GG, Gates J, Stuart K, et al. Hepatic chemoembolization: Effect of intra-arterial lidocaine on pain and postprocedure recovery. Cardiovasc & Interven Radiol, 1999; 22: 293–297.

45. Salem R. Yttrium-90: Concepts and principles. J Vasc Interv Radiol, Suppl (s1–s132) 2005; 16: p276–p280.

46. Kennedy AS, Coldwell D, Liu D, et al De Baere T. Liver directed radiotherapy with microspheres: Second Annual Clinical Symposium. Am J Oncol Rev, 2006; 4(Suppl 5): 1–8.

47. De Baere T. Complications after ablative therapy. J Vasc Interv Radiol, Suppl (s1–s132) 2005; 16: p18–p22.

48. Dluhy RG, Lawrence JE, and Williams GH. Pheochromocytoma: Incidence and importance. In: Larsen, Kronenberg, Melmed and Polonsky, eds. Williams' Textbook of Endocrinology, 10th ed, pp. 555–562. Philadelphia, PA: WB Saunders, 2003.

Chapter 26

INTERVENTIONAL RADIOLOGY FOR THE TREATMENT OF LIVER METASTASES FROM NEUROENDOCRINE TUMORS

Thierry de Baère

Neuroendocrine gut and pancreatic tumors are rather rare malignant diseases, but development of new diagnostic tools (somatostatin receptor scintigraphy) and therapeutic options (somatostatin analogs, radioactive-labeled octreotide, transarterial therapy, radiofrequency ablation) make them of great interest to the medical community. The term *neuroendocrine tumor* encompasses a variety of relatively different diseases:

- Carcinoid tumors, which are the most common, with an incidence of about 3 per 100,000 persons

- Islet cell carcinomas, also called pancreatic endocrine tumors, with an incidence of about 0.3 per 100,000 persons

Carcinoid tumors arise most often from the small bowel, sometimes from pancreas, lung and bronchi, and more rarely from other organs such salivary glands or uterus but can arise from nearly everywhere due to the widespread diffusion of neuroendocrine cells, which give rise to the disease. Most often, they induce high levels of serotonin or chromogranin A. Islet cell carcinomas or pancreatic endocrine tumors arise from the pancreas and can produce insulin,

glucagons, or vasoactive intestinal peptide (VIP). Production of various systemic hormones associated with specific immunohistochemical markers such as neurospecific enolase (NSE), synaptophysin, cytokeratin, chromogranin and CD 56 allows the diagnosis of these neuroendocrine tumors. For clinical considerations, the histopathologic grade of the tumor is an even more important factor than the histopathologic type. The grade obtained from the number of mitoses per microscope high-power field is linked to the aggressiveness of the disease and thus will influence therapeutic choices. Tumors with two or fewer mitoses are classified as low grade. Alternatively, Ki-67 can be used to quantify grade, and less than 2% up-take of Ki-67 will classify the tumor as a low grade.

Hepatic metastases are common in patients with neuroendocrine tumors, and these metastases can have a long, indolent history. The presence of metastases is a sign of worse prognosis, with around 40% survival at 5 years compared with 75% to 99% for patients free of metastases. Gastrointestinal carcinoid and pancreatic tumors tend to behave similarly, and both can produce hormones that induce various symptoms that may be the major clinical problem even though the disease is slow growing. In such cases, the first goal of treatment is to achieve symptom palliation.

SURGERY

Surgery obviously must be performed when the goal is complete cure of the disease, and in this setting it provides 5-year survival between 73% and 85% (1, 2). The role of palliative resection or surgical debulking remains controversial. It can improve symptoms but only one retrospective study compared intra-arterial therapy with surgical debulking (3). The authors reported greater and more prolonged symptomatic relief following surgery than for embolization – 59% versus 32% and 35 ± 22 months versus 22 ± 13.6 months respectively. However, this study is retrospective with probably some bias in terms of patient selection, with non-surgical patients referred to embolization. In addition, the rate and duration of palliation benefit after embolization is lower than usually reported in the literature in terms of percentage and duration of symptom palliation (4–6).

SYSTEMIC CHEMOTHERAPY

Systemic chemotherapy proved to have very low efficacy in these diseases. For carcinoid tumors, response rates remain below 20%, and best responses are obtained with a combination of streptozotocin, doxorubicin and fluorouracil (7). For islet cell carcinoma, response rates are higher, reaching 40% (8). Interferon-alpha has been used for carcinoid, but response remains below that of systemic chemotherapy. Antiangiogenic drugs such as vascular endothelial growth factor (VEGF) inhibitors or tyrosine kinase inhibitor are under evaluation and appear promising, at least theoretically, due to the usually hypervascular pattern of these tumors. Symptom palliation with systemic treatment relies on somatostatin analogs. Today, long-acting somatostatin analogs that can be injected every 2 to 4 weeks have replaced the need for two or three daily injections, as required by the first generation of somatostatin analogs due to their very short half-life. Symptomatic palliation with somatostatin analogs is achieved in more than 70% of patients, but efficacy can decrease with time. In addition, even though somatostatin analogs rarely produce tumor regression, stabilization of tumor growth has been observed in 36% of patients with initially progressive disease (9).

HEPATIC INTRA-ARTERIAL THERAPIES

Indications

Indications for intra-arterial hepatic therapies are tumor progression in the liver and palliation for homone-related symptoms uncontrolled with somatostain analogs. When tumor burden of the liver is low, progression of the tumor must be documented on two subsequent imaging studies before starting intra-arterial therapy (or any other treatment) for morphologic reasons, because liver metastases of neuroendocrine tumors are sometimes very slow growing and can stay stable for years. Extensive tumor involvement of the liver at the time of discovery of the disease is an indication to start aggressive therapy because it is now established in several studies that a major liver involvement limits the chances of success and increases the risk of complication of intra-arterial therapy. When disease is predominantly in the liver, intra-arterial therapy is usually the first-line treatment in our institution (4). Extra-hepatic disease to the lung or bones, or metastatic lymph nodes is not a contra-indication to intra-arterial therapy as long as the disease is predominant to the liver and the prognosis is linked to the liver disease. Intra-arterial therapy can be given in combination with systemic treatment in cases of distant disease.

Tumor grade according to histopathologic finding also influences therapeutic choices. Intra-arterial therapies are usually proposed as first-line treatment in low-grade tumors, whereas systemic chemotherapy is preferred in high-grade tumors. These high-grade tumors are usually fast growing, with high extra-hepatic tumor burden at diagnosis, and respond less to embolization than low-grade carcinoid. This lower response rate might be due to the usually lower arterialization in high-grade compared with low-grade tumors. Intra-arterial therapy is mainly a palliative treatment and is used for non-surgical candidates and patients not amenable to complete ablation with radiofrequency. Consequently, intra-arterial therapy is usually used for liver metastases larger than 3 cm or greater than five in number.

Rationale

Intra-arterial therapies have been used for many years for the treatment of liver metastases from neuroendocrine tumors because these tumors are highly vascularized and nearly 100% of their blood supply derives from the hepatic artery, inversely to the normal liver parenchyma, which receives two-thirds of its vascular supply from the portal branches. The arterial route can be used in two different ways – to deliver toxic drug preferentially to the tumor or to occlude the blood supply through the artery to induce ischemia and alter tumor cells. In the past, ischemia was the first treatment applied by performing transient or definitive ligation of arteries supplying the liver. Such surgical ischemia is largely obsolete, and intra-arterial therapies are nowadays performed by percutaneous approach and catheterization of the hepatic artery. However, such surgical maneuvers provided as high as 60% of response rate with duration up to 12 months (10, 11). This response was improved by systemic chemotherapy associated with vascular dearterialization, improving duration of response from 6.6 months to 19.8 months and survival from 27 to 49 months (10).

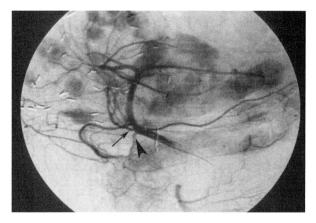

FIGURE 26.1. Angiogram obtained by injection of the hepatic artery of a patient bearing numerous hepatic metastases from carcinoid tumor that can be seen as blushes. Note that only the left lobe of the liver is opacified due to previous right hepatectomy. TACE will be performed selectively in the left branches and branch for segment IV (*arrow*), avoiding injecting chemotherapy and embols in the gastroduodenal artery (*arrowhead*).

Technique

Intra-arterial therapy can be bland transarterial embolization (TAE) or, more often, transarterial chemoembolization (TACE). However, today there is not clear evidence of superiority of one technique over the other, or evidence of increased toxicity and complication of one technique or the other. A series published by Gupta et al. found no differences in response rate between TACE and TAE in carcinoid tumors. In islet cell carcinoma, patients treated with TACE had a prolonged overall survival (31.5 months vs. 18.2 months) and improved response (50% vs. 25%), even if these differences did not reach significance (6). Ruutiainen et al. report a trend for superiority of TACE vs. TAE in terms of time to progression (49% vs. 0% at 12 months), mean duration of symptom relief (15 vs. 7.5 months) and survival (76% vs. 68% at 2 years) (12). All the studies comparing TACE and TAE are retrospective, with choice of treatment left to operator preferences. In our institution, we use TACE, which might be more efficient, because there is no difference reported in tolerance or complications. Indeed, Ruutiainen et al. found no differences in post-treatment toxicities or hospital stay for TACE or TAE. When TACE is performed, the drug used varies from center to center. Usually, doxorubicin alone (50 mg/m^2) or CAM [cisplatin 100 mg – doxorubicin (Adriamycin) 50 mg – mitomycin-C 10 mg] are the two most commonly used regimens. The use of streptozotocin, known to be an active drug against

neuroendocrine tumors after intravenous delivery, has not demonstrated superiority and is cumbersome to use due to the pain encountered during injection (13). Drug is injected mixed with iodized oil (10 ml) and then followed by particle embolization until stasis is achieved, or the three components are injected as a slurry. The drug is mixed with lipiodol to obtain an emulsion and provide a pharmacokinetic benefit and selectivity for tumor than can be seen as selective lipiodol uptake on follow-up computed tomography (CT) (Figures 26.1–26.4). In fact, it is not a real selectivity for tumors but a propensity of lipiodol to go through the largest vessels, which are, most often, the tumor-feeding vessels (14). In addition, lipiodol increases dwell time between tumor and drug due

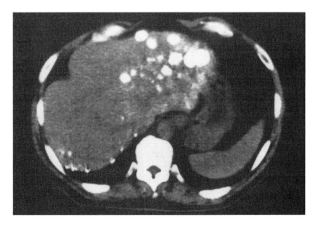

FIGURE 26.2. CT scan obtained 1 month after a first course of TACE demonstrates numerous spots of lipiodol up-take corresponding to carcinoid tumor metastases. Up-take is complete, and no further treatment is planned.

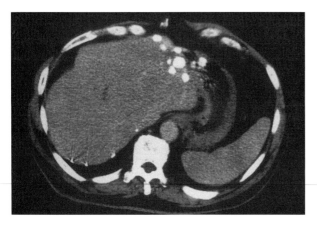

FIGURE 26.3.   CT scan at 6 months demonstrated persistent lipiodol up-take and morphologic response.

to vascular slackening induced by its viscosity (15). Finally, lipiodol goes through the abnormal vascular layers of tumoral vessels (16).

More recently, loadable embolic materials became available and are being investigated. Such spheres can be chosen from 100 to 900 μ in diameter and are loadable with up to 150 mg of doxorubicin for 4 ml of embolic material (Figures 26.5–26.9). The embolic beads are loaded with more than 95% of drug after 2 hours of contact in a vial. In this setting, lipiodol is not used. The loaded embolics are injected intra-arterially mixed with contrast medium to allow visualization of the product under fluoroscopy. If stasis is not reached after 4 g of embolics, the treatment can be completed with non-loaded embolics. From recent pharmacokinetic studies, the embolics release the drug over 14 days, with a peak intra-tumoral concentration at 3 days, which is 400 times higher than when drug is injected intra-arterially without loading (17). The exposure is thought to be at least four

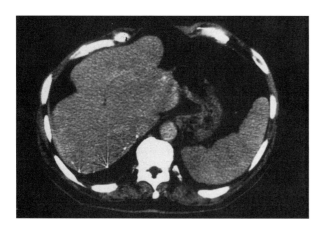

FIGURE 26.4.   CT scan 18 months after TACE demonstrated nearly complete response. This patient will benefit from a second TACE 28 months after the first one for new tumor occurrence.

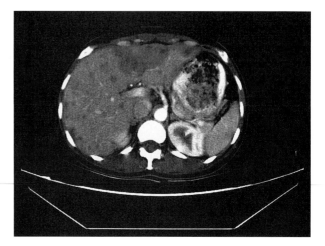

FIGURE 26.5.   CT scan of metastases from carcinoid tumor developed mostly in the left lobe of the liver. Despite the arterial phase, the tumor does not appear highly vascular, but it will demonstrate hyper-arterialization on the angiogram.

times greater than when a mixture of doxorubicin and lipiodol is used.

For TAE or TACE, patency of the portal vein must be verified first because hepatic artery embolization requires a patent portal system. For some authors, embolization can still be performed in case of portal thrombosis extended to two or fewer segments.

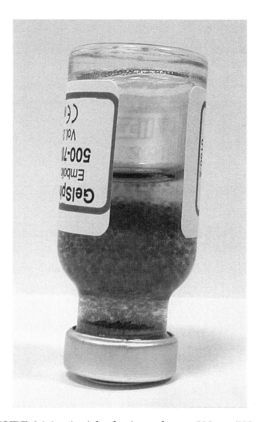

FIGURE 26.6.   A vial of microspheres 500 to 700 μm (Biocompatible, UK) before loading with doxorubicin. See Color Plate 23.

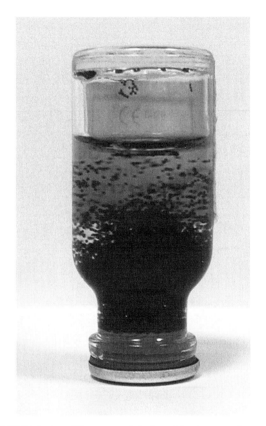

FIGURE 26.7. The same vial after 40 minutes of contact with 50 mg of doxorubicin diluted in 5 ml of isotonic contrast medium shows uptake of doxorubicin by the embols, which turn red. The solution is clear and does not contain any more doxorubicin. See Color Plate 24.

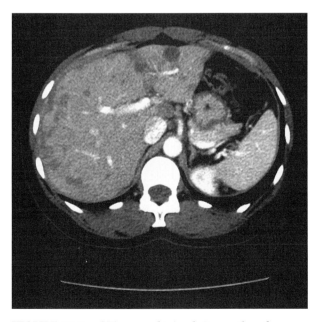

FIGURE 26.8. CT scan obtained 8 months after one course of TACE with drug-eluting beads in the left lobe of the liver demonstrates dramatic tumor response compared with Figure 26.5.

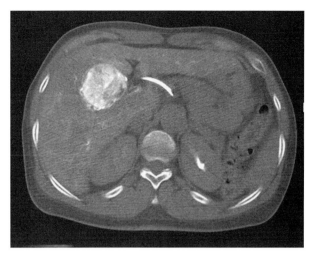

FIGURE 26.9. CT scan obtained during intra-arterial injection of contrast media in the hepatic artery demonstrated a highly enhanced tumor in segment IV of the liver. Note the 5F catheter in the hepatic artery.

TAE or TACE in patients with a compromised portal vein will induce liver failure. On the other hand, it is possible to perform injection of lipiodol mixed with drug without subsequent embolization. Obviously, therapeutic benefit will be lower. Extension and number of tumors will modify the technique accordingly. When selective catheterization of each tumor is possible, or all tumor is located in one-half of the liver, a single course aiming at all the tumors will be performed. When there is a bilateral disease with multiple tumors, half of the liver is treated in one session, repeated for the other half of the liver 4 to 8 weeks later.

Catheterization must be as distal as possible to target the tumors without embolization of non-target organs. Obviously, the origin of the gastroduodenal artery must be left behind. To avoid post-TACE ulcers, one should look carefully for the right gastric artery, which can arise anywhere from the hepatic artery proper or its left branches. An omental artery, usually arising from the left hepatic artery, must be recognized and embolized with steel coil to avoid severe post-TACE pain. Catheterization must try to go beyond the origin of the cystic artery in order to lower post-embolization pain. Patients with preserved liver function are not at risk of post-treatment liver insufficiency, whereas patients with more than 50% liver involvement, lactate dehydrogenase (LDH) greater than 425 IU/L, alanine aminotransferase (AST) greater than 100 IU/L or bilirubin greater than 2 mg/dl are at risk for post-treatment liver failure. These patients must be treated with sequential TAE or TACE, treating only a small part of the liver as a test. The treatment will be repeated according to clinical and biological tolerance until the goal (usually symptom palliation) is reached. Bile duct dilation is a relative contraindication to treatment due to the higher risk of sepsis.

Drainage of the involved segment must be performed before intra-arterial treatment. Patients with a bilioenteric anastomosis (which is not rare in islet cell carcinoma patients) are at high risk of severe infectious complications after hepatic artery embolization (18). Indeed, bile ducts are colonized by germs from the digestive tract due to the reflux of digestive liquid in the liver. If hepatic artery embolization is mandatory in patients with a bilioenteric anastomosis, a regimen of antibiotic prophylaxis should be tailored for them according to that reported by Geschwind (19) and Patel (20). Intravenous tazobactam sodium/piperacillin sodium at 10 g/day is started the day before the procedure and maintained for 3 days. It is associated with bowel preparation with 45 ml of oral Fleet phospho-Soda, 1 g neomycin and 3 g/day oral erythromycin. However, despite such prophylaxis, septic complications are more frequent than in patients without bilioenteric anastomosis (20). In patients without bilioenteric anastomosis, typical prophylaxis is 3 to 5 days of antibiotic therapy started immediately before the procedure. Clavulanate/amoxicillin or cefazoline + metronidazole are the most commonly used regimens. It is important to cover all patients with somatostatin analogs at the time of intra-arterial therapy due to the risk of inducing carcinoid crisis. Patient must receive vigorous intravenous hydration (200 ml/hour) and corticoid and anti-emetic medications that will help mitigate post-embolization syndrome.

Follow-up

Usually, a first follow-up imaging is performed 4 weeks after treatment. At this time point, it is usually too early to evaluate treatment response, but this first imaging follow-up will be used to assess completeness of the treatment and subsequently the part of the liver that must be treated during the next course if the first treatment targeted only a part of the liver. In addition, imaging will search for potential complications, such as hepatic necrosis or liver abscess, that can modify the location and type of subsequent treatment. CT is the most commonly used technique for follow-up of TACE and TAE, and is easy to use when lipiodol

has been injected. If lipiodol has been used, a high degree of lipiodol up-take by the tumors is linked with subsequent efficacy of the treatment. If TAE has been performed or drug-eluting beads have been used, devascularization must be evaluated because it will be the only sign of treatment at 4 weeks. In our short experience with drug-eluting beads, a CT perfusion study with dedicated software performed as early as 4 days after TACE with drug-eluting beads was predictive of later tumor response in 8 of 10 responders when treated tumors showed a significant elongation of the median transit time (MTT) from 3.2 seconds before treatment to 5.7 seconds, and a decrease of the mean blood flow from 476 ml/100g/min before treatment to 285 ml/100g/min after treatment (Figures 26.9–26.11) (21). Recent publications reporting magnetic resonance imaging (MRI) as the most sensitive cross-sectional imaging mode for depiction of liver metastases from neuroendocrine tumors (22) have associated good results of MRI in the follow-up of TACE of hepatocellular carcinomas (23). This will probably favor MRI in the future, particularly if lipiodol is abandoned for drug-eluting embolics. Indeed, Kamel et al. confirmed the interest in quantifying tumor enhancement in the arterial and venous phases but, more interestingly, demonstrated the value of diffusion imaging by demonstrating increase in

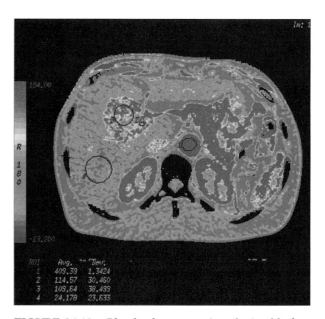

FIGURE 26.10. Blood volume mapping obtained before treatment from CT study at the same level as Figure 26.9 shows a high blood volume in the tumor compared with the normal liver parenchyma, 109.64 and 24.17 respectively. See Color Plate 25.

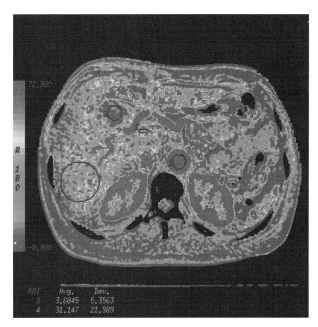

FIGURE 26.11.   Blood volume mapping at the same level as Figures 26.9 and 26.10 obtained 2 days after selective TACE of segment IV shows a decrease of blood volume in the tumor to 3.68, whereas blood volume in the liver does not differ much from pre-TACE values, at 31.14. See Color Plate 26.

apparent diffusion coefficient in hepatocellular carcinomas treated by TACE (23).

Results

Intra-arterial therapies seem to provide a better response rate and better survival than systemic chemotherapies. In patients with islet cell carcinomas and carcinoid tumors, Touzios et al. reported a significantly better 5-year survival rate after TACE (50%) than after medical therapies (25%) (24). After medical therapy, Chamberlain et al. reported 76% and 39% survival at 1 and 3 years respectively while it was 94%, 83%, and 50% at 1,3, and 5 years after TAE (2). For Chu et al., factors that had a significant favorable effect on survival included curative resection of the primary tumor, metachronous liver metastases, absence of liver metastases and aggressive treatment of the liver metastases. (25). In this report, aggressive treatments included surgery and TACE.

Our experience of TACE in 64 patients with carcinoid demonstrated complete symptom relief in 53 and partial in 40% (26). Sixty-four patients treated had proven tumor progression before treatment, and we obtained decrease in tumor burden in 74% of patients and disease remained stable in 15%. Better response was obtained when tumor burden was below 30% of liver volume. The best response to treat-

ment was obtained after one or two courses in 81% of patients. This fact emphasizes that if no response is obtained after one or two courses, treatment must be abandoned. Major complications occurred after 5.9% of TACE, including liver failure, liver abscess and renal failure. Prognostic factors for complications were tumor burden superior to 80% of liver volume and treatment of the complete liver in one session.

A recent report of a series of 69 non-randomized patients treated with TAE or TACE left to operator preferences demonstrated a significantly higher morphologic response rate for carcinoid tumors (66.7%) than for islet cell carcinoma (35.2%) (6). Progression-free survival was also significantly higher for carcinoid tumors (22.7 months) than for islet cell carcinoma (16.1 months). Most of the series of TACE that separate islet cell from carcinoid report such differences in response rate. Indeed, for Eriksson et al., median survival was 80 months for carcinoid tumors and 20 months for islet cell carcinomas (27). For Stokes et al., response rates were 66.7% vs. 35.2%, progression-free survival was 22.7 months vs. 16.1 months and overall survival was 33.8 months vs. 23.2 months for carcinoid tumors and islet cell carcinomas respectively (28). These results enhanced the major interest in intra-arterial therapies for carcinoid tumors but questioned the effectiveness of these therapies for islet cell carcinomas.

Because drug-loadable embolics are relatively new, and there is no report in the literature, we have only our short-term results to provide with this type of material (Figure 26.12). We have, so far, the follow-up

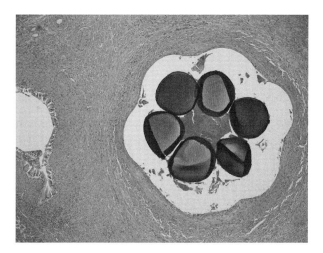

FIGURE 26.12.   Patient underwent liver resection after morphologic tumor response, and pathologic study shows the drug-eluting beads in an artery surrounded by necrosis and inflammation. See Color Plate 27.

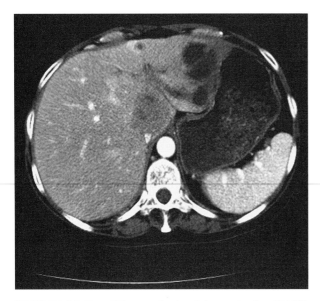

FIGURE 26.13. CT scan obtained 1 month after TACE of the left lobe of the liver with drug-eluting beads for metastases of carcinoid tumor. Post-embolization period has been painful with fever. There are some necrotic spots in segment II and III that will be managed with prolonged antibiotic therapy.

of 16 patients with gastrointestinal carcinoid tumors treated with drug-eluting embolics. We used DC beads (Bicompatible, London, UK), 4 ml loaded with 100 mg of doxorubicin. Liver involvement was below 30% in 4 patients, between 30% and 50% in 10 patients and over 50% in 2 patients. Twelve patients had bilateral disease, and a mean tumor diameter of 35 mm. Clinical tolerance was not really different from that observed with the more classical TACE regimen. Vomiting was less, but two patients had prolonged abdominal pain linked to peripheral necrosis of healthy liver discovered at 1-month follow-up CT (Figure 26.13). Increases in transaminases and bilirubin were usual for TACE, with a mean of 2-, 3- and 1.2-fold increases for AST, ALT and bilirubin respectively. Symptomatic response was observed at 2 months in four of four symptomatic patients. Among the 16 patients who had progressive disease before treatment, partial response according to Response Evaluation Criteria in Solid Tumors (RECIST) was observed in nine patients, minor response in four, stable disease in two and progressive disease in one.

SELECTIVE INTERNAL RADIATION THERAPY

Selectivity to the tumor in order to obtain internal radiation can be achieved in two different ways. (1) Radioactive microspheres loaded with [90]Yttrium are injected inside of the hepatic artery, and the rationale is similar to that discussed earlier for TAE or TACE, with selectivity due to the predominant arterial feeding of the tumors. (2) A beta-emitter loaded on a somatostatin analog is injected intravenously, taking advantage of the selective binding of the somatostatin analog for the tumor to deliver locally internal radiation therapy. Intravenous injection of beta-emitter loaded on a somatostatin analog is beyond the scope of this chapter. Trying to further enhance the selectivity of beta-emitter loaded on somatostatin analog by local delivery, some authors have recently tried intra-arterial injection. Some performed intra-arterial delivery of ^{131}I-labeled metaiodobenzylguanidine, which is an established treatment modality for neuroendocrine tumors. In another study, hepatic intra-arterial injection provided an up to fourfold higher tumor uptake than what is obtained after classical intravenous injection (29). Hepatic intra-arterial injection of [90]Yttrium-tetraazacyclododecane tetraacetic acid lanreotide provided partial response to treatment in 16% and stable disease in 63% (30). In the same study, clinical improvement was reported by 61% of 23 patients, while a reduction in biologic marker levels was observed in 60% of 15 patients.

The intra-arterial route with radioactive microspheres has been explored mainly for hepatocellular carcinomas and metastases from colorectal cancer. These are non-degradable microspheres, made of resin or glass, loaded with [90]Yttrium. Use of these products in neuroendocrine tumors is scarce, but it is noteworthy that it has been used in patients who developed progressive disease after use of other intra-arterial therapy, with relief of patient symptoms in 80%. (31)

PERCUTANEOUS ABLATIVE THERAPIES

The aim of ablative therapy is close to that of surgery, and nowadays these techniques are mainly used in a curative intent. They can be used alone or associated with liver resection to allow for complete resection/ablation of liver metastases. Most of the time, ablation is limited to fewer than five tumors with a size smaller than 4 cm due to the low efficacy of radiofrequency ablation (RFA) for larger tumors. An extensive pre-ablation imaging work-up is mandatory, and liver imaging must be of excellent quality to depict all metastases. MRI has been recently demonstrated as the most sensitive imaging technique for this goal (22). An interesting point about metastases from neuroendocrine tumor is that they demonstrated a very high sensitivity to local ablative technique, either by percutaneous injection of alcohol or by radiofrequency. Indeed, percutaneous injection of alcohol is known to be rarely effective for treatment of metastases; however, it was reported as effective in all treated tumors by Livraghi et al. (32). In the largest series of RFA for metastases of neuroendocrine tumors, Berber et al. reported a local efficacy of 97%, which is higher than that reported for other liver tumors (33). In this series, RFA was performed during laparoscopy in 34 patients bearing 234 metastases with a mean size of 2.3 cm. Symptom relief was complete in 63% and partial in 32%. Mean size of tumors that cannot be completely ablated was 4.2 cm, confirming the difficulty of obtaining compete ablation of large tumors with RF ablation. In a manner akin to TACE, when performing RFA of liver metastases from neuroendocrine tumors, the patient must be premedicated with somatostatin analogs to avoid a severe carcinoid crisis due to the demonstrated release of hormone during ablation (34). As is the case for TACE, bilioenteric anastomosis is a risk factor for liver abscess after RFA. Indeed, liver abscess has been reported to occur despite prolonged antibiotic therapy in four of nine patients bearing a bilioenteric anastomosis 13 to 62 days after RFA (35).

REFERENCES

1. Soreide O, Berstad T, Bakka A, et al. Surgical treatment as a principle in patients with advanced abdominal carcinoid tumors. Surgery, 1992; 111(1): 48–54.
2. Chamberlain RS, Canes D, Brown KT, et al. Hepatic neuroendocrine metastases: Does intervention alter outcomes? J Am Coll Surg, 2000; 190(4): 432–445.
3. Osborne DA, Zervos EE, Strosberg J, et al. Improved outcome with cytoreduction versus embolization for symptomatic hepatic metastases of carcinoid and neuroendocrine tumors. Ann Surg Oncol, 2006; 13(4): 572–581.
4. Roche A, Girish BV, de Baere T, et al. Trans-catheter arterial chemoembolization as first-line treatment for hepatic metastases from endocrine tumors. Eur Radiol, 2003; 13(1): 136–140.
5. Therasse E, Breittmayer F, Roche A, et al. Transcatheter chemoembolization of carcinoid progressive liver metastasis. Radiology, 1993; 189: 541–547.
6. Gupta S, Johnson MM, Murthy R, et al. Hepatic arterial embolization and chemoembolization for the treatment of patients with metastatic neuroendocrine tumors: Variables affecting response rates and survival. Cancer, 2005; 104(8): 1590–1602.
7. Sun W, Lipsitz S, Catalano P, et al. Phase II/II study of doxorubicin with fluorouracil compared with streptozocin with fluorouracil or dacarbazine in the treatment of advanced carcinoid tumors: Eastern Cooperative Oncology Group Study E1281. J Clin Oncol, 2005; 23(22): 4897–4904.
8. Kouvaraki MA, Ajani JA, Hoff P, et al. Fluorouracil, doxorubicin, and streptozocin in the treatment of patients with locally advanced and metastatic pancreatic endocrine carcinomas. J Clin Oncol, 2004; 22(23): 4762–4771.
9. Arnold R, Trautmann ME, Creutzfeldt W, et al. Somatostatin analogue octreotide and inhibition of tumour growth in metastatic endocrine gastroenteropancreatic tumours. Gut, 1996; 38(3): 430–438.
10. Moertel CG, Johnson CM, McKusick MA, et al. The management of patients with advanced carcinoid tumors and islet cell carcinomas. Ann Intern Med, 1994; 120(4): 302–309.
11. Nobin A, Mansson B, Lunderquist A. Evaluation of temporary liver dearterialization and embolization in patients with metastatic carcinoid tumour. Acta Oncologica, 1989; 28: 419–424.
12. Ruutiainen AT, Soulen MC, Tuite CM, et al. Chemoembolization and bland embolization of neuroendocrine tumor metastases to the liver. J Vasc Interv Radiol, 2007; 18: 847–855.
13. Dominguez S, Denys A, Madeira I, et al. Hepatic arterial chemoembolization with streptozotocin in patients with metastatic digestive endocrine tumours. Eur J Gastroenterol Hepatol, 2000; 12(2): 151–157.
14. de Baere T, Dufaux J, Roche A, et al. Circulatory alterations induced by intra-arterial injection of iodized oil and emulsions of iodized oil and doxorubicin: Experimental study. Radiology, 1995; 194: 165–170.
15. de Baere T, Denys A, Briquet R, et al. Modification of arterial and portal hemodynamic after injection of iodized oil in the hepatic artery: Experimental study. J Vasc Interv Radiol, 1998; 9: 305–310.
16. Imaeda T, Ymawaki Y, Seki M, et al. Lipiodol retention and massive necrosis after lipiodol-chemoembolization of hepatocellular carcinoma: Correlation between computed tomography and histopathology. Cardiovasc Intervent Radiol, 1993; 16: 209–213.
17. Hong K, Khwaja A, Liapi E, et al. New intra-arterial drug delivery system for the treatment of liver cancer: Preclinical assessment in a rabbit model of liver cancer. Clin Cancer Res, 2006; 12(8): 2563–2567.
18. de Baere T, Roche A, Amenabar JM, et al. Liver abscess formation after local treatment of liver tumors. Hepatology, 1996; 23(6): 1436–140.
19. Geschwind JF, Kaushik S, Ramsey DE, et al. Influence of a new prophylactic antibiotic therapy on the incidence of liver abscesses after chemoembolization treatment of liver tumors. J Vasc Interv Radiol, 2002; 13(11): 1163–1166.
20. Shalin Patel S, Tuite CM, Mondschein JI, et al. Effectiveness of an aggressive antibiotic regimen for chemoembolization in patients with previous biliary intervention. J Vasc Interv Radiol, 2006; 17: 1931–1934.
21. Coenegrachts K, de Baere T, Abdel-Rehim M, et al. TransArterial ChemoEmbolization (TACE) of neuroendocrine hepatic metastases using drug eluting beads (abstr). RSNA book of abstracts, 2005: 72.
22. Dromain C, de Baere T, Lumbroso J, et al. Detection of liver metastases from endocrine tumors: A prospective

comparison of somatostatin receptor scintigraphy, computed tomography, and magnetic resonance imaging. J Clin Oncol, 2005; 23(1): 70–78.

23. Kamel IR, Bluemke DA, Eng J, et al. The role of functional MR imaging in the assessment of tumor response after chemoembolization in patients with hepatocellular carcinoma. J Vasc Interv Radiol, 2006; 17(3): 505–512.

24. Touzios JG, Kiely JM, Pitt SC, et al. Neuroendocrine hepatic metastases: Does aggressive management improve survival? Ann Surg, 2005; 241(5): 776–783; discussion 83–85.

25. Chu QD, Hill HC, Douglass HO, Jr., et al. Predictive factors associated with long-term survival in patients with neuroendocrine tumors of the pancreas. Ann Surg Oncol, 2002; 9(9): 855–862.

26. Roche A, Girish BV, de Baere T, et al. Prognostic factors for chemoembolization in liver metastasis from endocrine tumors. Hepatogastroenterology, 2004; 51(60): 1751–1756.

27. Eriksson BK, Larsson EG, Skogseid BM, et al. Liver embolizations of patients with malignant neuroendocrine gastrointestinal tumors. Cancer, 1998; 83(11): 2293–2301.

28. Stokes KR, Stuart K, Clouse ME. Hepatic arterial chemoembolization for metastatic endocrine tumors. J Vasc Interv Radiol, 1993; 4(3): 341–345.

29. Brogsitter C, Pinkert J, Bredow J, et al. Enhanced tumor uptake in neuroendocrine tumors after intraarterial application of 131I-MIBG. J Nucl Med, 2005; 46(12): 2112–2116.

30. McStay MK, Maudgil D, Williams M, et al. Large-volume liver metastases from neuroendocrine tumors: Hepatic intraarterial ^{90}Y-DOTA-lanreotide as effective palliative therapy. Radiology, 2005; 237(2): 718–726.

31. Murthy R, Gupta S, Madoff DC, et al. Feasibility of hepatic arterial therapy with Yttrium-90 microspheres (SIR-Spheres) in metastatic dominant progression after failure of multiple systemic and hepatic artery therapies [abstr]. Radiology, 2005; 237(suppl): 410.

32. Livraghi T, Vettori C, Lazzaroni S. Liver metastases: Results of percutaneous ethanol injection in 14 patients. Radiology, 1991; 179: 709–712.

33. Berber E, Flesher N, and Siperstein AE. Laparoscopic radiofrequency ablation of neuroendocrine liver metastases. World J Surg, 2002; 26(8): 985–990.

34. Wettstein M, Vogt C, Cohnen M, et al. Serotonin release during percutaneous radiofrequency ablation in a patient with symptomatic liver metastases of a neuroendocrine tumor. Hepatogastroenterology, 2004; 51(57): 830–832.

35. Elias D, Di Pietroantonio D, Gachot B, et al. Liver abscess after radiofrequency ablation of tumors in patients with a biliary tract procedure. Gastroenterol Clin Biol, 2006; 30(6–7): 823–827.

Chapter 27

IMMUNOEMBOLIZATION FOR MELANOMA

Kevin L. Sullivan

IMMUNOTHERAPY

There is evidence to support the concept that the human immune system can be manipulated to elicit an immune response to cancer cells and, at least in some cases, lead to tumor regression (1). The goal of immune therapy is to identify cancer as targets for immune system destruction. The challenge is that tumors are not foreign, but self. Some tumors do have cell surface markers that are unique to tumors, are present in much larger numbers than on normal cells or are normally present only on fetal cells. Such differences are probably the products of normally unexpressed genes. In tumors of viral origin, viral antigens may be present on the cell surface. It is these differences that provide the rationale for cancer immune therapy.

RATIONALE FOR LOCAL IMMUNOTHERAPY OF LIVER METASTASES

There is considerable experience in the treatment of cancer with systemic cytokines; however, there are a number of reasons why local, rather than systemic, administration of cytokines should be considered. Cytokines are normally present at very low levels systemically, but high, non-physiologic levels are necessary for systemic therapy. Some cytokines delivered in this manner can induce severe toxicity. Tolerance is a major barrier to immunotherapy. Direct administration of immunostimulants may alter the local environment and break the immunotolerance created by the tumor cells. In addition, the ischemia-induced necrotic tumor cells from embolization with the concomitant delivery of immunostimulants supply activated antigen-presenting cells with tumor antigens, which may lead to the creation of an in situ cancer vaccine. Finally, the liver provides a unique opportunity for immunotherapy, as it is the largest organ of the reticuloendothelial system. It contains greater than 70% of all tissue macrophages (Kupffer cells).

IMMUNOEMBOLIZATION

The concept of immunoembolization was first proposed by Kanai et al. in the treatment of hepatocellular carcinoma (HCC) with a mixture of the streptococcal antigen OK-432, fibrinogen, ethiodized poppyseed oil and thrombin infused into the hepatic artery. They treated 19 patients with advanced HCC who failed conventional treatment, and 6 of 19 exhibited marked reduction in tumor size. A second series of six patients without prior treatment were also treated with this therapy. These patients underwent resection 6 to 48 days post immunoembolization, which revealed massive mononuclear cell infiltration of tumor, as well as tumor necrosis. Further experience by these investigators supported the efficacy of this therapy (2).

There have been many recent advances in the understanding of the immune system that have opened potential new approaches to immune therapy. One such discovery is the role of antigen presenting cells (APC) in immune function. Dendritic cells are probably the most important of the APC. All normal cells present cellular molecules on major histocompatibility complex (MHC) I molecules, which reside on the cell's surface and permit immune cell recognition. APC travel about the body and endocytose dead or dying cells, and place cellular antigens from these cells on MHC II molecules, which are unique to APC. In the proper stimulatory environment, these MHC II-antigen complexes are presented to CD4$^+$ T cells (helper cells), which stimulate CD8$^+$ T cells (killer cells), which, in turn, seek out and destroy cells presenting the antigen that the APC presented to the CD4$^+$ cell. Knowledge of this sequence of events, which is believed to play a key role in the immune response to cancer, provides points of intervention. For example, autologous APC have been exposed to known tumor antigens in vitro and returned to facilitate tumor destruction (3). Another approach is to utilize cytokines to stimulate immune cells in vivo. The cytokine granulocyte macrophage-colony stimulating factor (GM-CSF), a glycoprotein secreted by T cells, is known to increase production and maturation of the entire monocyte cell line, including dendritic cells. In a murine study, a tumor vaccine was created with irradiated melanoma cells (B16) transduced with the GM-CSF gene (4). New tumors were prevented or retarded and established tumors regressed in mice injected with irradiated cells containing the transduced GM-CSF gene. Irradiated cells alone were not protective. The immunity was long-lived and specific – that is, anti-tumor activity was present several months later, and there was no activity against murine lung cancer. The anti-tumor activity required both CD4$^+$ and CD8$^+$ T cells. Interleukin (IL)-4 and IL-6 had similar, but weaker, anti-tumor activity. B16 melanoma cells do not express detectable MHC II molecules, and yet the immune response depended upon CD4$^+$ cells, which must have been activated by APC. The anti-tumor activity observed in this study was therefore attributed to the influence of GM-CSF on the maturation and/or function of specialized APC.

Immunoembolization with GM-CSF is based upon the hypothesis that intra-arterial introduction of this cytokine into the region of the tumor will produce an environment similar to that of the tumor cells with the transduced GM-CSF gene, and elicit a similar immune response. Investigations of this technique for the treatment of uveal melanoma metastatic to liver

indicate that some patients experience a prolonged period of hepatic tumor regression (Figure 27.1). There is also limited evidence of systemic immune response based upon immune cell infiltration of extra-hepatic metastases (5). Another possible mechanism of intrahepatic tumor regression is activation of the innate (non-memory) component of the immune system. Hepatic Kupffer cells can be activated by GM-CSF, and secrete TNF (tumor necrosis factor)-alpha, which may be the mechanism by which Kupffer cells cause death of tumor cells (6). Such cells are short-lived, and not tumor specific. It is quite possible that both the innate and memory components of the cellular immune system are activated by immunoembolization with GM-CSF.

BARRIERS TO IMMUNOTHERAPY

Loss of Antigenicity

Loss of antigenic tumor cell markers during the course of disease is a documented phenomenon and has been identified as a cause of recurrence (7, 8). Such an event would lead to loss tumor control if immunoembolization is dependent upon T cell–mediated cell destruction. A better understanding of patients' tumor antigenicity, which may be dynamic, could provide therapeutic guidance.

Tolerance

Another possible cause of failure of immunotherapy is that of tolerance to autologous antigens. In one murine study of a tumor with viral surface antigens present from birth, infection with the same virus induced transient tumor immunity, but immunity subsided with resolution of the viral infection, despite the presence of tumor-specific cytotoxic T cells, and tumor cells with appropriate antigenic markers (9). Thus, the tumor cells were antigenic but not immunogenic, and were presumably protected by the strong tendency to suppress an immune response to self antigens. This work suggests that repeated vaccinations are necessary to maintain cytotoxic T cell activity. This may explain why repeated immunoembolizations have been necessary to maintain control of tumor.

There is also the risk that immune therapy can cause antigen presentation in a manner that could have the opposite effect from that intended, and induce immune tolerance to the tumor.

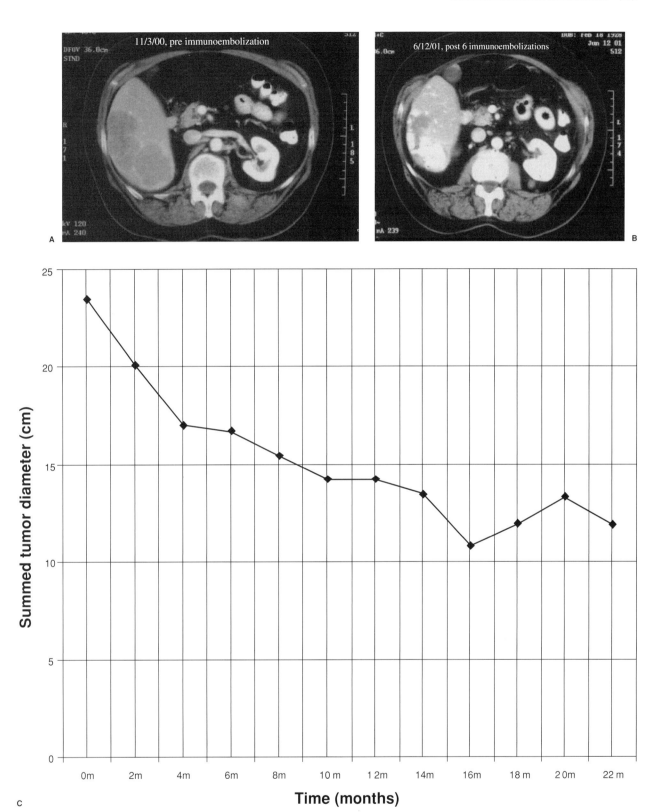

FIGURE 27.1. (A) CT scan of a patient with large uveal melanoma metastases occupying the caudal aspect of the right hepatic lobe. (B) CT scan of the same patient following six immunoembolization procedures. There is reduction in tumor diameter, as well as retention of iodized poppyseed oil within the hepatic tumor. Note soft tissue masses posterior to the left kidney, which are metastatic uveal melanoma. (C) Summed largest diameter of the hepatic metastases is dis-played on the vertical axis, and time since first immunoembolization on the horizontal axis, of the same patient. This patient elected to stop immunoembolization after six treatments, but there was continued decline in the summed tumor diameter without treatment until 16 months. The patient was retreated with immunoembolization at 20 months and again experienced regression of the intrahepatic metastases, but ultimately died of cardiac metastases at 44 months.

ASSESSMENT OF RESPONSE

Although traditional cross-sectional imaging methods should play a role in assessment of response, there are limitations with these techniques. One problem is that the response may be delayed. A study of spontaneous canine melanoma treated with local injection of GM-CSF and streptococcus endotoxin plasmids every 2 weeks for 12 weeks demonstrated an average time to tumor regression in responding animals of 7 weeks, or greater than three treatment sessions (10). One canine did not respond until 3 months after completion of the 12-week treatment session, with complete remission occurring at 28 weeks. In this canine study, tumor-infiltrating CD4 and CD8 T cells, not present on pre-treatment biopsies, were present 5 to 7 days post treatment, so the delay was not due to failed transfection or a delay in the proliferation of T cells. The slow tumor regression was attributed to the need for repeated stimulation of the immune system in order to induce a vigorous response. Thus, identification of immune responses that are positive predictors to tumor regression may be useful in conjunction with imaging.

Techniques exist to monitor the formation of antigen-specific cytotoxic lymphocytes (11). Peripheral blood monocytes can be harvested and tested for their ability to lyse autologous tumor cells. In addition, activated T lymphocytes secrete certain cytokines. The patient's T cells can be stimulated in vitro with tumor-specific antigens, and the production of cytokines measured as a means of assessing the presence of tumor-specific T cells. Biopsies of intra- and extra-hepatic tumors may also yield information that would predict patients' response to immunoembolization.

FUTURE DIRECTIONS

Although the precise role of the many cytokines in developing an anti-tumor response is incompletely understood, there is ample reason to believe that such a response is orchestrated by multiple cytokines (12). An animal model of immunoembolization might advance understanding of the role of multiple cytokines in this treatment. A challenge with this approach is that immune response is species-specific. For example, Sinclair mini-swine develop cutaneous melanoma, but unlike humans, experience a high rate of immune-mediated regression (13).

Reduction of tumor volume, with bland- or chemoembolization, or other local techniques, such as radiofrequency ablation or cryoablation, or surgical resection in selected patients, may be useful in patients with large tumor volumes.

There is limited experience that helps in understanding the role of immunoembolization with cytokines in the treatment of other hepatic tumors, both primary and metastatic, but this deserves further study. However, some caution should be exercised. The immune-mediated regression of cutaneous melanoma in Sinclair mini-swine can lead to cutaneous depigmentation and uveitis (14). Vitiligo has also been documented in prior human cutaneous melanoma trials. Concern about the possibility of immunoembolization-induced autoimmune hepatitis prompted a porcine study prior to human trials, which found no evidence of such a complication (15).

REFERENCES

1. Schott, M. Immune surveillance by dendritic cells: Potential implication for immunotherapy of endocrine cancers. Endocr Relat Cancer, 2006; 13 (3): 779–795.
2. Yoshida T, Sakon M, Umeshit K, et al. Appraisal of transarterial immunoembolization for hepatocellular carcinoma. J Clin Gastroenterol, 2001; 32: 59–65.
3. Lin AM, Hershberg RM, and Small EJ. Immunotherapy for prostate cancer using prostatic acid phosphatase loaded antigen presenting cells. Urol Oncol, 2006 Sep–Oct; 24(5): 434–441.
4. Dranoff G, Jafee E, Lazenby A, et al. Vaccination with irradiated tumor cells engineered to secrete murine granulocyte-macrophage colony stimulation factor stimulated potent, specific, and long lasting anti-tumor immunity. Proc Natl Acad Sci USA, 1993; 90: 3539–3543.
5. Shiloh A, Sullivan K, and Sato T. Response of melanoma metastatic to liver following immunoembolization. J Vasc Interv Radiol, 2003; 14: s93.
6. Schuurman B, Heuff G, Beelen RH, et al. Enhanced killing capacity of human Kupffer cells after activation with human granulocyte/macrophage-colony-stimulating factor and interferon gamma. Cancer Immunol Immunother, 1994 Sep; 39(3): 179–184.
7. Maeurer MJ, Gollin SM, Martin D, et al. Tumor escape from immune recognition: Lethal recurrent melanoma in a patient associated with down regulation of the peptide transporter protein TAP-1 and loss of expression of the immunodominant MART-1/Melan-A antigen. J Clin Invest, 1996 October 1; 98(7): 1633–1641.
8. Paschen A, Arens N, Sucker A, et al. The coincidence of chromosome 15 aberrations and β2-microglobulin gene mutations is causative for the total loss of human leukocyte antigen class I expression in melanoma. Clin Cancer Res, 2006; 12: 3297–3305.

9. Speiser DE, Miranda R, Zakarian A, et al. Self antigens expressed by solid tumors do not efficiently stimulate naive or activated T cells: Implications for immunotherapy. J Exp Med, August 29, 1997; 186(5): 645–653.

10. Dow SW, Elmslie RE, Willson AP, et al. In vivo tumor transfection with superantigen plus cytokine genes induces tumor regression and prolongs survival in dogs with malignant melanoma. J Clin Invest, June 1998; 101(11): 2406–2414.

11. Whiteside TL. Methods to monitor immune response and quality control. Dev Biol (Basel), 2004; 116: 219–228.

12. Mocellin S, Ohnmacht GA, Wang E, et al. Kinetics of cytokine expression in melanoma metastases classifies immune responsiveness. Int J Cancer, 2001 Jul 15; 93(2): 236–242.

13. Morgan CD, Measel JW Jr, Amoss MS Jr, et al. Immunophenotypic characterization of tumor infiltrating lymphocytes and peripheral blood lymphocytes isolated from melanomatous and non-melanomatous Sinclair miniature swine. Vet Immunol Immunopathol, 1996 Dec; 55(1–3): 189–203.

14. Lentz K, Burns R, Loeffer K, et al. Uveitis caused by cytotoxic immune response to cutaneous malignant melanoma in swine: Destruction of uveal melanocytes during tumor regression. Invest Opthalmol Vis Sci, 24: 1063–1069; 1983.

15. Sullivan KL, Aoyama T, Sato T, et al. Safety of immunoembolization of normal swine liver with human GM-CSF (granulocyte macrophage colony stimulating factor) and ethiodol. J Vasc Interv Radiol, 2001; 12: S132.

Chapter 28

PREOPERATIVE PORTAL VEIN EMBOLIZATION

David C. Madoff

With advances in perioperative care, major liver resections are being increasingly performed for primary and metastatic liver tumors. Although fatal liver failure and major technical complications are now rare after resection, complications associated with cholestasis, fluid retention and impaired synthetic function still contribute to protracted recovery time and extended hospital stay (1, 2). Although the risk for perioperative liver failure is multifactorial, one of the most important factors associated with this complication is the volume of the liver remaining after surgery. Patients considered at high risk are those with normal underlying liver in whom more than 80% of the functional liver mass will be removed or those with chronic liver disease who undergo resection of more than 60% of their functional liver mass (2–5).

One strategy used to improve the safety of extensive liver surgery in patients with small remnant livers is preoperative portal vein embolization (PVE) (5–15). PVE redirects portal flow to the intended future liver remnant (FLR) in an attempt to initiate hypertrophy of the non-embolized segments, and PVE has been shown to improve the functional reserve of the FLR before surgery. In appropriately selected patients, PVE can reduce perioperative morbidity and allow for safe, potentially curative hepatectomy for patients previously considered ineligible for resection based on anticipated small remnant livers (5–15). For this patient subset, PVE is now utilized as the standard of care at many comprehensive hepatobiliary centers prior to major hepatectomy.

The clinical use of PVE is based on experimental observations first reported in 1920 by Rous and Larimore (16), who studied the consequences of segmental portal venous occlusion in rabbits and found progressive atrophy of the hepatic segments with ligated portal veins and hypertrophy of the hepatic segments with patent portal veins. Later investigators reported clinical studies showing that portal vein or bile duct occlusion secondary to tumor invasion or ligation leads to ipsilateral liver atrophy (i.e., liver to be resected) and contralateral liver hypertrophy (i.e., liver to remain in situ after resection) (17–19). In the mid-1980s, Kinoshita et al. (20) used PVE to limit extension of segmental portal tumor thrombi from hepatocellular carcinoma (HCC) for which transcatheter arterial embolization (TAE) was ineffective. In 1990, Makuuchi et al. (10) first reported the use of PVE solely to induce left-liver hypertrophy prior to major hepatic resection in 14 patients with hilar cholangiocarcinoma.

Since these seminal publications, many investigators have described the usefulness of preoperative PVE in their multi-disciplinary management of patients with HCC, biliary cancer and liver metastases. Given this, considerable research efforts into the mechanisms of liver regeneration, indications for PVE, methods of measuring the FLR before and after PVE, technical aspects of PVE and potential surgical strategies are under way and in continual evolution. This chapter reviews the current indications for and technical aspects of PVE before hepatic

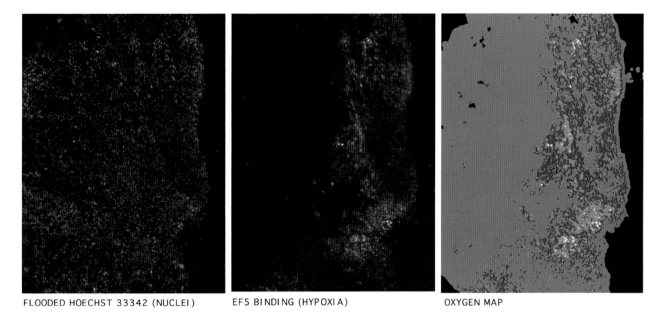

FLOODED HOECHST 33342 (NUCLEI)   EF5 BINDING (HYPOXIA)   OXYGEN MAP

PLATE 1. Generation of an oxygen map. These images represent the EF5 binding pattern and resultant oxygen map from a human extremity sarcoma. The image on the left demonstrates the location of all nuclei in the sample. Areas that are black on the EF5 image (*central image*) can represent absence of tissue, presence of oxic cells or presence of necrotic tissue. Comparison of the EF5 and Hoechst image allow these two possibilities to be distinguished from each other. In the oxygen map (*right image*), areas that are green–blue represent oxic regions, red–orange represent mild to moderate hypoxia and yellow–white represent severe hypoxia. The methods used to generate oxygen maps have been previously described in detail (24).

T1, Gd-enhanced MRI **18-F EF5 PET** **MRI-PET Fusion**

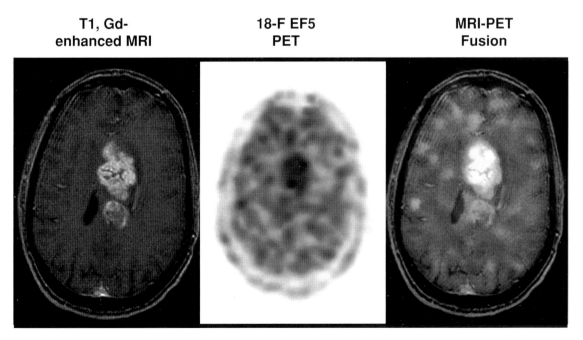

PLATE 2. Non-invasive imaging of hypoxia. MRI (T1, Gd-enhanced) and ^{18}F-EF5 PET scans from a patient with a glioblastoma multiforme (GBM). The MRI image demonstrates that this patient's tumor is contrast enhancing, compatible with the diagnosis of a GBM. There is EF5 binding in only a portion of the enhancing regions, demonstrating hypoxic heterogeneity within this mass.

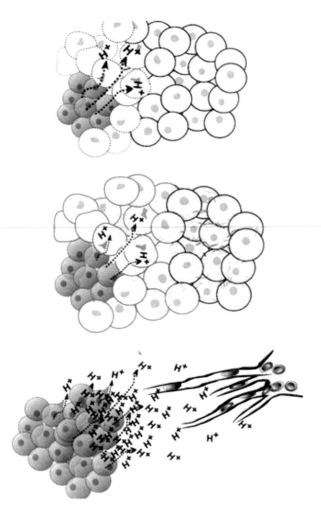

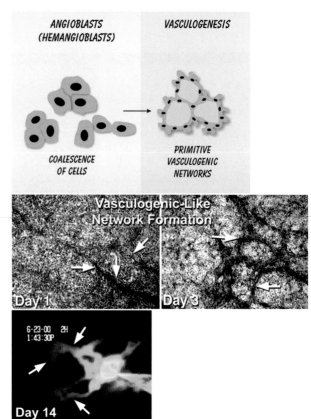

PLATE 3. Proposed mechanisms for acid-mediated tumor invasion. Increased acid in the tumor extracellular space due to glycolytic metabolism causes diffusion of H^+ along concentration gradients from the tumor (dark cells) into peritumoral normal tissues (light cells). The resulting decease in the extracellular pH causes normal cell death due to increased caspase activity, which triggers apoptosis via a *p53*-dependent pathway (*top panel*). In addition, the increased H^+ concentration results in extracellular matrix degradation due to release of cathepsin B and other proteolytic enzymes (*middle panel*) and induction of angiogenesis through release of IL-8 and VEGF (*lower panel*).

PLATE 5. Schematic overview of vasculogenesis. *Upper panel:* Schematic overview of vasculogenesis, showing how endothelial cell precursors (angioblasts and hemangioblasts) coalesce and differentiate into endothelial cells that form primitive vasculogenic networks (vasculogenesis). Remodeling of these networks occurs through angiogenesis. *Lower panel:* The unique ability of aggressive melanoma cells to form vasculogenic-like networks (*arrows*) in 3-D collagen I in vitro while simultaneously expressing genes associated with an endothelial-like cell type – called vasculogenic mimicry. The ECM-rich networks are perfusable (with a fluorescent dye) by day 14.

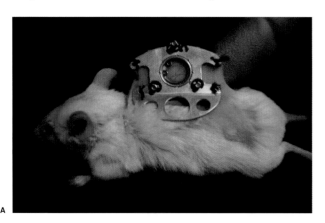

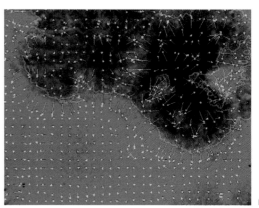

PLATE 4. Fluorescence imaging in a wound chamber tumor model. (A) demonstrates the dorsal wound chamber surgically implanted in a SCID mouse. GFP-transfected tumors implanted in the chamber can be continuously observed microscopically. Regional variations in pH$_e$ can be measured using fluorescent ratio imaging. (B) demonstrates the tumor–host interface defined by the irregular line. Because the tumor cells are GFP transfected, the tumor border can be precisely defined. The vectors demonstrate the flow of acid from the tumor into normal tissue based on gradients of pH$_e$ measurement.

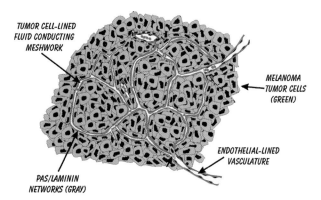

PLATE 6. The biological implications of melanoma vasculogenic mimicry have evolved to a "tumor cell–lined, fluid-conducting meshwork" corresponding to periodic acid-Schiff (PAS) and laminin-positive, patterned networks. This diagram represents the current interpretation of data generated from several studies involving the use of tracers and perfusion analyses of mice containing aggressive melanoma cells (green) during tumor development. The endothelial-lined vasculature is closely apposed to the tumor cell–formed fluid-conducting meshwork, and it is suggested that as the tumor remodels, the vasculature becomes leaky, resulting in the extravascular conduction of plasma. There is also evidence of a physiological connection between the endothelial-lined vasculature and the extravascular melanoma perfusion meshwork.

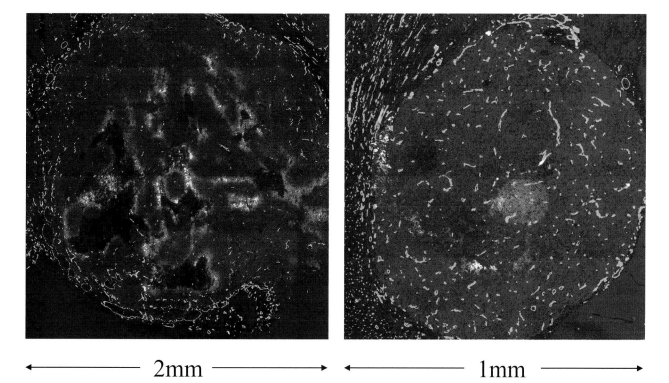

PLATE 7. Tumor heterogeneity. Images of two individual xenografts of human SiHa cervix cancer stained with fluorescent markers for hypoxia (EF5 – red), blood vessels (CD31 – green) and perfusion (Hoechst 33342 dye – blue). These tumors show considerable heterogeneity in these markers even though they were transplanted with cells from the same cell suspension into identical sites in two SCID mice. (*From* Vukovic V, Nicklee T, and Hedley DW. Multiparameter fluorescence mapping of nonprotein sulfhydryl status in relation to blood vessels and hypoxia in cervical carcinoma xenografts. Int J Radiat Oncol Biol Phys, 2002; 52: 837–843, with permission.)

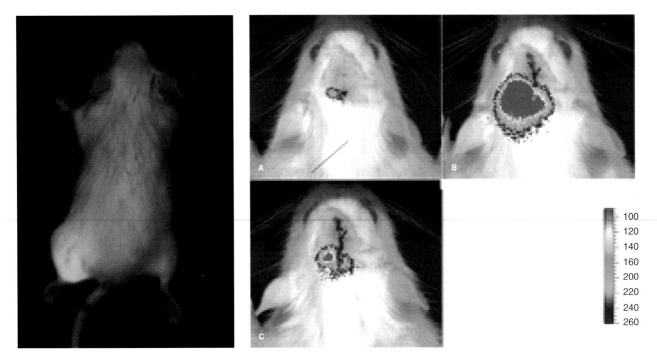

PLATE 8. Examples of fluorescence imaging of tumors and bioluminescence imaging of gene activity. The left panel illustrates a tumor labeled with green fluorescent protein, imaged with a charge couple device (CCD) camera. The right group of panels illustrate a tumor growing from cells containing a luciferase gene driven by a hypoxia-sensitive promoter implanted into the brain of a rat. Injecting luciferin into the rat allows the luciferase protein to produce a burst of light that can be imaged with a CCD camera. The animal was imaged prior to treatment with photodynamic therapy (PDT) and then at 4 and 24 hours. (A) Prior to treatment, there is little signal because the extent of hypoxia is limited. (B) The image at 4 hours demonstrates that hypoxia, induced by the PDT caused the production of luciferase, which was able to produce light. (C) By 24 hours, hypoxia was decreased and much of the luciferase protein had been degraded, resulting in a reduced signal. (Courtesy of Drs. Wilson and Moriyama, Ontario Cancer Institute.)

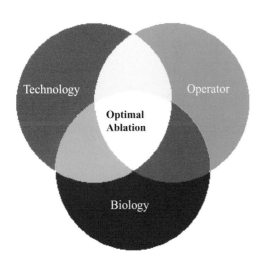

PLATE 9. Conceptualization of the key components necessary to achieve optimal ablation. The three key components for achieving successful RF ablation include *technology* (i.e., the RF generator and electrodes selected), the *biology* of the tumor and background tissue; and *operator* factors. Interfaces between technology and biology include *adjuvant therapies* that modulate these two factors. *Technique* defines the interface between technology and operator; whereas *patient selection* represents the operator interacting with tumor biology.

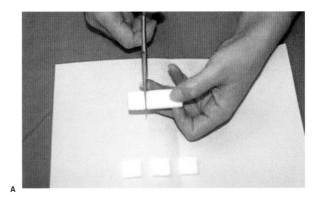

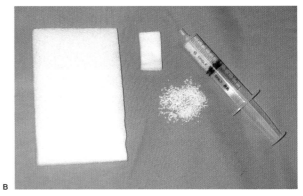

PLATE 10. Gelfoam particles. (A) A gelatin sponge sheet is easily cut into smaller size particles. (B) These particles, $2 \times 2 \times 2$ mm cubes, can be sterilized with ethylene oxide (EO) gas in a 10 cc syringe.

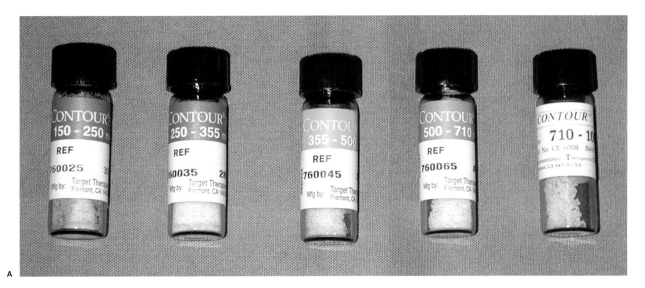

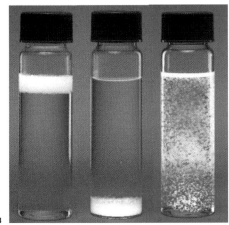

PLATE 11. PVA particles. (A) PVA particles (Contour®) are available commercially in different sizes (150–1000 μm). (B) Dilution of contrast media. Particles are suspended in contrast media (*left*) and precipitated in saline (*middle*) and then freely dispersed in the bottle of specific gravity–matched contrast media (*right*).

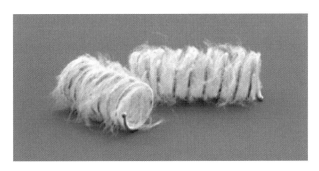

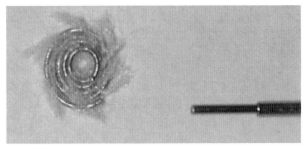

PLATE 12. Microcoils. Several different types of microcoils are currently available, i.e., spiral or Tornado types, with thrombogenic Dacron fibers.

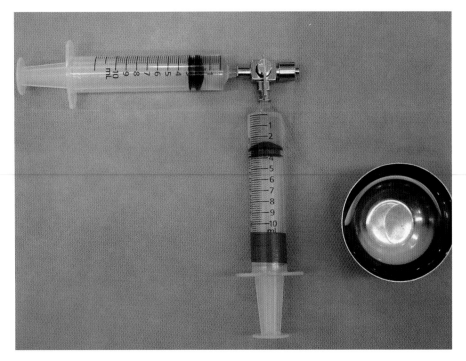
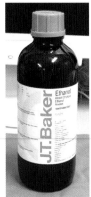
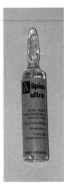

PLATE 13. A mixture of ethanol and lipiodol. Pumping method used to mix ethanol and lipiodol using two syringes connected via a three-way valve. The syringe marked with red tape contains absolute ethanol.

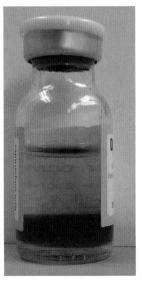
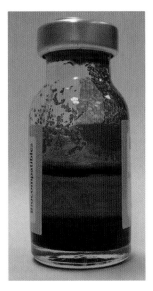
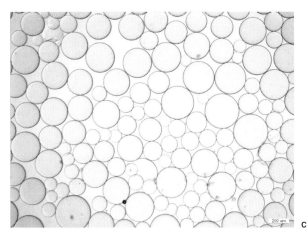

A, B

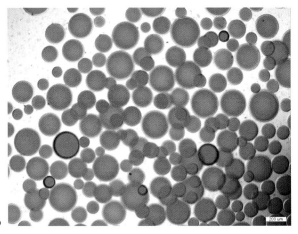

D

PLATE 14. DC bead spheres. (A) A bottle of DC bead spheres (doxorubicin-capable beads, Biocompatible, UK) of 100–300 mm size. (B) A bottle containing DC beads after mixing with doxorubicin solution for 1 hour. (C) Microscopic view of DC beads of 100–300 mm. (D) Microscopic view of red-tinged DC beads containing doxorubicin after soaking in drug solution.

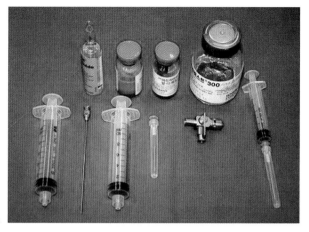

A

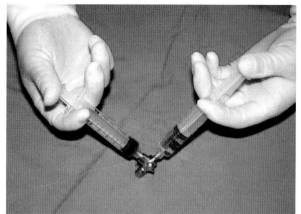

B

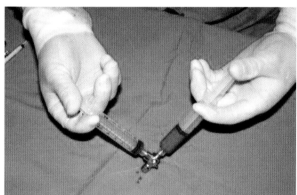

C

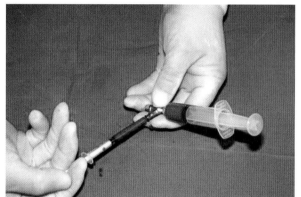

D

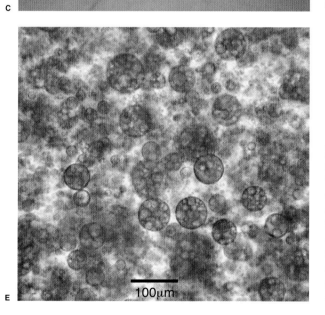

E

PLATE 15. Doxorubicin(Adriamycin)-lipiodol emulsion formation using the pumping technique. (A) Preparation. The materials used were a single 10-mL sample of lipiodol, two bottles of doxorubicin powder and a bottle of contrast media (iopamidol). (B) Mixing of doxorubicin solution with lipiodol using the three-way stopcock. (C) Manual pumping (more than 30 times) to produce a homogenous emulsion. (D) Ready to infuse chemoembolic material with 1 cc tuberculin syringe. (E) Microscopic view of lipiodol emulsion showing variably sized droplets containing red-colored doxorubicin after pumping.

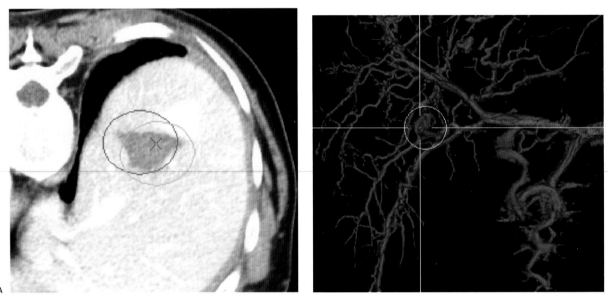

PLATE 16. (A) Imaging used for planning. Planning software is used to plan overlapping thermal ablations to fully cover the tumor volume. Each circle represents the theoretical volume of necrosis from a single radiofrequency ablation. (B) Planning software can segment the hepatic arterial tree from a rotational angiographic study. By pointing to the tumor target, the software can identify the feeding branches as depicted in red.

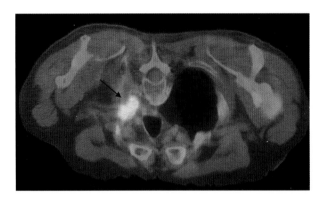

PLATE 17. Imaging used for guiding therapy. Fusion of PET and CT can indicate which part of the anatomic changes still contains viable tumor. This can then guide therapy to the incompletely treated tumor. Fusion allows capitalizing on the best features of CT (anatomy) with the best features of PET (physiology). The arrow indicates the FDG-avid part of the tumor.

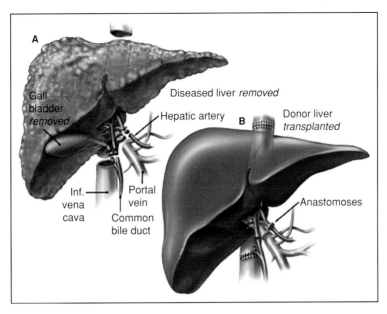

PLATE 18. Schematic of orthotopic liver transplantation. (Courtesy of Johns Hopkins University School of Medicine, Division of Gastroenterology.)

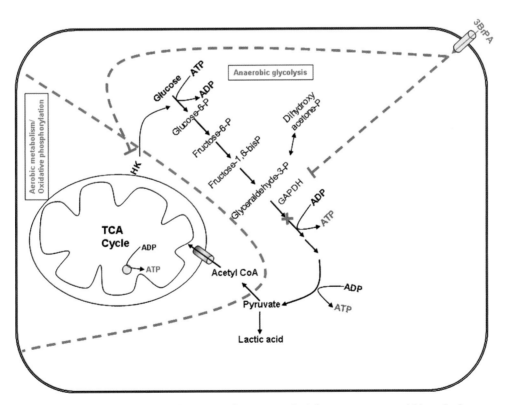

PLATE 19. Proposed mechanism of action of 3-bromopyruvate. (*Adapted from* Geschwind JF, et al. Novel therapy for liver cancer. Direct intraarterial injection of a potent inhibitor of ATP production. Cancer Res 62, 3909–3913, July 15, 2002; with permission.)

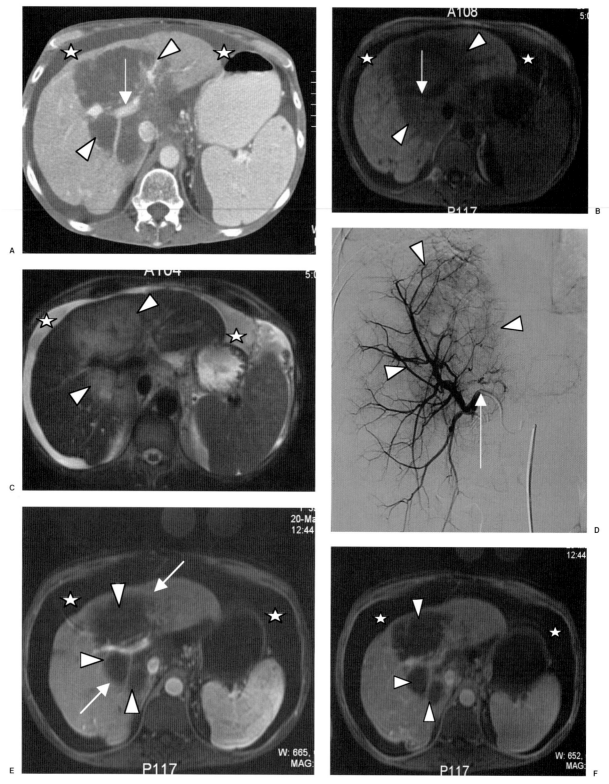

PLATE 20. Sixty-eight-year-old man with history of liver cirrhosis presented with a large (9 × 8 cm) mass on his first surveillance CT. Patient admitted to many-month history of vague abdominal pain, but attributed it to his known ascites (*asterisk*). Axial contrast-enhanced, venous-phase CT of the liver (A) and a non-contrast-enhanced, T1-weighted MRI (B), show a solid, hypovascular mass (*arrowheads*) that, as is the case in the patient in Figure 18.1, allows vessels (*arrows*) to traverse it with minimal distortion. Again as in Figure 18.1, T2-weighted MRI shows increased signal throughout the tumor but again low enough to exclude a hemangioma (C). Digital subtraction, right hepatic arteriogram using a micro-catheter (*arrow*) reveal the hypervascular nature of this ICC (*arrowheads*) (D). Repeat contrast-enhanced MRI of the liver was obtained 3 weeks after TACE. Arterial (E) and venous (F) phase images reveal near-complete necrosis and cystic transformation (*arrowheads*) of the tumor with minimal shrinkage. A thin rim of enhancement (*arrows*) is seen, representing either residual tumor or a hypervascular fibrotic, inflammatory capsule commonly seen after TACE. When response to TACE is above 75% necrosis, as in this case, a repeat MRI is planned in 6 weeks. Additional TACE is offered only if an enlarging tumor is again noted.

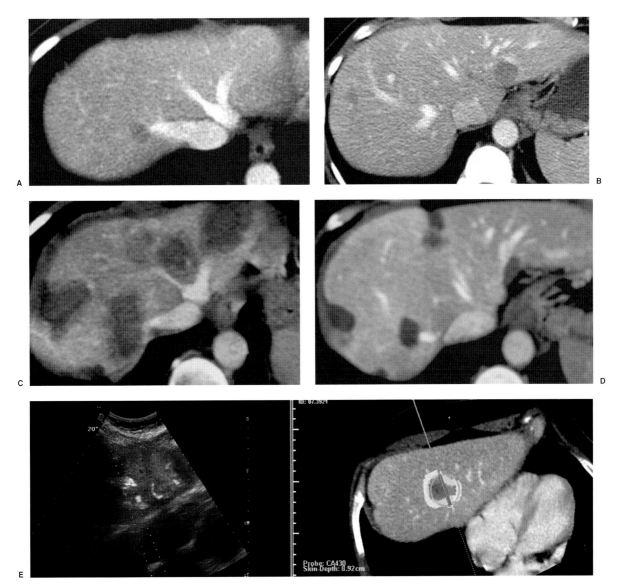

PLATE 21. A 43-year-old patient with history of colon carcinoma surgically resected and systemic chemotherapy. Follow-up CT scans show the presence of six small liver metastases (one is visible in A, two in B). (C) All the lesions are treated with cool-tip RFA in a single session and large necrotic areas are achieved. (D) Three years after ablation, all the necrotic areas show marked shrinkage, but a new metastasis appears in segment IV, adjacent to one of the areas of necrosis. (E) This new metastasis is precisely treated with real-time CT-US fusion imaging.

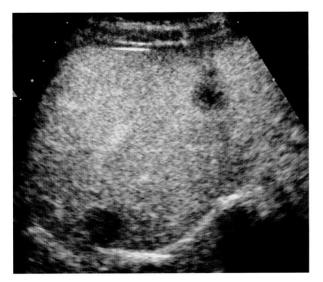

PLATE 22. Contrast-enhanced sonographic scan in early portal phase in a patient with history of colorectal metastasis in segment VII, treated with RFA. The completely necrotic area in segment VII appears avascular and well demarcated. A new metastasis is visible in segment IV and shows moderate peripheral enhancement and ill-defined margins.

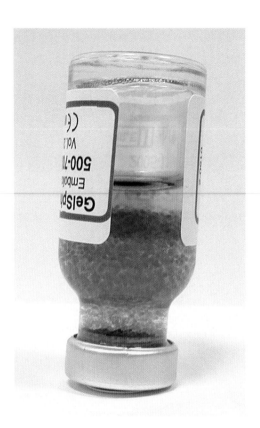

PLATE 23. A vial of microspheres 500 to 700 μm (Biocompatible, UK) before loading with doxorubicin.

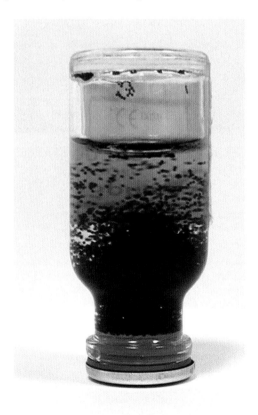

PLATE 24. The same vial after 40 minutes of contact with 50 mg of doxorubicin diluted in 5 ml of isotonic contrast medium shows uptake of doxorubicin by the embols, which turn red. The solution is clear and does not contain any more doxorubicin.

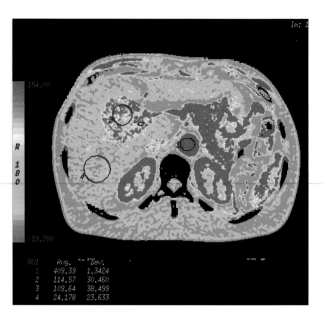

PLATE 25. Blood volume mapping obtained before treatment from CT study at the same level as Figure 26.9 shows a high blood volume in the tumor compared with the normal liver parenchyma, 109.64 and 24.17 respectively.

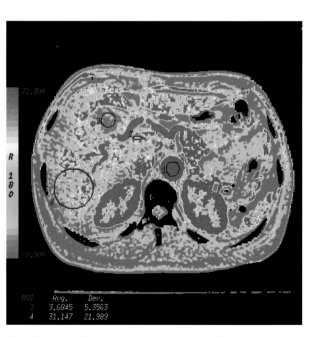

PLATE 26. Blood volume mapping at the same level as Figures 26.9 and 26.10 (Color Plate 25) obtained 2 days after selective TACE of segment IV shows a decrease of blood volume in the tumor to 3.68, whereas blood volume in the liver does not differ much from pre-TACE values, at 31.14.

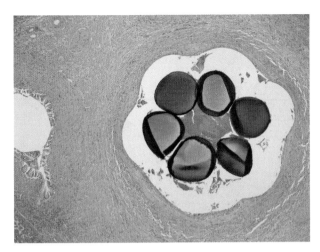

PLATE 27. Patient underwent liver resection after morphologic tumor response and pathologic study shows the drug-eluting beads in an artery surrounded by necrosis and inflammation.

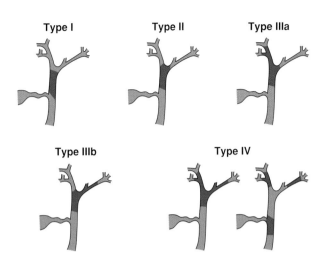

PLATE 28. Classification of (peri)hilar cholangiocarcinoma according to the Bismuth-Corlette system. (*From* Lazaridis KN and Gores GJ. Cholangiocarcinoma. Gastroenterology 2005; 128: 1655–1667; with permission.)

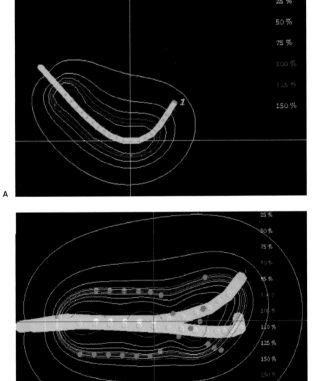

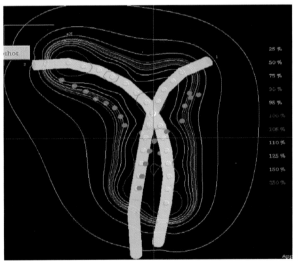

PLATE 29. The cumulative dose from the combination of the various dwell points are shown in the anteroposterior view for one-catheter technique (A). Two-catheter technique with both anteroposterior (B) and lateral (C) views also is shown.

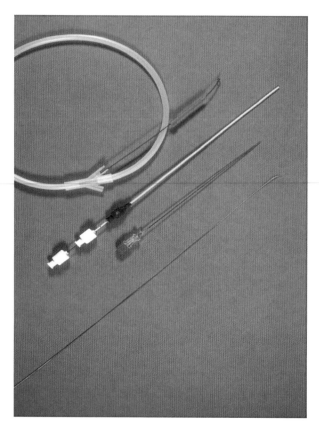

PLATE 30. Minimally invasive access set (Accustick, Boston Scientific).

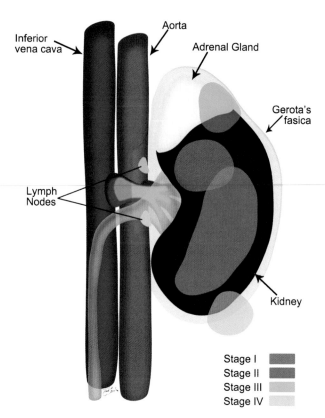

PLATE 32. Diagrammatic representation of staging of RCC. (*Adapted from* Cohen et al. with permission [2].)

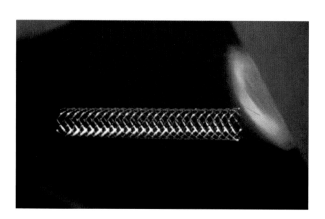

PLATE 31. Self-expanding metallic endoprostheses in a deployed state (10 mm diameter and 7 cm long).

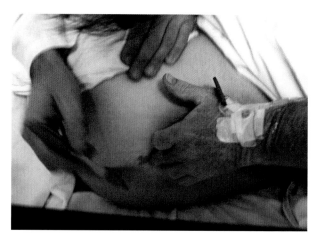

PLATE 33. Patients are physically examined prior to the cryoablation procedure for careful identification of the area of focal pain. The area is marked on the skin and correlated with imaging findings prior to the cryoablation procedure.

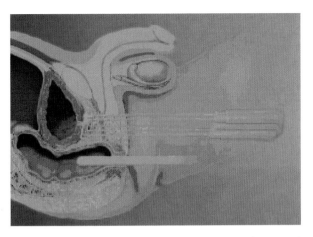

PLATE 34. Diagram showing the transperineal approach of prostate cryosurgery. The cryoprobes are placed percutaneously through the perineum using trans-rectal ultrasound for guidance. The approach is identical in concept to brachytherapy of the prostate. [Reproduced with permission from Endocare, Inc, Irvine, California (1-800-418-4677; http://www.endocare.com).]

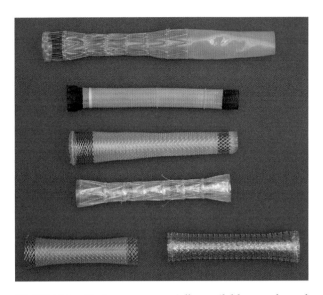

PLATE 36. Various commercially available esophageal stents in their fully deployed state. The uppermost stent has an anti-reflux valve.

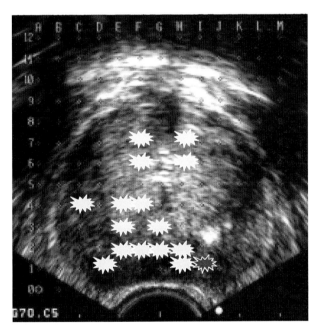

PLATE 35. Ultrasound of a patient who presented with a single core positive, Gleason 6 on his TRUS biopsy on the left side of the gland. The starburst patterns indicate all the locations he was positive on his 3D-PMB. The pink starburst indicates an area of extra-capsular extension.

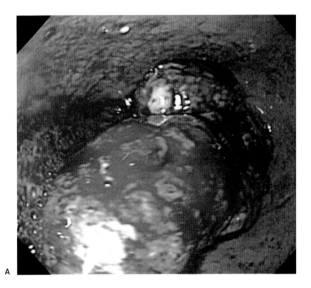

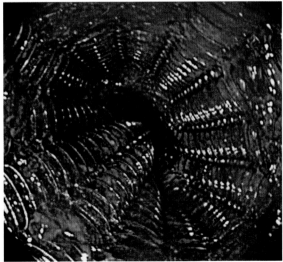

PLATE 37. Palliation of esophageal obstruction. (A) Endoscopic view of obstructing tumor. (B) Immediately after placement of partially covered stent.

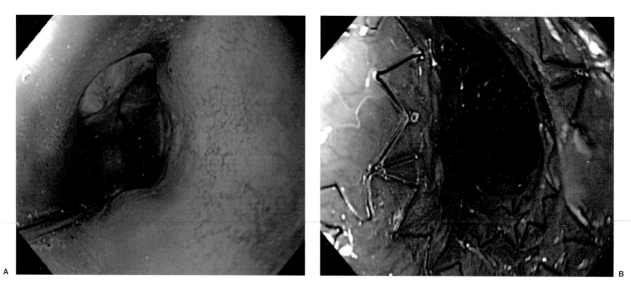

PLATE 38.   Closure of tracheoesophageal fistula. (A) Endoscopic view of fistula: Note
guidewire is in esophageal lumen. (B) Immediately after placement of covered stent.

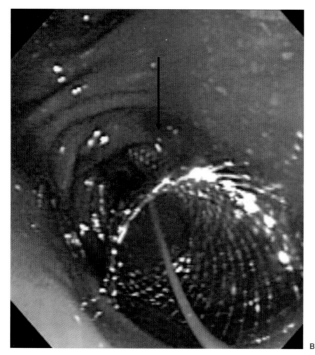

PLATE 39.   Double stenting of pancreatic cancer. (B)
Endoscopic view of both duodenal stent and biliary stent
(*arrow*) immediately after deployment.

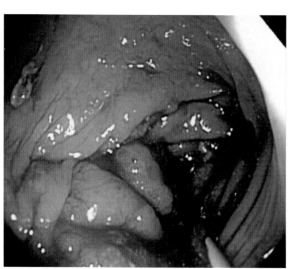

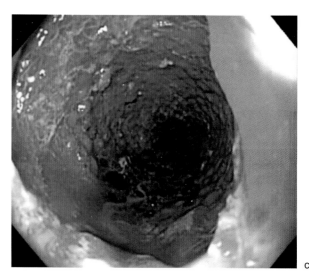

PLATE 40.   Palliative stent placement for obstructing mass
near splenic flexure. (B) Endoscopic view of obstructing

mass. (C) Endoscopic view of Wallstent immediately after
deployment.

resection, with an emphasis on strategies to improve outcomes.

MECHANISMS OF LIVER REGENERATION

The ability of the liver to regenerate following injury or resection has long fascinated scientists, physicians and laypersons. The earliest reference to the liver's capacity to regenerate is from classical Greek mythology, in Hesiod's *Theogony* (750–700 B.C.) (21). However, the human liver's regenerative ability was not documented scientifically until 1890 (22).

Despite its considerable metabolic load, the liver is essentially a quiescent organ in terms of hepatocyte replication, with only 0.0012% to 0.01% of hepatocytes undergoing mitosis at any time (21, 23, 24). However, this low cell turnover in healthy liver can be altered by toxic injury or surgical resection, which stimulates sudden, massive hepatocyte proliferation resulting in recovery of the functional liver mass within 2 weeks after the loss of up to two-thirds of the liver. This regenerative response is typically mediated by the proliferation of surviving hepatocytes within the acinar architecture of the remnant liver. Following resection, this response results in hypertrophy of the remnant liver rather than restoration of the resected lobes, a phenomenon that is correctly termed **compensatory hyperplasia** rather than true regeneration (24). The term *hypertrophy* actually means an increase in cell size and may be misleading because the primary mechanism of volume restitution after liver resection or embolization is more precisely termed hyperplasia, or an increase in cell number (25–27). However, studies also suggest that both hypertrophy and hyperplasia aid in restoring functional hepatic volume (28–30). The term **hypertrophy after PVE** or **resection** is used throughout this chapter since this is the term used throughout the published literature.

Most information about the molecular and cellular events during liver regeneration comes from studies of partial hepatectomy in animal models (21). In brief, the events that occur in hepatocytes result from growth-factor stimulation in response to injury. In regenerating liver, hepatocyte growth factor (HGF), transforming growth factor-α and epidermal growth factor are important stimuli for hepatocyte replication. HGF is the most potent mitogen for hepatocyte replication, and in combination with other mitogenic growth factors (i.e., transforming growth factor-α and epidermal growth factor), it can induce the production of cytokines, including tumor necrosis factor-α and interleukin-6, and activate immediate response genes that ready the hepatocytes for cell cycle progression and regeneration. Insulin is synergistic with HGF, resulting in slower regeneration rates seen in patients with diabetes (31, 32). Extrahepatic factors are transported primarily from the gut via the portal vein and not the hepatic artery (9, 22, 33, 34).

RATE OF LIVER REGENERATION

Hepatocyte regeneration occurs early following partial hepatectomy, PVE or liver injury. Soon after the stimulus, hepatocytes exit the resting stage of the cell cycle (G_0), enter G_1 phase, proceed to DNA synthesis or S phase, and ultimately undergo mitosis, with a first peak of DNA synthesis (as determined by the DNA index) occurring in the parenchymal cells (e.g., hepatocytes and biliary epithelial cells) at 24 and 40 hours after resection in rat and mouse models, respectively (35). In both species, non-parenchymal cells display a first peak of proliferation approximately 12 hours after the parenchymal cells (36). In large-animal models of regeneration after partial hepatectomy, DNA synthesis peaks later, at 72 to 96 hours in canines (37) and 7 to 10 days in primates (38). Notably, the degree of hepatocyte proliferation is directly proportional to the degree of injury (i.e., a minor liver insult will result in only a localized mitotic reaction, but any injury greater than 10% will result in proliferation of cells throughout the liver) (39). When more than 50% of the liver is resected, a second, less distinct wave of hepatocyte mitoses is observed. In rat and mouse models, this second peak is observed at 3 to 5 days; in larger animals, this second peak occurs over many days. Studies in other injury models have suggested that similar time courses of regeneration and cellular signaling are involved in the regenerative response. For example, examination of the regenerative response after PVE in swine demonstrated induction of hepatocyte proliferation at 2 to 7 days (40). Replication peaked at 7 days, occurring in approximately 14% of hepatocytes, and then decreased to baseline levels by day 12, a process similar to what is seen with PVE clinically. When compared with replication after resection, the peak replication after PVE is delayed approximately 3 to 4 days, suggesting that the stimulus of hepatocyte removal is superior to the stimulus of apoptosis seen with PVE (25).

Also important to the understanding of liver regeneration is the observation that the diseased (i.e., cirrhotic) liver has a lower capacity to regenerate than does the healthy liver (25). This may be the result of the diminished capacity of hepatocytes to respond to hepatotropic factors or because parenchymal damage such as fibrosis leads to slower portal blood flow rates (41). Lee et al. (25) evaluated rats with normal livers or chemically induced cirrhotic livers and found that the weight of the normal livers increased after 24 hours, tripled after 7 days and reached a plateau between 7 and 14 days, whereas the rate of regeneration of the cirrhotic livers was delayed and of a lesser magnitude. Findings in clinical studies have been similar. Non-cirrhotic livers in humans regenerate fastest, at rates of 12 to 21 cm^3/day at 2 weeks, 11 cm^3/day at 4 weeks, and 6 cm^3/day at 32 days after PVE (32, 42). The rates of regeneration are slower (9 cm^3/day at 2 weeks) in patients with cirrhotic livers, with comparable rates found in diabetics (32, 43).

Steatosis also seems to impair liver regeneration in animal models, but regeneration may still occur after PVE (44). Currently, however, the severity of clinically significant steatosis is unknown. In laboratory animals, exposure to a high-fat diet impairs liver regeneration after partial hepatectomy and is also associated with increased hepatocellular apoptosis. Thus, a high-fat diet may not only impair liver regeneration but may also increase the risk for hepatic injury (steatohepatitis) (45).

PATHOPHYSIOLOGY OF PREOPERATIVE PVE

Makuuchi et al. (10) published the initial experience using preoperative PVE to induce left-liver hypertrophy before right hepatectomy. The rationale for using PVE in this setting was to minimize the abrupt rise in portal pressure at resection that can lead to hepatocellular damage to the FLR, to dissociate portal pressure-induced hepatocellular damage from the direct trauma to the FLR during physical manipulation of the liver at the time of surgery and to improve overall tolerance to major resection by increasing hepatic mass prior to resection in order to reduce the risk of post-resection metabolic changes.

The rationale for PVE has also been based on data showing that increases in FLR volume are associated with improved function as demonstrated by increases in biliary excretion (46, 47) and technetium-99m-galactosyl human serum albumin uptake (48) and by significant improvements in the postoperative liver function tests following PVE compared with no PVE (3).

Following PVE, alterations in liver function tests are typically minor and transient. When transaminase levels rise, they usually peak at levels less than three times baseline 1 to 3 days after PVE and return to baseline within 10 days, regardless of the embolic agent used (10, 11, 32, 43, 49–51). Slight changes in white blood cell count and total serum bilirubin concentration may be seen after PVE, and prothrombin time is almost never affected.

Unlike arterial embolization, PVE is not associated with the post-embolization syndrome; nausea and vomiting are rare, and fever and pain are minimal (9). This is because PVE produces no distortion of the hepatic anatomy, minimal inflammation except immediately around the embolized vein, and little, if any, parenchymal or tumor necrosis (10, 52). Animal studies have shown that hepatocytes undergo apoptosis and not necrosis after portal venous occlusion (40, 53), which explains the relative lack of systemic symptoms following PVE.

Portal blood flow to the non-embolized hepatic segments measured by Doppler sonography increases significantly and then falls to near-baseline values after 11 days. The resultant hypertrophy rate correlates with the portal flow rate (9, 41).

FLR VOLUME MEASUREMENT AND PREDICTING FUNCTION AFTER PVE

Computed tomography (CT) with volumetry is used as an important tool to predict liver function after resection of the tumor-bearing liver, and many methods have been proposed (14, 54, 55). However, these volumes must be used within the context of the patient's underlying liver function and not as a stand-alone value upon which resection will be solely based.

Three-dimensional CT volumetric measurements are acquired by outlining the hepatic segmental contours and calculating the volumes from the surface measurements from each slice. Multiphasic contrast-enhanced CT must be performed to demarcate the vascular landmarks of the hepatic segments (55).

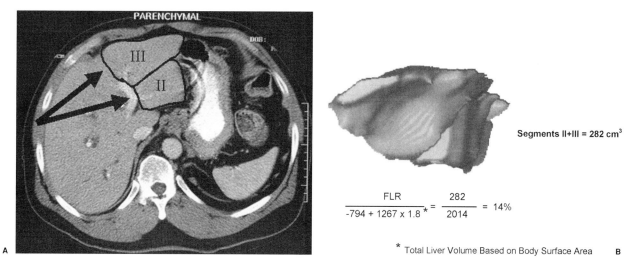

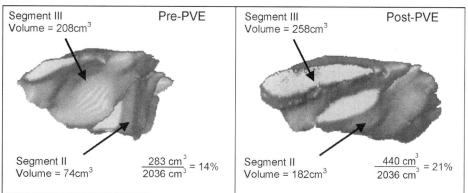

FIGURE 28.1. Hypertrophy of the future liver remnant after portal vein embolization as determined by three-dimensional reconstruction of CT images. (A) Three-dimensional volumetric measurements are determined by outlining the hepatic segmental contours and then calculating the volumes from the surface measurements of each slice. (B) The formula for calculating total liver volume is based on the patient's body surface area. (*Modified from* Vauthey JN, et al. Liver Transpl, 2002; 8: 233–240; with permission.) (C) Before embolization, the volume of segments II and III was 283 cm³, or 14% of the total liver volume (2,036 cm³). After embolization, the volume of segments II and III was 440 cm³, or 21% of the total liver volume (an increase of 7 percentage points). (B *modified from* Vauthey JN, et al. Liver Transpl 2002; 8:233–24; C modified from Vauthey JN, et al. Surgery 2000; 127:512–9; with permission.)

Using this technique, an accurate and reproducible FLR volume can be calculated within minutes of scanning, with an error less than ± 5% (56, 57). The FLR can then be standardized to the total liver volume (TLV) to determine the %TLV that will remain after resection.

Although measurement of the TLV is possible with CT, direct TLV measurements may not be relevant to surgical planning for several reasons. First, in patients with large tumors, the TLV is altered, and attempts to subtract tumor volume from the TLV require additional time to calculate, especially when multiple tumors are present, and may lead to additive mathematical errors in volume calculation (TLV minus tumor volume) (7, 58). Furthermore, this approach does not account for the actual functional liver volume when vascular obstruction, chronic liver disease or biliary dilatation is present in the liver to be resected. Patients with cirrhosis often have enlarged or shrunken livers such that the measured TLV may not be useful as an index to which FLR volume is standardized, leading some investigators to advocate clinical algorithms in which functional tests such as indocyanine green retention at 15 minutes (ICGR$_{15}$) are evaluated along with the extent of planned resection (59).

A simple, more accurate and reproducible method (Figure 28.1) standardizes liver remnant size to individual patient size to account for the reality that large patients need a larger liver remnant than do smaller patients. CT is used to directly measure the FLR, which is by definition disease free. The TLV is *estimated* by a formula derived from the close association between liver size and patient size based on body weight and body surface area (BSA): (estimated TLV or TELV = −794.41 + 1,267.28 × BSA) (3,14). The FLR/TELV ratio is then calculated to provide a volumetric estimate of FLR function. From this calculation method, called **standardized FLR measurement**, a correlation between the anticipated liver remnant and operative outcome has been established (3). Recently, this formula was evaluated in a meta-analysis comparing 12 different formulas and was recommended as one of the least biased and most precise for TLV estimation (60). At our institution, CT scans are performed before PVE and approximately 3 to 4 weeks after PVE to assess the degree of FLR hypertrophy.

Shirabe et al. (2) also recognized the importance of standardizing liver volume to BSA and found that no patient with underlying liver disease who had a standardized liver volume greater than 285 mL/m² BSA died of liver failure following liver resection. Given similar data in another study, the guideline for utilizing PVE in patients with cirrhotic livers has been set at a standardized FLR volume less than 40% (7).

Technological advances in nuclear imaging are being designed to measure both anatomical and functional differences in liver volume. Technetium-99m-labeled diethylenetriamine pentaacetic acid-galactosyl-human serum albumin binds specifically to asialoglycoprotein receptors on hepatocyte cell membranes. Agent distribution is monitored in real time with single-photon emission scintigraphy and has been shown to correlate with $ICGR_{15}$ (61). Another technique, axial image reconstruction, can be used to estimate the differential functions of the right and left liver. However, neither technique is, as of yet, sufficiently accurate in assessing segmental or bisegmental function during the planning for extended hepatectomy.

TECHNICAL CONSIDERATIONS FOR PVE

Standard Approaches

PVE is performed to redirect portal blood flow toward the hepatic segments that will remain after surgery (i.e., the FLR). To ensure adequate hypertrophy, embolization of portal branches must be as complete as possible so that recanalization of the occluded portal system is minimized. The entire portal system to be resected must be occluded to avoid the development of intrahepatic portoportal collaterals that may limit regeneration (62).

PVE can be performed by any of three standard approaches: the transhepatic contralateral (i.e., portal access via the FLR), the transhepatic ipsilateral (i.e., portal access via the liver to be resected), and the intraoperative transileocolic venous approach. These approaches are chosen based on operator preference, type of hepatic resection planned, extent of embolization (e.g., right PVE [RPVE] with or without extension to segment IV) and type of embolic agent used.

The transhepatic contralateral approach, developed by Kinoshita et al. (20), is currently the most commonly used technique worldwide (Figure 28.2). With this approach, a branch of the left portal system (usually segment III) is accessed, and the catheter is advanced into the right portal venous system for embolization (49). The major advantage of this approach is that catheterization of the desired right portal vein branches is more direct via the left system than via the right, making the procedure technically easier. However, the disadvantage of this technique is the risk of injury to the FLR parenchyma and the left portal vein. A recent multicenter European study of 188 patients who underwent contralateral PVE reported 24 (12.8%) adverse events including migration of embolic material to the FLR in 10 patients (5.3%), occlusion of a major portal branch requiring intervention in three patients (1.6%), bleeding in five patients (2.7%: one hemobilia, one hemoperitoneum, one rupture of gallbladder metastases, two

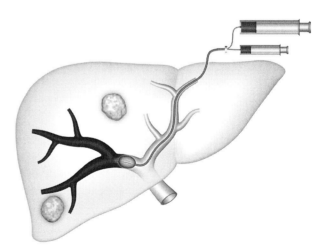

FIGURE 28.2. Schematic representation of the contralateral approach. An occlusion balloon catheter is placed from the left lobe into right portal branch, with delivery of the embolic agent in the antegrade direction.

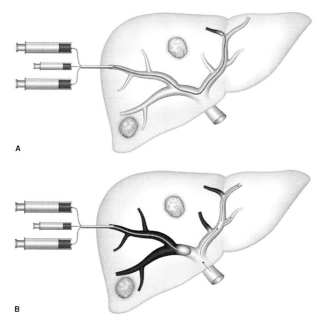

FIGURE 28.3. Schematic representation of the ipsilateral approach for RPVE and segment IV as described by Nagino et al. (12). Different portions of the balloon catheter are used for antegrade embolization of segment IV veins (A) and for retrograde delivery of the embolic agent into the right portal system (B). (A modified from Vauthey JN, et al. Liver Transpl 2002; 8:233–24; B modified from Vauthey JN, et al. Surgery 2000; 127:512–9; with permission.)

subcapsular hematomas) and transient liver failure in six patients (3.2%) (63). These adverse events may compromise the integrity of the FLR and may make the planned resection more difficult or impossible. Furthermore, embolization of segment IV, if needed, may prove difficult (15).

The transhepatic ipsilateral approach, first described by Nagino et al. (64) in the mid-1990s (Figure 28.3), is now advocated by additional investigators (65, 66). For this approach, a peripheral portal vein branch in the liver to be resected is accessed, through which the embolic material is administered. Because Nagino's ipsilateral approach requires the use of specialized catheters not available outside of Japan, modifications of the ipsilateral technique have been developed. At M.D. Anderson Cancer Center, standard angiographic catheters have been used for combined particulate and coil embolization (Figure 28.4) (54, 65, 66). When right heptatectomy is planned, RPVE is performed (Figure 28.5), and when extended right hepatectomy is planned, RPVE is extended to segment IV (RPVE + IV) (Figure 28.6). Ipsilateral RPVE ± IV is performed after a 5- or 6F sheath is placed into a distal right portal vein branch. When RPVE + IV is needed, segment IV embolization is performed first so as to not manipulate catheters through previously embolized

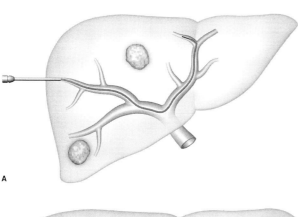

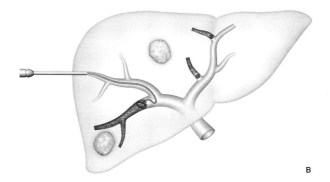

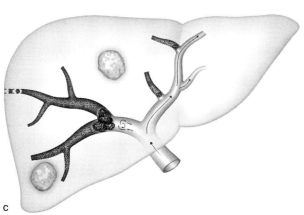

FIGURE 28.4. Schematic representation shows modification of the ipsilateral technique for RPVE extended to segment IV. (A) Placement of a 6F vascular sheath into the right portal branch An angled 5F catheter is placed into the left portal system with coaxial placement of a microcatheter into a segment IV branch. Particulate embolization is performed, followed by placement of coils, until all the branches are occluded. (B) After segment IV embolization is completely occluded, a 5F reverse-curve catheter is used for RPVE. (C) After PVE is complete, the access tract is embolized with coils and/or gelfoam to prevent subcapsular hemorrhage.

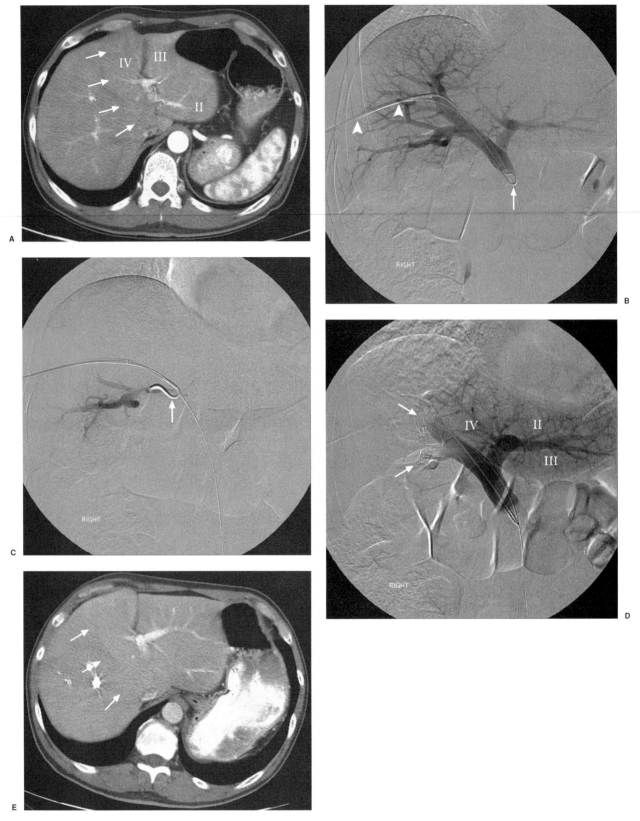

FIGURE 28.5. A 59-year-old man with colorectal liver metastases, status post-oxaliplatin-based chemotherapy, who had transhepatic ipsilateral RPVE with particles and coils prior to right hepatectomy. (A) Contrast-enhanced CT scan of liver shows small left liver (FLR/TELV of 18% [*arrows*]). (B) Anteroposterior flush portogram shows a 6F vascular sheath (*arrowheads*) in a right portal vein branch and a 5F flush catheter (*arrow*) in the main portal vein. (C) A selective right portogram is performed with 5F reverse-curve catheter (*arrow*) prior to administration of particles and coils. (D) Post-procedure portogram shows occlusion of the portal vein branches to segments V–VIII (*white arrows* point to coils within the proximal anterior and posterior sector right portal vein branches) with continued patency of the veins supplying the left lateral lobe (segments II, III and IV). (E) Contrast-enhanced CT scan of liver performed 1 month after RPVE shows hypertrophy of left liver (FLR/TELV of 32% [*arrows*]). The patient underwent successful right hepatectomy.

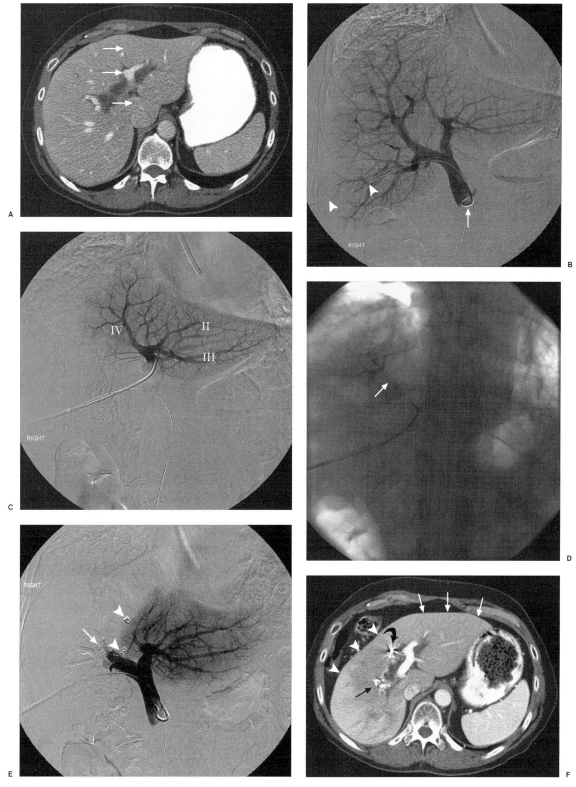

FIGURE 28.6. A 59-year-old woman with gallbladder carcinoma who underwent transhepatic ipsilateral RPVE extended to segment IV prior to an extended right hepatectomy. (A) A single image from pre-PVE contrast-enhanced CT scan shows small left lateral liver (*arrows*) and FLR/TELV of 17%. (B) Anteroposterior flush portogram from the ipsilateral approach shows a 6F vascular sheath (*arrowheads*) in a right portal vein branch and a 5F flush catheter (*arrow*) in the main portal vein. (C) Selective left portogram shows the veins that supply segments II, III and IV. (D) Superselective portogram shows a microcatheter (*arrow*) within a segment IVa branch. (E) Post-procedure portogram shows complete occlusion (with par-ticles and coils) of the portal vein branches to segments IV–VIII (*arrowheads* point to microcoils within segment IV portal vein branches; *arrow* points to coils within the right portal vein) with continued patency of the veins supplying the left lateral lobe (segments II and III). (F) Contrast-enhanced CT scan performed 4 weeks after PVE shows hypertrophy of the left lateral liver (FLR/TELV now 26%, an increase of 9 percentage points) with rounded margins (*straight white arrows*). Massive atrophy of the embolized liver is seen (*white arrowheads*). Coils within segment IV (*curved white arrow*) and the right lobe (*straight black arrow*) are seen. The patient underwent an uncomplicated extended right hepatectomy 4 weeks later.

segments. A microcatheter is advanced coaxially through an angled catheter into the portal vein branches in segment IV so that particulate embolics and coils can be delivered. Once segment IV embolization is completed, a reverse-curve catheter is often needed for RPVE. After complete occlusion of the right portal vein, embolization of the access tract is performed with coils and/or gelfoam to reduce the risk of perihepatic hemorrhage at the puncture site.

One advantage of the ipsilateral approach is that the anticipated liver remnant is not instrumented. However, catheterization of the right portal vein branches may be more difficult because of severe angulations between right portal branches, necessitating the use of reverse-curved catheters. Another potential disadvantage of this approach is that some embolic material could be displaced upon catheter removal, leading to non-target embolization, although this has not occurred in our experience with more than 100 RPVEs, most of which included extension to the segment IV branches. Similarly, in our experience, ipsilateral access has not been a problem even in patients with large liver tumors.

The transileocolic venous approach is performed during laparotomy by direct cannulation of the ileocolic vein and advancement of a balloon catheter into the portal vein for embolization (10). This approach, preferred by many Asian surgeons, is performed when an interventional radiology suite is not available, when a percutaneous approach is not considered feasible or when additional treatment is needed during the same surgical exploration (55, 67). Disadvantages of this method are the need for general anesthesia and laparotomy, with their inherent risks, and the inferior imaging equipment often (but not always) available in the operating room compared with the state-of-the-art imaging equipment available in most interventional radiology suites.

Non-standard Approaches

Other approaches for PVE have been used. The idea of combining PVE and TAE for complete portal venous and hepatic arterial occlusion has been described in patients with biliary tract cancer and colorectal metastases who did not have sufficient hypertrophy after PVE alone (68, 69). Nagino et al. (68) reported that one patient required an extended left hepatectomy, but the FLR volume (i.e., right posterior liver) did not change 51 days after PVE (pre-PVE: 485 cm^3, post-PVE: 470 cm^3). After TAE, the FLR volume rose to 685 cm^3, an increase of 215 cm^3. A second patient required a right hepatectomy, but after PVE no significant volume change was noted (pre-PVE: 643 cm^3, post-PVE: 649 cm^3). After TAE, the left lobe volume was 789 cm^3, an increase of 140 cm^3. Both patients underwent resection following staged PVE and TAE procedures. As both arterial and portal systems are blood deprived, the possibility of hepatic infarction exists so that only one-half the target segments were treated with TAE superselectively. Although this approach is effective, the downside is that two separate procedures are required, performed at different times, leading to substantially longer overall waiting periods. During these waiting periods, tumor progression may occur to the degree that tumors become unresectable.

In 2004, Aoki et al. (70) reported the use of sequential transcatheter arterial chemoembolization (TACE) followed within 2 weeks by PVE in 17 patients with HCC (Figure 28.7). The rationale for this approach is as follows: 1) The livers of most patients with HCC are compromised by underlying liver disease so that the liver's regenerative capacity after hepatic resection is impaired, making it difficult to predict whether sufficient FLR hypertrophy can be achieved after PVE. 2) Because most HCCs are hypervascular and fed primarily by arterial blood flow, cessation of portal flow induces a compensatory increase in arterial blood flow ("arterialization of the liver") in the embolized segments that may result in rapid tumor progression after PVE. 3) Arterioportal shunts often found in cirrhotic livers and HCC may attenuate the effects of PVE. To this end, sequential TACE and PVE were used to prevent tumor progression during the period between the PVE and planned hepatectomy and to strengthen the effect of PVE by embolizing arterioportal shunts with TACE. As a result, the investigators found that the procedures were safe, induced adequate FLR hypertrophy within 2 weeks and caused no deterioration in the basal hepatic functional reserve or increase in tumor progression. Importantly, when the explanted livers were evaluated, tumor necrosis was profound but without substantial injury to the non-cancerous liver, and they therefore encourage the aggressive application of this treatment strategy in patients with large HCC and chronically injured livers. However, similar to Nagino's TAE/PVE approach, the downside of this method is that two separate approaches are required.

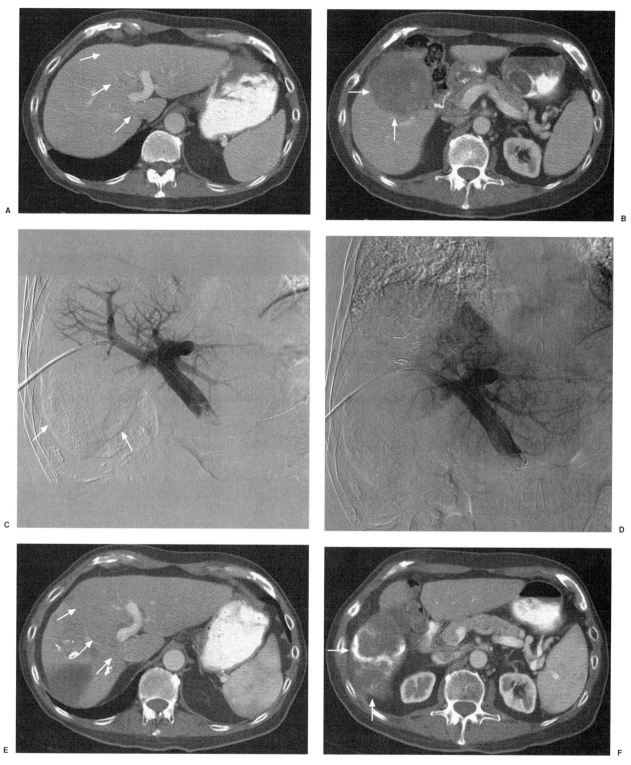

FIGURE 28.7. A 74-year-old man with an 8-cm solitary hepatocellular tumor and hepatitis C cirrhosis who underwent sequential transcatheter arterial chemoembolization (TACE) followed 1 month later by RPVE prior to a right hepatectomy. (A) A single image from pre-PVE contrast-enhanced CT scan shows small left liver (*arrows*) and FLR/TELV of 27%. (B) A single image caudal of (A) shows the solitary 8-cm tumor (*arrows*). (C) Pre-embolization portogram (after TACE) shows persistent iodized oil uptake within the right lobe (*arrows*). (D) Post-embolization portogram shows complete occlusion of all branches to right portal vein. The left portal vein remains patent. (E) A single image from post-PVE contrast-enhanced CT scan shows hypertrophy of the left liver (*arrows*). The FLR/TELV increased to 47%. (F) A single image from post-PVE contrast-enhanced CT scan more caudal to (E) shows massive atrophy of the right lobe with necrosis of the tumor (*arrows*). The patient underwent uncomplicated right hepatectomy. No viable tumor cells were found in the resected specimen.

In 2003, a pilot study of PVE using a transjugular approach was reported (71). This technique was attempted because of the large experience gained during the previous decade with transjugular intrahepatic portosystemic shunts (TIPS). Under sonographic guidance, the right internal jugular vein was accessed, and then with fluoroscopy, a right or left portal branch was punctured from a right, middle, or left hepatic vein. A catheter was placed near the portal bifurcation and used to perform right portal branch embolization with a mixture of n-butyl-2-cyanoacrylate (NBCA) and iodized oil. All 15 procedures performed were technically successful without any serious complication. FLR hypertrophy was adequate, and right hepatectomy was performed in 12 patients. Although this approach appears safe and effective, the series was small, and additional studies will be needed before this approach becomes widespread. For RPVE in patients with cirrhosis, this may be an attractive approach; however, the technical feasibility of RPVE extended to segment IV has not been explored.

At other centers, intraoperative portal vein ligation has been used during the first step of a planned two-stage hepatectomy (72). This approach is not recommended because regeneration is not optimized without segment IV occlusion (13) and tumor growth in segment IV may be accelerated (73, 74). Furthermore, PVE leads to superior FLR hypertrophy rates compared with portal vein ligation (75), and recanalization through portoportal collaterals has been reported (62).

Extent of Embolization

The optimal extent of PVE is currently a topic of debate. Left PVE is rarely necessary due to consistently large volumes of the right posterior liver (i.e., segments VI/VII) (12, 76, 77). Currently, several groups who use PVE to prepare for extended right hepatectomy occlude only branches of the right portal vein and leave the segment IV portal veins patent despite the need to resect segment IV (11, 78, 79). Although FLR hypertrophy occurs, full diversion of portal flow to segments II and III, with or without I, ensures the maximal stimulus for FLR hypertrophy (12, 13). Furthermore, incomplete embolization of the liver to be resected (i.e., RPVE only) leads to segment IV hypertrophy as well. Segment IV hypertrophy is not desired for extended right hepatectomy because of the larger area of intraoperative parenchymal transection across this hypertrophic

segment (12). Nagino et al. (13) first showed that a greater left lateral bisegment hypertrophy occurs after RPVE + IV (50% increase in FLR volume) than after RPVE only (31% increase, p < 0.0005) (32). Others have refined the ipsilateral approach for RPVE + IV using small particulate embolic agents and have shown further improvements in hypertrophy and operative outcomes (66).

A second potential benefit of RPVE + IV, from an oncological standpoint, is that the entire tumor-bearing liver is systematically embolized to reduce the risk of tumor growth that may result from increased portal blood flow and hepatotrophic factors. Tumor growth within the non-embolized liver has been discussed upon analysis of a very limited number of patients with primary and secondary liver tumors after RPVE alone (although no comparison to pre-PVE tumor growth rate was made so the true effect of PVE on tumor growth could not be proven) (73, 74). In contrast, a recent M.D. Anderson study analyzed reasons for failure to resect after PVE and found that change in tumor size after complete embolization of the entire tumor-bearing liver did not affect subsequent resectability (80). Furthermore, liver hypertrophy occurs quickly in patients with normal liver, and thus resection can be undertaken in most patients with multiple colorectal metastases within 3 to 4 weeks of PVE. Recent literature has shown that systemic chemotherapy administered in the interim between PVE and resection does not seem to affect FLR hypertrophy or outcome (81, 82).

Embolic Materials

Many embolic materials have been used for PVE without significant differences in degrees or rates of hypertrophy (9). In their initial report, Makuuchi et al. used gelatin sponge, but frequent recanalization was observed within 2 weeks after PVE (10). In comparison with other embolic agents, gelatin sponge seems to induce less hypertrophy at 4 weeks. Kaneko et al. (83) proposed a combination of gelatin sponge with the sclerosing agent polidocanol that produced portal occlusion for up to 8 weeks after PVE in canines.

Other investigators use NBCA mixed with ethiodized oil because this mixture leads to fast, reliable hypertrophy and minimizes the delay between PVE and definitive resection (49). This material ensures portal vein occlusion that persists beyond 4 weeks, whereas the combination of gelatin sponge and thrombin tends to recanalize (84). de Baere et al. (11)

reported that PVE with NBCA led to a 90% increase in liver volume after 30 days, whereas the combination of gelatin sponge and thrombin resulted in only a 53% volume increase after 43 days. Furthermore, Denys et al. (85) found NBCA effective in inducing hypertrophy in patients with underlying cirrhosis or advanced fibrosis. There are two potential drawbacks of NBCA for PVE: 1) it induces an inflammatory process (peribiliary fibrosis or casting of the portal vein) that may increase the difficulty of the subsequent resection and 2) it is difficult to use clinically, especially in patients with reduced hepatopetal portal flow as is often seen in patients with cirrhosis (49, 50). These altered flow dynamics can lead to non-target embolization in other segments with this agent (49).

Ethanol has been useful for PVE owing to its strong coagulation effect. Shimamura et al. (43) reported that 20 ml of ethanol was adequate to produce complete right portal vein occlusion, with a massive increase in FLR size (32% pre-PVE to 59% post-PVE). Ogasawara et al. (86) demonstrated near-doubling of the left liver volume within 4 weeks in patients with chronic liver disease and HCC who had PVE with ethanol. However, ethanol produces the greatest changes in liver function tests and thus poor patient tolerance may be found (87). Although ethanol causes considerable periportal fibrosis, endothelial destruction and necrosis, recanalization is rare.

Fibrin glue mixed with ethiodized oil is another commonly used agent for PVE that usually induces less than 75% portal occlusion at 2 weeks and less than 25% portal occlusion at 4 weeks (84). Nagino and colleagues reported increases in FLR volume of 10% to 20% after a mean of 18 days following PVE (12, 32, 88).

Recently, the use of particulate agents such as polyvinyl alcohol (PVA) particles for PVE has been proposed (40, 54, 65, 89). PVA particles are safe, cause little periportal reaction, and generate durable portal vein occlusion, especially when used in combination with coils (54, 66). Theoretically, the particles occlude the small "outflow" vessels (i.e., third-order portal branches and smaller), while the coils occlude the larger "inflow" vessels (i.e., second-order portal branches). In the first clinical report in a single patient, no recanalization of the right portal vein was observed 5 weeks after PVE with PVA particles alone (89). In 2003, results were reported for 26 patients who had PVE with PVA particles ranging in size from 300 to 1000 μm and coils; the mean FLR/TELV increased 7.8 percentage points (pre-PVE FLR/TELV, 17.6%; post-PVE FLR/TELV, 25.4%), and the mean absolute FLR increase was 47% (65). The recent development of spherical particulate embolics has led to further refinements in technique for RPVE + IV by using a step-wise infusion of very small (100 to 300 μm) tris-acryl microspheres followed by larger spheres (up to 700 μm) and coils. This approach led to an absolute increase in FLR volume of 69.0%, a FLR/TELV increase of 9.7 percentage points, and a subsequent resection rate of 86% and is a significant improvement over Madoff et al.'s (65, 66) previously described method.

Complications

As with all transhepatic procedures, complications can occur from PVE and include subcapsular hematoma, hemoperitoneum, hemobilia, pseudoaneurysm, arteriovenous fistula, arterioportal shunts, portal vein thrombosis, transient liver failure, pneumothorax and sepsis (63, 90). In 2002, Kodama et al. (90) reported a series in which 7 (15%) of 47 patients had complications: two pneumothoraces, two subcapsular hematomas, one arterial puncture, one pseudoaneurysm (in a patient who also had a subcapsular hematoma), one hemobilia, and one portal vein thrombosis. As most technical complications occurred in the punctured lobe, Kodama and colleagues recommended that the transhepatic ipsilateral approach be tried first.

Additional studies from experienced investigators (63, 66) have reiterated the low procedural complication rates (9.1% to 12.8%) for RPVE regardless of whether segment IV is embolized.

INDICATIONS AND CONTRAINDICATIONS FOR PVE

General Indications

To determine whether a patient will benefit from PVE, several factors must be considered (15). First, the presence or absence of underlying liver disease will have a major impact on the volume of liver remnant needed for adequate function. Second, patient size must be considered; larger patients require larger liver remnants than do smaller patients. Third, the extent and complexity of the planned resection and the possibility that associated non-hepatic surgery will be performed at the time of liver resection (e.g., hepatectomy plus pancreaticoduodenectomy) must be considered. These three factors are considered in the setting of the patient's age and comorbidities (e.g., diabetes) that may affect hypertrophy. Thus, once the procedure type and extent of resection necessary to treat the patient have been determined, appropriate liver volumetry is performed so that the standardized FLR volume expressed as a percentage of the estimated TLV can be used to determine the need for PVE.

As described earlier, a normal liver has a greater regenerative capacity than a cirrhotic liver, functions more efficiently and tolerates injury better. Patients can survive resection of up to 90% of the liver in the absence of underlying liver disease, but survival after resection beyond 60% of the functional parenchyma in patients with cirrhosis is unlikely (5). Lethal post-resection liver failure is more common after resection in patients with cirrhosis, and other complications of the poorly functioning liver remnant (e.g., ascites, fluid retention and wound breakdown from poor protein synthesis) occur more often after resection in patients with cirrhosis than in patients without cirrhosis. With regard to liver volume, there is a limit to how small a liver can remain after resection. If too little liver remains after resection, immediate post-resection hepatic failure leads to multisystem organ failure and death. If a marginal volume of liver remains, cirrhotic or not, the lack of reserve often leads to a cascade of complications, prolonged hospital and intensive-care unit stays, and slow recovery or slowly progressive liver failure over weeks to months, with eventual death (1–3).

Normal Underlying Liver

In patients with an otherwise normal liver, the indications for PVE have evolved with the greater accuracy of liver volumetric measurements and the use of standardized liver volumes. Although extended resections can be performed with a low likelihood of death from liver failure, small-for-patient-size normal liver remnants are associated with increased complications and slower postoperative recovery (3). A FLR/TELV of less than 20% is associated with a four-fold increase in complications compared with an FLR/TELV of 20% or more (5). This finding was validated in a retrospective study that revealed that residual liver volume, not resected volume, predicts post-hepatectomy course (4).

It is also important to recognize and individualize the indication for PVE with use of the standardized 20% cutoff for liver volume due to intrahepatic segmental variability. Liver volume analysis revealed that the lateral left liver (segments II/III) contributes less than 20% of the TLV in more than 75% of patients in the absence of compensatory hypertrophy. In addition, the left liver (segments II/III/IV) contributes 20% or less of the TLV in more than 10% of patients (76). Therefore, a FLR/TELV of less than 20% can be expected in most patients who do not develop compensatory hypertrophy from tumor growth and require an extended right hepatectomy. In these patients, RPVE extended to segment IV is indicated. However, left PVE is rarely needed; Nagino et al. (12) showed that an extended left hepatectomy with caudate lobectomy results in resection of only 67% of the liver, leaving a FLR of 33%, the same residual volume after right hepatectomy in a normal liver. Volumetric analysis of normal livers also confirms the consistently large volume of the posterior right liver (segments VI/VII) (77).

Recently, Farges et al. (78) showed that RPVE performed before right hepatectomy in patients with an otherwise normal liver showed no clinical benefit, and they concluded that in this setting, PVE may be unnecessary (except in the small subset of patients whose left liver is <20% of the TLV). Failure to follow these well-established guidelines may result in overuse of PVE.

Underlying Liver Disease

Major resection can be performed safely in some patients with cirrhosis, although extended hepatectomy is rarely an option. Unlike patients with normal liver, those with cirrhosis with marginal liver remnants are not only at risk for complications but are also at increased risk for death from liver failure (2). However, in carefully selected patients with cirrhosis with preserved liver function (Child-Pugh Class A) and normal $ICGR_{15}$ (<10%), major resection can be performed safely and PVE is indicated when the FLR volume is less than 40% of the TLV (7). This guideline is supported by the finding that when liver volume is standardized to BSA, standardized FLR volume predicts death from liver failure after hepatectomy in chronic liver disease (2).

These studies were corroborated by the only prospective study that evaluated the use of PVE before right hepatectomy. Farges et al. (78) showed that patients with chronic liver disease who underwent PVE before right hepatectomy had fewer complications and shorter intensive care unit and hospital stays than those with chronic liver disease who did not have PVE before right hepatectomy. This guideline has been expanded to include patients in whom the liver is compromised by prolonged biliary obstruction who require extended hepatectomy (3, 9, 10, 32).

Highly selected patients with advanced liver disease might also undergo safe resection. Specifically, in patients with cirrhosis with a moderately abnormal $ICGR_{15}$ (10%–20%) but with preserved liver function, sequential TACE and PVE have been used to maximize the atrophy/hypertrophy complex (70). Because of the continuum of "liver disease," the specific indications for PVE in patients with chronic liver disease remain to be defined precisely and require an individualized approach. It is anticipated that refined criteria will be developed with the accrual of more experience with the standardized measurement of FLR.

At M.D. Anderson Cancer Center, portal pressures are routinely measured before and after PVE in patients with chronic liver disease because of the lack of reliability of assessment of hepatic fibrosis by core needle biopsy (91). Patients with overt portal hypertension (splenomegaly, low platelets, imaging evidence of varices) are not candidates for major hepatectomy and therefore are not candidates for PVE. Mild portal hypertension, however, is not a contraindication to PVE followed by hepatectomy provided liver function test results are otherwise normal (Child-Pugh A+).

High-dose Chemotherapy

Retrospective data suggest an increased risk of surgical complications in patients after preoperative systemic or regional chemotherapy (92, 93), but no definite guidelines for a minimal FLR have been established. Patients with steatosis have an increased incidence of complications after resection, but the potential benefit and selection criteria for PVE in these patients is currently unknown (94). Furthermore, knowledge of a patient's specific chemotherapeutic regimen is essential as patients may develop hepatic injuries such as steatohepatitis and sinusoidal dilatation from oxaliplatin and irinotecan-based fluoropyrimidine chemotherapy regimens, with an increased 90-day mortality rate after resection (95). Thus, some investigators have advocated larger buffer zones (i.e., a larger FLR than required for normal underlying liver) when performing extended resection in selected patients who have received preoperative chemotherapy. Although such patients have been less well studied than patients with normal liver, PVE may be indicated when the FLR is 30% or less of the TLV (93, 96).

General Contraindications

Contraindications to PVE include an inadequate FLR volume based on the criteria discussed earlier, tumor invasion of the portal vein to be resected as portal flow is already diverted and disease progression that leads to overall unresectability (15, 54). Relative contraindications to PVE include tumor extension to the FLR, uncorrectable coagulopathy, biliary dilatation in the FLR (if the biliary tree is obstructed, drainage is recommended), portal hypertension and renal failure. The presence of an ipsilateral tumor may preclude safe transhepatic access if the tumor burden is great, but this is also unlikely, as there is no evidence that tumor spread occurs during PVE. If access to an adequate portal vein branch for PVE is not possible, the contralateral approach can be considered.

OUTCOMES FOLLOWING PVE AND HEPATECTOMY

Chronic Liver Disease

In patients with chronic liver disease such as chronic hepatitis, fibrosis or cirrhosis, the increase in nonembolized liver volumes after PVE varies (range, 28–46%), and hypertrophy after PVE may take more than 4 weeks because of slower regeneration rates (32, 43). The degree of parenchymal fibrosis is thought to limit regeneration, possibly as a result of reduced portal blood flow (94). The complication rates after PVE are higher in patients with chronic liver disease than in those with an otherwise normal liver because of the increased risk of secondary portal vein thrombosis, presumably from slow flow in the portal vein trunk after PVE (63, 93). The combination of TACE of the tumor followed by PVE within 2 weeks may optimize outcome for some patients who have HCC in the presence of chronic liver disease and require major resection (70). However, a 2005 study by Denys et al. (85), which included 40 patients with HCC in the setting of advanced liver fibrosis and cirrhosis, found that only two factors significantly affected hypertrophy: a lower degree of fibrosis, as indicated by a Knodell histological score (97) of less than F4, and a pre-PVE lower functional liver ratio as defined by the ratio between the left lobe (i.e., FLR) and the total liver volume minus tumor volume. Factors that did not correlate with improved hypertrophy included age, gender, history of diabetes and prior TACE.

In patients with chronic liver disease, hepatectomy outcomes, including the number and severity of complications and the incidence of postoperative liver failure and death, are better with PVE than without (25, 43, 78, 93, 98, 99). In 2000, Azoulay et al. (93) reported long-term outcomes after resection of three or more liver segments for HCC in patients with cirrhosis. PVE was performed when the FLR volume was predicted to be less than 40% and led to significant increases in the FLR volumes in all embolized patients. Importantly, none of 10 patients who underwent PVE had liver failure or death following resection, whereas 3 of 19 patients in the non-PVE group suffered liver failure and one patient died. Overall and disease-free survival rates were similar with or without PVE. Tanaka et al. (99) reported several benefits of PVE in a larger study of patients with HCC and cirrhosis. Disease-free survival rates were similar, but cumulative survival rates were significantly higher in the PVE group than in the non-PVE group. In addition, patients with recurrence following PVE plus resection were more often candidates for further treatments such as TACE, an additional benefit of PVE in the long term.

No Chronic Liver Disease

The outcome from PVE and subsequent resection may be even more closely linked to the PVE technique in patients with otherwise normal livers than in patients with chronically diseased livers. In patients with cirrhosis, RPVE (without segment IV) is the most common technique used since extended hepatectomy is rarely indicated or possible. In patients without cirrhosis who have hilar biliary duct cancer, liver metastases, or HCC (100), extended hepatectomy resection of the right liver + segment IV $\pm$ I (extended right hepatectomy) or, less often, the left liver + segments V + VIII $\pm$ I (extended left hepatectomy) – is often indicated. In the former case (i.e., extended right hepatectomy), owing to the consistently small volume of the left lateral bisegment (II + III), preoperative PVE is frequently needed (76).

A recent report from M.D. Anderson Cancer Center considered 127 consecutive extended hepatec-

tomies using standardized liver volume calculations to select patients for PVE (6). In this series, 31 (24.4%) of the patients underwent PVE prior to extended hepatectomy. Only six patients (5%) experienced significant postoperative liver insufficiency (total bilirubin level >10 mg/dl or international normalized ratio >2). The postoperative complication rate was 30.7% (39 of 127), and only one patient (0.8%) died after hepatectomy. The median survival was 41.9 months, and the overall 5-year survival rate was 26% for the entire group. The low mortality rate following extended hepatectomy in this series reflects many factors, among which was the systematic attention to FLR volume and the use of PVE based on the indications reviewed earlier.

Additional studies have validated residual volume as the key to prediction of postoperative liver function and post-hepatectomy course. In a retrospective analysis of outcome after resection of liver metastases from colorectal cancer, Shoup et al. (4) found that a FLR volume of 25% or less was an independent predictor of postoperative complications and increased duration of hospital stay, and they recommended FLR volume assessment prior to consideration of PVE. Elias et al. (101) showed that patients considered ineligible for resection due to inadequate liver volume at presentation could undergo complete resection after preparation with PVE, with an associated 5-year overall survival rate of 29%. Azoulay et al. (8) found that the 5-year overall survival rate after resection in patients who required PVE was similar to that in patients who did not have PVE (40% compared with 38%, respectively).

PVE has a major role in the preoperative preparation of patients with normal underlying liver and an inadequate FLR volume prior to extended hepatectomy. Understanding proper patient selection (FLR/TLV of <20%) and the technical aspects of PVE affects the degree and rate of hypertrophy of the FLR, and although changes in tumor size related to PVE seem not to have clinical significance, increases in tumor size can be avoided and FLR hypertrophy maximized if the entire tumor-bearing liver is systematically embolized, including the right liver and segment IV, prior to extended right hepatectomy.

CONCLUSION

PVE is now a validated technique to increase the volume and function of the remnant liver prior to resection of hepatobiliary cancer. PVE increases the safety of major resection in patients with liver disease and extends the option of resection to patients with multiple hepatic metastases and limited parenchymal sparing from metastatic disease. Careful attention to key factors, such as the presence or absence of underlying liver disease, adjustment of liver size to patient size using proper techniques to measure the liver remnant and recognition of the physiologic effect of the type of hepatic and extrahepatic procedure planned, permits the appropriate selection of patients for PVE. The FLR should be measured and standardized to the patient using the calculated FLR/TELV ratio, because this method produces a reproducible, accurate index of post-hepatectomy liver function. Currently recommended thresholds prompting consideration of preoperative PVE are FLR/TELV ratios of less than or up to 20% for patients with an otherwise normal liver, 30% or less for patients who have received high-dose chemotherapy, and less than 40% for patients with chronic liver disease. Continued critical analysis of the factors affecting liver hypertrophy in parallel with improvements in oncological treatments will further improve the selection and outcomes of patients with liver cancer considered for PVE.

REFERENCES

1. Tsao JI, Loftus JP, Nagorney DM, et al. Trends in morbidity and mortality of hepatic resection for malignancy: Matched comparative analysis. Ann Surg, 1994; 220: 199–205.

2. Shirabe K, Shimada M, Gion T, et al. Postoperative liver failure after major hepatic resection for hepatocellular carcinoma in the modern era with special reference to remnant liver volume. J Am Coll Surg, 1999; 188: 304–309.

3. Vauthey JN, Chaoui A, Do KA, et al. Standardized measurement of the future liver remnant prior to extended liver resection: Methodology and clinical associations. Surgery, 2000; 127: 512–519.

4. Shoup M, Gonen M, D'Angelica M, et al. Volumetric analysis predicts hepatic dysfunction in patients undergoing major liver resection. J Gastrointest Surg, 2003; 7: 325–330.

5. Abdalla EK, Barnett CC, Doherty D, et al. Extended hepatectomy in patients with hepatobiliary malignancies with and without preoperative portal vein embolization. Arch Surg, 2002; 137: 675–680.

6. Vauthey JN, Pawlik TM, Abdalla EK, et al. Is extended hepatectomy for hepatobiliary malignancy justified? Ann Surg, 2004; 239: 722–730.

7. Kubota K, Makuuchi M, Kusaka K, et al. Measurement of liver volume and hepatic functional reserve as a guide to decision-making in resectional surgery for hepatic tumors. Hepatology, 1997; 26: 1176–1181.

8. Azoulay D, Castaing D, Smail A, et al. Resection of non-resectable liver metastases from colorectal cancer after percutaneous portal vein embolization. Ann Surg, 2000; 231: 480–486.

9. Abdalla EK, Hicks ME, and Vauthey JN. Portal vein embolization: Rationale, technique and future prospects. Br J Surg, 2001; 88: 165–175.

10. Makuuchi M, Thai BL, Takayasu K, et al. Preoperative portal vein embolization to increase safety of major hepatectomy for hilar bile duct carcinoma: A preliminary report. Surgery, 1990; 107: 521–527.

11. de Baere T, Roche A, Vavasseur D, et al. Portal vein embolization: Utility for inducing left hepatic lobe hypertrophy before surgery. Radiology, 1993; 188: 73–77.

12. Nagino M, Nimura Y, Kamiya J, et al. Right or left trisegment portal vein embolization before hepatic trisegmentectomy for hilar bile duct carcinoma. Surgery, 1995; 117: 677–681.

13. Nagino M, Kamiya J, Kanai M, et al. Right trisegment portal vein embolization for biliary tract carcinoma: Technique and clinical utility. Surgery, 2000; 127: 155–160.

14. Vauthey JN, Abdalla EK, Doherty DA, et al. Body surface area and body weight predict total liver volume in Western adults. Liver Transpl, 2002; 8: 233–240.

15. Madoff DC, Abdalla EK, and Vauthey JN. Portal vein embolization in preparation for major hepatic resection: evolution of a new standard of care. J Vasc Interv Radiol, 2005; 16: 779–790.

16. Rous P and Larimore LD. Relation of the portal blood flow to liver maintenance: A demonstration of liver atrophy conditional on compensation. J Exp Med, 1920; 31: 609–632.

17. Schalm L, Bax HR, and Mansens BJ. Atrophy of the liver after occlusion of the bile ducts or portal vein and compensatory hypertrophy of the unoccluded portion and its clinical importance. Gastroenterology, 1956; 31: 131–155.

18. Honjo I, Suzuki T, Ozawa K, et al. Ligation of a branch of the portal vein for carcinoma of the liver. Am J Surg, 1975; 130: 296–302.

19. Takayasu K, Matsumura Y, Shima Y, et al. Hepatic lobar hypertrophy following obstruction of the ipsilateral portal vein from cholangiocarcinoma. Radiology, 1986; 160: 389–393.

20. Kinoshita H, Sakai K, Hirohashi K, et al. Preoperative portal vein embolization for hepatocellular carcinoma. World J Surg, 1986; 10: 803–808.

21. Koniaris LG, McKillop IH, Schwartz SI, et al. Liver regeneration. J Am Coll Surg, 2003; 197: 634–659.

22. Ponfick VA. Ueber Leberresection und Leberreaction. Verhandl Deutsch Gesellsch Chir, 1890; 19:28.

23. Michalopoulos GK and DeFrances MC. Liver regeneration. Science, 1997; 276: 60–66.

24. Black DM and Behrns KE. A scientist revisits the atrophy-hypertrophy complex: Hepatic apoptosis and regeneration. Surg Oncol Clin North Am, 2002; 11: 849–864.

25. Lee KC, Kinoshita H, Hirohashi K, et al. Extension of surgical indication for hepatocellular carcinoma

by portal vein embolization. World J Surg, 1993; 17: 109–115.

26. Mizuno S, Nimura Y, Suzuki H, et al. Portal vein branch occlusion induces cell proliferation of cholestatic rat liver. J Surg Res, 1996; 60: 249–257.

27. Takeuchi E, Nimura Y, Mizuno S, et al. Ligation of portal vein branch induces DNA polymerases alpha, delta, and epsilon in nonligated lobes. J Surg Res, 1996; 65: 15–24.

28. Kim RD, Stein GS, and Chari RS. Impact of cell swelling on proliferative signal transduction in the liver. J Cell Biochem, 2001; 83: 56–69.

29. Nagy P, Teramoto T, Factor VM, et al. Reconstitution of liver mass via cellular hypertrophy in the rat. Hepatology, 2001; 33: 339–345.

30. Komori K, Nagino M, and Nimura Y. Hepatocyte morphology and kinetics after portal vein embolization. Br J Surg, 2006; 93: 745–751.

31. Starzl TE, Francavilla A, Porter KA, et al. The effect of splanchnic viscera removal upon canine liver regeneration. Surg Gynecol Obstet, 1978; 147: 193–207.

32. Nagino M, Nimura Y, Kamiya J, et al. Changes in hepatic lobe volume in biliary tract cancer patients after right portal vein embolization. Hepatology, 1995; 21: 434–439.

33. Kock NG, Hahnloser P, Roding B, et al. Interaction between portal venous and hepatic arterial blood flow: An experimental study in the dog. Surgery, 1972; 72: 414–419.

34. Michalopoulos GK and Zarnegar R. Hepatocyte growth factor. Hepatology, 1992; 15:149–155.

35. Bucher NLR and Swaffield MN. Regulation of hepatic regeneration in rats by synergistic action of insulin and glucagon. Proc Natl Acad Sci USA, 1975; 72: 1157–1160.

36. Fabrikant JI. The kinetics of cellular proliferation in regenerating liver. J Cell Biol, 1968; 36: 551–565.

37. Francavilla A, Porter KA, Benichou J, et al. Liver regeneration in dogs: Morphologic and chemical changes. J Surg Res, 1978; 25: 409–419.

38. Gaglio PJ, Baskin G, Bohm R Jr, et al. Partial hepatectomy and laparoscopic-guided liver biopsy in rhesus macaques (Macaca mulatta): Novel approach for study of liver regeneration. Comp Med, 2000; 50: 363–368.

39. Bucher NLR and Swaffield MN. The rate of incorporation of labeled thymidine into the deoxyribonucleic acid of regenerating rat liver in relation to the amount of liver excised. Cancer Res, 1964; 24: 1611–1625.

40. Duncan JR, Hicks ME, Cai SR, et al. Embolization of portal vein branches induces hepatocyte hypertrophy in swine: A potential step in hepatic gene therapy. Radiology, 1999; 210: 467–477.

41. Goto Y, Nagino M, and Nimura Y. Doppler estimation of portal blood flow after percutaneous transhepatic portal vein embolization. Ann Surg, 1998; 228: 209–213.

42. Yamanaka N, Okamoto E, Kawamura E, et al. Dynamics of normal and injured liver regeneration after hepatectomy as assessed on the basis of computed tomography and liver function. Hepatology, 1993; 18: 79–85.

43. Shimamura T, Nakajima Y, Une Y, et al. Efficacy and safety of preoperative percutaneous transhepatic portal embolization with absolute ethanol: A clinical study. Surgery, 1997; 121: 135–141.

44. Anderson CD, Meranze S, Bream P Jr, et al. Contralateral portal vein embolization for hepatectomy in the setting of hepatic steatosis. Am Surg, 2004; 70: 609–612.

45. DeAngelis RA, Markiewski MM, Taub R, et al. A high-fat diet impairs liver regeneration in C57BL/6 mice through overexpression of the NF-κB inhibitor, IκBα. Hepatology, 2005; 42: 1148–1157.

46. Ijichi M, Makuuchi M, Imamura H, et al. Portal embolization relieves persistent jaundice after complete biliary drainage. Surgery, 2001; 130: 116–118.

47. Uesaka K, Nimura Y, Nagino M. Changes in hepatic lobar function after right portal vein embolization: An appraisal by biliary indocyanine green excretion. Ann Surg, 1996 223: 77–83.

48. Hirai I, Kimura W, Fuse A, et al. Evaluation of preoperative portal embolization for safe hepatectomy, with special reference to assessment of nonembolized lobe function with 99mTc-GSA SPECT scintigraphy. Surgery, 2003; 133: 495–506.

49. De Baere T, Roche A, Elias D, et al. Preoperative portal vein embolization for extension of hepatectomy indications. Hepatology 1996; 24: 1386–1391.

50. Imamura H, Shimada R, Kubota M, et al. Preoperative portal vein embolization: An audit of 84 patients. Hepatology, 1999; 29: 1099–1105.

51. Wakabayashi H, Okada S, Maeba T, et al. Effect of preoperative portal vein embolization on major hepatectomy for advanced-stage hepatocellular carcinomas in injured livers: A preliminary report. Surg Today, 1997; 27: 403–410.

52. Shibayama Y, Hashimoto K, Nakata K. Recovery from hepatic necrosis following acute portal vein embolism with special reference to reconstruction of occluded vessels. J Pathol, 1991; 165: 255–261.

53. Ikeda K, Kinoshita H, Hirohashi K, et al. The ultrastructure, kinetics and intralobular distribution of apoptotic hepatocytes after portal branch ligation with special reference to their relationship to necrotic hepatocytes. Arch Histol Cytol, 1995; 58: 171–184.

54. Madoff DC, Hicks ME, Vauthey JN, et al. Transhepatic portal vein embolization: Anatomy, indications, and technical considerations. Radiographics, 2002; 22: 1063–1076.

55. Denys A, Madoff DC, Doenz F, et al. Indications for and limitations of portal vein embolization prior to major hepatic resection for hepatobiliary malignancy. Surg Oncol Clin North Am, 2002; 11: 955–968.

56. Heymsfield SB, Fulenwider T, Nordlinger B, et al. Accurate measurement of liver, kidney, and spleen volume and mass by computerized axial tomography. Ann Intern Med, 1979; 90: 185–187.

57. Soyer P, Roche A, Elias D, et al. Hepatic metastases from colorectal cancer: Influence of hepatic volumetric analysis on surgical decision making. Radiology, 1992; 184: 695–697.

58. Ogasawara K, Une Y, Nakajima Y, et al. The significance of measuring liver volume using computed tomographic images before and after hepatectomy. Surg Today, 1995; 25: 43–48.

59. Makuuchi M, Kosuge T, Takayama T, et al. Surgery for small liver cancers. Semin Surg Oncol, 1993; 9: 298–304.

60. Johnson TN, Tucker GT, Tanner MS, et al. Changes in liver volume from birth to adulthood: A meta-analysis. Liver Transpl, 2005; 11: 1481–1493.

61. Mitsumori A, Nagaya I, Kimoto S, et al. Preoperative evaluation of hepatic functional reserve following hepatectomy by technetium-99m galactosyl human serum albumin liver scintigraphy and computed tomography. Eur J Nucl Med, 1998; 25: 1377–1382.

62. Denys AL, Abehsera M, Sauvanet A, et al. Failure of right portal vein ligation to induce left lobe hypertrophy due to intrahepatic portoportal collaterals: Successful treatment with portal vein embolization. AJR Am J Roentgenol, 1999; 173: 633–635.

63. Di Stefano DR, de Baere T, Denys A, et al. Preoperative percutaneous portal vein embolization: Evaluation of adverse events in 188 patients. Radiology, 2005; 234: 625–630.

64. Nagino M, Nimura Y, Kamiya J, et al. Selective percutaneous transhepatic embolization of the portal vein in preparation for extensive liver resection: The ipsilateral approach. Radiology 1996; 200: 559–563.

65. Madoff DC, Hicks ME, Abdalla EK, et al. Portal vein embolization with polyvinyl alcohol particles and coils in preparation for major liver resection for hepatobiliary malignancy: Safety and effectiveness – study in 26 patients. Radiology, 2003; 227: 251–260.

66. Madoff DC, Abdalla EK, Gupta S, et al. Transhepatic ipsilateral right portal vein embolization extended to segment IV: Improving hypertrophy and resection outcomes with spherical particles and coils. J Vasc Interv Radiol, 2005; 16: 215–225.

67. Azoulay D, Raccuia JS, Castaing D, et al. Right portal vein embolization in preparation for major hepatic resection. J Am Coll Surg, 1995; 181: 266–269.

68. Nagino M, Kanai M, Morioka A, et al. Portal and arterial embolization before extensive liver resection in patients with markedly poor functional reserve. J Vasc Interv Radiol, 2000; 11: 1063–1068.

69. Gruttadauria S, Luca A, Mandala' L, et al. Sequential preoperative ipsilateral portal and arterial embolization in patients with colorectal liver metastases. World J Surg, 2006; 30: 576–578.

70. Aoki T, Imamura H, Hasegawa K, et al. Sequential preoperative arterial and portal venous embolizations in patients with hepatocellular carcinoma. Arch Surg, 2004; 139: 766–774.

71. Perarnau JM, Daradkeh S, Johann M, et al. Transjugular preoperative portal embolization (TJPE): A pilot study. Hepatogastroenterology, 2003; 50: 610–613.

72. Kianmanesh R, Farges O, Abdalla EK, et al. Right portal vein ligation: A new planned two-step all-surgical approach for complete resection of primary gastrointestinal tumors with multiple bilateral liver metastases. J Am Coll Surg, 2003; 197: 164–170.

73. Elias D, de Baere T, Roche A, et al. During liver regeneration following right portal embolization the growth rate of liver metastases is more rapid than that of the liver parenchyma. Br J Surg, 1999; 86: 784–788.

74. Kokudo N, Tada K, Seki M, et al. Proliferative activity of intrahepatic colorectal metastases after preoperative hemihepatic portal vein embolization. Hepatology, 2001; 34: 267–272.

75. Broering DC, Hillert C, Krupski G, et al. Portal vein embolization vs. portal vein ligation for induction of hypertrophy of the future liver remnant. J Gastrointest Surg, 2002; 6: 905–913.

76. Abdalla EK, Denys A, Chevalier P, et al. Total and segmental liver volume variations: Implications for liver surgery. Surgery, 2004; 135: 404–410.

77. Leelaudomlipi S, Sugawara Y, Kaneko J, et al. Volumetric analysis of liver segments in 155 living donors. Liver Transpl, 2002; 8: 612–614.

78. Farges O, Belghiti J, Kianmanesh R, et al. Portal vein embolization before right hepatectomy: Prospective clinical trial. Ann Surg, 2003; 237: 208–217.

79. Capussotti L, Muratore A, Ferrero A, et al. Extension of right portal vein embolization to segment IV portal branches. Arch Surg, 2005; 140: 1100–1103.

80. Ribero D, Abdalla EK, Madoff DC, et al. Portal vein embolization before major hepatectomy and its effects on regeneration, resectability and outcome. Br J Surg, 2007; 94: 1386–1394.

81. Goere D, Farges O, Leporrier J, et al. Chemotherapy does not impair hypertrophy of the left liver after right portal vein obstruction. J Gastrointest Surg, 2006; 10: 365–370.

82. Beal IK, Anthony S, Papadopoulou A, et al. Portal vein embolisation prior to hepatic resection for colorectal liver metastases and the effects of periprocedure chemotherapy. Br J Radiol, 2006; 79: 473–478.

83. Kaneko T, Nakao A, Takagi H. Experimental study of new embolizing material for portal vein embolization. Hepatogastroenterology, 2000; 47: 790–794.

84. Matsuoka T. Experimental studies of intrahepatic portal vein embolization and embolic materials. Nippon Igaku Hoshasen Gakkai Zasshi, 1989; 49: 593–606.

85. Denys A, Lacombe C, Schneider F, et al. Portal vein embolization with N-butyl cyanoacrylate before partial hepatectomy in patients with hepatocellular carcinoma and underlying cirrhosis or advanced fibrosis. J Vasc Interv Radiol, 2005; 16: 1667–1674.

86. Ogasawara K, Uchino J, Une Y, et al. Selective portal vein embolization with absolute ethanol induces hepatic hypertrophy and makes more extensive hepatectomy possible. Hepatology, 1996; 23: 338–345.

87. Yamakado K, Takeda K, Nishide Y, et al. Portal vein embolization with steel coils and absolute ethanol: A comparative study with canine liver. Hepatology, 1995; 22: 1812–1818.

88. Nagino M, Nimura Y, Hayakawa N. Percutaneous transhepatic portal embolization using newly devised catheters: Preliminary report. World J Surg, 1993; 17: 520–524.

89. Brown K, Brody L, Decorato D, et al. Portal vein embolization with use of polyvinyl alcohol. J Vasc Interv Radiol, 2001; 12: 882–886.

90. Kodama Y, Shimizu T, Endo H, et al. Complications of percutaneous transhepatic portal vein embolization. J Vasc Interv Radiol, 2002; 13: 1233–1237.

91. Bedossa P, Dargere D, Paradis V. Sampling variability of liver fibrosis in chronic hepatitis C. Hepatology, 2003; 38: 1449–1457.

92. Elias D, Lasser P, Spielmann M, et al. Surgical and chemotherapeutic treatment of hepatic metastases from

carcinoma of the breast. Surg Gynecol Obstet, 1991; 172: 461–464.

93. Azoulay D, Castaing D, Krissat J, et al. Percutaneous portal vein embolization increases the feasibility and safety of major liver resection for hepatocellular carcinoma in injured liver. Ann Surg, 2000; 232: 665–672.

94. Kooby DA, Fong Y, Suriawinata A, et al. Impact of steatosis on perioperative outcome following hepatic resection. J Gastrointest Surg, 2003; 7: 1034–1044.

95. Vauthey JN, Pawlik TM, Ribero D, et al. Chemotherapy regimen predicts steatohepatitis and an increase in 90-day mortality after surgery for hepatic colorectal metastases. J Clin Oncol, 2006; 24: 2065–2072.

96. Adam R, Delvart V, Pascal G, et al. Rescue surgery for unresectable colorectal liver metastases downstaged by chemotherapy: A model to predict long-term survival. Ann Surg, 2004; 240: 644–657.

97. Knodell R, Ishak K, Black W, et al. Formulation and application of a numerical scoring system for assessing histological activity in asymptomatic chronic active hepatitis. Hepatology, 1981; 1: 431–435.

98. Wakabayashi H, Yachida S, Maeba T, et al. Indications for portal vein embolization combined with major hepatic resection for advanced-stage hepatocellular carcinomas: A preliminary clinical study. Dig Surg, 2000; 17: 587–594.

99. Tanaka H, Hirohashi K, Kubo S, et al. Preoperative portal vein embolization improves prognosis after right hepatectomy for hepatocellular carcinoma in patients with impaired hepatic function. Br J Surg, 2000; 87:879–882.

100. Nzeako UC, Goodman ZD, and Ishak KG. Hepatocellular carcinoma in cirrhotic and noncirrhotic livers: A clinico-histopathologic study of 804 North American patients. Am J Clin Pathol, 1996; 105: 65–75.

101. Elias D, Cavalcanti A, de Baere T, et al. Long-term oncological results of hepatectomy performed after selective portal embolization. Ann Chir, 1999; 53: 559–564.

Extrahepatic Biliary Cancer

Chapter 29

CANCER OF THE EXTRAHEPATIC BILE DUCTS AND THE GALLBLADDER: SURGICAL MANAGEMENT

Steven C. Cunningham

Richard D. Schulick

Cholangiocarcinoma is often divided into two types, intra- and extrahepatic – the latter group often classified into lesions of the proximal, middle and distal thirds of the extrahepatic ductal system. However, we (1, 2) and others (3, 4) have used a simpler and more surgically relevant three-tiered classification system: Intrahepatic lesions are those confined to the liver and not involving the extrahepatic biliary tree. Perihilar tumors are those involving or requiring resection of the hepatic duct bifurcation, typically arising in the extrahepatic biliary tree proximal to the origin of the cystic duct. Distal tumors are extrahepatic lesions located in the peripancreatic region. Intrahepatic cholangiocarcinoma is often considered to be a different disease than perihilar or distal cholangiocarcinoma, with distinct clinical, therapeutic and epidemiologic differences (2, 5), and is discussed elsewhere in this book. The present chapter focuses on the surgical treatment of extrahepatic cancers of the biliary system – namely, perihilar and distal cholangiocarcinoma and gallbladder cancer.

HISTORY

The history of biliary tract surgery begins at least as long ago as the Middle Ages, but documentation of early procedures is sparse. Animal experiments were common in the seventeenth century (6). The first case of extrahepatic cholangiocarcinoma was reported in 1840 by Durand-Fardel (7) in a series of six cases of cancer of the extrahepatic biliary tree: three cases of gallbladder cancer, two cases of intrahepatic cholangiocarcinoma and one case of cholangiocarcinoma of the common bile duct. The first description of cholangiocarcinoma of the hepatic ducts was attributed by Renshaw to Scheuppel in 1878 (8, 9). Nearly 120 years later, Altmeier in 1957 and Klatskin in 1965 described patients with adenocarcinoma of the hepatic duct at its bifurcation within the porta hepatis, describing in detail the clinical and pathological features, and leading to the eponym "Klatskin tumor" for a cholangiocarcinoma at this location (10, 11).

The gallbladder was first described circa 2000 B.C. by the Babylonians, and the first gallbladders were removed (from dogs) in the mid-1600s (6, 12). Gallbladder cancer was first described in 1777 (13). By the early 1900s, several series of patients with gallbladder cancer were reported in the literature (8, 9).

EPIDEMIOLOGY

Overall, the worldwide incidence of cholangiocarcinoma is increasing (5). This represents the net effect of a marked increase in the incidence of intrahepatic cholangiocarcinoma and what may be a more subtle decrease in extrahepatic cholangiocarcinoma. However, there are substantially fewer epidemiologic data available for extrahepatic cholangiocarcinoma compared with intrahepatic cholangiocarcinoma (5). In any case, extrahepatic biliary cancer is still a substantial worldwide problem, with an incidence in North America and Europe between 0.53 and 1.14 per 100,000 (14). Worldwide, perihilar and distal cholangiocarcinoma account for 1% to 2% of all cancers, and in the United States there are approximately 2500 new cases each year (5, 15–17). The risk for the development of cholangiocarcinoma is most strongly associated with sclerosing cholangitis (8% to 20%) and choledochal cysts (3% to 28%), followed by inflammatory bowel disease (7% to 8%) and viral hepatitis (2% to 3%) (5).

DIAGNOSIS

Unlike intrahepatic cholangiocarcinoma, which is significantly more likely to produce pain initially than perihilar or distal cholangiocarcinoma, and is typically associated with other nonspecific symptoms such as anorexia, weight loss, night sweats, malaise and fatigue, perihilar and distal lesions are significantly more likely to present with stigmata of biliary obstruction, especially jaundice, and commonly present with weight loss (Table 29.1) (1).

Initial assessment of patients with symptoms of biliary tract disease should include an examination of the right upper quadrant by ultrasound, which not only provides information about bile-duct and gallblad-

TABLE 29.1 Signs and Symptoms of Cholangiocarcinoma

	Intrahepatic	Perihilar	Distal
Abdominal pain	XX*	X	X
Anorexia	X	X	X
Weight loss	X	XX	XX
Pruritis	X	X	X
Jaundice	–*	XXX	XXX
Distended palpable GB	–	–	X
Abnormal AP/GGT	X	X	X

Number of Xs indicated approximate relative likelihood of finding indicated signs or symptoms.
*p < 0.05 in Nakeeb et al.
Abbreviations: GB, gallbladder; AP, alkaline phosphatase; GGT, gamma glutamyl transpeptidase.
Modified from Cunningham SC and Schulick RD. Bile-duct cancer. In: Cameron JL (ed.), Current Surgical Therapy, 9th ed. St. Louis: Elsevier, 2008; and from Nakeeb A, Pitt HA, and Sohn TA, et al. Cholangiocarcinoma. A spectrum of intrahepatic, perihilar, and distal tumors. Ann Surg, 1996; 224: 463–473; with permission.

der dilatation, thickening and masses but is increasingly able to diagnose gallbladder cancer, as discussed subsequently. Often, patients will be referred with preliminary imaging and a working diagnosis already in place. The choice of subsequent imaging modalities – both to further secure the diagnosis and to plan treatment – depends, in part, on the anatomic structures most of interest. There has been a general trend toward less-invasive imaging modalities. The biliary system is often best visualized by endoscopic retrograde cholangiopancreatography (ERCP) or percutaneous transhepatic cholangiography (PTC), but magnetic resonance cholangiopancreatography (MRCP) can provide nearly equivalent imaging information while being relatively non-invasive. If non-invasive modalities fail to sufficiently demonstrate the anatomy of the biliary tree, then PTC remains a viable option. The integrity of major blood vessels can be well studied by multidetector computed tomography (CT) with three-dimensional reconstructions, by magnetic resonance angiography (MRA), or by x-ray angiography, which has become exceedingly uncommon.

The differential diagnosis for extrahepatic cholangiocarcinoma includes benign biliary strictures, such as those that may result from primary sclerosing cholangitis (PSC), choledocholithiasis and Mirizzi's syndrome. Cholangiocarcinoma superimposed on PSC is especially challenging to diagnose, as there may not be a dominant biliary stricture.

For patients with suspected cancers of the extrahepatic biliary system who are potentially curable, biopsy is not required and, indeed, may cause tumor dissemination. If nonoperative management is planned, then percutaneous or endoscopic biopsy may be performed to establish the diagnosis.

Certain laboratory values, such as alkaline phosphatase, and tumor markers such as CEA and CA 19–9 may be elevated, but lack sensitivity and specificity for cholangiocarcinoma. Nehls et al. recently reviewed serum and bile markers for the diagnosis of cholangiocarcinoma and reported that CA 19–9 is the most important marker for cholangiocarcinoma, with serum, but not bile, levels greater than 100 U/ml in unexplained symptomatic biliary disease supporting a diagnosis of cancer (18). Although no evidence exists to support a role for use of CA 19–9 in screening non-PSC asymptomatic individuals, there may be a role for CA 19–9 determination in surveillance for PSC-related cholangiocarcinoma. In the setting of PSC, the sensitivity of serum CA 19–9 ranges from as low as 38% (19) to as high as 89% (20), and the specificity from 50% (19) to 98% (21). There is currently insufficient to evidence to support a role for other markers, such as CA 125 (18).

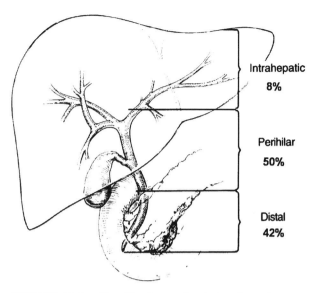

FIGURE 29.1. Classification of cholangiocarcinomas according to the Hopkins system. (*From* Nakeeb A, et al. Cholangiocarcinoma: A spectrum of intrahepatic, perihilar, and distal tumors. Ann Surg. 1996; 224: 463–475; with permission.)

(Figure 29.2), portal vein invasion, and hepatic lobar atrophy. Jarnagin and colleagues found this system to be able to predict resectability, metastasis and survival in a series of 219 patients (24). The AJCC staging system for gallbladder cancer is shown in Table 29.3.

CLASSIFICATION AND STAGING

Cholangiocarcinomas may be classified by various systems. Some systems separate tumors into intrahepatic and extrahepatic groups, with the extrahepatic groups being subdivided into proximal, middle and distal subgroups. At our institution, we have favored the simpler and more surgically relevant three-tiered classification shown in Figure 29.1. Tumors in the perihilar area have historically been subdivided by a system developed by Bismuth and Corlette (Figure 29.2) (22).

Regarding staging, the American Joint Committee on Cancer (AJCC) staging system correlates very well with survival for most gastrointestinal cancers (23). For extrahepatic cholangiocarcinoma, however, this staging system does not adequately account for resectability. Therefore, Jarnagin et al. recently proposed the Blumgart staging system (Table 29.2), which differs from the AJCC system by placing great emphasis on local tumor extent (24). Tumors are classified according to three factors: bile duct involvement (according to the Bismuth-Corlette system

PREOPERATIVE PREPARATION

Extrahepatic cholangiocarcinoma and gallbladder cancers are often diagnosed at late stages. Resection

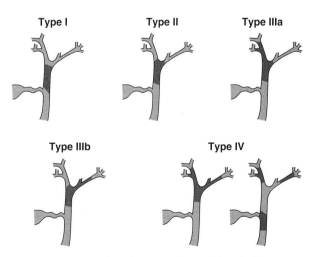

FIGURE 29.2. Classification of (peri)hilar cholangiocarcinoma according to the Bismuth-Corlette system. (*From* Lazaridis KN and Gores GJ. Cholangiocarcinoma. Gastroenterology 2005; 128: 1655–1667; with permission.) See Color Plate 28.

TABLE 29.2 Staging of Cholangiocarcinoma

Staging System	Stage	Tumor	Node	Metastasis
AJCC TNM (Extrahepatic)	0	Tis	N0	M0
	IA	T1	N0	M0
	IB	T2	N0	M0
	IIA	T3	N0	M0
	IIB	T1 to T3	N1	M0
	III	T4	Any N	M0
	IV	Any T	Any N	M1
		Tis, Carcinoma in situ; T1, confined to bile duct; T2, beyond bile duct; T3, invades liver, gallbladder, pancreas or unilateral HA or PV; T4, invades other adjacent organs or main HA or PV; N1, regional LN metastasis; M1, distant metastasis.		
		Criteria		
Blumgart T-Stage Criteria (Perihilar only)	T1	Tumor involving biliary confluence ± unilateral extension to second-order biliary radicles.		
	T2	Tumor involving biliary confluence ± unilateral extension to second-order biliary radicles **and** ipsilateral portal vein involvement ± ipsilateral hepatic lobar atrophy.		
	T3	Tumor involving biliary confluence + bilateral extension to second-order biliary radicles; or unilateral extension to second-order biliary radicles with contralateral portal vine involvement; or unilateral extension to second-order biliary radicles with contralateral hepatic lobar atrophy; or main or bilateral portal venous involvement.		

Abbreviations: HA, hepatic artery; PV, portal vein; LN, lymph node; AJCC, American Joint Committee on Cancer. *Modified from* Jarnagin WR, Fong Y, DeMatteo RP, et al. Staging, resectability, and outcome in 225 patients with hilar cholangiocarcinoma. Ann Surg, 2001; 234: 507–517; and American Joint Committee on Cancer: AJCC Cancer Staging Manual, 6th edition. 6th ed. New York: Springer, 2002; with permission.

TABLE 29.3 Staging of Gallbladder Cancer

Staging System	Stage	Tumor	Node	Metastasis
AJCC TNM	0	Tis	N0	M0
	IA	T1	N0	M0
	IB	T2	N0	M0
	IIA	T3	N0	M0
	IIB	T1 to T3	N1	M0
	III	T4	Any N	M0
	IV	Any T	Any N	M1
		Tis, Carcinoma in situ; T1a, tumor invades lamina propria; T1b, tumor invades the muscle layer; T2, tumor invades the perimuscular connective tissue; T3, tumor perforates the serosa and/or directly invades the liver and/or 1 other adjacent organ or structure; T4, tumor invades main PV or HA or invades multiple extrahepatic structures; N1, regional LN metastasis; M1, distant metastasis.		

Abbreviations: HA, hepatic artery; PV, portal vein; LN, lymph node; AJCC, American Joint Committee on Cancer. *Modified from* American Joint Committee on Cancer: AJCC Cancer Staging Manual, 6th edition. 6th ed. New York: Springer, 2002; with permission.

of these tumors is therefore associated with the potential for significant morbidity and mortality. All patients considered for resection should receive preoperative treatment to optimize their condition relative to all medical comorbidities, such as treatable cardiac, pulmonary, hepatic and renal disease and the malnutrition often attendant to these disease states.

Although preoperative stenting of cholangiocarcinoma patients used to be routine at some centers, it is now recognized that this is associated with increased risk of infectious complications. Nevertheless, biliary stenting may be useful in select cases. Potential advantages include decompressing an obstructed biliary system (e.g., in patients with a serum bilirubin >15 mg/dl, allowing hepatic function to improve) and providing a window of recovery to patients with significant malnutrition, biliary sepsis or other medical problems before an elective resection.

Because resection of cancers of the extrahepatic biliary system offers the only hope for a cure, all patients who are potentially resectable should be considered for operation unless prohibitive contraindications are present. Regarding cholangiocarcinoma, Blumgart and colleagues have recently proposed local tumor-related criteria for unresectability (Table 29.4). In brief, these tumor-related contraindications include involvement of bilateral secondary biliary radicles or unilateral extension to secondary radicles with contralateral vein branch encasement or occlusion; encasement or occlusion of the main portal vein; and hepatic lobe atrophy with contralateral compromise of the secondary biliary radicles or portal-vein branch. Patient-related contraindications include severe medical comorbidities that are refrac-

TABLE 29.4 Local Tumor-related Criteria for Unresectability

1. Hepatic duct involvement up to secondary biliary radicals bilaterally
2. Encasement or occlusion of the main portal vein proximal to its bifurcation*
3. Atrophy of one hepatic lobe with contralateral encasement of portal vein branch
4. Atrophy of one hepatic lobe with contralateral involvement of secondary biliary radicals
5. Unilateral tumor extension to secondary biliary radicals with contralateral vein branch encasement or occlusion

*Relative criterion. Portal vein resection and reconstruction may be possible.

Modified from Jarnagin WR, Fong Y, DeMatteo RP, et al. Staging, resectability, and outcome in 225 patients with hilar cholangiocarcinoma. Ann Surg, 2001; 234: 507–517; with permission.

tory to meaningful optimization, especially major cardiopulmonary disease and cirrhosis.

OPERATIONS

Many beautifully illustrated and detailed descriptions of operative technique exist (25–28). For the purpose of the present chapter, an abbreviated description of some common, relevant operations follows.

Operation for Perihilar Resection

Because of the close proximity of vital structures in the porta hepatis, resection of perihilar cholangiocarcinomas is often technically challenging. The first portion of the operation is devoted to determining resectability and to confirming the absence of metastatic disease. Resectability criteria are described earlier and in Table 29.4. In cases requiring concomitant hepatic resection (see later discussion), preoperative portal vein embolization of that portion of the liver that is to be resected is an option available to stimulate growth of the future liver remnant and thereby maximize post-resection hepatic function. Unlike resection of intrahepatic cholangiocarcinoma, resections of the extrahepatic biliary system are typically accompanied by resection of the bile-duct bifurcation, an extensive lymphadenectomy at the hilum of the liver and reconstruction of the biliary-enteric tract.

An extended right subcostal incision provides good exposure for dissection of the porta hepatis. Once metastatic disease is excluded, the gallbladder, if present, is separated from its fossa and the common bile duct is divided just proximal to the pancreas. If this margin is positive on frozen section, then a pancreaticoduodenectomy will be required to achieve complete resection. If the frozen-section margin is negative, then resection of the perihilar disease may proceed. The extrahepatic biliary tree is dissected away from surrounding structures, removing the perihilar lymphatic tissue en bloc, and exposing the bifurcation of the hepatic artery and the confluence of the portal vein. To gain access to the porta hepatis, the left hilar plate is dissected to expose the left bile duct (Figure 29.3). The left bile duct is then divided near the umbilical fissure of the liver, and a biopsy of the margin is sent frozen for pathologic analysis to confirm that the margin is negative for cancer. If so, then an extended right hepatectomy may be performed to resect the tumor. If,

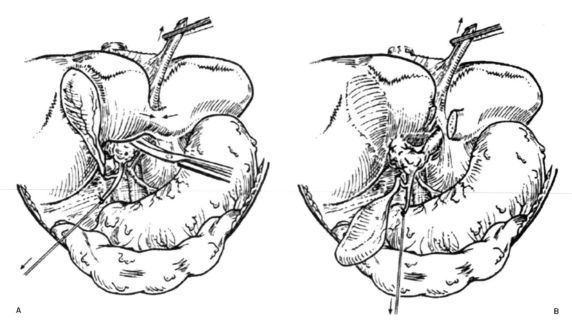

A   B

FIGURE 29.3.   Dissection of the hilus of the liver. (A) With firm upward traction on the ligamentum teres, dissection at the base of the quadrate lobe (scissors) lowers the hilar plate. (B) The bridge of tissue between segments III and IV (*arrows* in [A]) is divided, further exposing the hilar structures. (*From* Blumgart LH and Fong Y (eds), Surgery of the Liver and Biliary Tract, 3rd ed. Philadelphia: WB Saunders, 2003; with permission.)

however, this margin is positive, an attempt to dissect the right bile duct should be made in order to reach a negative margin on the main right bile duct or in the right posterior bile duct, in which case a left or extended left hepatectomy may proceed. The principles for performing the hepatectomy are described in detail in textbooks of surgical technique. Briefly, the right or left hepatic artery and portal vein are controlled in the hilum of the liver. Control of hepatic venous outflow can then be obtained by dividing the right or left hepatic vein. Alternatively, division of the hepatic vein may be delayed until later, but this may allow problematic hepatic venous back-bleeding to occur. Intermittent Pringle maneuver (compressing the portal triad at the foramen of Winslow) can further decrease bleeding. The parenchyma is then transected in any of various manners, including simple finger- or clamp-fracture techniques and devices using ultrasonic, stapling, tissue-sealing, and water-jet technologies. Reconstruction is typically performed using a Roux-en-Y limb of jejunum to the remnant bile duct(s).

Several studies have demonstrated a correlation between the rate of concomitant hepatectomy and the rate of margin-negative resection of perihilar cholangiocarcinoma (2, 29). Most experts now advocate liberal use of concomitant hepatectomy rather than simple excision of the bifurcation and extrahepatic

biliary tree because the survival benefit associated with attaining negative margins is widely thought to outweigh any potential increase in morbidity and mortality associated with these technically challenging resections (1, 15, 29, 30). Lesions requiring hepatic resection are considered resectable if localized and if 25% or more of unaffected liver remnant will be maintained with adequate hepatic portal and arterial inflow, hepatic venous outflow and biliary-enteric drainage. Many centers also advocate routine resection of segment I (the caudate lobe), as it often has one or more bile ducts joining the main biliary tree within 1 cm of the bifurcation. Some have advocated the routine resection of the portal venous bifurcation and anastomosis of the main and left portal vein, citing improved clearance of tumor (given that the venous bifurcation is often situated adjacent and posterior to the main tumor) and avoidance of dissecting the hilus with the resulting potential for tumor dissemination.

Operation for Distal Cholangiocarcinoma Resection

Distal cholangiocarcinoma is resected with a pancreaticoduodenectomy. Cancers in this location are considered resectable if there is no metastatic disease or involvement of the portal and superior mesenteric veins, the hepatic artery and the superior mesenteric artery. An upper midline incision provides good exposure for pancreaticoduodenectomy. As with operations for perihilar cholangiocarcinomas, these operations also begin with an exploration for metastatic disease and signs of nonresectability. In the absence of such signs, the duodenum is widely mobilized out of its retroperitoneal location (i.e., an extensive Kocher maneuver is performed) to manually and visually evaluate the lesion and to palpate its relationship to the portal and superior mesenteric veins and the superior mesenteric artery. Generally, at this point in the operation, a plane is dissected posterior to the neck of the pancreas and anterior to the portal and superior mesenteric veins proceeding in a caudad to cephalad direction. The gallbladder, if present, is mobilized from its fossa, and the common hepatic duct is divided proximal to the insertion of the cystic duct or where required to obtain a negative margin. Once the bile-duct margin is confirmed to be negative for cancer, the gastroduodenal artery should be divided to mobilize the specimen from the hepatic artery. The plane of dissection posterior to the neck of the pancreas and anterior to the portal and superior mesenteric veins can then be completed proceeding from the opposite direction – that is, cephalad to caudad. For a pylorus-preserving pancreaticoduodenectomy, the duodenum is divided 2 to 3 cm distal to the pylorus and for a classic pancreaticoduodenectomy, the pylorus is included in an antrectomy.

Despite numerous series comparing pylorus-preserving and classic Whipple operations, neither one has a clear advantage over the other with respect to survival or complications (31–33). Rather, the choice is generally dictated by the location and extent of the tumor and by surgeon preference and experience. Those tumors involving the pylorus or first few centimeters of the duodenum are most appropriately resected in a classic pancreaticoduodenectomy. After the neck of the pancreas is transected down to the previously dissected tunnel, the jejunum is divided 15 to 20 cm distal to the ligament of Treitz and the proximal jejunum and fourth portion of the duodenum are mobilized free of their ligamentous attachments. The proximal jejunum and fourth portion of the duodenum are then brought through the resultant defect in the transverse mesocolon into the lower abdomen. After the uncinate process of the pancreas and associated lymphatic tissues are dissected off of the portal and superior mesenteric veins and superior mesenteric artery, the specimen is removed.

There are multiple options for reconstruction of the pancreatico-biliary-enteric tract. Typically, the remnant jejunal limb is brought through a defect in the right transverse mesocolon created for this purpose. An end-to-side pancreaticojejunostomy is first performed, either with the cut end of the distal pancreas invaginated into the jejunum and sutured in place, pancreatic parenchyma to bowel wall, or in a duct-to-mucosa fashion in which the pancreatic duct in sutured directly to the jejunal mucosa. An end-to-side hepaticojejunostomy is performed in the several inches distal to the pancreaticojejunostomy. Finally, gastrointestinal continuity is re-established with an anastomosis of the duodenum (or stomach, depending on whether the pylorous was preserved) to the jejunum distal to the previous two anastomoses. The jejunal limb placed through the tranverse mesocolon is secured with sutures, and the defect at the ligament of Treitz is closed to prevent herniation. Closed-suction drains are often placed, although some groups prefer not to use them.

Operation for Gallbladder Resection

The operative strategy for resection of a gallbladder cancer depends on multiple variables, such as a history of a previous cholecystectomy after which the diagnosis of gallbladder cancer was made (either laparoscopically or open), and the degree to which other structures outside of the gallbladder are involved (e.g., liver, bile duct, hilar vessels, duodenum, colon). The diagnosis of gallbladder cancer is usually made in one of three ways. The lesion may be discovered incidentally during a laparoscopic or open cholecystectomy, discovered incidentally on pathological examination after laparoscopic or open cholecystectomy, or suspected or even biopsy-proven preoperatively after evaluation of a hilar or gallbladder mass.

If the lesion is discovered incidentally during a laparoscopic or open cholecystectomy, then consideration should be given to stopping the operation before or after removal of the gallbladder, awaking the patient and discussing options for further therapy, including rescheduling the patient at another time for definitive resection, especially for extensive lesions.

If the gallbladder was previously resected, then the depth of penetration of the cancer, the cystic duct margin status, and possibly status of Callot's node will be known. If the lesion has a T stage 1a, the cystic duct margin is negative, and if Callot's node was removed and is negative, then most surgeons would recommend observation and no operation. If the lesion has a T stage greater than 1a, a positive cystic duct margin or if Callot's node is positive, most surgeons would recommend further surgery to include exploratory laparotomy, excision of the extrahepatic biliary tree, portal lymphadenectomy and partial hepatectomy of the gallbladder bed (2-cm margin) with Roux-en-Y biliary reconstruction. If the cystic duct margin is negative, some surgeons will forego resection of the extrahepatic biliary tree and just perform portal lymphadenectomy and partial hepatectomy of the gallbladder bed (2-cm margin). If, on re-exploration, there appears to be significant involvement of the gallbladder bed, a central hepatectomy or even extended right or left hepatectomy may be required to remove the lesion. Often, it is difficult to distinguish tumor from scar tissue, and significant partial hepatectomy may be required to ensure adequate margins. If the gallbladder was previously resected via a laparoscopic cholecystectomy, some surgeons will also resect previous port sites to try to decrease the incidence of port-site metastases. However, it is often difficult to discern the actual trajectory of the port from the incision on the patient's abdomen.

If a patient presents without previous gallbladder surgery with a lesion that is highly suspicious for a gallbladder cancer, then the patient should be prepared for exploratory laparotomy and the appropriate resection. Very few of these patients will have only a T1a lesion, if a mass is evident on preoperative imaging. If a very early (T1a) lesion is suspected, intraoperative frozen section of the gallbladder can be performed to confirm. If jaundiced, the patient will likely require resection of the extrahepatic biliary tree. If the lesion is in the dome of the gallbladder and clearly not involving the cystic duct or main biliary ductal structures, some surgeons will not resect the extrahepatic biliary tree. The gallbladder should be removed with a partial hepatectomy en bloc to ensure adequate margin. If there appears to be no invasion of the liver or if the invasion appears relatively superficial, then a 2-cm rim of hepatic parenchyma should be resected. If there appears to be significant invasion of the liver or either the main right or left portal pedicle appears involved, then a central hepatectomy or even extended right or left hepatectomy may be required to remove the lesion. A portal lymphadenectomy should be performed to include the lymph nodes and lymphatic tissues surrounding the portal vein, including the portocaval, hepatic artery and bile duct nodes. Other involved structures or organs, including the

duodenum and colon, are also sometimes partially removed en bloc. Rarely, a pancreaticoduodenectomy will be required to resect a gallbladder cancer for negative margins.

Palliation of Unresectable Disease

According to recent estimates, approximately 80% of cholangiocarcinoma patients are eventually candidates for palliative management due to unresectability, either due to tumor- or patient-related issues (34). The main goals of palliative therapy are to provide biliary drainage and symptomatic relief. Obstructed bile ducts may be remedied either by stenting or bypass. Endoscopic placement of plastic biliary stents is associated with low rates of complications and high rates of symptomatic relief for patients with biliary obstruction caused by unresectable tumors. However, their utility may be limited by the need for frequent replacement for recurrent obstruction. This limitation has, in part, been addressed by the use of self-expanding metallic biliary stents, which have improved patency rates compared with plastic stents, the disadvantage being increased difficulty in exchanging the occasional metallic stents that do reocclude. An acceptable alternative to endoscopic stents is percutaneous biliary drainage, especially when endoscopic expertise is not available, has failed or is inappropriate for accessing multiple, isolated pockets that are infected or obstructed within the intrahepatic biliary tree. Revision of percutaneous drains is straightforward and provides a versatility not afforded by endostents, in that they can used for drainage of bile externally or be capped off to allow internal, physiologic drainage of bile into the small intestine. Biliary-enteric bypass effected via an open operation provides durable palliation of obstructive jaundice. This is commonly performed once a patient has been found at operative exploration to be unresectable. Due to a modest increase in mortality and morbidity, however, it is usually not the first choice in patients who are deemed clearly to have unresectable disease as determined by imaging studies.

OUTCOMES

In our series of 564 operations (2), 430 (76%) underwent resection and 134 (24%) underwent palliation initially. Distal lesions were more frequently resectable (96%) than perihilar lesions (61%) or intrahepatic lesions (66%). Similarly, the rate of complications (ranging in our series from 10% to 60%)

TABLE 29.5 Review of the Literature

Author, Location, Year (Ref)	Resected (N)	Liver Rx (%)	5-year Survival, R0 (%)	5-year Survival, All (%)	Mortality (%)
Intrahepatic					
Pichlmayr, Germany, 1995 (36)	32	100	NR	17	6
Jan, Taiwan, 1996 (37)	41	100	44	27	0
Casavilla, Pittsburgh, 1997 (38)	34	100	NR	31	7
Lieser, Rochester, 1998 (39)	32	100	45	NR	NR
Madariaga, Pittsburgh, 1998 (30)	34	100	51	35	6
Valverde, France, 1999 (40)	30	100	NR	22	3
Inoue, Japan, 2000 (41)	52	100	55	36	2
Weber, New York, 2001 (42)	33	100	NR[‡]	31	3
DeOliveira, Baltimore, 2006 (2)	34	100	63	40	2
Perihilar					
Sugiura, Japan, 1994 (43)	83	100	33	20	8
Su, China, 1996 (44)	49	50	34	15	10
Nagino, Japan, 1998 (45)	138	90	26	NR	10
Miyazaki, Japan, 1998 (46)	76	86	40	26	15
Madariaga, Pittsburgh, 1998 (30)	28	100	25	9	14
Kosuge, Japan, 1999 (47)	65	80	52	35	9
Neuhaus, Germany, 1999 (48)	95[†]	85	37	22	6
Jarnagin, New York, 2001 (24)	80	78	30	NR	10
Kondo, Japan, 2004 (49)	40	78	NR*	NR	0
Rea, Rochester, 2004 (50)	46	100	30	26	9
Nishio, Japan, 2006 (51)	301	95	27	22	8
Dinant, Netherlands, 2006 (52)	99	38	33	27	15
Wahab, Egypt, 2006 (53)	73	100	NR	13	11
DeOliveira, Baltimore, 2006 (2)	173	20	30	10	5
Distal					
Bortolasi, Rochester, 2000 (54)	15	0	NR	20	0
Yoshida, Japan, 2002 (55)	27	0	44	37	4
DeOliveira, Baltimore, 2006 (2)	229	0	27	23	3

NR = not reported.
*Three-year survival = 44%.
[†]Includes 15 hepatectomies with liver transplantation.
[‡]Three-year survival = 62%.
Modified from DeOliveira ML, Cunningham SC, Cameron JL, et al. Cholangiocarcinoma: 31-year experience with 564 patients at a single institution. In Press 2006; with permission.

also depended, in part, on the location of the tumor. Resection of intrahepatic tumors was associated with lower rates of complications, whereas perihilar resections were generally associated with the highest rates.

Table 29.5 compares mortality rates and the 5-year survivals reported in recent series. Operative mortality rates range from 0% to 15% and, as with complication rates, are highest for perihilar resections. In our series, the overall complication rate was 35%, and the operative mortality rate was 4%. Survival following resection of cholangiocarcinoma depends on several factors. In our series, margin status, followed by lymph node status, was the most robust predictor of patient survival. Tumor size and differentiation also predicted survival. When only R0 patients are analyzed, then lymph node status is the only one of the aforementioned factors that remains a significant predictor of survival.

Long-term survival rates for cholangiocarcinoma depend on tumor location and are highest for intrahepatic cancers and lowest for perihilar cancers (Table 29.5). In our series, the 5-year survivals for R0-resected intrahepatic, perihilar and distal tumors were 63%, 30% and 27%, respectively. Palliated patients have a median survival of less than 12 months.

It is intuitive that stage will correlate with survival, and indeed studies correlating survival not only with the AJCC staging system but also with the Blumgart staging system (24) have both found significant results. Nevertheless, other studies have not (35).

CONCLUSION

Cholangiocarcinoma and gallbladder cancer are often diagnosed at late stages, and therefore mortality is high. Resection is the only chance for long-term survival. The most reliable predictors of long-term survival are margin-negative resection and lymph-node status. Further improvements in survival will only be possible with earlier diagnosis and the development of effective adjuvant or neoadjuvant therapy.

REFERENCES

1. Nakeeb A, Pitt HA, Sohn TA, et al. Cholangiocarcinoma. A spectrum of intrahepatic, perihilar, and distal tumors. Ann Surg, 1996; 224: 463–473; discussion 473–475.

2. DeOliveira ML, Cunningham SC, Cameron JL, et al. Cholangiocarcinoma: 31-year experience with 564 patients at a single institution. Ann Surg, 2007; 245(5): 755–762.

3. Serafini FM, Sachs D, Bloomston M, et al. Location, not staging, of cholangiocarcinoma determines the role for adjuvant chemoradiation therapy. Am Surg, 2001; 67: 839–843; discussion 843–844.

4. Kelley ST, Bloomston M, Serafini F, et al. Cholangiocarcinoma: Advocate an aggressive operative approach with adjuvant chemotherapy. Am Surg, 2004; 70: 743–748; discussion 748–749.

5. Shaib Y, El-Serag HB. The epidemiology of cholangiocarcinoma. Semin Liver Dis, 2004; 24: 115–125.

6. Thorbjarnarson B. History of biliary tract surgery. In: Thorbjarnarson B (ed.), Surgery of the Biliary Tract, Vol. XVI, pp. 1–2. Philadelphia: WB Saunders, 1982.

7. Durand-Fardel M. Recherches anatomico-pathologiques sur la vesicule dt les canaux biliares: Premiere partie. Archives Generales de Medicine, 1840; 8: 167–188.

8. Renshaw K and Magoun JAH. Malignant neoplasia in the gall-bladder. Annals of Surgery, 1921; 74: 700–720.

9. Renshaw K. Malignant neoplasms of the extrahepatic biliary ducts. Ann Surg, 1922; 76: 205–221.

10. Klatskin G. Adenocarcinoma of the hepatic duct at its bifurcation within the porta hepatis. An unusual tumor with distinctive clinical and pathological features. Am J Med, 1965; 38: 241–256.

11. Altmeier WA, Gall EA, Zinninger MM, et al. Sclerosing carcinoma of the major intrahepatic bile ducts. Arch Surg, 1957; 75: 450–461.

12. Glenn F, Grafe WR, Jr. Historical events in biliary tract surgery. Arch Surg, 1966; 93: 848–852.

13. Stoll MD. Ratioonis Medendi in nosocomio practico vindobonensi. Quoted by Rolleston, HD and McNee, JS: Diseases of the Liver, Gallbladder, and Bile Ducts, 3rd ed., p 691. London, Macmillan, 1929.

14. Strom BL, Hibberd PL, Soper KA, et al. International variations in epidemiology of cancers of the extrahepatic biliary tract. Cancer Res, 1985; 45: 5165–5168.

15. Vauthey JN and Blumgart LH. Recent advances in the management of cholangiocarcinomas. Semin Liver Dis, 1994; 14: 109–114.

16. Kuwayti K, Baggenstoss AH, Stauffer MH, et al. Carcinoma of the major intrahepatic and the extrahepatic bile ducts exclusive of the papilla of Vater. Surg Gynecol Obstet, 1957; 104: 357–366.

17. Kirshbaum JD and Kozoll DD. Carcinoma of the gall bladder and extrahepatic bile ducts. Surg Gynecol Obstet, 1941; 73: 740–754.

18. Nehls O, Gregor M, and Klump B. Serum and bile markers for cholangiocarcinoma. Semin Liver Dis, 2004; 24: 139–154.

19. Bjornsson E, Kilander A, Olsson R. CA 19–9 and CEA are unreliable markers for cholangiocarcinoma in patients with primary sclerosing cholangitis. Liver, 1999; 19: 501–8.

20. Nichols JC, Gores GJ, LaRusso NF, et al. Diagnostic role of serum CA 19–9 for cholangiocarcinoma in patients with primary sclerosing cholangitis. Mayo Clin Proc, 1993; 68: 874–879.

21. Siqueira E, Schoen RE, Silverman W, et al. Detecting cholangiocarcinoma in patients with primary sclerosing cholangitis. Gastrointest Endosc, 2002; 56: 40–47.

22. Bismuth H and Corlette MB. Intrahepatic cholangioenteric anastomosis in carcinoma of the hilus of the liver. Surg Gynecol Obstet, 1975; 140: 170–8.

23. Greene FL, Page DL, Fleming ID, et al. AJCC Cancer Staging Manual, p. 435. New York: Springer-Verlag, 2002.

24. Jarnagin WR, Fong Y, DeMatteo RP, et al. Staging, resectability, and outcome in 225 patients with hilar cholangiocarcinoma. Ann Surg, 2001; 234: 507–517; discussion 517–519.

25. Cameron JL and Sandone C. Atlas of Gastrointestinal Surgery. B.C. Decker, 2006.

26. Jarnagin WR, Saldinger RF, Blumgart LH. Cancer of the bile ducts: The hepatic ducts and common bile duct. In: Blumgart LH and Fong Y (eds), Surgery of the Liver and Biliary Tract. New York: W.B. Saunders, 2000; pp. 1018–1058.

27. Dalton RR and Gadacz TR. Tumors of the biliary tract. In: Zuidema GD and Yeo CJ (eds.), Surgery of the Alimentary Tract. Philadelphia: W.B. Saunders, 2002, pp. 263–272.

28. Cunningham SC and Schulick RD. Bile-duct cancer. In: Cameron JL (ed.), Current Surgical Therapy, 9th ed. St. Louis: Elsevier, 2008.

29. Boerma EJ. Research into the results of resection of hilar bile duct cancer. Surgery, 1990; 108: 572–580.

30. Madariaga JR, Iwatsuki S, Todo S, et al. Liver resection for hilar and peripheral cholangiocarcinomas: A study of 62 cases. Ann Surg, 1998; 227: 70–79.

31. Horstmann O, Markus PM, Ghadimi MB, et al. Pylorus preservation has no impact on delayed gastric emptying after pancreatic head resection. Pancreas, 2004; 28: 69–74.

32. Seiler CA, Wagner M, Sadowski C, et al. Randomized prospective trial of pylorus-preserving vs. classic duodenopancreatectomy (Whipple procedure): Initial clinical results. J Gastrointest Surg, 2000; 4: 443–452.

33. Di Carlo V, Zerbi A, Balzano G, et al. Pylorus-preserving pancreaticoduodenectomy versus conventional Whipple operation. World J Surg, 1999; 23: 920–925.

34. Singhal D, van Gulik TM, Gouma DJ. Palliative management of hilar cholangiocarcinoma. Surg Oncol, 2005; 14: 59–74.

35. Zervos EE, Osborne D, Goldin SB, et al. Stage does not predict survival after resection of hilar cholangiocarcinomas promoting an aggressive operative approach. Am J Surg, 2005; 190: 810–815.

36. Pichlmayr R, Lamesch P, Weimann A, et al. Surgical treatment of cholangiocellular carcinoma. World J Surg, 1995; 19: 83–88.

37. Jan YY, Jeng LB, Hwang TL, et al. Factors influencing survival after hepatectomy for peripheral cholangiocarcinoma. Hepatogastroenterology, 1996; 43: 614–619.

38. Casavilla FA, Marsh JW, Iwatsuki S, et al. Hepatic resection and transplantation for peripheral cholangiocarcinoma. J Am Coll Surg, 1997; 185: 429–336.

39. Lieser MJ, Barry MK, Rowland C, et al. Surgical management of intrahepatic cholangiocarcinoma: A 31-year experience. J Hepatobiliary Pancreat Surg, 1998; 5: 41–47.

40. Valverde A, Bonhomme N, Farges O, et al. Resection of intrahepatic cholangiocarcinoma: A Western experience. J Hepatobiliary Pancreat Surg, 1999; 6: 122–127.

41. Inoue K, Makuuchi M, Takayama T, et al. Long-term survival and prognostic factors in the surgical treatment of mass-forming type cholangiocarcinoma. Surgery, 2000; 127: 498–505.

42. Weber SM, Jarnagin WR, Klimstra D, et al. Intrahepatic cholangiocarcinoma: Resectability, recurrence pattern, and outcomes. J Am Coll Surg, 2001; 193:384–91.

43. Sugiura Y, Nakamura S, Iida S, et al. Extensive resection of the bile ducts combined with liver resection for cancer of the main hepatic duct junction: A cooperative study of the Keio Bile Duct Cancer Study Group. Surgery, 1994; 115: 445–451.

44. Su CH, Tsay SH, Wu CC, et al. Factors influencing postoperative morbidity, mortality, and survival after resection for hilar cholangiocarcinoma. Ann Surg, 1996; 223: 384–394.

45. Nagino M, Nimura Y, Kamiya J, et al. Segmental liver resections for hilar cholangiocarcinoma. Hepatogastroenterology, 1998; 45: 7–13.

46. Miyazaki M, Ito H, Nakagawa K, et al. Aggressive surgical approaches to hilar cholangiocarcinoma: Hepatic or local resection? Surgery, 1998; 123: 131–136.

47. Kosuge T, Yamamoto J, Shimada K, et al. Improved surgical results for hilar cholangiocarcinoma with procedures including major hepatic resection. Ann Surg, 1999; 230: 663–671.

48. Neuhaus P, Jonas S, Bechstein WO, et al. Extended resections for hilar cholangiocarcinoma. Ann Surg, 1999; 230: 808–818; discussion, 819.

49. Kondo S, Hirano S, Ambo Y, et al. Forty consecutive resections of hilar cholangiocarcinoma with no postoperative mortality and no positive ductal margins: Results of a prospective study. Ann Surg, 2004; 240: 95–101.

50. Rea DJ, Munoz-Juarez M, Farnell MB, et al. Major hepatic resection for hilar cholangiocarcinoma: Analysis of 46 patients. Arch Surg, 2004; 139: 514–523; discussion 523–525.

51. Nishio H, Nagino M, Nimura Y. Surgical management of hilar cholangiocarcinoma: The Nagoya experience. HPB, 2006; 7: 259–262.

52. Dinant S, Gerhards MF, Rauws EA, et al. Improved outcome of resection of hilar cholangiocarcinoma (Klatskin tumor). Ann Surg Oncol, 2006; 13: 872–880.

53. Abdel Wahab M, Fathy O, Elghwalby N, et al. Resectability and prognostic factors after resection of hilar cholangiocarcinoma. Hepatogastroenterology, 2006; 53: 5–10.

54. Bortolasi L, Burgart LJ, Tsiotos GG, et al. Adenocarcinoma of the distal bile duct. A clinicopathologic outcome analysis after curative resection. Dig Surg, 2000; 17: 36–41.

55. Yoshida H, Onda M, Tajiri T, et al. Extreme left hepatic lobar atrophy in a case with hilar cholangiocarcinoma. J Nippon Med Sch, 2002; 69: 278–281.

Chapter 30

EXTRAHEPATIC BILIARY CANCER: HIGH DOSE RATE BRACHYTHERAPY AND PHOTODYNAMIC THERAPY

Eric T. Shinohara

James M. Metz

CAUSES OF MALIGNANT OBSTRUCTIVE JAUNDICE

Various types of malignancies, including pancreatic cancer, cholangiocarcinoma, hepatocellular carcinoma, gallbladder carcinoma and metastatic disease, can cause malignant obstruction of the biliary ducts. Cholangiocarcinomas represent approximately 3% of all gastrointestinal cancers (1). It was estimated that approximately 18,500 primary liver cancers would be diagnosed in the United States in 2006 (2) and of these, approximately 15% would be intrahepatic cholangiocarcinomas (3). An estimated 4,600 cases of extrahepatic cholangiocarcinoma were diagnosed in 2007 per estimates from the American Cancer Society. Risk factors include primary sclerosing cholangitis, ulcerative cholitis, choledochal cysts and biliary infections, such as in typhoid carriers. Chemical exposures to nitrosamines, dioxin, asbestos and polychlorinated biphenyls have also been linked to cholangiocarcinoma. Cholangiocarcinomas are usually adenocarcinomas (95% of the time) but rarely are found to be cystadenocarcinomas, hemangioendotheliomas or mucoepidermoid carcinomas. Patients commonly present with right upper quadrant pain, pruritis, anorexia, malaise and weight loss.

Up to 30% of patients may present with cholangitis. Elevated liver enzymes, alkaline phosphate and bilirubin can also be seen. Cholangiocarcinomas are usually discovered on ultrasound, computed tomography (CT), magnetic resonance imaging (MRI) or endoscopic retrograde cholangiopancreatography (ERCP). Percutaneous transhepatic cholangiography and laparoscopy can also be used for diagnosis. If the cholangiocarcinoma appears resectable, a Whipple resection or partial hepatectomy can be attempted; with complete resection, 5-year survival rates of up to 25% are seen. Palliative surgery with a biliary bypass can be done in the event that resection is not possible.

The majority (50%–90%) of patients with cholangiocarcinoma present with advanced disease and are unresectable (1, 4, 5). Generally, a tumor is unresectable if it involves the portal vein or hepatic artery, or invades adjacent liver or the biliary tree into the liver. Metastasis to lymph nodes, liver or peritoneum also renders the disease unresectable. Unresectable disease is generally approached with palliative intent with the goal of maintaining biliary drainage. It is important to maintain patency as most patients will die of liver failure. Studies have suggested that biliary stenting is as effective as surgical bypass in providing relief from obstructive jaundice (6). Biliary stenting can be used to relieve symptoms of jaundice in patients with an average patency of 5 to 6 months (7, 8). Recent studies have suggested that even in patients with unresectable pancreatic cancer or cholangiocarcinoma, approximately 21% will be alive at 1 year. Hence, long-term solutions for malignant obstruction are required, as patients often survive long enough that re-occlusion of stents will be a significant problem for them, even in patients with unresectable disease (9). Several studies have suggested that intraluminal brachytherapy (ILBT) is a safe way to improve the duration of stent patency, and when used in combination with external beam radiation therapy (EBRT) and chemotherapy, may have a role in improving survival.

ROLE OF LOW-DOSE ILBT IN MAINTAINING PATENCY OF BILIARY DUCTS

There are several advantages to brachytherapy in treating malignant biliary obstruction. EBRT is limited by toxicity to surrounding normal tissues. The liver, kidneys, spinal cord and bowel can all be in the EBRT field and can affect the total dose that can be safely delivered. The small source size used in brachytherapy allows close contact with ductal tissues, with a treatment range of 0.5 to 2 cm. The radiation quickly attenuates at a rate inversely proportional to the square of the distance from the source, which allows sparing of normal tissues.

There are several retrospective trials examining the effectiveness of ILBT in the treatment of malignant obstruction. One of the first publications regarding the treatment of malignant obstruction with brachytherapy was published in 1982, reporting results using radium needles placed for 3 days (10). A prospective, non-randomized Japanese study addressed the effectiveness of EBRT and low dose rate (LDR) brachytherapy without stenting (11). Twenty-five patients with extrahepatic cholangiocarcinoma were treated with a combination of EBRT to a dose of between 30 and 50 Gy and LDR brachytherapy to a dose of 24 to 40 Gy. Biliary tubes were removed after treatment, and no stents were placed. Seventy-six percent of patients achieved full patency after treatment and the median tube-free interval was 76 days. The median survival for these patients was

9.3 months, and eight patients were tube free until death.

A retrospective study examining 56 patients suggested that radiation may increase the need for repeat stenting. Patients were treated with stenting, followed by EBRT combined with LDR brachytherapy or no further treatment (12). Median survival for patients who had stenting alone was 7 months, and for those patients who received radiation and stenting, it was 10 months. This finding was not statistically significant and the radiation group was found to have more frequent stent changes and longer hospital stays.

ROLE OF LOW-DOSE BRACHYTHERAPY IN TREATING BILE DUCT MALIGNANCIES

A number of studies have examined the use of external beam radiation combined with LDR brachytherapy and chemotherapy to improve survival in patients with bile duct malignancies. There are case reports of patients with unresectable cholangiocarcinoma treated with EBRT and LDR brachytherapy, who have had long-term survival (13). A large study addressing the use of combined EBRT and LDR brachytherapy for treatment of unresectable extrahepatic cholangiocarcinoma came from Japan (14). This study also addressed prognostic factors associated with survival. Ninety-three patients with unresectable disease were treated with definitive radiation composed of 50 Gy of EBRT and 27 to 50 Gy (mean 39.2) of LDR brachytherapy. EBRT was given in 2 Gy fractions, 4 days a week with a 1 to 2 cm border. LDR brachytherapy was given using ^{192}Ir with the dose prescribed to 0.5 cm from the source. Eighty-eight patients then underwent stent placement. Median survival was 11.9 months and 4.3% were alive at 5 years. Obstruction developed in 49% of patients, with a mean time to obstruction of 11.6 months. Approximately one-third of patients experienced some gastroduodenitits, with 10 patients requiring a procedure to stop bleeding. Biliary complications, such as cholangitis, cholecystitis, intrahepatic abscess and biliary fistula, were noted in about one-third of patients, and five of these were life threatening. Hemobilia occurred in five patients, with one death. Previous studies from the University of California, San Francisco have suggested that age, T stage, N stage, degree of histologic differentiation, extent of surgery, residual tumor, radiation dose and the use of adjuvant radiotherapy (RT) are important prognostic factors for survival in biliary duct cancers (15). In the previously mentioned Japanese study, the length of duct involved with the tumor, hepatic involvement and M stage were found to be significantly prognostic factors for survival. Dose escalation did not appear to improve survival in this study, with patients treated with 90 to 100 Gy having no better survival than patients treated with 70 to 86 Gy.

Previous studies of radiation therapy for biliary cancer have suggested that for microscopic disease, a minimum dose of 45 to 50 Gy is required for sterilization, and in gross disease, 60 to 70 Gy is required for disease control (16). Recent studies in which LDR brachytherapy was used have suggested that higher doses may improve survival (17, 18). Studies by Smoron found that patients treated to a dose of greater than or equal to 40 Gy had a mean survival of 15 months, compared with patients who received less than 40 Gy, who had a mean survival of 2.5 months. Alden found that in the subgroup of patients treated with more than 55 Gy, there was 48% survival at 2 years, compared with those treated with less than 55 Gy, who had a survival of 0% at 2 years.

Alden et al. compared patients with extrahepatic bile duct malignancies treated with chemotherapy alone as opposed to chemotherapy with external beam radiation and LDR brachytherapy. There were a total of 48 patients in this study. Twenty-four patients received combined external beam radiation and LDR brachytherapy as a part of their treatment, and 24 had no radiation. EBRT was given to a mean dose of 46 Gy and LDR brachytherapy was given to a mean dose of 25 Gy to 1 cm from the source. Patients received 5-fluorouracil (5-FU) alone or in combination with doxorubicin (Adriamycin), or mitomycin-C. For the entire group, 2-year survival was 18%, with a median survival of 9 months. There was a significant improvement in overall survival in patients treated with radiation, with a survival at 2 years of 30% (median 12 months) in the radiation group and 17% (median 5.5 months) in the chemotherapy-alone arm.

A publication from Japan studied the management of extrahepatic bile duct cancer with brachytherapy with or without EBRT in 145 patients (19). A total of 103 of the 145 patients were found to be candidates for radiation, either with LDR brachytherapy alone (85 patients) or with EBRT (18 patients). LDR brachytherapy was given at a dose ranging from 20 to 95 Gy (mean 42.2), and for patients who had EBRT,

dose varied from 7.5 to 80 Gy (mean 42.2). Overall actuarial survival for all patients was 55%, 18% and 10% at 1, 3 and 5 years respectively, with a mean survival of 12 months. No patient in the palliative group survived more than 15 months, with a mean survival time of 4.3 months. Patients who received postoperative adjuvant therapy had an overall actuarial survival of 73%, 31% and 18% (1, 3 and 5 years), with a median survival of 21.5 months. The rate of severe complication was found to be 16.5% among all patients. There did not appear to be a benefit to dose escalation between doses of 70 to 135 Gy; however, doses greater than 90 Gy were associated with a higher incidence of complications. Ultimately, resectability was found to be the most important factor in overall survival, and the greatest advantage was seen in patients treated with postoperative radiation.

Memorial Sloan-Kettering Cancer Center published a retrospective review of 25 patients treated for malignant obstruction due to primary tumors of the biliary system or metastatic disease. This study compared the use of LDR brachytherapy as a boost after EBRT in 15 patients compared with 10 patients who had EBRT alone. EBRT was given to doses of between 2000 and 3000 cGy, followed by an LDR brachytherapy boost given over 29 to 177 hours to doses of 800 to 6000 cGy in patients who received combined treatment. Patients who received EBRT alone received between 1760 to 3000 cGy. Fifteen patients received various types of chemotherapy. Median survival from the initiation of radiation in patients treated with combined LDR brachytherapy and EBRT was 4.0 months for patients with metastatic disease and 4.5 months for patients with primary or recurrent biliary cancers. Patients with recurrent or primary disease treated with EBRT alone had a median survival after initiating radiation of 2.65 months and for the four patients with metastatic disease treated with EBRT alone, survival was 1, 1.25, 5 and 7 months. No further statistical analysis was done due to the small number of patients. No patient had long-term relief from malignant obstruction without stent placement. There were no significant toxicities associated with treatment (20).

A study from the Mayo Clinic compared LDR brachytherapy boost, intraoperative radiation and EBRT boost in patients treated to 45 Gy with EBRT. They studied 34 patients who had subtotal resection or unresectable extrahepatic bile duct carcinomas

(21). One-half the patients were treated with EBRT to 45 Gy followed by a 5 to 15 Gy EBRT boost; the other half received a boost using LDR brachytherapy (Ir192) or intraoperative radiation (IORT). Ten patients received LDR brachytherapy and seven received IORT. The median survival was 12 months for the entire cohort of patients. The only patients to survive more than 18 months were patients who had a total or subtotal resection and those who had LDR brachytherapy or IORT. A study from Washington University had similar results (22). This study examined patients with unresectable, gross residual or microscopically residual extrahepatic biliary cancer. They found a borderline significant difference (p = 0.06) in median survival between patients treated with EBRT alone (7 months) versus those treated with EBRT and brachytherapy (15 months).

However, other studies have demonstrated no difference in survival in patients treated with EBRT alone versus EBRT plus brachytherapy (23). One study examined the effects of brachytherapy in patients with both resectable (71 patients) and unresectable (38 patients) disease. In resectable patients, the 5-year survival was 24%, compared with unresectable patients, who had a 5-year survival of 10%. Brachytherapy was not found to be of benefit in either of these subgroups.

A recent study from Italy showed that survival was worse when EBRT was combined with LDR brachytherapy compared with treatment with EBRT alone. This study examined 22 patients with either unresectable extrahepatic cholangiocarcinoma or residual disease after resection (24). Seventeen patients had unresectable disease, and five patients had residual extrahepatic biliary carcinomas. Patients with unresectable tumor had stent placement with ERCP. Patients were treated with 39.6 (first three patients) or 50.4 Gy (in the remaining 19 patients) of EBRT using a three-field technique with a 1.5 cm margin. The majority of patients (n = 21) received 5-FU. Twelve patients received a boost using LDR brachytherapy with Ir192 to a dose of 30 to 50 Gy. Duration of local control, disease-free survival and overall survival for the entire cohort were 44.5, 16.3 and 22.0 months respectively. The addition of LDR brachytherapy to EBRT and 5-FU appeared to be detrimental, with a 5-year survival of 16.7% for patients treated without brachytherapy and 0% with brachytherapy, although this difference was not

statistically significant. The overall survival in this study appeared to be longer compared with survival from historical controls.

HIGH DOSE RATE (HDR) BRACHYTHERAPY

There are several benefits to HDR brachytherapy compared with LDR. Shorter treatment times may decrease the effects of organ motion and are easier for the patient. There is decreased radiation exposure to medical staff due to computerized remote afterloading, which also decreases treatment time, which may also limit the risk of infection. ^{192}Ir is usually used in HDR brachytherapy. It has an average energy of 0.38 MeV and a half-life of 74.2 days. Generally, the radioactive source needs to be changed every 3 months due to decay. HDR brachytherapy can be used as a boost after chemoradiation for unresectable cholangiocarcinoma. It has also been used postoperatively in patients who have a positive margin after resection or severe dysplasia after EBRT. HDR brachytherapy has also been used in the palliative setting to maintain stent or biliary tube patency. Table 30.1 shows the contraindications to HDR brachytherapy. Common complications of HDR include cholangitis, biliary stricture and duodenal ulcer.

A recent study of 13 patients with resected (5 patients) and unresected (8 patients) bile duct and gallbladder carcinomas found that HDR brachytherapy was a safe and effective means of treating icterus (25). Mean survival in this study was 275 days. Another study addressed the efficacy of HDR brachytherapy followed by stenting in controlling jaundice and pain (26). This study was a nonrandomized study of eight patients with inoperable extrahepatic bile duct carcinomas. All patients first underwent percutaneous transhepatic drainage of their biliary system and were then treated with HDR brachytherapy with ^{192}Ir. Patients were treated twice with brachytherapy, to a dose of 10 Gy to 1 cm from the source axis. Treatments were spaced 1 week

TABLE 30.1 Contraindications for HDR Brachytherapy

Active cholangitis
Inadequate biliary tube drainage
Inability to place at least a 10F catheter
Disease above the right and left hepatic ducts
Previous HDR above level at which retreatment is
 feasible in short intervals

apart. After treatment, patients had self-expanding metal stents placed. All eight patients tolerated the first treatment, and five out of eight completed both treatments. Mean and median survival from stent placement was 7.5 and 5.5 months respectively, mean and median survival from diagnosis was 11 and 8.4 months respectively. The mean and median stent patency was 6.9 and 5 months respectively, and 5 of 7 patients maintained stent patency until death. One patient was alive at follow-up with continued patency of the stent. Acute side effects from the first HDR brachytherapy treatment were generally mild, with five patients complaining of Radiation Therapy Oncology Group (RTOG) grade 2 nausea and vomiting and four patients with RTOG grade 1 or 2 abdominal pain. The second treatment was well tolerated, with only two patients having RTOG grade 2 abdominal pain. After completing treatment, two patients experienced fevers of unknown origin, which resolved with antibiotics; two patients experienced gastrointestinal bleeds, one requiring transfusion.

Few prospective trials have examined the use of HDR brachytherapy to maintain stent patency compared with controls. A recent study examined 233 patients with malignant obstruction treated with percutaneous transhepatic biliary drainage, followed by a variety of local treatments (27). Forty-nine of the 233 patients agreed to undergo further treatment with either EBRT (14 patients), transcatheter arterial chemoembolization (TACE) (22 patients) or HDR brachytherapy (13 patients). In this study, they compared patients who received local therapy and those who did not. Patients who received local therapy had a median survival of 10.5 months with a 12-month survival of 33%, compared with patients who did not receive local therapy, who had a 12-month survival of 6%. This difference was found to be significant (p < 0.001). The median patency time in patients who had local treatment was 14 months and patency at 12 months was 57%, as compared to 36% in the group which received no local treatment. However, this difference was not found to be significantly different (p = 0.123).

Another non-randomized prospective study examined stent patency in patients treated with HDR brachytherapy compared with patients who received no treatment (28). All had stent placement, after which they were given the option of HDR brachytherapy or no further therapy. HDR brachytherapy was elected by 14 patients and 20 patients elected

for no further therapy. Patients treated with HDR were treated with 4 to 7 Gy fractions, three or four times at 3- to 6-day intervals. Total dose ranged from 14 to 21 Gy. Dose was prescribed to 0.5 to 1 cm from the source. Nine patients in the HDR brachytherapy arm and ten in the control arm subsequently underwent TACE. RTOG grade 1 acute morbidity was seen in three patients and one patient developed RTOG grade 1 late morbidity. There was a significant improvement in the duration of stent patency with HDR brachytherapy. Patients who received HDR brachytherapy had a mean stent patency of 12.6 months, compared with controls, who had a mean stent patency of 8.3 months (p < 0.05). Stent patency was measured from stent placement to time of obstruction. In patients who had not reoccluded at the time of death, stent patency time was taken to be the survival time; however, these patients were then censored. Mean survival in patients who received brachytherapy was 9.4 months, as compared with untreated patients, who had a survival of 6.0 months. Taken together, these studies suggest that HDR ILBT is a safe and effective way to maintain stent patency.

COMBINED EXTERNAL BEAM TREATMENT WITH HDR BRACHYTHERAPY

Several studies have investigated the use of HDR brachytherapy concurrently with EBRT as a means both to palliate symptoms and increase survival. A cohort of 32 patients with Klatskin's tumor, gallbladder carcinoma and carcinoma of the ampulla of Vater were treated with EBRT and HDR brachytherapy, followed by metallic stent implantation (29). Mean survival was 457 days for patients with Klatskin's tumor, 237 days for patients with gallbladder tumors and 850 days in patients with tumors of the ampulla of Vater. Two-year survival for these patients was 27%, 0% and 50% respectively, which was found to be significantly different (p < 0.05). Stent patency was 418, 220 and 850 days respectively.

A prospective, non-randomized study from Korea compared EBRT alone with EBRT with HDR brachytherapy (30). Patients received treatment based on physician preference. After external drainage had been established, EBRT was administered in doses ranging from 36 to 55 Gy with a median dose of 50.4 Gy. HDR brachytherapy was given using ^{192}Ir after the insertion of an expandable intrabiliary prosthesis. Dose was prescribed to 1.5 cm from the source and three fractions of 5 Gy for a total of 15 Gy were given. Complete response was better in the group treated with EBRT and HDR brachytherapy (43%) compared with those treated with EBRT alone (29%). Overall response rate was 86% in the combined group as compared with 65% in the EBRT-only group. Patterns of failure were also different between the two groups. Local failure, regional failure and distant failure were 58%, 12% and 6% respectively for the EBRT-alone group and 36%, 21% and 21% for the EBRT and HDR brachytherapy group. There was a significant difference in locoregional recurrence rates between EBRT (53%) and EBRT with HDR brachytherapy (36%) ($p > 0.05$). There was a marginally significant difference in time to tumor recurrence seen between EBRT (5 months) and HDR brachytherapy (9 months; $p = 0.06$). Overall 2-year survival was significantly better for patients receiving combined EBRT and HDR brachytherapy (21%) compared with those who received radiation alone (0%; $p < 0.015$). Toxicity from both treatment arms was similar.

Another recent study by Fritz et al. also looked at combining HDR with EBRT and various stenting techniques in treating patients with bile duct carcinomas. Thirty patients with bile duct carcinomas were treated with combined HDR brachytherapy and EBRT, 21 definitively and 9 palliatively (31). Twenty-five patients were able to complete treatment. Doses of 30 to 45 Gy were used for EBRT and 20 to 45 Gy for HDR brachytherapy. Percutaneous drains, stents or endoprostheses were used to maintain patency after radiation treatment. Median survival for the entire group was 10 months, with 34%, 18% and 8% actuarial survival at 1, 3 and 5 years respectively. Stents provide the longest relief from malignant obstruction, and replacing percutaneous drains with stents or endoprosthesis reduced the rate of cholangitis from 37% to 28%. Frequency of radiation-induced ulcer was reduced from 23% to 7.3% when HDR brachytherapy boost was reduced to 20 Gy. The findings from this study suggest that 40 Gy of EBRT with HDR brachytherapy boost to 20 Gy is well tolerated and, when combined with stenting, effectively palliates malignant obstruction.

A recent Phase I/II study investigated whether dose escalation can improve survival in patients treated with HDR brachytherapy (32). Eighteen patients

with unresectable or partially resected extrahepatic biliary duct carcinoma received 5-FU and EBRT to 45 Gy. Patients were then divided into three groups for HDR brachytherapy treatments at doses of 7 Gy, 14 Gy and 21 Gy. Median survival for each of these groups was 9, 12 and 20 months respectively, but this difference was not statistically significant. However, when comparing the rate of partial and complete responses between patients who received 7 Gy (25% response rate) of HDR brachytherapy, and those who received either 14 Gy or 21 Gy (80% response rate), there was a statistically significant difference ($p = 0.05$). One patient in the 14-Gy boost group had Eastern Oncology Cooperative Group (ECOG) grade 3 toxicity, and none had Grade 4 toxicity. Other studies have investigated the use of local chemotherapy with hepatic arterial infusion combined with brachytherapy and EBRT, which also appeared to be effective at prolonging survival (33).

The Mayo Clinic has investigated the use of hepatic transplantation after neoadjuvant chemoradiation in patients with unresectable but relatively localized cholangiocarcinoma. They found survival rates of 92% at 1 year and 82% at 5 years. This study compared neoadjuvant therapy followed by transplantation with resection alone. A total of 71 patients were randomized to transplantation, but ultimately only 38 patients could undergo transplantation. Patients were treated with 45 Gy of EBRT with a boost of 20 to 30 Gy using LDR ^{192}Ir. Patients received 5-FU during radiation treatment followed by oral capcitabine or continuous 5-FU until transplantation. Sixteen of 38 livers were found to be tumor free at explantation; however, it is difficult to draw strong conclusions because this is a very select subset of the initial patients enrolled in the study.

DIFFERENT TECHNIQUES FOR DELIVERING HDR BRACHYTHERAPY

Generally, percutaneous transhepatic biliary tubes are used to introduce brachytherapy catheters for the delivery of radiation. There have been limited studies of different approaches for implantation of brachytherapy catheters, generally using a transduodenal approach. Some investigators have used nasobiliary tubes (34). The Mayo Clinic has recently published a study in which they stented the biliary duct and an ^{192}Ir-embedded ribbon was directly cannulated into the stent without use of a nasobiliary tube (35). Studies have also examined the use of the nasobiliary approach in HDR brachytherapy. In one study, 11 patients were treated with nasobiliary HDR brachytherapy with a mean survival of 284 days (36).

Generally, for malignant obstruction, patency of the biliary ducts with adequate drainage is required prior to treatment. Radiation treatments rarely facilitate the opening of obstructed ducts but can be used to maintain patency. Usually, when disease is primarily extraluminal, EBRT is the preferred method of radiation treatment, with consideration of a brachyther-

apy boost. When the disease is primarily intraluminal, brachytherapy is usually preferred if the catheter can be advanced across the lesion. Percutaneous transhepatic placement of biliary drains by interventional radiology is usually performed first. In patients with disease involving one hepatic duct or the common duct, a single drain may be adequate for treatment (Figure 30.1A and B). In patients with disease extending along both the right and left hepatic ducts, two drains are required for adequate drainage (Figure 30.1C and D). At minimum, a 10F drainage catheter is required for treatment, as this is the

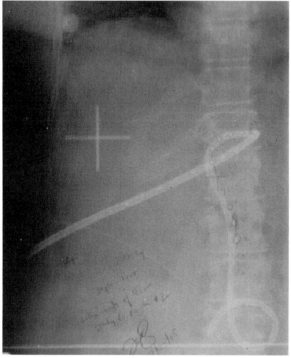

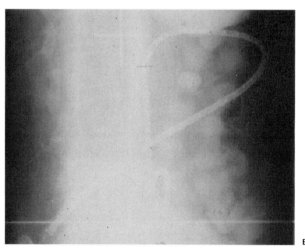

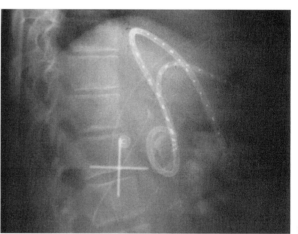

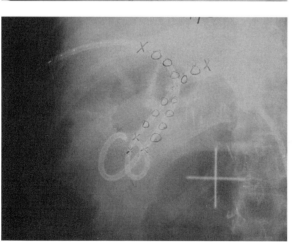

FIGURE 30.1. Anteroposterior (A) and lateral film (B) for a patient being treated with one catheter for cholangiocarcinoma, and anteroposterior (C) and lateral film (D) from a patient being treated for cholangiocarcinoma with two catheters. Note the two drains on the anteroposterior film of the patient being treated with two catheters; the left side shows the right biliary tube entering into the right hepatic duct. A centrally placed drain enters the left hepatic duct. The various dwell points can be seen as radiopaque dots within the drains. The selected dwell points have been circled.

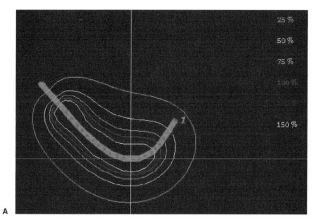

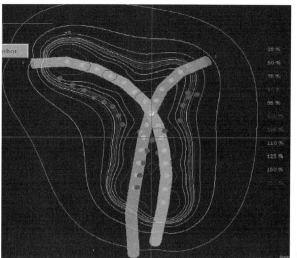

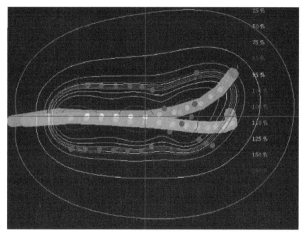

FIGURE 30.2.   The cumulative dose from the combination of the various dwell points is shown in the anteroposterior view for one-catheter technique (A). Two-catheter technique with both anteroposterior (B) and lateral (C) views also is shown. See Color Plate 29.

minimum diameter that will allow insertion of the HDR brachytherapy catheter.

Prior to treatment, CT or MR imaging is used to determine the areas of obstructions that are to be treated. During the interventional procedure, a cholangiogram under fluoroscopy can be used to define areas of stricture. After establishing the areas to be treated, HDR catheters are inserted into the biliary drains across the region to be treated by the radioactive source. The catheters contain radiopaque dummy seeds, so that the radiolucent catheter can be visualized along with the potential dwell positions for the radioactive source. The fenestrations in the biliary drains make it challenging to insert the catheter and may require manipulations by the interventional radiologist to get the HDR catheter in the proper position. The catheter and dummy source are secured and, after recovery, the patient is transported to the fluoroscopy simulator room in the radiation oncology department. An anteroposterior and lateral film are taken such that the dummy seeds can be visualized (Figure 30.1). The desired dwell points are marked next to the dummy seeds on the films. In the event that two drains are present and both drains are to be treated, two distinct dummy seed strands are used.

Once the desired dwell points have been selected based on the areas of obstruction seen on imaging, the dwell points on both the lateral and anteroposterior films are digitized into the treatment planning system. This allows the precise three-dimensional location of each dwell point to be calculated. Dwell times are then calculated by the treatment planning system and optimized by the physics team (Figure 30.2). Generally, lesions are treated to 1 cm from the source axis in depth and to 1 cm proximally and distally to the lesion. At the University of Pennsylvania, 7 Gy fractions are usually used for each treatment. When combined with EBRT (median dose of 50.4 Gy), a single treatment of 7 Gy is used. When the treatment is done without EBRT, three separate treatments spaced 1 week apart for a total dose of 21 Gy is delivered. The HDR catheter is removed after the treatment, and the patient returns to interventional radiology for attachment of any appliances for drainage. For each treatment, the HDR catheter needs to be placed in interventional radiology and the plan is recalculated based on the position of the catheters and dummy sources that day. After the brachytherapy treatment course is completed, stents may be placed to maintain patency. Generally, it is recommended that stents are placed after completion of brachytherapy, although studies suggest that stents do not attenuate or scatter radiation (37). However, placement through drainage catheters allows more uniform centering of the source within the malignant stricture, whereas the source can lie eccentrically inside expanded metal stents.

PHOTODYNAMIC THERAPY

Photodynamic therapy (PDT) involves the use of a photosensitizing drug that preferentially accumulates in tumor compared with normal tissues. Photosensitizers are not active until the area to be treated is exposed to specific wavelengths of light generated by a laser. The photosensitizer absorbs the light, and a photochemical process takes place. The photosensitizer goes to an excited state, which can then transfer the energy to oxygen, generating oxygen free radicals. This causes tumor destruction through direct cell kill, disruption of the vascular supply to the tumor and stimulation of an immune response.

Currently, the most commonly used photosensitizers are those derived from haematoporphyrin, such as Photofrin II. Generally, the optimal ratio of Photofrin is reached 48 hours after the initial administration with a tumor-to-normal tissue ratio of approximately 2:1 (38). Photofrin is activated by a laser-generated light with a wavelength of 630 nm. Photofrin can be used to treat to a depth of a few millimeters up to a centimeter based on the depth the 630 nm light penetrates the tissue and the absorptive properties of the tissue being treated. Because the sun has the complete spectrum of wavelengths of light, a major side effect of photosensitizers is sensitivity to natural sunlight that can last for up to 6 weeks after treatment. A second photosensitizer, 5-aminolevulinic acid (ALA) causes an increase in protoporphyrin IX, the immediate precursor to heme, via a negative feedback loop. Advantages of using ALA is that the photosensitivity only lasts a few days and it preferentially accumulates in the mucosa, resulting in a shallower treatment depth, which may limit complications. However, the shallower treatment depth also limits its utility in tumors that extend beyond 2 mm in depth. ALA is also less specific for tumor tissue and has other systemic side effects, such as nausea, vomiting and hypotension, and may cause abnormal liver function tests. Preclinical trials with ALA have been disappointing, largely due to the poor depth of penetration (39).

PDT is currently approved for a variety of conditions worldwide. Approvals for specific disease processes and sites are related to specific photosensitizing drugs.

There have been several studies addressing the effectiveness of PDT in unresectable cholangiocarcinoma. A pilot study from the Mayo Clinic studied the use of PDT in eight patients with unresectable cholangiocarcinoma. A mean of 2.4 treatments were given per patient, and biliary stents were placed after PDT (40). There was an improvement in bilirubin levels, from a mean initial value of 7.7 mg/dl prior to treatment to 1.1 mg/dl prior to the third and fourth PDT treatments. However, elevated bilirubin levels were considered a contraindication for further PDT treatment, and only three patients had a third and a four treatment. Median survival from the first PDT treatment was 276 days.

Ortner et al. also published a pilot study of nine patients with unresectable cholangiocarcinomas treated with PDT (41). They found a significant reduction in serum bilirubin levels, from 318 to 103 μmol/L (p < 0.0039), and an improvement in performance status. Median survival was 439 days. This was followed by a randomized study of patients with unresectable cholangiocarcinomas (53). Patients with unresectable, histologically confirmed cholangiocarcinomas were divided randomly into two groups, one in which patients were stented followed by PDT (n = 20) and the second group undergoing stenting alone (n = 19). The study also included data on patients who either refused to consent for the study or those who did not meet the selection criteria, who were treated with stenting followed by PDT (n = 31). Median survival time in the stenting followed by PDT group was 493 days and in the stenting-alone group, 98 days (p < 0.0001). PDT also appeared to improve cholestasis and quality of life. Patients in the non-randomized group that received PDT after stenting tended to have worse functional status compared with the randomized patients; however, they still had improved overall survival compared with patients who had stenting alone, with a median survival of 426, compared with 98 days (p < 0.0001), and were similar to patients treated in the randomized PDT group (p > 0.05). However, there were more fatalities associated with infection in the PDT group (n = 6) versus the stenting-alone group (n = 2). Possible explanations for the large difference in median survival between the Mayo study and the Ortner studies include different inclusion criteria and the use of a more flexible scope in Ortner's studies, which allowed treatment of multiple hepatic branches.

A second randomized trial studied PDT in 32 patients with unresectable cholangiocarcinoma (43). Patients were randomized to either placement of endoprosthesis followed by PDT vs. endoprosthesis placement alone. Median survival in patients with endoprosthesis placement and PDT was 21 months, versus 7 months in those with endoprosthesis alone (p = 0.0109). This is slightly longer than in Ortner studies; however, the Karnofsky performance statuses were higher and the initial bilirubin levels were lower in patients in the present study compared with Ortner's study. There was improvement in bilirubin levels after PDT and stenting, which appears superior to stenting alone. In this study, there was also an increase in infectious complication, with 4 of 16 patients in the PDT group having infectious complications and 1 of 16 in the control, which trended toward significance (p = 0.166); however, there were no deaths related to cholangitis. After the first eight patients were treated with PDT, antibiotic coverage was increased to 10 days and there were no further infectious complications. Nine of sixteen patients underwent two treatments with PDT and one had three treatments.

A third study examining PDT in uresectable cholangiocarcinoma now has 5-year data available (44, 45). In this study, 23 unresectable patients were treated with one or two treatments of PDT followed by stent placement. All patients had Bismuth type III or IV tumors, and all were pathologically confirmed. Median survival was 9.3 months in all patients and 11.2 months in those without metastasis. Bilirubin levels were well controlled after treatment. All patients died of either progression of disease (74%, n = 17) or infectious causes (26%) (cholangitis [n = 4], septic shock [n = 1], appendicitis/peritonitis [n = 1]).

These studies of PDT treatment of unresectable cholangiocarcinoma suggest that PDT effectively palliates symptoms and appears to improve survival. However, there also appears to be an increased risk of infection, and prophylactic antibiotics may be warranted both during and after treatment with PDT. A few studies have addressed the use of PDT in the adjuvant and neoadjuvant setting.

A recent study from Japan investigated eight patients treated with adjuvant PDT after surgery (46).

None of the patients had had previous chemotherapy or radiation therapy, and all underwent en bloc resection with nodal dissection. Five patients had to be reresected, and six had positive margins at the hepatic bile duct stump. Results of treatment were assessed using cholangioscope and intraductal ultrasound, which showed ductal mucosal degeneration 1 day after PDT and fibrotic scar formation along the duct on day seven after PDT. One of the eight patients died at 2 months due to causes unrelated to their cholangiocarcinoma. Two patients were alive with recurrence at 9 and 33 months and four are alive without recurrence at 6, 12, 12 and 17 months.

A study conducted in Germany examined neoadjuvant PDT in seven patients (47). Patients were treated with one or two sessions of PDT followed by stent placement. One patient had Bismuth-Corlette stage II disease, with the rest of the patients being either stage III or IV. The patients then underwent en bloc resection, and all seven had R0 resections. Initially, after treatment with PDT, bilirubin levels were found to increase, but within 3 to 7 days there was a statistically significant decrease. Of the seven patients, two died due to cholangiocarcinoma at 9 and 36 months. The remaining five patients were alive at last follow-up, with survivals of 12, 15, 16, 29 and 40 months.

A recent large study examined 184 resectable and unresectable patients with cholangiocarcinoma (48). Unresectable patients underwent either PDT followed by stenting (n = 68) or stenting alone (n = 56). Sixty patients were surgically resectable. Overall survival for resected patients was 69%, 30% and 22% at 1, 3 and 5 years. R0, R1 and R2 resections resulted in 5-year survivals of 27%, 10% and 0%, respectively. Multivariant analysis demonstrated that R0 resection (p < 0.01) and tumor grade (p < 0.05) were significantly associated with survival. Unresectable patients treated with PDT and stenting had significantly improved median survival (12 versus 6.4 months; p < 0.01), lower bilirubin levels (p < 0.05) and improved Karnofsky performance status (p < 0.01) compared with patients treated with stenting alone. Median survival after PDT and stenting was comparable to median survival after R1 and R2 resections.

REFERENCES

1. Vauthey JN and Blumgart LH. Recent advances in the management of cholangiocarcinomas. Semin Liver Dis, 1994; 14: 109–114.

2. Jemal A, Siegel R, Ward E, et al. Cancer statistics, 2006. CA Cancer J Clin, 2006; 56: 106–130.

3. Patel T. Increasing incidence and mortality of primary intrahepatic cholangiocarcinoma in the United States. Hepatology, 2001; 33: 1353–1357.

4. Tompkins RK, Thomas D, Wile A, et al. Prognostic factors in bile duct carcinoma: Analysis of 96 cases. Ann Surg, 1981; 194: 447–457.

5. Erickson BA and Nag S. Biliary tree malignancies. J Surg Oncol, 1998; 67: 203–210.

6. Andersen JR, Sorensen SM, Kruse A, et al. Randomised trial of endoscopic endoprosthesis versus operative bypass in malignant obstructive jaundice. Gut, 1989; 30: 1132–1135.

7. Freeman ML and Overby C. Selective MRCP and CT-targeted drainage of malignant hilar biliary obstruction with self-expanding metallic stents. Gastrointest Endosc, 2003; 58: 41–49.

8. Cheng JL, Bruno MJ, Bergman JJ, et al. Endoscopic palliation of patients with biliary obstruction caused by nonresectable hilar cholangiocarcinoma: Efficacy of self-expandable metallic wallstents. Gastrointest Endosc, 2002; 56: 33–39.

9. Kawamoto H, Ishii Y, Nakagawa M, et al. Analysis of long-term survivors with expandable metallic stent inserted for malignant biliary stenosis. J Hepatobiliary Pancreat Surg, 2003; 10: 95–100.

10. Conroy RM, Shahbazian AA, Edwards KC, et al. A new method for treating carcinomatous biliary obstruction with intracatheter radium. Cancer, 1982; 49: 1321–1327.

11. Ishii H, Furuse J, Nagase M, et al. Relief of jaundice by external beam radiotherapy and intraluminal brachytherapy in patients with extrahepatic cholangiocarcinoma: Results without stenting. Hepatogastroenterology, 2004; 51: 954–957.

12. Bowling TE, Galbraith SM, Hatfield AR, et al. A retrospective comparison of endoscopic stenting alone with stenting and radiotherapy in non-resectable cholangiocarcinoma. Gut, 1996; 39: 852–855.

13. Chan SY, Poon RT, Ng KK, et al. Long-term survival after intraluminal brachytherapy for inoperable hilar cholangiocarcinoma: A case report. World J Gastroenterol, 2005; 11: 3161–3164.

14. Takamura A, Saito H, Kamada T, et al. Intraluminal low-dose-rate ^{192}Ir brachytherapy combined with external beam radiotherapy and biliary stenting for unresectable extrahepatic bile duct carcinoma. Int J Radiat Oncol Biol Phys, 2003; 57: 1357–1365.

15. Schoenthaler R, Phillips TL, Castro J, et al. Carcinoma of the extrahepatic bile ducts. The University of California at San Francisco experience. Ann Surg, 1994; 219: 267–274.

16. Pilepich M. (Semin ed.), Hepatic and Biliary Cancer. New York: Marcel Dekker; 1987.

17. Smoron GL. Radiation therapy of carcinoma of gallbladder and biliary tract. Cancer, 1977; 40: 1422–1424.

18. Alden ME and Mohiuddin M. The impact of radiation dose in combined external beam and intraluminal Ir-192 brachytherapy for bile duct cancer. Int J Radiat Oncol Biol Phys, 1994; 28: 945–951.

19. Kamada T, Saitou H, Takamura A, et al. The role of radiotherapy in the management of extrahepatic bile duct cancer: An analysis of 145 consecutive patients treated with intraluminal and/or external beam radiotherapy. Int J Radiat Oncol Biol Phys, 1996; 34: 767–774.

20. Molt P, Hopfan S, Watson RC, et al. Intraluminal radiation therapy in the management of malignant biliary obstruction. Cancer, 1986; 57: 536–544.

21. Buskirk SJ, Gunderson LL, Schild SE, et al. Analysis of failure after curative irradiation of extrahepatic bile duct carcinoma. Ann Surg, 1992; 215: 125–131.

22. Fields JN and Emami B. Carcinoma of the extrahepatic biliary system – results of primary and adjuvant radiotherapy. Int J Radiat Oncol Biol Phys, 1987; 13: 331–338.

23. Gonzalez Gonzalez D, Gouma DJ, Rauws EA, et al. Role of radiotherapy, in particular intraluminal brachytherapy, in the treatment of proximal bile duct carcinoma. Ann Oncol, 1999; 10 Suppl 4: 215–220.

24. Deodato F, Clemente G, Mattiucci GC, et al. Chemoradiation and brachytherapy in biliary tract carcinoma: Long-term results. Int J Radiat Oncol Biol Phys, 2006; 64: 483–488.

25. Dvorak J, Jandik P, Melichar B, et al. Intraluminal high dose rate brachytherapy in the treatment of bile duct and gallbladder carcinomas. Hepatogastroenterology, 2002; 49: 916–917.

26. Kocak Z, Ozkan H, Adli M, et al. Intraluminal brachytherapy with metallic stenting in the palliative treatment of malignant obstruction of the bile duct. Radiat Med, 2005; 23: 200–207.

27. Qian XJ, Zhai RY, Dai DK, et al. Treatment of malignant biliary obstruction by combined percutaneous transhepatic biliary drainage with local tumor treatment. World J Gastroenterol, 2006; 12: 331–335.

28. Chen Y, Wang XL, Yan ZP, et al. HDR-192Ir intraluminal brachytherapy in treatment of malignant obstructive jaundice. World J Gastroenterol, 2004; 10: 3506–3510.

29. Bruha R, Petrtyl J, Kubecova M, et al. Intraluminal brachytherapy and self-expandable stents in nonresectable biliary malignancies – the question of long-term palliation. Hepatogastroenterology, 2001; 48: 631–637.

30. Shin HS, Seong J, Kim WC, et al. Combination of external beam irradiation and high-dose-rate intraluminal brachytherapy for inoperable carcinoma of the extrahepatic bile ducts. Int J Radiat Oncol Biol Phys, 2003; 57: 105–112.

31. Fritz P, Brambs HJ, Schraube P, et al. Combined external beam radiotherapy and intraluminal high dose rate brachytherapy on bile duct carcinomas. Int J Radiat Oncol Biol Phys, 1994; 29: 855–861.

32. Lu JJ, Bains YS, Abdel-Wahab M, et al. High-dose-rate remote afterloading intracavitary brachytherapy for the treatment of extrahepatic biliary duct carcinoma. Cancer J, 2002; 8: 74–78.

33. Nomura M, Yamakado K, Nomoto Y, et al. Clinical efficacy of brachytherapy combined with external-beam radiotherapy and repeated arterial infusion chemotherapy in patients with unresectable extrahepatic bile duct cancer. Int J Oncol, 2002; 20: 325–331.

34. Urban MS, Siegel JH, Pavlou W, et al. Treatment of malignant biliary obstruction with a high-dose rate remote afterloading device using a 10 F nasobiliary tube. Gastrointest Endosc, 1990; 36: 292–296.

35. Simmons DT, Baron TH, Petersen BT, et al. A novel endoscopic approach to brachytherapy in the management of hilar cholangiocarcinoma. Am J Gastroenterol, 2006; 101: 1792–1796.

36. Dvorak J, Petera J, Papik Z, et al. Transduodenal intraluminal high dose rate brachytherapy in the treatment of carcinomas of the subhepatic region. Hepatogastroenterology, 2002; 49: 1045–1047.

37. Mayo-Smith WW, Dawson SL, Mauceri T, et al. Attenuation effects of biliary endoprostheses on therapeutic radiation. Radiology, 1996; 199: 571–572.

38. Nishioka NS. Drug, light, and oxygen: A dynamic combination in the clinic. Gastroenterology, 1998; 114: 604–606.

39. Ortner MA. Photodynamic therapy in cholangiocarcinomas. Best Pract Res Clin Gastroenterol, 2004; 18: 147–154.

40. Harewood GC, Baron TH, Rumalla A, et al. Pilot study to assess patient outcomes following endoscopic application of photodynamic therapy for advanced cholangiocarcinoma. J Gastroenterol Hepatol, 2005; 20: 415–420.

41. Ortner MA, Liebetruth J, Schreiber S, et al. Photodynamic therapy of nonresectable cholangiocarcinoma. Gastroenterology, 1998; 114: 536–542.

42. Ortner ME, Caca K, Berr F, et al. Successful photodynamic therapy for nonresectable cholangiocarcinoma: A randomized prospective study. Gastroenterology, 2003; 125: 1355–1363.

43. Zoepf T, Jakobs R, Arnold JC, et al. Palliation of nonresectable bile duct cancer: Improved survival after photodynamic therapy. Am J Gastroenterol, 2005; 100: 2426–2430.

44. Berr F, Wiedmann M, Tannapfel A, et al. Photodynamic therapy for advanced bile duct cancer: Evidence for improved palliation and extended survival. Hepatology, 2000; 31: 291–298.

45. Wiedmann M, Berr F, Schiefke I, et al. Photodynamic therapy in patients with non-resectable hilar cholangiocarcinoma: 5-year follow-up of a prospective phase II study. Gastrointest Endosc, 2004; 60: 68–75.

46. Nanashima A, Yamaguchi H, Shibasaki S, et al. Adjuvant photodynamic therapy for bile duct carcinoma after surgery: A preliminary study. J Gastroenterol, 2004; 39: 1095–1101.

47. Wiedmann M, Caca K, Berr F, et al. Neoadjuvant photodynamic therapy as a new approach to treating hilar cholangiocarcinoma: A phase II pilot study. Cancer, 2003; 97: 2783–2790.

48. Witzigmann H, Berr F, Ringel U, et al. Surgical and palliative management and outcome in 184 patients with hilar cholangiocarcinoma: Palliative photodynamic therapy plus stenting is comparable to R1/R2 resection. Ann Surg, 2006; 244: 230–239.

Chapter 31

EXTRAHEPATIC BILIARY CANCER/BILIARY DRAINAGE

Tarun Sabharwal

Manpreet Singh Gulati

Andy Adam

In the early 1970s, Molnar and Stockum introduced nonsurgical biliary intervention in the form of percutaneous transhepatic biliary drainage (PTBD) (1). Percutaneous transhepatic cholangiography (PTC) had been performed for several years prior to this, but therapeutic biliary interventions had been outside the radiologists' domain. In the past 30 years, improved diagnostic imaging techniques and significant developments in interventional radiology and experience gained by clinical trials have revolutionized and clearly defined the role of percutaneous biliary interventions.

The role of PTC has progressively diminished in the face of noninvasive imaging techniques such as ultrasonography (US), three-dimensional (3D) computer tomography and magnetic resonance cholangiography (MRC). Endoscopic retrograde cholangiography has further reduced its diagnostic role in the recent years. PTC is now reserved only for problematic cases and as an evaluation immediately prior to percutaneous intervention.

PTBD, which was initially proposed as a routine preoperative measure for those with severe obstructive jaundice, is now more of a palliative procedure in patients with inoperable malignant obstruction. This has been brought about by improved preoperative patient preparation, good antibiotic therapy, improved surgical techniques and easy availability of endoscopic biliary drainage expertise. One of the most important recent advances has been the introduction of self-expanding metallic stents for use in malignant obstructions.

In this chapter, we discuss all of the aforementioned percutaneous interventional radiological techniques, their indications and the other issues involved.

PALLIATIVE BILIARY DRAINAGE FOR MALIGNANT STRICTURES

In clinical gastrointestinal practice, malignant biliary obstruction is not an infrequent occurrence. The most important causes of malignant biliary obstruction include carcinoma of the head of the pancreas and ampulla, cholangiocarcinoma, metastatic hilar and peripancreatic adenopathy, carcinoma of the gallbladder (which frequently involves the bile ducts at the hepatic hilum) and carcinoma of the duodenum.

Percutaneous drainage of the biliary tract is indicated for the relief of biliary obstruction, as biliary obstruction is potentially fatal because of the adverse pathological effects, including depressed immunity, impaired phagocytic activity, reduced Kupffer cell function and paucity of bile salts reaching the gut, with consequent endotoxemia, septicemia and renal failure. The majority of malignant hepatic tumors, such as carcinoma of the gallbladder, carcinoma of the pancreas and cholangiocarcinoma, are unresectable (2, 3), and only 20% to 30% of these tumors are resectable at the time of diagnosis (2, 4). Palliation of the malignant obstruction relieves the patient of itching and jaundice, reduces the risk of infection and septicemia and generally improves the quality of life. Surgical, endoscopic and interventional radiological percutaneous techniques are available for palliation. Non-surgical techniques are preferred because they are associated with lower morbidity and mortality.

Endoscopic insertion of biliary endoprostheses is performed more often than percutaneous drainage. This is often because most patients undergo endoscopic retrograde cholangiopancreaticogram (ERCP) during the diagnostic work-up for obstructive jaundice. If ERCP demonstrates a malignant stricture, an endoprosthesis can be inserted immediately after cholangiography. In patients with strictures below the hilum of the liver, endoscopic drainage is less invasive than percutaneous biliary drainage (PBD), has reduced complications and avoids the discomfort of a percutaneous biliary catheter.

The majority of strictures of the mid- and lower common bile ducts, which are mainly due to carcinoma of the head of the pancreas, can be drained effectively by the endoscopic approach (5). Percutaneous drainage is performed when the stricture cannot be crossed endoscopically. Malignant strictures at the liver hilum are difficult to treat effectively endoscopically and are best dealt with by interventional radiological techniques (6). Hilar lesions may cause obstruction of a single lobe or may cause atrophy of a lobe and the radiologist is better able than the endoscopist to choose the appropriate liver lobe for drainage. If a hilar lesion obstructs both the right and the left hepatic ducts, it is not necessary to drain both lobes if only ducts of one lobe are demonstrated by the PTC. The lobar ducts outlined by the PTC should be drained; the unopacified lobe may be left undrained. Unilateral drainage usually relieves jaundice and pruritus. Drainage of the other side is required only in the minority of patients who develop cholangitis in the undrained lobe or if drainage of only one lobe does not relieve the jaundice. If the initial cholangiogram shows communication between the right and left sides of the liver in a patient with a hilar lesion, both lobes should be drained, as there is a significant likelihood of infection of the contralateral lobe if unilateral drainage is performed.

In clinical practice, a cohesive team consisting of a gastroenterologist, a surgeon, an oncologist and an interventional radiologist should participate in a multi-disciplinary approach to the management of the patient before treatment is initiated.

ROLE OF IMAGING BEFORE PALLIATIVE BILIARY DRAINAGE

Management of malignant biliary obstruction depends on the resectability of the underlying tumor. Therefore, patients should undergo accurate staging following the diagnosis. One of the important goals of preoperative imaging is to identify vascular invasion by the tumor at the hepatic hilum. Hitherto, angiography was used to identify the vascular anatomy prior to surgery in carcinoma of the gallbladder (7) and hilar cholangiocarcinoma (8–10). Recently, dual-phase helical CT has been used to evaluate vascular invasion in hilar tumors (11, 12). As a single modality, it cannot only detect the malignancy but also has the potential of comprehensively evaluating each patient for criteria of unresectability (2).

High-quality 3D reconstruction images made possible by helical CT are uniquely suitable for the depiction of the complex anatomy of the biliary tract. 3D reconstructions can be produced successfully by taking advantage of the negative contrast effect of low-attenuation bile in the dilated ducts relative to the adjacent enhanced liver (13). 3D CT cholangiography with minimum intensity projection can determine the level and cause of biliary obstruction (14, 15). With CT, not only is the resectability of the tumor better defined (2) but also the identification of variant ductal anatomy is possible. Additionally, it helps in choosing the appropriate duct for drainage (Figure 31.1).

MRI performs as well as CT for direct spread of the tumor to the liver and hepatic metastases. Visualization of intrahepatic bile ducts on MRI depends on the size of the ducts, concentration of bile, pulse sequence used, motion artifact and periportal high signal. CT and US are more sensitive than MRI for detecting intrahepatic bile duct dilatation. The advent of magnetic resonance cholangio-pancreaticography (MRCP) has been a very useful development for

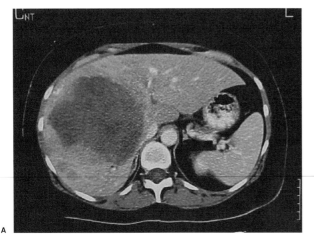

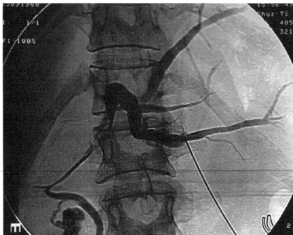

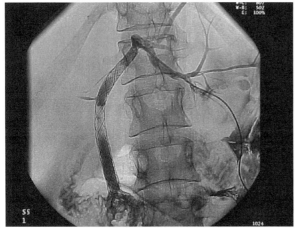

FIGURE 31.1. (A) CT scan shows large right-sided tumor and therefore the left lobe was chosen for PTC. (B) Long stricture of left common hepatic duct. (C) Adequate drainage of liver following stenting left common hepatic duct.

imaging of biliary disease (16–18). MRCP is highly accurate for defining extent of ductal involvement in patients with malignant hilar and perihilar obstruction (19). Ductal dilatation, strictures and anatomical variation are well depicted by this technique, and this ability makes this modality well suited for planning the optimal therapeutic approach for patients with biliary obstruction.

PERCUTANEOUS INTERVENTION IN MALIGNANT BILIARY OBSTRUCTION

Biliary Cytology and Biopsy Procedures

In suspected malignant biliary obstructions, the percutaneous tract can be used for cytologic or histologic confirmation. Bile collected from the external drainage bag is more likely to yield positive cytology than fluid obtained at PTC alone. Cytologic study is positive in roughly 50% of the patients with cholangiocarcinoma, although the reported sensitivity varies widely. The positive cytology rate is lower for primary pancreatic tumors.

If cytology is negative, percutaneous biopsy can be done by cholangiographic or US guidance. Alternatively, the cholangiographic tract could also be used to obtain brushings or biopsy using forceps, bioptome, myocardial biopsy needle (Figure 31.2) or a needle biopsy through a transhepatic sheath.

PREOPERATIVE PERCUTANEOUS TRANSHEPATIC BILIARY DRAINAGE

The practice of PTBD prior to surgery is controversial and is generally not recommended. It has not been shown to decrease surgical morbidity or mortality. It is, however, advocated by some surgeons in select situations before curative resection, to correct metabolic derangements produced by biliary obstruction and decrease the complications of biliary surgery in the jaundiced patient. Either internal or external biliary drainage catheters or, more preferably, plastic stents are inserted 2 to 6 weeks prior to elective surgery. Other surgeons may advise preoperative PTBD because the biliary catheters are easy to locate

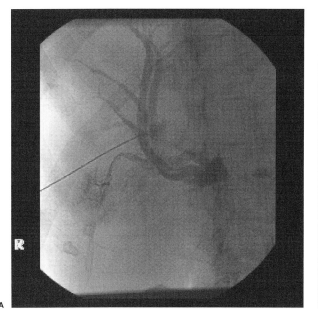

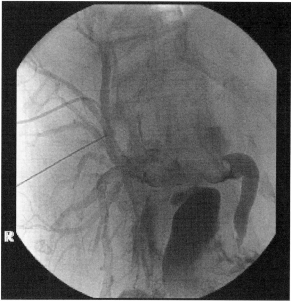

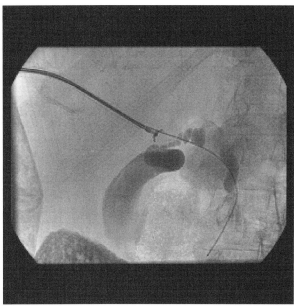

FIGURE 31.2.   Seventy-year-old patient with proximal biliary obstruction but no mass lesion seen on US or CT. (A) PTC image with ductal occlusion. (B) PTC image showing intraductal filling defect. (C) Myocardial biopsy needle used via PTC route and through 7F sheath. Biopsy result was highly suggestive of cholangiocarcinoma.

at surgery, particularly during difficult dissections of lesions at the hepatic hilum (6).

PALLIATION OF MALIGNANT BILIARY OBSTRUCTION USING PTBD

PTBD is now standard management for patients with incurable malignant biliary obstruction, particularly in certain specific situations.

Indications for PTBD

- To treat cholangitis secondary to obstruction.

- To treat symptomatic obstructive jaundice when an endoscopic retrograde approach fails or is not possible (as discussed earlier).

- Preoperative decompression and stent placement to assist in surgical manipulation (controversial).

- To gain access to the biliary system to perform transhepatic brachytherapy for cholangiocarcinoma.

Relative Contraindications for PTBD

- Incorrectable bleeding diathesis.

- Large volume of ascites (relative; procedure may be difficult, with potential for bile peritonitis. Consider a left-sided approach or insert an ascitic drain).

- Segmental isolated intrahepatic obstructions that do not cause significant symptoms should not be drained. Bacterial contamination usually occurs when an isolated ductal system is accessed. As a consequence of this contamination, it is often impossible to withdraw drainage even if the drainage is not required clinically. Thus, a patient could be left with a permanent, unwanted and potentially problematic drainage catheter.

- Totally uncooperative patient (may require general anesthesia or heavy conscious sedation).

Preparation for PTBD

Blood Tests

Coagulation profile: The international normalized ratio (INR) should be less than 1.5. Vitamin K, fresh-frozen plasma and platelets (as needed) should be administered to correct any coagulopathy.

Liver function tests: Serum bilirubin and alkaline phosphatase levels should be checked to obtain baseline values (an elevated alkaline phosphatase level, even in the setting of a near-normal bilirubin, indicates a low-grade obstruction).

Baseline renal function: Blood urea and creatinine should be checked, especially before administering preprocedure nephrotoxic antibiotics.

Informed Consent

The procedure should be explained completely to the patient, outlining the risks with specific attention to sepsis and bleeding.

Prophylactic Antibiotics

Appropriate antibiotics are administered 1 to 2 hours before the procedure to avoid biliary sepsis. The spectrum of antibiotic coverage must include both gram-positive and gram-negative organisms, and therefore a combination of antibiotics as appropriate, is needed. The antibiotics should be continued for 24 to 72 hours following the procedure. A regular appraisal should be done to identify the prevalent infectious organisms and their drug resistance pattern in the local setting.

Sedation/Analgesia

Biliary procedures are most often performed with the patient under conscious sedation (midazolam and fentanyl) with liberal infiltration of local anesthetic at the site and up to the capsule of the liver. Use of longer-acting local anesthetics may help provide long post-procedure pain relief. Intercostal blocks have also

been used, and in some cases general anesthetic is required.

Skin Preparation

It is best to prepare a wide area, which will permit access to the biliary system from the left and right sides, as needed.

Procedure

Technical Approach: Entry from Right or Left Side

According to the Bismuth classification system (20): a type 1 obstruction occurs distal to the confluence of the right and left hepatic ducts (primary confluence); type 2 involves the primary confluence but not the secondary confluence; type 3 involves the primary confluence and, additionally, either right (3a) or left (3b) secondary confluence; and type 4 involves the secondary confluence of both the right and left hepatic ducts. Whether to use a right- or left-sided approach must be decided on a case-by-case basis. Extensive right-sided disease with sparing of the left side makes the decision easy (left-approach) (Figure 31.1), as does a patient with an atrophic left lobe (right approach).

In the case of a type 1 lesion, there are two advantages in approaching from the right side (especially right anterior): the angle of approach to the point of obstruction is 90° or greater, making for easy catheter insertion, and the radiologist's hands are well away from the primary X-ray beam. One needs to be careful of the pleural reflection, however, to avoid breaching the pleural space. The advantage of using the left-sided approach is that US can be utilized for the initial puncture, avoids the accidental breach of pleural space and also the patient has less catheter-related discomfort (the right intercostal approach being more painful). This approach is also preferable when there is ascites. The patient relatively easily manages the catheter when it exits out from the midline, rather than the mid-axillary line. The operator needs to ensure that the catheter enters the medial rather than the lateral ducts. The lateral ducts are more posterior and therefore the catheter pathway will be directed posteriorly and then anteriorly, thus affecting the pushability, while negotiating the more distal obstruction.

When the obstruction is at the confluence, the situation is more complex. It is important to be aware of the anatomy of the right and left hepatic ducts. The right hepatic duct is short, unlike the left, which is 2 to 3 cm long until its bifurcation into the segmental ducts. Thus, a catheter placed in the right system initially drains a greater part of the liver because of the size difference between the lobes. However, once the tumor grows, the situation reverses because the catheter placed in the right side now drains only one segment, whereas the left-sided catheter drains the entire left lobe. Thus, for type 2 lesions, either the right anterior system or the left system is chosen (left is chosen if the left lobe of the liver is of good size). For type 3a lesions, if there is extensive involvement of the right secondary confluence, we do either a single left-sided drainage or, ideally, combine it with right anterior or posterior drainage (keeping in mind the cost of the procedure, life expectancy and the subjective assessment of the amount of liver to be drained as seen on CT). It has been shown that drainage of 25% of the liver volume using a single catheter/endoprosthesis may be sufficient (21). However, an endoscopic study has shown that draining both lobes in patients with hilar lesions prolongs life expectancy (22). For type 3b lesions, the approach is similar. For type 4 lesions, one should use at least two drains. Lobes and segments that are atrophic are excluded from the proposed drainage plan. A duct suspected to be already infected or contaminated due to the procedure is always drained. Another approach in type 4 lesions is to perform T (chi-configuration) stenting (Figure 31.3), which allows drainage of the entire major segmental ducts (23). One stent extends from the left duct through the hilar stricture to the right anterior duct; the other stent is placed across the right posterior segmental duct through the hilar stricture into the common bile duct or transpapillary duodenum. Stent deployment should be performed simultaneously. Ultimately, the two stents form a chi-shaped configuration (23).

Technique

External Drainage

A PTC is performed prior to biliary drainage to define the biliary anatomy. A 22-gauge needle is inserted into the liver immediately anterior to the mid-axillary line and advanced horizontally to the lateral border of the vertebral column. (Figure 31.4) Dilated ducts are located by withdrawing the needle and injecting contrast medium or aspirating until bile is obtained. The aspiration method has the advantage of avoiding

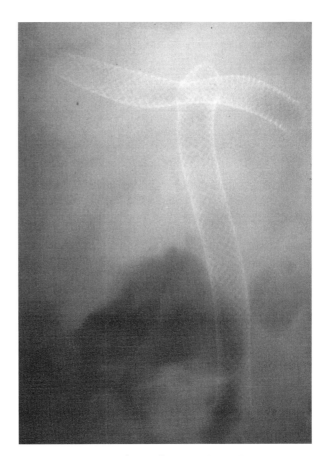

FIGURE 31.3. T (chi-configuration) stenting.

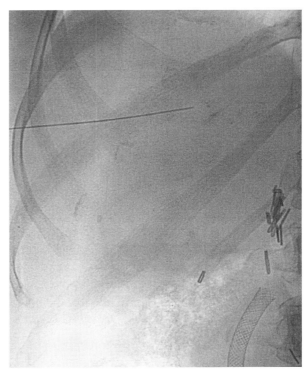

FIGURE 31.4. PTC with 22-gauge needle placed immediately anterior to mid-axillary line and advanced horizontally to the lateral border of the vertebral column.

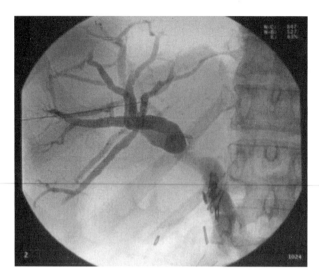

FIGURE 31.5. Undiluted contrast medium injected until obstructed biliary system is outlined.

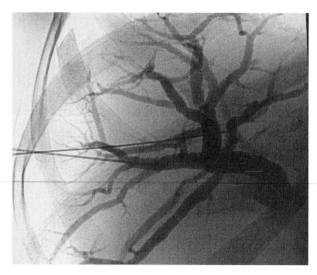

FIGURE 31.6. Second puncture of a more peripheral and better-angled duct was performed.

a large stain of parenchymal contrast if several passes are required. If the ducts are not dilated, the aspiration method is less effective, and the injection method should be used. Some radiologists puncture the bile ducts using ultrasound guidance. Once a duct has been located, undiluted contrast medium is injected until the obstructed biliary system is outlined (Figure 31.5). A tilting table is helpful to convey contrast to the lower common bile duct. In many patients with obstruction of the common bile duct, flow of contrast medium may appear to stop immediately below the hilum, creating a false impression of hilar obstruction; tilting the fluoroscopy table is the best way of demonstrating the lower common bile duct (CBD) in such cases.

Although it may be possible to use the duct catheterized by the PTC needle for drainage, the duct is usually at an angle to the needle track, which causes difficulty in catheter manipulations, or is close to the liver hilum, which increases the risk of complications. In most cases, it is best to perform a second, peripheral puncture of a suitable duct with a horizontal course (Figure 31.6). Lateral screening using a C-arm is very helpful, although not essential, for localization of the duct in the anterior-posterior plane.

Although bile duct catheterization can be achieved with standard 18-gauge needles and guidewires, most radiologists use one of several minimally invasive access sets such as the Accustick set (Meditech, Boston Scientific Corp., MA) (Figure 31.7) or the Neff set (William Cook, Europe) for this purpose. These systems allow the radiologist to drain the biliary tree using an initial puncture with a 21- or 22-gauge

needle followed by sequential changes of increasingly larger guidewires and catheters (9). The use of such systems enables small ducts to be selected for drainage and probably reduces the risk of complications such as hemobilia and bile leakage. The final result of either method is the placement of a catheter with several side holes deep in the biliary tree. At this stage, the

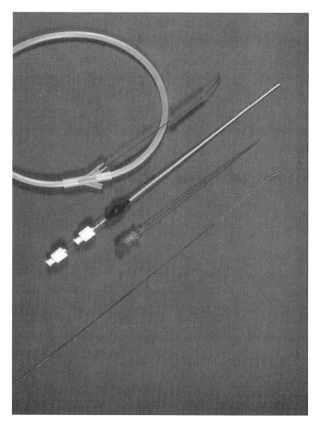

FIGURE 31.7. Minimally invasive access set (Accustick, Boston Scientific). See Color Plate 30.

tip of the catheter lies above the obstructing lesion, which is referred to as external biliary drainage. The catheter is connected to a gravity drainage bag and the tube is secured to the skin to prevent inadvertent removal.

Most radiologists puncture the ducts in the right lobe for PBD. This is partly historical, although right-sided drainage keeps the operator's hands out of the beam and achieves drainage of a larger volume of liver when there is obstruction at the liver hilum. However, left biliary drainage is not technically difficult. The left-sided ducts can be punctured easily using ultra-sound guidance, which reduces radiation to patient and operator. In addition, left biliary catheters are usually more comfortable for patients than right biliary catheters, mainly because they do not traverse the intercostal space.

External-internal Drainage

External-internal drainage refers to percutaneous catheter drainage of the bile ducts with the catheter passed through the stricture so that side-holes are placed above and below the obstructing lesion. This offers increased stability compared with external drainage and also allows drainage of bile into the duodenum with the advantages of improved fluid and electrolyte balance. For these reasons, most radiologists aim for internal-external drainage if possible at the time of initial PBD. Most strictures can be catheterized with modern angled-tip catheters and hydrophilic guidewires. Occasionally, a stricture is so tight that it cannot be traversed. In this situation, an external catheter should be inserted. After a few days of external drainage, a channel through the stricture usually appears due to resolution of tissue edema, which can be negotiated by the radiologist at a second session.

Some patients are managed for long periods of time with internal-external catheters. However, this type of biliary drainage is associated with bile leaks, infection, patient discomfort and psychological problems connected with catheters protruding through the skin. If possible, internal-external catheters should be exchanged for endoprostheses.

Internal Drainage

Endoprostheses

Endoprostheses enable internal drainage of bile across the obstructing lesion and avoid the need for

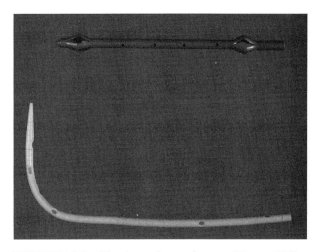

FIGURE 31.8. Plastic endoprostheses. (*Top* – Miller stent, Cook, with double mushroom either end; *bottom*, the Carey-Coons stent, Boston Scientific.)

external catheters. There are two types of endoprostheses available for use in the biliary tract – plastic and metallic. Both types may be inserted using either the percutaneous or endoscopic route.

Plastic endoprostheses consist of plastic or Teflon hollow tubes 8 to 14 cm long with end-holes (e.g., Carey-Coons, Boston Scientific Corp., Galway, Ireland) and, in some cases, side-holes (Cook prosthesis, W. Cook, Europe) (Figure 31.8) to allow drainage of bile from above a stricture to the duodenum. The caliber of plastic stents varies from 8 to 12F. Ideally, the largest size should always be used to provide optimal biliary drainage and reduce problems of occlusion by bile encrustation. As a result, a relatively large transhepatic track is required for percutaneous insertion of most plastic endoprostheses. Because of the increased risk of pain, bleeding and perihepatic bile leakage, which may be caused by the creation of a 12F hole in the liver, insertion of plastic endoprostheses is generally carried out as a two-stage procedure. PBD is performed and an 8F biliary drainage catheter is inserted. After a few days, the patient is brought back to the interventional radiology suite and the biliary catheter is removed over a guidewire. The transhepatic track is dilated from 8F to 12F followed by insertion of the plastic endoprosthesis across the stricture so that the upper end is above the stricture and the lower end projects through the ampulla into the duodenum. It is usual to insert a temporary external biliary catheter, which is removed 24 hours later, after check cholangiography (Figure 31.9).

Self-expanding metallic endoprostheses are metallic springs 7 to 10 cm long, which are introduced into

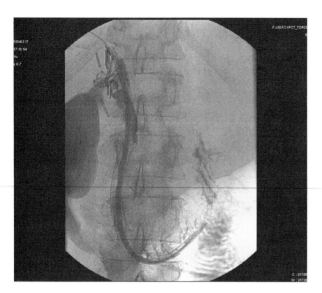

FIGURE 31.9. Check cholangiography shows satisfactory position of Carey-Coons stent with proximal end lying above stricture and distal end projects through the ampulla into the duodenum.

the bile ducts in a compressed state and expand to a much larger diameter (8 to 12 mm) when the stents are released from their introducer (Figure 31.10). The Wallstent endoprosthesis (Boston Scientific Corp.) is the most common stent used in the biliary tract. The main advantage of metallic stents is that they achieve a much larger diameter than plastic stents when deployed, which allows more efficient biliary drainage. In addition, because they are inserted in a compressed state, the transhepatic track required for metallic stent insertion is generally smaller (5F to 7F) than for plastic stents (10F to 12F). This means that metallic stents can be inserted during the same procedure as PBD, which avoids the necessity for a period of external biliary drainage.

Percutaneous biliary drainage is performed and a catheter is manipulated across the stricture. Instead

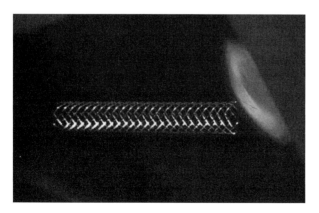

FIGURE 31.10. Self-expanding metallic endoprostheses in a deployed state (10 mm diameter and 7 cm long). See Color Plate 31.

of inserting a biliary drainage catheter, the stricture is pre-dilated to 10 mm using a balloon catheter to facilitate rapid expansion of the metallic stent. After pre-dilation, the stent, on its introducer system, is advanced across the lesion and is deployed so that the lower end projects through the ampulla and the upper end is well above the stricture. After stent deployment, a temporary small catheter is inserted for access in case of complications and is removed the next day after cholangiography

Internal Biliary Drainage: Principles

Mid and lower common bile duct strictures can be treated by a single stent. Hilar strictures may be treated by a single stent or by bilateral stents, depending on the pattern of biliary obstruction (see earlier discussion). If there is free communication between the left and right systems, unilateral stenting is sufficient. If both the right and left ducts are obstructed, bilateral stents may be necessary (Figure 31.11). As for PBD, if only one lobe is opacified at PTC, the operator may elect to stent that lobe alone (25). Bilateral stenting is performed, usually using a side-by-side or Y configuration. If only unilateral biliary drainage has been performed, but it is necessary to drain both lobes, bilateral drainage can still be accomplished if metallic stents are used. A metallic stent is placed from one hepatic duct to the other across the hepatic duct confluence, followed by placement of a second long stent from the ipsilateral lobe to the duodenum (Figure 31.12). Although this T configuration achieves drainage of both liver lobes, the Y configuration is preferable because it allows easier intervention if the stents become occluded.

Metallic or Plastic Stents?

Both types of stent provide good palliation of malignant obstructive jaundice. Metallic stents are more expensive than plastic endoprostheses and there has been considerable debate since metallic stents were introduced as to whether the results of metallic stents compared with plastic devices justify their additional costs. Although most retrospective studies suggest that both types of stents produce acceptable palliation (26), the results of randomized trials indicate that metallic stents have significantly longer patency rates than plastic stents (27–29). In addition, these trials reported that metallic stents are, in fact, more cost effective than plastic devices because of the reduced

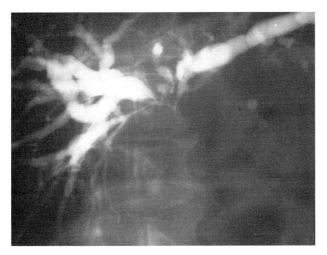

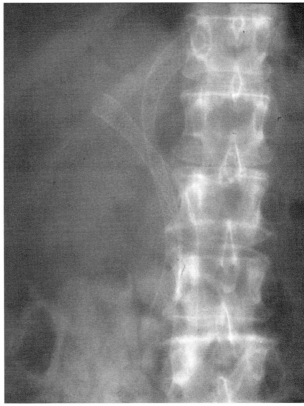

FIGURE 31.11.   Right and left hepatic duct to CBD metallic stents (Y configuration).

number of re-interventions required for the patients with metallic stents compared with plastic stents and the shorter stay in hospital (27–29) (Table 31.1). As a result of these data and the smaller introducer systems of metallic stents, most interventional radiologists choose metallic endoprosteses for internal biliary drainage (30). However, if there is evidence of involvement of the duodenum by infiltrating tumor, a metallic stent is contraindicated, and a plastic stent should be used.

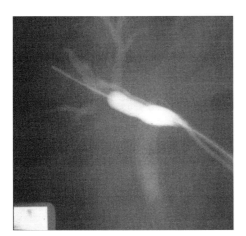

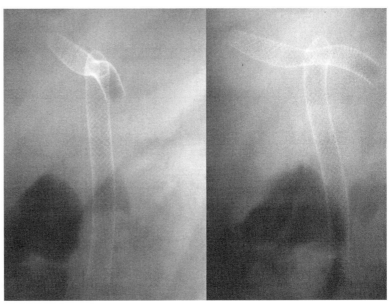

FIGURE 31.12.   A metallic stent is placed from one hepatic duct to the other across the hepatic duct confluence, followed by placement of a second long stent from the ipsilateral lobe to the duodenum.

TABLE 31.1 Obstruction Rate of Plastic and Metallic Stents in Malignant Biliary Obstruction

Authors	Number of Patients	Obstruction Rate: Plastic Stent (%)	Obstruction Rate: Metal Stent (%)	Median Duration of Plastic Stent Patency (days)	Median Duration of Metallic Stent Patency (days)
Davids et al. (63)	105	54	33	126	273
Knyrim et al. (64)	62	43	22	–	–
Lammer et al. (56)	101	27	19	96	272

Plastic stents are still placed by many endoscopists because of their acceptable patency rates, low cost and the ability of the endoscopist to insert plastic stents in a single-stage procedure.

Percutaneous Management of the Occluded Stent

Plastic stents are prone to occlusion by bile encrustation. The main cause of occlusion of metallic stents is tumor ingrowth or overgrowth; bile encrustation seldom occurs. The best method of treatment of blocked biliary stents is endoscopic replacement, in the case of plastic endoprostheses, or endoscopic insertion of a plastic stent inside a metallic endoprosthesis. Percutaneous evaluation and therapy of occluded stents is usually reserved for patients in whom endoscopy has been unsuccessful or is not possible. The percutaneous method involves an initial PTC to confirm stent occlusion and to define the biliary anatomy, followed by catheterization of a suitable duct. If the occluded stent is plastic, the stent must be removed before a new endoprosthesis is inserted. Plastic stents can be removed either by withdrawing them through the transhepatic track by grasping them with a wire loop snare or balloon catheter, or by pushing them into the duodenum and allowing them to pass through the digestive tract (Figure 31.13).

Most metallic stents cannot be removed (there is a new generation of retrievable metallic stents now available). Occlusion of metallic stents is managed percutaneously by inserting a new metallic endoprosthesis coaxially within the first stent. If the cause of occlusion is overgrowth of tumor, the new device must extend beyond the upper limit of the tumor (Figure 31.14).

Access Loops

Surgeons often affix the afferent loop of jejunum to the parietal peritoneum at the time of the creation

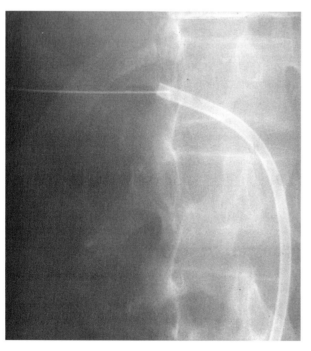
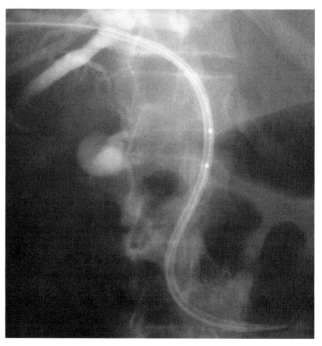

FIGURE 31.13. Pusher displacing an occluded Carey-Coons stent into the duodenum.

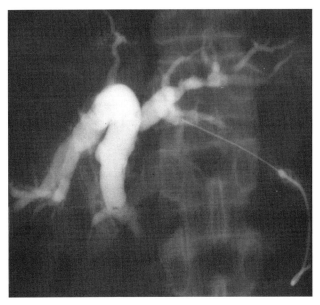

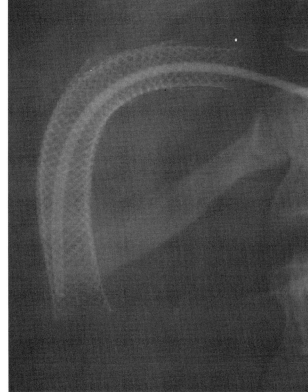

FIGURE 31.14. Occlusion of metallic stents is managed percutaneously by inserting a new metallic endoprosthesis coaxially within the first stent.

of the bilioenteric anastomosis to allow easy percutaneous access to the biliary tree if a stricture occurs at a later date. The apex of the loop is marked by a circle of metallic clips enabling the entry site of the loop to be visualised on fluoroscopy. If an access loop is present, it can be punctured with a fine needle under fluoroscopic guidance. Contrast medium is injected to opacify the loop and identify the route to the bilioenteric anastomosis. A minimally invasive access set (e.g., Accustick) is used to dilate the percutaneous track, and to pass a catheter and guidewire to the site of the anastomosis. The catheter is advanced across the stricture into the biliary tree and a stiff guidewire inserted into the intrahepatic ducts. This method of access allows repeated percutaneous dilatation of the stricture without the discomfort of the transhepatic route.

Covered Biliary Stents

Covered stents represent an evolution of bare stents and are aimed mainly to prevent obstruction caused by tumor ingrowth within the stent lumen (31). The first clinical studies of polyurethane-covered Wallstents showed that these stents can be safely implanted (31, 32). However, the 6-month patency rate was found to be inferior to that of noncovered Wallstents (46.8% vs. 67%), partly because of a breach in the covering membrane that allowed tumor ingrowth (32). It was concluded that such a type of covered stent had no significant advantages vs. bare stents (32, 33). Now, polytetrafluoroethylene and fluorinated ethylene propylene (ePTFE/FEP)-covered metallic stents have been introduced. The stent consists of an inner ePTFE/FEP lining and an outer supporting structure of nitinol wire. Multiple wire sections elevated from the external surface provide anchoring. Stents are available in two versions, with or without holes in the proximal stent lining. Holes should provide drainage of the cystic duct or biliary side branches when covered by the proximal stent end. They are more effective than polyurethane-covered Wallstents (34, 35). However, in 10% of cases, one can still get branch duct obstruction (35). These early studies are promising; however, significant improvements in patency still would be desirable.

It is generally advisable to have the distal end of the stent project just through the ampulla into the duodenum (6). This is because the rigid nature of the stent can sometimes cause kinking of the lower part of the

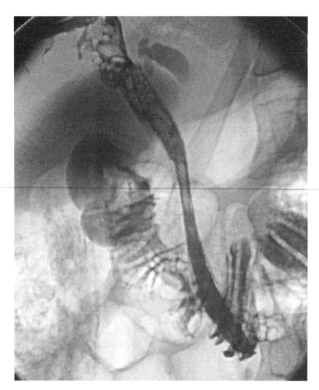

FIGURE 31.15. A Wallstent is seen to be deployed, too, across the ampulla such that it is abutting the duodenal wall. This later caused erosion of the duodenum, leading to a perforation.

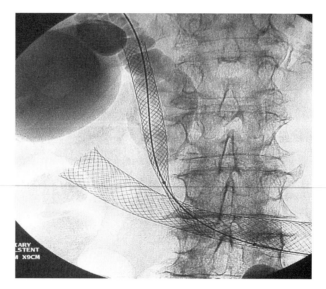

FIGURE 31.16. Patient with pancreatic carcinoma who developed both duodenal and biliary obstruction. Transoral placement of a duodenal stent and percutaneous placement of biliary stent.

common bile duct, which may cause obstruction (with the newer flexible Nitinol stents, this may probably be unnecessary). Additionally, it is easier to cannulate them endoscopically for clearance or for additional endoprosthesis insertion. If the stent projects too far into the duodenum, it can cause erosion of the opposite wall (Figure 31.15). Side branches covered by the uncovered stents during placement are not associated with branch occlusion (36).

Combined Biliary and Duodenal Obstruction

In some advanced cases of pancreatic cancer, metastasis or malignant lymphadenopathy patients can present with both biliary and duodenal obstruction. As a palliative procedure, the combined stenting of both the biliary stricture and duodenal stricture can be performed in one sitting by the radiologist. The biliary stent is placed from the percutaneous route as described earlier, whereas the duodenal stent can be placed via the transoral route. There are essentially two ways for these placements – that is, placing the duodenal stent first and then the biliary stent just through the mesh of the duodenal stent (Figure 31.16) or placing both stents side to side within the duodenal lumen.

COMBINED TRANSHEPATIC ENDOSCOPIC APPROACH (RENDEZVOUS PROCEDURE)

Transhepatic placement of a catheter of small diameter across the obstructed duct and into the duodenum offers a second chance for the endoscopist. This arrangement is very useful when the endoscopist has initially failed to negotiate the obstruction at an earlier attempt (37), and it is not advisable to create a large transhepatic track because of the risk of bile leakage into the peritoneum, or in patients with coagulopathy. With a transhepatically inserted 4F or 5F catheter negotiated across the obstruction into the duodenum, a 450-cm exchange guidewire such as Zebra (Microvasive) is inserted into the catheter. The patient is placed in the prone oblique position for the insertion of the endoscope. The endoscopist grasps the lower end of the guidewire with a snare or biopsy forceps and brings it out of the proximal end of the endoscope biopsy channel, while the radiologist keeps feeding the wire at the skin entry site. The transhepatic catheter is now withdrawn so that its tip lies in the intrahepatic portion of the biliary tree above the malignant stricture. The endoscopist now proceeds with the placement of a large-bore biliary endoprosthesis in the standard fashion, while the guidewire is held taut between the endoscopic and percutaneous ends. When the endoprosthesis is in position and free egress of bile is documented, the transhepatic catheter can be removed. However, if adequacy of decompression is questionable, the tran-shepatic catheter may be retained for observation and re-intervention, if required.

POST-PROCEDURE MANAGEMENT FOLLOWING BILIARY DRAINAGE

- Patients should be hospitalized for at least 24 hours following biliary drainage and monitored for sepsis and vital signs.

- An appropriate antibiotic combination should be continued after drainage is established.

- The internal-external biliary drainage catheter should be used for external drainage for the first 12 to 24 hours. If the catheter permits drainage of bile into the bowel, then the drainage catheter can be capped to allow internal drainage. If the patient is able to tolerate internal drainage for 8 to 12 hours, then he or she can be discharged. If internal drainage is not possible, then external bag drainage must be maintained. Bile output can range from 400 to 800 ml/day. With external drainage, dehydration can occur unless adequate steps are taken to replace the lost fluids.

- Biliary drainage catheters should be forward flushed with normal saline every 48 hours. This helps prevent debris from accumulating in the catheter and causing it to occlude.

- If the patient is to be sent home on internal drainage, they should not be sent until the ability to have their bile drained internally is demonstrated adequately without evidence of sepsis or peri-catheter leakage.

- Complete instructions for tube care are given prior to discharge. They should be instructed to flush the tube gently with 10 ml of saline once or twice per day to keep it debris free. They are instructed to call if they experience pain, chills, fever or nausea or vomiting. Any malposition of the tube, bleeding within it or leakage around the tube should also be taken seriously.

- The dressing around the drainage catheter should be changed at least every 48 hours and bathing avoided. Also, the biliary drainage catheters should be changed every 3 to 4 months.

- Pericatheter leakage is the result of catheter kink-ing, occlusion or displacement. Fluoroscopic eval-uation is essential for determining and correcting this problem depending on the causes as mentioned. Sometimes upsizing the catheter is the only solu-tion.

- Serum bilirubin values may be followed as an indi-cator of adequate drainage. Depending on the size and type of drain, it takes, on average, 10 to 15 days for the bilirubin levels to drop by 50%. If the biliru-bin level starts rising, catheter occlusion should be suspected.

- After adequate drainage, biliary sepsis should be relieved. If sepsis remains a problem, then addi-tional studies should be performed to determine the cause, which can be catheter occlusion or undrained biliary ducts. A thorough cholangiogram with spe-cial attention to the ductal anatomy can sometimes identify a missing ductal segment, indicating an iso-lated undrained system. Alternatively, a MRCP or CT cholangiogram can be performed.

- Late sepsis, manifesting as fever several days or weeks after the patient has been adequately drained, is usually indicative of obstruction of the drainage catheter. If the patient has a capped biliary catheter, the tube should be uncapped to allow the bile to drain externally. If externalizing the drainage catheter resolves the infection, then fluoroscopic evaluation of the catheter can be performed elec-tively. However, if fever persists after externaliza-tion, then an emergency catheter evaluation should be performed. If catheter obstruction is not the source of sepsis, then the patient should be eval-uated for undrained ductal segments.

COMPLICATIONS

Complications of percutaneous biliary interventions can be divided into early – that is, procedural com-plications – and late complications (6). Most proce-dural complications are related to the initial biliary drainage, with mortality ranging from 0% to 2.8% (38, 39) and major complications occurring in 3.5% to 9.5% (40, 41). Also, higher rates of procedure-related deaths have been reported for malignant dis-eases (3%) compared with benign diseases (0%) (42, 43). This is also true of procedure-related compli-cations (7% vs. 2%). Minor complications such as mild, self-limiting hemobilia, fever and transient bac-teremia occur in up to 66% of patients (44).

Immediate Complications

These may be

1. Sedation: Problems may occur if care is not taken to constantly monitor patients during and after the procedure for complications of cardiorespiratory depression. Pulse oximetry should be used for monitoring all patients undergoing procedures involving conscious sedation.

2. Hemorrhage: Mild hemobilia is common, occurring in up to 16% of cases (39). More severe bleeding requiring transfusion occurs in approximately 3% of patients (45). Hemorrhage is minimized by the correction of coagulation defects and avoidance of percutaneous intervention in patients with severe, incorrectable coagulopathies. It is usually self-limited and seldom requires treatment. If bleeding is mild and venous in origin, repositioning the catheter so that the trailing side holes are located within the biliary tree and not within the hepatic parenchyma and, if required, upsizing the catheter to tamponade the bleeding point usually suffice. The catheter should be regularly irrigated with saline to maintain its patency and to clear any thrombus from the bile ducts (Figure 31.17). If hemobilia does not resolve with these measures or is severe, vascular embolization should be performed through the transhepatic track or by hepatic arteriography (Figure 31.18) (6).

3. Sepsis: Manipulation of catheters and guidewires within an infected biliary tract can produce rapid

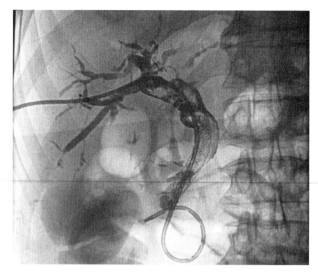

FIGURE 31.17.   Biliary catheter in situ. Cholangiogram demonstrating significant filling defects consistent with hemobilia.

bacteremia, which may progress to septicemic shock if antibiotic coverage is not administered prior to the procedure. Intravenous antibiotics should be continued following biliary drainage until the catheter is removed.

4. Pericatheter leak in approximately 15% of the patients (46).

5. Pancreatitis (0% to 4%) (46).

6. Pneumothorax, hemothorax, bilothorax (<1%) (47, 48).

7. Contrast reaction (<2%) (46).

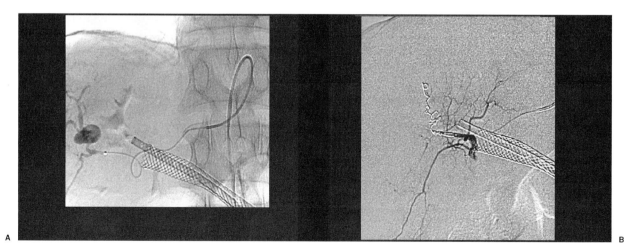

A

B

FIGURE 31.18.   (A) Selective angiography demonstrating bleeding site in right-lobe liver. (B) Coils placed through a microcatheter. Note that coiling is performed beyond and proximal to pseudoaneurysm/hemorrhage site in order to "close the front and back doors."

TABLE 31.2 Methods of Reducing Frequency of Common Complications

Sepsis	Antibiotic prophylaxis
Hemorrhage	Minimal manipulation
Bile leak	Restrict volume of contrast injected and aspirate bile prior to contrast injection
Cholangitis	Normalize coagulation factors
Catheter dislodgment	Fine-needle coaxial technique
	Peripheral duct puncture
	Careful positioning of side holes to avoid communication with an intrahepatic vessel
	Avoid puncture of extra-hepatic ducts
	Single puncture site in liver capsule
	Careful positioning of side holes
	Ensure adequate drainage by careful positioning of side holes
	Irrigation of catheter with sterile saline
	Large-diameter catheters (12F) for long drainage
	Routine tube exchange every 2 to 3 months
	Safety stitch method
	Self-retaining (pigtail) catheter

Delayed Complications

These include the following:

1. Cholangitis: Approximately 50% of bile cultures will be positive when obtained at initial puncture (42). When an internal-external drainage is performed with an 8F catheter, recurrent cholangitis secondary to inadequate drainage is possible. The rate of sepsis will decrease if this is replaced by a 10F to 12F drain (45).

2. Catheter dislodgment (approximately 15% to 20%) (39, 49).

3. Peritonitis (1% to 3%) (46).

4. Hypersecretion of bile (0% to 5%) (43): This can cause significant fluid and electrolyte imbalance and is usually seen within several days of drainage.

5. Cholecystitis – due to blockage of the cystic duct by covered stents. To address this complication, holes in the proximal stent lining are made, which should hypothetically allow for drainage of cystic or branch biliary ducts when their orifice is covered by the stent (40, 41). This complication still may be seen, for which percutaneous cystic duct stent placement (50), percutaneous cholecystostomy or cholecystectomy may be required.

6. Bilio-pleural fistula (47).

7. Skin infection, irritation.

8. Intrahepatic or perihepatic abscess.

9. Metastatic seeding of the serosa or tract with cholangiocarcinoma (43) and pancreatic carcinoma (39, 51) has been reported.

Some routine precautions that help in significantly reducing the incidence of complications are provided in Table 31.2 (52).

CLINICAL RESULTS

PTBD

The results of various series are tabulated in Table 31.3 (49, 53–58). In general, the technical success rate has varied from 86% to 100% with successful drainage rates of 81% to 96%. The 30-day mortality rate has been 1% to 49% and complication rate, 6% to 58%. This marked variation in results is probably due to differences in the criteria for patient selection, the experience and expertise of different operators and the criteria used to define success and complications.

PATIENT SURVIVAL

Patient survival after metallic stent placement is difficult to estimate and compare among various reports and this would be attributable to variations in population, additional treatment, patient selection and the stage of the tumor. In the literature, patients receiving this treatment have been reported to live 93 to 420 days longer (59, 60). In patients with hilar obstruction, longer survival rates have been observed after both lobes have been drained as compared with those

TABLE 31.3 Results of PTBD in Malignant Obstruction

Author	Number of Patients	Technical Success (%)	Drainage Success (%)	30-Day Mortality Rate (%)	Complication Rate (%)
Pereiras et al. (53)	12	100	83	–	58
Voegeli et al. (54)	76	97	92	27	20
Joseph et al. (55)	39	90	–	49	53
Lammer and Neumayer (56)	162	100	96	15	9
Schild et al. (57)	220	–	92	1	22
Gazzaniga et al. (49)	362	97	81	–	15
Murai et al. (58)	92	86	–	–	–
Schoder et al. (35)	42	100	100	20	5
Bezzi et al. (34)	26	100	100	11.5	19

who had one lobe drained (61, 62). This may be attributable to the higher septic complications that may occur in patients with unilateral drainage. However, the drawbacks for multi-segment drainage are increased cost, longer procedure time and greater technical difficulty.

REFERENCES

1. Molnar W and Stockum AE. Transhepatic dilatation of choledochoenterostomy strictures. Radiology, 1978 Oct; 129(1): 59–64.
2. Kumaran V, Gulati MS, Paul SB, et al. The role of dual phase helical CT in assessing resectability of carcinoma of the gallbladder. Eur Radiol, 2002; 12: 1993–1999.
3. Blumgart LH. Cholangiocarcinoma. In: Blumgart LH (ed.), Surgery of the Liver and Biliary Tract, pp. 721–753. Edinburgh: Churchill Livingstone, 1998.
4. Pillai VAK, Shreekumar KP, Prabhu NK, et al. Utility of MR cholangiography in planning transhepatic biliary interventions in malignant hilar obstructions. Indian J Radiol Imaging, 2002; 12: 37–42.
5. Speer AG, Russel CG and Hatfield ARW. Randomised trial of endoscopic versus percutaneous stent insertion in malignant obstructive jaundice. Lancet, 1987; 11: 57–62.
6. Morgan RA and Adam A. Percutaneous management of biliary obstruction. In: Gazelle GS, Saini S, Mueller PR (eds.): Hepatobiliary and Pancreatic Radiology Imaging and Intervention, pp. 677–709. Thieme: Verlag, 1998.
7. Kersjes W, Koster O, Heuer M, et al. A comparison of imaging procedures in the diagnosis of gallbladder and bile duct carcinomas. Rofo Fortschr Geb Rontgenstr Neuen Bildgeb Verfahr, 1990; 153: 174–180.
8. Gulliver DJ, Baker ME, Cheng CA, et al. Malignant biliary obstruction: Efficacy of thin section dynamic CT in determining resectability. AJR Am J Roentgenol, 1992; 159: 503–507.
9. Choi BI, Lee JH, Han MC, et al. Hilar cholangiocarcinoma: Comparative study with sonography and CT. Radiology, 1989; 172: 689–692.
10. de Aretxabala X, Roa I, Burgos L, et al. Gallbladder cancer in Chile. A report on 54 potentially resectable tumors. Cancer, 1992; 69: 60–65.
11. Cha JH, Han JK, Kim TK, et al. Preoperative evaluation of Klatskin tumor: Accuracy of spiral CT in determining vascular invasion as a sign of unresectability. Abdom Imaging, 2000; 25: 500–507.
12. Feydy A, Vilgrain V, Denys A, et al. Helical CT assessment in hilar cholangiocarcinoma: Correlation with surgical and pathologic findings. AJR Am J Roentgenol, 1999; 172: 73–77.
13. Van Beers BE, Lacrosse M, Trigaux JP, et al. Noninvasive imaging of the biliary tree before or after laparoscopic cholecystectomy: Use of three dimensional spiral CT cholangiography. AJR Am J Roentgenol, 1994; 162: 1331–1335.
14. Kwon AH, Uetsuji S, Yamada O, et al. Three dimensional reconstruction of the biliary tract using spiral computed tomography. Br J Surg, 1995; 82: 260–263.
15. Zeman RK, Berman PM, Silverman PM, et al. Biliary tract: Three dimensional helical CT without cholangiographic contrast material. Radiology, 1995; 196: 865–867.
16. Rao NDLV, Gulati MS, Paul SB, et al. Three-dimensional helical CT cholangiography with minimum intensity projection in gallbladder carcinoma patients with obstructive jaundice: Comparison with magnetic resonance cholangiography and percutaneous transhepatic cholangiography. J Gastroenterol Hepatol, 2005; 20: 304–308.
17. Park SJ, Han JK, Kim TK, et al. Three-dimensional spiral CT cholangiography with minimum intensity projection in patients with suspected obstructive biliary disease: Comparison with percutaneous transhepatic cholangiography. Abdom Imaging, 2001; 26(3): 281–286.
18. Adamck HE, Albert J, Lietz M, et al. A prospective evaluation of magnetic resonance cholangiography in patients with suspected bile duct obstruction. Gut, 1998; 43: 680–683.
19. Lopera JE, Soto JA, and Múnera F. Malignant hilar and perihilar biliary obstruction: Use of MR cholangiography to define the extent of biliary ductal involvement and plan percutaneous interventions. Radiology, 2001; 220: 90–96.
20. Bismuth H and Corlette MB. Intrahepatic cholangioenteric anastomosis in carcinoma of the hilus of the liver. Surg Gynecol Obstet, 1975; 140: 170–178.

21. Polydorou AA, Chisholm EM, Romanos AA, et al. A comparison of right versus left hepatic duct endoprosthesis insertion in malignant hilar biliary obstruction. Endoscopy, 1989; 21: 266–271.

22. Chang WH, Kortan P, and Haber GB. Outcome in patients with bifurcation tumors who undergo unilateral versus bilateral hepatic duct drainage. Gastrointest Endosc, 1998; 47: 354–362.

23. Lee KH, Lee DY, and Kim KW. Biliary intervention for cholangiocarcinoma. Abdom Imaging, 2004; 29: 581–589.

24. Cope C. Conversion from small (0.018 inch) to large (0.038 inch) guide wires in percutaneous drainage procedures. Am J Roentgenol, 1982; 138: 170–171.

25. Morgan RA and Adam A. Metallic stents in the treatment of patients with malignant biliary obstruction. Semin Intervent Radiol, 1996; 13: 229–240.

26. Rossi P, Bezzi M, Rossi M, et al. Metallic stents in malignant biliary obstruction: Results of a multicenter European study of 240 patients. J Vasc Interv Radiol, 1994; 5: 279–285.

27. Davids PHP, Groen AK, Rauws EAJ, et al. Randomised trial of self-expanding metal stents versus polyethylene stents for distal malignant biliary obstruction. Lancet, 1992; 340: 1488–1492.

28. Knyrim K, Wagner H-J, Pausch J, et al. A prospective, randomised controlled trial of metal stents for malignant obstruction of the common bile duct. Endoscopy, 1993; 25: 207–212.

29. Lammer J, Hausegger KA, Fluckiger F, et al. Common bile duct obstruction due to malignancy: Treatment with plastic versus metal stents. Radiology, 1996; 201: 167–172.

30. Adam A, Roddie ME, Jackson JE, et al. Wallstent endoprostheses for biliary malignancy: What is the verdict after 7 years use? Radiology, 1994; 193(P): 327.

31. Shim CS, Lee JH, Cho JD, et al. Preliminary results of a new covered biliary metal stent for malignant biliary obstruction. Endoscopy, 1998; 30: 345–350.

32. Rossi P, Bezzi M, Salvatori FM, et al. Clinical experience with covered Wallstents for biliary malignancies: 23-month follow-up. Cardiovasc Intervent Radiol, 1997; 20: 441–447.

33. Hausegger KA, Thurnher S, Bodendorfer G, et al. Treatment of malignant biliary obstruction with polyurethane-covered Wallstents. Am J Roentgenol Am J Roentgenol, 1998; 170: 403–408.

34. Bezzi M, Zolovkins A, Cantisani V, et al. New ePTFE/FEP-covered stent in the palliative treatment of malignant biliary obstruction. J Vasc Interv Radiol, 2002; 13: 581–589.

35. Schoder M, Rossi P, Uflacker R, et al. Malignant biliary obstruction: Treatment with ePTFE-FEP – covered endoprostheses – initial technical and clinical experiences in a multicenter trial. Radiology, 2002; 225: 35–42.

36. Nicholson DA, Cheety N, and Jackson J. Patency of side branches after peripheral placement of metallic biliary endoprosthesis. J Vasc Interv Radiol, 1992; 3: 127–130.

37. Wayman J, Mansfield JC, Mathewson K, et al. Combined percutaneous and endoscopic procedures for bile duct obstruction: Simultaneous and delayed techniques compared. Hepatogastroenterology, 2003; 50: 915–918.

38. Ferrucci JT Jr, Mueller PR, and Harbim WP. Percutaneous transhepatic biliary drainage: Technique, results and applications. Radiology, 1980; 135: 1–13.

39. Hamlin JA, Friedman M, Stein MG, et al. Percutaneous biliary drainage: Complications of 118 consecutive catheterizations. Radiology, 1986; 158: 199–202.

40. Lamaris JS, Stoker J, Dees J, et al. Nonsurgical palliative treatment of patients with malignant biliary obstruction – the place of endoscopic and percutaneous drainage. Clin Radiol, 1987; 38: 603–608.

41. Clark RA, Mitchell SE, Colley DP, et al. Percutaneous catheter biliary decompression. Am J Roentgenol, 1981; 137: 503–509.

42. Yee AC, Ho CS. Complications of transhepatic biliary drainage: Benign vs malignant diseases. Am J Roentgenol, 1987; 148: 1207–1209.

43. Carrasco CH, Zornoza J, and Bechtel WJ. Malignant biliary obstruction: Complications of percutaneous biliary drainage. Radiology, 1984; 152: 343–346.

44. Berquist TH, May GR, Johnson CM, et al. Percutaneous biliary decompression: Internal and external drainage in 50 patients. Am J Roentgenol, 1981; 136: 901–906.

45. Mueller PR, van Sonnenberg E, Ferrucci JT Jr. Percutaneous biliary drainage: Technical and catheter related problems in 200 procedures. Am J Roentgenol, 1982; 138: 17–23.

46. Rosenblatt M, Aruny JE, and Kandarpa K. Transhepatic cholangiography, biliary decompression, endobiliary stenting, and cholecystostomy. In: Kandarpa K, Aruny JE (eds), Handbook of Interventional Radiology Procedures, pp. 302–331. Philadelphia: Lippincott Williams & Wilkins, 2002.

47. Strange C, Allen ML, Freedland PN, et al. Biliopleural fistula as a complication of percutaneous biliary drainage: Experimental evidence for pleural inflammation. Am Rev Respir Dis, 1988; 137: 959–961.

48. Dawson SL, Neff CC, Mueller PR, et al. Fatal hemothorax after inadvertent transpleural biliary drainage. Am J Roentgenol, 1983; 141: 33–34.

49. Gazzaniga GM, Faggioni A, Bondanza G, et al. Percutaneous transhepatic biliary drainage – twelve years experience. Hepatogastroenterology, 1991; 38: 154–159.

50. Sheiman RG and Stuart K. Percutaneous cystic duct stent placement for the treatment of acute cholecystitis resulting from common bile duct stent placement for malignant obstruction. J Vasc Interv Radiol, 2004; 15: 999–1001.

51. Cutherell L, Wanebo HJ, Tegtmeyer CJ. Catheter tract seeding after percutaneous biliary drainage for pancreatic cancer. Cancer, 1986; 57: 2057–2060.

52. Wittich GR, Van Sonnertberg E, Simeone JF. Results and complications of percutaneous drainage. Semin Interv Radiol, 1985; 2: 39–49.

53. Pereiras RV Jr, Rheingold OJ, Huston D, et al. Relief of malignant obstructive jaundice by percutaneous insertion of a permanent prosthesis. Ann Intern Med, 1978; 89: 589–593.

54. Voegeli DR, Crummy AB, and Weese JL. Percutaneous transhepatic cholangiography, drainage and biopsy in patients with malignant biliary obstruction. An alternative to surgery. Am J Surg, 1985; 150: 243–247.

55. Joseph PK, Bizer LS, Sprayregan SS, et al. Percutaneous transhepatic biliary drainage. Results and complications in 81 patients. JAMA, 1986; 255: 2763–2767.

56. Lammer J, Neumayer K, and Steiner HK. Biliary drainage endoprosthesis: Experience with 201 patients. Radiology, 1986; 159: 625–629.

57. Schild H, Klose KJ, Staritz M, et al. The results and complications of 616 percutaneous transhepatic biliary drainages. Rofo Fortschr Geb Rontgenstr Neuen Bildgeb Verfahr, 1989 Sep; 151(3): 289–293.

58. Murai R, Hashiguchi F, Kusuyama A, et al. Percutaneous stenting for malignant biliary stenosis. Surg Endosc, 1991; 5: 140–142.

59. Rieber A and Brambs HJ. Metallic stents in malignant biliary obstruction. Cardiovasc Intervent Radiol, 1997; 20: 43–49.

60. Cowling MG and Adam AN. Internal stenting in malignant biliary obstruction. World J Surg, 2001; 25: 355–361.

61. Deviere J, Baize M, de Toeuf J, et al. Long-term follow-up of patients with hilar malignant stricture treated by endoscopic internal biliary drainage. Gastrointest Endosc, 1988; 34: 95–101.

62. Motte S, Deviere J, Dumonceau JM, et al. Risk factors for septicemia following endoscopic biliary stent. Gastroenterology, 1991; 101: 1374–1381.

63. Davids PH, Groen AK, Rauws EA, et al. Randomised trial of self expanding metallic stents versus polyethylene stents for distal malignant biliary obstruction. Lancet, 1992; 340: 1488–1492.

64. Knyrim K, Wagner HJ, Pausch J, et al. A prospective, randomized, controlled trial of metal stents for malignant obstruction of the common bile duct. Endoscopy, 1993 Mar; 25(3): 207–212.

Renal Cell Carcinoma

Chapter 32

SURGICAL AND MEDICAL TREATMENT

Surena F. Matin

INCIDENCE AND DIAGNOSIS

Renal cell carcinoma (RCC) is the most common malignancy of the kidney. In 2007, there were more than 51,100 new cases of RCC in the United States, and 12,890 patients died from the disease (1). The incidence of RCC has been on the rise since the latter part of the twentieth century, independent of advances in abdominal imaging that have improved diagnostic potential (2). According to the National Cancer Institute's 1975 to 1995 Surveillance, Epidemiology, and End Results database, this increase has been seen in both women and men and across racial boundaries (3).

RCC is associated with older age and is increasingly diagnosed in patients past the fifth decade of life. In addition to age, the only risk factors for RCC are smoking and tobacco exposure. Other factors that may be associated with a high risk of RCC include obesity, diabetes mellitus, hypertension, diuretic use, high alcohol intake, high fat intake and high red meat intake; however, the causative potential of these factors is yet unproven (4).

The kidney is a well-protected, markedly silent organ. It is sheltered within the rib cage and is often surrounded by a thick rind of fat, and it is innervated to respond to only acute visceral distension. Thus, small renal tumors typically develop asymptomatically. The classic symptoms of RCC are abdominal mass, pain and hematuria. This presentation is rare, but when these symptoms do occur, they are a signal for advanced-stage disease. A typical contemporary scenario is the incidental discovery of a renal mass on diagnostic imaging in a patient who presents with non-specific abdominal pain or discomfort. The symptoms are often unrelated to the renal mass.

Abdominal imaging is an absolute necessity in diagnosing RCC, and a variety of imaging tools can be utilized. Ultrasound is an effective initial screening tool, but it does not provide enough detail with which to plan surgical therapy. It is sometimes valuable in differentiating cysts from solid lesions when the computed tomography (CT) or magnetic resonance imaging (MRI) is inconclusive. CT performed with a renal protocol is the most useful imaging modality. It provides non-contrast scans that can be used to look for calcifications in the collecting system, parenchyma and vessels and is critical in the identification of hyperdense cysts. Multiphasic, post-contrast, thin-cut imaging is useful in evaluating the vascular anatomy; quantifying enhancement of a renal mass; evaluating the parenchymal and collecting system anatomy; and surveillance and staging of metastatic disease by evaluating abdominal lymph nodes, liver, bone, adrenals and the inferior vena cava. Aside from the lungs, these sites represent the most common areas of locoregional and disseminated disease.

In addition to a renal protocol CT scan, the standard work-up for patients presenting with localized disease consists of a chest X-ray and laboratory studies, including urinalysis, complete blood count, serum creatinine, calcium and liver function tests. If the patient has low-stage disease, no further analyses are done. In the absence of bone-related symptoms, an elevated calcium level or an elevated alkaline phosphatase level, a bone scan yields very little information about most incidentally detected, low- to intermediate-stage renal tumors and thus is not routinely used (5). When metastatic disease is suspected, a bone scan, skeletal survey and other imaging analyses, such as a brain MRI, may be required, depending on the patient's clinical presentation.

RCC is notorious for its association with paraneoplastic syndromes, which can occur in up to 20% of patients. These syndromes result from oversecretion by the tumor of renal hormones, such as erythropoietin, 1,25 dihydroxycholecalciferol and renin (6–10). Polycythemia is also associated with RCC and may be caused by the oversecretion of erythropoietin. Hypercalcemia, in the absence of metastatic bone disease, is an uncommon but clinically important finding, because it requires prompt medical therapy with saline hydration, diuresis, and, occasionally, steroid administration. Another clinically important syndrome is Stauffer's syndrome, which is seen with hepatic dysfunction in the absence of metastatic disease (9, 11, 12). Typical findings include elevation of liver function and coagulopathy with elevation of prothrombin time. In all cases of anemia, hypercalcemia or Stauffer's syndrome, it is critical to rule out metastatic disease as a source of the abnormality, especially with hepatic dysfunction, to ensure there is no obstruction of the hepatic veins by a vena caval tumor thrombus, causing Budd-Chiari syndrome. Most of these syndromes are reversed following nephrectomy or systemic therapy; if the abnormality persists after surgery, the patient should be followed closely to monitor for metastatic disease. The presence of paraneoplastic syndromes may portend a poor prognosis, particularly when cachexia is present (7).

STAGING

RCC staging has transitioned from the classic Robson staging system to the more contemporary tumor-node-metastasis (TNM) system developed by the American Joint Commission on Cancer (13). The most recent TNM staging schema is shown in Table 32.1. Stage T1 and T2 tumors are considered

TABLE 32.1 American Joint Committee on Cancer, 2002 TNM Staging System for Renal Cell Carcinoma

Primary Tumor (T)	Description
Tx	Primary tumor cannot be assessed
T1	Tumor 7 cm or less in greatest dimension, limited to kidney
T1a	Tumor 4 cm or less
T1b	Tumor greater than 4 cm
T2	Tumor more than 7 cm in greatest dimension, limited to kidney
T3	Tumor extends into major veins, or invades adrenal, sinus fat or perinephric fat, but not beyond Gerota's fascia
T3a	Tumor invades adrenal gland*
T3b	Tumor grossly extends into renal vein or vena cava but below diaphragm
T3c	Tumor grossly extends into the vena cava above the diaphragm
T4	Tumor invades beyond Gerota's fascia
Regional Lymph Nodes (N)†	
Nx	Regional lymph nodes cannot be assessed
N0	No regional lymph node metastases
N1	Metastasis to a single regional lymph node
N2	Metastasis to more than 1 regional lymph node
Metastasis (M)	
Mx	Distant metastasis cannot be assessed
M0	No distant metastasis
M1	Distant metastasis
Histopathologic Fuhrman Grade (G)	
Gx	Grade cannot be assessed
G1	Well differentiated
G2	Moderately differentiated
G3–4	Poorly differentiated or undifferentiated

* Non-contiguous involvement of the adrenal gland is considered M1 (metastatic) disease.
† Involvement of non-regional lymph nodes is considered M1 disease.

localized disease, whereas stage T3 and T4 tumors are considered locally advanced disease. According to the Fuhrman grading system, grades 1–2 are considered low-grade tumors, whereas grades 3–4 are considered high grade. In addition to the TNM and Fuhrman systems, several new findings have pointed to the prognostic value of other factors, such as the presence of symptoms, tumor necrosis, sarcomatoid histology and laboratory findings. Risk stratification has been particularly problematic in RCC, because multiple clinical, pathologic and laboratory factors can influence prognosis and risk of recurrence after therapy beyond what is described in the TNM system.

HISTOLOGIC SUBTYPES

Malignant Renal Tumors

Table 32.2 lists the most common histologic subtypes of RCC and their incidence, cell of origin and known associated genetic defects. These subtypes represent the most common malignant forms of the disease. Despite their common origin in the kidney, it is increasingly recognized that these phenotypically dissimilar tumors are likewise genetically dissimilar and represent different diseases. The most common histologic subtype of RCC is the "clear-cell" or conventional tumor. Papillary (types 1 and 2), chromophobe, collecting duct, medullary and unclassified are the other histologic subtypes.

Papillary RCC generally carries a favorable prognosis when it is localized. The risk of multi-focality in the same or opposite kidney is high with this histologic subtype and, indeed, higher than with the other subtypes. Treatment of metastatic papillary RCC,

on the other hand, is much more problematic and carries a poor prognosis. Although immunotherapy and chemotherapy are largely ineffective, the evolution of targeted therapies may hold some promise for patients with this histologic subtype. Papillary RCC types 1 and type 2 are histologically and genetically distinct entities and are differentiated on the same basis as hereditary syndromes (see "Genetic Syndromes Associated with Real Cell Carcinoma"). Differentiating type 2 papillary RCC from type 1 is clinically important because type 2 RCC may have a more aggressive course than type 1, so patients with type 2 may need to be followed more carefully after surgery.

The prognosis for patients with chromophobe RCC appears to be better than that of patients with any of the other histologic subtypes, and its prognosis is excellent even in cases of locally advanced disease.

Collecting-duct RCC is rare, highly infiltrative and very aggressive. No chemotherapeutic regimen has been developed for this entity. Most patients present with locally advanced or metastatic disease (14). Medullary RCC is also rare and aggressive, and it is suspected in patients with sickle-cell disease or sickle trait who have an infiltrative central renal mass (Figure 32.1). Collecting-duct and medullary RCC metastasize early, and many of the patients die soon after diagnosis (15–17).

Sarcomatoid RCC was once considered a separate subtype but actually represents dedifferentiation of one of the other primary subtypes, as other epithelial elements are usually found intermixed in these cases (18). Sarcomatoid RCC is usually associated with a grim prognosis, and this entity is generally

TABLE 32.2 Characteristics of the Histologic Subtypes of Renal Cell Carcinoma

Histology	Frequency (%)	Cell of Origin	Gene	Comment
Clear cell	75	Proximal tubule	*VHL*	The *VHL* gene is implicated in the majority of sporadic cases of conventional RCC.
Papillary Type 1	10–15	Proximal tubule	*C-Met*	Familial cases are associated with hereditary papillary renal cell carcinoma.
Type 2			*Fumarate hydratase*	Familial cases are associated with the leimyomatosis RCC and multiple cutaneous leiomyoma complex.
Chromophobe	4–5	Distal tubule	*BHD*	Familial cases are associated with the syndrome.
Medullary	<1	Calyceal epithelium	–	Aggressive and infiltrative tumor associated with sickle-cell trait.
Collecting duct	<1	Collecting duct	–	Aggressive and infiltrative tumor
Unclassified	2–4	–	–	Histologic diagnosis of exclusion

Adapted from Linehan et al (34).

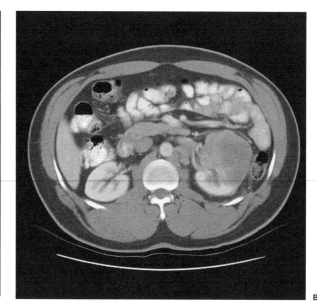

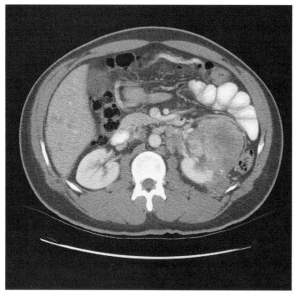

FIGURE 32.1. **(A) CT scan of the abdomen from a 35-year-old man with sickle-cell trait and left flank pain, showing infiltrative central renal mass and hilar adenopathy. CT of the chest showed pulmonary nodules. Renal biopsy confirmed medullary RCC. The patient deferred therapy. (B) The abdominal CT scan 3 months after diagnosis, showing enlarging retroperitoneal lymph nodes. The chest scan also showed rapidly progressive parenchymal and mediastinal disease. The patient succumbed to disease within 8 months of the original presentation. (Copyright Surena F. Matin, 2006.)**

resistant to most forms of chemotherapy (Figure 32.2) (19). Unclassified RCC is a histologic diagnosis of exclusion, when the tumor is dedifferentiated to such a degree that no distinct epithelial classification can be assigned. Similar to cases of sarcomatoid dedifferentiation, unclassified cases are associated with a poor prognosis and poor responses to systemic therapy.

Benign Renal Tumors

Oncocytomas and angiomyolipomas (AML) are the most common benign renal tumors. Histologically, oncocytomas are well-circumscribed masses composed of uniform cells with eosinophilic cytoplasm. Oncocytomas may be bilateral and multi-focal, and in a substantial number of cases, they co-exist with RCC. Oncocytoma is nearly indistinguishable from RCC

on radiologic examination (20), and distinguishing between these tumors without surgery remains a challenge. Preoperative biopsy may not be helpful because of sampling error or false-negative or non-diagnostic results resulting from insufficient tissue sample size (21). Nephron-sparing surgery (NSS) may be planned on the basis of preoperative radiographic suspicion, such as a well-encapsulated, homogeneous tumor with central scarring. Frozen-section analysis at the time of surgery is usually not sensitive enough to differentiate the eosinophilic appearance of oncocytomas from eosinophilic clear-cell or chromophobe RCCs and thus is not used to guide surgical strategy. For confirmation of the diagnosis, permanent-section analysis with electron microscopy is often required. Therefore, surgery must be performed

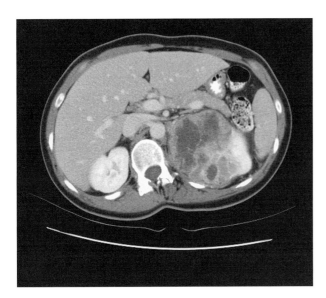

FIGURE 32.2. CT scan from a 55-year-old patient with a large renal mass, multiple small pulmonary lesions and single bony metastasis. Patient underwent nephrectomy, revealing pathologic T3a, high-grade RCC with sarcomatoid dedifferentiation. Two months after surgery, the patient died of fulminant metastatic disease. (Copyright Surena F. Matin, 2006)

with the assumption that it is a malignant tumor, as it is only in rare cases that oncocytomas are confidently diagnosed preoperatively without definitive intervention (Figures 32.3 and 32.4).

AML is the only benign renal tumor confidently diagnosed on CT scans. AMLs are typically recognized on CT due to the presence of fat in the tumor,

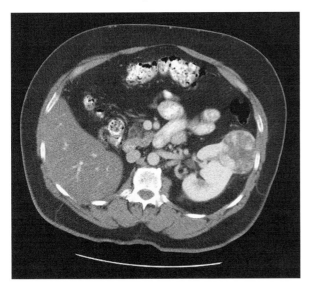

FIGURE 32.3. A preoperative CT scan showing an enhancing left upper pole renal mass suspicious for RCC. There was suggestion of a spoke-wheel pattern on CT. Percutaneous biopsy was inconclusive, showing only oncocytic cells, consistent with RCC or oncocytoma. A left partial nephrectomy was performed with preservation of 85% of the kidney. Pathology confirmed oncocytoma. (Copyright Surena F. Matin, 2006)

in which case thin sectioning may be required (22). When AMLs become large, they can be confused with liposarcomas; however, liposarcomas are extremely rare. Also, some AMLs contain minimal fat and thus may not be radiographically distinguishable from RCC. A variety of radiographic findings can help distinguish AML from malignancy, such as intratumoral calcification, irregular borders, loco-regional invasion, necrosis, adenopathy and vascular invasion (23). These features should alert the clinician to the possibility of malignancy. AML is also distinguishable by the presence of a discrete parenchymal defect at its origin. AMLs are usually sporadic but may occur in association with the tuberous sclerosis complex (TSC). This presentation usually occurs in younger patients (second or third decade of life) and frequently occurs in multiples, is bilateral, and is symptomatic (24). Due to the variable penetrance of the TSC mutation, the classic triad of seizures, adenoma sebaceum, and mental retardation may not be present (24). The typical sporadic presentation is that of a woman, 40 to 50 years old, with a single, asymptomatic tumor. Intervention for an asymptomatic tumor less than 4 cm in size is rarely needed, although surveillance is undertaken. Larger tumors appear to be associated with a higher risk of complications such as pain and hemorrhage, which can be acute and severe (24). In such cases, selective angioembolization offers good temporary symptomatic control, whereas NSS represents the best form of long-term therapy (25–27). Embolization can also provide satisfactory long-term results but is frequently associated with the need for secondary procedures (26, 27).

The recently described epithelioid AML is a very rare variant that has an aggressive, malignant natural history and may account for some of the published case reports of aggressive AML (28).

Renal Metastasis

Metastasis to the kidneys is rare and is most commonly seen with melanoma, lymphoma and cancers of the lung and breast. In such cases, metastatic disease is frequently present at other sites in addition to the kidney; isolated metastasis to the kidney is exceptionally uncommon. In these instances, renal biopsy is valuable and can distinguish metastasis from a primary renal tumor, which can dramatically alter the treatment plan. This is a situation in which renal biopsy can play an important role in patient management (Figure 32.5) (29).

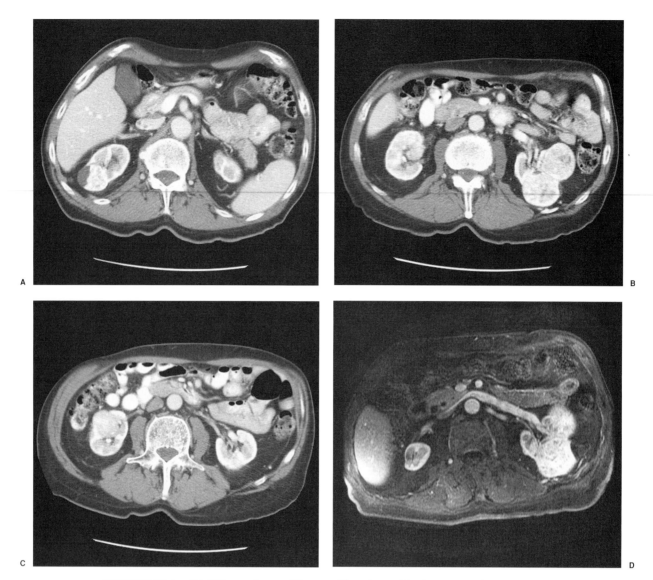

FIGURE 32.4. (A) CT scan from a 77-year-old patient with chronic renal insufficiency (creatinine 1.8 mg/dl) showing bilateral multifocal enhancing renal tumors suspicious for RCC. The patient underwent right partial nephrectomy with complete resection of two tumors and preservation of 50% of the renal parenchyma. Pathology of both specimens showed oncocytoma. Plans for a staged left partial nephrectomy were put on hold. A percutaneous biopsy of both left renal lesions was performed and revealed histology similar to his contralateral kidney. (B) After observation for 3 years, there was some growth in the left renal oncocytomas on MRI. Serum creatinine was stable at 3.1 mg/dl, and the patient remained off dialysis. (Copyright Surena F. Matin, 2006)

GENETIC SYNDROMES ASSOCIATED WITH RENAL CELL CARCINOMA

The majority of cases of RCC are sporadic in origin. Rarely, RCC may occur in association with a genetic syndrome, such as von Hippel Lindau (VHL), hereditary papillary RCC (HPRCC), and Birt-Hogg-Dube (BHD).

VHL, which occurs in 1 in approximately 36,000 people, is the most common genetic syndrome associated with development of RCC (30). It is a heritable, autosomal-dominant disease with a high penetrance.

Patients with VHL develop clear-cell RCC; retinal angiomas; cerebellar and spinal hemangioblastomas; pheochromocytomas; pancreatic neuroendocrine tumors; endolymphatic sinus tumors; and cysts of the pancreas, kidney and epididymis. This genetic lesion is found on the short arm of chromosome 3. The VHL protein is primarily involved in the regulation of hypoxia-inducible factors that control oxygen-sensing and upregulate pro-angiogenic factors, such as vascular endothelial growth factor (VEGF) and platelet-derived growth factor (PDGF) (Figure 32.6)

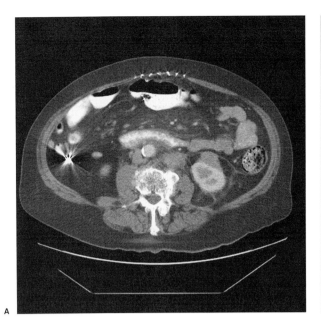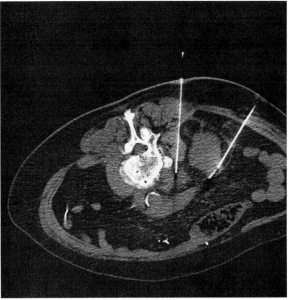

A   B

FIGURE 32.5. Illustration of the role of renal biopsy in a female patient with history of locally advanced breast cancer, referred because of a renal mass and retroperitoneal adenopathy found during staging of the breast cancer. (A) Abdominal CT scan showing a left renal and perinephric mass and retroperitoneal adenopathy. (B) Percutaneous biopsies of the perinephric/renal mass and the adenopathy were performed. Both showed lymphoma, prompting referral to an oncologist for chemotherapy. (Copyright Surena F. Matin, 2006)

(30). The majority of sporadic conventional RCCs also exhibit a mutation in the *VHL* gene, and this finding has led to much progress in the treatment of advanced RCC. Patients with VHL tend to develop multiple, bilateral RCC as young adults (Figure 32.7). In the past, the primary source of morbidity and mortality from VHL has been RCC, with patients frequently dying in their 30s and 40s.

HPRCC is associated with two separate genetic defects that manifest as different phenotypes, which are recapitulated in sporadic type 1 and type 2 papillary RCCs. Most sporadic type 1 papillary RCCs are associated with a somatic mutation of the *C-MET* gene on chromosome 7, the protein product that is a ligand for hepatocyte-derived growth factor (31). This growth factor is also inherited as an autosomal-dominant syndrome characterized by multi-focality and bilaterality that occurs in young adults (32–34). Type 2 papillary RCC is associated with a defect in the gene encoding for fumarate hydratase, an enzyme in the Krebs cycle encoded on the long arm of chromosome 1. Type 2 papillary RCC occurs with hereditary leiomyomatosis RCC, which is seen in patients with cutaneous and uterine leiomyomas.

With both VHL and HPRCC, the risk of metastasis increases when tumor size reaches or exceeds 3 cm. At this point, treatment, usually a nephron-sparing approach, is initiated because these patients frequently require multiple procedures over their lifetime (34).

BHD was recently found to be associated with RCC. Patients with BHD develop chromophobe RCC, cutaneous fibrofolliculomas and pulmonary cysts (35, 36). The renal tumors are also bilateral and multifocal, with many of them being oncocytomas or a mix of oncocytoma and chromophobe RCC (37).

PROGNOSTIC FACTORS

Prognostication of RCC has historically been problematic. Efforts are continuously being made to improve our ability to accurately stratify patients with localized disease on the basis of risk of recurrence and patients with metastatic disease on the basis of response to therapy and survival duration. Pathologic tumor stage, tumor grade, performance status (PS) and presence of symptoms seem to be predictive of recurrence and survival in patients with localized disease. The histologic tumor subtypes also provide some prognostic information; however, the independent predictive ability of histologic subtype has been questioned (38). Clear-cell RCC, for example, has been associated with the highest risk of

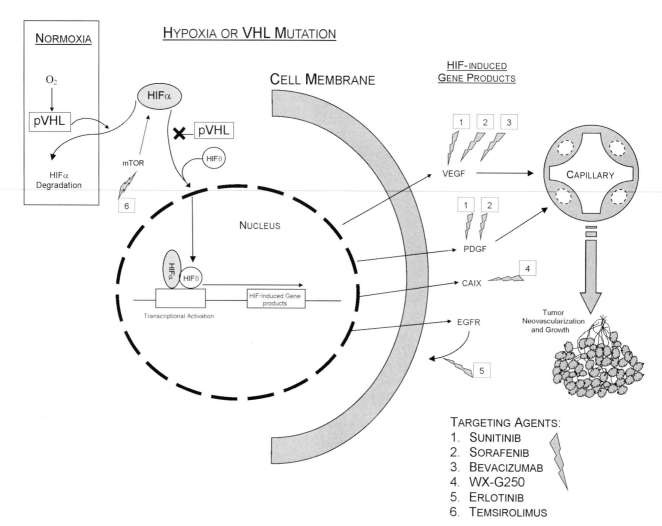

FIGURE 32.6. Mechanism of VHL neoplasia and current strategies for medical intervention. Under normal oxygen levels, the VHL protein allows breakdown of hypoxia inducible factor (HIF). In the presence of hypoxia or a dysfunctional VHL protein, HIF dimerizes, allowing transcriptional activation of HIF-inducible genes that drive responses to hypoxia, including promotion of neovascularization. Current medical regimens used to target these pathways are listed. (Copyright Surena F. Matin, 2006)

recurrence of all other histologic subtypes, whereas chromophobe RCC displays a reluctance to metastasize and arguably has a better survival prognosis than the other subtypes (38). Unclassified and sarcomatoid RCC are ominous findings and can overtake any other favorable prognostic features present.

Laboratory findings also play a role in risk stratification, particularly in patients with locally advanced and metastatic disease. The presence of anemia, hypercalcemia and elevated metabolic markers (e.g., lactate dehydrogenase, alkaline phosphatase, aspartate aminotransferase or alanine aminotransferase) heighten the suspicion of advanced disease in those without radiographic evidence of metastases, although these findings may sometimes be related to paraneoplastic syndromes known to occur with RCC. Considering the heterogeneity of RCC and all of the

possible variables affecting a patient's prognosis, it is no wonder that the development of predictive tools has been troublesome. Tumor stage has been known to play an important role in risk stratification and estimating risk of recurrence but does not seem to suffice as a single predictor (39). Several institutions have used large databases to construct prediction tables for patients undergoing surgery for localized disease. One of the first was the University of California at Los Angeles Integrated Staging System (UISS). This system used the risk factors of tumor stage, tumor grade and PS to construct low-, intermediate-, and high-risk groups (40). In an international multicenter study, investigators evaluated the ability of the UISS to predict survival (41). The UISS stratified both localized and metastatic RCC into low-, intermediate-, and high-risk groups. For localized

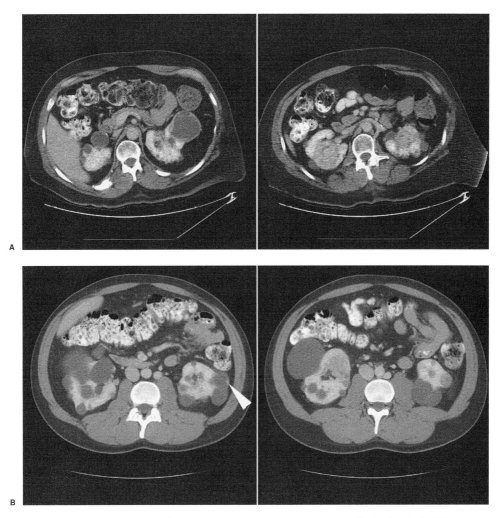

FIGURE 32.7. CT scan of patients with VHL renal tumors. (A) Abdominal CT scan from a patient with VHL and history of cerebellar and spinal hemangioblastomas and retinal hemangiomas. Multiple bilateral solid RCCs are seen as well as multiple renal cysts. (B) Abdominal CT scan from another patient with a recent diagnosis of VHL, showing multiple bilateral cysts and RCCs. In contradistinction to cysts seen in the general population, the renal cysts of VHL patients can be pre-malignant and some will form solid nodules within their walls (*arrowhead*). (Copyright Surena F. Matin, 2006)

RCC, the 5-year survival rates were 92%, 67% and 44%, respectively. The UISS was found to be less accurate for patients with metastatic disease (41). A predictive tool developed by investigators at the Mayo Clinic that used stage, size, grade and necrosis (SSIGN) as predictive factors recently underwent external validation (42, 43). Investigators at Memorial Sloan-Kettering developed a predictive nomogram on the basis of their use of similar models in other cancers (44). In a study evaluating different predictive models, those that considered postoperative data, such as the Memorial Sloan-Kettering nomogram, performed best, but the predictive accuracy for individual patients remains suboptimal (45).

For patients with metastatic disease, the heterogeneity of findings also makes accurate predictions problematic. PS seems to be an important predictor of survival in patients with metastatic RCC, as are laboratory findings, and the number of and sites of metastases. For example, patients with a PS of 0 (no symptoms and no limitations in activities of daily living) and only minimal pulmonary metastases generally respond well to systemic therapy and have a favorable prognosis within the metastatic cohort; however, at the other extreme, patients with a PS of 3 (confined to bed or chair more than 50% of the time) and visceral metastases to the liver and lymph nodes will likely have a poor prognosis as well as poor response to cytokine therapy.

The prognostic model proposed by Motzer et al. is widely used due to its accuracy, simplicity and reliability in predicting survival in patients with metastatic

TABLE 32.3 Motzer Criteria for Risk Stratification of Patients with Metastatic Renal Cell Carcinoma

Risk Factors	1. Low performance status 2. High LDH (>1.5 times the upper limit of normal) 3. Low serum hemoglobin, high corrected serum calcium (>10 mg/dl) 4. Time from initial diagnosis to treatment of less than 1 year		
Risk Group	Number of Risk Factors*	Progression-free Survival (Months)	Median Survival Time (Months)
Favorable	0	8.3	30
Intermediate	1–2	5.1	14
Poor	3–5	2.5	5

Adapted from Motzer et al (163).

disease (46). The Motzer model considers both clinical and laboratory risk factors in its prediction analysis. This tool allows standardization of risk groups and appropriate allocation of patients to suitable clinical trials, as shown in Table 32.3. The model was recently validated by a group from the Cleveland Clinic and was expanded to include prior radiation therapy and number of metastatic sites as independent prognosticators of survival (47).

Ultimately, molecular markers may simplify and improve the reliability of strategies to risk-stratify patients with localized and metastatic RCC. Results from recent studies highlighting the potential usefulness of tumor markers such as carbonic anhydrase IX are preliminary. Further analysis in larger patient datasets and external validation are needed to confirm these findings (48, 49).

EXPECTANT MANAGEMENT OF LOCALIZED DISEASE

In 1995, Bosniak reported the growth rate of small (<3 cm), incidentally detected tumors in high-risk patient groups or patients who refused surgery (50). The patients were followed for 2 to 8 years, with the majority of tumors growing minimally. These data led to the suggestion that expectant management or "watchful waiting" might be an appropriate initial intervention for some patients with small renal masses. Since then, other retrospective studies have confirmed these findings, with approximately 120 patients observed over 2 years (51, 52). These small, asymptomatic tumors appear to grow an average 0.5 cm/year, with rare or no cases of metastasis. After an initial period of watchful waiting, approximately one-third of patients have reportedly undergone treatment because of the apparent rapid growth

of the tumor or per the patient's choice. As a result of these emerging data, an increasing number of elderly patients in whom small, asymptomatic renal tumors are diagnosed incidentally undergo a course of expectant management with serial radiographic follow-up as an alternative to active therapy. If accelerated growth (greater than the observed average of 0.5 cm/year) is seen, intervention is usually offered.

SURGICAL MANAGEMENT OF RENAL CELL CARCINOMA

Surgery remains the only proven curative treatment for localized RCC and also plays an important role in the treatment of metastatic RCC when it is integrated with medical therapy. Surgical treatments have undergone tremendous changes since the 1990s, with the availability of minimally invasive techniques and increasing acceptance of nephron-sparing approaches.

Surgery for Localized Disease

Open and Laparoscopic Radical Nephrectomy

Robson and colleagues, in the early 1960s, were the first to show that radical nephrectomy provided a superior survival advantage for patients with RCC compared with other diverse forms of intervention used in that era, even though nearly two-thirds of patients had locally advanced disease (53). Radical nephrectomy thus became the gold standard therapy for RCC. In the nearly half century since this finding, no other treatment has had such an impact on survival for patients with RCC. The classic radical nephrectomy approach, as defined by Robson, involved the following: early vascular ligation, extrafascial dissection of the kidney (outside Gerota's fascia), en bloc resection of the adrenal gland and extensive lymph-adenectomy from the crus of the diaphragm to the aortic bifurcation (54).

The majority of surgery-outcomes research since the initial reports by Robson and Skinner has focused on reducing the morbidity associated with surgery and limiting the amount of tissue removed (54, 55). The need to routinely resect the ipsilateral adrenal gland has been questioned by several investigators, because the overall incidence of adrenal metastasis is low, generally less than 5% (56). The risk of adrenal metastasis appears to correlate with large, upper-pole and high-stage tumors (57, 58). Contemporary radiographic imaging has been found to be a very sensitive tool for detecting adrenal metastasis (59). In an analysis of the UCLA data, Tsui et al. reported a 99.4% negative predictive value of preoperative CT scan (60). In practice, when the adrenal gland appears normal on CT scan, an adrenal-sparing radical nephrectomy appears appropriate for a clinical T1–2 tumor that does not abut or encroach upon the adrenal gland.

A similar shift has occurred regarding the necessity of lymphadenectomy. The overall incidence of lymph node metastases ranges from 3% to 15% and correlates with the number of lymph nodes removed (61–63), tumor stage and tumor grade (62, 64). In a Phase III randomized trial conducted by the European Organization for Research and Treatment of Cancer that compared the complications of radical nephrectomy with (n = 389) and without (n = 383) lymphadenectomy in patients with resectable localized disease, no added risk was associated with lymphadenectomy (65). In a large study conducted at UCLA, patients with Tany, N0, M1 disease were more likely to respond to systemic immunotherapy than patients with N+, M1 disease (66). This phenomenon has also been observed by others (67).

Extensive lymph node mestastasis is an independent predictor of survival, and it generally portends poor survival as well as reduced response to therapy (67). Lymphadenectomy in this setting is considered to have little therapeutic value, but select patients with minimal lymph node disease and no other sites of metastatic disease represent a subgroup who may benefit from more extensive lymph node dissection (68). Other, more recent, data have also challenged the traditional notion, and have suggested that, at least in a subset of patients, a clinically relevant improvement in recurrence-free survival may be seen with aggressive resection of nodal metastasis (69). Lymph nodes smaller than 2 cm on CT scan or MRI are not always malignant and may just be reactive (70). Thus, visible enlargement on preoperative imaging or palpable enlargement at surgery warrant resection for diagnostic purposes, but the therapeutic benefit in this setting remains unclear (71). At present, lymphadenectomy appears to be a safe adjunct to radical nephrectomy that can aid in staging and risk stratification of disease.

Open radical nephrectomy remains indicated for locally advanced RCC, but the majority of low-to-intermediate clinical stage tumors are now removed laparoscopically as a standard practice (Table 32.4). Laparoscopic radical nephrectomy (LRN) was first reported in 1991 (72), but due to concerns regarding cancer spillage, port-site seeding and other oncologic issues, acceptance of this approach by the urologic community was slow. Several 5-year follow-up studies and a 10-year follow-up study have shown the

TABLE 32.4 Reported Survival Outcomes after Laparoscopic and Open Radical Nephrectomy

First Author and Reference	No. of Patients	Tumor Stage	Follow-up (Months)	5-year DFS (%)*	5-year OS (%)*
Saika et al. (76)	Open 68	T1	65	87	94
	Lap 168	T1	40	91	94
Chan et al. (74)	Open 54	T1–2	44	86	75
	Lap 67	T1–2	36	95	86
Portis et al. (75)	Open 69	T1–2	69	91	89
	Lap 64	T1–2	54	92	81
Permpongkosol et al.† (73)	Open 54	T1–2	80	87	72
	Lap 67	T1–2	73	94	85

* p = ns for all.
† Additional 10-year data also show no difference in survival data.
DFS, disease-free survival; OS, overall survival; Lap, laparoscopic.

TABLE 32.5 Indications for Laparoscopic and Open Radical Nephrectomy

Indications for laparoscopic radical nephrectomy	Clinical stage T1–2 disease
	Tumor size <14 cm
	M+ disease fulfilling above criteria, with good performance status
Relative contraindications for laparoscopic surgery	Extension outside Gerota's fascia
	Prior renal surgery
	Hilar adenopathy
Indications for open radical nephrectomy	Tumor thrombus within vena cava
	Extensive hilar or interaortocaval adenopathy
	Invasion of surrounding organs

survival advantages of LRN and open radical nephrectomy to be equivalent (Table 32.5) (73–76). The well-documented benefits of LRN compared with the open approach include reduced blood loss, less need for pain and narcotic analgesics, quicker ambulation, quicker resumption of an oral diet, shorter duration of hospitalization and shorter period of convalescence (77, 78). Nearly all clinical T1, most T2, and some T3 tumors are amenable to LRN. Complication rates are equivalent to, if not better than, those of open surgery (overall average, approximately 12% to 15% (79, 80). In the hands of an experienced urologist, the operative time of LRN is also equivalent or less to that of open surgery, and the cost is less (81). Thus, LRN is an accepted treatment approach for the majority of clinically localized RCCs, and an increasing number of urologists in the community have become facile at this operation.

LRN can be performed by many different techniques, such as conventional transperitoneal, conventional retroperitoneal and hand-assisted laparoscopy (82, 83). Hand-assisted laparoscopic nephrectomy (HALN) was developed as a consequence of the need to perform intact specimen extraction and to improve the learning curve of laparoscopy. The primary advantage of HALN compared with conventional LRN appears to be a shorter operative time. HALN also has several advantages over open nephrectomy (84–86).

Some institutions perform specimen morcellation in order to minimize the size of the surgical incision. Morcellation is performed solely for cosmesis and presumably to lessen postoperative pain. The short-sighted argument has also been made that, because no active therapy exists, pathologic information has no use in treatment. Our own data show that, on pathologic evaluation of the intact specimen, upward of

26% of patients with clinical T1–2 tumors are found to harbor high-risk disease undetected on preoperative imaging, warranting a more intensive follow-up regimen or enrollment in an adjuvant trial. Such information is likely lost with morcellation (87). Specimen morcellation is not performed at our institution or at most other institutions with a dedicated and active cancer program.

Port-site metastasis is another oncologic concern with regard to laparoscopic surgery. Data thus far suggest that port-site metastasis is an unusual event that appears to occur with the same frequency as implantation into an open incision and likely reflects the biology of disease (88). The carbon dioxide used to establish pneumoperitoneum does not facilitate tumor seeding as had initially been suspected (89). Very few cases of port-site metastases have been reported (90, 91).

Nephron-sparing Surgery (NSS)

Partial nephrectomy, or NSS, is now standard practice for the treatment of most small tumors. The ability to offer partial nephrectomy is in large part due to advances in imaging technology, improved surgical techniques and an improved understanding of the biology of RCC. In 1978, Palmer and Swanson were among the first to suggest that partial nephrectomy, when technically feasible, be considered in the setting of solitary kidneys, which was one of the first accepted indications for this approach (92). However, controversy persisted over more elective indications for partial nephrectomy (i.e., a small tumor with a normal contralateral kidney). In more recent years, several long-term studies have shown equivalent overall survival rates in patients undergoing NSS and those undergoing radical nephrectomy for a unilateral renal tumor less than 4 cm in size and a normal contralateral kidney, as well as comparable 5- and

TABLE 32.6 Indications for Nephron-sparing Surgery

Elective	Single renal tumor <4 cm, normal contralateral kidney
Relative	Systemic condition threatening but not yet affecting contralateral kidney or global renal function (e.g., diabetes mellitus, stone disease)
	Tumor 4–7 cm, well-demarcated, no local infiltration, minimal or no central extension
Imperative	Bilateral renal tumors
	Chronic renal insufficiency
	Solitary functioning kidney

10-year recurrence-free survival rates (93–95). The risk of recurrence increases with larger tumors, bilateral tumors, multi-focality, symptoms and certain histologies, such as papillary RCC (96). Results of a recent large-scale, multi-institutional study support the safety and efficacy of partial nephrectomy in patients with small (<4 cm) T1 tumors and select patients with larger (4–7 cm) T1 tumors (97). Contemporary indications for NSS are listed in Table 32.6. Recent data have also shown better quality of life for patients undergoing NSS compared with radical nephrectomy in addition to a lower long-term risk of renal failure (98–101). From a technical perspective, a 1-cm margin of normal tissue around the tumor has historically been deemed necessary during partial nephrectomy; however, recent data have shown that it is not necessary to specify an exact margin width as long as some margin is present (102–104).

The next generation of kidney surgery will be the integration of minimally invasive techniques with a nephron-sparing strategy. The increasing detection of small, incidentally discovered tumors, the advancements in minimally invasive techniques, the application of new ablative technologies and an improved understanding of the natural history of RCC have made minimally invasive nephron-sparing procedures possible. This is a rapidly evolving field, for which little multi-institutional data and virtually no long-term oncologic data are yet available. Current clinically utilized modalities and their roles in current management will be discussed briefly. Laparoscopic partial nephrectomy (LPN) has been shown to be an effective, minimally invasive nephron-sparing approach for select small renal tumors (105). LPN largely adheres to principles of open surgery, including hilar clamping, sharp dissection of the renal tumor

with a margin of normal tissue, suture ligation of the pelvicalyceal collecting system, ligation of central renal vessels and parenchymal reconstruction (105). However, it remains a challenging surgical endeavor that requires extensive laparoscopic experience and careful patient selection. Laparoscopic or percutaneous energy-ablative therapies, such as cryoablation and radiofrequency ablation (RFA), are discussed elsewhere in this textbook and are only reviewed here from a general urologic perspective (see Chapter 5, Image-guided Interventions: Fundamentals of Radiofrequency Tumor Ablation). These minimally invasive, nephron-sparing modalities are usually reserved for small (<4 cm) tumors and patients for whom surgery poses a risk. The greatest advantages of a percutaneous approach are the ease of repeat therapy and minimal patient morbidity. RFA may be performed under MRI or CT guidance for removal of tumors that are posteriorly or laterally located. Lesions that are anterior or in close approximation to the ureter, bowel or other critical structures may be approached laparoscopically or using adjunctive percutaneous measures such as hydrodissection. Small, exophytic tumors can most likely be treated efficaciously with cryoablation or RFA. Both techniques have a favorable adverse-outcome profile. A 3-year recurrence rate of approximately 4% has been reported following cryoablation (106). Incomplete treatment has been reported more frequently after RFA than after cryoablation, but there are factors that are clearly associated with improved outcomes, such as exophytic location, small size and improvements in the technology (107). With all energy-ablative therapies, intensive postoperative follow-up imaging is required to determine the effectiveness of treatment, because no pathology report nor long-term data are available to confirm cure. It is critical that patients understand this issue and adhere to a systematic follow-up regimen that involves evaluation by a care team composed of a urologist as well as the treating interventionalist. In a recent multi-institutional study, most cases of residual and recurrent disease were detected within 3 months, although many were also detected until 2 years following treatment. On the basis of the kinetics of detection, it was determined that patients should, at minimum, undergo contrast-enhanced imaging analysis at 1 month, 3 or 6 months and 12 months and then semiannually or annually after energy-ablative therapy (108).

Surgery for Locally Advanced Disease

Locally advanced RCC is identified by the presence of either a tumor thrombus in the venous system, local invasion of perinephric fat or surrounding structures. The presence of a tumor thrombus is not uncommon in RCC and is further defined by its level of extension, with 0 indicating the thrombus is limited to the renal vein; I, extension to less than or equal to 2 cm above the renal vein; II, extension greater than 2 cm above the renal vein but below the hepatic veins; III, extension to or above the level of the hepatic veins but below the diaphragm; and IV, extension above the diaphragm (right atrium) (109). MRI provides for accurate localization and excellent angiographic images and has largely replaced inferior venacavography as a noninvasive alternative (110). Transesophageal echocardiography (TEE) is useful as a presurgery adjunct for accurately defining the level of tumor thrombus if non-invasive studies are inconclusive, because extension at or above the hepatic veins may require a thoracotomy for complete extraction, and atrial tumor thrombi require cardiopulmonary bypass with hypothermic circulatory arrest. During surgery, TEE can aid in the detection of tumor embolization (111). The level of tumor thrombus may have an impact on survival, which, overall, has improved with modern imaging and surgical techniques, and can even result in satisfactory long-term outcomes when no metastatic disease is present and complete resection of disease is achieved, even with tumor thrombi extending to the atrium (109, 111–114). In patients with no perinephric fat invasion, a completely resected vena caval tumor thrombus and no evidence of metastatic disease, 5-year survival rates can exceed 60% (109, 112, 115). Prior data have suggested that survival was worse for those with tumor thrombi above the diaphragm compared with those in whom the tumor thrombi was below. Recent data, however, have shown that a clearer distinction in survival may be seen in those with a renal vein tumor thrombus (level 0) versus any in the vena cava (109, 112, 115).

Locally invasive disease can be manifested by direct tumor extension into the perinephric fat and into surrounding structures, such as the adrenal gland, psoas muscle, paraspinal muscles, liver, spleen, duodenum, colon and pancreas. Invasion of the liver, spleen, pancreas and duodenum is unusual. Direct invasion of the adrenal gland is technically stage T3a disease, but some have argued that survival in these cases is worse and these cases should more appropriately be classified as T4 disease (116). Disease invading other organs is classified as stage T4 disease. When there is no evidence of metastatic disease, the goal of therapy in these cases is complete surgical excision of the tumor. A less aggressive treatment inevitably results in local recurrence, and resection of recurrent tumor post-nephrectomy is difficult and results in reduced survival. Unfortunately, stage T4 disease is associated with significantly reduced survival, but there are patients who will enjoy a prolonged disease-free survival with complete resection of disease (116). Systemic therapy or radiation has not shown any benefit as salvage treatments following substandard surgery. Although this policy might be revised in the future as studies evaluating newer targeted agents are completed, the importance of an aggressive surgical approach to resect all disease remains paramount.

Surgery for Metastatic Disease

Cytoreductive Nephrectomy

Surgery has long played a role in the treatment of metastatic RCC (MRCC); however, results from two similarly designed Phase 3 randomized trials, one by the Southwest Oncology Group and the other by the European Organization for Research and Treatment of Cancer, which were subsequently published as a combined study, showed a clear survival advantage for patients who underwent surgery plus immunotherapy versus immunotherapy alone (117, 118). It is worth noting several misconceptions arising from these trials. First, the immunotherapeutic agent used in theses studies, interferon-alpha (IFNα), is not as active as interleukin-2 (IL-2), such that better overall responses may have been obtained if the latter agent was used. Second, these studies were performed prior to the availability of the newer targeted agents, which have shown more promising and possibly more durable responses than with either IFNα or IL-2. Third, these studies did not prove that surgery *prior to* systemic therapy was better than systemic therapy followed by surgery, only that the *addition of* surgery improved survival. It is common to hear arguments that surgery should be performed first based on these data, but no study has yet shown one particular order of treatment to be superior over the other. Determining the optimal multidisciplinary care plan for patients with MRCC remains unresolved.

It has become increasingly clear that the patients with good PS and in whom the bulk of the cancer is in the kidney benefit most from the addition of cytoreductive surgery. Those with decreased PS or in whom the bulk of the cancer is in metastatic sites usually undergo systemic therapy first and then, depending on the results, re-evaluation to determine the need for consolidative surgery. Laparoscopic cytoreductive nephrectomy can be done safely and with good outcomes with proper patient selection, and it allows earlier administration of systemic therapy as well as improved quality-of-life outcomes associated with the laparoscopic procedure (119, 120).

Resection of Local Recurrence

Select patients with recurrent RCC enjoy long-term survival after surgical resection, particularly those with an isolated recurrence and those with a disease-free interval of more 1 year before recurrence (121). A patient presenting with a single metastatic site years after surgery is the ideal candidate for resection of the metastasis. Patients with adrenal metastases may not derive curative benefit from adrenalectomy in general; however, select patients, particularly those presenting with an isolated metastasis after a long progression-free period, are most likely to benefit from resection (58). The advent of percutaneous ablative therapies for treatment of lesions in multiple organ systems, such as bone and lung, may allow for a change in this paradigm and a reassessment of the risk-benefit ratio of the morbidity of intervention with its potential incremental benefit to survival.

MEDICAL MANAGEMENT OF HIGH-RISK AND METASTATIC RENAL CELL CARCINOMA

Nearly 30% to 40% of patients undergoing surgery will have metastases, and some of them will survive a long period of time despite the development of metastases. The treatment of MRCC often requires a multi-disciplinary approach with involvement of a urologist and medical oncologist and frequently other specialists, such as an interventional oncologist. This strategy is required for the development of a treatment plan that can combine surgery, systemic therapy and possibly additional local therapies to impact survival or for palliation of symptoms. Multi-modality strategies are typically used for patients with a good PS and minimal metastatic dis-

ease, with surgery historically performed first followed by systemic therapy. As discussed previously, whether this treatment-administration sequence is superior to systemic therapy followed by surgery is unclear. Performing nephrectomy first, however, facilitates the most rapid way of reducing the tumor bulk. For patients presenting with advanced disease in which there are few or no symptoms from the primary, those in whom the large majority of disease burden is outside the kidney and those for whom surgery is deemed risky, our typical approach is initial systemic therapy followed by nephrectomy or another treatment when there is a reasonable response to initial treatment (Figure 32.8). This strategy spares patients who are unlikely to benefit from surgery and maximizes the benefit of surgery for those who are likely to respond. Those with dramatic responses in metastatic sites and who have a good PS may even undergo additional metastasectomy of residual sites.

It is important to keep in mind that the overwhelming majority of clinical research and medical treatment are focused on conventional, or clear-cell, RCC, which accounts for the majority of the different forms of RCC. Most of this discussion therefore focuses on conventional RCC, with a brief discussion of the treatment of non-conventional histologies to follow.

Adjuvant Therapy

Despite high cure rates with surgery alone for patients with low- to intermediate-stage disease, a significant proportion (40% to 60%, depending on risk status) will eventually develop recurrence due to the presence of clinically undetected micrometastases prior to surgery (39, 87, 122). To date, many therapies have been used in adjuvant fashion in an attempt to reduce the risk of recurrence after surgery, with randomized studies showing no benefit with radiation, medroxyprogesterone acetate, IFN or IL (123–126). One randomized study using an autologous tumor vaccine has shown a statistically improved progression-free survival, but this study was limited by significant patient attrition after randomization and absence of any estimates of survival (127). More recently, a heat-shock protein (HSPPC-96; Antigenics, New York, NY) has been used as a patient-specific tumor vaccine. Data from a multi-center randomized Phase II trial showed that HSPPC-96 was potentially beneficial and was associated with minimal patient toxicity; however, a Phase III confirmatory trial was closed

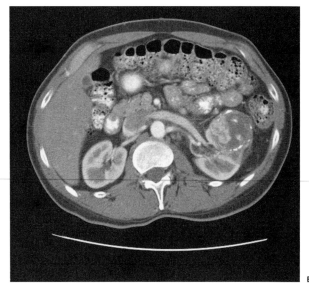

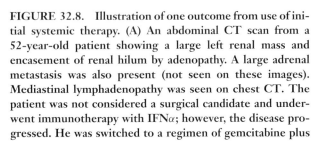

FIGURE 32.8. Illustration of one outcome from use of initial systemic therapy. (A) An abdominal CT scan from a 52-year-old patient showing a large left renal mass and encasement of renal hilum by adenopathy. A large adrenal metastasis was also present (not seen on these images). Mediastinal lymphadenopathy was seen on chest CT. The patient was not considered a surgical candidate and underwent immunotherapy with IFNα; however, the disease progressed. He was switched to a regimen of gemcitabine plus capecitabine. (B) A significant response is seen to this regimen, with a nearly complete response in the hilar adenopathy, rendering him a candidate for surgery, and with shrinkage of the primary lesion. A complete response in the chest was likewise seen. Nephrectomy and lymphadenectomy were subsequently performed. At 2 years post surgery, the patient still had no evidence of recurrence. (Copyright Surena F. Matin, 2006)

soon after enrollment began (128). Interest in the use of thalidomide as an adjuvant agent resulted from data showing that this drug produced some response, primarily disease stability, in the metastatic setting, and that its once-daily oral regimen was advantageous (129–131). In a Phase II randomized study, thalidomide significantly improved disease-specific survival but had no impact on time to recurrence and caused significant toxicity that limited tolerability (132). A Phase II, double-blind, randomized study is currently enrolling patients who have undergone nephrectomy and who are at high risk of recurrence. Patients will be randomized to sorafenib (BAY43–9006; Bayer Pharmaceuticals, West Haven, CT) or sunitinib malate (SU11248; Pfizer, New York, NY) or placebo, with a target enrollment of 1332 patients. When this study reaches its accrual goal, it will be one of the largest trials ever of adjuvant therapy for RCC (133).

Cytotoxic Chemotherapy

Traditionally, MRCC has been considered chemoresistant. Select agents have been intermittently used in the past but responses overall have been discouraging. Despite initial enthusiasm for vinblastine, when used alone, this agent did not appear to have any significant activity in patients with MRCC, with a reported response rate of 2.5% (134). Vinblastine in combination with IFNα produced slightly higher responses, but this effect was likely due primarily to the effect of IFNα (134). A Phase II trial of gemcitabine plus fluorouracil showed this combination to have an objective response rate of 17% with a tolerable toxicity profile (135). Gemcitabine plus fluorouracil also improved progression-free survival in patients with MRCC compared with historical controls and became a promising salvage regimen (135). More recently, capecitabine, which is converted to fluorouracil after ingestion, has been used in combination with gemcitabine with modest responses being observed in patients who had failed immunotherapy (136). Targeted therapies, although technically considered chemotherapy in the classic sense, have a unique and more specific mechanism of action than cytotoxic regimens and are therefore discussed in a separate section.

Cytokine and Biologic Therapy

The infiltration of tumor by lymphocytes, the modest responses to immunotherapy and the rare case of spontaneous tumor regression have contributed to the designation of RCC as an immunogenic tumor (137). IL-2, a growth factor that promotes the function and proliferation of T cells, was one of the first treatments approved by the Food and Drug Administration for treatment of MRCC (138). It is associated with a 15% overall response rate and a 7% complete response rate, which is durable in some patients. The most satisfactory responses come from administration of high-dose IL-2, a toxic regimen that can lead to respiratory distress, capillary leak syndrome and renal failure, and that requires hospitalization in a dedicated intensive care unit. IFNα, an immunomodulatory factor with a wide range of biologic activities, was never approved for use in MRCC but gained popularity in this application, likely due to its lower toxicity profile and reported 12% to 18% response rates, although complete responses were obtained in fewer than 5% of patients. Combination regimens using IFNα with other cytokines (e.g., IL-2) or with cytotoxic agents (e.g., vinblastine and medroxyprogesterone) have been tried with variable responses (134, 139). The combination of IL-2 with IFNα appears to induce better response rates than either agent alone, although with a higher toxicity profile and unclear benefit with regard to survival (140). It is important to note that these combinations are relevant only for patients with conventional RCC and cannot be translated to those with non-conventional histologies, which do not respond to immunotherapy.

Targeted Therapy

For more than two decades, no significant improvement in the treatment of MRCC was seen. Several discoveries, however, paved the way for the use of targeted therapies. The understanding of the relationship between cancer progression and VEGF along with the discovery of VHL mutations in the majority of tumors of patients with clear-cell RCC was a critical milestone in the development of targeted therapies (141). VEGF and a variety of other pro-angiogenic factors, such as PDGF, are induced when hypoxia-inducible factor (HIF), which is directly regulated by the VHL protein, is activated (Figure 32.6) (141). One of the initial strategies for targeting the VEGF pathway was accomplished with a humanized recombinant anti-VEGF antibody, bevacizumab (Genentech, San Francisco, CA). In a randomized Phase II trial, bevacizumab significantly prolonged time to progression of disease in patients with MRCC but had no effect on survival (142). This prompted the design of a Phase II

randomized study comparing bevacizumab in combination with IFNα and IFNα alone to determine their effects on survival (143).

In December 2005 and January 2006, two drugs were approved by the Food and Drug Administration for use in patients with MRCC – sorafenib and sunitinib malate. Both compounds are small-molecule, tyrosine kinase inhibitors directly targeting the VEGF receptor as well as the PDGF receptor (Figure 32.6). Because they affect multiple targets to varying degrees, these compounds are considered "dirty" targeting agents, which may be a positive factor in the observed clinical responses. A Phase III randomized trial of the use of sorafenib in 769 patients with advanced RCC who had received one prior therapy was recently presented (144). The median progression-free survival duration was 24 weeks for patients on sorafenib versus 12 weeks for those receiving a placebo, with 12-week, progression-free survival rates of 79% and 50%, respectively. These data add to the growing body of literature supporting the use of multi-targeted inhibitors such as sorafenib in prolonging survival of patients with advanced RCC at the cost of a reasonable safety profile. In another recently published study, sunitinib malate was shown to be superior to IFNα as first-line treatment for MRCC (145).

Given these data and additional data from other studies, it is anticipated that targeted therapies will increasingly become considered the standard first-line treatment for MRCC, with immunotherapy held in reserve for non-responders and those who may not tolerate these compounds. Other promising areas of clinical research include studies of combination therapies, such as anti-VEGF receptor plus anti-epithelial growth factor receptor (EGFR). This combination has shown activity in a variety of other tumor types (146). EGFR blockade as single therapy has not been shown to have any benefit, but as a multi-targeted approach, may be beneficial (147, 148). Another promising target uses inhibition of mTOR, a signaling protein regulating cell growth and angiogenesis. Hudes et al. recently reported results of an interim analysis of data from an ongoing Phase III trial of the use of temsirolimus (CCI-779; Wyeth Pharmaceuticals, Madison, NJ), an inhibitor of mTOR, in the treatment of advanced MRCC. As a single agent, temsirolimus, compared with INFα, significantly increased overall survival rates of patients who had failed first-line therapy (149). It has been approved by the FDA for treatment of poor prognosis patients.

Non-myeloablative Stem Cell Transplantation

The basis for non-myeloablative allogeneic stem cell transplantation is to induce a graft-versus-tumor response rather than relying on direct cytotoxicity. In contrast to myeloablative stem cell transplantation, in the non-myeloablative setting, chemotherapy is given to only partially suppress the immune system, allowing for engraftment of human leukocyte antigen (HLA)-matched donor tissue, which, in time, chimerizes with the host T cells. With recovery of the host immune system, immunosuppressant agents are given at a dose at which graft-versus-host (GVH) response is controlled to produce a selective graft-versus-tumor effect (150). Initial results of this treatment regimen showed an impressive 30% complete response rate in the first 10 patients treated. A recent update showed a 45% objective response rate (151, 152). These responses may not be seen until 8 months after transplantation, and initial tumor growth can be seen in the first few months. Unfortunately, this strategy is also associated with a high, and perhaps unacceptable, mortality rate (up to 20%) as a result of toxicity from GVH disease and opportunistic infections (150). A donor, usually a HLA-compatible sibling, is also needed. Due to these limitations and notably the high toxicity, non-myeloablative stem cell transplantation has been applied very selectively and sparingly.

Treatment of Non-conventional Histologic Subtypes

Metastatic sarcomatoid, papillary, collecting-duct, medullary and unclassified RCC are notoriously unresponsive to most agents. RCC with sarcomatoid elements represents a dedifferentiated form of conventional, papillary or other distinct histologies as opposed to being an actual renal sarcoma, which is quite rare (18). Sarcomatoid MRCC generally carries a poor prognosis, with a median survival duration of less than 1 year (19). Sarcoma regimens have had some activity against sarcomatoid RCC but are highly toxic (153). In a Phase II trial with 23 evaluable patients, there were no objective responses, and one patient death due to toxicity (153). Occasional case reports, however, show more favorable responses with this regimen, which is occasionally used for lack of other rational options (154). Regimens used to treat transitional-cell carcinoma have been used in patients with collecting-duct RCC with some activity being seen, probably because these two neoplasms may be closely associated (155, 156).

The use of chemotherapy will likely continue to be explored in experimental settings for treatment of non-conventional histologic subtypes, because options are so limited. Randomized trials in these populations are difficult to complete because of small sample sizes.

Local Treatment of Metastatic Disease

The most valuable role for radiation therapy appears to be that of palliation of bony metastasis and treatment of brain metastasis (157–159). Radiation therapy offers good palliation of painful bony metastases and usually results in stabilization, without any improvement in survival. This is still meaningful for these patients, who are usually quite limited by their symptoms (158). Stereotactic radiosurgery for brain metastases is a relatively low-risk option and minimally invasive, and it is especially advantageous as multiple lesions can be treated, and treatment can be repeated for local recurrences (157). At present, there is no role for the use of conventional radiation therapy in the treatment of primary renal tumors or as adjuvant to surgery for prevention of local recurrence.

Angioembolization plays an important role in prenephrectomy angioinfarction in select cases, as well as for vascular infarction of bony metastasis prior to surgery or as a palliative measure (160–162) but will not be discussed further as it is covered elsewhere in this text. (See Chapter 34, Embolotherapy in the Management of Renal Cell Carcinoma.)

REFERENCES

1. Jemal A, Siegel R, Ward E, et al. Cancer statistics, 2007. CA Cancer J Clin, 2007; 57(1): 43–66.
2. Lightfoot N, Conlon M, Kreiger N, et al. Impact of noninvasive imaging on increased incidental detection of renal cell carcinoma. Eur Urol, 2000; 37(5): 521–527.
3. Chow WH, Devesa SS, Warren JL, et al. Rising incidence of renal cell cancer in the United States. JAMA, 1999; 281(17): 1628–1631.
4. Murai M and Oya M. Renal cell carcinoma: Etiology, incidence and epidemiology. Curr Opin Urol, 2004; 14(4): 229–233.
5. Campbell RJ, Broaddus SB, and Leadbetter GW. Staging of renal cell carcinoma: Cost-effectiveness of routine preoperative bone scans. Urology, 1985; 25(3): 326–329.

6. Gold PJ, Fefer A, and Thompson JA. Paraneoplastic manifestations of renal cell carcinoma. Semin Urol Oncol, 1996; 14(4): 216–222.

7. Kim HL, Belldegrun AS, Freitas DG, et al. Paraneoplastic signs and symptoms of renal cell carcinoma: Implications for prognosis. J Urol, 2003; 170(5): 1742–1746.

8. Rosenblum SL. Paraneoplastic syndromes associated with renal cell carcinoma. J SC Med Assoc, 1987; 83(7): 375–378.

9. Sufrin G, Chasan S, Golio A, et al. Paraneoplastic and serologic syndromes of renal adenocarcinoma. Semin Urol, 1989; 7(3): 158–171.

10. Blay JY, Rossi JF, Wijdenes J, et al. Role of interleukin-6 in the paraneoplastic inflammatory syndrome associated with renal-cell carcinoma. Int J Cancer, 1997; 72(3): 424–430.

11. Hanash KA. The nonmetastatic hepatic dysfunction syndrome associated with renal cell carcinoma (hypernephroma): Stauffer's syndrome. Prog Clin Biol Res, 1982; 100: 301–316.

12. Stauffer MH. Nephrogenic hepatosplenomegaly. Gastroenterology, 1961; 40: 694.

13. AJCC Cancer Staging Manual, 6th edition. New York: Springer-Verlag; 2002.

14. Tokuda N, Naito S, Matsuzaki O, et al. Collecting duct (Bellini duct) renal cell carcinoma: A nationwide survey in Japan. J Urol, 2006; 176(1): 40–43.

15. Davis CJ, Jr., Mostofi FK, and Sesterhenn IA. Renal medullary carcinoma. The seventh sickle cell nephropathy. Am J Surg Pathol, 1995; 19(1): 1–11.

16. Figenshau RS, Basler JW, Ritter JH, et al. Renal medullary carcinoma. J Urol, 1998; 159(3): 711–713.

17. Avery RA, Harris JE, Davis CJ Jr, et al. Renal medullary carcinoma: Clinical and therapeutic aspects of a newly described tumor. Cancer, 1996; 78(1): 128–132.

18. de Peralta-Venturina M, Moch H, Amin M, et al. Sarcomatoid differentiation in renal cell carcinoma: A study of 101 cases. Am J Surg Pathol, 2001; 25(3): 275–284.

19. Mian BM, Bhadkamkar N, Slaton JW, et al. Prognostic factors and survival of patients with sarcomatoid renal cell carcinoma. J Urol, 2002; 167(1): 65–70.

20. Morra MN and Das S. Renal oncocytoma: A review of histogenesis, histopathology, diagnosis and treatment. J Urol, 1993; 150(2 Pt 1): 295–302.

21. Campbell SC, Novick AC, Herts B, et al. Prospective evaluation of fine needle aspiration of small, solid renal masses: Accuracy and morbidity. Urology, 1997; 50(1): 25–29.

22. Bosniak MA, Megibow AJ, Hulnick DH, et al. CT diagnosis of renal angiomyolipoma: The importance of detecting small amounts of fat. AJR Am J Roentgenol, 1988; 151(3): 497–501.

23. Helenon O, Merran S, Paraf F, et al. Unusual fat-containing tumors of the kidney: A diagnostic dilemma. Radiographics, 1997; 17(1): 129–144.

24. Steiner MS, Goldman SM, Fishman EK, et al. The natural history of renal angiomyolipoma. J Urol, 1993; 150(6): 1782–1786.

25. Fazeli-Matin S and Novick AC. Nephron-sparing surgery for renal angiomyolipoma. Urology, 1998; 52(4): 577–583.

26. Hamlin JA, Smith DC, Taylor FC, et al. Renal angiomyolipomas: Long-term follow-up of embolization for acute hemorrhage. Can Assoc Radiol J, 1997; 48(3): 191–198.

27. Han YM, Kim JK, Roh BS, et al. Renal angiomyolipoma: Selective arterial embolization – effectiveness and changes in angiomyogenic components in long-term follow-up. Radiology, 1997; 204(1): 65–70.

28. Eble JN, Amin MB, and Young RH. Epithelioid angiomyolipoma of the kidney: A report of five cases with a prominent and diagnostically confusing epithelioid smooth muscle component. Am J Surg Pathol, 1997; 21(10): 1123–1130.

29. Sanchez-Ortiz RF, Madsen LT, Bermejo CE, et al. A renal mass in the setting of a nonrenal malignancy: When is a renal tumor biopsy appropriate? Cancer, 2004; 101(10): 2195–2201.

30. Lonser RR, Glenn GM, Walther M, et al. von Hippel-Lindau disease. Lancet, 2003; 361: 2059–2067.

31. Sweeney P, El-Naggar AK, Lin SH, et al. Biological significance of c-met over expression in papillary renal cell carcinoma. J Urol, 2002; 168(1): 51–55.

32. Zbar B, Tory K, Merino M, et al. Hereditary papillary renal cell carcinoma. J Urol, 1994; 151(3): 561–566.

33. Schmidt L, Duh FM, Chen F, et al. Germline and somatic mutations in the tyrosine kinase domain of the MET proto-oncogene in papillary renal carcinomas. Nat Genet, 1997; 16(1): 68–73.

34. Linehan WM, Walther MM, and Zbar B. The genetic basis of cancer of the kidney. J Urol, 2003; 170(6 Pt 1): 2163–2172.

35. Birt AR, Hogg GR, Dube WJ. Hereditary multiple fibrofolliculomas with trichodiscomas and acrochordons. Arch Dermatol, 1977; 113(12): 1674–1677.

36. Nickerson M, Warren M, Toro J, et al. Mutations in a novel gene lead to kidney tumors, lung wall defects, and benign tumors of the hair follicle in patients with the Birt-Hogg-Dube syndrome. Cancer Cell, 2002; 2(2): 157.

37. Pavlovich CP, Walther MM, Eyler RA, et al. Renal tumors in the Birt-Hogg-Dube syndrome. Am J Surg Pathol, 2002; 26(12): 1542–1552.

38. Patard JJ, Leray E, Rioux-Leclercq N, et al. Prognostic value of histologic subtypes in renal cell carcinoma: A multicenter experience. J Clin Oncol, 2005; 23(12): 2763–2771.

39. Levy DA, Slaton JW, Swanson DA, et al. Stage specific guidelines for surveillance after radical nephrectomy for local renal cell carcinoma. J Urol, 1998; 159(4): 1163–1167.

40. Zisman A, Pantuck AJ, Wieder J, et al. Risk group assessment and clinical outcome algorithm to predict the natural history of patients with surgically resected renal cell carcinoma. J Clin Oncol, 2002; 20(23): 4559–4566.

41. Patard JJ, Kim HL, Lam JS, et al. Use of the University of California Los Angeles integrated staging system to predict survival in renal cell carcinoma: An international multicenter study. J Clin Oncol, 2004; 22(16): 3316–3322.

42. Frank I, Blute ML, Cheville JC, et al. An outcome prediction model for patients with clear cell renal cell carcinoma treated with radical nephrectomy based on tumor stage, size, grade and necrosis: The SSIGN score. J Urol, 2002; 168(6): 2395–2400.

43. Ficarra V, Martignoni G, Lohse C, et al. External validation of the Mayo Clinic Stage, Size, Grade and Necrosis (SSIGN) score to predict cancer specific survival using a European series of conventional renal cell carcinoma. J Urol, 2006; 175(4): 1235–1239.

44. Sorbellini M, Kattan MW, Snyder ME, et al. A postoperative prognostic nomogram predicting recurrence for patients with conventional clear cell renal cell carcinoma. J Urol, 2005; 173(1): 48–51.

45. Cindolo L, Patard JJ, Chiodini P, et al. Comparison of predictive accuracy of four prognostic models for nonmetastatic renal cell carcinoma after nephrectomy: A multicenter European study. Cancer, 2005; 104(7): 1362–1371.

46. Motzer RJ, Mazumdar M, Bacik J, et al. Survival and prognostic stratification of 670 patients with advanced renal cell carcinoma. J Clin Oncol, 1999; 17(8): 2530–2540.

47. Mekhail TM, Abou-Jawde RM, Boumerhi G, et al. Validation and extension of the Memorial Sloan-Kettering prognostic factors model for survival in patients with previously untreated metastatic renal cell carcinoma. J Clin Oncol, 2005; 23(4): 832–841.

48. Bui MH, Visapaa H, Seligson D, et al. Prognostic value of carbonic anhydrase IX and KI67 as predictors of survival for renal clear cell carcinoma. J Urol, 2004; 171(6 Pt 1): 2461–2466.

49. Kim HL, Seligson D, Liu X, et al. Using tumor markers to predict the survival of patients with metastatic renal cell carcinoma. J Urol, 2005; 173(5): 1496–1501.

50. Bosniak MA, Birnbaum BA, Krinsky GA, et al. Small renal parenchymal neoplasms: Further observations on growth. Radiology, 1995 Dec.; 197(3): 589–597.

51. Volpe A, Panzarella T, Rendon RA, et al. The natural history of incidentally detected small renal masses. Cancer, 2004; 100(4): 738–745.

52. Kassouf W, Aprikian AG, Laplante M, et al. Natural history of renal masses followed expectantly. J Urol, 2004; 171(1): 111–113; discussion, 113.

53. Robson CJ, Churchill BM, Anderson W. The results of radical nephrectomy for renal cell carcinoma. Transactions of the American Association of Genito-Urinary Surgeons, 1968; 60: 122–129.

54. Robson CJ, Churchill BM, Anderson W. The results of radical nephrectomy for renal cell carcinoma. J Urol, 1969; 101(3): 297–301.

55. Skinner DG, Vermillion CD, Colvin RB. The surgical management of renal cell carcinoma. J Urol, 1972; 107(5): 705–710.

56. Sagalowsky AI, Kadesky KT, Ewalt DM, et al. Factors influencing adrenal metastasis in renal cell carcinoma. J Urol, 1994; 151(5): 1181–1184.

57. Shalev M, Cipolla B, Guille F, et al. Is ipsilateral adrenalectomy a necessary component of radical nephrectomy? J Urol, 1995; 153(5): 1415–1417.

58. Kozak W, Holtl W, Pummer K, et al. Adrenalectomy – still a must in radical renal surgery? Brit J Urol, 1996; 77(1): 27–31.

59. Kletscher BA, Qian J, Bostwick DG, et al. Prospective analysis of the incidence of ipsilateral adrenal metastasis in localized renal cell carcinoma. J Urol, 1996; 155(6): 1844–1846.

60. Tsui KH, Shvarts O, Barbaric Z, et al. Is adrenalectomy a necessary component of radical nephrectomy? UCLA experience with 511 radical nephrectomies. J Urol, 2000; 163(2): 437–441.

61. Pizzocaro G, Piva L, Salvioni R. Lymph node dissection in radical nephrectomy for renal cell carcinoma: Is it necessary? Eur Urol, 1983; 9(1): 10–12.

62. Tsukamoto T, Kumamoto Y, Miyao N, Yet al. Regional lymph node metastasis in renal cell carcinoma: Incidence, distribution and its relation to other pathological findings. Eur Urol, 1990; 18(2): 88–93.

63. Terrone C, Guercio S, De Luca S, et al. The number of lymph nodes examined and staging accuracy in renal cell carcinoma. BJU International, 2003; 91(1): 37–40.

64. Ditonno P, Traficante A, Battaglia M, et al. Role of lymphadenectomy in renal cell carcinoma. Prog Clin Biol Res, 1992; 378: 169–174.

65. Blom JH, van Poppel H, Marechal JM, et al. Radical nephrectomy with and without lymph node dissection: Preliminary results of the EORTC randomized Phase III protocol 30881. EORTC Genitourinary Group. Eur Urol, 1999; 36(6): 570–575.

66. Pantuck AJ, Zisman A, Dorey F, et al. Renal cell carcinoma with retroperitoneal lymph nodes: Role of lymph node dissection. J Urol, 2003; 169(6): 2076–2083.

67. Vasselli JR, Yang JC, Linehan WM, et al. Lack of retroperitoneal lymphadenopathy predicts survival of patients with metastatic renal cell carcinoma. J Urol, 2001; 166(1): 68–72.

68. Giuliani L, Giberti C, Martorana G, et al. Radical extensive surgery for renal cell carcinoma: Long-term results and prognostic factors. J Urol, 1990; 143(3): 468–473; discussion, 473–474.

69. Canfield SE, Kamat AM, Sanchez-Ortiz RF, et al. Renal cell carcinoma with nodal metastases in the absence of distant metastatic disease (clinical stage TxN1–2M0): The impact of aggressive surgical resection on patient outcome. J Urol, 2006; 175(3Pt 1): 864–869.

70. Studer UE, Scherz S, Scheidegger J, et al. Enlargement of regional lymph nodes in renal cell carcinoma is often not due to metastases. J Urol, 1990; 144(2 Pt 1): 243–245.

71. Minervini A, Lilas L, Morelli G, et al. Regional lymph node dissection in the treatment of renal cell carcinoma: Is it useful in patients with no suspected adenopathy before or during surgery? BJU Int, 2001; 88(3): 169–172.

72. Clayman RV, Kavoussi LR, Figenshau RS, et al. Laparoscopic nephroureterectomy: Initial clinical case report. J Laparoendosc Surg, 1991; 1(6): 343–349.

73. Permpongkosol S, Chan DY, Link RE, et al. Long-term survival analysis after laparoscopic radical nephrectomy. J Urol, 2005; 174(4 Pt 1): 1222–1225.

74. Chan DY, Cadeddu JA, Jarrett TW, et al. Laparoscopic radical nephrectomy: Cancer control for renal cell carcinoma. J Urol, 2001; 166(6): 2095–2100.

75. Portis AJ, Yan Y, Landman J, et al. Long-term followup after laparoscopic radical nephrectomy. J Urol, 2002; 167(3): 1257–1262.

76. Saika T, Ono Y, Hattori R, et al. Long-term outcome of laparoscopic radical nephrectomy for pathologic T1 renal cell carcinoma. Urology, 2003; 62(6): 1018–1023.

77. Gill IS, Meraney AM, Schweizer DK, et al. Laparoscopic radical nephrectomy in 100 patients. Cancer, 2001; 92(7): 1843–1855.

78. Janetschek G, Jeschke K, Peschel R, et al. Laparoscopic surgery for stage T1 renal cell carcinoma: Radical nephrectomy and wedge resection. Eur Urol, 2000; 38(2): 131–138.

79. Matin SF, Abreu S, Ramani A, et al. Evaluation of age and comorbidity as risk factors after laparoscopic urological surgery. J Urol, 2003; 170(4 Pt 1): 1115–1120.

80. Fazeli-Matin S, Gill IS, Hsu TH, et al. Laparoscopic renal and adrenal surgery in obese patients: Comparison to open surgery. J Urol, 1999; 162(3 Pt 1): 665–669.

81. Meraney AM, Gill IS. Financial analysis of open versus laparoscopic radical nephrectomy and nephroureterectomy. J Urol, 2002; 167(4): 1757–1762.

82. Matin SF and Gill IS. Laparoscopic radical nephrectomy: Retroperitoneal versus transperitoneal approach. Curr Urol Reports, 2002; 3(2): 164–171.

83. Gill IS, Strzempkowski B, Kaouk JH, et al. Prospective randomized comparison: Transperitoneal vs retropritoneal laparoscopic radical nephrectomy [abstract]. J Endourol, 2002; 167(4): 19.

84. Wolf JS, Jr., Moon TD, Nakada SY. Hand assisted laparoscopic nephrectomy: Comparison to standard laparoscopic nephrectomy [see comments]. J Urol, 1998; 160(1): 22–27.

85. Matin SF, Dhanani N, Acosta M, et al. Conventional and hand-assisted laparoscopic radical nephrectomy: A comparative analysis of 271 cases. J Endourol, 2006; 20: 891–894.

86. Wolf JS, Jr., Marcovich R, Merion RM, et al. Prospective, case matched comparison of hand assisted laparoscopic and open surgical live donor nephrectomy. J Urol, 2000; 163(6): 1650–1653.

87. Cohen DD, Matin SF, Steinberg JR, et al. Evaluation of the intact specimen in patients who undergo laparoscopic radical nephrectomy for clinically localized renal cell carcinoma identifies a subset of patients at increased risk for recurrence. J Urol, 2005;173(5): 1487–1491.

88. Pearlstone DB, Feig BW, and Mansfield PF. Port site recurrences after laparoscopy for malignant disease. Semin Surg Oncol, 1999; 16(4): 307–312.

89. Tsivian A, Shtabsky A, Issakov J, et al. The effect of pneumoperitoneum on dissemination and scar implantation of intra-abdominal tumor cells. J Urol, 2000; 164(6): 2096–2098.

90. Tsivian A, Sidi AA. Port site metastases in urological laparoscopic surgery. J Urol, 2003; 169(4): 1213–1218.

91. Chen Y-T, Yang SSD, Hsieh C-H, et al. Hand portsite metastasis of renal-cell carcinoma following hand-assisted laparoscopic radical nephrectomy: Case report. J Endourol, 2003; 17(9): 771–775.

92. Palmer JM, Swanson DA. Conservative surgery in solitary and bilateral renal carcinoma: Indications and technical considerations. J Urol, 1978; 120(1): 113–117.

93. Novick AC, Gephardt G, Guz B, et al. Long-term follow-up after partial removal of a solitary kidney [see comments]. N Engl J Med, 1991; 325(15): 1058–1062.

94. Belldegrun A, Tsui KH, de Kernion JB, et al. Efficacy of nephron-sparing surgery for renal cell carcinoma: Analysis based on the new 1997 tumor-node-metastasis staging system. J Clin Oncol, 1999; 17(9): 2868–2875.

95. Herr HW. Partial nephrectomy for unilateral renal carcinoma and a normal contralateral kidney: 10-year followup. J Urol, 1999; 161(1): 33–34; discussion, 34–35.

96. Fergany AF, Hafez KS, Novick AC. Long-term results of nephron sparing surgery for localized renal cell carcinoma: 10-year followup. J Urol, 2000; 163(2): 442–445.

97. Patard JJ, Shvarts O, Lam JS, et al. Safety and efficacy of partial nephrectomy for all T1 tumors based on an international multicenter experience. J Urol, 2004; 171(6 Pt 1): 2181–2185.

98. Clark PE, Schover LR, Uzzo RG, et al. Quality of life and psychological adaptation after surgical treatment for localized renal cell carcinoma: Impact of the amount of remaining renal tissue. Urology, 2001; 57(2): 252–256.

99. Ficarra V, Novella G, Sarti A, et al. Psycho-social well-being and general health status after surgical treatment for localized renal cell carcinoma. Int Urol Nephrol, 2002; 34(4): 441–446.

100. Shinohara N, Harabayashi T, Sato S, et al. Impact of nephron-sparing surgery on quality of life in patients with localized renal cell carcinoma. Eur Urol, 2001; 39(1): 114–119.

101. Lau W, Blute M, and Zincke H. Matched comparison of radical nephrectomy versus elective nephron-sparing surgery for renal cell carcinoma (RCC): evidence for increased renal failure rate on long term followup (>10 years). J Urol, 2000; 163(4): S153.

102. Castilla EA, Liou LS, Abrahams NA, et al. Prognostic importance of resection margin width after nephron-sparing surgery for renal cell carcinoma. Urology, 2002; 60(6): 993–997.

103. Sutherland SE, Resnick MI, Maclennan GT, et al. Does the size of the surgical margin in partial nephrectomy for renal cell cancer really matter? J Urol, 2002; 167(1): 61–64.

104. Piper NY, Bishoff JT, Magee C, et al. Is a 1-cm margin necessary during nephron-sparing surgery for renal cell carcinoma? Urology, 2001; 58(6): 849–852.

105. Gill IS, Matin SF, Desai MM, et al. Comparative analysis of laparoscopic versus open partial nephrectomy for renal tumors in 200 patients. J Urol, 2003; 170(1): 64–68.

106. Steinberg AP, Gill IS, Strzempkowski B, et al. 3-year follow-up of laparoscopic renal cryoablation in 25 patients (abstract). J Urol, 2001; 167(4): 166.

107. Gervais DA, McGovern FJ, Arellano RS, et al. Renal cell carcinoma: Clinical experience and technical success with radio-frequency ablation of 42 tumors. Radiology, 2003; 226(2): 417–424.

108. Matin SF, Ahrar K, Cadeddu JA, et al. Residual and recurrent disease following renal energy-ablative therapy: Implications for management – a multi-institutional study. J Urol, 2006; 176: 1973–1977.

109. Blute ML, Leibovich BC, Lohse CM, et al. The Mayo Clinic experience with surgical management, complications and outcome for patients with renal cell carcinoma and venous tumour thrombus. BJU Int, 2004; 94(1): 33–41.

110. Kallman DA, King BF, Hattery RR, et al. Renal vein and inferior vena cava tumor thrombus in renal cell carcinoma: CT, US, MRI and venacavography. J Comput Assist Tomogr, 1992; 16(2): 240–247.

111. Glazer A and Novick AC. Preoperative transesophageal echocardiography for assessment of vena caval tumor thrombi: A comparative study with venacavography and magnetic resonance imaging. Urology, 1997; 49(1): 32–34.

112. Glazer AA and Novick AC. Long-term followup after surgical treatment for renal cell carcinoma extending into the right atrium. J Urol, 1996; 155(2): 448–450.

113. Naitoh J, Kaplan A, Dorey F, et al. Metastatic renal cell carcinoma with concurrent inferior vena caval invasion: Long-term survival after combination therapy with radical nephrectomy, vena caval thrombectomy and postoperative immunotherapy. J Urol, 1999; 162(1): 46–50.

114. Nesbitt JC, Soltero ER, Dinney CP, et al. Surgical management of renal cell carcinoma with inferior vena cava tumor thrombus. Ann Thorac Surg, 1997; 63(6): 1592–1600.

115. Moinzadeh A and Libertino JA. Prognostic significance of tumor thrombus level in patients with renal cell carcinoma and venous tumor thrombus extension. Is all T3b the same? J Urol, 2004; 171(2 Pt 1): 598–601.

116. Han KR, Bui MH, Pantuck AJ, et al. TNM T3a renal cell carcinoma: Adrenal gland involvement is not the same as renal fat invasion. J Urol, 2003; 169(3): 899–903.

117. Flanigan RC, Mickisch G, Sylvester R, et al. Cytoreductive nephrectomy in patients with metastatic renal cancer: A combined analysis. J Urol, 2004; 171(3): 1071–1076.

118. Wood CG. The role of cytoreductive nephrectomy in the management of metastatic renal cell carcinoma. Urol Clin North Am, 2003; 30(3): 581–588.

119. Walther MM, Lyne JC, Libutti SK, et al. Laparoscopic cytoreductive nephrectomy as preparation for administration of systemic interleukin-2 in the treatment of metastatic renal cell carcinoma: A pilot study. Urology, 1999; 53(3): 496–501.

120. Matin SF, Madsen L and Wood CG. Laparoscopic cytoreductive nephrectomy: The M.D. Anderson cancer center experience. Urol, 2006; 68: 528–532.

121. Kavolius JP, Mastorakos DP, Pavlovich C, et al. Resection of metastatic renal cell carcinoma. J Clin Oncol, 1998; 16(6): 2261–2266.

122. Lam JS, Shvarts O, Leppert JT, et al. Postoperative surveillance protocol for patients with localized and locally advanced renal cell carcinoma based on a validated prognostic nomogram and risk group stratification system. J Urol, 2005; 174(2): 466–472.

123. Clark JI, Atkins MB, Urba WJ, et al. Adjuvant high-dose bolus interleukin-2 for patients with high-risk renal cell carcinoma: A cytokine working group randomized trial. J Clin Oncol, 2003; 21(16): 3133–3140.

124. Lam JS, Leppert JT, Belldegrun AS, et al. Adjuvant therapy of renal cell carcinoma: Patient selection and therapeutic options. BJU Int, 2005; 96(4): 483–488.

125. Messing EM, Manola J, Wilding G, et al. Phase III study of interferon alfa-NL as adjuvant treatment for resectable renal cell carcinoma: An Eastern Cooperative Oncology Group/Intergroup trial [see comment]. J Clin Oncol, 2003; 21(7): 1214–1222.

126. Pizzocaro G, Piva L, Colavita M, et al. Interferon adjuvant to radical nephrectomy in Robson stages II and III renal cell carcinoma: A multicentric randomized study. J Clin Oncol, 2001; 19(2): 425–431.

127. Jocham D, Richter A, Hoffmann L, et al. Adjuvant autologous renal tumour cell vaccine and risk of tumour progression in patients with renal-cell carcinoma after radical nephrectomy: Phase III, randomised controlled trial. Lancet, 2004; 363(9409): 594–599.

128. Wood CG, Escudier B, Gorelov S, et al. A multicenter randomized study of adjuvant heat-shock protein peptide-complex 96 (HSPPC-96) vaccine in patients with high-risk of recurrence after nephrectomy for renal cell carcinoma (RCC) – a preliminary report. J Clin Oncol, 2004; 22(14S): 2618.

129. Daliani DD, Papandreou CN, Thall PF, et al. A pilot study of thalidomide in patients with progressive metastatic renal cell carcinoma. Cancer, 2002; 95(4): 758–765.

130. Clark PE, Hall MC, Miller A, et al. Phase II trial of combination interferon-alpha and thalidomide as first-line therapy in metastatic renal cell carcinoma. Urology, 2004; 63(6): 1061–1065.

131. Amato RJ. Thalidomide therapy for renal cell carcinoma. Crit Rev Oncol Hematol, 2003; 46(65): 27.

132. Sanchez-Ortiz R, Tamboli P, Lozano ML, et al. Adjuvant thalidomide improves disease specific survival for patients with renal cell carcinoma at high risk for relapse following surgery. J Clin Oncol, 2006; 24(18S): 14586.

133. Clinical Trials Support Unit C. ECOG2805: A randomized, double blind Phase III trial of adjuvant sunitinib versus sorafenib versus placebo in patients with resected renal cell carcinoma. http://www.ctsu.org; accessed Aug. 8, 2006.

134. Pyrhonen S, Salminen E, Ruutu M, et al. Prospective randomized trial of interferon alfa-2a plus vinblastine versus vinblastine alone in patients with advanced renal cell cancer. J Clin Oncol, 1999; 17(9): 2859–2867.

135. Rini BI, Vogelzang NJ, Dumas MC, W et al. Phase II trial of weekly intravenous gemcitabine with continuous infusion fluorouracil in patients with metastatic renal cell cancer. J Clin Oncol, 2000; 18(12): 2419–2426.

136. Waters JS, Moss C, Pyle L, et al. Phase II clinical trial of capecitabine and gemcitabine chemotherapy in patients with metastatic renal carcinoma. Br J Cancer, 2004; 91(10): 1763–1768.

137. Freed SZ, Halperin JP and Gordon M. Idiopathic regression of metastases from renal cell carcinoma. J Urol, 1977; 118(4): 538–542.

138. Fyfe G, Fisher RI, Rosenberg SA, et al. Results of treatment of 255 patients with metastatic renal cell carcinoma who received high-dose recombinant interleukin-2 therapy. J Clin Oncol, 1995; 13(3): 688–696.

139. Medical Research Council Renal Cancer Collaborators. Interferon-alpha and survival in metastatic renal carcinoma: Early results of a randomised controlled trial [see comments]. Lancet, 1999; 353(9146): 14–17.

140. Negrier S, Caty A, Lesimple T, et al. Treatment of patients with metastatic renal arcinoma with a combination of subcutaneous interleukin-2 and interferon alfa with or without fluorouracil. J Clin Oncol, 2000; 18(24): 4009–4015.

141. George DJ and Kaelin WG Jr. The von Hippel-Lindau protcin, vascular endothelial growth factor, and kidney cancer. N Engl J Med, 2003; 349(5): 419–421.

142. Yang JC, Haworth L, Sherry RM, et al. A randomized trial of bevacizumab, an anti-vascular endothelial growth

factor antibody, for metastatic renal cancer. N Engl J Med, 2003; 349(5): 427–434.

143. Rini BI, Halabi S, Taylor J, et al. Cancer and Leukemia Group B 90206: A randomized Phase III trial of interferon-alpha or interferon-alpha plus anti-vascular endothelial growth factor antibody (bevacizumab) in metastatic renal cell carcinoma. Clin Cancer Res, 2004; 10(8): 2584–2586.

144. Escudier B, Eisen T, Stadler WM, et al. Sorafenib in advanced clear-cell renal-cell carcinoma. N Engl J Med, 2007; 356(2): 125–134.

145. Motzer RJ, Hutson TE, Tomczak P, et al. Sunitinib versus interferon alfa in metastatic renal-cell carcinoma. N Engl J Med, 2007; 356(2): 115–124.

146. Herbst RS, Johnson DH, Mininberg E, et al. Phase I/II trial evaluating the anti-vascular endothelial growth factor monoclonal antibody bevacizumab in combination with the HER-1/epidermal growth factor receptor tyrosine kinase inhibitor erlotinib for patients with recurrent non-small-cell lung cancer. J Clin Oncol, 2005; 23(11): 2544–2555.

147. Druker BJ, Schwartz L, Marion S, et al. Phase II trial of ZD 1839 (Iressa), and EGF receptor inhibitor, in patients with renal cell carcinoma. Proc Am Soc Clin Oncol, 2002; 21: 720.

148. Dawson NA, Guo C, Zak R, et al. A phase II trial of gefitinib (Iressa, ZD1839) in stage IV and recurrent renal cell carcinoma. Clin Cancer Res, 2004; 10: 7812–7819.

149. Hudes G, Carducci M, Tomczak P, et al. Global ARCC Trial. Temsirolimus, interferon alfa, or both for advanced renal-cell carcinoma. N Engl J Med, 2007; 356(22): 2271–2281.

150. Drachenberg D, Childs RW. Allogeneic stem cell transplantation as immunotherapy for renal cell carcinoma: From immune enhancement to immune replacement. Urol Clin North Am, 2003; 30: 611–622.

151. Childs R, Chernoff A, Contentin N, et al. Regression of metastatic renal-cell carcinoma after nonmyeloablative allogeneic peripheral-blood stem-cell transplantation. N Engl J Med, 2000; 343(11): 750–758.

152. Childs RW, Clave E, Tisdale J, et al. Successful treatment of metastatic renal cell carcinoma with a nonmyeloablative allogeneic peripheral-blood progenitor-cell transplant: Evidence for a graft-versus-tumor effect. J Clin Oncol, 1999; 17(7): 2044–2049.

153. Escudier B, Droz JP, Rolland F, et al. Doxorubicin and ifosfamide in patients with metastatic sarcomatoid renal cell carcinoma: A Phase II study of the Genitourinary Group of the French Federation of Cancer Centers. J Urol, 2002; 168(3): 959–961.

154. Rashid MH, Welsh CT, Bissada NK, et al. Complete response to Adriamycin and ifosfamide in a patient with sarcomatoid renal cell carcinoma. Am J Clin Oncol, 2005; 28(1): 107–108.

155. Nanus DM, Garino A, Milowsky MI, et al. Active chemotherapy for sarcomatoid and rapidly progressing renal cell carcinoma. Cancer, 2004; 101(7): 1545–1551.

156. Milowsky MI, Rosmarin A, Tickoo SK, et al. Active chemotherapy for collecting duct carcinoma of the kidney: A case report and review of the literature. Cancer, 2002; 94(1): 111–116.

157. Muacevic A, Siebels M, Tonn JC, et al. Treatment of brain metastases in renal cell carcinoma: Radiotherapy, radiosurgery, or surgery? World J Urol, 2005; 23(3): 180–184.

158. Fakih M, Schiff D, Erlich R, et al. Intramedullary spinal cord metastasis (ISCM) in renal cell carcinoma: A series of six cases. Ann Oncol, 2001; 12(8): 1173–1177.

159. Goyal LK, Suh JH, Reddy CA, et al. The role of whole brain radiotherapy and stereotactic radiosurgery on brain metastases from renal cell carcinoma. Int J Radiat Oncol Biol Phys, 2000; 47(4): 1007–1012.

160. Wallace S, Granmayeh M, deSantos LA, et al. Arterial occlusion of pelvic bone tumors. Cancer, 1979; 43(1): 322–328.

161. Sweeney P, Wood CG, Pisters LL, et al. Surgical management of renal cell carcinoma associated with complex inferior vena caval thrombi. Urol Oncol, 2003; 21(5): 327–333.

162. Swanson DA, Johnson DE, von Eschenbach AC, et al. Angioinfarction plus nephrectomy for metastatic renal cell carcinoma – an update. J Urol, 1983; 130(3): 449–452.

163. Motzer RJ, Bacik J, Murphy BA, et al. Interferon-alfa as a comparative treatment for clinical trials of new therapies against advanced renal cell carcinoma. J Clin Oncol, 2002; 20(1): 289–296.

Chapter 33

PERCUTANEOUS RENAL ABLATION

Mansi A. Saksena

Debra Gervais

Peter R. Mueller

Approximately 38,890 new cases of renal cell carcinoma (RCC) were estimated to be diagnosed in the United States in 2006, with 12,840 cancer-related deaths attributed to cancers of the kidneys and the renal pelvis (1). More than one-half of these patients were diagnosed incidentally on cross-sectional imaging performed for non-related conditions (2). Increased incidental detection of small renal masses as well as advances in surgical techniques have led to development of nephron-sparing procedures for treatment in order to preserve renal function. Over the past decade, the options for the treatment of RCC have evolved to include radical nephrectomy as well as partial nephrectomy, laparoscopic nephrectomy and, in selected cases, percutaneous radiofrequency ablation (RFA) and cryotherapy. Each therapy has unique clinical applications and benefits. This article illustrates various treatment modalities used in the therapy of RCC with special emphasis on percutaneous ablative techniques.

CLINICAL OVERVIEW

RCC accounts for 85% of all renal tumors and is slightly more common in men than in women (1.6 to 1.0) (2). Symptomatic RCC usually presents with a triad of flank pain, hematuria and a palpable abdominal mass. Hematuria, either gross or microscopic, in any patient usually warrants evaluation by a computed tomographic (CT) scan. Other nonspecific symptoms include weight loss, anemia or fatigue. However, almost one-half the patients are asymptomatic at diagnosis and have incidentally detected tumors on cross-sectional imaging. Certain genetic syndromes such as von Hipple-Lindau (VHL) disease increase the incidence of RCC (accounting for approximately 2% of cases of RCC). Other risk factors include smoking, hypertension, obesity and end-stage renal disease resulting in dialysis.

Clear-cell RCC is the most common histological subtype and is associated with VHL syndrome and end stage renal disease (ESRD, Table 33.1). Other inherited forms include familial clear-cell RCC. Papillary RCC, when sporadic, has a prominent male preponderance and is associated with almost 90% 5-year survival rates prior to metastatic spread. Papillary RCC has a lesser incidence of metastases than clear-cell but, when metastatic, is harder to treat. Papillary RCC is also seen in ESRD and in several familial syndromes. Other less common cell types include chromophobe RCC and collecting-duct RCC.

One-quarter of patients with RCC have metastatic disease at diagnosis and have a poor 5-year survival rate (2). This underscores the importance of a robust initial metastatic work-up, which should include a chest X-ray and abdomen computerized tomography (CT) scan, with bone scan being optional to evaluate for bone metastases if needed. A head CT scan may be obtained in case the patient demonstrates any neurological symptoms. Moreover, one-third of patients

TABLE 33.1 Incidence of Various Histological Types of Sporadic RCC (2)

Histological Appearance	Incidence (%)
Conventional	75
Papillary	12
Chromophobe	4
Oncocytoma	4
Collecting duct	<1
Unclassified	3–5

RCC, renal cell carcinoma.

undergoing treatment develop metastatic disease on follow-up. Hence, the goal is to develop effective surgical or ablative therapies, bearing in mind that, for some patients, multiple treatments may be indicated.

The presence of multiple renal masses usually suggests a genetic predisposition, and patients are screened for various hereditary syndromes. Conditions such as VHL have unique extra-renal manifestations. Patients with these genetic syndromes are closely monitored with either contrast-enhanced CT or magnetic resonance imaging (MRI). In these patients, small masses are usually low grade and can occasionally be monitored with surgical or ablative therapy initiated for any mass as tumors enlarge (3, 4). The exact size at which therapy is generally initiated for a particular tumor in VHL patients is generally accepted to be 3 cm (3, 4) for surgical resection based on the low metastatic potential of small RCC. However, for percutaneous ablative therapies, some have advocated treating smaller tumors, starting at 2.5 to 3 cm (5–7).

STAGING

Like most cancers, the prognosis of RCC is largely dependent on the stage of disease. The tumor-node-metastasis (TNM) classification is a commonly used staging system wherein stage I disease is associated with a 95% 5-year survival rate, whereas survival in stage IV disease is 20% (Figure 33.1; Table 33.2) (2).

DIAGNOSIS

Any enhancing renal mass on a CT study of the abdomen is generally considered to be RCC unless proven otherwise. Ninety percent of masses greater than 3 cm are RCC and warrant surgical resection. However, 25% of small renal masses (<3 cm in size)

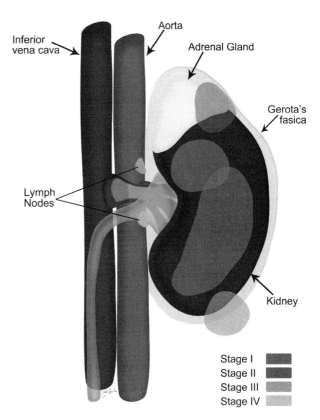

FIGURE 33.1. Diagrammatic representation of staging of RCC. (*Adapted from* Cohen et al. with permission [2].) See Color Plate 32.

TABLE 33.2 TNM staging of RCC

Primary Tumor (T):	
TX	Primary tumor cannot be assessed.
T0	No evidence of primary tumor.
T1	Tumor 7 cm or less, limited to the kidney.
T2	Tumor more than 7 cm, limited to the kidney.
T3	Tumor extension into major veins, adrenal gland or surrounding tissue, but limited within the Gerota's fascia.
	T3a – Tumor invades the adrenal gland or surrounding tissue.
	T3b – Tumor grossly extends into the renal vein or vena cava.
T4	Tumor extends beyond Gerota's fascia.
Regional Lymph nodes (N):	
NX	Regional lymph nodes cannot be assessed.
N0	No regional node metastasis.
N1	Metastasis in a single regional lymph node.
N2	Metastasis in more than one regional lymph node.
Distant Metastasis (M):	
MX	Presence of metastasis cannot be assessed.
M0	No distant metastasis present.
M1	Distant metastasis present.

TNM, tumor-node-metastasis; RCC, renal cell carcinoma.

are benign in nature (2). Thus, some physicians prefer biopsy confirmation prior to resection in order to avoid performing a nephrectomy for benign disease.

TREATMENT OPTIONS

Surgery

Stage I RCC is curable by complete resection and patients who have no contraindication to surgery generally undergo resection. The historical standard, radical nephrectomy, involves en bloc resection of the kidney along with the ipsilateral adrenal gland, Gerota's fascia and regional lymph nodes. Radical nephrectomy can be either open or laparoscopic with decreased postoperative pain and earlier recovery being the advantages of a laparoscopic procedure. Masses smaller than 3 to 4 cm may be amenable to nephron-sparing partial nephrectomy. The clinical indications for nephron-sparing surgery or partial nephrectomy include patient factors such as (6, 8, 9):

- Bilateral or multifocal tumors

- RCC in a solitary kidney

- Poor function of the unaffected kidney

- Significant comorbidities such as chronic renal failure or hypertension.

Additional tumor-related factors include a tumor less than 4 cm in size and polar lesions. These tumor features are not absolute but make partial nephrectomy technically less difficult.

Partial nephrectomy, which can also be performed laparoscopically, does bear the burden of a 3% to 6% rate of local recurrence, a result similar to radical nephrectomy (10). Given similar recurrence and survival rates, partial nephrectomy has become an acceptable alternative to radical nephrectomy.

Percutaneous Techniques

Small renal masses are increasingly being detected, particularly in patients with significant comorbid conditions. These patients are usually not ideal surgical candidates and can be treated by various minimally invasive therapies – namely, percutaneous RFA and cryoablation (11, 12). These techniques have shown promising early results and that in turn has generated enthusiasm for their application. Although other technologies such as high-intensity focused ultrasound (HIFU) have been proposed, percutaneous RFA and cryoablation are the most widely available and the most extensively evaluated and will be reviewed in this chapter.

Radiofrequency Ablation

Background

RF ablation of a tumor involves the delivery of an electrical current via needle electrodes to create high tissue temperatures and cause cell death. Cell death occurs at temperatures higher than 45°C, with complete tumor necrosis being achieved at 60° to 100°C (13). The needle electrode placed within a tumor is connected to a RF generator, and the circuit is completed by placement of grounding pads on the patient's thighs, which are also connected to the generator. As an electrical current is applied in this circuit, it causes ion agitation at the electrode tip, leading to an increase in tissue temperatures. The maximal diameter of a zone of ablation created by a 17-gauge needle electrode in liver experiments is 1.6 cm. The limitation in the size of the zone of ablation created by an electrode tip is caused by vaporization and carbonization of tissue as temperatures rise above 100°C (13). This leads to an increase in tissue impedance to the flow of electrical current. Hence, most recent technical innovations in RF ablation technology are aimed at achieving larger burns – that is, increasing the maximal diameter of the zone of ablation created by an electrode. Such innovations include the development of multi-tined electrodes, cluster arrangement of multiple electrodes, pulsing of the electrical current, internal cooling of the electrode and interstitial saline infusion (14–17).

Histology of RFA

Currently, RFA of normal porcine kidneys and ablation treatment of VX2 tumors implanted in rabbit kidneys are the primary animal tumor models utilized for determining the immediate and short-term histopathological renal changes brought about by RFA. Immediately after a RFA treatment, the zone of ablation has been found to be gray-white in VX2 rabbit tumors and well-circumscribed yellowish white in normal porcine kidneys (18, 19). Minimal hemorrhage may be seen at the electrode insertion site. Microscopically, treated cells demonstrate loss of cell border integrity, nuclear chromatin blurring, interstitial hemorrhage and cytoplasmic eosinophilia (18). By the third day post treatment, cellular nuclei become pyknotic and lysed, suggestive of coagulative necrosis. Early fibroblastic infiltration and inflammation are seen at the boundary between the region of treatment and normal renal parenchyma. By 14 days post treatment, as nuclear degeneration is completed, four zones are identified from the center to the periphery: namely, central necrosis, inflammatory infiltrate, hemorrhage and fibrosis and regeneration. Complete architectural distortion within the zone of necrosis is identified by the 30th day, and the necrotic focus is resorbed approximately 90 days after treatment (18). Initial studies in humans revealed similar results (20, 21), but the claim of complete tumor necrosis was soon challenged as Michaels et al. reported incomplete tumor necrosis in 17 tumors treated prior to nephrectomy (22). This and other studies suffered from limitations pertaining to technique and technology available at that time (23). For example, in the study by Michaels et al., only one ablation was performed per tumor without repositioning the electrode for overlapping ablations. The importance of meticulous technique with close attention to performing multiple ablations for adequate coverage of the entire tumor has since been promoted (8, 24).

Cryoablation

Background

Cryoablation operates on the conversion of high-pressure argon gas to cold low-pressure liquid by using the Joule-Thomson effect (25). The system comprises a computer workstation, a gas distribution apparatus and needle-like cryoprobes. Cryoprobes are equipped with a thermocouple, which is used to monitor tissue temperature during both freezing and thawing. Renal cryoablation can be performed via open, laparoscopic or percutaneous approaches (26–29). Percutaneous cryoablation has the advantage of allowing visualization of the iceball by imaging. This provides for intraprocedural monitoring and rough prediction of regions of cryonecrosis. This may prevent unwanted damage to normal structures and facilitate effective coverage of tumor tissue. Repetitive freeze-thaw cycles are used during cryoablation, with temperatures reaching a nadir of $-130°C$ during the freeze. Temperatures at the edge of the iceball are about $0°C$ and are considered non-lethal.

Histology of Cryoablation

Cryoablation achieves cell death by direct cryothermic and indirect ischemic cell injury. These two synergistic mechanisms are sequential, with direct cytotoxicity secondary to intracellular ice crystal formation occurring during the freeze phase and indirect ischemic injury due to local tissue microvasculature occlusion occurring during the thaw phase (30, 31). The threshold temperature at which irreversible cell death occurs is between $-19.4°C$ and $-40°C$ (32). Although such temperatures are easily achieved in the center of the iceball, the temperature at the periphery is $0°C$, and hence the iceball must extend approximately 3.1 mm beyond the tumor margins to achieve complete treatment (33). A double freeze-thaw cycle has been found to increase the region of cryonecrosis compared with a single freeze-thaw cycle (34). Histological examination of cryoablated tissue demonstrates signs of cell death such as vascular congestion, nuclear pyknosis, mitochondrial damage and coagulative necrosis, with central zones demonstrating complete cell death and transitional zones, incomplete cellular injury at the periphery (31).

Indications for Percutaneous Ablation

Patient Factors

Until robust 5-year survival and disease-free survival rates are available, percutaneous ablation is limited to treatment of patients who are not ideal candidates for other well-established treatments such as nephrectomy. These include the following conditions:

- Elderly patients (less than 10-year life expectancy)
- Multiple renal tumors, as in a VHL patient
- Solitary kidney
- Limited renal function
- Comorbid conditions precluding surgery

Additionally, RFA is generally reserved for patients with greater than 1-year life expectancy, as a small RCC is unlikely to cause clinically significant morbidity before 1 year.

Tumor-specific Factors

Tumor location and size are primary considerations when assessing a lesion for percutaneous ablation. As stated earlier, smaller tumors are more amenable to complete ablation. Although different reports use various size limits to define an ablatable RCC, the range of a small tumor is 2.5 to 4 cm (5, 6, 11, 35–40). Gervais et al. have shown that complete tumor necrosis at imaging can be achieved for tumors 4 cm or smaller (9, 24). In addition to size, tumor location also plays a significant role in the suitability of a lesion for ablation. For thermal ablation, an exophytic lesion surrounded by perirenal fat is ideal, as the insulation afforded by perirenal fat allows for achievement and maintenance of higher temperatures. A study by Gervais et al. demonstrated less complete necrosis in centrally located tumors (9). This can be attributed to a heat sink effect seen in tumors close to large hilar vessels. Blood flow in large vessels causes a perfusion-mediated cooling of tumor tissue, limiting the temperatures that can be achieved and hence inhibiting complete ablation. In addition, the rate of complications may be higher for more central tumors.

Preablation Imaging

Adequate preablation imaging provides vital information about the margins and extent of the tumor, which allows for effective treatment planning. Preablation imaging can be performed by contrast-enhanced CT or MRI regardless of the method of percutaneous ablation being used. Additionally, pretreatment images serve as a baseline for future evaluation on follow-up.

Adjunctive Procedures

A biopsy is usually performed prior to percutaneous ablation as the tumor is left in situ, unlike surgical resection, wherein specimens undergo pathological evaluation. In case of benign disease, one may not treat and, if treated, the follow-up may differ. The biopsy can be performed either on the same day as the ablation or tissue diagnosis may be obtained some time prior to ablation (24).

Technique
Anesthesia

Most patients can undergo RFA under conscious sedation as an outpatient procedure (9). Some patients may require an overnight admission. General anesthesia is usually reserved for those who do not meet institutional criteria for sedation or have failed sedation, although some operators prefer to perform all renal ablation under general anesthesia.

Cryoablation is far less painful than RFA, but takes longer to perform and requires breath holding for adequate intraprocedural imaging. Some practitioners prefer general anesthesia for cryoablation; however, it can be performed under conscious sedation as well.

Modality for Guidance

Cryoablation or RFA can be performed using ultrasound, CT or MRI guidance. The ease of tumor visualization, availability of imaging equipment and operator experience usually dictate the choice of modality. Ultrasound provides real-time visualization as the needle electrode is placed in the tumor for either technique. The disadvantage of ultrasound is that as thermal ablation is performed, tumors are often rendered highly echogenic due to formation of bubbles of water vapor or iceball formation. This makes tumor visualization for electrode repositioning to perform overlapping treatments particularly challenging. CT allows for adequate preprocedure planning and intraprocedure electrode repositioning as it produces consistent, easily reproducible images. Neither unenhanced CT nor ultrasound allows for intraprocedure precise delineation of the exact zone of ablation. MRI affords this luxury by providing accurate monitoring of treatment effects during an ablation as the iceball formed during cryoablation has a very short T2 relaxation time and is seen as a region of signal void on T2-weighted images. Limited interventional MRI units, MRI-compatible thermal ablation equipment and patient-monitoring equipment preclude widespread use of MRI guidance. Additionally, patients with a history of active ischemic heart disease cannot undergo MRI-guided cryoablation as the magnetic field of an MRI scanner precludes electrocardiographic monitoring during the procedure.

RF Ablation

Once adequate anesthesia and patient position are set up, the needle is placed within the tumor under image guidance. The value of overlapping ablations is well recognized, and multiple ablations involving repositioning the needle between sequential ablations are usually performed, with the ablation plan to cover the entire tumor. Thus, overlapping ablations are performed based on tumor size and geometry (Figure 33.2). RF electrodes allow the option of track ablation upon electrode removal. This is performed by

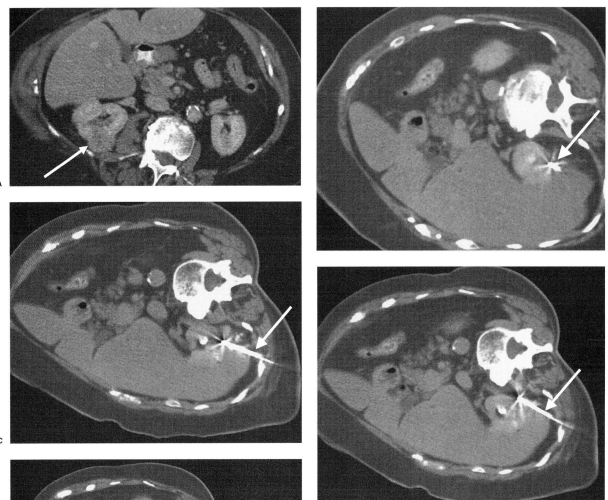

FIGURE 33.2. Seventy-eight-year-old woman with incidental detection of a right renal mass. (A) Axial section from a contrast-enhanced CT scan performed prior to RFA shows a 3 cm exophytic mass (*arrow*) in the middle pole of the right kidney. This mass was found to be an RCC after biopsy. (B–E) Axial CT images at RFA with the patient in right lateral decubitus position demonstrate multiple placements of a needle electrode (*arrow*) in order to perform overlapping ablations. Multiple treatments are often essential to ensure treatment of all regions of the tumor. The patient recovered uneventfully.

slow removal during application of current to cauterize any small bleeding vessels and to minimize the likelihood of track seeding. Once the tumor is satisfactorily covered, the patient undergoes routine post-procedure care depending on the type of anesthesia used.

Cryoablation

Unlike most RF systems, multiple cryoprobes can be used at one ablation. Typically, one cryoprobe generates an iceball that is 2 cm in the short axis (25). Tumors that measure 2 to 3 cm can be treated with two or three cryoprobes, whereas larger tumors require four or five probes (12). Thus, the treatment plan is determined by tumor size and geometry, and the number of cryoprobes is selected. Multiple (two or three) freeze-thaw cycles involving a 15-minute freeze and a 10-minute thaw can be used with temperatures reaching up to –130°C (12, 41). Intraprocedural iceball monitoring by CT or MRI can allow rough prediction of the region of cryonecrosis. If the iceball does not encompass the entire tumor and a 3.1 mm margin of tissue beyond the tumor, additional cryoprobes can be placed.

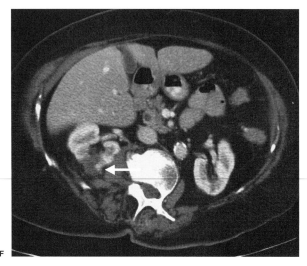

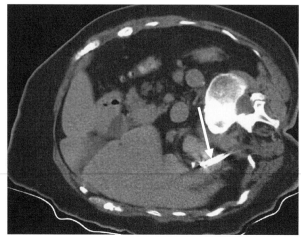

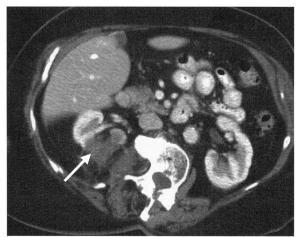

FIGURE 33.2. (*Continued*) **(F) Axial image from a contrast-enhanced CT scan performed 1 month after the ablation demonstrates an abnormal region of residual enhancement (*arrow*) along the medial margin of the ablated tumor. This appearance is consistent with residual disease. (G) Patient underwent re-ablation of the residual portion of the tumor. Axial CT image obtained at the second ablation demonstrates needle electrode (*arrow*) within the region of residual disease seen on prior image. (H) Axial image from a contrast-enhanced CT scan performed 1 month after the second ablation demonstrates expected post-ablation stranding in the region of treatment (*arrow*). There is no evidence of residual disease. No abnormal enhancement was seen on follow-up studies performed 3 and 6 months after the second ablation (*not shown*).**

Historically, cryoprobe size required open surgical exposure for placement (41–43). Advancements in cryoprobe technology have made probes small enough for percutaneous placement, enabling cryoablation to compete with percutaneous RFA (12).

Adjacent Structures

During thermal ablation, tissue injury may extend to adjacent normal organs such as the ureters or bowel. When planning ablation, note position of nearby structures to minimize risk. Techniques such as change in patient position and hydrodissection can be used to displace contiguous structures and protect them from thermal injury (44). Hydrodissection involves instillation of sterile 5% dextrose in the tissue planes between the tumor and any adjacent organ, such as bowel (Figure 33.3). This separates the tumor from nearby organs and allows ablation to be performed safely. Other agents such as carbon dioxide may also be used for organ separation (45, 46). Alternatively, laparoscopic exposure may allow retraction of bowel or ureter for safe ablation (5).

Post Procedure Follow-up

Because ablated tumor is left in situ, no histopathological information is available to assess adequacy of treatment. Imaging, therefore, is the mainstay of follow-up both for initial assessment of efficacy and for monitoring for local progression after ablation. Tumor regions that do not demonstrate any enhancement on follow-up CT or MRI are considered to be regions of complete necrosis, whereas residual foci of enhancement are interpreted to represent residual disease (Figure 33.2) (47). Residual disease can undergo retreatment by percutaneous ablation, assuming it remains within the limits of suitable size and location.

The initial post-ablation scan is generally performed between 1 and 5 weeks, depending on operator preference (9, 36–39). If no viable tumor is seen on the first follow-up study, repeat imaging can be performed at 3 months followed by 6 months and 1 year. If no new or residual disease is detected, the patient can then undergo long-term annual follow-up. In most cases, a small non-enhancing mass is

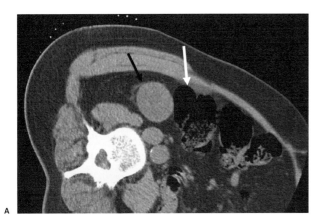

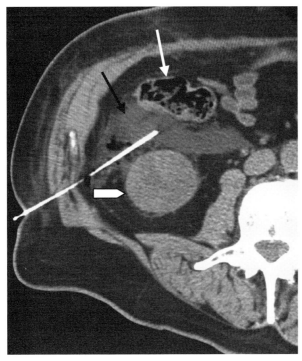

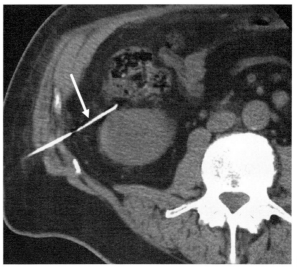

FIGURE 33.3. Seventy-year-old man presented with a right lower pole renal mass, which was amenable to RFA. **(A)** Axial CT image at RFA shows the mass (*black arrow*) lies within 1 mm of the colon (*white arrow*) increasing the risk of colonic injury during ablation. Hence, hydrodissection was performed to displace the colon and minimize risk of injury. **(B)** A 20-gauge chiba needle (*arrow*) was placed between the kidney and the colon. **(C)** Sterile 5% dextrose (*black arrow*) was instilled within the tissue planes to separate the colon (*white arrow*) from the kidney (*arrowhead*).

persistently seen at the ablation site. The zone of ablation is known to regress more after cryoablation than after RFA. However, the keystone of diagnosing residual disease remains enhancement.

Clinical Efficacy

As available RF equipment has improved, so have the results (Table 33.3). Earlier studies reported inferior treatment rates (79%) (48), probably attributable to weaker generators, which failed to achieve adequate treatment temperatures. Later studies using 150 to 200 W generators have shown 88% to 100% successful treatment rates in tumors 2.5 to 4 cm in size (5, 8, 24, 36–40, 48–50). Larger tumors (>3 cm) have predictably been harder to treat. McDougal et al. followed 16 patients treated with renal RFA for 4 years and found renal RFA of lesions less than 5 cm in diameter to be comparable to surgery (7). Although

renal RFA has been established as an effective therapy for small renal masses in non-surgical candidates, 5- to 10-year survival data are currently lacking. Once sufficient cohorts of post-ablation patients are available to assess 5-year survival, percutaneous ablation outcomes can be compared to surgical standards of resection.

Three-year follow-up data on laparoscopic renal cryoablation are encouraging, with a 3-year cancer-specific survival rate of 98% in 56 patients with a mean tumor size of 2.3 cm (51). However, percutaneous renal cryoablation is relatively newer, and there is a scarcity of efficacy data in the literature. In an initial report by Shingleton et al., 22 tumors in 20 patients were treated, with a mean tumor size of 3 cm. Only one patient required re-treatment at a mean follow-up of 9.1 months (43). A recent study of 23 patients by Silverman et al. reported complete ablation in 24 of 26

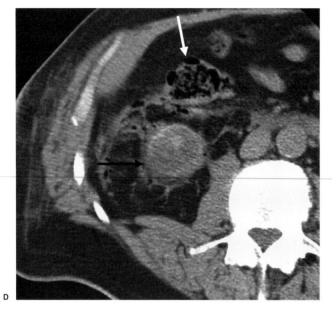
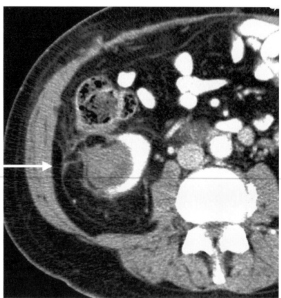

FIGURE 33.3. (*Continued*) (D) Axial image from a contrast-enhanced CT scan performed immediately following ablation shows dissolution of instilled dextrose. However, the colon (*white arrow*) and the kidney (*black arrow*) remain separated. (E) Axial image from a contrast-enhanced CT performed 1 month after ablation demonstrates a region of non-enhancement (*arrow*) at the site of ablation consistent with treated tumor. There are no regions of abnormal enhancement to suggest residual disease.

tumors, with only one patient needing re-treatment (12). These studies are limited by lack of long-term follow-up and small sample size. Larger trials with long-term follow-up are needed before accurate efficacy of cryoablation can be determined.

Complications

Compared with resection, percutaneous ablative techniques are relatively safe, with a lower rate of major complications. The most common minor complication is pain or paresthesia related to the probe insertion site (52). Other minor complications include self-limited paresthesias, transient hematuria and subcapsular hematomas (Figure 33.4) (52).

Hemorrhage necessitating blood transfusion or ureteral stent placement is the most common major complication and is more often seen in central tumors, where the proximity of large hilar vessels predisposes them to injury and bleeding. Other complications such as ureteral strictures and urinoma formation secondary to urine leaks are rare but more often seen in central tumor ablations (9, 36, 37, 52). Ureteral strictures are more common with medial tumors in the lower pole. Inadvertent injury can also

TABLE 33.3 Summary of Results Reported in Various Larger Trials of RCC Treated with Percutaneous RF Ablation

Author (Ref.)	Number of Tumors	Tumors Treated Completely after RF Ablation		
		Size	%	No.
Zagoria et al. (40)	24	<3 cm	100	(11/11)
		>3 cm	69	(9/13)
Gervais et al. (24)	100	<3 cm	100	(52/52)
		3–5 cm	92	(36/39)
		>3 cm	25	(2/8)
Mayo Smith et al. (37)	32		97	(31/32)
Farrell et al. (36)	35		100	(35/35)
Su et al. (38)	35		94	(33/35)
Pavlovich et al. (48)	21		79	(19/24)
Ogan et al. (39)	16		93	(12/13)
Total	263		91.2	(240/263)

RCC, renal cell carcinoma; RF, renal failure.

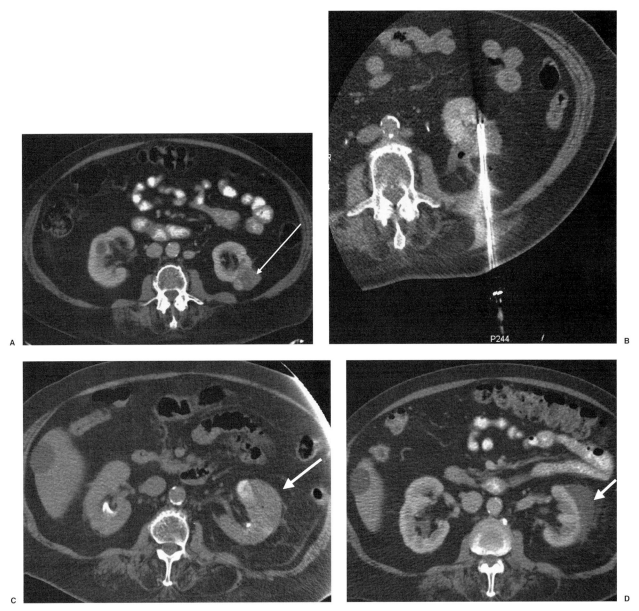

FIGURE 33.4. Sixty-seven-year-old woman underwent contrast-enhanced CT scan for evaluation of abdominal pain. (A) Axial image demonstrates a 3.5 cm exophytic mass (*arrow*) arising from the middle pole of the left kidney. Due to significant heart disease, the patient was not an ideal candidate for surgery and underwent treatment by percutaneous RFA. (B) Axial CT image at RFA shows the needle electrode placed within the mass. Multiple overlapping ablations were performed (*not shown*). (C) Post ablation, the patient was transferred to a recovery area, where she complained of increasing left-sided abdominal pain. Axial image from a repeat CT scan performed 4 hours after ablation demon-strates a left subcapsular hematoma (*arrow*) causing mass effect on the left renal parenchyma. She was admitted for overnight observation. Her hematocrit was stable, and the pain responded to medication. One day after treatment, the pain had decreased in intensity, and the patient was discharged in stable condition. (D) Axial image from a contrast-enhanced CT scan performed 1 month after ablation showed no evidence of residual disease and minimal decrease in size of hematoma (*arrow*). The patient was pain free. Follow-up scans performed 3 and 6 months after treatment (not shown) showed no residual disease and gradual decrease in size of the hematoma.

be inflicted upon adjacent organs, particularly the colon, which can result in abscess and/or fistula formation (12). Tumor seeding of electrode track has been reported as a rare complication in the treatment of liver tumors (53, 54). A single case of skin seeding was reported in the series by Mayo-Smith et al. (37).

TREATMENT OF METASTATIC DISEASE

Surgical and RFA Options

Palliative treatment with RFA, although rare, has been performed in patients with debilitating hematuria due to invasion of the collecting system (55).

The role of local therapies like percutaneous ablation in patients with metastatic RCC is limited due to the disseminated nature of the disease. Although cytoreductive nephrectomy is sometimes performed even in the setting of metastatic disease, the role of percutaneous ablation in the treatment of the primary mass is limited by the larger size of most primary renal masses once metastases have appeared. In isolated cases, focal ablation of a single painful osseous metastasis that has failed conventional pain management may result in substantial pain relief (56). A detailed review of ablation of bone metastases is beyond the scope of this chapter (56, 57). In addition, for those patients with limited metastases such as one or two small pulmonary metastases, RFA has been effective in achieving local control (58). Likewise, Gervais et al. reported two cases of isolated lymph node metastases in which complete necrosis was achieved by RFA (59). The number of patients with metastatic RCC suitable for percutaneous ablation is a small minority of all patients with stage IV disease, and ablation in these cases is palliative rather than potentially curative.

Medical Therapies

RCC is notoriously resistant to medical therapies, and these are offered only for locally, advanced or widely metastatic RCC. Response to chemotherapy is poor, and a number of immunomodulatory therapies are currently being evaluated. Prominent among these is interferon-α, being used for clear-cell RCC. It has a response rate of about 14% and few side effects (26). High-dose interleukin-2 is approved by the FDA for treating advanced-stage RCC; however, limited availability and debilitating side effects (capillary leak syndrome) compromise the effectiveness of interleukin-2.

One of several molecular pathways implicated in the pathogenesis of RCC is VHL gene inactivation leading to vascular endothelial growth factor (VEGF) expression. This has generated interest in anti-VGEF drugs such as bevacizumab (Avastin), which is an anti-VEGF monoclonal antibody that is FDA approved for use in metastatic colorectal carcinoma (61). A preliminary study evaluating bevacizumab in combination with an epidermal growth factor receptor tyrosine kinase inhibitor (erlotinib) in patients with metastatic clear-cell renal carcinoma demonstrated a 60% survival at 18 months (62). Another promising therapy is sunitinib, which is an oral multi-targeted tyrosine kinase inhibitor. In a recent trial evaluating patients with metastatic clear-cell RCC, Motzer et al.

demonstrated a median progression free-survival of 8.3 months (63). Currently, most of these results are at best encouraging, and early clinical trials remain to be substantiated in large studies (64). One recent development is the FDA approval in late 2005 of sorafenib for metastatic RCC based on prolongation of progression-free survival to 24 weeks compared to placebo (65). Alternative therapies such as tumor vaccines and stem cell transplantation are being researched, although none is available for clinical use yet.

CONCLUSION

Therapeutic options for RCC continue to expand with percutaneous techniques being the latest newcomers. Each modality has specific clinical applications, and reaching the right therapeutic decision is a complex process. This requires close collaboration between urologists and interventional radiologists in order to appropriately guide patients while providing adequate information about all viable treatment options available. Percutaneous ablation is safe, with proven short-term success. Long-term survival and disease-free data are awaited, and until then it is best suited for patients who are not ideal candidates for surgery. Small exophytic tumors up to 4 cm are best suited for treatment with percutaneous ablation.

REFERENCES

1. Jemal A, Siegel R, Ward E, et al. Cancer Statistics, 2006. CA Cancer J Clin, 2006; 56: 106–130.
2. Cohen HT and McGovern FJ. Renal-cell carcinoma. N Engl J Med, 2005; 353: 2477–2490.
3. Walther MM, Choyke PL, Glenn G, et al. Renal cancer in families with hereditary renal cancer: Prospective analysis of a tumor size threshold for renal parenchymal sparing surgery. J Urol, 1999; 161: 1475–1479.
4. Herring JC, Enquist EG, Chernoff A, et al. Parenchymal sparing surgery in patients with hereditary renal cell carcinoma: 10-year experience. J Urol, 2001; 165: 777–781.
5. Gervais DA, Arellano RS, and Mueller PR. Percutaneous radiofrequency ablation of renal cell carcinoma. Eur Radiol, 2005; 15: 960–967.
6. Gervais DA, Arellano RS, and Mueller P. Percutaneous ablation of kidney tumors in nonsurgical candidates. Oncology (Williston Park), 2005; 19: 6–11.
7. McDougal WS, Gervais DA, McGovern FJ, et al. Long-term followup of patients with renal cell carcinoma treated with radio frequency ablation with curative intent. J Urol, 2005; 174: 61–63.
8. Gervais DA, Arellano RS, McGovern FJ, et al. Radiofrequency ablation of renal cell carcinoma: Part 2, lessons

learned with ablation of 100 tumors. AJR Am J Roentgenol, 2005; 185: 72–80.

9. Gervais DA, McGovern FJ, Arellano RS, et al. Renal cell carcinoma: Clinical experience and technical success with radio-frequency ablation of 42 tumors. Radiology, 2003; 226: 417–424.

10. Novick AC. Nephron-sparing surgery for renal cell carcinoma. Annu Rev Med, 2002; 53: 393–407.

11. Chiou YY, Hwang JI, Chou YH, et al. Percutaneous radiofrequency ablation of renal cell carcinoma. J Chin Med Assoc, 2005; 68: 221–225.

12. Silverman SG, Tuncali K, vanSonnenberg E, et al. Renal tumors: MR imaging-guided percutaneous cryotherapy – initial experience in 23 patients. Radiology, 2005; 236: 716–724.

13. Goldberg SN, Gazelle GS, Mueller PR. Thermal ablation therapy for focal malignancy: A unified approach to underlying principles, techniques, and diagnostic imaging guidance. AJR Am J Roentgenol, 2000; 174: 323–331.

14. Tacke J, Mahnken A, Roggan A, et al. Multipolar radiofrequency ablation: First clinical results. Rofo, 2004; 176: 324–329.

15. Tacke J, Mahnken AH, Gunther RW. Percutaneous thermal ablation of renal neoplasms. Rofo, 2005; 177: 1631–1640.

16. Lee JM, Han JK, Choi SH, et al. Comparison of renal ablation with monopolar radiofrequency and hypertonic-saline-augmented bipolar radiofrequency: In vitro and in vivo experimental studies. AJR Am J Roentgenol, 2005; 184: 897–905.

17. Lee FT Jr., Haemmerich D, Wright AS, et al. Multiple probe radiofrequency ablation: Pilot study in an animal model. J Vasc Interv Radiol, 2003; 14: 1437–1442.

18. Hsu TH, Fidler ME, Gill IS. Radiofrequency ablation of the kidney: Acute and chronic histology in porcine model. Urology, 2000; 56: 872–875.

19. Munver R, Threatt CB, Delvecchio FC, et al. Hypertonic saline-augmented radiofrequency ablation of the VX-2 tumor implanted in the rabbit kidney: A short-term survival pilot study. Urology, 2002; 60: 170–175.

20. Zlotta AR, Wildschutz T, Raviv G, et al. Radiofrequency interstitial tumor ablation (RITA) is a possible new modality for treatment of renal cancer: Ex vivo and in vivo experience. J Endourol, 1997; 11: 251–258.

21. Walther MC, Shawker TH, Libutti SK, et al. A Phase 2 study of radio frequency interstitial tissue ablation of localized renal tumors. J Urol, 2000; 163: 1424–1427.

22. Michaels MJ, Rhee HK, Mourtzinos AP, et al. Incomplete renal tumor destruction using radio frequency interstitial ablation. J Urol, 2002; 168: 2406–2409; discussion, 2409–2410.

23. Rendon RA, Kachura JR, Sweet JM, et al. The uncertainty of radio frequency treatment of renal cell carcinoma: Findings at immediate and delayed nephrectomy. J Urol, 2002; 167: 1587–1592.

24. Gervais DA, McGovern FJ, Arellano RS, et al. Radiofrequency ablation of renal cell carcinoma: Part 1, indications, results, and role in patient management over a 6-year period and ablation of 100 tumors. AJR Am J Roentgenol, 2005; 185: 64–71.

25. Silverman SG, Tuncali K, Adams DF, et al. MR imaging-guided percutaneous cryotherapy of liver tumors: Initial experience. Radiology, 2000; 217: 657–664.

26. Delworth MG, Pisters LL, Fornage BD, et al. Cryotherapy for renal cell carcinoma and angiomyolipoma. J Urol, 1996; 155: 252–4; discussion, 254–255.

27. Gill IS, Novick AC, Meraney AM, et al. Laparoscopic renal cryoablation in 32 patients. Urology, 2000; 56: 748–753.

28. Nadler RB, Kim SC, Rubenstein JN, et al. Laparoscopic renal cryosurgery: The Northwestern experience. J Urol, 2003; 170: 1121–1125.

29. Uchida M, Imaide Y, Sugimoto K, et al. Percutaneous cryosurgery for renal tumours. Br J Urol, 1995; 75: 132–136; discussion, 136–137.

30. Hoffmann NE, Bischof JC. The cryobiology of cryosurgical injury. Urology, 2002; 60: 40–49.

31. Rupp CC, Hoffmann NE, Schmidlin FR, et al. Cryosurgical changes in the porcine kidney: Histologic analysis with thermal history correlation. Cryobiology, 2002; 45: 167–182.

32. Chosy SG, Nakada SY, Lee FT, Jr., et al. Monitoring renal cryosurgery: Predictors of tissue necrosis in swine. J Urol, 1998; 159: 1370–1374.

33. Campbell SC, Krishnamurthi V, Chow G, et al. Renal cryosurgery: Experimental evaluation of treatment parameters. Urology, 1998; 52: 29–33; discussion, 33–34.

34. Woolley ML, Schulsinger DA, Durand DB, et al. Effect of freezing parameters (freeze cycle and thaw process) on tissue destruction following renal cryoablation. J Endourol, 2002; 16: 519–522.

35. Ahrar K, Matin S, Wood CG, et al. Percutaneous radiofrequency ablation of renal tumors: Technique, complications, and outcomes. J Vasc Interv Radiol, 2005; 16: 679–688.

36. Farrell MA, Charboneau WJ, DiMarco DS, et al. Imaging-guided radiofrequency ablation of solid renal tumors. AJR Am J Roentgenol, 2003; 180: 1509–1513.

37. Mayo-Smith WW, Dupuy DE, Parikh PM, et al. Imaging-guided percutaneous radiofrequency ablation of solid renal masses: Techniques and outcomes of 38 treatment sessions in 32 consecutive patients. AJR Am J Roentgenol, 2003; 180: 1503–1508.

38. Su LM, Jarrett TW, Chan DY, et al. Percutaneous computed tomography-guided radiofrequency ablation of renal masses in high surgical risk patients: Preliminary results. Urology, 2003; 61: 26–33.

39. Ogan K, Jacomides L, Dolmatch BL, et al. Percutaneous radiofrequency ablation of renal tumors: Technique, limitations, and morbidity. Urology, 2002; 60: 954–958.

40. Zagoria RJ, Hawkins AD, Clark PE, et al. Percutaneous CT-guided radiofrequency ablation of renal neoplasms: Factors influencing success. AJR Am J Roentgenol, 2004; 183: 201–207.

41. Shingleton WB and Sewell PE Jr. Cryoablation of renal tumours in patients with solitary kidneys. BJU International, 2003; 92: 237–239.

42. Shingleton WB and Sewell PE, Jr. Percutaneous renal cryoablation of renal tumors in patients with von Hippel-Lindau disease. J Urol, 2002; 167: 1268–1270.

43. Shingleton WB and Sewell PE, Jr. Percutaneous renal tumor cryoablation with magnetic resonance imaging guidance. J Urol, 2001; 165: 773–776.

44. Farrell MA, Charboneau JW, Callstrom MR, et al. Paranephric water instillation: A technique to prevent bowel injury during percutaneous renal radiofrequency ablation. AJR Am J Roentgenol, 2003; 181: 1315–1317.

45. Kariya Z, Yamakado K, Nakatuka A, et al. Radiofrequency ablation with and without balloon occlusion of the renal artery: An experimental study in porcine kidneys. J Vasc Interv Radiol, 2003; 14: 241–245.

46. Raman SS, Aziz D, Chang X, et al. Minimizing diaphragmatic injury during radiofrequency ablation: Efficacy of intraabdominal carbon dioxide insufflation. AJR Am J Roentgenol, 2004; 183: 197–200.

47. Goldberg SN, Gazelle GS, Compton CC, et al. Treatment of intrahepatic malignancy with radiofrequency ablation: Radiologic-pathologic correlation. Cancer, 2000; 88: 2452–2463.

48. Pavlovich CP, Walther MM, Choyke PL, et al. Percutaneous radio frequency ablation of small renal tumors: Initial results. J Urol, 2002; 167: 10–15.

49. Roy-Choudhury SH, Cast JE, Cooksey G, et al. Early experience with percutaneous radiofrequency ablation of small solid renal masses. AJR Am J Roentgenol, 2003; 180: 1055–1061.

50. Veltri A, De Fazio G, Malfitana V, et al. Percutaneous US-guided RF thermal ablation for malignant renal tumors: Preliminary results in 13 patients. Eur Radiol, 2004; 14: 2303–2310.

51. Gill IS, Remer EM, Hasan WA, et al. Renal cryoablation: Outcome at 3 years. J Urol, 2005; 173: 1903–1907.

52. Johnson DB, Solomon SB, Su LM, et al. Defining the complications of cryoablation and radio frequency ablation of small renal tumors: A multi-institutional review. J Urol, 2004; 172: 874–877.

53. Llovet JM, Vilana R, Bru C, et al. Increased risk of tumor seeding after percutaneous radiofrequency ablation for single hepatocellular carcinoma. Hepatology, 2001; 33: 1124–1129.

54. Liu C, Frilling A, Dereskewitz C, et al. Tumor seeding after fine needle aspiration biopsy and percutaneous radiofrequency thermal ablation of hepatocellular carcinoma. Dig Surg, 2003; 20: 460–463.

55. Wood BJ, Grippo J, and Pavlovich CP. Percutaneous radio frequency ablation for hematuria. J Urol, 2001; 166: 2303–2304.

56. Callstrom MR, Charboneau JW, Goetz MP, et al. Image-guided ablation of painful metastatic bone tumors: A new and effective approach to a difficult problem. Skeletal Radiol, 2006; 35: 1–15.

57. Goetz MP, Callstrom MR, Charboneau JW, et al. Percutaneous image-guided radiofrequency ablation of painful metastases involving bone: A multicenter study. J Clin Oncol, 2004; 22: 300–306.

58. Zagoria RJ, Chen MY, Kavanagh PV, et al. Radio frequency ablation of lung metastases from renal cell carcinoma. J Urol, 2001; 166: 1827–1828.

59. Gervais DA, Arellano RS, Mueller PR. Percutaneous radiofrequency ablation of nodal metastases. Cardiovasc Intervent Radiol, 2002; 25: 547–549.

60. Dillman RO, Wiemann MC, Tai DF, et al. Phase II trial of subcutaneous interferon followed by intravenous hybrid bolus/continuous infusion interleukin-2 in the treatment of renal cell carcinoma: Final results of cancer biotherapy research group 95–09. Cancer Biother Radiopharm, 2006; 21: 130–137.

61. Rini BI. VEGF-targeted therapy in renal cell carcinoma: Active drugs and active choices. Curr Oncol Rep, 2006; 8: 85–89.

62. Hainsworth JD, Sosman JA, Spigel DR, et al. Treatment of metastatic renal cell carcinoma with a combination of bevacizumab and erlotinib. J Clin Oncol, 2005; 23: 7889–7896.

63. Motzer RJ, Rini BI, Bukowski RM, et al. Sunitinib in patients with metastatic renal cell carcinoma. JAMA, 2006; 295: 2516–2524.

64. Nathan P, Chao D, Brock C, et al. The place of VEGF inhibition in the current management of renal cell carcinoma. Br J Cancer, 2006; 94: 1217–1220.

65. Hampton T. Trials probe new agents for kidney cancer. JAMA, 2006 Jul 12; 296 (2): 155–157.

Chapter 34

EMBOLOTHERAPY IN THE MANAGEMENT OF RENAL CELL CARCINOMA

Armeen Mahvash

Sanaz Javadi

Kamran Ahrar

Renal cell carcinoma (RCC) is an uncommon tumor, accounting for only 3% of all adult malignancies (1), yet of all urological malignancies, it is the most lethal (2). Diagnosis and treatment of RCC have changed dramatically since the 1950s, when the disease was usually diagnosed at an advanced stage on the basis of clinical symptoms of palpable mass, flank pain and hematuria (3). In recent years, routine use of cross-sectional abdominal imaging has resulted in earlier diagnosis (4, 5).

Radical nephrectomy, once believed to be the standard for treatment of RCC, is now used only to treat large tumors that are locally advanced or metastatic at diagnosis. Today, the treatment of choice for smaller tumors (<4 cm in diameter) is partial nephrectomy (6). Energy-ablative techniques such as cryoablation and radiofrequency ablation (RFA) are promising, minimally invasive treatment options for smaller tumors in patients who may not be suitable surgical candidates (7–9).

Embolotherapy has been used as an adjunctive therapy in the management of RCC since the 1970s, although its role has evolved over the years (Table 34.1). At one time, it was thought that preoperative embolization of RCC would result in an immunologic response – that is, a form of autovaccination;

therefore, some investigators advocated routine use of preoperative embolization (10). The initial enthusiasm for this practice was dampened by a lack of scientific evidence that embolization of RCC did, in fact, induce a significant immunologic response, and the practice was abandoned. Today, preoperative embolization is reserved for large tumors and those tumors that have invaded the renal vein and the inferior vena cava (IVC) (Figure 34.1) (11). Surgical dissection and removal of these hypervascular tumors, which are often associated with hilar lymphadenopathy and perinephric extension of the tumor, are technically challenging. During the course of these procedures, large volumes of blood are lost, and multiple transfusions are necessary. Preoperative embolization has been reported to lower the need for transfusion in selected patients (12). In addition, preoperative embolization may lead to a decrease in the size of the tumor thrombus, facilitating resection of the tumor from the renal vein or the IVC (13, 14).

Unfortunately, selected patients with advanced disease may not qualify for curative or cytoreductive surgery. These patients may continue to suffer from a variety of tumor-related and paraneoplastic complications of RCC. In such cases, palliative embolization is an important adjunctive therapy for the

TABLE 34.1 Indications for Embolotherapy for Renal Cell Carcinoma

Indication	Benefits
Preoperative	Decreased blood loss, fewer transfusions
Palliative	Control of tumor-related and paraneoplastic symptoms
Preablative	Reduced perfusion-mediated cooling of the tumor, more effective ablation

management of symptoms such as pain, hematuria, and hypercalcemia (15–17).

More recently, energy-ablative therapies have been used to treat RCC in patients who may be at high risk for surgical complications, in patients who have limited renal function and in patients who are predisposed to the development of recurrent and multifocal RCC (7–9). Tumors less than 3 cm in diameter are relatively easy to treat with percutaneous RFA,

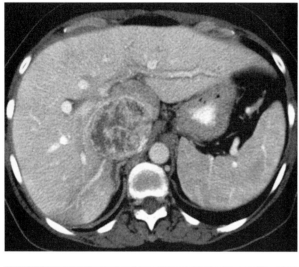
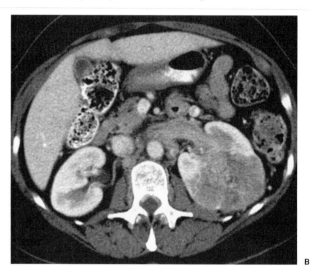
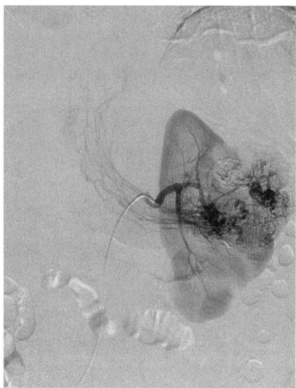
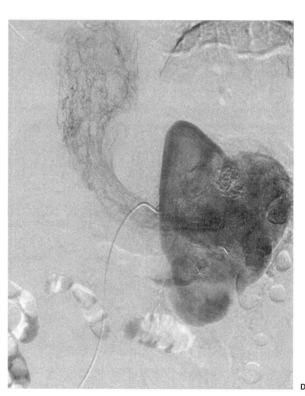

FIGURE 34.1. Axial computed tomography (CT) and angiographic images of a 57-year-old woman with RCC who was referred for preoperative embolization. Axial CT images of the abdomen demonstrate a large tumor thrombus within the IVC (A) and a large mass in the left kidney that has invaded the renal vein (B). A selective digital subtraction angiogram of the left renal artery in the arterial phase (C) shows neovascularity and tumor staining in the mid-portion of the left kidney. A later image from the same angiographic study (D) shows tumor thrombus within the renal vein and the IVC.

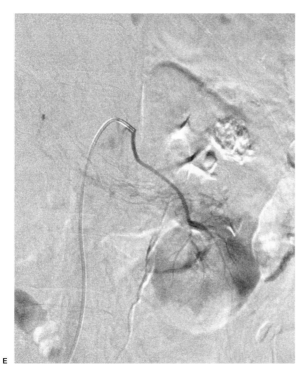

FIGURE 34.1. (*Continued*) **After embolization of the main renal artery, a search for other tumor-feeding arteries revealed a small accessory renal artery supplying the inferior pole of the left kidney (E). This branch was then embolized to achieve complete devascularization of the left renal unit. The patient underwent left radical nephrectomy and IVC thrombectomy. Pathology demonstrated a T3N0M0 renal cell carcinoma. At 6-month follow-up, there was no evidence of disease.**

as evidenced by a technical success rate of nearly 100%; larger tumors are more difficult to treat in this way (8). Perfusion-mediated cooling of the tumor is a major cause of technical failure in larger tumors treated with energy-ablative techniques (18). Preablation embolization of these tumors may help decrease this cooling effect and result in more effective thermal ablation (19).

This chapter reviews technical aspects and expected results of embolotherapy in the management of RCC.

TECHNICAL ASPECTS

Anatomy

The arterial anatomy of the kidneys varies significantly among individuals. This picture is further complicated by the presence of hypervascular tumors such as RCC. In most patients, each kidney is supplied by a single renal artery arising from the abdominal aorta at the level of the L1–L2 disk space, but mul-

tiple renal arteries supplying individual kidneys have been detected in 12% to 32% of the population (20). The main renal artery frequently divides into anterior and posterior branches. The posterior division is the smaller of the two and appears as a branch of the main renal artery, whereas the anterior division appears as a continuation of the main renal artery. The anterior branch divides into segmental arteries and provides blood supply to four of the five vascular segments in the kidney. In a two-dimensional angiographic image, the lateral border of the kidney is often supplied by the anterior branch (21). The segmental renal arteries further branch off to form lobar, interlobar, arcuate and interlobular arteries (22).

Perforating arteries, an important collateral pathway to the kidney, arise from the intraparenchymal branches of the renal artery and exit from the kidney to anastomose with various retroperitoneal arteries, including the renal capsular arteries (22). The superior capsular artery may arise from the inferior adrenal artery, main renal artery or aorta. The middle capsular artery, which may consist of one or more branches, arises from the main renal artery. The inferior capsular artery may originate from the gonadal artery, an accessory or aberrant lower pole or even the main renal artery. These vessels form a rich capsular network that anastomoses freely with perforating arteries and other retroperitoneal (especially lumbar) arteries and also with internal iliac, intercostal and mesenteric arteries (22).

Angiography

A careful angiographic examination is necessary to plan and execute successful embolization of RCC. Initially, an abdominal aortogram is performed to determine the number and location of various arterial branches that may supply the kidney, the tumor, or both. Each arterial branch is then selectively catheterized and evaluated angiographically to determine the extent of neovascularity, the extent of arteriovenous shunting (if any), and the risk of non-target embolization. Incomplete embolization may result in suboptimal tumor necrosis and increased intraoperative blood loss at nephrectomy (12). Incomplete embolization in the palliative setting is associated with recurrent hematuria and the need for repeat embolization (23).

Almost 80% of RCCs are shown to be hypervascular on angiography. In the other 20%, hypovascularity may be related to necrosis or cystic degeneration of

TABLE 34.2 Embolic Agents Used in Embolotherapy for Renal Cell Carcinoma

Class	Examples
Liquid agents	Absolute ethanol
Particulate agents	Polyvinyl alcohol
	EmboGold microspheres (BioSphere Medical, Inc., Rockland, MA)
Large-vessel occluders	Metallic coils

the tumor. Similarly, RCC arising within a cyst may appear hypovascular. Hypervascular tumors characteristically exhibit one or more of the following angiographic features: enlarged, tortuous, poorly tapering feeding arteries; coarse neovascularity and formation of small aneurysms; parasitization of adjacent vessels; tumor staining or puddling of contrast medium; and arteriovenous shunting. Tumor thrombus within the renal vein or the IVC may obstruct these venous channels and lead to the development of collateral draining veins. However, even in the absence of tumor thrombus, collateral veins may develop in response to extreme hypervascularity.

Embolic Agents and Embolization Techniques

Over the past three decades, more than 20 different embolic agents have been utilized for the devascularization of hypervascular renal tumors (24). These embolic agents can be divided into three major categories (Table 34.2): liquid agents (e.g., absolute ethanol), particulate materials (e.g., polyvinyl alcohol particles) and large-vessel occluders (e.g., metallic coils).

Among liquid agents, absolute ethanol is readily available and inexpensive. Because it is non-viscous, ethanol injected in the renal artery may diffuse into the distal vascular bed of the tumor, causing tumor necrosis rather than simple occlusion of the embolized artery (25). Embolization of renal tumors with absolute ethanol can be performed with or without an occlusion balloon catheter (Figures 34.2 and 34.3) (12, 23, 25). Ellman and associates (25) first described ablation of renal tumors with absolute ethanol in 1981. They recommended selective injection of ethanol at a rate of 2 ml/s in as many tumor arteries as possible. They hypothesized that injection of ethanol at a rate of 1 to 5 ml/s would result in tissue toxicity, thereby leading to necrosis in perivascular areas, sludging of erythrocytes in small arter-

ies and glomeruli, and spasm of these small arteries; subsequently, the endothelium would be damaged and slough off over several hours, resulting in complete occlusion of damaged vessels. In practice, injection of ethanol (0.1 ml/s) resulted in little direct tissue toxicity; instead, the formation of small clumps of damaged erythrocytes and denatured proteins led to proximal occlusion of the arteries. The desired angiographic endpoints were occlusion of all arteries smaller than major segmental branches, stagnation of flow in patent major arteries and extravasation of contrast material into the renal parenchyma.

There are several advantages to using an occlusion balloon catheter during ethanol perfusion: 1) The balloon interrupts renal blood flow, markedly prolonging the contact of ethanol with the endothelium and thereby reducing the volume of ethanol needed for complete ablation of the target tissue. 2) The balloon inhibits reflux into the aorta. 3) Use of the balloon catheter allows the main renal artery to be injected with ethanol and eliminates the need for selective catheterization of segmental branches (Figure 34.2). For embolization of the entire kidney, an occlusion balloon catheter is placed in the main renal artery (12, 23). A test injection of contrast medium is performed to determine the volume of ethanol needed to fill the whole tumor (12). A predetermined volume of ethanol is injected at a fairly rapid rate of 1 to 5 ml/s. Slow infusion of ethanol may lead to early thrombus formation and premature closure of the main renal artery, whereas rapid injection of ethanol theoretically allows for its rapid diffusion into the tumor bed. After injection of ethanol, the balloon is left inflated for 5 minutes. As the balloon is deflating, gentle suction through the distal endhole of the catheter prevents reflux of residual ethanol or thrombus into the aorta. This sequence is repeated until the renal arteries are totally occluded. Complete ablation of large, hypervascular tumors with absolute ethanol is associated with a significantly reduced requirement for blood transfusion at nephrectomy; in contrast, partial ablation is associated with higher transfusion requirement (12). Therefore, all other tumor-feeding arteries are selectively catheterized and embolized with either particulate embolic agents or absolute ethanol (Figure 34.1).

Absolute ethanol by itself is not radiopaque, which makes its use as an embolic agent under fluoroscopic monitoring somewhat challenging. Reflux of ethanol can lead to non-target embolization of the inferior

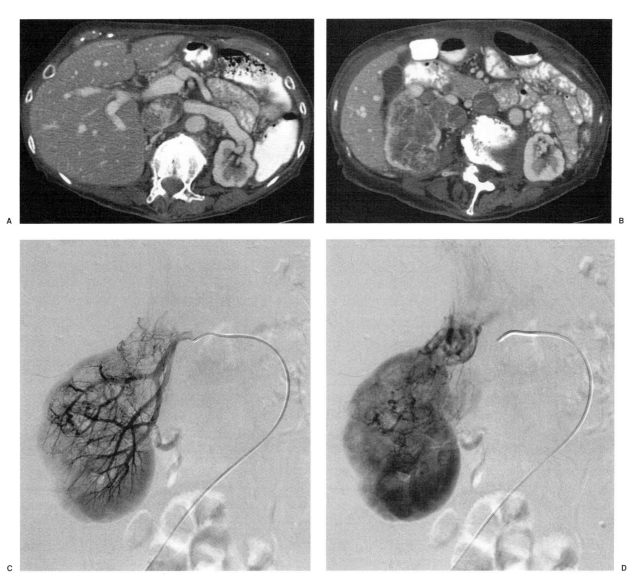

FIGURE 34.2. Axial computed tomography (CT) and angiographic images of a 78-year-old woman with a history of RCC who was referred for preoperative embolization. Axial CT images of the abdomen show tumor thrombus within the IVC (A) and a large tumor involving the right kidney (B). A selective digital subtraction angiogram of the right renal artery demonstrates the tumor in both arterial phase (C) and venous phase (D).

mesenteric artery and the lumbar arteries (16, 26–29). Mixing ethanol with a radiographic contrast medium may result in precipitation of the mixture (23). However, radiopacity may be achieved by mixing ethanol with iodized oil (lipiodol). The use of a 1:3 mixture of lipiodol and ethanol for successful embolization of RCC was described by Park et al. (30).

Particulate materials, such as absorbable gelatin sponge (Gelfoam, Pfizer, New York, NY) and polyvinyl alcohol foam (Ivalon, Unipoint Industries, High Point, NC) as an inert biocomp, have been used alone and with metallic coils (10). Newer embolic agents such as EmboGold microspheres (BioSphere Medical, Inc., Rockland, MA) and Contour SE (Boston Scientific; Natick, MA) are also used for embolization of renal masses. Theoretically, these spherical particles do not clump and therefore travel farther distally, resulting in embolization of smaller arteries in the tumor bed. Selecting an appropriate range of particle sizes for embolization of renal tumors warrants the following two considerations: first, distal embolization of tumor vessels at the tissue level is more desirable than proximal occlusion of the parent arteries; second, arteriovenous shunting, which is present in most hypervascular RCCs, may result in non-target embolization of the pulmonary vascular bed. In tumors characterized by rapid arteriovenous shunting, the use of larger particles or a liquid embolic agent in conjunction with a balloon occlusion catheter may be prudent; otherwise,

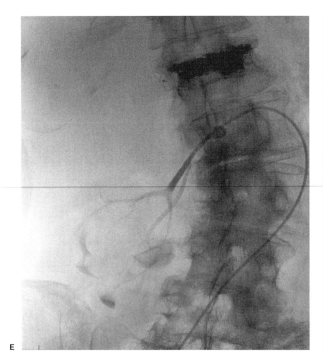
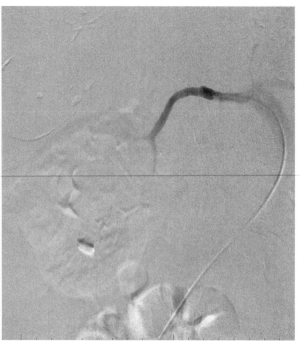

E

F

FIGURE 34.2. (*Continued*) **An occlusion balloon catheter was placed and inflated in the main renal artery (E). A fixed volume of contrast medium was injected to confirm isolation of the renal arterial circulation without any reflux into** the aorta or rapid arteriovenous shunting. A subsequent angiogram, obtained after absolute ethanol administration and balloon removal, shows complete devascularization of the right renal unit (F).

embolization should commence with the injection of small particles for distal embolization and occlusion of arteries in the tumor bed.

Large-vessel occluders such as metallic coils are often used for proximal occlusion of larger arteries. Their use for the palliation of tumor-related symptoms is discouraged because advanced renal tumors often have an extensive collateral blood supply, which makes proximal occlusion of the feeding arteries ineffective. Furthermore, many tumors require additional interventions, which requires that arterial access to the neoplasm remain intact (31). If coils are used for preoperative embolization, they should be appropriately sized and placed in order to minimize the risk of dislodgment during surgery and to avoid difficulties with renal artery clamping or ligation (10).

Overall, most RCCs are hypervascular and may recruit additional blood supply from other sources. The choice of agent used for embolization of each feeding artery partly depends on the size and location of the vessel. Even though absolute ethanol appears to be the embolic agent of choice (24), many interventional radiologists use a combination of agents to achieve complete devascularization of target tumors. Therefore, it seems appropriate for operators to be familiar with various techniques and have access to a full complement of different embolic agents.

RESULTS

Preoperative Embolization

In patients with RCC, preoperative embolization may help reduce intraoperative blood loss, decrease transfusion requirements, facilitate surgical resection and improve overall survival. Earlier studies of intraoperative blood loss were based on subjective estimates only (32–34). In a case-control study, 35 patients who underwent preoperative embolization were compared with a similar group of patients who did not (35). In that study, embolization did not reduce perioperative blood loss. Bakal et al. (12) demonstrated that estimated blood loss is an unreliable measurement and instead used the transfused volume as a measure of successful preoperative embolization. They demonstrated that the transfusion volume was statistically significantly lower after complete embolization in patients with large, hypervascular RCCs (volume >250 ml, diameter >7.8 cm) than it was in patients with smaller or hypovascular tumors.

Some reports have suggested that resection of RCC is facilitated by preoperative embolization (36, 37). Infarction of the tumor secondary to embolization creates a plane of edema that makes dissection of the tumor easier. In addition, in the case of larger tumors extending to the renal hilum and perihilar

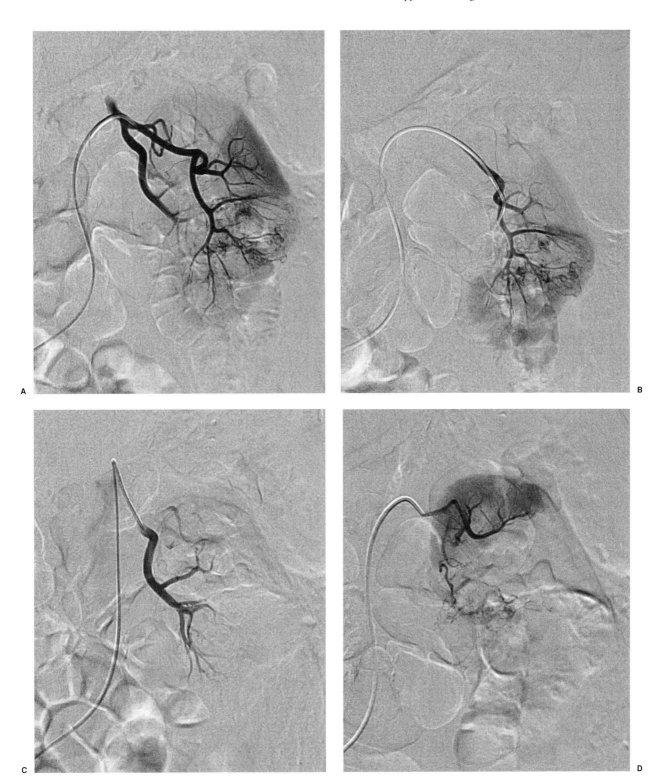

FIGURE 34.3. Angiographic images of a 69-year-old man with metastatic RCC and hematuria, who was referred for palliative embolization. A selective digital subtraction angiogram of the left renal artery (A) shows early branching of the main renal artery, which precluded placement of a balloon occlusion catheter. (B–D) demonstrate superselective catheterization and angiogram of the anterior, posterior and upper polar branches of the left renal artery, respectively. Because early branching of the renal artery precluded the placement of a balloon occlusion catheter, selective catheterization and embolization of each branch were warranted in order to prevent reflux of embolic agents into the aorta, reduce the risk of non-target embolization, and prevent rapid dilution of alcohol in the main renal artery. A selective angiogram of the left renal artery obtained after embolization shows devascularization of the left kidney and the tumor (E).

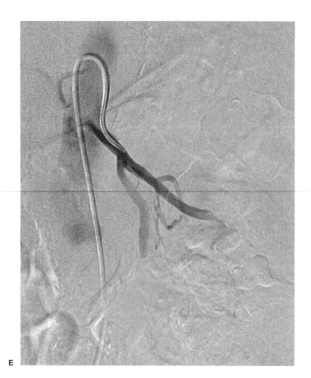

E

FIGURE 34.3. *(Continued)*

lymph nodes, preoperative embolization allows for ligation of the renal vein before the renal artery, alleviating some of the technical difficulties associated with resection of these bulky tumors (36). In the case of tumors that extend into the IVC, embolization causes the tumor to shrink and facilitates its resection from the vena cava (11, 13, 14).

In the published literature, the reported time between embolization and nephrectomy varies significantly (24), from 8 hours (36) to 183 days (38). In one study, a planned delay in performing a nephrectomy was thought to allow the development of edema and facilitate dissection (14), whereas in another study, dissections performed 3 days or more after embolization were reportedly made more difficult because of increasing collateral circulation (37). Although solid scientific evidence is lacking, the optimal delay between embolization and operation appears to be less than 48 hours (24).

In addition to facilitating surgical resection and lowering the need for blood transfusion, preoperative embolization may improve survival after nephrectomy. In a retrospective study comparing preoperative embolization and nephrectomy versus nephrectomy alone, Zielinski and colleagues demonstrated that survival improved after preoperative embolization. The overall 5- and 10-year survival rates were 62% and 47% for 118 patients embolized before

nephrectomy and 35% and 23% for a matched group of 116 patients treated with nephrectomy alone (p = 0.01) (39). Although promising, the results of this retrospective study should be interpreted with caution and confirmed in a prospective randomized trial.

Palliative Embolization

Palliative embolization has been described for patients with tumor-related symptoms including pain, hematuria, or life-threatening endocrine activity (16, 27, 40–43). In addition, palliative embolization has been used as an alternative therapy for patients with advanced disease who may not be surgical candidates (27).

In one study, severe hematuria resolved in 11 of 14 cases, and incomplete embolization of the tumor blood supply from parasitized lumbar arteries resulted in persistent hematuria in 3 of 14 cases (16). In another, Munro and coworkers reported on palliative embolization of 25 patients with RCC who were not surgical candidates (44). Presenting symptoms included hematuria or flank pain in 12 and 5 cases, respectively. After a median follow-up of 27 months for patients with advanced (stage IV) disease and 39 months for patients with less advanced (stage I–III) disease, 68% remained asymptomatic and 12% required brief hospital admission for treatment of recurrent hematuria. Onishi and associates reported resolution of tumor-related symptoms (i.e., hematuria, flank pain and ureteral obstruction) in 75% of patients who underwent embolotherapy (17). In another report, malignant hypercalcemia resolved after embolization (15).

In a study in which embolization and palliative care were compared in 54 patients with metastatic disease, the median survival for the embolized group was 229 days versus 116 days for the palliative group (17). The 1-, 2- and 3-year survival rates were 29%, 15% and 10%, respectively, for patients treated with embolization versus 13%, 7% and 3%, respectively, for those who received palliative care only (p = 0.016). The authors of that study concluded that embolization in patients with unresectable disseminated RCC was well tolerated, effectively devascularized the primary tumor and improved survival.

Embolization as Adjunct to Ablation Therapy

Percutaneous RFA is an alternative treatment option for RCC in patients who are not suitable surgical candidates (8). Successful eradication of the tumor by means of RF ablation is adversely affected by tumor size. In one study, the success rate for ablation of tumors 3 cm or smaller in diameter was 100%, as opposed to 92% for tumors 3.1 to 5 cm in diameter and 25% for those larger than 5 cm (8). In addition, 45% of tumors 3.1 to 5 cm in diameter required more than one ablation session for their eradication. In an effort to improve the primary technical success rate of RF ablation in larger RCCs, Yamakado and colleagues treated patients with renal artery embolization shortly before treating them with RFA (19). Overall, 12 patients with RCC tumors having a mean diameter of 5.2 cm (range, 3.5–9 cm) were treated in this study. Tumors were eradicated after a single RF session in nine cases (75%), after two sessions in two cases (17%) and after four sessions in one case (8%). These preliminary results indicate that renal artery embolization and RFA can be safely combined for treatment of larger RCC tumors in patients who are at high risk for surgical complications. Technical success rates and disease-free survival data remain to be determined in larger studies.

Complications

In reviewing the complication rates associated with renal artery embolization, technical advances and developments in the field of embolotherapy must be considered. In older studies using first-generation angiography equipment and catheters, serious complications resulted from non-target embolization of the large bowel, spinal cord, contralateral kidney or gonadal artery (26–29). Since the advent of digital subtraction angiography and modern angiographic equipment, these complications have nearly been eliminated. In 1985, Lammer and coworkers (27) reported a 9.9% overall complication rate and a mortality rate of 3.3% in 121 cases of renal tumor embolization. The most frequent complications in this series were renal failure and non-target embolization. The complication rate was four times higher during the palliative embolizations than during the preoperative embolizations. The authors attributed this discrepancy to the relatively larger mass of the tumors in patients who underwent embolization and the severely impaired health of patients who underwent palliative embolization (27). A decade later, Bakal and colleagues (12) reported a puncture-site hematoma as the sole complication in a group of 24 patients who underwent preoperative embolization. Even more recently, in a group of 24 patients

with advanced disease who underwent palliative embolotherapy, there were no major complications (17).

The most common toxicity of renal artery embolization is post-embolization syndrome, which lasts 24 to 96 hours after treatment. Post-embolization syndrome consists of flank pain, fever, nausea and vomiting, and nearly all patients will experience at least one or more of these symptoms (13, 33, 37, 45). The syndrome is self-limiting, and all that is required for its resolution is symptomatic management. Some studies suggest that ablation of tumors with ethanol versus particles results in a milder post-embolization syndrome (25, 42, 46). However, this finding has been disputed in other reports (23). Transient leukocytosis has also been observed but usually resolves in 3 to 5 days. Contrast-induced nephropathy, renal abscess and hypertension have also been reported (37). In their initial description of the technique, Rabe and associates (23) recommended the use of broad-spectrum antibiotics before and after embolization to prevent superinfection of necrotic tumors, and several reports have described renal abscesses in patients with recurrent urinary tract infections (27, 37). It is prudent in this select group of patients to provide pre- and postoperative antibiotics. In otherwise routine cases, the need for prophylactic antibiotics is not universally accepted. A common finding of intra-tumoral gas on post-procedural imaging has been postulated to be due to carbon dioxide formation due to anaerobic metabolism or oxygen formation from oxyhemoglobin. This finding, however, has not been associated with secondary bacterial infections (47).

CONCLUSIONS

Preoperative embolization is helpful for the management of large and hypervascular RCCs and those extending into the renal vein or IVC. Preoperative embolization facilitates resection of these tumors and decreases the amount of blood transfusion required during surgery. Embolization also effectively palliates tumor-related symptoms such as hematuria, flank pain or paraneoplastic symptoms in patients who experience them. Finally, embolization may be used as an adjunct to ablative therapies in treating larger tumors. As such, it reduces perfusion-mediated tissue cooling and allows for more effective thermal ablation of these hypervascular tumors.

The preferred technique for embolization of renal tumors is the perfusion of absolute ethanol with or without a balloon occlusion catheter. However, the use of other embolic agents alone or in combination with various agents may be needed to achieve complete devascularization of the tumor. Incomplete or partial embolization of tumors results in higher intraoperative blood loss in surgical patients and recurrence of symptoms in those treated palliatively.

When performed by experienced operators using modern angiographic techniques, embolotherapy is associated with very low rates of morbidity and mortality. Several recent reports have suggested a modest survival advantage for patients undergoing embolotherapy, although larger prospective trials are necessary to confirm these promising findings. Nevertheless, at the moment, embolotherapy appears to be a safe and effective treatment option for selected patients with RCC.

REFERENCES

1. American Cancer Society. Cancer Facts and Figures 2006. [http://www.cancer.org/downloads/STT/CAFF2006PW Secured.pdf.] 2006 [cited June 12, 2006].
2. Novick AC, Anderson CM, Campbell MF. Renal tumors. In: Campbell MF (ed.), Campbell's Urology, 8th edition, pp. 2672–2731. Philadelphia: WB Saunders, 2002.
3. Pantuck AJ, Zisman A, and Belldegrun AS. The changing natural history of renal cell carcinoma. J Urol, 2001 Nov; 166(5): 1611–1623.
4. Jayson M, Sanders H. Increased incidence of serendipitously discovered renal cell carcinoma. Urology, 1998 Feb; 51(2): 203–205.
5. Lightfoot N, Conlon M, Kreiger N, et al. Impact of noninvasive imaging on increased incidental detection of renal cell carcinoma. Eur Urol, 2000 May; 37(5): 521–527.
6. Uzzo RG, Novick AC. Nephron sparing surgery for renal tumors: Indications, techniques and outcomes. J Urol, 2001 Jul; 166(1): 6–18.
7. Ahrar K, Wallace MJ, and Matin SF. Percutaneous radiofrequency ablation: Minimally invasive therapy for renal tumors. Expert Rev Anticancer Ther, 2006 Dec; 6(12): 1735–1744.
8. Gervais DA, McGovern FJ, Arellano RS, et al. Radiofrequency ablation of renal cell carcinoma: Part 1, Indications, results, and role in patient management over a 6-year period and ablation of 100 tumors. AJR Am J Roentgenol, 2005 Jul; 185(1): 64–71.
9. Gill IS, Remer EM, Hasan WA, et al. Renal cryoablation: Outcome at 3 years. J Urol, 2005 Jun; 173(6): 1903–1907.
10. Wallace S, Charnsangavej C, Carrasco CH, et al. Therapeutic angiographic techniques, renal tumors: Clinical results. In: Dondelinger RF, Rossi P, Kurdziel JC, et al (eds.). Interventional Radiology, pp. 468–477. New York: Thieme Medical Publishers, 1990.
11. Sweeney P, Wood CG, Pisters LL, et al. Surgical management of renal cell carcinoma associated with complex inferior vena caval thrombi. Urol Oncol, 2003 Sep–Oct; 21(5): 327–333.
12. Bakal CW, Cynamon J, Lakritz PS, et al. Value of preoperative renal artery embolization in reducing blood transfusion requirements during nephrectomy for renal cell carcinoma. J Vasc Interv Radiol, 1993 Nov–Dec; 4(6): 727–731.
13. Bono AV, Caresano A. The role of embolization in the treatment of kidney carcinoma. Eur Urol, 1983; 9(6): 334–337.
14. Craven WM, Redmond PL, Kumpe DA, et al. Planned delayed nephrectomy after ethanol embolization of renal carcinoma. J Urol, 1991 Sep; 146(3): 704–708.
15. Jacobs JA, Ring EJ, Wein AJ. New indications for renal infarction. J Urol, 1981 Feb; 125(2): 243–245.
16. Nurmi M, Satokari K, Puntala P. Renal artery embolization in the palliative treatment of renal adenocarcinoma. Scand J Urol Nephrol, 1987; 21(2): 93–96.
17. Onishi T, Oishi Y, Suzuki Y, et al. Prognostic evaluation of transcatheter arterial embolization for unresectable renal cell carcinoma with distant metastasis. BJU Int, 2001 Mar; 87(4): 312–315.
18. Goldberg SN, Hahn PF, Tanabe KK, et al. Percutaneous radiofrequency tissue ablation: Does perfusion-mediated tissue cooling limit coagulation necrosis? J Vasc Interv Radiol, 1998 Jan–Feb; 9(1 Pt 1): 101–111.
19. Yamakado K, Nakatsuka A, Kobayashi S, et al. Radiofrequency ablation combined with renal arterial embolization for the treatment of unresectable renal cell carcinoma larger than 3.5 cm: Initial experience. Cardiovasc Intervent Radiol, 2006 May–Jun; 29(3): 389–394.
20. Kadir S. Diagnostic Angiography, pp. 445–495. Philadelphia: WB Saunders Company; 1986.
21. Boijsen E. Renal angiography. In: Baum S (ed.). Abram's Angiography, 4th edition, pp. 1101–1131. New York: Little, Brown and Company; 1997.
22. Kadir S. Atlas of normal and Variant Angiographic Anatomy, pp. 387–428. Philadelphia: WB Saunders; 1991.
23. Rabe FE, Yune HY, Richmond BD, et al. Renal tumor infarction with absolute ethanol. AJR Am J Roentgenol, 1982 Dec; 139(6): 1139–1144.
24. Kalman D, Varenhorst E. The role of arterial embolization in renal cell carcinoma. Scand J Urol Nephrol, 1999 Jun; 33(3): 162–170.
25. Ellman BA, Parkhill BJ, Curry TS 3rd, et al. Ablation of renal tumors with absolute ethanol: A new technique. Radiology, 1981 Dec; 141(3): 619–626.
26. Cox GG, Lee KR, Price HI, et al. Colonic infarction following ethanol embolization of renal-cell carcinoma. Radiology, 1982 Nov; 145(2): 343–345.
27. Lammer J, Justich E, Schreyer H, et al. Complications of renal tumor embolization. Cardiovasc Intervent Radiol, 1985; 8(1): 31–35.
28. Mulligan BD and Espinosa GA. Bowel infarction: Complication of ethanol ablation of a renal tumor. Cardiovasc Intervent Radiol, 1983; 6(1): 55–57.
29. Teertstra IIJ, Winter WA, and Frensdorf EL. Ethanol embolization of a renal tumor, complicated by colonic infarction. Diagn Imaging Clin Med, 1984; 53(5): 250–254.

30. Park JH, Kim SH, Han JK, et al. Transcatheter arterial embolization of unresectable renal cell carcinoma with a mixture of ethanol and iodized oil. Cardiovasc Intervent Radiol, 1994 Nov–Dec; 17(6): 323–327.

31. Ray CE and Waltman AC. General principles of embolization and chemoembolization. In: Bakal CW, Silberzweig JE, Cynamon J, et al (eds.). Vascular and Interventional Radiology Principles and Practice, pp. 89–100. New York: Thieme, 2002.

32. Mobilio G, Cavalli A, and Bianchi G. Preoperative arterial occlusion in renal tumors: 3 years' experience. Int Urol Nephrol, 1981; 13(1): 25–33.

33. Frasson F, Fugazzola C, Bianchi G, et al. Selective arterial embolization in renal tumors. Radiol Clin (Basel), 1978; 47(4): 239–251.

34. Frasson F, Roversi RA, Simonetti G, et al. Embolization of renal tumors. A survey of the Italian experience: 282 patients. Ann Radiol (Paris), 1981 Jun–Jul; 24(5): 396–399.

35. Lanigan D, Jurriaans E, Hammonds JC, et al. The current status of embolization in renal cell carcinoma – a survey of local and national practice. Clin Radiol, 1992 Sep; 46(3): 176–178.

36. Klimberg I, Hunter P, Hawkins IF, et al. Preoperative angioinfarction of localized renal cell carcinoma using absolute ethanol. J Urol, 1985 Jan; 133(1): 21–24.

37. Wallace S, Chuang VP, Swanson D, et al. Embolization of renal carcinoma. Radiology, 1981 Mar; 138(3): 563–570.

38. Kato T, Sato K, Abe R, et al. The role of embolization/chemoembolization in the treatment of renal cell carcinoma. In: Alan R (ed.). Therapeutic Progress in Urological Cancers, pp. 697–705. Wilmington, DE: Liss Inc., 1989.

39. Zielinski H, Szmigielski S, and Petrovich Z. Comparison of preoperative embolization followed by radical nephrectomy with radical nephrectomy alone for renal cell carcinoma. Am J Clin Oncol, 2000 Feb; 23(1): 6–12.

40. Kurth KH, Debruyne FM, Hall RR, et al. Embolization and postinfarction nephrectomy in patients with primary metastatic renal adenocarcinoma. Eur Urol, 1987; 13(4): 251–255.

41. Leinonen A. Embolization of renal carcinoma. Comparison between the early results of Gelfoam and absolute ethanol embolization. Ann Clin Res, 1985; 17(6): 299–305.

42. Ekelund L, Ek A, Forsberg L, et al. Occlusion of renal arterial tumor supply with absolute ethanol. Experience with 20 cases. Acta Radiol Diagn (Stockh), 1984; 25(3): 195–201.

43. Gottesman JE, Crawford ED, Grossman HB, et al. Infarction-nephrectomy for metastatic renal carcinoma. Southwest Oncology Group Study. Urology, 1985 Mar; 25(3): 248–250.

44. Munro NP, Woodhams S, Nawrocki JD, et al. The role of transarterial embolization in the treatment of renal cell carcinoma. BJU Int, 2003 Aug; 92(3): 240–244.

45. Kurth KH, Cinqualbre J, Oliver RT, et al. Embolization and subsequent nephrectomy in metastatic renal cell carcinoma. Prog Clin Biol Res, 1984; 153: 423–436.

46. Nakano H, Nihira H, Toge T. Treatment of renal cancer patients by transcatheter embolization and its effects on lymphocyte proliferative responses. J Urol, 1983 Jul; 130(1): 24–27.

47. Weckermann D, Schlotmann R, Tietze W, et al. Gas formation after renal artery embolisation: Genesis and clinical relevance. Urol Int, 1992; 49(4): 211–214.

Chest

Chapter 35

EPIDEMIOLOGY, DIAGNOSIS, STAGING AND THE MEDICAL-SURGICAL MANAGEMENT OF LUNG CANCERS

Rex Yung

Lung cancer (LC) is the leading cause of cancer mortality, and even as the annual incidence of LC may have reached a plateau in the United States, making it the second most prevalent cancer for both men and women. LC mortality continues to exceed the deaths from breast, prostate and colon cancers combined (1). Of note, LC mortality as a single cause of death is even greater than deaths due to cerebral vascular accidents, hence making it the second single cause of death in the United States, after heart diseases. The widespread availability of high-speed multi-slice detector computer-axial tomography (MDCT) scanners, implementation of prospective controlled and uncontrolled LC screening studies (2, 3), unwarranted proprietary "screening" services and incidental findings on scans performed for other thoracoabdominal indications have led to the frequent finding of lung nodules. If experience with other early detection tests such as mammography and

prostate-specific antigen is any indication, there will be an expected increase in the diagnosis of "early stage" LCs (1), although whether this would lead to meaningful reduction in disease-specific mortality remains to be seen as there is much debate about the potential efficacy of such screenings (4–6). Parallel with the improvement in diagnostic imaging are advances made in the fields of cancer diagnosis, including real-time image-guided tissue biopsies and molecular characterization of thoracic malignancies. Within the past 5 years, we have confirmation of the value of postoperative multi-modality adjuvant therapy and introduction of a number of biologic therapies; however, we have yet to detect a clear trend toward the reduction in LC mortality. With the many fields of LC care in rapid development, LC should be managed by a dedicated multi-disciplinary care team. The preferred practice in clinical medicine, as will be emphasized in this chapter, is therefore a careful consideration of updated diagnosis and treatment guidelines based on the best evidence-based practices (EBP) (7–9).

EPIDEMIOLOGY OF PRIMARY BRONCHOGENIC AND THORACIC MALIGNANCIES

Primary bronchogenic carcinomas, or LC were a rarely reported entity at the turn of the twentieth century, and the burgeoning incidence and subsequent cancer-related morbidity and mortality can be traced to increased exposure to known, modifiable risk factors (10). Foremost among these are tobacco-related carcinogens, with direct deposition in the tracheal-bronchial tree from both primary exposure (direct inhalation) and secondary exposure (environmental tobacco smoke). The route of exposure and excretion also explains the increased incidence of the other tobacco-related aerodigestive tract malignancies (head and neck, esophageal) and bladder cancers. The age of industrialization has also increased exposure to other compounds known to promote bronchial carcinogenesis, including inhalation of radon, asbestos fibers and outdoor air pollution, and other routes of exposure to nickel, chromate and polycyclic aromatic hydrocarbons (PAH) compounds. Outside of the United States and developed countries, there has been an observed increase in incidence of LC associated with exposure to certain methods of cooking, such as using wood and charcoal stoves (11). Exposures to multiple lung carcinogens have been observed to exert a synergistic (multiplicative) effect on the risk of developing LC, an example being smokers who are also exposed to asbestos. As with other disease entities, it can be expected that genetic determinants will interact with risk exposures to modify the likelihood of carcinogenesis and progression. Emerging data on specific populations and molecular epidemiology will lead to further refinements in risk assessment (12, 13).

There has been a stabilization in the LC incidence among males in the United States, likely attributable to a gradual reduction of smoking prevalence in the adult population, with a peaking and consequent 1.1% annual reduction in LC mortality among males over the past decade (1, 7, 11). However, the LC mortality for women continued to rise 0.3% per annum between 1987 and 2002, the last period with com-

plete survival data (7). It is important to remember that for every active smoker, there is an ex-smoker who will continue to harbor increased risk for an additional 15 to 20 years. The data from Western Europe, Japan and other developed countries show a similar trend of stabilizing incidence in males, but an increase in females, and as yet without proof of significant improvement in case fatalities and certainly not in population LC mortality, despite the gradual adoption of second and third generations of combination chemotherapies. Furthermore, approaching primary LC as a worldwide epidemic, the anticipated expanding global disease burden is alarming. The World Health Organization (WHO) predicts that 70% of smoking related mortality shall occur in low- and middle-income countries by 2020 (14). Countries such as China, with rapid industrial and economic development, have seen associated increasing environmental pollution that will compound the grave risk of increasing tobacco consumption. The 600,000 annual LCs and greater than 1 million tobacco-induced deaths in China are expected to double by 2025, with especially vulnerable females expanding the pool of 500 million people already at high-risk. The situation is not helped by inadequate health care awareness, advocacy and actual smoking by health care providers (15). Data for other developing countries may vary but the eager adoption of a "middle-class mass consumption" lifestyle by these societies points toward the same trend. Early detection and intervention by advanced imaging modalities and sophisticated but expensive technologies are unlikely to be available widely, and only primary prevention by education and multi-factorial risk-reduction through national policy changes are likely to be truly effective in reducing the global disease burden and its attendant human and economic costs.

In addition to primary bronchogenic carcinomas, other intra-thoracic malignancies include mediastinal tumors (thyroid, thymic, neurogenic tumors, teratomas, lymphomas), primary pulmonary parenchymal lymphomas and cancers metastatic to the thoracic cavity. Comprehensive data on the exact incidence of metastatic carcinomas are scant, and often based on selected series based on location or on therapies (16–19). With the introduction of new anti-cancer therapies, the overall 5-year survival for all cancers diagnosed is averaging 60%, with a number of common cancers such as breast, colorectal and melanoma now approaching 80% or better. Conversely, being able to maintain a number of non-resectable cancers in a stable or slowly progressive state with multiple and sequential therapies means that more cancers will eventually present as metastatic disease, including spread to the lungs. The primary sites from which pulmonary metastases originate include colorectal, breast, various sarcomas, renal, other uroepithelial cancers, melanoma, thyroid, head and neck and esophageal, and from primary LCs to other parts of the lung, although virtually all primary-site tumors have been reported to metastasize to the lungs due to the position of the pulmonary circulation in receiving all systemic venous return. Sites of tumor dissemination within the pulmonary system include lung parenchyma, mediastinal and hilar lymph nodes, endobronchial passages and the pleural space.

DIAGNOSIS AND STAGING OF THORACIC MALIGNANCIES

The clinical presentation of intra-thoracic malignancies may be protean in its manifestations. The symptoms depend on the size and location of a tumor, and central lesions causing tracheal-bronchial irritation or obstruction will likely cause earlier noticeable symptoms, such as hemoptysis, wheezing, intractable cough or stridor. Pleural involvement may lead to chest wall pain, and accumulation of an effusion may cause dyspnea. Conversely, isolated parenchymal lesions, even when sizable, may be missed because afferent sensory pain fibers are relatively scant in the lung parenchyma. Symptoms such as cough, dyspnea, fatigue, sputum production and signs of bronchial infections, including a postobstructive pneumonia, may be dismissed as chronic findings common in the middle-aged to elderly smoker population. Sometimes, extra-pulmonary signs such as seizures or alteration in mental status, jaundice or right upper quadrant pain, focal bone pain or pathologic fractures may be the presenting finding of a primary LC that has already metastasized. Also not uncommonly, an intra-thoracic lesion may be the sentinel finding of a cancer that has metastasized to the lungs. Typically, multiple thoracic lesions may originate from cancers of the thyroid, breast, kidney and sarcomas, whereas solitary pulmonary metastases, whether parenchymal or nodal, can often be seen with head and neck, esophageal or colon cancers. In practice, however, there can be no hard and

fast rules for such predictions. Indeed, with the frequent practice of pan thoracoabdominal-pelvic imaging with high-resolution computed tomography (CT) or positron emission tomography (PET)-CT scanners, metastatic lesions are being detected earlier, when only a single focus of metastasis is seen. Patients with a non-lung primary cancer can also develop a primary LC; this is especially true for patients who already have a tobacco-related cancer of the head and neck, esophagus and lung, or those who may have the genetic predisposition for multiple malignancies with well-described entities such as Fanconi anemia or, more recently, molecular genetic and epigenetic defects (20, 21). In summary, with the development of ever-more-targeted therapies specific for selected cancers, accurate tissue acquisition to diagnose cancer and to guide therapy is a top priority.

As stated, the first principle in LC diagnosis and staging is for accurate pathologic staging, as this is of prognostic and treatment significance. The same principle can be applied toward diagnosing cancers metastatic to the lungs; hence, the rest of the discussion will focus on the approach to a presumed bronchogenic primary LC. At the present time, even with the gradual shift toward finding more early stage lesions detected radiographically, only around 25% to 30% of LC are potentially resectable stage I or stage II disease at diagnosis. Although complete lobar resection and lymph node dissection for complete pathologic staging and for directing adjuvant therapy provide the best hope for cure, many cancers are found to have regional nodal metastasis at surgery or even distant metastasis shortly thereafter, and hence such patients would have undergone very invasive but futile procedures. An appreciation of the current LC staging system, the strengths and limitations of clinical staging by imaging, and diagnostic and therapeutic options will ideally provide tissue diagnosis and staging information in the most expedient fashion while limiting the number of invasive procedures.

Lung Cancer Staging

LC staging follows the TNM staging system adopted for all tumor types by both the American Joint Cancer Commission and the UICC (International Union for the Control of Cancer). The LC staging system currently in place has been in use for more than 11 years and is based on a relatively small cohort of around 5600 patients in several largely surgical series

(22). Starting in mid-2008 to early 2009, a sixth revision, as proposed by the International Association for the Study of Lung Cancer (IASLC) and based on 100,869 cases of LC diagnosed and treated worldwide between 1990 and 2000, will be adopted (23). Proposed changes to the current TNM criteria are based on observations of the clinical outcome of patients treated in the decade ending 2000.

Three changes will take place in the T-descriptors (24). There will be sub-classifications of T1 (primary tumor ≤3 cm) into T1a (≤2cm) and T1b (2 cm to 3 cm); and sub-classifications of T2 (primary tumor >3 cm) into T2a (>3 cm to 5 cm), T2b (>5 cm to 7 cm) and T2c (>7 cm) based on survival differences. In particular, large primary cancers (T2c >7 cm) have a prognosis worse than other T2 cancer patients, even when there is no pathologic nodal involvement, and therefore T2c will be regarded prognostically as a T3, thereby warranting treatment, including systemic chemotherapy. Previously, satellite tumor nodule(s) found in the same lobe as the primary tumor had been designated as T4 lesions; however, the data suggest that these patients have survival data similar to other pathologic T3 patients and hence they shall now be downgraded to T3. Previously, satellite nodule(s) found outside of the primary tumor lobe were uniformly designated as M1 metastatic disease, but in this much larger cohort database, a distinction can be made between those with satellite nodule(s) outside of the primary node but still within the ipsilateral lung, henceforth designated T4, versus those in the contralateral lung, which will remain as M1 (24). Another significant change is the transition of a malignant pleural or pericardial effusion, henceforth staged as IIIB to stage IV metastatic status, thus confirming what most clinicians in this field have felt – that a "wet IIIB" usually portended a poor prognosis similar to those patients with metastatic disease. The practical impact of these upcoming changes shall be discussed more in the section on therapeutic options and treatment paradigm.

In the area of nodal staging, the current N-descriptors for N0, N1, N2 and N3 will be maintained (25), with suggestion for clearer separation of the intra-thoracic nodes into six distinctive nodal zones, and a consensus between the principal American and Japanese systems on the naming and numbering of nodes (25, 27–29). Although there is no recommendation to change the current nodal designations, the expanded database demonstrates a trend toward

different long-term survival in patients who undergo surgical resection without induction chemotherapy. They can be separated into three groups depending on whether they have a single-station N1 node (stage II patient), multiple-zone N1 nodes (still stage II), single-stage N2 (stage IIIA) and those with multiple-zone N2 nodes (bulky stage IIIA). The impact these observations have on best evidence-based clinical practice may be that, in addition to initially aiming to sample the highest stage potentially involved lymph node either by mediastinoscopy or by endoscopy needle aspiration, we should also strive to sample all potentially involved nodal stations within a nodal class for prognostic purposes. Practically speaking, however, because adjuvant postoperative chemotherapy is already recommended for all stage II and III patients, it may not change the overall treatment plan. Still in development, the advent of molecular analysis of resected and needle aspirate samples of tumor and lymph node for so-called micro-metastasis detection and molecular staging may change our ability to predict who should receive which type of therapy as an adjuvant therapy, in which case the attention called on fine cataloguing of all lymph nodes may be part of individualized therapy in the future.

With regard to the M-descriptor for metastatic diseases in LCs, the downgrading of ipsilateral lung satellite tumor nodules found away from the primary tumor lobe from M1 to T4 (stage IIIB) status, and the upstaging of malignant effusions to M (stage IV) status have been discussed. However, a further subdivision will be introduced that recognizes malignant effusions as having a prognosis similar to satellite tumor nodules found in the contralateral lung, but designating these cases as M1a is, nevertheless, somewhat more favorable than patients with extra-thoracic metastasis to the central nervous system (CNS), liver, adrenals and bone, which will be designated as M1b (26).

A summary of all the proposed changes has yet to be published as a single paper, but extensive details of the changes, supporting data and method of analysis, including for small cell LCs, have been published as a series of papers (23–26, 30, 31).

Clinical Diagnosis

The initial presumption of a LC diagnosis may be based on classic clinical symptoms such as worsening dyspnea with hemoptysis in a smoker who, on examination, may be found to have new-onset clubbing and cachexia. However, given the lack of both sensitivity and specificity in symptoms and physical findings, the clinical diagnosis and presumptive clinical staging of LC and thoracic malignancies rely on imaging studies.

Plain radiographs will show a parenchymal lung mass, and pleural effusions sufficient in size to cause blunting of the costal-phrenic angle, but the overall sensitivity is suboptimal and planar radiographs provide inadequate information about nodal involvement or even the exact segmental or sub-segmental location to guide bronchoscopic examination or lobar resection.

Hence, at present, a CT scan of the chest, preferably with intravenous contrast unless contraindicated by allergies or renal insufficiency, would be a standard for imaging the primary lesion, the mediastinum, liver and adrenal glands (8, 32). Introduced for clinical mediastinal staging in the early 1990s (33, 34), the diagnostic accuracy of the contrast-enhanced CT scan is still imperfect, because using greater than 1 cm short axis as the definition for an abnormal lymph node misses 38% to 46% of pathologic nodes and has specificities of only 0.62 to 0.69 (33, 34). Advances in CT imaging but with adherence to the same diagnostic criteria have not significantly improved the overall accuracy, as demonstrated by the pooled diagnostic sensitivity and specificity of 51% and 85% respectively, as analyzed in the recent evidence-based guidelines for LCs (32). Nevertheless, a good-quality contrast CT scan is indispensable in the assessment of a suspected LC and for follow-up assessment after therapy, as the high resolution provides characterization of the primary mass, presence of obvious regional adenopathy, presence of any satellite nodules and presence of pleural abnormalities. A CT scan can also provide much more information about the exact lobar, segmental and sub-segmental location of a lesion, which will be valuable for diagnostic procedures such as bronchoscopic biopsies and therapeutic procedures such as placement of brachytherapy catheters or for surgical resections when a tumor may have crossed fissural or pleural planes (35, 36).

With the current generation of MDCT capable of very-high-resolution multi-planar reconstruction and three-dimensional reconstruction, the primary lesion's relationships to vital vascular, spinal and mediastinal structures can be further clarified, and this information is very useful in the multi-disciplinary discussion and planned management of thoracic cancers. In addition to directing biopsies of the highest staged nodal or extra-thoracic lesions to simultaneously diagnose and stage a patient, these imaging details may inform the team to engage the involvement of other services such as neurosurgeons when there may be vertebral-spinal invasion of otherwise potentially resectable cancers, or radiation oncologists for the placement of brachytherapy seeds and meshes at resection lines in cases of questionable resection margins. With advanced software, the standard DICOM dataset from high-resolution CT scans can generate pre-procedural "virtual bronchoscopic" fly-throughs of the central toward the peripheral airway segments, and may provide information about unsuspected endobronchial tumor involvement and extent of endobronchial narrowing in anticipation of endobronchial therapies such as local tumor débridement and stent placements (37–39). Of particular interest to the interventional oncologist and radiologist is the integration of high-resolution imaging with proprietary hardware that has led to the development of electromagnetic bronchoscopy guidance systems that are expanding applications of real-time image-guided interventions in the field of minimally invasive thoracic surgical and interventional bronchoscopy (39–43). These systems improve the accuracy of locating smaller peripheral lung lesions by providing real-time steering directions and, when combined with the placement of fiducial markers, will improve the targeting of high-dose external beam radiotherapy and lung-sparing surgeries in patients with marginal physiologic reserve (44–46).

Given the recognized limitations of the CT scan in predicting the presence of nodal disease and, indeed, its ability to fully characterize a solitary pulmonary nodule, the emergence of advances in metabolic imaging, especially with [18]fluoro-2-deoxy-D-glucose (FDG), has led to the studies and validation of PET as a useful imaging modality for the clinical diagnosis and staging of LC. Starting in the early 1990s, initial studies with FDG-PET metabolic studies focused on isolated solitary pulmonary nodules (SPNs) (47–49), subsequently expanding toward the more challenging and critical clinical staging of the mediastinum (50, 51). In recent analysis of the accuracy of FDG-PET scan in clinical staging of the mediastinum, the pooled sensitivity and specificity are 74% and 85% respectively (32). With the superior performance of

PET, and with the increasing availability and improving performance of combined PET-CT scanners that can provide fused metabolic-anatomic imaging, it is the recommendation by the American College of Chest Physicians writing panel that best evidence-based practice guidelines include the use of PET scanning in clinically staged IB to IIIB potentially resectable LCs (32). In clinical practice, the use of preoperative PET scans in this group of patients has reduced the likelihood of performing futile non-curative LC surgeries (51). Although not currently recommended as a routine modality for the detection of distant metastases in patients without focal symptoms (32), FDG-PET scans have detected asymptomatic pleural and extrathoracic metastasis between 10% and 15% of the time in case series, and have been specifically studied in pleural (52) and distant (53, 54) metastasis.

The availability of combined PET-CT imaging has improved the clinical staging of LCs; however, it is important to stress that the dictum, "tissue is the issue" remains true, and PET-CT and other advanced imaging modalities are to be a guide to tissue sampling and generally must not be regarded as a substitute to tissue staging. This is especially important as false-positive findings may be due to tissue inflammation and reaction, most often seen in the mediastinal nodes of large and necrotic tumors or in individuals with a postobstructive pneumonia. Granulomatous adenopathy, including fungal, mycobacterial and sarcoid lymph nodes, can be strongly positive by PET. Therefore, much as we caution against performing futile surgeries as a result of inadequate tissue staging, it is unfair to deny patients the sole treatment known to offer long-term cure if they are inaccurately upstaged by an imaging study. There are several conditions in which false-negative readings are encountered. The standardization of dedicated PET scanners has largely eliminated false-negative readings as a result of the use of single photon emission-computed tomography (SPECT) scanners for [18]FDG studies. A number of malignant lesions with relatively low proliferation rates, including carcinoid tumors, bronchioloalveolar-cell carcinomas (BAC) and metastatic cancers from hypernephromas, hepatocellular carcinomas, prostate carcinomas and mucinous carcinomas, may all be falsely negative or indeterminate by PET. Finally, tumors smaller than 0.8 to 1.0 cm may have insufficient metabolic activity to

register at above the commonly accepted standardized uptake value (SUV) threshold of 2.5. A small lesion that is very metabolically active should prompt further diagnostic action. As yet uncertain also is whether the intensity of the metabolic activity as measured by the SUV is prognostic of a tumor's biologic behavior, or whether and how to use FDG-PET for post-therapy follow-up assessment.

Magnetic resonance imaging (MRI) of the chest has no role in the routine staging of LCs. Where it may be indicated is when there is a question of local extension of the tumor into vital mediastinal vascular, cardiac and posterior neural and spinal structures that may affect resectability for cure (32). In patients with small cell carcinoma with known high risk for CNS dissemination, and in selected patients with non-small cell LCs (NSCLC) with focal neurologic findings, MRI of the brain with contrast is preferred over standard CT scans for detection of CNS metastasis.

Ventilation-perfusion scan is another nuclear medicine imaging modality that has been used in LC studies. Initially used for the detection of pulmonary thromboembolism, an event that is increased in patients with malignancies, it is now specifically most useful for assessing the potential resectability of LCs in patients with limited pulmonary reserve. A quantitative split-lung perfusion ^{99}Tc lung scan is used to calculate the predicted residual postoperative lung functions (55, 56). Whereas this may, at first glance, seem unrelated to the tissue diagnosis of a suspected LC, for patients with borderline pulmonary reserve, the predicted residual function may determine whether a patient with an otherwise isolated lesion would go forward with a diagnostic and potentially curative lobar resection, a sub-lobar resection with increased risk for recurrence, or be referred for an alternative tissue diagnosis, including possible trans-thoracic needle biopsy, followed by therapeutic procedures such as radiofrequency ablation of a diagnosed tumor.

Radionuclide bone scans may localize and characterize skeletal lesions in patients with focal skeletal pain, or those who have suspicious serum laboratory values such as hypercalcemia or hyperphosphatemia with an elevated alkaline phosphatase. FDG-PET scans are as sensitive as bone scans in the detection of metastatic lesions, and the increasing use of FDG-PET may obviate the need for most bone scans for this purpose. Unless the PET scan is combined with a CT scan, planar long-bone films or a CT scan may still be needed to assess the risks for a pathologic fracture that may warrant more urgent interventions.

Selective pulmonary arteriograms have relatively few indications given the ease and efficacy of conducting contrast-enhanced CT scans in the evaluation for pulmonary thromboembolism. Arteriograms occasionally are helpful in therapeutic situations in which selective pulmonary or, more frequently, bronchial arterial embolizations are performed to control life-threatening hemoptysis secondary to tumor erosion into thoracic vasculature.

Standard laboratory studies include a complete blood count and coagulation studies to ensure acceptable bleeding risks for biopsy procedures. A comprehensive metabolic panel is drawn to assess for adequacy of renal function before intravenous contrast exposure and will occasionally reveal hepatic transaminitis or elevation of alkaline phosphatase and calcium, which may indicate hepatic and skeletal metastases, but these findings are nonspecific and of no prognostic value. At present, there is no blood marker for LC that is of sufficient sensitivity or of proven prognostic value.

Tissue for Pathologic Diagnosis and Staging

There are many modalities of acquiring tissue for the diagnosis of a LC or cancers metastatic to the lungs and mediastinum. The ideal would be an approach that is non-invasive or only minimally invasive with high sensitivity and specificity. Given the heterogeneity of the types of "LCs" (57), their predominant location within the central airways (example being the central squamous or small cell carcinoma) or lung parenchyma often toward the periphery (example being the small adenocarcinoma), degree of differentiation and radiographic opacity (example being the faint ground-glass opacities that are the foci of atypical adenomatous hyperplasia in transition into a BAC), there is no single approach that is ideal in all circumstances (58, 59).

Sputum cytology, when read as positive for cancer, has a very high specificity, and both primary LC and even metastatic cancers have been diagnosed in this manner (60). The major limitation of sputum cytology is in its relatively low sensitivity, especially for tumors located in the periphery of the lung or in the mediastinum without direct exfoliation into the central conducting airways. The other limitation is the lack of any staging information when one is presented only with a positive sputum cytology. At the present time, sputum diagnosis is often an incidental finding in a sample sent for multiple studies, including cultures for infectious organisms. As a completely non-invasive test, it is reasonable to send a sputum sample for cytologic examination when the functional status of the patient is very marginal and other clinical diagnostic studies, including CT and or PET scans, suggest that disease has disseminated beyond a surgical stage, and tissue diagnosis is only needed to initiate definitive systemic therapy or palliative care.

At the other end of the diagnostic procedural spectrum, surgical excision of the primary lesion and dissection of lymph nodes will provide the most complete information regarding tumor cell types, which, in the case of small cell LCs, may show mixed cell histology in 10% to 15% of specimens. Completely resected specimens, with lobar resection being the standard procedure, will also provide information regarding tumor extension to the pleural surface, bronchial margins, and presence or absence of lympho-vascular dissemination. Lymph nodes dissected at the time of surgery will stage nodal spread of disease, which occasionally skip N1 stations and appear at higher, stage N2 stations. Finally, surgical specimens will provide adequate tissue to conduct corollary molecular diagnostic "biomarker" studies that are becoming the norm in some other tumor types such as breast cancer and may have therapeutic implications in the choice of adjuvant systemic chemo- and biologic therapies. Based on integrating information from radiologic staging with CT scans that show an isolated suspicious solitary pulmonary nodule with the absence of any regional adenopathy, or an isolated FDG-PET–positive parenchymal lesion, patients with sufficient physiologic reserve may be referred for direct surgical resection as the definitive diagnostic and therapeutic procedure (61).

Because the majority of LCs present at a stage other than stage I without any evidence of nodal enlargement, some other method of tissue biopsy or biopsies usually is selected for the initial tissue diagnosis and staging.

Trans-thoracic needle aspiration (TTNA) under uni- or bi-planar fluoroscopy, and currently, most often under real-time CT-fluoroscopic guidance, have a high diagnostic sensitivity targeting peripheral lung lesions (58, 59, 62, 63). Depending on operator experience and location of lesions, TTNA can also target mediastinal lesions and lymph nodes

(64). Pooled analyses of published series suggest a high diagnostic sensitivity of 88% for fluoroscopy-guided and 92% for CT-guided biopsies of peripheral pulmonary nodules, and the consensus guidelines would recommend a CT-guided biopsy of the primary peripheral lesion, especially if it is smaller than 2 cm and there is a reason to confirm malignancy before proceeding with a surgical excision (59, 63).

The alternative approach to sampling a parenchymal lesion is via bronchoscopy, through which tissue samples can be collected by a variety of techniques, including trans-bronchial brushing, trans-bronchial needle aspiration (TBNA), trans-bronchial forceps or curette biopsies, and a broncho-alveolar lavage of the bronchial segment from which the culprit lesion is suspected to arise. These methods are complementary and can be performed in sequence (58,59). Although bronchoscopy is the diagnostic method of choice for central lesions, especially when there are signs of bronchial obstruction and the need to evaluate for endobronchial interventions, the historical yield from trans-bronchial sampling of peripheral lesions smaller than 2 cm is only around 30%. A number of approaches have been used to improve on this yield, including the development of smaller bronchoscopes, down to 2.8 mm diameter, that can be steered out through greater number of airway generations that previously would not be permitted the passage of a 5-mm bronchoscope (65), the concomitant use of 3D-CT software to develop a pathway to guide the steering of the bronchoscopes, and performing the bronchoscopy in a CT scanner to engage real-time CT guidance to locate otherwise planar-fluoroscopy-invisible lesions (66, 67). When CT-fluoroscopy is not available, radial endobronchial ultrasound (EBUS) probes are extended through the working channels of bronchoscopes and assist in confirming the correct location for biopsy by the recognizable abnormal EBUS signals of a peripheral lung lesion (68–71). The development of electromagnetic navigation bronchoscopy has added yet another modality to target the peripheral lesion, such that diagnostic sensitivities of nearly 80% are achievable for lesions less than 2 cm in size (42, 43, 71) when performed with either fluoroscopic guidance or under EBUS guidance (72).

The other major indication for bronchoscopy is in the sampling of mediastinal and hilar pathology, including mediastinal tumors, metastatic or primary LC, and suspected tumor metastasis to these regional lymph nodes. Although mediastinoscopy, left-sided median sternotomy (Chamberlain procedure) and video-assisted thoracic surgery (VATS)-directed mediastinal biopsies have been the gold standards for sampling these regions, they do not usually provide access to all of the N1 station peribronchial, hilar and segmental nodes (73, 74). Furthermore, significant scarring usually results from the first mediastinoscopy and, as a result, it is difficult to repeat a mediastinoscopy to confirm successful down-staging of cancer by induction neo-adjuvant chemotherapy given to stage IIIA NSCLC patients, who are then considered for definitive resection. Mediastinoscopy is still recommended for the diagnosis of certain tumors such as lymphomas, for which TBNA seldom provides sufficient material for a definitive diagnosis. It is also recommended as a repeat procedure when a less invasive bronchoscopic TBNA is non-diagnostic, and before thoracotomy and definitive lung resection if there is a concern for residual cancer that will make cure unlikely after induction therapy.

TBNA can sample most of the mediastinal nodal stations except for stations 5 and 6 (the aortopulmonary and para-aortic nodes) and 8 (the subcarinal node) (75, 76). The diagnostic yield depends on the size of the nodes, availability of bedside cytopathology to provide "rapid on-site evaluation" (ROSE) (77) and operator experience. Many pulmonologists and thoracic surgeons in practice today who perform diagnostic bronchoscopy may not have received training in TBNA in their training programs, although this situation is improving as TBNA is becoming a routine requirement in most programs. The expanding interest in learning and practice of this technique is driven by the importance attached to lymph node staging of LCs and by the introduction of EBUS devices, initially as radial balloon probes for the visualization of bronchial walls, but now available as a convex probe device that facilitates real-time-image–guided TBNA of nodes down to the sub-centimeter range (78, 79). The ability to visualize the peri-bronchial structures, including with Doppler reading of blood flow, reduces the risk of vascular puncture and has increased the accuracy of TBNA to the 90% range. An alternative but less-tested approach is to use electromagnetic navigation bronchoscopy that can locate the entry point for accurate TBNA sampling of extramural structures. TBNA, and especially EBUS-TBNA, during a single bronchoscopy session, can be used to sample multiple nodal stations, including on both sides of the mediastinum, starting with the potentially highest staged node, to provide the diagnostic and potentially prognostic information about extent of disease spread.

An adjunctive ultrasound-guided endoscopic biopsy technique is the use of endoscopic ultrasound (EUS) during upper-gastrointestinal endoscopy (80, 81). The same radial probe with angled needle set-up permits real-time-image–guided sampling of mediastinal lymph nodes. EUS can visualize the left-sided paraesophageal lymph nodes of 2L, sub-carinal station 7 equally well compared with EBUS via the trachea and bronchus. EUS provides superior visualization of station 8, the sub-subcarinal node, and allows concomitant examination of some structures below the diaphragm, including the occasional LC metastasis to lower esophageal, paragastric, paraduodenal structures. EUS is, however, inferior to EBUS-directed sampling of the right-sided 2R,4R, 10R and 11R lymph nodes.

The presence of a pleural effusion, even in the absence of pleural thickening, loculation, or symptoms of pain or dyspnea, may indicate pleural dissemination and, if confirmed, will be designated stage IV M1a disease. There are many other causes of pleural effusions in LC patients, including congestive heart failure, hypoalbuminemia and other causes of a transudative effusion, infectious parapneumonic or frank empyema or effusions associated with thromboembolism that are more common in patients with cancer. Malignancies remain the third most common cause of pleural effusions overall, with primary LC and metastases from breast and other solid tumors being the leading causes. Hence, in the initial evaluation of a case of suspected lung or metastatic cancer, finding a pleural effusion that does not rapidly disappear warrants sampling of the fluid. Diagnostic thoracentesis is rapid and, when guided by real-time ultrasound, is extremely safe. Pneumothoraces result more often from blind insertions or the use of larger-gauge aspiration needles. But even when pneumothoraces occur, they may often be observed with the patient breathing supplemental oxygen and may not require tube thoracostomy for drainage. The sensitivity of thoracentesis for cancer detection varies between 40% and 70%, depending on the quantity of fluid withdrawn and the number of times the fluid is tested. Blind pleural biopsies with the Cope or Abrams needle add only a small percentage to the overall diagnostic yield, as this biopsy technique sampling error is greater with

metastatic cancers to the pleural space than it is for diffuse inflammatory processes such as a granulomatous infection. Therefore, a non-diagnostic thoracentesis that reveals an exudative effusion should be followed up by a definitive pleural diagnostic procedure such as medical pleuroscopy or VATS, the distinction being that the former usually involves only a single, or at most two, port entry in a spontaneously breathing patient and does not require general anesthesia or split lung ventilation. In either method, the use of optical instruments facilitates endoscopic-image-guided biopsies of suspicious lesions. The choice between the two approaches depends on the operator's preference and also whether the visceral pleura and underlying lung parenchyma is to be biopsied, or if the pleural space is already complicated by loculations as suggested by baseline CT imaging studies, in which case VATS is needed. If it is obvious at the time of pleuroscopy that there is pleural dissemination of cancer, then simultaneous pleuradesis by talc poudrage or mechanical pleuradesis may prevent future re-accumulation of fluid or the eventual development of a complicated pleural space.

In summary, the clinical and pathologic diagnoses of LC and other intrathoracic malignancies are best accomplished in a multi-disciplinary setting, with input from diagnostic and interventional radiologists, pulmonologists, thoracic surgeons and medical and radiation oncologists. Pre-procedural planning, whether for initial tissue diagnosis and staging, or in anticipation of definitive resection that most often is to be followed by adjuvant local or systemic therapies, will ensure for the patients and their supporting family a smooth transition through the otherwise bewildering array of alien tests, sub-specialists with incomprehensible jargons and treatments that should be complementary and well integrated.

MANAGEMENT OF THORACIC MALIGNANCIES

Surgical Management

Complete resection of LC with lobectomy and complete lymph node dissection remain the standard procedures of choice and offer patients the best chance of a long-term disease-free survival (82). The Lung Cancer Study Group (LCSG) randomized stage IA patients to lobar resection versus an anatomic sub-segmental resection and found in the latter group higher rates of disease recurrence (three times local recurrence, 75% greater combined local and distance recurrences) and a trend toward lower survival (83). Hence, the standard dictum is to evaluate patients, even those with marginal lung reserve, for a lobar resection. Subsequent to the LCSG randomized controlled trial (RCT), there have been other single-institution studies that offer somewhat different results (84, 85), suggesting that stage IA T1N0 patients may not have a worse outcome with lesser resections but that stage IB T2N0 cases should be treated by standard lobectomy. However, the frequent coexistence of moderate to severe chronic obstructive pulmonary disease, pulmonary hypertension or other comorbidities in patients with LC results in only perhaps two-thirds of patients with otherwise resectable, limited stage I and II disease having the physiologic reserve to tolerate a standard lobectomy. The current EBP guidelines suggest that whereas lobectomy is the preferred surgery of choice, it is still preferable for a patient to undergo a sub-lobar resection rather than no resection at all (61). The separation of T1 lesions less than 1 cm into T1a ($\leq$2 cm) and T1b (>2 cm to 3 cm) sub-divisions recognizes a continuum in survival and prognosis (24), such that with the expected proliferation of smaller lesions (certainly 1 cm and sub-centimeter) being detected on CT scans, there may well be new prospective RCTs to look at the efficacy of sub-lobar resections for lesions within the T1a category.

The presentation of multi-focal lesions, when at least one is proven to be a bronchogenic LC primary, also raises difficult diagnostic, prognostic and management issues. Occasionally, the lesions are detected in the context of an evaluation of a diagnosed aerodigestive tract cancer in the head and neck or esophagus. Patients with one LC or another tobacco-related cancer are at increased risk for synchronous and metachronous second primary LCs (SPLC). If assuming only LCs are under consideration, and there appears to be a dominant "primary" mass, these satellite nodule(s) have heretofore been regarded, at a minimum, as stage IIIB disease (T4 if in the same lobe) or stage IV (M1 if in another lobe in the ipsilateral lung or contralateral lung). As noted in the section on staging (24), and in multiple large surveys (86, 87), such patients, when offered surgical resections, have a much better outcome when compared with other "medical" stage IIIB, IV patients. The new T-staging system should encourage a more aggressive approach in the management of patients with multiple

nodules, including resection for those with adequate physiologic reserve, and consideration of aggressive adjuvant local therapy including modalities such as radio-frequency ablation (RFA) or high-dose focused radiation for those not suitable for lobectomies or even sub-lobar resections.

Surgical management of stage IIIA and lymph-node-diagnosed stage II (N1 nodes) patients is the area that highlights most the importance of a coordinated multi-disciplinary approach to the diagnosis, evaluation and management of LC. Whereas most N1 nodal involvement in stage II cancers is confirmed at the time of surgery, the increasing use of PET scans for clinical staging followed by TBNA and EBUS-guided TBNA, and nodal sampling guided by VATS is resulting in a number of patients with a tissue diagnosis of N1 disease pre-surgery. Whether these patients should receive preoperative induction chemotherapy is undecided, and these patients should be enrolled in controlled clinical trials. Patients with stage II N1 disease found at the time of surgery should routinely be referred for adjuvant therapy, and this will be discussed in greater detail in the section on medical management that follows. For the patients with clinical and preoperative tissue-confirmed IIIA LCs, the recent EBP guidelines for LCs stress the importance of regarding these as systemic disease with the need for multi-modal therapy (82). Patients with documented IIIA LC, most often diagnosed by mediastinal lymph node sampling, again should be enrolled in prospective studies to evaluate the unanswered question of the value of induction neoadjuvant therapy versus the accepted administration of postoperative adjuvant therapy. Whether combination chemo-radio induction therapy is superior to chemotherapy alone is unknown, but experiences with surgical complications post induction therapy caution against pneumonectomies, especially after combined therapy including radiation (82). Thorough lymph node sampling or complete dissection, whether performed preoperatively by mediastinoscopy or during surgery, should be the rule to provide detailed information regarding the true pathologic staging, especially as metastasis to LNs are known to "skip" more peripheral N2 stations (82, 88–90). The presentation of skipped metastasis may confer different prognosis and is one reason why the new nodal N-staging system has separated lymph nodes into distinct zones, with the recommendation for multi-nodal sampling (25, 88, 91). Other general guidelines regarding surgical management of stage IIIA LC cases include the exclusion of surgery for "bulky" mediastinal disease or attempts at surgical debulking of these patients, as they are unlikely to benefit from aggressive surgical interventions that will not be curative. Recovering from their major surgeries may only delay the administration of systemic chemotherapy, combined with radiotherapy as the definitive combination therapy for truly unresectable cancers. Finally, for those who have undergone surgery with finding of N2 nodal involvement, whether suspected clinically or detected only on final pathology, surgery alone is never sufficient, and these patients should be referred back to the multi-disciplinary team for adjuvant systemic therapies (82). A discussion of special circumstances, including performing bronchoplasties and sleeve resection versus a pneumonectomy, is beyond the scope of this chapter, but the general philosophy is to promote a lung-sparing approach as long as it should not compromise long-term disease-free survival (82, 92, 93).

Stage IV M1b metastatic disease, as a rule, portends very poor prognosis, and surgery is not warranted for either the primary cancer or the metastatic lesions for this stage of disease. The exception may be for T1N0 intrathoracic LC with a single focus of distant disease in the brain, liver or, perhaps, the adrenal gland in patients with good functional status. Single-center series outcomes suggest that up to 20% 5-year survival may be experienced in such select subgroups who undergo primary cancer lobar resection and metastectomy (94). These patients have, by definition, systemic disease and should receive adjuvant systemic chemotherapy postoperatively, but it is less certain about the value of concomitant adjuvant radiotherapy. There is no set recommendation regarding management of those who are of poor functional status or who clearly cannot tolerate even a sub-lobar resection.

Medical Management

The medical management of LCs with systemic chemotherapies and so-called biologic or targeted therapies have made significant progress in the past decade, reflected in the pivitol trials and subsequent approval of a number of second- or third-generation chemotherapies used in combination and in sequence for LCs of all stages, as definitive therapy or in an adjuvant therapy setting (95–98). The individual compounds and combinations are too numerous to discuss in detail, but suffice to say, the current guidelines for the management of advanced stage LC suggest that based on best current evidence, treatment with cancer-specific active agents may improve functional status as well as lengthen survival time compared with providing only best supportive care. There has not been demonstrated any combination of chemotherapies that is superior to another, although a platinum-based agent (platinol or carboplatin) is included unless there is contraindication to its use (96–98). Giving a third agent (triplet) does not add to the response seen with the standard "doublet" therapy and may increase toxicities. The decision to treat, especially in the aged, with cut-offs for age 70 and 80, and individuals with poor functional status will have to be individualized; a single agent may be selected in such cases. Palliative and supportive care, including the recognition that most cases of LC presently diagnosed are ultimately incurable, will lead to a timely consideration of end of life discussions and hospice care.

Throughout the continuum of LC stages and evolution of an individual's disease, there is a growing recognition that LC should be regarded as a systemic disease with frequent and often early dissemination, if albeit microscopic, even in clinically "early stage" disease. Hence, in the medical oncology field, there is also the call for a multi-disciplinary approach to the evaluation and management of LC patients, with cases ideally presented at a tumor board, with coordinated planning and timing for multi-modal concurrent or sequential therapies. One of the major focuses is, again, on stage II and IIIA diseases, those who have potentially resectable cancers. Multi-national and consortium trials have documented the benefit of adjuvant platinum-based therapies, given initially only to stage IIB and IIIA patients (82, 99, 100), with subsequent studies showing benefit in earlier, stage IB and II, diseases (101). Data on giving induction chemotherapy or chemo-radiotherapy in patients with known stages II (N1) or IIIA (N2) involvement are unclear, as is the role for adjuvant therapy post surgery for this subset of patients who may have received preoperative treatment (61, 82); ongoing studies may provide answers in the future.

The number of "biologic" or "targeted" therapies using non-traditional cytotoxic drugs are growing at a pace that is difficult to monitor. For primary LCs, most are still at the clinical investigation phase. Several compounds representing two drug classes have demonstrated efficacy as second-line agents or used in combination with current standard chemotherapeutic agents (102–104). Epidermal growth factor receptors (EGFR) have been targeted in a large number of malignancies, and multiple EGFR antagonists have shown promise, some only to fail demonstration of benefit in pivotal Phase III trials. Currently, the tyrosine kinase inhibitor (TKI) erlotonib is the only EGFR agent approved for LC as a second-line agent (102), although a number of other agents in the same class may gain approval based on further validation studies. Vascular endothelial growth factor (VEGF) inhibitors represent another class of agent with a rational therapeutic target and mode of action, and currently bevacizumab is approved for combination therapy in advanced LC (103, 104). More interesting than the specific agents is the recognition that the very selective mechanism of targeting and antiproliferative action makes it important to incorporate selection criteria that will predict response or exclusion criteria that should predict failure or toxicities. The presence of EGFR mutations and absence of K-ras mutation predicts a positive response to the EGFR antagonists. Patients with large central squamous cell cancers and endobronchial lesions that bleed are excluded from VEGF inhibitor use to prevent the life-threatening hemoptysis and exsanguination that were seen with VEGF inhibitors in clinical trials.

The expansion in targeted biologic therapies, at a time when there is recognition of the need for better individual disease-specific prognostication, has led researchers to explore why patients with the same stage LC, especially early stage cancers, may have such varied outcomes (105–108). The focus is shifting from consideration of clinical factors such as location of tumors (105) to the consideration of genotype that is associated with tumor aggressiveness (107) and, ultimately, response to adjuvant therapies (106). The goal is to develop usable panels or arrays of genetic studies that will shift the prognostication and prediction to therapy to all stages of disease such that multi-modality assessment and planning for treatment will become the paradigm of LC management (108).

CONCLUSION

In summary, thoracic malignancies, including primary bronchogenic carcinomas and cancers metastatic to the lung parenchyma and airways, are important causes of pulmonary pathology, and LC is and shall remain the leading cause of cancer mortality. Advancements in diagnostic radiology, including combined multi-modality metabolic-anatomic imaging techniques, are constantly improving in the detection of smaller, potentially more curable and certainly more treatable, lesions. Advanced imaging is also guiding the diagnosis of the highest staged lesion, as accurate staging is paramount in formulating appropriate therapy. It is important to remember, however, that tissue or pathologic staging is the preferred aim, and clinical staging by imaging modalities is no substitute except in cases of clearly unresectable lesions. Real-time image guidance is increasingly being used to achieve an accurate diagnosis of otherwise difficult-to-approach lesions and may also serve to assist in the placement of fiducial markers that are used to guide follow-up treatment. In therapy, the goal is aimed toward achieving cure but, at the same time, avoiding unnecessarily aggressive but futile treatment. The advances in therapeutic options have also pointed toward sequential or concurrent multi-modal treatments with the goal of extending quality survival even for those with incurable disease. Finally, recognition of palliation of symptoms has led to more attention toward quality supportive and palliative care. Management of these often complex conditions is best achieved by adopting a multi-disciplinary approach in which diagnostic and therapeutic options are discussed at a tumor board to ensure timely incorporation of evidence-based medical advances and the continuum of efficient and humane patient care.

REFERENCES

1. Jemal A, Siegal R, Ward E, et al. Cancer statistics, 2007. CA Cancer J Clin, 2007; 57: 43–66.
2. Henschke CI, Shaham D, Yankelevitz DF, et al. CT screening for lung cancer: Past and ongoing studies. Semin Thorac Cardiovasc Surg, 2005; 17: 99–106.
3. National Lung Screening Trial (NLST). National Cancer Institute Web site. http://www.cancer.gov/nlst. Accessed May 21, 2007.
4. International Early Lung Cancer Action Program Investigators: Henschke CI, Yankelevitz DF, Libby DM, et al. Survival of patients with stage I lung cancer detected on CT screening. N Engl J Med, 2006; 355: 1763–1771.
5. Bach PB, Jett JR, Pastorino U, et al. Computed tomography screening and lung cancer outcomes. JAMA, 2007; 297: 953–961.
6. Welch HG, Woloshin S, Schwartz LM, et al. Overstating the evidence for lung cancer screening: The International Early Lung Cancer Action Program (I-ELCAP) study. Arch Intern Med, 2007; 167: 2289–2295.

7. Edwards BK, Brown ML, Wingo PA, et al. Annual report to the nation on the status of cancer, 1975–2002, featuring population-based trends in cancer treatment. J Natl Cancer Inst, 2005; 97: 1407–1427.

8. Alberts WM. Diagnosis and management of lung cancer executive summary: ACCP Evidence-Based Clinical Practice Guidelines (2nd edition). Chest 2007; 132 (3 Suppl): 1S–19S.

9. McCrory DC, Zelman-Lewis S, Heitzer J, et al. Methodology for lung cancer evidence review and guideline development: ACCP Evidence-based Clinical Practice Guidelines (2nd edition). Chest, 2007; 132(3 Suppl): 23S–28S.

10. Alberg AJ, Yung RC, Samet J. Epidemiology of lung cancer. In: Murray J, Nadel J, Broaddus C, et al (eds.), Textbook of Respiratory Medicine, 4th edition. Philadelphia, Elsevier, 2004, pp. 1328–1356.

11. Alberg AJ, Ford JG, Samet JM. Epidemiology of lung cancer: ACCP Evidence-based Clinical Practice Guidelines (2nd edition). Chest, 2007; 132(3 Suppl): 29S–55S.

12. Haiman CA, Stram DO, Wilkens LR, et al. Ethnic and racial differences in the smoking-related risk of lung cancer. N Engl J Med, 2006; 354: 333–442.

13. Zheng YL, Harris C, Alberg A, et al. Less efficient G2/M checkpoint is associated with an increased risk of lung cancer in African-Americans. Cancer Research, 2005; 65: 9566–9573.

14. Wright AA, Katz IT. Tobacco tightrope – balancing disease prevention and economic development in China. N Engl J Med, 2007; 356: 1493–1496.

15. Jiang Y, Ong, MK, Tong EK, et al. Chinese physicians and their smoking knowledge, attitudes, and practices. Am J Prev Med, 2007; 33: 15–22.

16. Kiryu T, Hoshi H, Matsui E, et al. Endotracheal/endobronchial metastases: Clinicopathologic study with special reference to developmental modes. Chest, 2001; 119: 768–75.

17. Katsimbri PP, Bamias AT, Froudrakis ME, et al. Endobronchial metastases secondary to solid tumors: Report of eight cases and review of the literature. Lung Cancer, 2000; 28: 163–70.

18. Akoglu S, Ucan ES, Celik G, et al. Endobronchial metastases from extrathoracic malignancies. Clin Exp Metastasis, 2005; 22: 587–591.

19. Pastorino U, Buyse M, Friedel G, et al. Long-term results of lung metastasectomy: Prognostic analyses based on 5206 cases. J Thorac Cardiovasc Surg, 1997; 113: 37–49.

20. Hittelman WN. Genetic instability in epithelial tissues at risk for cancer. Ann N Y Acad Sci. 2001; 952: 1–12.

21. Estellar M and Herman JG. Cancer as an epigenetic disease: DNA methylation and chromatin alterations in human tumours. J Pathol, 2002; 196: 1–7.

22. Mountain CF. A new international staging system for lung cancer. Chest 1986; 89 (4 Suppl): 225S–233S.

23. Goldstraw P, Crowley JJ, Chansky K, et al. The IASLC Lung Cancer Staging Project: Proposals for the revision of the TNM stage groupings in the forthcoming (7th) edition of the TNM classification of malignant tumours. J Thorac Oncol, 2007; 2: 706–714.

24. Rami Porta R, Ball D, Crowley J, et al. The IASLC Lung Cancer Staging Project: Proposals for the revision of the T descriptors in the forthcoming (7th) edition of the TNM classification for lung cancer. J Thorac Oncol, 2007; 2: 593–602.

25. Rusch VW, Crowley J, Giroux DW, et al. The IASLC Lung Cancer Staging Project: Proposals for the revision of the N descriptors in the forthcoming (7th) edition of the TNM classification for lung cancer. J Thorac Oncol, 2007; 2: 603–612.

26. Postmus PE, Brambilla E, Chansky K, et al. The IASLC Lung Cancer Staging Project: Proposals for revision of the M descriptors in the forthcoming (7th) edition of the TNM classification of lung cancer. J Thorac Oncol, 2007; 2: 686–693.

27. Mountain CF and Dresler CM. Regional lymph node classification for lung cancer staging. Chest 1997; 111: 1718–1723.

28. Naruke T, Suemasu K, and Ishikawa S. Lymph node mapping and curability at various levels of metastasis in resected lung cancer. J Thorac Cardiovasc Surg, 1978; 76: 833–39.

29. The Japan Lung Cancer Society. Classification of Lung Cancer, 1st English edition. Tokyo: Kanehara & Co.; 2000.

30. Groome PA, Bolejack V, Crowely JJ, et al. The IASLC Lung Cancer Staging Project: validation of the proposals for revision of the T, N, and M descriptors and consequent stage groupings in the forthcoming (7th) edition of the TNM classification of malignant tumours. J Thorac Oncol, 2007; 2: 694–705.

31. Shepherd FA, Crowley J, Van Houtte P, et al. The International Association for the Study of Lung Cancer lung cancer staging project: Proposals regarding the clinical staging of small cell lung cancer in the forthcoming (7th) edition of the tumor, node, metastasis classification for lung cancer. J Thorac Oncol, 2007; 2: 1067–1077.

32. Silvestri GA, Gould MK, Margolis ML, et al. Noninvasive staging of non-small cell lung cancer: ACCP Evidence-based Clinical Practice Guidelines (2nd edition). Chest. 2007; 132(3 Suppl): 178S–201S.

33. Webb W, Gatsonis C, Zerhouni E, et al. CT and MR imaging in staging non-small cell bronchogenic carcinoma: Report of the Radiologic Diagnostic Oncology Group. Radiology, 1991; 178: 705–713.

34. McLoud T, Bourgouin P, Greenberg R, et al. Bronchogenic carcinoma: Analysis of staging in the mediastinum with CT by correlative lymph node mapping and sampling. Radiology, 1992; 182: 319–323.

35. Naidich DP, Sussman R, Kutcher WL, et al. Solitary pulmonary nodule: CT-bronchoscopic correlation. Chest, 1988; 93: 595–598.

36. Bilaceroglu S, Kumcuoglu Z, Alper H, et al. CT bronchus sign-guided bronchoscopic multiple diagnostic procedures in carcinomatous solitary pulmonary nodules and masses. Respiration, 1988; 65: 49–55.

37. Shitrit D, Valdsislav P, Grubstein A, et al. Accuracy of virtual bronchoscopy for grading tracheobronchial stenosis. Correlation with pulmonary function test and fiberoptic bronchoscopy. Chest, 2005; 128: 3545–3550.

38. Finkelstein SE, Summers RM, Nguyen DM, et al. Virtual bronchoscopy for evaluation of malignant tumors of the thorax. J Thorac Cardiovasc Surg, 2002; 123: 967–972.

39. Kiraly AP, Helferty JP, Hoffman EA, et al. Three-dimensional path planning for virtual bronchoscopy. IEEE

Transactions on Medical Imaging, 2004; 23: 1365–1379.

40. Solomon SB, White P, Wiener CM, et al. Three-dimensional CT-guided bronchoscopy with a real-time electromagnetic position sensor: A comparison of two image registration methods. Chest, 2000; 118: 1783–1787.

41. Hautmann H, Schneider A, Pinkau T, et al. Electromagnetic catheter navigation during bronchoscopy. Validation of a novel method by conventional fluoroscopy. Chest, 2005; 128: 382–387.

42. Schwarz Y, Greif J, Becker HD, et al. Real-time electromagnetic navigation bronchoscopy to peripheral lung lesions using overlaid CT images: The first human study. Chest, 2006; 129: 988–994.

43. Gildea TR, Mazzone PJ, Karnak D, et al. Electromagnetic navigation diagnostic bronchoscopy: A prospective study. AJRCCM, 2006; 174: 982–989.

44. McGuire FR, Kerley M, Ochran T, et al. Radiotherapy monitoring device implantation into peripheral lung cancers: A therapeutic utility of electromagnetic navigational bronchoscopy. J Bronchology, 2007; 14: 173–176.

45. McLemore TL and Bedekar AR. Accurate diagnosis of peripheral lung lesions (PLL) in a private community hospital employing electromagnetic guidance bronchoscopy (EMB) coupled with a radial endobronchial ultrasound (EBUS). Chest Meeting Abstracts, 2007; 132: 452S.

46. Krimsky K, Sethi S, and Cicernia J. Tattooing of pulmonary nodules for localization prior to VATS. Chest, 2007; 132: 425S.

47. Gupta NC, Frank AR, Dewan NA, et al. Solitary pulmonary nodules: Detection of malignancy with PET with 2-[F-18]-fluoro-2-deoxy-D-glucose. Radiology, 1992; 184: 441–444.

48. Minn H, Sasadny KR, Quint LE, et al. Lung cancer: Reproducibility of quantitative measurements for evaluating 2-[F-18]-fluoro-2-deoxy-D-glucose uptake at PET. Radiology, 1995; 196: 167–173.

49. Gould MK, Fletcher J, Iannettoni MD, et al. Evaluation of patients with pulmonary nodules: When is it lung cancer? ACCP Evidence-based Clinical Practice Guidelines (2nd edition). Chest, 2007; 132(3 Suppl): 108S–130S.

50. Wahl RL, Quint LE, Greenough RL, et al. Staging of mediastinal non-small cell lung cancer with FDG PET, CT, and fusion images: Preliminary prospective evaluation. Radiology, 1994; 191: 371–377.

51. van Tinteren H, Hoekstra OS, Smit EF, et al. Effectiveness of positron emission tomography in the preoperative assessment of patients with suspected non-small-cell lung cancer: The PLUS multicentre randomised trial. Lancet, 2002; 359: 1388–1393.

52. Erasmus JJ, McAdams HP, Rossi SE, et al. FDG PET of pleural effusions in patients with non-small cell lung cancer. AJR Am J Roentgenol, 2000; 175: 245–249.

53. Kumar R, Xiu Y, Yu JQ, et al. 18F-FDG PET in evaluation of adrenal lesions in patients with lung cancer. J Nucl Med 2004; 45: 2058–2062.

54. Rodríguez Fernández A, Gómez Río M, Llamas Elvira JM, et al. Diagnosis efficacy of structural (CT) and functional (FDG-PET) imaging methods in the thoracic and extrathoracic staging of non-small cell lung cancer. Clin Transl Oncol, 2007; 9: 32–39.

55. Giordano A, Calcagni ML, Meduri G, et al. Perfusion lung scintigraphy for the prediction of postlobectomy residual pulmonary function. Chest, 1997; 111: 1542–1547.

56. Colice GL, Shafazand S, Griffin JP, et al. Physiologic evaluation of the patient with lung cancer being considered for resectional surgery: ACCP Evidenced-based Clinical Practice Guidelines (2nd edition). Chest, 2007; 132(3 Suppl): 161S–177S.

57. Brabilla E, Travis WD, Colby TV, et al. The new World Health Organization classification of lung tumours. Eur Respir J, 2001; 18: 1059–1068.

58. Yung RC. Tissue diagnosis of suspected lung cancer: Selecting between bronchoscopy, transthoracic needle aspiration, and resectional biopsy. Respir Care Clin North Am, 2003 Mar; 9(1): 51–76.

59. Rivera MP and Mehta AC. Initial diagnosis of lung cancer: ACCP evidence-based clinical practice guidelines (2nd edition). Chest, 2007; 132(3 Suppl): 131S–5148S.

60. Barach A, Bickerman H, Beck G, et al: Induced sputum as a diagnostic technique for cancer of the lungs. Arch Intern Med, 1960; 106: 120–126.

61. Scott WJ, Howington J, Feigenberg S, et al. Treatment of non-small cell lung cancer stage I and stage II: ACCP evidence-based clinical practice guidelines (2nd edition). Chest, 2007; 132(3 Suppl): 234S–242S.

62. Lacasse Y, Wong E, Guyatt GH, et al. Transthoracic needle aspiration biopsy for the diagnosis of localised pulmonary lesions: A meta-analysis. Thorax, 1999; 54: 884–893.

63. Schreiber G and McCrory D. Performance characteristics of different modalities for diagnosis of suspected lung cancer. Chest, 2003; 123(suppl): 115S–128S.

64. Protopapas Z and Westcott JL. Transthoracic needle biopsy of mediastinal lymph nodes for staging lung cancer and other cancers. Radiology, 1996; 199, 489–496.

65. Shinagawa N, Yamazaki K, Onodera Y, et al. CT-guided transbronchial biopsy using an ultrathin bronchoscope with virtual bronchoscopic navigation. Chest, 2004; 125: 1138–1143.

66. Tsushima K, Sone S, Hanaoka T, et al. Comparison of bronchoscopic diagnosis for peripheral pulmonary nodule under fluoroscopic guidance with CT guidance. Respiratory Medicine, 2006; 100: 737–745.

67. Heyer CM, Kagel T, Lemburg SP, et al. Transbronchial biopsy guided by low-dose MDCT: A new approach for assessment of solitary pulmonary nodules. AJR Am J Roentgenol, 2006; 187: 933–939.

68. Asahina H, Yamazaki K, Onodera Y, et al. Transbronchial biopsy using endobronchial ultrasonography with a guide sheath and virtual bronchoscopic navigation. Chest, 2005; 128: 1761–1765.

69. Herth FJF, Eberhardt R, Becker HD, et al. Endobronchial ultrasound-guided transbronchial lung biopsy in fluoroscopically invisible solitary pulmonary nodules. A prospective trial. Chest, 2006; 129: 147–150.

70. Kurimoto N, Murayama M, Yoshioka S, et al. Analysis of the internal structure of peripheral pulmonary lesions using endobronchial ultrasonography. Chest, 2002; 122: 1887–1894.

71. Eberhardt R, Anantham D, Ernst A, et al. Multimodality bronchoscopic diagnosis of peripheral lung lesions: A randomized controlled trial. Am J Respir Crit Care Med, 2007; 176: 36–41.

72. Wilson DS, Bartlett RJ. Improved diagnostic yield of bronchoscopy in a community practice: Combination of electromagnetic navigation system and rapid on-site evaluation. J Bronchol, 2007; 14: 227–232.

73. Detterbeck FC, Jantz MA, Wallace M, et al. Invasive mediastinal staging of lung cancer: ACCP Evidence-based Clinical Practice Guidelines (2nd edition). Chest, 2007; 132(3 Suppl): 202S–220S.

74. Vallières E, Pagé A, and Verdant A. Ambulatory mediastinoscopy and anterior mediastinotomy. Ann Thorac Surg, 1991; 52: 1122–1126.

75. Wang K, Brower R, Haponik E, et al. Flexible transbronchial needle aspiration for staging of bronchogenic carcinoma. Chest, 1983; 84: 571–576.

76. Bilaçeroglu S, Cagiotariotaciota U, Günel O, et al. Comparison of rigid and flexible transbronchial needle aspiration in the staging of bronchogenic carcinoma. Respiration, 1998; 65: 441–449.

77. Diette G, White P, Terry P, et al. Utility of on-site cytopathology assessment for bronchoscopic evaluation of lung masses and adenopathy. Chest, 2000; 117: 1186–1190.

78. Yasufuku K, Chiyo M, Sekine Y, et al. Real-time endobronchial ultrasound-guided transbronchial needle aspiration of mediastinal and hilar lymph nodes. Chest, 2004; 126: 122–128.

79. Herth FJF, Eberhardt R, Vilmann P, et al. Real-time endobronchial ultrasound guided transbronchial needle aspiration for sampling mediastinal lymph nodes. Thorax, 2006; 61: 795–798.

80. Fritscher-Ravens A, Bohuslavizki KH, Brandt L, et al. Mediastinal lymph node involvement in potentially resectable lung cancer: Comparison of CT, positron emission tomography, and endoscopic ultrasonography with and without fine-needle aspiration. Chest, 2003; 123: 442–451.

81. Annema JT, Veersteegh MI, Veselic M, et al. Endoscopic ultrasound added to mediastinoscopy for preoperative staging of patients with lung cancer. JAMA, 2005; 294: 931–936.

82. Robinson LA, Ruckdeschel JC, Wagner H, et al. Treatment of non-small cell lung cancer-stage IIIA: ACCP Evidence-based Clinical Practice Guidelines (2nd edition). Chest, 2007; 132(3 Suppl): 243S–265S.

83. Ginsberg RJ and Rubinstein L. The comparison of limited resection to lobectomy for T1N0 non-small cell lung cancer. LCSG 821. Chest. 1994; 106(Suppl): 318S–319S.

84. Martin-Ucar AE, Nakas A, Pilling JE, et al. A case-matched study of anatomical segmentectomy versus lobectomy for stage I lung cancer in high-risk patients. Eur J Cardiothorac Surg, 2005; 27: 675–679.

85. El-Sherif A, Gooding WE, Santos R, et al. Outcomes of sublobar resection versus lobectomy for stage I non-small cell lung cancer: A 13-year analysis. Ann Thorac Surg, 2006; 82: 408–415.

86. Zell JA, Ou SH, Ziogas A, et al. Survival improvements for advanced stage nonbronchioloalveolar carcinoma-type nonsmall cell lung cancer cases with ipsilateral intrapulmonary nodules. Cancer, 2008; 112: 136–143.

87. Battafarano RJ, Meyers BF, Guthrie TJ, et al. Surgical resection of multifocal non-small cell lung cancer is associated with prolonged survival. Ann Thorac Surg, 2002; 74: 988–993.

88. Prenzel KL, Mönig SP, Sinning JM, et al. Role of skip metastasis to mediastinal lymph nodes in non-small cell lung cancer. J Surg Oncol, 2003; 82: 256–260.

89. Riquet M, Assouad J, Bagan P, et al. Skip mediastinal lymph node metastasis and lung cancer: A particular N2 subgroup with a better prognosis. Ann Thorac Surg, 2005; 79: 225–233.

90. Ilic N, Petricevic A, Arar D, et al. Skip mediastinal nodal metastases in the IIIa/N2 non-small cell lung cancer. J Thorac Oncol, 2007; 2: 1018–1021.

91. Pisters KM and Darling G. The IASLC Lung Cancer Staging Project: "The nodal zone." J Thorac Oncol, 2007; 2: 583–584.

92. Yildizeli B, Fadel E, Mussot S, et al. Morbidity, mortality, and long-term survival after sleeve lobectomy for non-small cell lung cancer. Eur J Cardiothorac Surg, 2007; 31: 95–102.

93. Tronc F, Grégoire J, Rouleau J, et al. Long-term results of sleeve lobectomy for lung cancer. Eur J Cardiothorac Surg, 2000 May; 17(5): 550–556.

94. Billing PS, Miller DL, Allen MS, et al. Surgical treatment of primary lung cancer with synchronous brain metastases. J Thorac Cardiovasc Surg, 2001; 122: 548–553.

95. Chu Q, Vincent M, Logan D, et al. Taxanes as first-line therapy for advanced non-small cell lung cancer: A systematic review and practice guideline. Lung Cancer, 2005; 50: 355–374.

96. Schiller JH, Harrington D, Belani CP, et al. Comparison of four chemotherapy regimens for advanced non-small-cell lung cancer. N Engl J Med 2002; 346: 92–98.

97. Jett JR, Schild SE, Keith RL, et al. Treatment of non-small cell lung cancer, stage IIIB: ACCP Evidence-based Clinical Practice Guidelines (2nd edition). Chest, 2007; 132(3 Suppl): 266S–276S.

98. Socinski MA, Crowell R, Hensing TE, et al. Treatment of non-small cell lung cancer, stage IV: ACCP Evidence-based Clinical Practice Guidelines (2nd edition). Chest, 2007; 132(3 Suppl): 277S–289S.

99. Arriagada R, Bergman B, Dunant A, et al. The International Adjuvant Lung Cancer Trial Collaborative Group. Cisplatin-based adjuvant chemotherapy in patients with completely resected non-small-cell lung cancer. N Engl J Med, 2004; 350: 351–360.

100. Douillard JY, Rosell R, De Lena M, et al. Adjuvant vinorelbine plus cisplatin versus observation in patients with completely resected stage IB-IIIA non-small-cell lung cancer (Adjuvant Navelbine International Trialist Association [ANITA]): A randomised controlled trial. Lancet Oncol, 2006; 7: 719–727.

101. Winton T, Livingston R, Johnson D, et al. Vinorelbine plus cisplatin vs. observation in resected non-small-cell lung cancer. N Engl J Med 2005; 352: 2589–2597.

102. Shepperd FA, Perira JR, Ciuleanu T, et al. Erlotinib in previously treated non-small-cell lung cancer. N Engl J Med, 2005; 353: 123–132.

103. Johnson DH, Fehrenbacher L, Novotny WF, et al. Randomized phase II trial comparing bevacizumab plus carboplatin and paclitaxel with carboplatin and paclitaxel alone in previously untreated locally advanced or metastatic non-small-cell lung cancer. J Clin Oncol, 2004; 22: 2184–2191.

104. Sandler A, Gray R, Perry MC, et al. Paclitaxel-carboplatin alone or with bevacizumab for non-small-cell lung cancer. N Engl J Med, 2006; 355: 2542–2550.

105. Ou SH, Zell JA, Ziogas A, et al. Prognostic factors for survival of stage I nonsmall cell lung cancer patients: A population-based analysis of 19,702 stage I patients in the California Cancer Registry from 1989 to 2003. Cancer, 2007; 110: 1532–1541.

106. Olaussen KA, Dunant A, Fouret P, et al. DNA repair by ERCC1 in non-small-cell lung cancer and cisplatin-based adjuvant chemotherapy. N Engl J Med, 2006; 355: 983–991.

107. Ahrendt SA, Hu Y, Buta M, et al. p53 mutations and survival in stage I non-small-cell lung cancer: Results of a prospective study. J Natl Cancer Inst, 2003; 95: 961–970.

108. Potti A, Mukherjee S, Petersen R, et al. A genomic strategy to refine prognosis in early-stage non-small-cell lung cancer. N Engl J Med, 2006 Aug 10; 355(6): 570–570.

Chapter 36

IMAGE-GUIDED ABLATION IN THE THORAX

Ryan A. McTaggart

Damian E. Dupuy

Thomas DiPetrillo

Surgical resection has been the mainstay of treatment for the minority of patients diagnosed with primary lung cancer and for selected patients with pulmonary metastatic disease. However, most patients with thoracic malignancies have little recourse other than the modest therapeutic benefits of chemotherapy or radiotherapy, which offer little chance for quality, prolonged survival.

Thermal ablation is an exciting new technique that offers clinicians and patients new hope with a repeatable, effective, low-cost, and safe treatment to effectively palliate and, in some cases, cure both primary and metastatic thoracic malignancies either before or concurrent with systemic therapy and radiotherapy.

The natural history of thoracic malignancies is of locoregional treatment failure and distant recurrence, except for non-small cell, primary lung cancers less than 2 cm in diameter, for which the likelihood of regional (extra-segmental) spread is small and surgery may be most appropriate. Although thermal ablation strategies have been used in patients with primary lung cancer who are too sick or have disease burdens that are too great for surgical therapy, most thoracic oncologists now recognize that primary lung cancer, like metastatic lung cancer, is a systemic disease with bewildering heterogeneity at the start, and that effective, local palliation and systemic therapy for both primary and metastatic thoracic cancer is the goal.

In this chapter, we discuss the basic physics of thermal ablation, applications for thermal ablation therapy in the thorax and technical considerations for thermal ablation. As of the time of this writing, there exists no randomized and controlled clinical trial that compares thermal ablation therapies alone or in combination to other established treatments for thoracic malignancies. At the conclusion of this chapter, we hope the reader will be as eager as the authors to participate in and see the inception of such trials.

BASIC PHYSICS OF ABLATION THERAPY

Cells and tissues can be destroyed by extreme heating or cooling. Thermal ablation is a descriptive term for the controlled, thermal destruction of cells and tissue. The three techniques to be discussed in this chapter are radiofrequency ablation (RFA), microwave ablation (MWA), and cryoablation (CA).

Radiofrequency Ablation

In RFA, an alternating current is created between an electrode and grounding pads placed on the patient. More specifically, an insulated RF electrode with a conducting tip is placed into the target tissue and when an electric current (about the frequency of radio waves – 460 to 480 KHz) is applied, tissue heating results from resistive energy loss (friction) as electrons agitate ionic molecules in tissues as they move toward the reference electrodes (grounding pads) placed on the patient. The concentration of electrons at the RF electrode tip thereby heats the tissue to 50° to 100°C, leading to thermal injury and cell death in a controlled and predictable manner [reviewed in (1)].

RF energy is efficiently deposited in lung masses for two reasons. First, the surrounding air in the normal parenchyma of the lung acts as an insulator and concentrates RF energy in the targeted tissue, requiring less energy deposition (2). Second, the high vascular flow of the lung results in a "heat sink" effect, dissipating heat away from normal adjacent tissue and concentrating the effective energy deposition within the solid component of the lesion; albeit this same effect can limit successful ablation of larger tumors.

Microwave Ablation

For a microwave oscillating at 9.2×10^8 Hz, the charge of the electromagnetic wave changes polarity nearly 2 billion times a second (9.2×10^8 Hz). When an oscillating electric charge from this electromagnetic wave interacts with a water molecule, it causes the molecule to flip. Microwave radiation can be specifically tuned to the natural frequency of water molecules to maximize this interaction, and the water molecules flip back and forth 2 to 5 billion times a second, depending on the frequency of the microwave energy. Because temperature is a measure of how fast molecules move in a substance, the vigorous movement of the water molecules as they oscillate with microwaves generates heat. Therefore, electromagnetic microwaves heat matter by agitating water molecules in the surrounding tissue, producing friction and heat, thus inducing cellular death via thermal injury.

Early "ablate and resect" data suggest that MWA produces greater diameters of thermocoagulation, possibly due to its higher intra-tumoral temperatures, increased affinity for water-based tissues and decreased "heat sink" effect (3, 4). During RFA, the zone of active tissue heating is limited to a few millimeters surrounding the active electrode; the remainder of the ablation zone is heated via thermal conduction (5). Owing to the much broader field of power density deposition (up to 2 cm surrounding the antenna), MWA results in a much larger zone of active heating (6). This has the potential to allow for a more uniform tumor kill in the ablation zone

than RFA produces, both within the targeted zone and next to blood vessels. RFA is also limited by the increase in impedance with tissue boiling and charring (7), because water vapor and char act as electrical insulators. Due to the electromagnetic nature of MW, ablations performed do not seem to be subject to this limitation, thereby allowing the intra-tumoral temperature to be driven considerably higher, which results in a considerably larger ablation zone within a shorter ablation time period.

Cryoablation

Cryoablation exploits a simple experiment performed by Joule and Thompson (Lord Kelvin) in which they allowed gas in a region at a constant temperature to seep through a porous plug of cotton into an area of lower pressure. As the gas expanded, it became cooler. This is known as the Joule-Thompson (J-T) effect. Ultra-cold temperatures on the order of −160°C result when argon gas is allowed to expand from high pressure to low pressure through a constricted orifice (J-T port) within a cryoprobe. Helium gas has the opposite J-T effect and is used to warm the probe to facilitate its removal at the end of the procedure. A freeze-thaw-freeze technique is generally used for cryoablation. The osmotic shifts accompanying these cycling temperatures are largely responsible for the cellular membrane rupture and eventual cell death brought about by the procedure. Cryotherapy exerts its ablative effects via a number of proposed tumoricidal pathways. These include direct cytolysis via intracellular and extracellular ice crystal formation, which causes protein denaturation, intracellular dehydration and pH changes, ischemic necrosis via vascular injury, cellular edema and vessel disruption (during the thaw phase), activation of anti-tumor immune responses and induction of cellular apoptosis. The resulting endothelial damage leads to platelet aggregation and microthrombosis.

PERFORMING ABLATION THERAPY

RFA Technique

Patients referred for RFA of the lung are initially evaluated in a clinic setting, where the patient's history and pertinent imaging studies are reviewed. At this time, the appropriateness for RFA and the risks and benefits of the procedure are discussed, and any additional pre-procedural studies are ordered. This pre-procedural evaluation is very similar to a surgical evaluation, whereby any possible risks of bleeding or serious cardiopulmonary issues are addressed. Side effects from RFA are also discussed, including post-ablation syndrome – a transient (days to 1 week) systemic response to circulating factors such as tumor necrosis factor that results in fever, malaise and anorexia. In general, most patients who are healthy enough to undergo computed tomography (CT)-guided needle biopsy are good candidates for pulmonary RFA. In fact, patients with only one lung can safely undergo pulmonary RFA as long as provisions for rapid deployment of a chest catheter are made. Patients with severe emphysema requiring supplemental oxygen can also be treated. However, patients with emphysema who may retain carbon dioxide may lose their respiratory drive when given higher percentages of supplemental oxygen under conscious sedation during an RFA. Patients with underlying idiopathic pulmonary fibrosis should be considered poor candidates for pulmonary RFA because exacerbation of the underlying disease my lead to serious respiratory failure and, possibly, death after pulmonary RFA.

To reduce potential complications of sedation-induced nausea and aspiration of gastric contents, all patients are treated after an overnight fast. Patients on extensive medications – in particular anti-hypertensive and cardiac medications – may take these medications in the morning with a small quantity of water. Insulin-dependent diabetic patients should administer one-half of their usual morning insulin dose. An abridged physical examination is performed outside the procedure suite, and an intravenous line is placed. At our institution, we do not routinely administer prophylactic antibiotics.

Patients are then brought to the CT scanner, wherein the technical staff place the appropriate grounding pads on the opposite chest wall from the skin entry site (e.g., the anterior chest wall for a patient lying prone) in order to direct the RF current and thus prevent damage to adjacent structures in the target area. After the initial scout images are taken, a skin mark is placed on the patient that corresponds to the skin entry site as determined by the computer grid at the appropriate table position. Horizontal and vertical laser lights in the CT gantry correspond to the x- and y-axes from the computer grid on the screen, and a ruler can be placed to match the desired skin entry site as determined on the computer screen. The area is prepped and draped in sterile fash-

ion and local buffered lidocaine anesthesia is administered both intradermally and to the level of the pleura with a 25-gauge skin needle and 22-gauge spinal needle, respectively. CT fluoroscopy is initiated and an image is taken with the spinal needle in place to identify proper table position and needle angle. Repositioning can be performed with the spinal needle if necessary. A small skin incision is made at the correct skin entry site by plunging a #11 scalpel blade 1 to 2 cm into the subcutaneous tissues. The RF electrode is placed through the skin and pleura to a length corresponding to one-half to two-thirds the distance to the target lesion. A CT fluoroscopic image is obtained, and the RF electrode angle in the x, y and z planes is corrected as necessary. For pleural-based masses, a shorter RF electrode is used. Placement of the electrode within the target tumor in these cases may need to be performed without initial superficial positioning because superficial placement from a lateral position may result in protrusion of the electrode, thereby obstructing patient placement into the gantry. A coaxial guiding catheter could also be used in this situation, whereby the RF electrode is placed into the mass all at once after the outer cannula position has been confirmed. For lesions smaller than 2 cm in diameter, central and distal positioning of the RF electrode is usually adequate for the first ablation, with subsequent tandem ablation zones performed during more proximal positioning. When at all possible, the target lesion should be entered along its longitudinal axis to allow for this type of sequential, overlapping, tandem ablations during electrode withdrawal. For lesions larger than 2 cm in diameter, larger electrodes or several overlapping ablation zones may need to be performed to insure adequate thermocoagulation of the target lesion.

Ablation of the liver may be used as a comparison to that of the lung. In a similar way to liver tumor ablation, working around the periphery of larger tumors in the lung helps ensure adequate ablation of the soft-tissue margins. However, lung tumor ablation, in contrast to liver ablation, tends to require less time and current to achieve adequate thermocoagulation. The baseline circuit impedance of small parenchymal masses surrounded by aerated lung may not allow the same amount of current deposition as with a liver ablation. Depending upon the RF equipment used, each ablation should be carried out according to the manufacturer's specifications regarding temperature (e.g., Talon and Starburst electrodes, RITA Medical Systems, Mountainview, CA) impedance

(Leveen electrode, Radiotherapeutics-Boston Scientific, Watertown, MA) or both (e.g., Cool-tip, Valley-Lab, Boulder, CO).

Just before and during RF heating, patients are given intravenous conscious sedation with midazolam (0.5- to 1-mg doses) and fentanyl (25- to 50-μcg doses). Continuous vital sign and electrocardiographic monitoring is essential to provide adequate and safe conscious sedation. The RF heating of small parenchymal masses located away from the visceral pleura may require less sedation and may not produce any pain to the patient. In contrast, pleural-based masses can be quite painful during RF heating. Therefore, it is important to instill 10 to 20 ml of local anesthetic into the extrapleural space. Some institutions perform creative adjunctive procedures to either optimize targeting, prevent complications (8) or lessen pain by creating a controlled pneumothorax to move the peripheral mass away from the parietal pleura. Given the somatic innervation of the parietal pleura (via the intercostal and phrenic nerves), irritation may result in pain felt either on the body wall or in the corresponding dermatomes, for which multiple doses of sedation during the procedure may be needed. RF heating of central lesions adjacent to bronchi elicits a prominent cough response from patients that may require sedation to reduce patient motion. Vagal nerve stimulation may produce referred pain to the jaw, teeth, chest or upper extremity similar to pain that results from myocardial ischemia. In addition, bradycardia may result from vagal nerve stimulation that is easily controlled with 0.5-mg doses of atropine. Occasionally, general anesthesia may need to be used in pediatric patients or patients who may not tolerate the RF heating with conscious sedation alone. Dual-lumen endotracheal tubes are not necessary as the pulmonary bleeding from RFA is not any different from a CT-guided biopsy and in fact may be less, given the coagulating effect of the RF current.

After the target tumor is treated, the RF electrode is removed and a CT fluoroscopic image is obtained to evaluate for a pneumothorax. Large pneumothoraces can be evacuated at this time with chest catheters and wall suction. Smaller, asymptomatic pneumothoraces can be monitored with chest radiographs. We put such patients on 100% oxygen via a non-rebreathing mask and obtain an immediate chest radiograph and 2-hour follow-up radiograph. An increasing pneumothorax on the follow-up radiograph typically necessitates placement of a chest catheter. Once a chest catheter has been placed and there is radiographic documentation of pneumothorax resolution, the patient may be discharged home with a Heimlich valve placed on the end of the catheter; a 24-hour follow-up chest radiograph is scheduled. Hospitalization may be required if a patient has pain or is apprehensive about outpatient management of the chest catheter. If the pneumothorax is resolved on follow-up, the tube is checked for an air leak by having the patient cough with the tube end in a container of sterile water. If no air bubbles are seen, then the tube is removed with petroleum jelly-based gauze to provide an airtight seal upon removal. In patients with air leaks, prolonged chest catheter drainage may be required, including the placement of a surgical chest tube that will require prolonged hospitalization. All patients are observed for at least 2 hours after the procedure, and interval follow-up imaging is scheduled upon discharge.

Contraindications are few and include uncontrollable bleeding diathesis and recent use of anticoagulants. Because many elderly patients have implanted cardiac devices such as pacemakers and defibrillators, caution must be used. Pacemakers are susceptible to interference by energy in the radiofrequency and microwave spectrum (10^9 to 10^{11} Hz). According to manufacturers, pacemakers can sense electrical activity more than 15 cm from their leads and are at risk to electrically reset from activity within 15 cm. Careful positioning of grounding pads may be able to direct the flow of current away from the cardiac device. It is important to note that ablation using MW energy does not require the use of grounding pads and thus may result in less extraneous current flow. We suggest the following preliminary guidelines for patients with pacemakers and defibrillators undergoing tumor ablation procedures: coordinate treatment with cardiac electrophysiologists to interrogate and program pacemakers to automatic pacing modes, and turn off defibrillators during the ablation procedure; provide an external pacing or defibrillation system for emergency use; place grounding pads to guide current flow away from the pacemaker or defibrillator; and, when possible, position electrodes and antennae more than 5 cm from pacemaker or defibrillator leads.

Potential treatment complications include mild to moderate intraprocedural pain (usually controlled with adequate analgesics), mild pyrexia (usually self-limiting and lasting up to 1 week), pneumothorax, hemorrhage, hemoptysis, broncho-pleural fistulas, acute respiratory distress syndrome, reactive pleural effusion (usually self-limiting), damage to adjacent anatomic structures, skin burns (secondary to inappropriate grounding pad placement) and infection or abscess formation.

Currently in the United States, there are three commercially available RF tumor ablation systems. Two of the systems (Radiotherapeutics-Boston Scientific, Watertown, MA and RITA Medical Systems Inc., Mountain View, CA) utilize a deployable-array RF electrode that consists of 10 to 16 small wires (tines) deployed through a 14- to 17-gauge needle. Because the tines curve backward toward the handle, the Radiotherapeutics-Boston Scientific Device (Leveen electrode) is initially deployed at the deep aspect of the tumor. In contrast, the RITA electrode tines course forward and lateral so the probe is deployed on the near surface of the tumor. The third RF system (ValleyLab, Boulder, CO) utilizes a single or triple "cluster" (no tines) perfused electrode and the tip is positioned at the deep aspect. This internally cooled RF electrode can increase the volume of the induced thermocoagulation by up to 4 to 7 cm in diameter, as reported in the liver (9), but may be greater in lung due to the insulative effect of aerated tissue (10). The single or cluster RF electrode contains a thermocouple embedded in its tip, used to measure intra-tumoral temperature. The effective local control and safety profile of percutaneous RFA have been firmly established in the treatment of numerous solid malignancies, including those in liver, bone, lung, breast, kidney and adrenals (2). As of this writing, there is no discernable difference between these devices.

Microwave Technique

Like RFA, MWA allows for flexible approaches to treatment, including percutaneous, laparoscopic and open surgical access. The preprocedural work-up is similar to that for RFA. Percutaneous MWA is usually performed with the patient under conscious sedation (achieved with intravenous administration of midazolam and fentanyl, for example), although in certain situations, when procedural pain is problematic, a general anesthetic may be required. Patients undergo monitoring with continuous pulse oximetry and electrocardiography and measurement of blood pressure every 5 minutes. Standard surgical preparation and draping are performed. Local anesthesia is achieved with injection of 1% lidocaine hydrochloride solution both intradermally and into deeper tissues. With either CT or ultrasound (US) guidance, the tumor is localized, and the optimal approach is determined. A thin (14.5-gauge) microwave antenna is then placed directly into the tumor. When the antenna is attached to the microwave generator with a coaxial cable, an electromagnetic microwave is emitted from the exposed, non-insulated portion of the antenna. Each generator is capable of producing 60 W of power at a frequency of 915 MHz. Because of the inherent properties of the electromagnetic wave, the device does not need to be grounded, thus alleviating the problem of grounding pad burns. Intratumoral temperatures can be measured with a separately placed thermocouple.

Several groups have successfully applied microwave ablation in the treatment of hepatic malignancies (4, 11–13). For tumors larger than 2 cm, it is prudent to use three MWA applicators to create larger areas of thermocoagulation. Spacing of the applicators 2 cm apart is optimal and, depending upon the length of the active tip (1.6 or 3.7 cm), spherical zones of ablation measuring approximately 4.5 to 6 cm can be achieved in a single 7- to 10-minute treatment. To our knowledge, there is currently only one percutaneous MWA system (Valley Lab, Boulder, CO) available for use in humans in the United States. Single microwave antennas may be used individually or combined to give a triple-cluster configuration to achieve greater ablation volumes.

Cryoablation (Cryotherapy) Technique

Percutaneous CA may be performed under CT guidance in order to exploit the readily visible intraprocedural ice formation as a marker for ablative margin estimation. However, US guidance and magnetic resonance imaging (MRI) can also demonstrate such "ice-balls." At our institution, percutaneous CA is performed under CT fluoroscopic guidance using an argon-based CA system (Endocare, Irvine, CA) and 1.7- to 2.4-mm diameter percutaneous cryotherapy applicators. Freeze lengths are consistent for probes (about 4.5 cm), with diameters varying according to tissue type and surrounding structures (14). As with RFA and MWA procedures, the pretreatment placement of the cryotherapy applicators is planned according to the site and size of the tumor, and tumor margins, taking into account any involved adjacent structures.

Typically, each patient undergoes a 10-minute freeze of the tumor site, followed by an 8-minute active helium thaw followed by another 10-minute freeze. The number of freeze-thaw-freeze cycles remains dependent upon the individual clinical case. A CT scan is typically performed after treatment, with the low density changes within the targeted tumor tissue measured and approximated to the size of the ablated region. Since the margin of the freeze zone is variable and cytotoxic temperatures may not have been achieved, a 3- to 5-mm margin is subtracted from the diameter of the low-density ablated region in order to better approximate the true volume of tissue necrosis.

COMPARISON OF THERMAL ABLATION TECHNIQUES

The goals of all thermal ablation strategies are to (1) obtain a negative margin, (2) avoid injury to adjacent structures and (3) create large ablation areas quickly. There is no study that compares either the three available RFA devices or RFA with MWA or CA in lung. Therefore, any comparisons between systems or ablation strategies are speculative at best.

The greatest advantage of RFA is experience. Nearly all studies on thermal ablation for lung cancer employ this ablation strategy. There are three companies (five if one includes devices outside the United States) competing to provide low-profile devices that will efficiently maximize volumes of tissue necrosis. The main disadvantage of the RFA systems are that they are to be avoided in the mediastinum and high in the lung apex as they can cause mechanical and thermal injury to blood vessels, central airways and nerves. However, some groups have reported clever ways to employ RFA in these areas (8, 15). Tissue charring (burned tissue) and cavitation also are limitations of RFA because when this happens, tissue peripheral to the charred area is insulated from the electrode tip and therefore may escape thermal injury – good for normal tissue, bad for destroying tumor. A more theoretical disadvantage discussed by some authors (16, 17) is the risk of systemic embolism, including stroke, when gas microbubbles during charring and "roll-off" impedance occurs. However, we have no documented embolic events after nearly 200 cases, and there is only one reported acute stroke in the literature (18). Furthermore, animal studies on lung RFA and its effects on brain circulation failed to identify any changes attributable to the act of lung tissue heating with RFA (19).

Practically speaking, MWA may be superior to RFA because microwave technology can provide consistently higher intra-tumoral temperatures, larger tumor ablation volumes, faster ablation times, the ability to use multiple applicators, more effective heating of cystic masses and less procedural pain (6, 20–22). In addition, MWA does not require the placement of grounding pads, thereby eliminating the problem of grounding pad injuries.

MWA has another theoretical, yet clinically unproven in lung, advantage that may result in improved tumor thermocoagulation, with greater energy deposition in aerated lung and greater heating near blood vessels. Unlike RFA, in which the zone of active tissue heating is limited to a few millimeters surrounding the active electrode (5), MWA has a much broader field of power density deposition (up to 2 cm surrounding the antenna), which results in a much larger zone of active heating (6). This has the potential to allow for a more uniform tumor kill in the ablation zone, both within the targeted zone and next to blood vessels. RFA is also limited by tissue boiling and charring (7) because water vapor and char act as electrical insulators. Because the physical nature of the of the electromagnetic wave is not limited by tissue charring, MW ablations do not seem to be subject to this limitation, thereby allowing the intra-tumoral temperature to be driven considerably higher, which may result in a considerably larger ablation zone within a shorter ablation time period. Based on imaging findings that correlate with pathological findings ("ablate and resect" data from liver), it appears that MWA produces greater diameters of thermocoagulation, possibly as result of its higher intra-tumoral temperatures, increased affinity for water-based tissues and decreased "heat sink" effect (3, 4).

Like MWA, CA may be superior to RFA because of larger tumor ablation volumes, the ability to use multiple applicators, and less procedural pain. In addition, CA does not require the placement of grounding pads, thereby eliminating the problem of grounding pad injuries. A frequently mentioned benefit of cryoablation over other heat-based thermal ablative methods such as RFA and MWA is the apparent ability to preserve collagenous and other structural cellular architecture in virtually any frozen tissue (23–25). Another potential benefit is the ability to see lower attenuation ice as it covers a soft-tissue mass during the freeze cycles (26). Percutaneous CA systems (argon-based and with small cryotherapy probe diameters) allow for its use in solid tumors in varying anatomic locations, including liver (27, 28), kidney (29) and, more recently, extrabdominal (30) and lung tumors (14).

One report discusses that complication rates may be higher with CA than with RFA (31). However, this was in a sub-group analysis of patients with multiple (more than three) lesions and did not appear to be valid for the group as a whole. Thus, theoretical problems with percutaneous CA include bleeding requiring additional maneuvers such as tract coagulation with fibrin glue.

IMAGING FEATURES POST-ABLATION

Follow-up imaging immediately after the procedure and during follow-up is necessary to measure the success of thermal ablation. These imaging studies allow one to measure the success or failure of the initial ablation, interval growth and need for repeat ablation, and metachronous tumor development. As of this writing, there is no proven imaging modality or time interval for subsequent imaging that most accurately detects treatment failure, recurrent disease or new tumor. As one might expect, as thermal ablation technology improves, such protocols will require revision and may largely depend on tumor biology (initial size of lesion and histology). In addition, given the paucity of data for CA and MWA, our discussion must be limited to RFA. Here we discuss peri- and post-procedural imaging findings and current follow-up strategies.

At the time of ablation procedure and up to 48 to 72 hours after the procedure, the appearance of the ablated lesion usually changes, demonstrating vaporization and wrinkling at the edges. There may be a "cockade phenomenon" (Gadaleta and coworkers, 32), which consists of concentric rings with varying densitometric characteristics. However, the most commonly described appearance is that of surrounding ground-glass opacification representing the ablated zone (33, 34). In fact, a 24- to 48-hour ratio of ground-glass opacity area to pretreatment tumor area greater than 4 may predict complete treatment (35). Cavitation can occur in 25% of lesions and is seen more frequently when the size of the lesion 1 week after treatment exceeds pretreatment size by more than 200% (36). At 1 week to 1 month post-RFA,

the lesion appears as an area of consolidation or nodules, the mean diameter of which is larger than the preablation size. There may be some cavitation and "bubble lucencies" associated with it (32, 33, 36, 37). CT scans obtained 2 to 6 months after the ablation demonstrate no change or decreased size from the post-RFA baseline study in patients with complete response. Jin and colleagues demonstrated that completely ablated lesions were larger immediately after RFA but decreased in size by 5.7%, 11.4%, 14.3%, 40% and 40% at 3, 6, 9, 12 and 15 months, respectively. Similar findings were confirmed by Steinke and coworkers (36). The partially ablated lesions in the Jin et al. cohort showed similar changes immediately after ablation and until 6 months. In contrast to completely ablated lesions, the partially ablated lesions showed an increase in diameter (18% and 20%) at 9 and 12 months (38).

Nodule CT densitometry has been applied to RFA-treated nodules. This technique involves measurement of nodule enhancement after administration of contrast and relies on the difference in vasculature of benign versus malignant lesions (39). Berber and coworkers reported that successfully treated liver tumors have decreased enhancement after RFA (40). Suh applied the same principle to RFA-treated pulmonary malignancies and found that there was marked diminution of mean contrast material up-take at 1- to 2-month follow-up. At 3-month follow-up, there was an increase in contrast material up-take, but it still remained less than the preablation levels (41). Enhancement patterns were also evaluated by Jin and colleagues and were used to define their complete versus partial ablation study groups. Interestingly, 55% and 44.4% of lesions that were defined as completely ablated had complete and peripheral pretreatment enhancement, whereas 83% and 17% of the partial ablation group had complete and peripheral enhancement. As such, perhaps complete pretreatment enhancement may allow one to better predict the completeness of ablation. Notably, however, one lesion showed no enhancement post-ablation but increased in size during follow-up (38). Thus, lesion size, along with the level of enhancement, may be used to follow up lesions post-RFA. The only caveat is that most RFA-treated tumors are heterogeneous, and lesion enhancement may fail to accurately reflect tumor activity. There may be viable areas within the lesion that do not demonstrate enhancement. These areas are frequently found at the periphery of the zone of ablation in a punctuated or crescen shape (42).

Complete disappearance of [18]fluorodeoxyglucose (FDG) accumulation is an indicator of less local recurrence and better prognosis after any treatment such as surgery, radiation therapy and chemotherapy in patients with lung cancer (43, 44). It follows, then, there is a potential role for positron emission tomography (PET) scan in follow-up of tumors after RFA (Figure 36.1), with residual or recurrent tumors appearing as increased up-take, usually at the periphery of the lesion (8, 42, 45–50). Akeboshi and coworkers have found that the preablation increased FDG uptake on PET is eliminated in tumors post-RFA (42). In a study unique in the fact that it used biopsy data to compare the sensitivity and specificity of CT and PET to detect residual tumor, these same authors stated PET was more sensitive than contrast-enhanced CT to detect early tumor progression (42). Given our discussion of the reactive changes seen on CT early after treatment, it is no surprise that Kang and coworkers reported PET to be superior to CT in evaluating effectiveness of ablation shortly after the procedure (49). Additional data are required in post-RFA patients to evaluate the role of PET imaging for detection of residual tumors.

It is difficult to evaluate the therapeutic response on lesion size alone. At our institution, an overall increase in size of the soft-tissue ablation zone 1.25 times that of the greatest diameter noted on initial baseline CT is considered to represent local progression, as is the presence of any soft-tissue focus larger than 9 mm in greatest dimension showing significant enhancement (>15 HU greater than the non-contrast series). An enhancing rim of soft tissue surrounding the ablation zone is considered reactive if it is uniform in thickness and 5 mm or less in thickness. PET scans are performed when CT findings are suggestive of disease progression.

APPLICATIONS FOR THERMAL ABLATION THERAPIES

Thermal ablation can be applied to treat any thoracic malignancy: primary lung cancers, recurrent primary lung cancers, metastatic disease, chest wall masses and painful bony metastases. Since it was first reported (51), the goal of thermal ablation has been to fill a void in treatment of lung cancer for patients who are unable to tolerate surgical resection;

who require palliation for pain, cough, dyspnea, and hemoptysis; who require treatment for recurrence (particularly recurrences in an irradiated field); who require cytoreduction; and those who refuse surgery. Worldwide experience with image-guided ablation of thoracic maligancies has grown rapidly (Table 36.1) (8, 32, 33, 35–38, 41, 42, 45–60).

The literature is diverse. Not only are the study groups heterogeneous, but comparisons are difficult because of very different follow-up periods, reporting and evaluations. To be fair, outcome reporting is difficult because no standardized system has been proposed or validated. Successes could be documented by "gold-standard" biopsy (37, 52), but this is too invasive and unrealistic and, unfortunately, the Response and Evaluation Criteria in Solid Tumors (61) are ineffective because even completely ablated tumors may not shrink. Thus, it is impossible to compare studies because of the different patients and methods used to measure outcomes. However, some conclusions can be drawn, such as adequacy of tumor ablation depends on size (42, 49, 52, 55, 58), adequacy of tumor ablation predicts survival (47, 58), PET is superior to CT for follow-up (42), palliation is effective (8, 52, 58), adjuvant therapy may improve results (46, 48), and RFA successfully palliates colorectal cancer metastases to lung (50, 62). Thermal ablation therapies have proven themselves to be safe. In addition, their success, primarily in very sick patients who would be excluded from surgical trials and perhaps even most adjuvant therapy trials, leads us to speculate that their role in the treatment of lung cancer and pulmonary metastases may extend well beyond medically inoperable patients and those requiring palliation.

PRIMARY LUNG CANCER

Primary lung cancer is the leading cause of worldwide cancer mortality, with 1.2 million diagnosed each year. It is anticipated that 215,020 new cases of lung cancer will be diagnosed in the United States in 2008, and that lung cancer will be responsible for more cancer deaths in the United States than colorectal, breast and prostate cancer combined (63).

With non-small cell lung cancer (NSCLC), 30% of patients present with the disease confined to the lung parenchyma, 30% with spread to the intra-thoracic lymph nodes, and 40% with metastatic disease (64). Surgery is regarded as the best treatment option

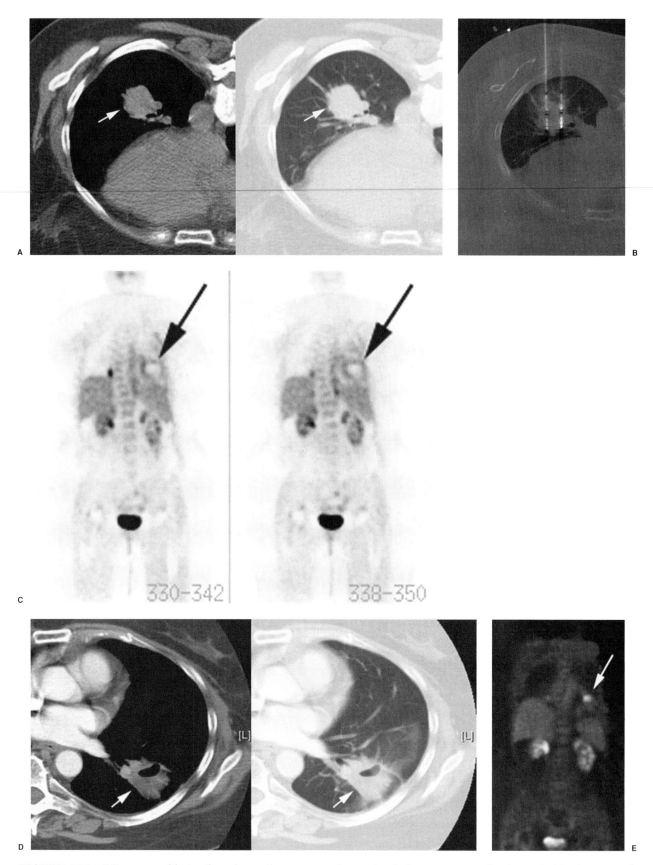

FIGURE 36.1. Microwave ablation for colorectal metastasis adjacent to the left lower lobe pulmonary artery branches. (A) A 64-year-old woman with three CRC metastases in the lungs s/p resection on right with dominant mass abutting left lower lobe pulmonary artery branches (*arrows*). (B) MWA was performed to decrease heat sink effect. Twenty-four-hour PET was performed to identify any residual mass. PET shows ring inflammatory uptake (*arrows*). (C) Four-month follow-up CT with contrast shows lack of nodular enhancement and cavitation. (D) Seven-month follow-up PET shows new activity adjacent to vessels consistent with recurrent tumor (*arrows*). Patient is being referred for external beam radiotherapy for additional treatment.

TABLE 36.1 Worldwide Experience with Image-guided Ablation of Thoracic Malignancies

Author	Title	Journal	Study Group	Ablation Strategy	PTX	Number of Ablations	F/U Assessment	Significant Findings
Primary Lung Study Groups								
Grieco CA, Simon CJ, Mayo-Smith WW, DiPetrillo TA, Ready NE, Dupuy DE	Percutaneous image-guided thermal ablation and radiation therapy: Outcomes of combined treatment for 41 patients with inoperable Stage I/II non-small-cell lung cancer	J Vasc Interv Radiol (July 2006); 17(7): 1117–1124	41 Patients Primary lung n = 41 T1 n = 21 T2 n = 17 T3 n = 3	RFA n = 37 Microwave n = 4	any ptx – 36.6% tx ptx – 22%	1 ablation session per patient	CT/PET	This study did not directly compare RF with XRT to RF alone. Unlike prior reports, survival was not predicted by tumor size, suggesting XRT may assist in the the ablation of larger tumors (independent of its peritumoral effect). Survival of this cohort dramatically exceeded historical reports for patients treated with XRT alone.
Dupuy DE, DiPetrillo T, Gandhi S, Ready N, Ng T, Donat W, Mayo-Smith WW	RFA followed by conventional radiotherapy for medically inoperable Stage I non-small-cell lung cancer	Chest (March 2006); 129(3): 738–745	24 Patients T1 n = 10 T2 n = 10 No PET n = 4	All RFA	any ptx – 29% tx ptx – 12.5%	1 ablation session per patient	CT/PET	Since XRT has poor local control, the possibility of a synergistic effect of both XRT and RFA was explored. This study demonstrated the safety and adequate local control with this combined therapy.
Wang H, Littrup PJ, Duan Y, Zhang Y, Feng H, Nie Z	Thoracic masses treated with percutaneous cryotherapy: Initial experience with more than 200 procedures	Radiology (April 2005); 235(1): 289–298	187 Patients 234 Tumors Primary lung = 196 Metastases = 38 Stage I n = 5 Stage II n = 17 Stage IIIA n = 20 Stage IIIB n = 60 Stage IV n = 63	Cryoablation	any ptx – 12% tx ptx – 1.6%	217 CA sessions 178 masses (76%) were treated with a single CA session	CT By 6 months (86%) of treated areas were stable or smaller than the original tumor (based on 56 available CTs).	A landmark technical report documenting the safety and feasibility of the procedure. Although ice coverage for peripheral lesions less than 4 cm was nearly complete, only 80% coverage was achieved for central masses larger than 4 cm. The KPS improved significantly for those with advanced stage disease.

449

(continued)

TABLE 36.1 (*Continued*)

Author	Title	Journal	Study Group	Ablation Strategy	PTX	Number of Ablations	F/U Assessment	Significant Findings
Fernando HC, Hoyos AD, Lanreneau RJ, Gilbert S, Gooding WE, Nuenaventura PO, Christie NA, Belani C, Luketich JD	RFA for the treatment of non-small-cell lung cancer in marginal surgical candidates	J Thorac Cardiovasc Surg (March 2005); 129(3): 639–644	18 Patients 21 Tumors Stage I n = 9 Stage II n = 2 Stage III n = 3 Stage IV n = 4	All RFA	any ptx – 38% tx ptx – 38%	One patient had repeat RFA.	CT/PET	This study demonstrates the feasibility of RFA for small, peripheral NSCLC tumors. Local control is comparable to, if not better than, that provided by XRT. Overall mean survival was 20.97 months; median survival not reached. Disease progression was seen in 8 nodules (38%) in 6 patients (33%). Mean progression free interval for Stage I versus other stages was 17.6 months versus 14.98 months (NS).
Belfiore G, Moggio G, Tedeschi E, Greco M, Cioffi R, Cincotti F, Rossi R	CT-guided RFA: A potential complementary therapy for patients with unresectable primary lung cancer – a preliminary report of 33 patients	AJR Am J Roentgenol (October 2004); 183: 1003–1011	33 Patients 33 Tumors Primary lung n = 33 NSCLC n = 32 Small CLC n = 1	All RFA	any ptx – 10% tx ptx – 0%	35 RFA sessions	CT and biopsy Performed biopsies at 6 months in 19 patients; 7 (36%) had complete necrosis, most of whom had lesions smaller than 3 cm. Viable tumor seen in 12 patients; all had tumors >3 cm.	Contrast-enhanced CT at 6-month follow-up showed 4 cases of complete, 13 cases of partial ablation, 11 cases of stabilized lesion size, and 1 case of increased lesion size. Contrast-enhanced CT at 1-year follow-up (n = 10) showed unchanged lesion size in 6 cases and reduction in 4 cases. RFA can be used successfully in unresectable lung cancer as an alternative or complementary treatment to radio- or chemotherapy.
Jin GY, Lee JM, Lee YC, Ha YM, Lim YS	Primary and secondary lung malignancies treated with percutaneous RFA: Evaluation with follow-up CT	AJR Am J Roentgenol (October 2004); 183(4): 1013–1020	21 Patients 21 Tumors Primary lung n = 17 Mestastases n = 4	All RFA	any ptx – 38.1% tx ptx – 4.2%	unknown	CT In both the complete and partial ablation groups lesions were bigger within 30 minutes of RFA.	In the complete ablation group (n = 9), ablated lesions were completely without contrast enhancement on follow-up CT and got smaller. In the partial ablation group (n = 12), the ablated lesions had varying degrees of enhancement, and the mean lesion size gradually increased during follow-up.

Pulmonary Metastases Study Groups

Authors	Title	Publication	Patients/Tumors	Treatment	Complications	Procedures	Follow-up	Results
Yan T, King J, Sjarif A, Glenn D, Steinke K, Morris D	Percutaneous RFA of pulmonary metastases from colorectal carcinoma: Prognostic determinants for survival	Ann Surg Oncol (November 2006); 13(11): 1529–1537	55 Patients with a mean number of 2 ± 1 CRC pulmonary metastases.	All RFA with and without adjuvant therapies	any ptx – 27% tx ptx – 17%	70 RFAs 13 repeat 2 third-time	CT 1 week 1 month 3 months thereafter	Even though 30 of 55 patients had previously resected liver metastases, overall median survival was 33 months. One-, 2-, and 3-year actuarial survival was 85%, 64%, and 46%. In univariate analysis lesion size, location, and need for repeat RFA were predictive of survival. In a multivariate model only lesion size remained predictive.
Yan T, King J, Sjarif A, Glenn D, Steinke K, Morris D	Learning curve for RFA of pulmonary metastases from colorectal carcinoma: A prospective study of 70 consecutive cases	Ann Surg Oncol (December 2006); 13(12): 1588–1595	55 Patients with a mean number of 2 ± 1 CRC pulmonary metastases.	All RFA with and without adjuvant therapies	any ptx – 27% tx ptx – 17%	70 RFAs 13 repeat 2 third-time	CT 1 week 1 month 3 months thereafter	A comparison between the initial 35 and subsequent 35 procedures was made. The number of metastases and experience (treatment period) were independent risk factors for overall morbidity, ptx, and need for tube thoracostomy.
de Baere T, Palussiere J, Auperin A, Hakime A, Abdel-Rehim M, Kind M, Dromain C, Ravaud A, Tebboune N, Boige V, Malka D, Lafont C, Ducreux M	Midterm local efficacy and survival after RFA of lung tumors with minimum follow-up of 1 year: Prospective evaluation	Radiology (August 2006); 240(2): 587–589	60 Patients 100 Tumors Primary lung n = 9 Metastatic n = 51	All RFA	any ptx – 54% tx ptx – 9%	163 RFAs	CT	All patients had tumors 4 cm or smaller. RFA local treatment success was 93% per tumor and 88% per patient. An ablation area at least 4 times larger than the initial tumor was predictive of complete ablation treatment.
Kawamura M, Izumi Y, Tsukada N, Asakura K, Sugiura H, Yashiro H, Nakano K, Nakatsuka S, Kuribayashi S, Kobayashi K	Percutaneous cryoablation of small pulmonary malignant tumors under CT guidance with local anesthesia in nonsurgical candidates	J Thorac Cardiovasc Surg (May 2006); 131(5): 1007–1013	20 Patients 35 Tumors All had metastatic tumors.	Cryoablation	any ptx – 50% tx ptx – 4.5%	22 sessions of cryoablation	CT	Cryoablation was safe. Local recurrence occurred in 20% of tumors with 1 year survival of 90%.

(continued)

TABLE 36.1 (*Continued*)

Author	Title	Journal	Study Group	Ablation Strategy	PTX	Number of Ablations	F/U Assessment	Significant Findings
Steinke K, Glenn D, King J, Clark W, Zhao J, Clingan P, Morris DL	Percutaneous imaging-guided RFA in patients with colorectal pulmonary metastases: 1-year follow-up	Ann Surg Oncol (February 2004);11(2): 207–212	23 Patients 52 CRC metastases	All RFA	any ptx – 43% tx ptx – 26.1%	6 patients had a second RF session	CT Serum CEA	Eighteen patients with CT scan follow-up at 1 year have 40 lesions classified as disappeared (n = 17), decreased (n = 5), stable/same size (n = 4), or increased (n = 14).
King J, Glenn D, Clark W, Zhao J, Steinke K, Clingan P, Morris DL	Percutaneous RFA of pulmonary metastases in patients with colorectal cancer	Br J Surg (February 2004); 91(2): 217–233	19 Patients 44 CRC metastases	All RFA	any ptx – 52% tx ptx – 32%	25 RFA sessions 2 patients retx at 12 and 22 months 5 patients had retx for new mets	CT Serum CEA	Six months after treatment, CT demonstrated 3 lesions had progressed, 25 were stable or smaller, and 11 were no longer visible. At 12 months, 5 had progressed, 11 were stable or smaller, and 9 were not visible.
Steinke K, King J, Glenn D, Franz CR, Morris DL	Radiologic appearance and complications of percutaneous CT-guided RFA pulmonary metastases from colorectal carcinoma	J Comput Assist Tomogr (September/ October 2003); 27(5): 750–757 [Abstract only available]	20 Patients 41 CRC metastases	All RFA	any ptx – 50% tx ptx – 25%	Not reported	CT	At 3 months after RFA, the lesion was approximately the same size as at baseline. The lesion subsequently shrank within the following 3 months, usually with a small scar remaining. Ablated lesion size usually exceeds the dimensions of the initial tumor for the first 3 months after ablation and continuously shrinks thereafter.
Mixed Primary Lung and Pulmonary Metastases Study Groups								
Simon CJ, Dupuy DE, DiPetrillo TA, Safran HP, Grieco CA, Ng T, Mayo-Smith WW	Pulmonary RFA: Long-term safety and efficacy in 153 patients	Radiology (April 2007); 243(1): 268–275	153 Patients 189 Tumors 122 Lung 67 Metastatic	RFA	any ptx – 27.5% tx ptx – 9.5%	602 RFAs	CT/PET	Initial technical success was 98%. Survival for Stage I NSCLC patients was reported and did not differ among patients with tumors less than or greater than 3 cm. For 18 patients with colorectal metastases: 1-, 2-, and 3-year survival was 86.8%, 77.5%, and 57%, respectively.

452

				Microwave			CT/USG	
He W, Hu X, Wu D, Guo L, Zhang L, Xiang D, Ning B	Ultrasonography-guided percutaneous microwave ablation of peripheral lung cancer	Clin Imaging (July/August 2006); 30: 234–241	12 Patients 16 Tumors Primary lung n = 9 Metastatic n = 7		any ptx – 8.3% tx ptx – 0%	21 treatments in 16 patients	CT/USG	Safety and feasibility study. There were no complications. By CT all tumors had area reduction ("remarkable" in 10 and mild in 6). By color Doppler all tumors were visible before ablation and 10 were invisible afterward.
Ambrogi MC, Lucchi M, Dini P, Melfi F, Fontanini G, Faviana P, Fanucchi O, Mussi A	Percutaneous RFA of lung tumors: Results in the midterm	Eur J Cardiothorac Surg (July 2006); 30(1): 177–183	54 Patients 64 Tumors Primary lung n = 40 Metastasis n = 24	All RFA	any ptx – 12.7% tx ptx – 11.1%	79 RFAs	CT/PET	At a mean follow-up of 2 years, there were 62% complete responses with higher response rates for metastatic lesions (71%) and those smaller than 3 cm (70%).
Bojarski JD, Dupuy DE, Mayo-Smith WW	CT imaging findings of pulmonary neoplasms after treatment with RFA results in 32 tumors	AJR Am J Roentgenol (August 2005); 185: 466–471	26 Patients 32 Tumors Primary lung n = 14 Metastases n = 18	All RFA	not reported	an average of 3.1 RFAs were performed	CT CT immediately after and at 1, 3, and 6–12 months and 18–24 months after the procedure.	Many (66%) treated neoplasms increased in size from baseline on 1–3 month follow-up CT scans. A report on important observations and what to expect on post-treatment CT scans.
VanSonnenberg E, Shankar S, Morrison PR, Nair RT, Silverman SG, Jaklitsch MT, Liu F, Cheung L, Tuncali K, Skarin AT, Sugarbaker DJ	RFA of thoracic lesions: Part 2 initial clinical experience – technical and multidisciplinary considerations in 30 patients	AJR Am J Roentgenol (February 2005); 184(2): 381–390	30 Patients 36 Tumors Primary lung n = 18 Metastases n = 11 Mesothelioma n = 1	All RFA	any – 26.7% tx PTX – 3.3%	2nd RFA done immediately in 18 patients; 1 delayed RFA	CT and PET	All ablations were technically successful. No periprocedural mortality occurred. Necrosis of tumor was greater than 90% in 26 of 30 lesions based on short-term follow-up imaging (CT, PET, MRI). In the 11 patients who underwent ablation for pain, relief was complete in 4 and partial in the other 7. RFA for a variety of thoracic tumors can be performed safely and with a high degree of efficacy for pain control and tumor killing.

(continued)

TABLE 36.1 (*Continued*)

Author	Title	Journal	Study Group	Ablation Strategy	PTX	Number of Ablations	F/U Assessment	Significant Findings
Gadaleta C, Catino A, Ranieri G, Armenise F, Colucci G, Lorusso V, Cramarossa A, Fiorentini G, Mattioli V	Radiofrequency thermal ablation of 69 lung neoplasms	J Chemother (November 2004); 16(suppl 5): 86–89	34 Patients 69 Tumors Primary lung n = 6 Metastases n = 28	All RFA	any ptx – not reported tx ptx – 16%	45 sessions of treatment were performed and 100 electrode-needle placements were performed	CT and MRI CT and MRI performed at one month and every three months thereafter CT only for first 8 patients	The rate of complete necrosis of lung neoplasms was high (92%). Lung RFA is an attractive technique suitable for patients not otherwise eligible for surgery.
Kang S, Luo R, Liao W, Wu H, Zhang X, Meng Y	Single group study to evaluate the feasibility and complications of RFA and usefulness of post-treatment positron emission tomography in lung tumors	World J Surg Oncol (September 2004); 2: 30	50 Patients 120 Tumors Primary lung n = 23 Metastases n = 27 17 Patients had single lesions	All RFA	any ptx – 18% tx ptx – 8%	No repeat RFA	CT and PET	Tumors smaller than 3.5 cm were completely killed after RFA. In tumors larger than 3.5 cm, the part within 3.5 cm was killed. While CT showed that tumors became larger 1 to 2 weeks after RFA procedure, PET demonstrated tumor destruction in 70% cases, compared with 38% in CT.
Gadaleta C, Mattiolo V, Colucci G, Cramarossa A, Lorusso V, Canniello E, Timurian A, Ranieri G, Fiorentini G, De Lena M, Catino A	RFA of 40 lung neoplasms: Preliminary results	AJR Am J Roentgenol (August 2004); 183: 361–368	18 Patients 40 Tumors Primary lung n = 4 Metastases n = 14	All RFA	any ptx – 12.5% tx ptx – 4.2%	24 RFA sessions with 65 insertions	CT/MRI	The authors of the article emphasized the safety of lung RFA. It is a conservative, minimally invasive treatment that can be administered multiple times; it could be especially effective in patients not eligible for surgery or with slow-growing lesions.

454

Authors	Title	Citation	Treatment	Complications	Tumors	Imaging/Assessment	Results
Yasui K, Kanazawa S, Sano Y, Fujiwara T, Kagawa S, Mimura H, Dendo S, Mukai T, Fujiwara H, Iguchi T, Hyodo T, Shimizu N, Tanaka N, Hiraki Y	Thoracic tumors treated with CT-guided RFA: Initial experience	Radiology (June 2004); 231: 850–857	35 Patients 99 Tumors Primary lung n = 3 Metastases n = 96	All RFA	any ptx – 35.2% tx ptx – 7.2%	1 for n = 63 tumors 2 for n = 22 tumors 3 for n = 8 tumors 4 for n = 4 tumors 5 for n = 1 tumors	CT and biopsy 60% no viable tumor 40% viable tumor CT at 2 months show target zone increases in size 50–100%	Ninety tumors showed no growth progression at follow-up CT. Probable complete coagulation necrosis obtained with initial RFA was achieved in 91% (90 of 99) of the tumors. There was no size or histological reason that 9 tumors were not controlled.
Akeboshi M, Yamakado K, Nakatsuka A, Hataji O, Taguchi O, Takao M, Takeda K	Percutaneous RFA of lung neoplasms, initial therapeutic response	J Vasc Interv Radiol (May 2004); 15: 463–470	31 Patients 54 Tumors Primary lung n = 13 Metastases n = 41	All RFA	any ptx – 29% tx ptx – 16.1%	There were 22 residual tumors and 13 were treated by RF again	CT, PET, biopsy Biopsy data showed PET was more sensitive and specific to determine residual viable tumor.	Complete necrosis was achieved in 32 of 54 tumors (59%) after initial RF session. There was a significant difference in necrosis success based on tumor size smaller or larger than 3 cm (69% vs. 39%).
Lee JM, Jin GY, Goldberg SN, Lee YC, Chung GH, Han YM, Lee SY, Kim CS	Percutaneous RFA for inoperable non-small cell lung cancer and metastases: Preliminary report	Radiology (January 2004); 230: 125–134	30 Patients 32 Tumors Primary lung = 27 Metastases = 5	All RFA	any ptx – 23% tx ptx – 7%	Not reported	CT	Complete necrosis was attained in 12 (38%) of 32 lesions; partial (>50%) necrosis in the remaining 20 (62%) lesions. Complete necrosis was attained in all 6 (100%) tumors smaller than 3 cm, but only in 6 (23%) of 26 larger tumors (P < 0.05). Mean survival of patients with complete necrosis (19.7 months) was significantly better than that of patients with partial necrosis (8.7 months) (P < 0.01).

(continued)

TABLE 36.1 (*Continued*)

Author	Title	Journal	Study Group	Ablation Strategy	PTX	Number of Ablations	F/U Assessment	Significant Findings
Suh RD, Wallace AB, Sheehan RE, Heinze SB, Goldin JG	Unresectable pulmonary malignancies: CT-guided percutaneous RFA – and preliminary results	Radiology (December 2003); 229: 821–829	12 Patients 19 Tumors Primary lung n = 9 Metastatic n = 10	All RFA	any ptx – 100% tx ptx – 20%	Not reported	CT	RFA was well tolerated by all patients. In the 8 patients with 3-month follow-up, lesion size increased in 2 and remained stable in 6. Mean contrast enhancement decreased from 46.8 HU (range, 19–107 HU) at baseline to 9.6 HU (range, 0–32 HU) at 1- to 2-month follow-up. In the 1 patient with 12-month CT densitometry follow-up, lesion enhancement was less than 50% of that at baseline, and lesion diameter remained stable.
Jain S, Dupuy DE, Cardarelli GE, Zheng Z, DiPetrillo T	Percutaneous RFA of pulmonary malignancies: Combined treatment with brachytherapy	AJR Am J Roentgenol (September 2003);181: 711–715	3 Patients 3 Tumors Primary lung n = 2 Metastasis n = 1	All RFA Plus brachytherapy	any ptx – 33% tx ptx – 0%	No additional tx's	CT	Percutaneous RFA in conjunction with brachytherapy is a promising minimally invasive combination modality. It may be a treatment option for patients with primary, recurrent, or metastatic malignancies of the lung that are not amenable to surgery or further external beam radiotherapy.
Herrera LJ, Fernando HC, Perry Y, Gooding WE, Buenaventura PO, Christie NA, Luketich JD	RFA of pulmonary malignant tumors in nonsurgical candidates	J Thorac Cardiovasc Surg (April 2003);125(4): 929–936	18 Patients (13 from a percutaneous approach) 33 Tumors Metastases n = 13 Primary lung n = 5	All RFA	any ptx – 53.8% tx ptx – 53.8%	2 patients underwent a second RFA	CT Response: complete (6%) partial (44%) stable (33%) progressed (17%)	RFA achieved a radiographically determined response (67%) in 8 of 12 patients with treated tumors smaller than 5 cm. The response was less robust for lesions larger than 5 cm (33.3%). This pilot study demonstrates the feasibility of RFA for small peripheral lung tumors.

Authors	Title	Citation	Tumors	Modality	Pneumothorax	Repeat	Imaging	Results
Nishida, T, Inoue K, Kawata Y, Izumi N, Nishiyama N, Kinoshita H, Matsuoka T, Toyoshima M	Percutaneous RFA of lung neoplasms: A minimally invasive strategy for inoperable patients	J Am Coll Surg (September 2002); 195(3): 426–430	6 Patients 8 Tumors Primary lung n = 2 Metastases n = 4	All RFA	Any ptx – 75% tx ptx – not reported	Not reported	CT	Safety and feasibility study. Five of 6 patients were alive at followup, ranging from 195 to 658 days. In 1 patient with 3 renal cell metastases: 1 lesion disappeared and 2 others did not grow. A biopsy of these 2 lesions at 9 months revealed fibrous tissue with no evidence of malignancy.
Dupuy DE, Zagoria RJ, Akerley W, Mayo-Smith WW, Kavanagh PV, Safran H	Percutaneous RFA of malignancies in the lung	AJR Am J Roentgenol (January 2000); 174(1): 57–59	3 Patients 3 Tumors Primary lung n = 2 Metastasis n = 1	All RFA	Any ptx – 33% tx ptx – 0%	1 repeat session in 1 patient	Not reported	RFA is a promising new minimally invasive technique for the treatment of solid malignancies. Unlike other percutaneous techniques, RFA can provide controlled regions of coagulation necrosis with a single application to an area as large as 3–5 cm depending on the blood flow in the treated tissue. RFA may result in reduced tumor burden when combined with external beam radiation or systemic chemotherapy.

Thoracic Wall Malignancy Study Group

Authors	Title	Citation	Tumors	Modality	Pneumothorax	Repeat	Imaging	Results
Grieco CA, Simon CJ, Mayo-Smith WW, DiPetrillo TA, Ready NE, Dupuy DE	Percutaneous thermoablation as a palliative treatment for chest wall masses	J Vasc Interv Radiol (2006); 17: S61 Abstract 168	52 Patients 58 Thoracic wall masses	RFA n = 51 MWA n = 5 Cryo n = 2	None	Not reported	CT	Improvement in pain symptoms occurred in 70.5%. There was no change in 18.2% and worsening of pain symptoms in 11.4%. None of the patients with more than 1 tumor showed improvement. Ablations done within 90 days of XRT yielded a 100% response, versus 57.7% in those who received XRT greater than 90 days prior to ablation. No comparisons could be made among thermal ablation strategies.

for the minority of patients with localized disease (i.e., no mediastinal invasion), but even 20% of these patients are not suitable candidates for potentially curative resection (65, 66). Given that the projected 5-year survival rate is 15% for all stages of NSCLC combined (63), optimizing the nonoperative treatments for these patients and all patients with cancer remains the most compelling application of image-guided thermal ablation.

Radiofrequency Ablation

Currently, there are two basic rationales for performing RFA for primary lung malignancies. The first is to use it with the intention of achieving definitive therapy in early-stage lung cancer patients who are not candidates for surgery because of comorbid medical conditions (Figure 36.2). This cohort could potentially derive significant benefit – even a cure – from

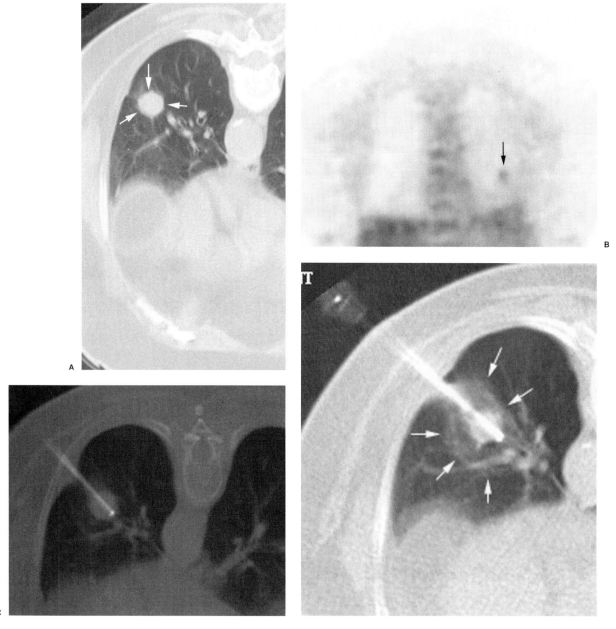

FIGURE 36.2. RFA for early-stage lung cancer. A 72-year-old woman with CAD and COPD who has a biopsy-proven 2-cm NSCLC in the right lower lobe (*arrows*). (A) Medical comorbidities deemed surgery a poor option. (B) Corresponding coronal FDG PET image shows mild uptake within the tumor (*arrow*) and no evidence of regional or distant disease. (C) CT-fluoroscopic image with the patient lying prone shows the optimal positioning of the RF electrode within the mass. (D) CT-fluoroscopic image after 10 minutes of RF energy application shows the corresponding thermal changes with the adjacent lung (*arrows*) referred to as the "halo sign."

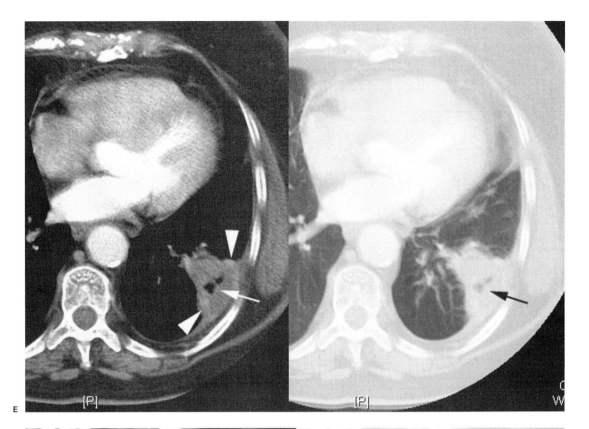

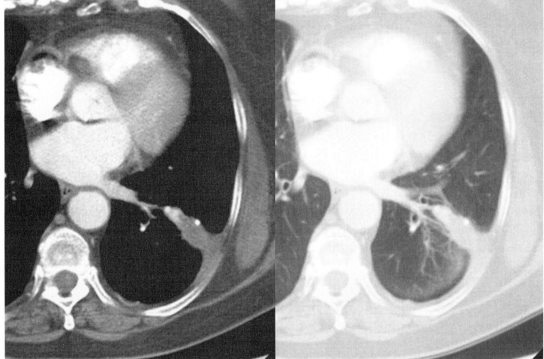

FIGURE 36.2.   (*Continued*) (E) Contrast-enhanced CT 1 month after RFA shows the large area of thermocoagulation with central bubble lucencies (*arrows*) and adjacent perilesional enhancement (*arrowhead*). (F) Contrast-enhanced CT 6 months after RFA shows contraction of the region of thermocoagulation into a wedge-shaped defect with resolution of enhancement and cavitation.

a minimally invasive alternative therapy. The second rationale is to use it as a palliative measure to achieve tumor reduction before chemotherapy; palliate local symptoms related to aggressive tumor growth, chest wall pain or dyspnea; palliate painful bony metastatic disease; or as salvage therapy for disease recurrence in patients who are not suitable candidates for repeat radiotherapy or surgery.

Given that surgical data show a greater than two-fold increase in locoregional recurrence rate with regard to limited resections (67–70), pulmonary RFA alone for the treatment of early-stage primary lung cancer has not been validated. The purported reasons for recurrence in anything less than a lobectomy include inadequate resection of the primary tumor and presence of microscopic lymphatic disease within the ipsilateral hilar nodes. However, for stage IA NSCLC less than 2 cm, several studies comparing limited resection (segmentectomy) and lymph node (LN) assessment versus lobectomy have shown equivalent 5-year survival rates (87.1% vs. 93%) and local recurrence (71–77). These recent studies and the RFA study by Lee et al. (58) led us to speculate that for tumors less than 2 cm in size, RFA might provide an alternative for local disease control. RFA of these lesions could be inexpensive outpatient procedures, unlike much more costly and painful thoracotomies. Therefore, a comparison of the two treatments in this select group of early-stage lung cancer patients seems reasonable. Unfortunately, detection of microscopic lymphatic disease is not possible by the current imaging methods, and RF technology does not allow the treatment regimen to extend extensively into the normal lung parenchyma. However, until either such detection methods becomes available or RFA, is proven to effectively ablate regions that include such disease, RFA can continue to be a highly effective treatment for patients who are not candidates for surgery because they have co-morbid conditions, poor cardiopulmonary reserve or prior radiation therapy (RT) with recurrence in the treatment field.

Even with current technology, survival benefits can be realized with RFA, and ablation success appears to be related to the size of the target lesion. Fernando (47) demonstrated the feasibility of RFA for small, peripheral NSCLC tumors, finding that local control was comparable to, if not better than, that provided by RT, especially when one considers their study included higher-stage patients than the

historical XRT data they cited. Overall mean survival in 18 patients (of all stages) was 20 months, median survival not reached. Disease progression was seen in only eight nodules (38%) in six patients (33%). The mean progression-free interval was 17.6 months for stage I cancers; a median progression-free interval could not be calculated. The mean progression-free interval for stage I versus other stages was 17.6 months versus 15 months (NS). Another success with small, early stage NSCLC was reported in a 2004 study of 32 patients with malignant lung cancers (27 NSCLC) treated with CT-guided RFA (58). Tumors less than 3 cm had higher complete necrosis, rates than larger tumors (100% vs. 8%). Mean survival in patients with complete necrosis was higher than in those with partial necrosis (19.7 vs. 8.7 months). Size also mattered in a study of 40 primary lung cancers with a mean follow-up of 2 years (45). There were 62% complete responses and higher response rates for lesions less than 3 cm (70%). Belfiore confirmed the size/response observations with histopathological data (52). In this primary lung cancer study, Belfiore performed 6-month biopsies in 19 of the 33 study group patients. Seven patients (36%), most of whom had tumors smaller than 3 cm, had complete necrosis, and of the 12 with viable tumor at biopsy, all had tumors larger than 3 cm. In the largest single-center analysis of 80 patients with stage I NSCLC, Dupuy et al. (50) estimated a 29-month median survival for all stage 1 patients. The 1-, 2- and 3-year survival rates were 78.3%, 56.5% and 36.4%. These stage 1 NSCLC patients were then further subdivided according to the diameter of index tumor ablated: 74.7% (56/75) stage 1A patients with tumors less than 3 cm and 25.3% (19/75) stage 1B patients with tumors greater than 3 cm in greatest diameter or involvement of the visceral pleura. The estimated median survival for stage 1A patients was 30 months (95% CI; 22–38 months). The estimated median survival for stage 1B patients was 25 months (95% CI; 14–36 months). Survival differences between stage 1A and 1B patients were not statistically different (p = 0.58). Tumor size greater than 3 cm did predict recurrence (p = 0.04) but the 162 tumors used for this analysis included metastatic lesions and were not limited to NSCLC.

In keeping with the observations discussed earlier, it is valuable to consider other selected studies of RFA, even though they include a heterogeneous cohort of lung cancer patients that includes both those with primary and with metastatic lung cancer. Gadaleta et al. (53) treated a mixed cohort of 69 primary and metastatic lung cancer patients with percutaneous CT-guided RFA, achieving a complete tumor necrosis response rate in 92% after a median follow-up period of 9 months. In a similar cohort of patients, Yasui et al. (37) percutaneously ablated 99 malignant thoracic tumors (mean diameter 2 cm) with a reported probable complete coagulation necrosis rate of 91% over a mean follow-up period of 7 months. Akeboshi et al. (42) percutaneously ablated 54 mixed primary and secondary lung neoplasms (mean diameter 2.7 cm) and obtained a 59% complete tumor necrosis rate after the initial RFA. All of these investigators concluded that a significant difference in the complete tumor necrosis rate existed between tumors less than 3 cm and tumors greater than 3 cm in diameter (69% vs. 39%; $p < 0.05$). PET scanning of ablated lung tumors has shown lesions less than 3.5 cm to dissipate 1 to 2 weeks after RFA, but not in areas outside of this 3.5-cm region in larger tumors (49), suggesting that RFA may be inadequate for treating tumors greater than 3.5 cm in greatest diameter.

Given the potential limitations of RFA for treating larger lesions and those with unfavorable locations within or near the mediastinum and in the lung apex, RFA can also be used in conjunction with other treatments (Figure 36.3). At our institution, we completed a Phase II trial comparing the combination therapy of up-front RFA followed by conventional radiation therapy (dose of 66 Gy) (46). Although we did not directly compare RFA with RT versus RFA alone, our survival data at 6 months (97.6%), 1 year (86.8%), 2 years (70.4%) and 3 years (57.1%) compared favorably with both historical controls for RT (78) and similar cohorts (79–81) and studies of RFA alone (58), especially considering that our patients, even with tumors greater than 3 cm, had an average survival time of 34.6 ± 7 months. An important contrast with previous reports is that we did not observe a significant difference in survival based on tumor size greater than 3 cm. This suggests that RT may improve the efficacy of RFA for larger tumors.

Other ongoing studies are combining RFA with brachytherapy in patients with either metastatic lung malignancies or prior treatment that precludes additional external beam RT (33, 48, 56). The rationale is to enhance local control by magnifying the cytoreductive and radiation effect by destroying the central hypoxic area of the target tumor. CT can be used for brachytherapy catheter placement (after the RFA has been performed), and the entire treatment can be accomplished in 1 day. That said, tumors that tend to be more encapsulated and have a sharp lung/tumor interface (e.g., well-differentiated squamous cell carcinoma) may have a natural history more suitable for local therapy alone.

Microwave Ablation

Published experience with MWA for the treatment of primary lung cancer is limited. However, at our institution, we have performed several successful percutaneous lung MWA procedures (Figure 36.4) (3, 48). The largest published series (82) reported their experience with MWA of 16 thoracic tumors, 9 of which were NSCLC. On CT, all tumors had area reductions after treatment, and no enhancement was seen in 9 of 16. As a surrogate for assessing postablation tumor viability, color Doppler sonography was used to assess intra-tumoral blood flow. Ten tumors that were visible before treatment were invisible afterward; the other six were only less visible. Tumors ranged between 3 and 6 cm in diameter; comparisons were not made based on tumor size or volume. The mean follow-up period was 20 months; seven patients were alive.

Cryoablation

The use of cryoablation during rigid bronchoscopy in the treatment of endobronchial neoplasms has been extensively reported (35–25). It was only recently, however, in a landmark report by Wang et al., that the technique, feasibility, and safety of the procedure for thoracic malignancy were reported (14). In their experience with 217 percutaneous cryotherapy sessions in 187 patients (89% had advanced-stage cancer for which prior treatment had failed), ice coverage for peripheral lesions less than 4 cm was complete and was 80% for lesions greater than 4 cm. Tumor size and location were highly predictive of tumor ice coverage even when controlled for tumor stage and type. By 6 months, 86% of the CT scans available showed tumors stable or smaller than the original tumor. A short follow-up period precluded any accurate survival estimates, but palliative benefits of cryoablation were noted in terms of the Karnofsky Performance Status scale and general health status (e.g., increased dietary intake and weight

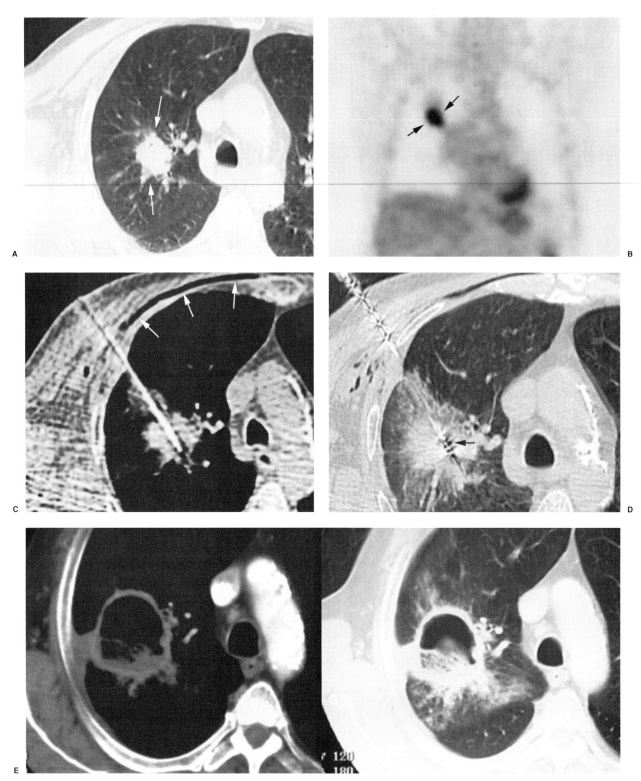

FIGURE 36.3. Combined radiofrequency ablation/brachytherapy with microwave ablation salvage. A 75-year-old man with severe COPD and CAD with biopsy-proven 3-cm right upper lobe adenocarcinoma (*arrows*). The patient was deemed a poor surgical candidate. (A) Based upon the size, RFA followed by high dose rate brachytherapy was planned. (B) Coronal PET image shows the intense FDG accumulation (*arrows*) without evidence of metastatic disease. (C) CT-fluoroscopy image during RFA shows the electrode in the mass and associated extra-pleural air (*arrows*) consistent with an air leak. (D) CT image after placement of brachytherapy catheter with internal "dummy" seeds (*arrow*) used to generate three-dimensional dosimetry for the iridium wire placement. (E) Contrast-enhanced CT images on soft-tissue (*left*) and lung windows (*right*) 2 months after RFA/brachytherapy shows the appearance of a large cavity with internal debris and surrounding parenchymal air-space disease.

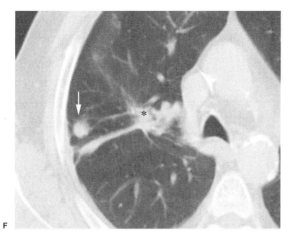

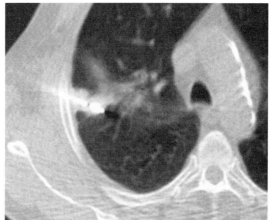

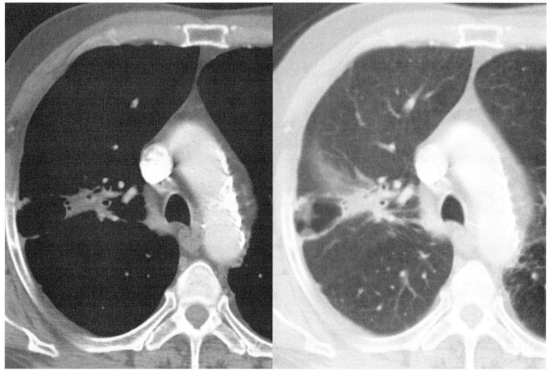

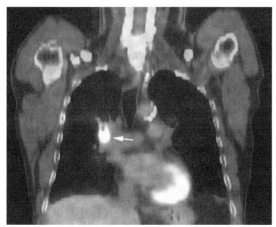

FIGURE 36.3. (*Continued*) (F) Follow-up CT image 24 months after initial RFA shows the growth of a new tumor nodule (*arrow*) separate from the previous treatment. Note resolution of cavity (*). (G) CT scan of MW applicator placed within the new tumor nodule. (H) Contrast-enhanced CT images on soft-tissue (*left*) and lung windows (*right*) 24 months after RFA/brachytherapy and 1 month after MWA shows the appearance of a new cavity with internal debris at the site of MWA. Note lack of solid enhancing tumor. (I) Coronal FDG PET/CT fused image at 27 months S/P RFA/brachytherapy and 3 months S/P MWA shows a new right hilar lymph node with intense metabolic activity (*arrows*) consistent with tumor.

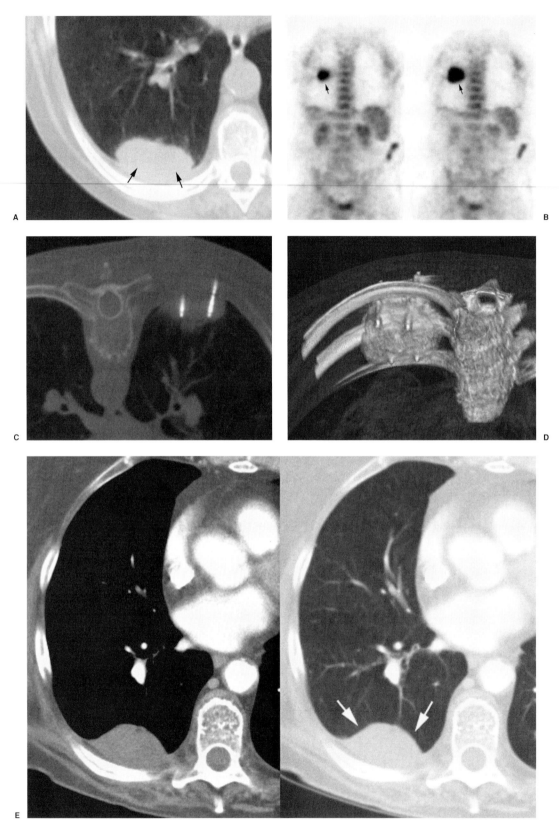

FIGURE 36.4. Microwave ablation of primary lung cancer. An 83-year-old woman with a large squamous cell carcinoma in the right lower lobe with probable extension into the pleura (*arrows*). (A) Underlying COPD, age, and baseline dementia deemed the patient a poor risk for surgical treatment. (B) Coronal FDG PET images show intense metabolic activity within the mass (*arrows*), but no regional or distant disease. (C) CT-fluoroscopic image shows two MW applicators spaced 2 cm apart centered within the mass. (D) Three-dimensional shaded surface display reconstruction image shows the placement of the four MW applicators within the mass. (E) Contrast-enhanced CT images on soft-tissue (*left*) and lung windows (*right*) 6 months after MWA shows lack of enhancement, tumor shrinkage and a sharp interface with the normal lung (*arrows*). Note lack of chest wall extension.

gain). Technological advances however, may already make the coverage rate data for larger lesions historical.

METASTATIC LUNG CANCER

In a report of the International Registry of Lung Metastasis (83), based on 5206 cases, the distribution of major primary malignancies was as follows: soft-tissue sarcoma, 751; osteosarcoma, 734; colorectal cancer, 645; breast cancer, 396; renal cancer, 372; melanoma, 282; and head and neck, 247. Although pulmonary metastatic disease tends to be an indicator of widespread disease, in certain tumors and certain patients, pulmonary metastatic disease may exist in isolation. In these patients, who have a finite number of metastatic deposits in the lung, and in a tumor with favorable biological characteristics (e.g., soft tissue sarcoma, renal cell carcinoma, colorectal carcinoma and pulmonary carcinoma), resection is considered a viable treatment option (84–89) that improves prognosis, depending on the nodule size, completeness of resection and LN status. In colorectal metastases, for example, studies have shown overall 5-year and 10-year survival rates to increase from 22% to 62% and 42% to 47% and a 3-year survival benefit after resection of pulmonary metastases (85, 86). Indications for surgical treatment include exclusion of other distant disease, no tumor at the primary site, probability of complete resection, and adequate cardiopulmonary reserve to withstand the procedure. Surgical treatment of metastatic lung cancer remains controversial given the lack of randomized, controlled clinical trials comparing surgery with non-surgical treatments, but its use is becoming more widely accepted because of studies showing better long-term survival (83, 90). Pulmonary metastasectomy for isolated pulmonary metastases of different tumor types results in an overall 5-year survival rate of approximately 36% (83) and is associated with a mortality rate of less than 2% (91). Five-year survival rates range as follows for pulmonary metastasectomy: osteogenic sarcoma, 20% to 50% (92); soft-tissue sarcoma, 18% to 28% (93, 94); head and neck carcinoma, 40.9% to 47% (95); colon carcinoma, 21% to 48% (86, 96–105), breast carcinoma, 31% to 49.5% (106–109); and renal cell carcinoma, 20% to 44% (87, 110–112). Repeat resection is supported (90) in select patients who are free of disease at the primary location but have recurrent metastatic disease of the lung.

Because of their natural history, patients with metastatic deposits from renal cell carcinoma, sarcoma (Figure 36.5) and colorectal carcinoma seem to be the types who will benefit from thermal ablation strategies (reviewed in 113). This is important as, at least historically before the incidental detection of smaller tumors by multi-detector CT, a significant percentage of patients with renal cell carcinoma have pulmonary metastases (89, 114). Furthermore, nearly 10% of colorectal cancer patients will have pulmonary metastases at autopsy (100). For patient populations at high risk of morbidity secondary to a potential thoracotomy or for those who refuse surgery, the only treatment alternatives have been systemic chemotherapy or local therapy with external beam radiation. Unfortunately, many secondary tumors are not sensitive to radiation or comprise a large radiation field, thus requiring alternative treatments to improve survival or provide palliation. However, thermal ablation may be applied both to these patients and to certain patients in whom a small number of slowly growing metastases are identified. Patients who have volunteered for thermal ablation with or without adjuvant therapy are not typically in as robust health as surgical candidates, but their survival outcomes compare favorably and even surpass those in surgical cohorts (50, 60, 62, 115).

The exact size and number of lesions appropriate for thermal ablation therapies has yet to be defined, but it is not unreasonable to use parameters similar to those applied for RFA of liver tumors (i.e., four or fewer metastases). The maximum size for effective treatment has not been established, but Kang et al. (49) found lack of heat dissipation to tumor cells outside of a 3.5-cm diameter providing further evidence that lesions fewer than 3 cm in size (as in the liver) are optimal candidates given the treatment regions achievable with current thermal ablation technology. These data are supported clinically by the recent report by Yan et al. (62) in which 70% of patients with lesions greater than 3 cm in size died within 14 months of treatment, whereas the median survival of the entire cohort was 33 months. Histologic evidence of complete lethal thermal injury in pulmonary metastases has been shown (116). However, and similar to the findings of Belfiore with primary lung cancer, Yasui found in his study of pulmonary metastases that residual tumor cells were noted in 13 (40%) of 33 specimens (37). Yan et al. (62, 117) report the following exclusion

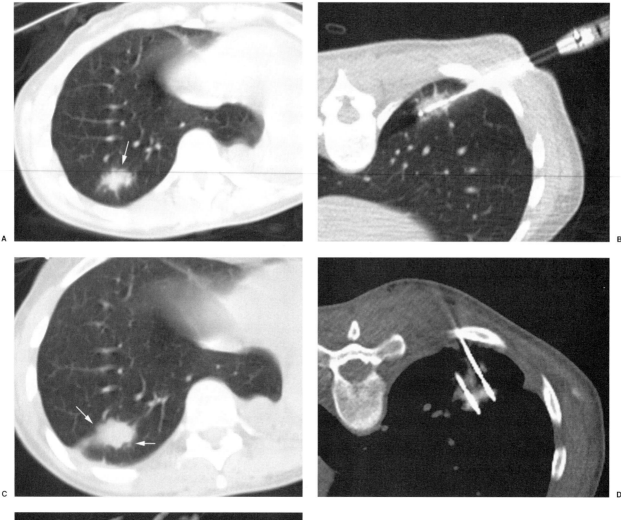

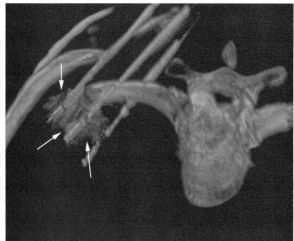

FIGURE 36.5. Radiofrequency ablation for metastatic sarcoma. A 43-year-old woman with a history of previous left pneumonectomy for metastatic leiomyosarcoma of the uterus presents with new metastasis in the right lower lobe (*arrow*). (A) RFA was felt to be the best option because of previous pneumonectomy and the patient's unwillingness for repeat surgery. (B) CT fluoroscopic image shows a cluster RF electrode well positioned within the metastasis. (C) Follow-up CT scan 10 months after the initial RFA shows some interval growth of the metastasis (*arrows*). PET scan confirmed residual metabolic activity consistent with tumor. (D) CT fluoroscopic image shows two of the three MW applicators positioned within the lesion. (E) Three-dimensional shaded surface display of tumor (*arrows*) including the ribs and vertebral body shows the three MW applicators in satisfactory position.

criteria for their metastatic colorectal group: 1) more than six lesions per hemithorax; 2) diameter of metastases greater than 5 cm; 3) international normalized ratio (INR) greater than 1.5 and platelets less than 100 × 10^9 g/L; 4) extra-pulmonary systemic metastases. This same group has also reported that there is a real learning curve for the procedure, as experience significantly reduces the incidence of overall morbidity,

pneumothorax and chest drain requirement. Furthermore, the distribution of lung metastases (unilateral vs. bilateral) is an independent risk factor for overall morbidity and pneumothorax (117).

Radiofrequency Ablation

Although most studies of RFA for metastatic pulmonary disease have inadequate sample sizes for subset analyses of specific tumor types, some treatment centers have begun to examine data for metastatic colorectal cancer. In 2004, a group from the University of New South Wales reported their follow-up on RFA for 23 patients with 53 colorectal cancer metastases (57). After 1 year, CT findings showed that 40 lesions were classified as disappeared (n = 17), decreased (n = 5), same size (n = 4), or increased (n = 14). The group judged RFA to provide safe and successful (but not terrific) local control. More recently, this same group (62) has reported more follow-up and predictors for survival in their cohort of 55 patients with colorectal pulmonary metastases. After a univariate analysis found largest size of lung metastasis, location of lung metastasis (hilar or non-hilar) and need for repeat RFA to predict survival, only size (>3 cm) of lung metastasis remained predictive in the multivariate model (HR = 4.456; p = 0.003). Overall median survival was 33 months, with 1-, 2- and 3-year actuarial survival rates of 85%, 64% and 46%, respectively. Interestingly, this survival was achieved even though 55% of the patients had undergone a prior hepatectomy for liver metastases. Furthermore, and unlike pulmonary metastasectomy study groups, patients with bilateral pulmonary metastases had similar survival to those with unilateral pulmonary metastases. Our own data suggest a survival benefit in a cohort of 18 patients with colorectal cancer metastases to the lungs (50), with 1-, 2- and 5-year survival rates of 87%, 78% and 57% respectively. In our study and others, including those from the University of New South Wales, the sole effect of RFA cannot be reliably estimated because it would be unethical to withhold systemic therapy in patients with colorectal cancer. It must also be considered that a synergistic effect of chemotherapy plus RFA is playing a role similar to that in colorectal liver metastases, where the addition of RFA to chemotherapy may double survival time (118).

Cryoablation

At the time of this writing, the only study of CA in patients with pulmonary metastases is a report by Kawamura and colleagues, who recently performed CA on 35 tumors in 20 patients (115). The primary tumors were colorectal (30%), lung cancer (25%), liver cancer (10%), soft-tissue sarcomas (10%), head and neck cancer (10%), uterine cancer (10%) and renal cancer (5%) The mean hospital stay was 2.6 days. There was local recurrence of seven tumors in seven patients (20%), and the 1-year survival rate was 89.4%.

Microwave Ablation

No meaningful data are available.

PALLIATION

The cytoreductive effect of RFA may be used in symptom palliation. Patients with an inoperable lung cancer and tumor size too large for radical radiotherapy have a poor prognosis, with limited therapeutic options. Symptom palliation is therefore an important part of the management of a cancer patient, yet the current medical literature reflects our failure to accomplish this (119), as 50% of patients die without adequate pain relief (71).

Conventional treatment of osseous metastatic disease involves RT and chemotherapy. RT has been shown to palliate respiratory symptoms and improve quality of life in NSCLC patients (120), yet extension of tumor into the chest wall and osseous metastatic disease can be difficult to treat this way because previous treatment fields may have encompassed the symptomatic region. Therefore, current treatment is often ineffective in patients with complex disease. Newer alternatives such as percutaneous ethanol injection, embolization of bone tumor vasculature and RFA may be viable salvage therapies because they provide, at minimum, palliative relief to patients for whom conventional treatment fails.

Most lung cancer patients die from their disease, and the most common clinical symptoms are cough, dyspnea, hemoptysis and pain (121). Three main causes of malignancy-related pain in lung cancer are osseous metastatic disease (34%), Pancoast tumor (31%) and chest wall disease (21%) (122).

For palliation of symptoms related to a focal lesion, the ablation size or coverage is less important; larger tumors with chest wall and osseous involvement can be treated with attention given to the tumor/bone interface. Current studies confirm the palliative results of RFA in musculoskeletal, gastrointestinal, pulmonary and neurologic-associated lesions, presumably via cytoreduction, destruction of adjacent sensory neural fibers and decreased neural stimulation secondary to debulking (123–128). The resultant improved quality of life illustrates the dynamic use of this procedure, but more controlled studies need to be done.

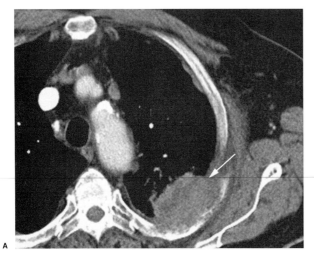

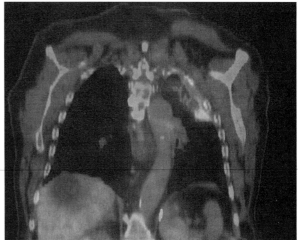

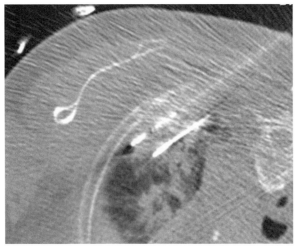

FIGURE 36.6. MWA for chest wall mass. A 74-year-old man with a large NSCLC eroding into the chest wall (*arrows*) underwent chemoradiation. **(A)** Coronal FDG PET/CT fused image 6 months after completion of chemoradiation shows persistent FDG accumulation within the mass. **(B)** Image-guided ablation was requested for additional therapy. **(C)** CT-fluoroscopic image shows two MW applicators positioned within the region of most intense FDG uptake.

Pain relief was reported by all 11 patients (complete 36%, partial 64%) who were symptomatic in one study (8). In a more objective study of 15 patients with chest pain, 5 patients (33%) and 4 patients (27%) enjoyed complete and partial pain relief. Pain scores reduced from 1.73 to 1.38 on a scale of 1 to 4 (52). The same authors reported that cough and dyspnea scores also improved: 1.45 to 1.17 and 1.48 to 1.14, respectively. Lee et al. (58) demonstrated that RF ablation offered relief in 80% of patients with mild hemoptysis, but less-than-ideal relief of chest pain, dyspnea and coughing. RFA has provided a substantial decrease in pain from skeletal metastasis from primary tumors other than lung, subsequently improving quality of life (126, 129). Although their analysis was performed only 1 week after CA, Wang et al. (14) calculated the palliative benefits of CA in a sub-group of 143 patients with advanced-stage cancer. The mean Karnofsky Performance Score increased from 75.2 to 82.6 (p < 0.01).

In the only study of its kind, Grieco and colleagues (54) administered palliative thermal ablation specifically to painful tumors of the chest wall; 52 patients with 58 tumors were treated (Figures 36.6 and 36.7). All three thermal ablation strategies were used: RFA, n = 50; MWA, n = 5; and CA, n = 3. Follow-up data were available for 44 procedures: 70.5% reported improvement in pain, 18.2% reported no change and 11.4% had progression. Among those reporting an improvement, the benefit was maintained in 100% at 1 month, 95.8% at 3 months, 73.9% at 6 months, and 64.3% at 1 year. Interestingly, RT done within 90 days before RFA yielded a 100% response, whereas only 57.7% reported improvement if RT was done more than 90 days before ablation.

It is important to note that pleural-based masses can be quite painful during RF heating. Given the somatic innervation of the parietal pleura via the intercostal and phrenic nerves, irritation may result in pain felt either on the body wall or in the

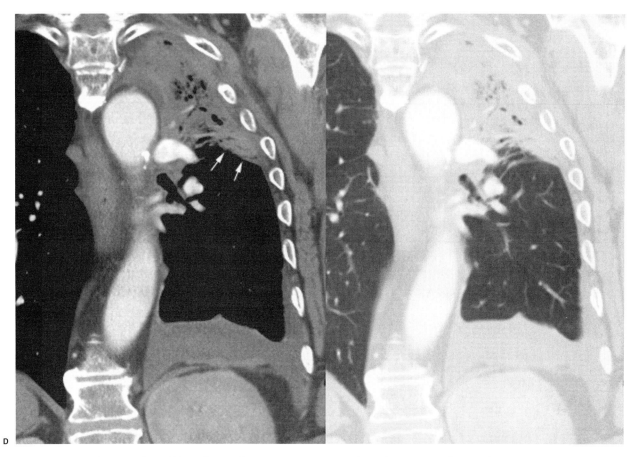

D

FIGURE 36.6. (*Continued*) (D) Coronal contrast-enhanced CT reformations on soft-tissue (*left*) and lung windows (*right*) 1 month after MWA show a large area of parenchymal opacity without enhancing tumor in the area of concern (*arrows*).

corresponding dermatomes, for which multiple doses of sedation during the procedure may be needed.

CONCLUSIONS

Since the first reported use of thermal ablation for lung cancer in 2000, there has been an explosive use of the procedure, and by 2010, the number of procedures to treat thoracic malignancy is expected to exceed 150,000 per year. Presently, thermal ablation is best used for patients with early-stage lung cancers who are not surgical candidates, patients with small and favorably located pulmonary metastases, and patients in whom palliation of tumor-related symptoms is the goal. Because percutaneous thermal ablation is repeatable and may have synergistic effects when combined with other cancer treatments, thermal ablation may, in fact, answer a call for the larger group of about 140,000 inoperable patients diagnosed each year with primary lung cancer and a similarly astounding number of patients with secondary pulmonary cancers. Without this treatment, patients face limited therapeutic options (chemotherapy and radiation) and, in the case of lung cancer, a 5-year survival rate of 15%.

Investigators must now organize and focus single- and multi-institutional efforts to address specific questions in specific, well-matched study groups. In so doing, we must develop specific methods for reporting our data, including tumor size, cell type, morphology and location; the type of probe and ablation strategy performed for each lesion; the size of the ablation field; concurrent or antecedent therapies; adequate follow-up and accurate disease-free reporting for both primary and metastatic lung cancer; new criteria to best determine the histological success of ablation and determine recurrence (ablation failure); and indices to quantify improvement in pain, cough, hemoptysis and respiratory performance. Furthermore, we need to further define the role of RFA, MWA, and CA in the laboratory and in patients; we simply do not know which thermal ablation technique is best.

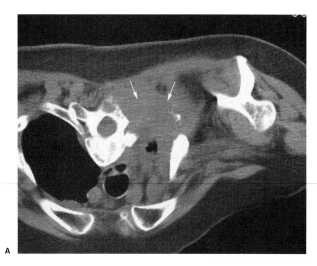

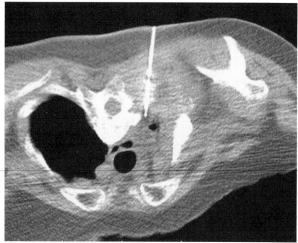

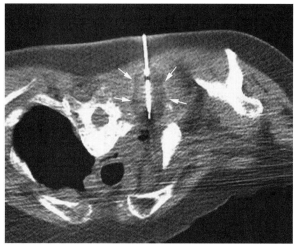

FIGURE 36.7. Cryoablation for a painful primary lung cancer. Prone CT image of a 75-year-old woman with a recurrent Pancoast tumor in the left lung S/P external beam radiotherapy with associated pain from brachial plexus involvement. (A) Cryoablation was planned because of involvement of the brachial plexus. (B) CT image of a single cryoprobe positioned along the interface of destroyed costovertebral junction. (C) CT-image of a second placement of cryoprobe into the more central mass. Note visibility of low-density iceball (*arrows*).

At the same time, we must continue to develop the technology and provide solutions where it has limitations. To enhance our ability to obtain reliable margins and complete necrosis we need to optimize ablation monitoring with imaging and employ adjunctive therapies, including external radiation and, perhaps in combination, radiation-inducible, gene-therapy vectors such as TNFerade (130) or other radiotherapy-sensitizing gene-targeting strategies like TNF-related apoptosis-inducing ligand (TRAIL) (131). We must continue to develop separation techniques that will allow us to provide adequate thermal ablation without injuring critical structures in the mediastinum or lung apex. Finally, we must work with our engineering colleagues to develop systems that provide for larger and faster ablations with multiple applicators, favorable and perhaps customized probe geometry and more powerful devices.

While we wait for 5-year data from the studies discussed earlier and the recruitment of patients in newly opened trials, we must become more integrated in the management of these patients. We should participate in tumor boards and develop close relationships with the patients and the cancer specialists who have traditionally called on thermal ablation as a last resort. Only through education and research can we enable this technology to help patients in a timely manner and more successfully lobby insurers to cover this cost-effective procedure that improves the quality of life for patients.

Thermal tumor ablation is a young, exciting science. Now that the safety and efficacy of these procedures have been validated, carefully designed multi-institutional studies and advances in engineering and biological technologies will allow us to successfully treat and replace surgical treatments for lung cancer and pulmonary metastatic disease.

REFERENCES

1. Nahum Goldberg S and Dupuy DE. Image-guided radiofrequency tumor ablation: Challenges and opportunities Part I. J Vasc Interv Radiol, 2001; 12(9): 1021–1032.

2. Dupuy DE, Goldberg SN. Image-guided radiofrequency tumor ablation: Challenges and opportunities Part II. J Vasc Interv Radiol, 2001; 12(10): 1135–1148.

3. Simon CJ, Dupuy DE, Mayo-Smith WW. Microwave ablation: Principles and applications. Radiographics, 2005; 25(Suppl 1): S69–83.

4. Yu NC, Lu DS, Raman SS, et al. Hepatocellular carcinoma: Microwave ablation with multiple straight and loop antenna clusters – pilot comparison with pathologic findings. Radiology, 2006; 239(1): 269–275.

5. Organ LW. Electrophysiologic principles of radiofrequency lesion making. Appl Neurophysiol, 1976; 39(2): 69–76.

6. Skinner MG, Iizuka MN, Kolios MC, et al. A theoretical comparison of energy sources – microwave, ultrasound and laser – for interstitial thermal therapy. Phys Med Biol 1998; 43(12): 3535–3547.

7. Goldberg SN, Gazelle GS, Solbiati L, et al. Radiofrequency tissue ablation: Increased lesion diameter with a perfusion electrode. Acad Radiol, 1996; 3(8): 636–644.

8. VanSonnenberg E, Shankar S, Morrison PR, et al. Radiofrequency ablation of thoracic lesions: Part 2, initial clinical experience – technical and multidisciplinary considerations in 30 patients. AJR Am J Roentgenol, 2005; 184(2): 381–390.

9. Goldberg SN, Solbiati L, Hahn PF, et al. Large-volume tissue ablation with radio frequency by using a clustered, internally cooled electrode technique: Laboratory and clinical experience in liver metastases. Radiology, 1998; 209(2): 371–379.

10. Ahmed M, Liu Z, Afzal KS, et al. Radiofrequency ablation: Effect of surrounding tissue composition on coagulation necrosis in a canine tumor model. Radiology, 2004; 230(3): 761–767.

11. Lu MD, Chen JW, Xie XY, et al. Hepatocellular carcinoma: US-guided percutaneous microwave coagulation therapy. Radiology, 2001; 221(1): 167 –172.

12. Seki T, Tamai T, Nakagawa T, et al. Combination therapy with transcatheter arterial chemoembolization and percutaneous microwave coagulation therapy for hepatocellular carcinoma. Cancer, 2000; 89(6): 1245–1251.

13. Shibata T, Iimuro Y, Yamamoto Y, et al. Small hepatocellular carcinoma: Comparison of radio-frequency ablation and percutaneous microwave coagulation therapy. Radiology, 2002; 223(2): 331–337.

14. Wang H, Littrup PJ, Duan Y, et al. Thoracic masses treated with percutaneous cryotherapy: Initial experience with more than 200 procedures. Radiology, 2005; 235(1): 289–298.

15. Hiraki T, Yasui K, Mimura H, et al. Radiofrequency ablation of metastatic mediastinal lymph nodes during cooling and temperature monitoring of the tracheal mucosa to prevent thermal tracheal damage: Initial experience. Radiology, 2005; 237(3): 1068–1074.

16. Rose SC, Fotoohi M, Levin DL, et al. Cerebral microembolization during radiofrequency ablation of lung malignancies. J Vasc Interv Radiol, 2002; 13(10): 1051–1054.

17. Yamamoto A, Matsuoka T, Toyoshima M, et al. Assessment of cerebral microembolism during percutaneous radiofrequency ablation of lung tumors using diffusion-weighted imaging. AJR Am J Roentgenol, 2004; 183(6): 1785–1789.

18. Jin GY, Lee JM, Lee YC, et al. Acute cerebral infarction after radiofrequency ablation of an atypical carcinoid pulmonary tumor. AJR Am J Roentgenol, 2004; 182(4): 990–992.

19. Ahrar K, Stafford RJ, Tinkey PT, et al. Evaluation of cerebral microemboli during radiofrequency ablation of lung tumors in a canine model. J Vasc Interv Radiol, 2006; 17: S63.

20. Shock SA, Meredith K, Warner TF, et al. Microwave ablation with loop antenna: In vivo porcine liver model. Radiology, 2004; 231(1): 143–149.

21. Stauffer PR, Rossetto F, Prakash M, et al. Phantom and animal tissues for modelling the electrical properties of human liver. Int J Hyperthermia, 2003; 19(1): 89–101.

22. Wright AS, Lee FT Jr, and Mahvi DM. Hepatic microwave ablation with multiple antennae results in synergistically larger zones of coagulation necrosis. Ann Surg Oncol, 2003; 10(3): 275–283.

23. Maiwand MO. The role of cryosurgery in palliation of tracheo-bronchial carcinoma. Eur J Cardiothorac Surg, 1999; 15(6): 764–768.

24. Maiwand MO and Homasson JP. Cryotherapy for tracheobronchial disorders. Clin Chest Med, 1995; 16(3): 427–443.

25. Sanderson DR, Neel HB 3rd, Fontana RS. Bronchoscopic cryotherapy. Ann Otol Rhinol Laryngol, 1981; 90(4 Pt 1): 354–358.

26. Lee FT Jr, Chosy SG, Littrup PJ, et al. CT-monitored percutaneous cryoablation in a pig liver model: Pilot study. Radiology, 1999; 211(3): 687–692.

27. Mala T, Edwin B, Samset E, et al. Magnetic-resonance-guided percutaneous cryoablation of hepatic tumours. Eur J Surg, 2001; 167(8): 610–617.

28. Silverman SG, Tuncali K, Adams DF, et al. MR imaging-guided percutaneous cryotherapy of liver tumors: Initial experience. Radiology, 2000; 217(3): 657–664.

29. Shingleton WB and Sewell PE Jr. Percutaneous renal cryoablation of renal tumors in patients with von Hippel-Lindau disease. J Urol, 2002; 167(3): 1268–1270.

30. Beland MD, Dupuy DE and Mayo-Smith WW. Percutaneous cryoablation of symptomatic extraabdominal metastatic disease: Preliminary results. AJR Am J Roentgenol, 2005; 184(3): 926–930.

31. Bilchik AJ, Wood TF, Allegra D, et al. Cryosurgical ablation and radiofrequency ablation for unresectable hepatic malignant neoplasms: A proposed algorithm. Arch Surg, 2000; 135(6): 657–662; discussion 62–64.

32. Gadaleta C, Mattioli V, Colucci G, et al. Radiofrequency ablation of 40 lung neoplasms: Preliminary results. AJR Am J Roentgenol, 2004; 183(2): 361–368.

33. Bojarski JD, Dupuy DE, and Mayo-Smith WW. CT imaging findings of pulmonary neoplasms after treatment with radiofrequency ablation: Results in 32 tumors. AJR Am J Roentgenol, 2005; 185(2): 466–471.

34. Goldberg SN, Gazelle GS, Compton CC, et al. Radiofrequency tissue ablation in the rabbit lung: Efficacy and complications. Acad Radiol, 1995; 2(9): 776–784.

35. de Baere T, Palussiere J, Auperin A, et al. Midterm local efficacy and survival after radiofrequency ablation of lung tumors with minimum follow-up of 1 year: Prospective evaluation. Radiology, 2006; 240(2): 587–596.

36. Steinke K, King J, Glenn D, et al. Radiologic appearance and complications of percutaneous computed tomography-guided radiofrequency-ablated pulmonary metastases from colorectal carcinoma. J Comput Assist Tomogr, 2003; 27(5): 750–757.

37. Yasui K, Kanazawa S, Sano Y, et al. Thoracic tumors treated with CT-guided radiofrequency ablation: Initial experience. Radiology 2004; 231(3): 850–857.

38. Jin GY, Lee JM, Lee YC, et al. Primary and secondary lung malignancies treated with percutaneous radiofrequency ablation: Evaluation with follow-up helical CT. AJR Am J Roentgenol, 2004; 183(4): 1013–1020.

39. Swensen SJ, Viggiano RW, Midthun DE, et al. Lung nodule enhancement at CT: Multicenter study. Radiology, 2000; 214(1): 73–80.

40. Berber E, Foroutani A, Garland AM, et al. Use of CT Hounsfield unit density to identify ablated tumor after laparoscopic radiofrequency ablation of hepatic tumors. Surg Endosc, 2000; 14(9): 799–804.

41. Suh RD, Wallace AB, Sheehan RE, et al. Unresectable pulmonary malignancies: CT-guided percutaneous radiofrequency ablation – preliminary results. Radiology, 2003; 229(3): 821–829.

42. Akeboshi M, Yamakado K, Nakatsuka A, et al. Percutaneous radiofrequency ablation of lung neoplasms: Initial therapeutic response. J Vasc Interv Radiol, 2004; 15(5): 463–470.

43. Akhurst T, Downey RJ, Ginsberg MS, et al. An initial experience with FDG-PET in the imaging of residual disease after induction therapy for lung cancer. Ann Thorac Surg, 2002; 73(1): 259–264; discussion 64–66.

44. Patz EF, Jr., Connolly J, and Herndon J. Prognostic value of thoracic FDG PET imaging after treatment for non-small cell lung cancer. AJR Am J Roentgenol, 2000; 174(3): 769–774.

45. Ambrogi MC, Lucchi M, Dini P, et al. Percutaneous radiofrequency ablation of lung tumours: Results in the mid-term. Eur J Cardiothorac Surg, 2006; 30(1): 177–183.

46. Dupuy DE, DiPetrillo T, Gandhi S, et al. Radiofrequency ablation followed by conventional radiotherapy for medically inoperable stage I non-small cell lung cancer. Chest, 2006; 129(3): 738–745.

47. Fernando HC, De Hoyos A, Landreneau RJ, et al. Radiofrequency ablation for the treatment of non-small cell lung cancer in marginal surgical candidates. J Thorac Cardiovasc Surg, 2005; 129(3): 639–644.

48. Grieco CA, Simon CJ, Mayo-Smith WW, et al. Percutaneous image-guided thermal ablation and radiation therapy: Outcomes of combined treatment for 41 patients with inoperable stage I/II non-small-cell lung cancer. J Vasc Interv Radiol, 2006; 17(7): 1117–1124.

49. Kang S, Luo R, Liao W, et al. Single group study to evaluate the feasibility and complications of radiofrequency ablation and usefulness of post treatment position emission tomography in lung tumours. World J Surg Oncol, 2004; 2(1): 30.

50. Simon CJ, Dupuy D, Safran H, et al. Pulmonary radiofrequency ablation: Long-term safety and efficacy in 153 patients. Radiology, 2006.

51. Dupuy DE, Zagoria RJ, Akerley W, et al. Percutaneous radiofrequency ablation of malignancies in the lung. AJR Am J Roentgenol, 2000; 174(1): 57–59.

52. Belfiore G, Moggio G, Tedeschi E, et al. CT-guided radiofrequency ablation: A potential complementary therapy for patients with unresectable primary lung cancer – a preliminary report of 33 patients. AJR Am J Roentgenol, 2004; 183(4): 1003–1011.

53. Gadaleta C, Catino A, Ranieri G, et al. Radiofrequency thermal ablation of 69 lung neoplasms. J Chemother, 2004; 16 Suppl 5: 86–89.

54. Grieco CA, Simon CJ, Mayo-Smith WW, et al. Percutaneous thermoablation as a palliative treatment for chest wall masses. J Vasc Interv Radiol, 2006; 17: S61.

55. Herrera LJ, Fernando HC, Perry Y, et al. Radiofrequency ablation of pulmonary malignant tumors in nonsurgical candidates. J Thorac Cardiovasc Surg, 2003; 125(4): 929–937.

56. Jain SK, Dupuy DE, Cardarelli GA, et al. Percutaneous radiofrequency ablation of pulmonary malignancies: Combined treatment with brachytherapy. AJR Am J Roentgenol, 2003; 181(3): 711–715.

57. King J, Glenn D, Clark W, et al. Percutaneous radiofrequency ablation of pulmonary metastases in patients with colorectal cancer. Br J Surg, 2004; 91(2): 217–223.

58. Lee JM, Jin GY, Goldberg SN, et al. Percutaneous radiofrequency ablation for inoperable non-small cell lung cancer and metastases: Preliminary report. Radiology, 2004; 230(1): 125–134.

59. Nishida T, Inoue K, Kawata Y, et al. Percutaneous radiofrequency ablation of lung neoplasms: A minimally invasive strategy for inoperable patients. J Am Coll Surg, 2002; 195(3): 426–430.

60. Steinke K, Glenn D, King J, et al. Percutaneous imaging-guided radiofrequency ablation in patients with colorectal pulmonary metastases: 1-year follow-up. Ann Surg Oncol, 2004; 11(2): 207–212.

61. Therasse P, Arbuck SG, Eisenhauer EA, et al. New guidelines to evaluate the response to treatment in solid tumors. European Organization for Research and Treatment of Cancer, National Cancer Institute of the United States, National Cancer Institute of Canada. J Natl Cancer Inst, 2000; 92(3): 205–216.

62. Yan T, King J, Sjarif A, et al. Percutaneous radiofrequency ablation of pulmonary metastases from colorectal carcinoma: Prognostic determinants for survival. Ann Surg Oncol, 2006; 13(11): 1529–1537.

63. Jemal A, Siegel R, Ward E, et al. Cancer statistics, 2006. CA Cancer J Clin, 2006; 56(2): 106–130.

64. Rajdev L, Keller SM. Neoadjuvant and adjuvant therapy of non-small cell lung cancer. Surg Oncol, 2002; 11(4): 243–253.

65. American Joint Committee on Cancer: AJCC Cancer Staging Manual, 6th edition. New York: Springer, 2002.

66. Bach PB, Cramer LD, Warren JL, et al. Racial differences in the treatment of early-stage lung cancer. N Engl J Med, 1999; 341(16): 1198–1205.

67. Ginsberg RJ and Rubinstein LV. Randomized trial of lobectomy versus limited resection for T1 N0 non-small cell lung cancer. Lung Cancer Study Group. Ann Thorac Surg, 1995; 60(3): 615–622; discussion 22–23.

68. Martini N, Bains MS, Burt ME, et al. Incidence of local recurrence and second primary tumors in resected stage I lung cancer. J Thorac Cardiovasc Surg, 1995; 109(1): 120–129.

69. Miller DL, Rowland CM, Deschamps C, et al. Surgical treatment of non-small cell lung cancer 1 cm or less in diameter. Ann Thorac Surg, 2002; 73(5): 1545–1550; discussion 50–51.

70. Warren WH, Faber LP. Segmentectomy versus lobectomy in patients with stage I pulmonary carcinoma. Five-year survival and patterns of intrathoracic recurrence. J Thorac Cardiovasc Surg, 1994; 107(4): 1087–1093; discussion 93–94.

71. A controlled trial to improve care for seriously ill hospitalized patients. The study to understand prognoses and preferences for outcomes and risks of treatments (SUPPORT). The SUPPORT Principal Investigators. JAMA, 1995; 274(20): 1591–1598.

72. Errett LE, Wilson J, Chiu RC, et al. Wedge resection as an alternative procedure for peripheral bronchogenic carcinoma in poor-risk patients. J Thorac Cardiovasc Surg, 1985; 90(5): 656–661.

73. Kodama K, Doi O, Higashiyama M, et al. Intentional limited resection for selected patients with T1 N0 M0 non-small-cell lung cancer: A single-institution study. J Thorac Cardiovasc Surg, 1997; 114(3): 347–353.

74. Koike T, Yamato Y, Yoshiya K, et al. Intentional limited pulmonary resection for peripheral T1 N0 M0 small-sized lung cancer. J Thorac Cardiovasc Surg, 2003; 125(4): 924–928.

75. Landreneau RJ, Sugarbaker DJ, Mack MJ, et al. Wedge resection versus lobectomy for stage I (T1 N0 M0) non-small-cell lung cancer. J Thorac Cardiovasc Surg, 1997; 113(4): 691–698; discussion 698–700.

76. Okada M, Yoshikawa K, Hatta T, et al. Is segmentectomy with lymph node assessment an alternative to lobectomy for non-small cell lung cancer of 2 cm or smaller? Ann Thorac Surg, 2001; 71(3): 956–960; discussion 961.

77. Read RC, Yoder G, and Schaeffer RC. Survival after conservative resection for T1 N0 M0 non-small cell lung cancer. Ann Thorac Surg, 1990; 49(3): 391–398; discussion 399–400.

78. Talton BM, Constable WC, and Kersh CR. Curative radiotherapy in non-small cell carcinoma of the lung. Int J Radiat Oncol Biol Phys, 1990; 19(1): 15–21.

79. Kupelian PA, Komaki R, and Allen P. Prognostic factors in the treatment of node-negative nonsmall cell lung carcinoma with radiotherapy alone. Int J Radiat Oncol Biol Phys, 1996; 36(3): 607–613.

80. Bradley JD, Wahab S, Lockett MA, et al. Elective nodal failures are uncommon in medically inoperable patients with Stage I non-small-cell lung carcinoma treated with limited radiotherapy fields. Int J Radiat Oncol Biol Phys, 2003; 56(2): 342–347.

81. Zierhut D, Bettscheider C, Schubert K, et al. Radiation therapy of stage I and II non-small cell lung cancer (NSCLC). Lung Cancer, 2001; 34 Suppl 3: S39–43.

82. He W, Hu XD, Wu DF, et al. Ultrasonography-guided percutaneous microwave ablation of peripheral lung cancer. Clin Imaging, 2006; 30(4): 234–241.

83. Long-term results of lung metastasectomy: Prognostic analyses based on 5206 cases. The International Registry of Lung Metastases. J Thorac Cardiovasc Surg, 1997; 113(1): 37–49.

84. Hamy A, Baron O, Bennouna J, et al. Resection of hepatic and pulmonary metastases in patients with colorectal cancer. Am J Clin Oncol, 2001; 24(6): 607–609.

85. Labow DM, Buell JE, Yoshida A, et al. Isolated pulmonary recurrence after resection of colorectal hepatic metastases – is resection indicated? Cancer J, 2002; 8(4): 342–347.

86. Okumura S, Kondo H, Tsuboi M, et al. Pulmonary resection for metastatic colorectal cancer: Experiences with 159 patients. J Thorac Cardiovasc Surg, 1996; 112(4): 867–874.

87. Piltz S, Meimarakis G, Wichmann MW, et al. Long-term results after pulmonary resection of renal cell carcinoma metastases. Ann Thorac Surg, 2002; 73(4): 1082–1087.

88. Temple LK and Brennan MF. The role of pulmonary metastasectomy in soft tissue sarcoma. Semin Thorac Cardiovasc Surg, 2002; 14(1): 35–44.

89. van der Poel HG, Roukema JA, Horenblas S, et al. Metastasectomy in renal cell carcinoma: A multicenter retrospective analysis. Eur Urol, 1999; 35(3): 197–203.

90. Kandioler D, Kromer E, Tuchler H, et al. Long-term results after repeated surgical removal of pulmonary metastases. Ann Thorac Surg, 1998; 65(4): 909–912.

91. Todd TR. The surgical treatment of pulmonary metastases. Chest, 1997; 112(4 Suppl): 287S–290S.

92. Tsuchiya H, Kanazawa Y, Abdel-Wanis ME, et al. Effect of timing of pulmonary metastases identification on prognosis of patients with osteosarcoma: The Japanese Musculoskeletal Oncology Group study. J Clin Oncol, 2002; 20(16): 3470–3477.

93. Choong PF, Pritchard DJ, Rock MG, et al. Survival after pulmonary metastasectomy in soft tissue sarcoma. Prognostic factors in 214 patients. Acta Orthop Scand, 1995; 66(6): 561–568.

94. Kawai A, Fukuma H, Beppu Y, et al. Pulmonary resection for metastatic soft tissue sarcomas. Clin Orthop Relat Res, 1995; (310): 188–193.

95. Liu D, Labow DM, Dang N, et al. Pulmonary metastasectomy for head and neck cancers. Ann Surg Oncol, 1999; 6(6): 572–578.

96. Girard P, Ducreux M, Baldeyrou P, et al. Surgery for lung metastases from colorectal cancer: Analysis of prognostic factors. J Clin Oncol, 1996; 14(7): 2047–2053.

97. Goya T, Miyazawa N, Kondo H, et al. Surgical resection of pulmonary metastases from colorectal cancer. 10-year follow-up. Cancer, 1989; 64(7): 1418–1421.

98. Inoue M, Kotake Y, Nakagawa K, et al. Surgery for pulmonary metastases from colorectal carcinoma. Ann Thorac Surg, 2000; 70(2): 380–383.

99. Mansel JK, Zinsmeister AR, Pairolero PC, et al. Pulmonary resection of metastatic colorectal adenocarcinoma. A ten year experience. Chest, 1986; 89(1): 109–112.

100. McCormack PM and Attiyeh FF. Resected pulmonary metastases from colorectal cancer. Dis Colon Rectum, 1979; 22(8): 553–556.

101. McCormack PM, Burt ME, Bains MS, et al. Lung resection for colorectal metastases. 10-year results. Arch Surg, 1992; 127(12): 1403–1406.

102. Pfannschmidt J, Muley T, Hoffmann H, et al. Prognostic factors and survival after complete resection of pulmonary metastases from colorectal carcinoma: Experiences in 167 patients. J Thorac Cardiovasc Surg, 2003; 126(3): 732–739.

103. Saito Y, Omiya H, Kohno K, et al. Pulmonary metastasectomy for 165 patients with colorectal carcinoma: A prognostic assessment. J Thorac Cardiovasc Surg, 2002; 124(5): 1007–1013.

104. Sakamoto T, Tsubota N, Iwanaga K, et al. Pulmonary resection for metastases from colorectal cancer. Chest 2001; 119(4): 1069–1072.

105. van Halteren HK, van Geel AN, Hart AA, et al. Pulmonary resection for metastases of colorectal origin. Chest, 1995; 107(6): 1526–1531.

106. Friedel G, Pastorino U, Ginsberg RJ, et al. Results of lung metastasectomy from breast cancer: Prognostic criteria on the basis of 467 cases of the International Registry of Lung Metastases. Eur J Cardiothorac Surg, 2002; 22(3): 335–344.

107. Lanza LA, Natarajan G, Roth JA, et al. Long-term survival after resection of pulmonary metastases from carcinoma of the breast. Ann Thorac Surg, 1992; 54(2): 244–247; discussion 248.

108. Livartowski A, Chapelier A, Beuzeboc P, et al. Surgical excision of pulmonary metastasis of cancer of the breast: Apropos of 40 patients. Bull Cancer, 1998; 85(9): 799–802.

109. Ludwig C, Stoelben E, and Hasse J. Disease-free survival after resection of lung metastases in patients with breast cancer. Eur J Surg Oncol, 2003; 29(6): 532–535.

110. Cerfolio RJ, Allen MS, Deschamps C, et al. Pulmonary resection of metastatic renal cell carcinoma. Ann Thorac Surg, 1994; 57(2): 339–344.

111. Fourquier P, Regnard JF, Rea S, et al. Lung metastases of renal cell carcinoma: Results of surgical resection. Eur J Cardiothorac Surg, 1997; 11(1): 17–21.

112. Pfannschmidt J, Hoffmann H, Muley T, et al. Prognostic factors for survival after pulmonary resection of metastatic renal cell carcinoma. Ann Thorac Surg, 2002; 74(5): 1653–1657.

113. Kondo H, Okumura T, Ohde Y, et al. Surgical treatment for metastatic malignancies. Pulmonary metastasis: Indications and outcomes. Int J Clin Oncol, 2005; 10(2): 81–85.

114. Dekernion JB, Ramming KP, and Smith RB. The natural history of metastatic renal cell carcinoma: A computer analysis. J Urol, 1978; 120(2): 148–152.

115. Kawamura M, Izumi Y, Tsukada N, et al. Percutaneous cryoablation of small pulmonary malignant tumors under computed tomographic guidance with local anesthesia for nonsurgical candidates. J Thorac Cardiovasc Surg 2006; 131(5): 1007–1013.

116. Steinke K, Habicht JM, Thomsen S, et al. CT-guided radiofrequency ablation of a pulmonary metastasis followed by surgical resection. Cardiovasc Intervent Radiol, 2002; 25(6): 543–546.

117. Yan TD, King J, Sjarif A, et al. Learning curve for percutaneous radiofrequency ablation of pulmonary metastases from colorectal carcinoma: A prospective study of 70 consecutive cases. Ann Surg Oncol, 2006; 13(12): 1588–1595.

118. Berber E, Pelley R, and Siperstein AE. Predictors of survival after radiofrequency thermal ablation of colorectal cancer metastases to the liver: A prospective study. J Clin Oncol, 2005; 23(7): 1358–1364.

119. Griffin JP, Nelson JE, Koch KA, et al. End-of-life care in patients with lung cancer. Chest, 2003; 123(1 Suppl): 312S–331S.

120. Langendijk JA, ten Velde GP, Aaronson NK, et al. Quality of life after palliative radiotherapy in non-small cell lung cancer: A prospective study. Int J Radiat Oncol Biol Phys, 2000; 47(1): 149–155.

121. Kvale PA, Simoff M, and Prakash UB. Lung cancer. Palliative care. Chest, 2003; 123(1 Suppl): 284S–311S.

122. Watson PN and Evans RJ. Intractable pain with lung cancer. Pain, 1987; 29(2): 163–173.

123. Kishi K, Nakamura H, Sudo A, et al. Tumor debulking by radiofrequency ablation in hypertrophic pulmonary osteoarthropathy associated with pulmonary carcinoma. Lung Cancer, 2002; 38(3): 317–320.

124. Ohhigashi S, Nishio T, Watanabe F, et al. Experience with radiofrequency ablation in the treatment of pelvic recurrence in rectal cancer: Report of two cases. Dis Colon Rectum, 2001; 44(5): 741–745.

125. Patti JW, Neeman Z, and Wood BJ. Radiofrequency ablation for cancer-associated pain. J Pain, 2002; 3(6): 471–473.

126. Posteraro AF, Dupuy DE, and Mayo-Smith WW. Radiofrequency ablation of bony metastatic disease. Clin Radiol, 2004; 59(9): 803–811.

127. Simon CJ and Dupuy DE. Image-guided ablative techniques in pelvic malignancies: Radiofrequency ablation, cryoablation, microwave ablation. Surg Oncol Clin North Am, 2005; 14(2): 419–431.

128. Simon CJ and Dupuy DE. Percutaneous minimally invasive therapies in the treatment of bone tumors: Thermal ablation. Semin Musculoskelet Radiol, 2006; 10(2): 137–144.

129. Callstrom MR, Charboneau JW, Goetz MP, et al. Painful metastases involving bone: Feasibility of percutaneous CT- and US-guided radio-frequency ablation. Radiology, 2002; 224(1): 87–97.

130. Senzer N, Mani S, Rosemurgy A, et al. TNFerade biologic, an adenovector with a radiation-inducible promoter, carrying the human tumor necrosis factor alpha gene: A phase I study in patients with solid tumors. J Clin Oncol, 2004; 22(4): 592–601.

131. Zhang X, Cheung RM, Komaki R, et al. Radiotherapy sensitization by tumor-specific TRAIL gene targeting improves survival of mice bearing human non-small cell lung cancer. Clin Cancer Res, 2005; 11(18): 6657–6668.

Chapter 37

INTERVENTIONAL TREATMENT METHODS FOR UNRESECTABLE LUNG TUMORS

Thomas J. Vogl

Stefan Zangos

Christopher Herzog

Sebastian Lindemayr

Malignant lung diseases are a major topic in community health. The incidence for lung cancer rapidly increased in the last century (1), and today it is the most common malignant disease worldwide. In the United States, bronchial carcinoma is the leading malignant disease for both genders, and in 2000, the incidence was 164,000 with a morbidity of 157,000 (2). Pulmonary metastases are also a challenge and occur in patients with a variety of cancers. Between 20% and 30% of patients afflicted with cancer generate pulmonary metastases (3).

The prognoses for bronchial carcinomas and metastases remain poor. Resection of stage I and II carcinomas offers the best chance in long-term survival (4–7), but only 25% to 30% of these tumors are resectable (4–6). Survival rates for bronchial carcinomas and pulmonary metastases are similar, with a mean survival for all bronchial carcinomas of 12 months (4) and a mean survival after diagnosis of non-resectable lung metastases of less than 1 year (8). Five-year survival rates of 10% for all bronchial carcinomas (5) have been reported, with a mean 5-year survival rate of 23% to 50% after resection (4, 9–11) and 1% (4) for unresectable carcinomas. In patients with lung metastases who undergo pulmonary resection, a 5-year survival rate of 20% to 46% (12–19) has been reported.

As an alternative to resection or as a neoadjuvant therapeutic option, various therapies such as radiotherapy or chemotherapy have been developed (1), and in particular, systemic chemotherapy has shown encouraging results (16, 20). However, the overall response rate remained disappointing (1), with 20% to 30% for doxorubicin and 20% to 50% for combination chemotherapy (19–22). Besides, intravenous chemotherapy has a number of disagreeable adverse effects, which limit its use (23).

A promising alternative to systemic chemotherapy might be isolated lung perfusion (ILuP), an experimental clinical technique to improve treatment results in the therapy of pulmonary metastases from certain tumors (24). This method emerged at the end of the 1950s and experienced a renaissance at the beginning of the 1980s (25). The idea behind ILuP is to create a closed circuit by cannulation of the pulmonary arteries and veins, which permits a selective delivery of high-dose chemotherapy into the lungs while systemic toxicity remains limited (8, 23, 26,

27). It was reported that with this procedure, cytostatic drug concentrations were twice as high as those obtained with systemic administration, using only one fourth of the dose (28). This correlates well with findings of various animal studies that report tumor levels (23, 29) and efficacy (30) to be significantly higher after ILuP when compared with systemic administration. Between 2001 and 2003, isolated lung perfusion was performed in 16 patients, which showed this method to be suitable for humans (11). This was also supported by several studies (23, 31); however, despite positive and promising results in humans, ILuP is not used clinically today. The reasons for this are the intricacy of this method, insufficient cognition regarding technical necessities of this procedure (32) and limited human trials (8). Another disadvantage of ILuP is its dependence on cannulation of pulmonary vessels achieved either by minimally invasive operative and catheter technology (33) or via thoracotomy (8). This means it cannot be repeated indefinitely; moreover it requires extracorporeal cardiovascular circulation (31, 34–36). In contrast to ILuP, transpulmonary chemoembolization (TPCE) can be performed percutaneously in a much less invasive manner, making invasive schemes obsolete. In 2002, a survey was published that compared intravenous administration versus isolated lung perfusion and chemoembolization in a CC531 rat model. Chemoembolization turned out to be superior to intravenous therapy and equal to ILuP in efficacy (37).

Transarterial chemoembolization is already established in the treatment of primary and secondary hepatic tumors (38). The aim of this procedure is to achieve a desarterialization of nutritive vessels by injection of embolizing particles leading to tumor necrosis. In addition, high levels of cytostatic agents can be delivered close to the tumor, prolonging the contact time between cancer cells and the agents (39). Finally, leakage of cytotoxic agents into the systemic circulation is avoided, which reduces systemic side effects of the chemotherapy drugs. Because of the special anatomical blood supply through the pulmonary artery (40), this concept can be applied to the treatment of lung tumors.

Under local anesthesia, access into the groin can be obtained via a 7F sheath, which is inserted into the femoral vein. Then, a 5F headhunter catheter (Terumo, Frankfurt/Main, Germany) is positioned into the right or left pulmonary artery subject to tumor localization. After imaging of the pulmonary arterial system of the side of interest by contrast-enhanced angiography, a hydrophilic guidewire (Terumo, Frankfurt, Germany) is inserted into the segmental pulmonary artery, and the headhunter catheter is pushed forward. Then, an Amplatz superstiff guidewire (Boston Scientific, Stuttgart, Germany) is inserted and a balloon catheter (diameter, 7 mm; length, 110 mm) is positioned into the relevant segmental pulmonary artery. According to dimension, position and supply of the arteries, the catheter tip is maneuvered into subsegmental pulmonary arteries with the help of the guidewire.

In order to prevent arteriovenous shuntings, the balloon catheter is blocked and contrast-enhanced angiography is performed. Once the catheter is deemed to be in good position, 5 mg/m^2 mitomycin C as the cytostatic drug and up to 10 ml lipiodol, followed by 200 to 450 mg of microspheres, are slowly administered under fluoroscopic guidance until stasis of the blood flow is achieved (Figures 37.1–37.3).

In 2005, a preliminary study was published that evaluated TPCE for the treatment of patients with lung metastases (41). In this study, 23 patients suffering from unresectable lung metastases underwent chemoembolization several times. In total, 26 metastases were treated; treatment was repeated between two and four times per patient at intervals of 2 to 4 weeks. For tumor volume calculation and assessment of tumor sizes, contrast-enhanced as well as non-enhanced computed tomographies were performed before the initial treatment and every 3 months thereafter. Follow-up was performed between 6 and 12 months after therapy.

This study showed that TPCE was, indeed, technically feasible and applicable for the treatment of lung tumors in humans and, moreover, it was well tolerated by the patients, with a low complication rate. No major complications or procedure-related mortality were recorded; all patients were discharged on the day of treatment. Laboratory parameters, such as leukocyte or platelet count, hemoglobin, bilirubin or creatinine levels and others were not significantly affected by the procedure. In 35% (8/23) of the treated patients, tumor volume was reduced according to the World Health Organization criteria, which means a reduction of at least 25% of the target lesion. In 26% (6/23), tumor volume remained unchanged under therapy ("stable disease"). In 39% (9/23) tumor growth of at least 10% was observed ("progressive disease").

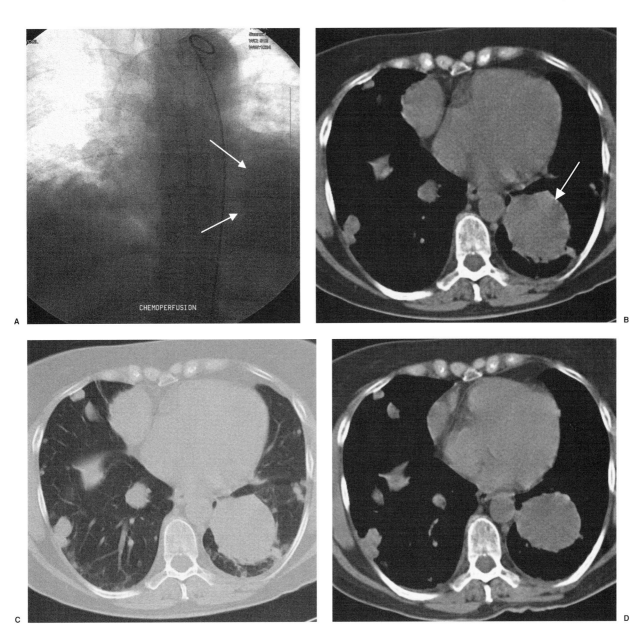

FIGURE 37.1. A 54-year-old woman patient suffering from multiple lung metastases of a leiomyosarcoma. Verification of a moderate degree of lipiodol uptake and a measurable response to treatment. (A) Final angiogram after the first course of chemoperfusion of the left tumor-supplying pulmonary arteries. Note the increased opacity of the tumor (*arrows*). (B,C) Unenhanced axial CT scan after first course of chemoperfusion. Documentation of a moderate peripheral lipiodol uptake in the periphery of the metastasis (*arrow*). (D,E) CT scan 2 months after the first treatment. A volume reduction from 96.05 ml to 83.62 ml (–12.0%) had been achieved at that point of time. After that, the patient underwent six sessions of TPCE. (F) Angiogram after the first course of TPCE. Stasis of lipiodol in the tumor-supplying vessels (*arrow*). (G,H) CT scan after the first course of TPCE. Again, documentation of lipiodol uptake in the periphery of the lesion (*arrows*). (I,K) Unenhanced axial CT scan after three sessions of chemoperfusion and six courses of TPCE, 8 months after the initial treatment. A volume reduction from initially 96.05 ml to 23.43 ml was accomplished, which means a reduction of 75%.

Tumors with a distinctive vascular supply, such as metastases from thyroid carcinoma, leiomyosarcoma, renal cell carcinoma and carcinoid tumors, showed maximum lipiodol uptake and responded best to the treatment.

In addition to this study, clinical trials involving drug-eluting beads exist (42). These beads are micro-spheres produced for embolization, but they can also be loaded with chemotherapeutic agents such as doxorubicin (43). An improvement of the therapy by providing a simplified procedure, a more target-oriented and accurate chemotherapy and, finally, a better controlled drug release over a longer period of time are anticipated advantages. In comparison with

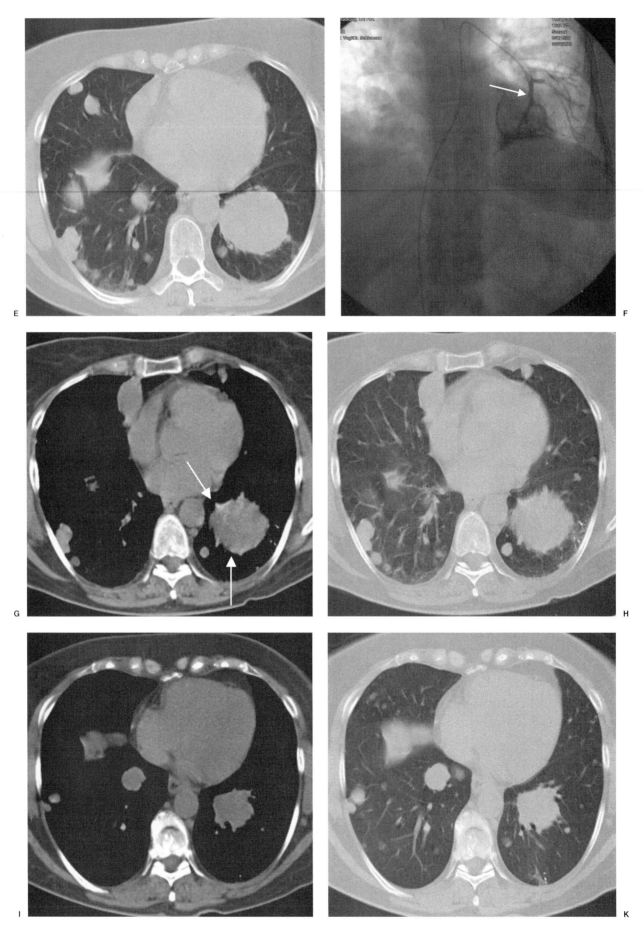

FIGURE 37.1. (*Continued*)

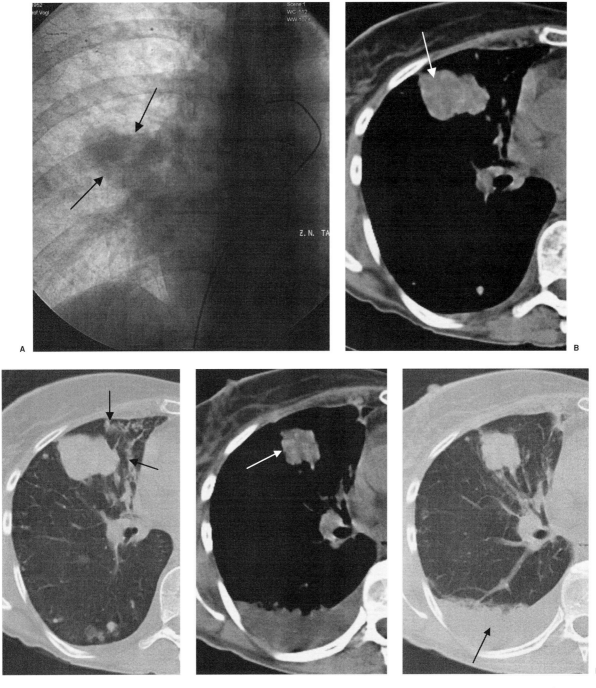

FIGURE 37.2. A 54-year-old woman with metastases of breast cancer. (A) Final angiogram after the first course of TPCE. Illustration of the tumor (*arrows*). (B,C) CT scan after the first treatment. Verification of the metastasis (*white arrow*). Note the small adjacent lung infarction verified as an area with lung consolidation (*black arrows*).

(D,E) CT scan 3 months after the first course of treatment. Note the lipiodol uptake (*white arrow*) and the measurable response to treatment. A volume reduction from 23.9 ml to 9.7 ml has been achieved. Note the pleural effusion (*black arrow*).

standard chemoembolization, the application of the beads should decrease systemic side effects by reducing peak systemic blood plasma levels of doxorubicin. Furthermore, the increased local delivery of cytostatic agents as well as the prolonged exposure of the tumor to the chemotherapy achieved by these beads might result in better tumor response rates (44).

Treatment of pulmonary metastases is still an enormous challenge today. As already emphasized, long-term survival has been reported to be only 46% (12–19) of treated patients at best and systemic chemotherapy did not fulfill desired expectations (1, 19–22). For this reason, multi-modality therapy regimens have been postulated (45). In 2005, a

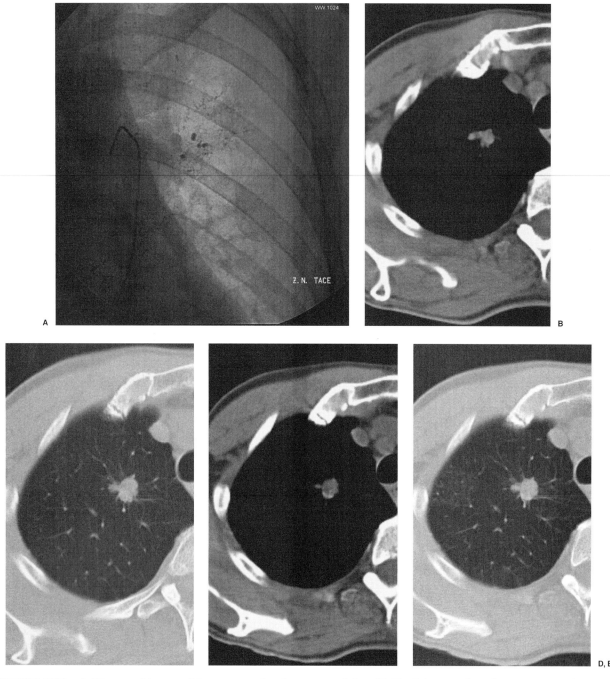

FIGURE 37.3. A 52-year-old man with a metastasis of a colorectal carcinoma. Tumor growth has been successfully avoided by the treatment. (A) Final angiogram after the first treatment. (B,C) CT scan after the initial TPCE. Documentation of the moderate lipiodol-absorbing lesion in the right upper lobe. (D,E) CT scan after three courses of TPCE 3 months after the first treatment. Reduction of the tumor volume from 2.07 ml to 1.76 ml. According to the RECIST criteria, it was classified as "stable disease."

retrospective study comparing multi-modality therapy – including modified pharmacokinetic modulating chemotherapy (PMC), radiation and radiofrequency ablation (RFA) – versus single chemotherapy was published, which showed a significant survival advantage for patients treated with multi-modality therapy: 3-year survival rate of patients in the multimodality group was 87.5% versus 33.3% in the chemotherapy group (46). Another promising alternative might be the combination of surgical ablation and chemotherapy (18, 47). Surgical intervention could excise the macroscopic portion while chemotherapy could annihilate residual microscopic components (18). As already mentioned, TPCE of the lung has the advantages of ILuP over systemic chemotherapy (23, 29, 30) without the disadvantages of ILuP. This means TPCE of the lung could be even more attractive when combined with surgery (Figure 37.2). However, it should be considered that only around 30% of the patients are suitable for surgical intervention (37). In these cases, TPCE of the lung could be performed without the surgical element of the combined therapy, whereas ILuP should be reserved for "patients already scheduled for metastasectomy" (31) because, in this case, a thoracotomy is required anyway. Another advantage of TPCE over ILuP is that TPCE can be repeated as often as necessary, whereas ILuP "is a single-course treatment, [with an] effectiveness [...] which remains unknown" (31). Furthermore, extracorporal circulation, required for IluP, (37) is not necessary for TPCE.

The findings of the study involving TPCE might have been affected by four basic facts: First, a balloon catheter was used to avoid outflow of the embolization solution (suspension, particles) into the pulmonary artery and to prevent arteriovenous shunting. Second, medication was administered superselectively. Third, lipiodol was used as a drug carrier (48) and fourth, microspheres (Embocept, Pharmacia & Upjohn, Erlangen, Germany) were used to retard drug elimination.

There are still some limitations to the study: First, quantity of treated patients is still limited and a control group is missing. Thus, no conclusions can be drawn about the clinical effectiveness of TPCE and whether treated patients benefit in terms of survival. Second, no conclusion can be drawn from this study regarding whether tumor reduction is attributed to the application of mitomycin C or microspheres, because they were administered simultaneously, and the ischemia achieved by the application of microspheres may be the only reason for tumor regression.

In summary, local chemoperfusion or chemoembolization of the lung are promising techniques for patients who suffer from unresectable primary or secondary lung tumors. Both therapy regimens are applicable in palliative or even neoadjuvant oncological settings.

REFERENCES

1. Zutic H. Bronchial carcinoma – an overview. Med Arh, 1999; 53(3 Suppl 1): 27–31; PMID: 10546465.
2. De Vita Jr VT, Hellmann S, and Rosenburg SA. Cancer: Principles and Practice of Oncology, vol. 1, 6th edition. Philadelphia, PA: Lippincott/Williams and Wilkins, 2001.
3. Weiss W, Boucot KR, and Cooper DA. The Philadelphia pulmonary neoplasm research project. Survival factors in bronchogenic carcinoma. JAMA 1971; 216(13): 2119–2123. PMID: 5108675.
4. Müller M. Chirurgie für Studium und Praxis: Unter Berücksichtigung des Gegenstandskataloges und der mündlichen Examina in den ärztlichen Prüfungen 2002/03/ Markus Müller und Mitarb. – 6. Aufl. – Breisach /Rh.: Med.Verl.– und Informationsdienste, 2001, S. 101.
5. Frommhold W and Gerhardt P. Klinisch-radiologisches Seminar, Band 17, Tumoren der Lunge. Stuttgart and New York: Georg-Thieme-Verlag, 1987, S. 93.
6. Mc Cormack P. Surgical resection of pulmonary metastases. Semin Surg Oncol, 1990; 6: 297–302.
7. Herth FJF. Epidemiologie, Symptomatik und Diagnostik des Bronchialkarzinoms. Klinikarzt, 2005; 34 (7): 202–205.
8. Brown DB, Ma MK, Battafarano RJ, et al. Endovascular lung perfusion using high-dose cisplatin: Uptake and DNA adduct formation in an animal model. Oncol Rep 2004 Jan; 11(1): 237–243. PMID: 14654932.
9. American Cancer Society. Facts and Figures 2004.
10. Plickova K, Spidlen V, Pesek M, et al. Patient survival analysis in surgery of bronchogenic carcinoma from 1986 to 1997. Rozhl Chir, 2003 Jun; 82(6): 293–299. PMID: 12898778.
11. Hendriks JM, Grootenboers MJ, Schramel FM, et al. Isolated lung perfusion with melphalan for resectable lung metastases: A phase I clinical trial. Ann Thorac Surg, 2004 Dec; 78(6): 1919–1927. PMID: 15561001.
12. Vogt-Moykopf I, Bulzebruck H, Krysa S, et al. Results in surgery of pulmonary metastases. Chirurgie, 1992; 118: 263–271.
13. Friedel G, Pastorino U, Buyse M, et al. Resection of lung metastases: Long-term results and prognostic analyses based on 5.206 cases. The International Registry of Lung Metastases. Zentralbl Chir, 1999; 124: 96–103.
14. Hendriks JM, Romijn S, Van Putte B et al. Long-term results of surgical resection of lung metastases. Acta Chir Belg, 2001; 101: 267–272.
15. Abecasis N, Cortez F, Bettencourt A, et al. Surgical treatment of lung metastases: Prognostic factors for long-term survival. J Surg Oncol 1999; 72: 193–198.
16. Lanza LA, Putnam JB, Benjamin RS, et al. Response to chemotherapy does not predict survival after resection of sarcoma pulmonary metastases. Ann Thorac Surg, 1991; 51: 219–224.
17. Casson AG, Putnam JB, Natarajan G, et al. Five year survival after pulmonary metastasectomy for adult soft-tissue sarcoma. Cancer, 1992; 69: 662–668.
18. Ueda T, Uchida A, Kadama K, et al. Aggressive pulmonary metastasectomy for soft tissue sarcoma. Cancer, 1993; 72: 1919–1925.
19. Weksler B, Ng B, Lenert JT, Burt ME. Isolated single-lung perfusion with doxorubicin is pharmacokinetically superior to intravenous injection. Ann Thorac Surg, 1993; 56: 209–214.
20. Mentzer SJ, Antman KH, Attinger C, et al. Selected benefits of thoracotomy and chemotherapy for sarcoma metastatic to the lung. J Surg Oncol, 1993; 53: 54–59.
21. Greenall MJ, Magill GB, De Cosse JJ, et al. Chemotherapy for soft tissue sarcoma. Surg Gynecol Obstet, 1986; 162: 193–198.

22. Dirix LJ, Oosterom AT. Diagnosis and treatment of soft tissue sarcomas in adults. Curr Opin Oncol, 1994; 6: 372–383.

23. Van Schil PE. Surgical treatment for pulmonary metastases. Acta Clin Belg, 2002 Nov–Dec; 57(6): 333–339. PMID: 12723252.

24. Romijn S, Hendriks JM, Van Putte BP, et al. Anterograde versus retrograde isolated lung perfusion with melphalan in the WAG-Rij rat. Eur J Cardiothorac Surg, 2005 Jun; 27(6): 1083–1085. Epub 2005 Apr 2. PMID: 15896622.

25. Hendriks JM, Romijn S, Van Putte B, et al. Isolated lung perfusion for the treatment of pulmonary metastatic disease: A review. Acta Chir Belg, 2005 Aug; 105(4): 338–343. PMID: 16184713.

26. Pan Y, Krueger T, Tran N, et al. Evaluation of tumour vascularisation in two rat sarcoma models for studying isolated lung perfusion. Injection route determines the origin of tumour vessels. Eur Surg Res, 2005 Mar–Apr; 37(2): 92–99. PMID: 15905614.

27. Van Putte BP, Hendriks JM, Romijn S, Van Schil PE., Isolated lung perfusion for the treatment of pulmonary metastases current mini-review of work in progress. Surg Oncol, 2003 Nov; 12(3): 187–193. PMID: 12957622.

28. Muller H, Hilger R. Curative and palliative aspects of regional chemotherapy in combination with surgery. Support Care Cancer, 2003 Jan; 11(1): 1–10. Epub 2002 Jun 8. PMID: 12527948.

29. Van Putte BP, Hendriks JM, Romijn S, et al. Single-pass isolated lung perfusion versus recirculating isolated lung perfusion with melphalan in a rat model. Ann Thorac Surg, 2002 Sep; 74(3): 893–898; discussion, 898. PMID: 12238857.

30. Romijin S, Hendriks JM, Van Putte BP, et al. Regional differences of melphalan lung levels after isolated lung perfusion in the rat. J Surg Res, 2005 May 15; 125(2): 157–160. PMID: 15854668.

31. Ratto GB, Toma S, Civalleri D, et al. Isolated lung perfusion with platinum in the treatment of pulmonary metastases from soft tissue sarcomas. J Thorac Cardiovasc Surg, 1996 Sep; 112(3): 614–622. PMID: 8800147.

32. Franke UF, Wittwer T, Lessel M, et al. Evaluation of isolated lung perfusion as neoadjuvant therapy of lung metastases using a novel in vivo pig model: I. Influence of perfusion pressure and hyperthermia on functional and morphological lung integrity. Eur J Cardiothorac Surg, 2004 Oct; 26(4): 792–799. PMID: 15450575.

33. Demmy TL, Wagner-Mann C, Allen A. Isolated lung chemotherapeutic infusions for treatment of pulmonary metastases: a pilot study. J Biomed Sci, 2002 Jul–Aug; 9(4): 334–338. PMID: 12145531.

34. Burt ME, Liu D, Abolhoda A, et al. F. Isolated lung perfusion for patients with unresectable metastases from sarcoma: A Phase I trial. Ann Thorac Surg, 2000; 69: 1542–1549.

35. Johnston MR, Minchin R, Dawson CA. Lung perfusion with chemotherapy in patients with unresectable metastatic sarcoma to the lung or diffuse bronchioloalveolar carcinoma. J. Thorac Cardiovasc Surg, 1995; 110: 368–373.

36. Pass HI, Mew DJ, Kranda KC, et al. Isolated lung perfusion with tumor necrosis factor for pulmonary metastases. Ann Thorac Surg, 1996; 61: 1609–1617.

37. Schneider P, Kampfer S, Loddenkemper C, et al. Chemoembolization of the lung improves tumor control in a rat model. Clin Cancer Res, 2002 Jul; 8(7): 2463–2468. PMID: 12114454.

38. Vogl TJ, Trapp M, Schroeder H, et al. Transarterial chemoembolization for hepatocellular carcinoma: volumetric and morphologic CT criteria for assessment of prognosis and therapeutic success – results from a liver transplantation center. Radiology, 2000; 214: 349–357.

39. Huppert PE, Geissler F, Duda SH, et al. Chemoembolisation des hepatozellulären Karzinoms: Computertomographische Befunde und klinische Resultate bei prospektiver repetitiver Therapie. Fortschr Roentgenstr, 1994; 160: 425–432.

40. Miller BJ, Rosenbaum AS. The vascular supply to metastatic tumors of the lung. Surg Gynecol Obstet, 1967; 125: 1009–1012.

41. Vogl TJ, Wetter A, Lindemayr S, et al. Treatment of unresectable lung metastases with transpulmonary chemoembolization: Preliminary experience. Radiology, 2005 Mar; 234(3): 917–922. Epub 2005 Jan 28. PMID: 15681689.

42. Start of trial to evaluate drug eluting bead in lung cancer announced. Lung Cancer, 2006, March 20; http://www.newsrx.com/newsletters/Clinical-Oncology-Week/2006–03–20/03202006333205CO.html.

43. Lewis AL, Gonzalez MV, Lloyd AW, et al. DC bead: In vitro characterization of a drug-delivery device for transarterial chemoembolization. J Vasc Interv Radiol, 2006 Feb; 17(2 Pt 1): 335–342.

44. http://www.biocompatibles.co.uk/content.asp?pid = 9.

45. Mountain CF, Khalil KG, Hermes KF, et al. The contribution of surgery to the management of carcinomatous pulmonary metastases. Cancer 1978; 41: 833–840.

46. Inoue Y, Miki C, Hiro J, et al. Improved survival using multi-modality therapy in patients with lung metastases from colorectal cancer: A preliminary study. Oncol Rep, 2005 Dec; 14(6): 1571–1576. PMID: 16273258.

47. Wagner W, von Eiff M, Klinke F, et al. [Neoadjuvant radiochemotherapy in locally advanced non-small cell bronchial carcinoma. Initial results of a prospective multicenter study]. Strahlenther Onkol, 1995 Jul; 171(7): 390–397. PMID: 7631260.

48. Bhattacharya S, et al. Human liver cells and endothelial cells incorporate iodised oil. Br J Cancer, 1996; 73: 877–881.

Head and Neck Tumors

Chapter 38

INTERVENTIONAL NEURORADIOLOGY IN HEAD AND NECK ONCOLOGY

John B. Weigele

Robert W. Hurst

Interventional neuroradiologic procedures are integral to the management of patients with head and neck tumors. Preoperative embolization of vascular neoplasms is used at many centers to minimize intraoperative hemorrhage and facilitate surgical resection. Also, balloon test occlusion provides a valuable preoperative assessment of an artery that may undergo surgical sacrifice. In some cases, preoperative permanent arterial occlusion facilitates radical tumor resection. In addition, endovascular techniques are critically important for the control of intractable hemorrhage due to vascular erosion from tumor or complications of therapy (carotid blowout syndrome). Finally, selective intra-arterial infusion of chemotherapeutic agents contributes to the multidisciplinary management of malignant head and neck carcinomas. The role of interventional neuroradiology in head and neck oncology promises to expand as new devices and techniques are developed.

EMBOLIZATION OF VASCULAR HEAD AND NECK TUMORS

Vascular head and neck tumors frequently are referred for preoperative embolization. Most common are juvenile nasopharyngeal angiofibromas (JNAs) and paragangliomas. Various other vascular head and neck tumors also have been embolized (1–3). Preoperative embolization is widely believed to improve surgical outcomes by decreasing surgical blood loss, minimizing operative time, and facilitating the tumor resection. Nonetheless, no level I evidence exists. Many case series have been published supporting preoperative embolization; a minority of conflicting reports concludes preoperative embolization only adds risk without significantly improving surgical morbidity and mortality (4).

Technique

Two techniques have been developed for preoperative embolization of vascular head and neck tumors:

transarterial embolization with small particulates and direct-puncture embolization with liquid embolic agents (1–7). Transarterial embolization is employed much more commonly and is usually safe and effective. However, in selective cases (e.g., numerous tiny feeders, dangerous collaterals) direct-puncture embolization may be preferable (2, 3, 5–7).

The safe performance of endovascular interventions in the head and neck requires an advanced knowledge of relevant vascular anatomy. There are a number of potential collateral pathways between the external and internal carotid territories that must be identified to prevent inadvertent embolization of the central nervous system. Similarly, anatomic variants and collateral pathways involving the ophthalmic artery can cause ischemic damage to the retina during embolization. In addition, embolization of normal external carotid territories may cause ischemic damage to normal tissues (e.g., the mucosa, larynx, tongue, cranial nerves) (1, 4).

At our institution, external carotid territory embolizations are usually performed with the patient under conscious sedation. Selective angiograms of the common, internal and external carotid arteries are obtained, with special attention directed to the orbital and intracranial supply in addition to the arterial supply to the tumor. A 5F or 6F (Fr) Envoy guide catheter (Cordis, Miami Lakes, FL) is placed into the proximal external carotid artery. A roadmap is obtained; a microcatheter (e.g., Prowler Plus [Cordis], Prowler 14 [Cordis], or Echelon 14 [EV3, Plymouth, MN]) then is advanced with a Synchro 14 microguidewire (Boston Scientific, Natick, MA) through the guide catheter into the appropriate external carotid artery branch. A superselective microcatheter angiogram is carefully evaluated for supply to the tumor, supply to normal structures and dangerous anastamoses. Once the microcatheter is optimally positioned within the arterial feeder to the tumor, the supply is embolized to near hemostasis with 150- to 250-μ polyvinyl alcohol (PVA) particles (Contour, Boston Scientific) during subtracted fluoroscopic monitoring. The particles are suspended in non-heparinized Omnipaque 300 (GE Healthcare, Princeton, NJ) in a 1-ml syringe and injected through the microcatheter in small (0.05 to 0.1 ml) aliquots. The injection of each aliquot is assessed for free flow and for sequential decreases in the flow rate as the embolization progresses. Extreme care is taken to avoid a wedged microcatheter position that could force the particles through unseen collaterals. The pattern of contrast flow is continuously evaluated for the opening of dangerous new collateral pathways. As hemostasis is approached, the rate and volume of PVA injections are decreased, and care is taken to avoid reflux into normal vascular territories. Final angiograms are obtained, and additional feeders are embolized in the same fashion. A separate working surface is used during the embolization. Care is taken to avoid contamination of the angiographic working surface, syringes and solutions with PVA particles. Gloves are changed after each feeder has been embolized. Attention to detail is essential to prevent avoidable complications.

Juvenile Nasopharyngeal Angiofibroma

JNAs compose fewer than 0.5% of all head and neck tumors, occurring almost exclusively in young males between the ages of 14 and 25 years old. Patients typically present with painless unilateral nasal obstruction and recurrent epistaxis. The tumor usually arises near the sphenopalatine foramen, occupying the nasopharynx and the posterior nasal cavity. The cell of origin is unknown. Although the JNA is a benign tumor, it typically displays aggressive local growth and commonly extends through the sphenopalatine foramen into the pterygopalatine fossa. Additional tumor spread may occur into the ipsilateral sphenoid, ethmoid and maxillary sinuses, across the midline into the contralateral nasal cavity and paranasal sinuses, posteriorly into the central skull base or laterally from the pterygopalatine fossa into the infratemporal fossa, as well as intraorbitally and intracranially. The tumor is markedly hypervascular, consisting of a fibrovascular stroma with endothelial-lined vascular spaces containing little or no smooth muscle (1, 8, 9).

It is generally accepted that the imaging appearance of a JNA on computed tomography (CT), magnetic resonance imaging (MRI) and digital subtraction angiography (DSA) in the usual clinical context is sufficiently diagnostic to preclude the need for a biopsy prior to definitive surgical resection. Widening of the sphenopalatine foramen, erosion of the medial pterygoid plate and anterior bowing of the posterior maxillary wall are characteristic findings on CT. The tumor typically displays marked, diffuse or patchy enhancement on both MRI and CT. MRI accurately displays the extent of the tumor, distinguishes tumor from mucoperiosteal thickening and fluid in the paranasal sinuses and detects intracranial extension (8).

JNAs typically display an intense, inhomogeneous blush persisting into the venous phase without arteriovenous shunting on DSA (1). The sphenopalatine branch of the internal maxillary artery typically is a major source of blood supply to the tumor given that it supplies the lateral aspect of the posterior nasal cavity and nasopharynx, the site of tumor origin (Figure 38.1). Other branches of the external carotid artery –

in particular, the ascending pharyngeal artery – are recruited as the tumor grows. Branches of both external carotid arteries may feed large tumors. Extensive tumors may also recruit supply from branches of the internal carotid and vertebral arteries (8, 9).

The standard treatment for a JNA is surgical excision. Because of the tumor's highly vascular nature, significant blood loss may occur during surgery. Preoperative embolization was first reported in 1972 and has been widely accepted to decrease intraoperative

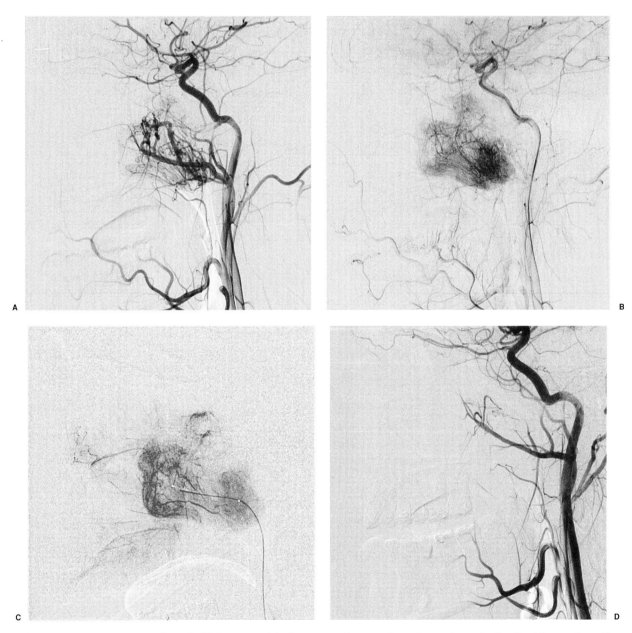

FIGURE 38.1. JNA (A) Early and (B) late arterial phase lateral common carotid angiogram images demonstrate a hypervascular tumor supplied by sphenopalatine and other branches of the internal maxillary artery. (C) Superselective angiogram via a microcatheter in the distal internal maxillary artery. (D) Post-embolization common carotid angiogram demonstrates complete obliteration of the tumor neovascularity.

blood loss and operative time, resulting in improved morbidity and mortality, supported by the results of many case series (Figure 38.1) (4, 10–14). Nonetheless, some studies have not found a benefit for preoperative embolization (4, 15–17). Although serious complications from JNA embolization are rare, monocular blindness caused by central retinal artery occlusion and an ischemic stroke due to a paradoxical embolus through a patent foramen ovale have been reported (18, 19).

Paraganglioma

Paragangliomas (also known as glomus tumors and chemodectomas) are uncommon vascular tumors originating from neural crest cells of the autonomic nervous system. Most head and neck paragangliomas occur spontaneously; 15% are familial, with autosomal dominant inheritance. Multicentric tumors occur in 10% of spontaneous and 30% of familial cases. Spontaneous tumors typically present in mid-life (after 40 years of age), whereas familial tumors usually are found in younger patients (10 to 30 years old). There is a 2:1 female-to-male ratio. Signs and symptoms depend on the location and size of the tumor; typical clinical presentations include a painless, enlarging neck mass, cranial nerve (IX–XII) dysfunction and pulsatile tinnitus (1, 20).

In the head and neck, paragangliomas occur in four common locations: 35% originate within the carotid body at the carotid bifurcation (carotid body tumor), 11% arise within the perineureum of the vagus nerve adjacent to the cervical internal carotid artery (glomus vagale tumor), and 50% occur in the temporal bone, arising either within the adventitia of the jugular bulb in the jugular foramen (glomus jugulare tumor) or within the mucosa of the cochlear promontory (glomus tympanicum tumor). Glomus jugulare tumors arise from Arnold's nerve, an auricular branch of the vagus nerve, whereas glomus tympanicum tumors arise from Jacobsen's nerve, a tympanic branch of the glossopharyngeal nerve. Larger temporal bone paragangliomas involve both regions (glomus jugulotympanicum tumors) and the site of origin may be uncertain. Rare head and neck paragangliomas also occur in the orbit, nasal cavity, nasopharynx and larynx. Malignant transformation occurs in 10% to 18% of glomus vagale and carotid body tumors but only 3% of temporal paragangliomas. The tumors are encapsulated and composed of a highly vascular stroma with sinusoidal spaces (1, 20).

Both CT and MRI play important roles in the evaluation of head and neck paragangliomas. On MRI, the tumors are hypointense on T1-weighted images and hyperintense on T2-weighted images. A characteristic "salt-and-pepper" appearance may be seen on T2-weighted images, representing enlarged vessels with varied low and high flow rates, particularly in larger paragangliomas. Intense, homogeneous enhancement is the rule following contrast administration. Coronal fat-suppressed T2-weighted and fat-suppressed post-contrast T1-weighted images are useful for characterization of skull base tumors. High-resolution CT is useful to detect invasion of adjacent bony structures; it can demonstrate expansion and "moth-eaten" destruction of the jugular foramen by glomus jugulare tumors, as well as evaluate potential superior extension into the tympanic cavity and possible destruction of the facial canal or ossicular chain. CT can also confirm the presence of a small glomus tympanicum on the cochlear promontory and exclude clinical mimics such as an aberrant internal carotid artery (1, 20).

On angiography, the paraganglioma displays an early, intense and mildly inhomogeneous blush. Enlarged feeding arteries and early draining veins are present. Paragangliomas in all locations receive blood supply from branches of the ascending pharyngeal artery; the musculospinal branch supplies carotid body and glomus vagale tumors; the neuromeningeal branch supplies glomus jugulare tumors; and the inferior tympanic branch supplies glomus tympanicum tumors (1, 21). Other branches of the external carotid artery, including the superior thyroid, occipital, internal maxillary and posterior auricular arteries, may provide additional blood supply, depending upon the location of the tumor. Muscular branches of the vertebral artery, the ascending cervical branch of the thyrocervical trunk and the deep cervical branch of the costocervical trunk can also contribute supply. Carotid body tumors splay the carotid bifurcation, displacing the external carotid artery anteromedially and the internal carotid artery posterolaterally. Arterial encasement can occur (Figure 38.2). In comparison, glomus vagale tumors do not splay the carotid bifurcation; the internal and external carotid arteries are both displaced anteriorly (1, 20).

Similar to the JNA, the primary treatment for paragangliomas is surgical excision, and intraoperative hemorrhage can be massive. Preoperative embolization has been widely accepted to decrease intraoperative

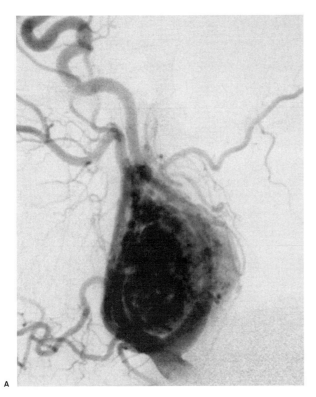
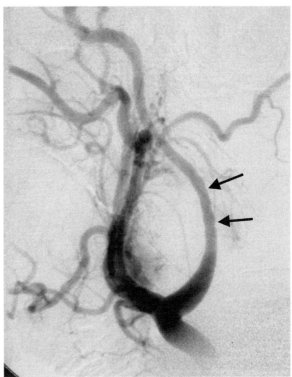

FIGURE 38.2. Carotid body tumor. (A) Lateral common carotid neck angiogram demonstrates typical hypervascular tumor splaying the internal and external carotid arteries. (B) Post-embolization angiogram reveals obliteration of the majority of the tumor neovascularity. Note mild irregularity and narrowing of the proximal internal carotid artery (*arrows*) suggesting tumor encasement.

blood loss and operative time, resulting in improved morbidity and mortality, supported by a number of case series (Figures 38.2 and 38.3) (4, 21–25). Some studies have found more benefit from preoperative embolization of glomus vagale and jugulare tumors than carotid body tumors, but other studies have found preoperative embolization of carotid body tumors also is effective (4, 20, 22). Reported complications from preoperative embolization are rare, but they include ischemic stroke and cranial nerve injuries. When carotid artery encasement is present, a preoperative balloon occlusion test provides useful information about the safety of potential surgical sacrifice.

PREOPERATIVE BALLOON TEST OCCLUSION AND ELECTIVE PERMANENT CAROTID OCCLUSION

Preoperative Balloon Test Occlusion

Advanced tumors of the neck and skull base often encase the cervical, petrous or cavernous segments of the internal carotid artery. Surgical resection of these tumors may require sacrifice of the carotid artery or dissection of the tumor away from the artery, risk-

ing iatrogenic vascular occlusion. The clinical consequences are highly variable. Depending on the potential collateral pathways, permanent carotid occlusion may be well tolerated without development of a clinical deficit or may result in a severe ischemic stroke. Without any preoperative testing, high incidences of stroke (17% to 30%) following permanent carotid occlusion have been reported (26). In a review of the literature, Linskey et al. found a cumulative 26% rate of stroke with a 12% mortality rate for permanent carotid occlusion without prior testing (27).

Carotid balloon test occlusion (BTO) was developed to predict the risk for stroke following permanent arterial occlusion. Initially described by Serbinenko in 1974, this technique employs the inflation of a low-pressure, compliant balloon in the distal cervical or intracranial internal carotid artery to arrest blood flow temporarily, usually for 20 to 30 minutes (28). The patient is anticoagulated during the BTO to prevent thromboembolic complications. Neurological examinations are performed immediately prior to and continuously throughout the BTO. If the patient develops a new neurological deficit (weakness, sensory loss, visual deficit, aphasia or decreased level of consciousness) the balloon is immediately deflated,

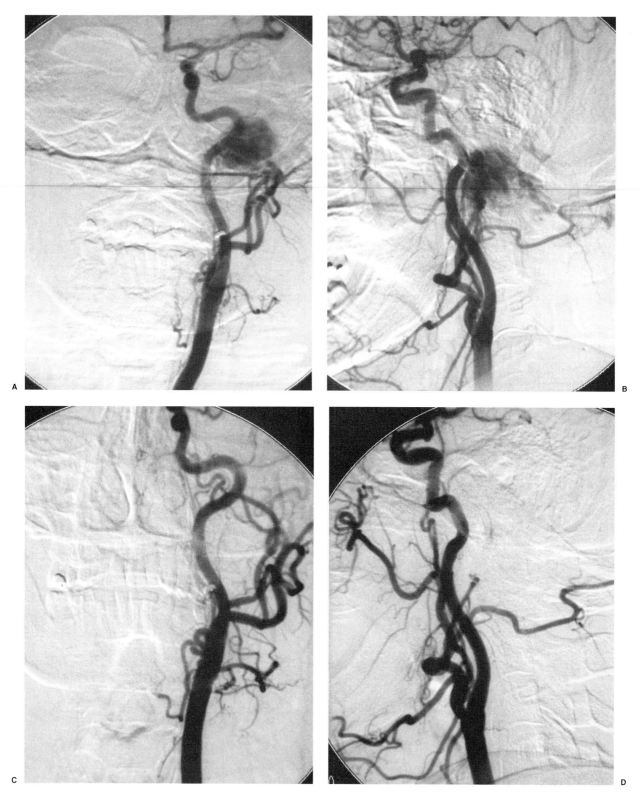

FIGURE 38.3. Glomus jugulare tumor. AP (A,C) and lateral (B,D) left common carotid neck angiograms prior to (A,B) and following (C,D) transarterial embolization with PVA particles revealing total obliteration of the tumor neovascularity.

and the test is considered a clinical failure. Virtually all patients who clinically fail a BTO will develop an ischemic stroke if the internal carotid artery is permanently occluded without revascularization (29). The test is considered clinically passed if the neurological examination remains unchanged (26).

The BTO is a safe procedure when performed in a cooperative patient by an experienced physician.

The complication rate is only slightly greater than the rate for diagnostic angiography. In a retrospective evaluation of 500 BTOs using a variety of balloon-catheter systems, Mathis et al. identified 16 complications (3.2%). Eight (1.6%) were asymptomatic. Neurological deficits occurred in eight (1.6%). Of those, six (1.2%) were transient; only two (0.4%) were permanent. Nonetheless, complications included carotid dissections and a pseudoaneurysm, emphasizing the potential for iatrogenic injury of the carotid artery and the necessity for careful technique. Inadequate anticoagulation was associated with an increased risk for thromboembolic ischemic events (29). A subsequent review of 103 BTOs performed with a non-detachable silicone balloon mounted on a microcatheter combined with a 0.010-inch microguidewire revealed no carotid injury or neurological complication, suggesting microcatheter-based compliant silicone balloons may confer increased safety over larger, more rigid balloon-catheter systems (30).

The incidence of stroke caused by permanent carotid occlusion is significantly reduced when the BTO has been passed on the basis of the neurological examination; however, it is not completely eliminated. Numerous efforts to increase the sensitivity and specificity of BTO by measuring various parameters directly or indirectly related to cerebral blood flow (CBF) or perfusion have been reported. These include qualitative or quantitative measurements of CBF during BTO, induced hypotension to measure cerebral perfusion reserve during BTO, and indirect indicators of cerebral perfusion during BTO, including angiography with evaluation for venous phase asymmetry, measurement of the arterial stump pressure, electroencephalography and transcranial Doppler ultrasonography. These add to the complexity, cost and potentially in some cases, to the risks of the procedure (26).

The value of these adjunctive tests is controversial. Outcomes data in many of the published reports are limited or absent. A literature review in 1995 found that 192 patients in five case series who underwent permanent carotid occlusion without bypass after passing a BTO based only on the clinical examination experienced a 4.7% incidence of permanent stroke, none fatal (29). Another retrospective analysis published in 2001 found that 198 patients in three case series who underwent permanent carotid occlusion without bypass after passing a BTO based on the clinical examination alone experienced a 3% inci-

dence of permanent neurological deficits. By comparison, the same review found 120 patients in six case series that underwent permanent carotid occlusion without bypass after passing a BTO based on examination and adjunctive CBF analysis or induced hypotension experienced a 6.7% incidence of permanent neurological deficits. This study noted the difficulties in comparing case series with small numbers of subjects, low complication rates and widely varying techniques and concluded it was not possible to prove superiority for a specific BTO protocol (26).

Nonetheless, efforts to improve the positive and negative predictive values of BTO continue. Marshall et al. reported outcomes on 33 patients who underwent permanent carotid occlusion following BTO with standard neurological testing, sustained-attention testing and quantitative CBF analysis using intracarotid ^{133}Xe injections. The only variable that predicted stroke following permanent carotid occlusion was a CBF during BTO less than or equal to 30 ml/100 g/minute (log rank = 5.87, p = 0.015) (31). Van Rooij et al. recently reported that synchronous venous opacification on angiography during BTO corresponded with a 98% positive predictive value for tolerance of permanent carotid occlusion in 51 patients (95% CI: 89% to 100%), however, a negative predictive value for venous phase asymmetry was not established (32). Ultimately, prospective multicenter trials may be necessary to definitively establish an optimal BTO method.

Elective Permanent Carotid Occlusion

The surgical management of an internal carotid artery in the operative field during resection of a tumor of the neck or skull base is challenging, particularly when the tumor encases the artery. Surgical options can include arterial skeletonization, subperiosteal or subadventitial dissection, vascular bypass and sacrifice of the artery during an en bloc resection with the tumor. Each approach has unique advantages and disadvantages. Surgical manipulation may weaken, dissect or thrombose the carotid artery. Revascularization is associated with significant morbidity and mortality and is often not feasible in the previously operated neck (33, 34). Permanent carotid occlusion (PCO) is frequently performed prior to an en bloc surgical resection in patients who have demonstrated adequate collateral blood flow by passing a BTO. A number of case series in the literature have reported low major morbidity (0% to 6.7%) and negligible mortality rates for preoperative PCO prior to tumor resection (1, 34–39). By comparison, Zane et al. reported a 50% complication rate from intra-operative carotid occlusion (35).

Detachable balloons are the most popular devices for PCO because they provide rapid, safe and pre-cisely located vascular occlusion. These balloons are constructed out of latex or silicone, are highly com-pliant and have self-sealing valves. For deployment, a balloon is mounted on a microcatheter, advanced through a guide catheter and positioned in the desired location. Partial inflation of the balloon can be used to "flow-direct" the system. The balloon is inflated with radiopaque media until the artery is occluded and the balloon is firmly fixed against the endothelium; then the balloon is detached by gentle traction on the microcatheter.

Typically, an initial balloon is deployed in the cav-ernous segment of the internal carotid artery between the origins of the inferolateral trunk and ophthalmic artery. This positioning limits the length of thrombus that forms distal to the balloon because the supracli-noid internal carotid artery usually remains patent due to collateral inflow from the ophthalmic artery; therefore, this placement theoretically limits the risk of thromboembolic complications. A second balloon is immediately deployed in the distal cervical internal carotid artery as a backup for the unlikely event that the first balloon is defective and deflates (1).

At our institution, patients are fully anticoagulated during and 24 to 48 hours after the procedure to prevent propagation of thrombus. We keep patients supine for 24 hours in an intensive care unit and avoid hypotension. This is followed by gradual mobiliza-tion. It has been suggested that a 3-week interval after PCO before proceeding to tumor resection may min-imize both hemodynamic and thromboembolic com-plications by providing time for the collateral path-ways to fully develop and for the distal surface of the occluded segment to mature and become less throm-bogenic (40).

Unfortunately, detachable balloons are currently unavailable in the United States. Although the Food and Drug Administration approved a detachable sil-icone balloon in 1998, the product recently was withdrawn from the market. Most U.S. interven-tional neuroradiologists currently use coils for PCO, a technique that is more tedious, time-consuming and expensive. To occlude the intracranial internal carotid artery, we typically begin by placing two or

three fibered GDC coils (GDC 18-Fibered VortX Shape, Boston Scientific), using the detachable coils to achieve optimal positioning and stability of the ini-tial coil mass, and then complete the occlusion with less expensive "pushable" fibered minicoils (Tornado Embolization Coils, Cook, Bloomington, IN). Full anticoagulation is essential during coil embolization to prevent thromboembolic events because the coils are thrombogenic and there is progressive stagna-tion of blood flow during the procedure. In some cases, we have used proximal flow arrest with an occlusion balloon guide catheter to prevent poten-tial distal migration of the initially deployed coils and also when anticoagulation is not feasible. Rapid, precise parent artery occlusion requiring fewer coils has been described using Hydrocoils (detachable plat-inum microcoils coated with a hydrophilic, expansile polymer; MicroVention, Aliso Viejo, CA) (41). Effi-cient, quick occlusion of the cervical internal carotid artery recently was reported with the Amplatzer vas-cular plug (AGA Medical, Golden Valley, MN); how-ever, this device is too stiff to be advanced into the intracranial internal carotid artery (42).

An intriguing alternative to PCO followed by en bloc resection recently has been developed using a self-expanding stent to facilitate subsequent subad-ventitial dissection while preserving the parent artery. The stent is deployed across the segment of carotid artery encased by tumor. Following 4 to 6 weeks to allow the stent to be covered with a mature neoin-timal lining, aggressive surgical resection with dis-section down to the struts of the stent has resulted in complete removal of a malignant fibrous histio-cytoma encasing the cervical internal carotid artery and three cases of jugular paragangliomas encasing the petrous internal carotid artery while maintaining vascular patency in every case (43, 44). Covered stents have been used in a similar fashion to resect a jugu-lar paraganglioma, an endolymphatic sac tumor and a carotid body tumor (45–47).

MANAGEMENT OF CAROTID BLOWOUT SYNDROME

Carotid blowout syndrome (CBS) is defined as impending or actual hemorrhage from rupture of the one of the extracranial carotid arteries or its primary branches. Four categories have been described: 1) Threatened carotid blowout refers to evidence for imminent hemorrhage on physical examination (e.g., an exposed, desiccated carotid artery within an open wound) or radiographic imaging (e.g., carotid artery pseudoaneurysm with necrotic tumor encasement). 2) Impending carotid blowout is indicated by a sentinel hemorrhage (either transoral or transcervical through an open wound or fistula) that either resolves spontaneously or is controlled with packing or pressure. 3) Acute carotid blowout refers to active hemorrhage that cannot be controlled well by packing or pressure. 4) Recurrent carotid blowout represents threatened, impending or acute carotid blowout in a patient who has had a prior episode of CBS (48–50).

CBS can be caused by any pathologic process that damages the structural integrity of the extracranial carotid system, including various tumors, trauma, functional endoscopy and infection. However, the most common causes for CBS are squamous cell carcinoma of the head and neck and complications from its treatment. In one series of 394 radical neck dissections, CBS occurred in 4.3% and was strongly associated with previous radiotherapy and wound dehiscence. Radiation therapy increased the risk for CBS by a factor of seven (51).

A summary of several case series found the most common site for CBS was the cervical internal carotid artery (43.6%), followed by the external carotid artery (23.4%) and the common carotid artery (11.7%) (50). Although not included within the strict definition of CBS, hemorrhage from the tumor and from jugular vein disruption also occurs in patients with head and neck cancers.

Prior to the advent of endovascular techniques, surgical management of CBS with neck exploration and ligation was associated with very high rates of major neurological morbidity and mortality (60% and 40% averages, respectively) (48). More recent results with endovascular management have been more favorable; however, as many as 15% to 20% of patients with CBS who are treated with PCO develop immediate or delayed cerebral ischemia (48).

The approach to the endovascular treatment of CBS depends on the clinical presentation and the anatomic site. In all cases, initial clinical management includes control of the airway, control of any active hemorrhage with pressure and fluid resuscitation. The interventional neuroradiology suite is equipped and managed similarly to an operating room. An anesthesiologist and an interventional neuroradiology nurse care for the patient during the procedure. Intravenous access is secured with multiple large-bore

peripheral catheters or with a central line. An arterial line is placed for continuous blood pressure monitoring. The electrocardiogram and pulse oximeter are also continuously monitored (1, 50).

Management of CBS involving the external carotid artery or its branches is relatively straightforward because permanent arterial occlusion is generally well tolerated, without the risk of cerebral ischemia. Following the diagnostic angiogram, a 5F or 6F guide catheter is advanced into the proximal aspect of the external carotid artery. An appropriate microcatheter such as a Prowler Plus (Cordis) is advanced and positioned across the injured site, which is then embolized with fibered minicoils (Tornado Embolization Coils, Cook). It is important to occlude the parent vessel on both sides of the injury in order to prevent continued blood flow to the injured site through collaterals (48, 50).

Management of CBS involving the common or cervical internal carotid artery is more challenging because permanent occlusion of these arteries is associated with a risk of cerebral ischemia. In threatened or impending CBS where there is not active hemorrhage, a BTO can be considered. If the patient cannot cooperate for a clinical examination, or if the requisite full heparinization is considered too dangerous, angiographic evaluation of the contralateral carotid artery and the dominant vertebral artery can be performed during the BTO, and the angiogram can be assessed for venous phase symmetry as well as for the quality of the circle of Willis collaterals (32). Balloon test occlusion is generally not feasible in patients who are actively hemorrhaging (acute CBS). Patients who pass this assessment can be treated with PCO using detachable balloons or coils (Figure 38.4). Similar to external carotid embolizations, it is essential to embolize the parent artery on both sides of the injury to prevent continued supply to the injured site by collateral blood flow (Figure 38.5) (48, 50).

There is controversy over the optimal endovascular technique to manage head and neck cancer patients with common or internal carotid injuries who are actively hemorrhaging or who have failed a BTO. Until recently, the only endovascular option was PCO, and this was certainly preferable to fatal exsanguination or the very high morbidity and mortality of surgery despite the 15% to 20% risk of causing brain ischemia. Recently, several small case series have described reconstructive techniques to treat internal and common CBS using stents and covered

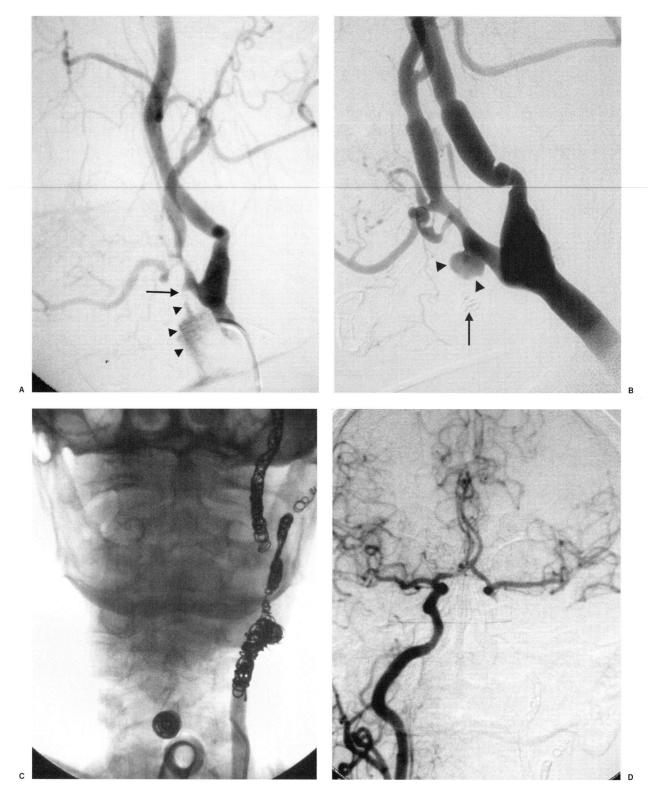

FIGURE 38.4. CBS. (A) Lateral common carotid neck angiogram demonstrates frank hemorrhage (*arrowheads*) from the origin of the superior thyroid artery (*arrow*) in a patient with advanced head and neck carcinoma. A single coil was placed at another medical center. (B) A follow-up angiogram after recurrent hemorrhage demonstrates coil migration (*arrow*) and a new pseudoaneurysm (*arrowheads*) at the site of the previous hemorrhage. Extensive tumor encasement of the internal and external carotid arteries and branches is evident. (C) Following confirmation of adequate collateral circulation, coil embolization of the distal common, internal and external carotid arteries was performed (AP view). (D) AP right common carotid angiogram following embolization confirming robust collateral supply to the left anterior circulation.

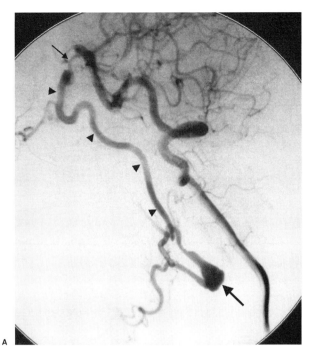

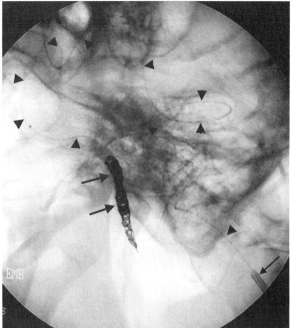

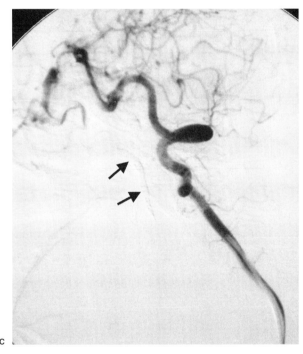

FIGURE 38.5. CBS via intracranial collateral supply in a patient with a common carotid artery previously occluded by tumor. (A) Lateral left vertebral angiogram demonstrates collateral flow from the vertebrobasilar system through the right posterior communicating artery (*small arrow*) with retrograde flow through the intracranial and cervical right internal carotid artery (*arrowheads*) into a fusiform aneurysm of the right internal carotid artery origin (*large arrow*). (B) Coils (*large arrows*) deployed via a microcatheter (*arrowheads*) that was advanced from a guide catheter (*small arrow*) in the vertebral artery through the posterior communicating artery and retrograde through the intracranial and cervical right internal carotid artery. (C) Final left vertebral angiogram confirms successful obliteration of the carotid pseudoaneurysm by the coils (*arrows*).

stents (52–58). Although their initial technical success rates have been high and acute hemorrhage has been successfully controlled, multiple delayed complications have been reported, including rebleeding, delayed thromboses, thromboembolic strokes, brain abscesses secondary to infected emboli and extrusion of stents into open wounds (52, 53, 56–58). The presence of recurrent tumor, radiation damage, pharyngocutaneous fistula, chronic non-healing wound or infection in the treatment field probably contributes

to these failures. Although reconstructive techniques with stents and stent-grafts appear useful for acute control of active hemorrhage from the common or internal carotid arteries, their long-term value compared with PCO in patients with head and neck cancer remains to be determined. In some cases of acute CBS, it may be reasonable to control the acute hemorrhage with a stent-graft with the intention to perform an elective BTO and possible PCO once the patient has stabilized.

SELECTIVE INTRA-ARTERIAL CHEMOTHERAPY FOR HEAD AND NECK CARCINOMAS

Head and neck carcinoma is the fifth most common cancer in the world, with an estimated annual global incidence of 533,100 cases (59). In the United States, approximately 44,600 new patients are diagnosed each year; 30% to 40% eventually die from the disease. Ninety percent to ninety-five percent of all head and neck cancers are squamous cell carcinomas (HNSCC). Locally advanced HNSCC (stages III and IV) represents more than 50% of cases, and historically it has had a poor prognosis when treated with conventional surgery and/or radiotherapy (40% 5-year survival; 10% to 30% 5-year survival for stage IV disease) (60). In addition, patients undergoing surgery for advanced local disease often undergo extensive resections, leading to functional and cosmetic disabilities.

Selective intra-arterial chemotherapy for advanced HNSCC has been investigated since the 1960s (61, 62). The interest in intra-arterial chemotherapy arose from the pharmacokinetic advantage of achieving a much higher first-pass concentration of the drug within the tumor compared with an intravenous administration. Nonetheless, the early results were limited by high complication rates and long infusion times (63).

In the late 1980s and early 1990s, a novel intra-arterial chemotherapy technique combined with local radiotherapy (RADPLAT) was developed at the University of California, San Diego and the University of Tennessee that solved many of the early problems. This protocol combined the infusion of an extremely high-dose intensity of cisplatin directly into the tumor bed through a selective arterial catheter during the simultaneous intravenous administration of sodium thiosulfate, a neutralizing agent that limited systemic toxicity. The tumor was exposed to dose intensities up to 10 times higher than standard intravenous chemotherapeutic regimens (63–66).

The technical details of the intra-arterial infusion were described by Kerber et al. (63). Common and external carotid artery angiograms were obtained with a 5F catheter. Placement of the catheter for the chemoinfusion was determined by the location of the tumor on cross-sectional imaging given that the tumor was usually avascular on angiography. Typically, the superior thyroid artery was infused for laryngeal carcinoma, the lingual artery was infused for tongue base carcinomas and the proximal external carotid artery was infused for pharyngeal carcinomas. For tumors crossing the midline, bilateral infusions were performed through catheters in both external carotid systems with the dose divided proportionate to the tumor volume on each side. Coaxial micro-catheters were used as necessary. Once the catheter was in position, the optimal infusion rate was determined by sequential power injections of contrast at increasing rates until slight proximal reflux during diastole was visible. This infusion rate conferred several advantages: the dose intensity of cisplatin delivered to the tumor was maximized, cisplatin was not exposed to the neutralizing agent during the first pass because all of the blood flow was displaced from the vascular bed by the infusion, and the selective infusion of only a portion of the vascular bed due to poor mixing (streaming) was eliminated. The infusion volume was typically 300 ml given over 3 to 5 minutes. During 323 infusions, only three patients could not be treated, two due to atherosclerosis and one due to hypotension. There were six cerebral ischemic events, three permanent (63).

A Phase I study determined cisplatin could be administered at a dose intensity of 150 mg/m^2/week and a total of 600/m^2 in four doses over 22 days. Higher doses resulted in reversible nephrotoxicity (67). A Phase II study determined that three or four weekly intra-arterial infusions of cisplatin combined with local radiation therapy (1.8 to 2.0 Gy/day in 35 fractions over 7 weeks) were safe and effective. Cisplatin is a potent radiosensitzer. Ninety-one percent of patients had a complete response (CR). The estimated 1-year survival rate was 67%. There were 32 events of National Cancer Institute scale grade 3 or 4 toxicity in 25 of 60 patients; there were no deaths (68).

The investigators continued to treat all eligible candidates over an 8-year period while maintaining a prospective database. In 2000, Robbins et al. reported their results in 213 patients. The overall CR rate in the primary site was 80%. The projected rate of locoregional disease control was 78%; projected 5-year disease-specific and overall survival rates were 53.6% and 38.8%, respectively. There were 95 episodes of grade 3 or 4 toxicity, and six deaths (2.8%). For a patient population with such a poor prognosis, the results suggested improved outcomes with respect to organ preservation and locoregional disease control, and possibly improved overall survival (69).

RADPLAT was subsequently evaluated in a multicenter trial in 53 patients with T4 HNSCC (66).

The CR rate was 85% at the primary site and 88% at nodal regions; the overall CR rate was 80%. The estimated 1-year and 2-year locoregional tumor control rates were 66% and 57%, respectively. The estimated 1-year and 2-year survival rates were 72% and 63%, respectively. The estimated 1-year and 2-year disease-free survival rates were 62% and 46%, respectively. The RADPLAT protocol was feasible and effective at inexperienced centers, although the inexperienced centers had higher rates of grade 4 and 5 toxicities than experienced centers. The investigators concluded there did not seem to be a significant learning curve associated with the technical aspects of the intra-arterial infusion; however, there was a significant learning curve associated with the clinical management of side effects and toxicities.

Many centers have investigated RADPLAT as well as other intra-arterial chemoradiation protocols; almost all report positive results that support further investigations (64, 65). Nonetheless, favorable results have also been reported for a number of combined intravenous chemoinfusion and radiation protocols for locally advanced HNSCC (60). It remains to be determined whether intra-arterial infusion of the chemotherapeutic agent provides a definitive advantage over systemic administration for chemoradiation.

The early results from a Phase III randomized trial comparing RADPLAT to intravenous chemoradiation at five centers in the Netherlands recently were reported (70). Between 2000 and November 2005, 236 patients with advanced, inoperable HNSCC were randomized to intra-arterial or intravenous cisplatin with concomitant radiation therapy. Completion of the treatment plan and toxicities were similar in both groups. There were no significant differences between the intra-arterial and the intravenous groups in 2-year locoregional control (62% vs. 68%, respectively) or survival (61% vs. 63%). The significance of these early data depends on the final analysis of the completed study. Nonetheless, the pharmacokinetic advantage of intra-arterial chemoinfusion, with its highly active anti-tumoral effects and demonstrated technical feasibility and safety, will continue to motivate further investigations into this approach.

CONCLUSION

Interventional neuroradiology contributes a number of valuable diagnostic and therapeutic procedures to the management of patients with head and neck tumors. This dynamic subspecialty will likely offer additional multidisciplinary treatment options for these challenging patients in the future through continuing innovations.

REFERENCES

1. Valavanis A and Christoforidis G. Applications of interventional neuroradiology in the head and neck. Semin Roentgenol, 2000; 35(1): 72–83.
2. Chaloupka JC, Mangla S, Huddle DC, et al. Evolving experience with direct puncture therapeutic embolization for adjunctive and palliative management of head and neck hypervascular neoplasms. Laryngoscope, 1999; 109(11): 1864–1872.
3. Casasco A, Houdart E, Biondi A, et al. Major complications of percutaneous embolization of skull-base tumors. AJNR Am J Neuroradiol, 1999; 20(1): 179–181.
4. Smith TP. Embolization in the external carotid artery. J Vasc Interv Radiol, 2006; 17(12): 1897–1912; quiz 1913.
5. Casasco A, Herbreteau D, Houdart E, et al. Devascularization of craniofacial tumors by percutaneous tumor puncture. AJNR Am J Neuroradiol, 1994; 15(7): 1233–1239.
6. Abud DG, Mounayer C, Benndorf G, et al. Intratumoral injection of cyanoacrylate glue in head and neck paragangliomas. AJNR Am J Neuroradiol, 2004; 25(9): 1457–1462.
7. Gobin YP, Murayama Y, Milanese K, et al. Head and neck hypervascular lesions: Embolization with ethylene vinyl alcohol copolymer – laboratory evaluation in swine and clinical evaluation in humans. Radiology, 2001; 221(2): 309–317.
8. Schick B and Kahle G. Radiological findings in angiofibroma. Acta Radiol, 2000; 41(6): 585–593.
9. Scholtz AW, Appenroth E, Kammen-Jolly K, et al. Juvenile nasopharyngeal angiofibroma: Management and therapy. Laryngoscope, 2001; 111(4 Pt 1): 681–687.
10. Siniluoto TM, Luotonen JP, Tikkakoski TA, et al. Value of pre-operative embolization in surgery for nasopharyngeal angiofibroma. J Laryngol Otol, 1993; 107(6): 514–521.
11. Mistry RC, Qureshi SS, and Gupta S. Juvenile nasopharyngeal angiofibroma: A single institution study. Indian J Cancer, 2005; 42(1): 35–39.
12. Moulin G, Chagnaud C, Gras R, et al. Juvenile nasopharyngeal angiofibroma: Comparison of blood loss during removal in embolized group versus nonembolized group. Cardiovasc Intervent Radiol, 1995; 18(3): 158–161.
13. Li JR, Qian J, Shan XZ, et al. Evaluation of the effectiveness of preoperative embolization in surgery for nasopharyngeal angiofibroma. Eur Arch Otorhinolaryngol, 1998; 255(8): 430–432.
14. Glad H, Vainer B, Buchwald C, et al. Juvenile nasopharyngeal angiofibromas in Denmark 1981–2003: Diagnosis, incidence, and treatment. Acta Otolaryngol, 2007; 127(3): 292–299.
15. da Costa DM, Franche GL, Gessinger RP, et al. Surgical experience with juvenile nasopharyngeal angiofibroma. Ann Otolaryngol Chir Cervicofac, 1992; 109(5): 231–234.
16. Duvall AJ 3rd and Moreano AE. Juvenile nasopharyngeal angiofibroma: Diagnosis and treatment. Otolaryngol Head Neck Surg, 1987; 97(6): 534–540.

17. Petruson K, Rodriguez-Catarino M, Petruson B, et al. Juvenile nasopharyngeal angiofibroma: Long-term results in preoperative embolized and non-embolized patients. Acta Otolaryngol, 2002; 122(1): 96–100.

18. Onerci M, Gumus K, Cil B, et al. A rare complication of embolization in juvenile nasopharyngeal angiofibroma. Int J Pediatr Otorhinolaryngol, 2005; 69(3): 423–428.

19. Horowitz MB, Carrau R, Crammond D, et al. Risks of tumor embolization in the presence of an unrecognized patent foramen ovale: Case report. AJNR Am J Neuroradiol, 2002; 23(6): 982–984.

20. van den Berg R. Imaging and management of head and neck paragangliomas. Eur Radiol, 2005; 15(7): 1310–1318.

21. Persky MS, Setton A, Niimi Y, et al. Combined endovascular and surgical treatment of head and neck paragangliomas – a team approach. Head Neck, 2002; 24(5): 423–431.

22. Wang SJ, Wang MB, Barauskas TM, et al. Surgical management of carotid body tumors. Otolaryngol Head Neck Surg, 2000; 123(3): 202–206.

23. Tikkakoski T, Luotonen J, Leinonen S, et al. Preoperative embolization in the management of neck paragangliomas. Laryngoscope, 1997; 107(6): 821–826.

24. Liu DG, Ma XC, Li BM, et al. Clinical study of preoperative angiography and embolization of hypervascular neoplasms in the oral and maxillofacial region. Oral Surg Oral Med Oral Pathol Oral Radiol Endod, 2006; 101(1): 102–109.

25. Kasper GC, Welling RE, Wladis AR, et al. A multidisciplinary approach to carotid paragangliomas. Vasc Endovascular Surg, 2006; 40(6): 467–474.

26. American Society of Interventional and Therapeutic Neuroradiology. Carotid artery balloon test occlusion. AJNR Am J Neuroradiol, 2001; 22(8 Suppl): S8–S9.

27. Linskey ME, Jungreis CA, Yonas H, et al. Stroke risk after abrupt internal carotid artery sacrifice: accuracy of preoperative assessment with balloon test occlusion and stable xenon-enhanced CT. AJNR Am J Neuroradiol, 1994; 15(5): 829–843.

28. Serbinenko FA. Balloon catheterization and occlusion of major cerebral vessels. J Neurosurg, 1974; 41(2): 125–145.

29. Mathis JM, Barr JD, Jungreis CA, et al. Temporary balloon test occlusion of the internal carotid artery: Experience in 500 cases. AJNR Am J Neuroradiol, 1995; 16(4): 749–754.

30. Meyers PM, Thakur GA, and Tomsick TA. Temporary endovascular balloon occlusion of the internal carotid artery with a nondetachable silicone balloon catheter: Analysis of technique and cost. AJNR Am J Neuroradiol, 1999; 20(4): 559–564.

31. Marshall RS, Lazar RM, Young WL, et al. Clinical utility of quantitative cerebral blood flow measurements during internal carotid artery test occlusions. Neurosurgery, 2002; 50(5): 996–1004; discussion, 1004–1005.

32. van Rooij WJ, Sluzewski M, Slob MJ, et al. Predictive value of angiographic testing for tolerance to therapeutic occlusion of the carotid artery. AJNR Am J Neuroradiol, 2005; 26(1): 175–178.

33. Adams GL, Madison M, Remley K, et al. Preoperative permanent balloon occlusion of internal carotid artery in patients with advanced head and neck squamous cell carcinoma. Laryngoscope, 1999; 109(3): 460–466.

34. Sanna M, Piazza P, Ditrapani G, et al. Management of the internal carotid artery in tumors of the lateral skull base: Preoperative permanent balloon occlusion without reconstruction. Otol Neurotol, 2004; 25(6): 998–1005.

35. Zane RS, Aeschbacher P, Moll C, et al. Carotid occlusion without reconstruction: A safe surgical option in selected patients. Am J Otol, 1995; 16(3): 353–359.

36. de Vries EJ, Sekhar LN, Janecka IP, et al. Elective resection of the internal carotid artery without reconstruction. Laryngoscope, 1988; 98(9): 960–966.

37. Kotapka MJ, Kalia KK, Martinez AJ, et al. Infiltration of the carotid artery by cavernous sinus meningioma. J Neurosurg, 1994; 81(2): 252–255.

38. Browne JD, Fisch U, and Valavanis A. Surgical therapy of glomus vagale tumors. Skull Base Surg, 1993; 3(4): 182–192.

39. de Vries EJ, Sekhar LN, Horton JA, et al. A new method to predict safe resection of the internal carotid artery. Laryngoscope, 1990; 100(1): 85–88.

40. Sekhar LN and Patel SJ. Permanent occlusion of the internal carotid artery during skull-base and vascular surgery: Is it really safe? Am J Otol, 1993; 14(5): 421–422.

41. Kallmes DF and Cloft HJ. The use of hydrocoil for parent artery occlusion. AJNR Am J Neuroradiol, 2004; 25(8): 1409–1410.

42. Ross IB and Buciuc R. The vascular plug: A new device for parent artery occlusion. AJNR Am J Neuroradiol, 2007; 28(2): 385–386.

43. Nussbaum ES, Levine SC, Hamlar D, et al. Carotid stenting and "extarterectomy" in the management of head and neck cancer involving the internal carotid artery: Technical case report. Neurosurgery, 2000; 47(4): 981–984.

44. Sanna M, Khrais T, Menozi R, et al. Surgical removal of jugular paragangliomas after stenting of the intratemporal internal carotid artery: A preliminary report. Laryngoscope, 2006; 116(5): 742–746.

45. Tripp HF, Jr., Fail PS, Beyer MG, et al. New approach to preoperative vascular exclusion for carotid body tumor. J Vasc Surg, 2003; 38(2): 389–391.

46. Cohen JE, Ferrario A, Ceratto R, et al. Covered stent as an innovative tool for tumor devascularization and endovascular arterial reconstruction. Neurol Res, 2003; 25(2): 169–172.

47. Cohen JE, Spektor S, Valarezo J, et al. Endolymphatic sac tumor: Staged endovascular-neurosurgical approach. Neurol Res, 2003; 25(3): 237–440.

48. Chaloupka JC, Putman CM, Citardi MJ, et al. Endovascular therapy for the carotid blowout syndrome in head and neck surgical patients: Diagnostic and managerial considerations. AJNR Am J Neuroradiol, 1996; 17(5): 843–852.

49. Chaloupka JC, Roth TC, Putman CM, et al. Recurrent carotid blowout syndrome: Diagnostic and therapeutic challenges in a newly recognized subgroup of patients. AJNR Am J Neuroradiol, 1999; 20(6): 1069–1077.

50. Cohen J and Rad I. Contemporary management of carotid blowout. Curr Opin Otolaryngol Head Neck Surg, 2004; 12(2): 110–115.

51. Maran AG, Amin M, and Wilson JA. Radical neck dissection: A 19-year experience. J Laryngol Otol, 1989; 103(8): 760–764.

52. Chang FC, Lirng JF, Tai SK, et al. Brain abscess formation: A delayed complication of carotid blowout

syndrome treated by self-expandable stent-graft. AJNR Am J Neuroradiol, 2006; 27(7): 1543–1545.

53. Chang FC, Lirng JF, Luo CB, et al. Carotid blowout syndrome in patients with head-and-neck cancers: Reconstructive management by self-expandable stent-grafts. AJNR Am J Neuroradiol, 2007; 28(1): 181–188.

54. Desuter G, Hammer F, Gardiner Q, et al. Carotid stenting for impending carotid blowout: Suitable supportive care for head and neck cancer patients? Palliat Med, 2005; 19(5): 427–429.

55. Kim HS, Lee DH, Kim HJ, et al. Life-threatening common carotid artery blowout: Rescue treatment with a newly designed self-expanding covered nitinol stent. Br J Radiol, 2006; 79(939): 226–231.

56. Lesley WS, Chaloupka JC, Weigele JB, et al. Preliminary experience with endovascular reconstruction for the management of carotid blowout syndrome. AJNR Am J Neuroradiol, 2003; 24(5): 975–981.

57. Warren FM, Cohen JI, Nesbit GM, et al. Management of carotid "blowout" with endovascular stent grafts. Laryngoscope, 2002; 112(3): 428–433.

58. Simental A, Johnson JT, and Horowitz M. Delayed complications of endovascular stenting for carotid blowout. Am J Otolaryngol, 2003; 24(6): 417–419.

59. Parkin DM, Bray F, Ferlay J, et al. Estimating the world cancer burden: Globocan 2000. Int J Cancer, 2001; 94(2): 153–156.

60. Seiwert TY, Salama JK, and Vokes EE. The chemoradiation paradigm in head and neck cancer. Nat Clin Pract Oncol, 2007; 4(3): 156–171.

61. Sullivan RD. Continuous intra-arterial infusion chemotherapy of head and neck cancer. Trans Am Acad Ophthalmol Otolaryngol, 1962; 66: 111–117.

62. Klopp CT, Smith DF, and Alford TC. Palliation achieved in carcinoma of the head and neck with intra-arterial chemotherapy. Am J Surg, 1961; 102: 830–834.

63. Kerber CW, Wong WH, Howell SB, et al. An organ-preserving selective arterial chemotherapy strategy for head and neck cancer. AJNR Am J Neuroradiol, 1998; 19(5): 935–941.

64. Alkureishi LW, de Bree R, and Ross GL. RADPLAT: An alternative to surgery? Oncologist, 2006; 11(5): 469–480.

65. Robbins KT. Is high-dose intensity intraarterial cisplatin chemoradiotherapy for head and neck carcinoma feasible? Cancer, 2005; 103(3): 447–450.

66. Robbins KT, Kumar P, Harris J, et al. Supradose intra-arterial cisplatin and concurrent radiation therapy for the treatment of stage IV head and neck squamous cell carcinoma is feasible and efficacious in a multi-institutional setting: Results of Radiation Therapy Oncology Group Trial 9615. J Clin Oncol, 2005; 23(7): 1447–1454.

67. Robbins KT, Storniolo AM, Kerber C, et al. Phase I study of highly selective supradose cisplatin infusions for advanced head and neck cancer. J Clin Oncol, 1994; 12(10): 2113–2120.

68. Robbins KT, Kumar P, Regine WF, et al. Efficacy of targeted supradose cisplatin and concomitant radiation therapy for advanced head and neck cancer: The Memphis experience. Int J Radiat Oncol Biol Phys, 1997; 38(2): 263–271.

69. Robbins KT, Kumar P, Wong FS, et al. Targeted chemoradiation for advanced head and neck cancer: Analysis of 213 patients. Head Neck, 2000; 22(7): 687–693.

70. Rasch CR SC, Schornagel JH, et al. Intra-arterial versus intravenous chemoradiation for advanced head and neck cancer, early results of a multi-institutional trial [abstract]. Int J Radiat Oncol Biol Phys, 2006; 66: 51–52.

Musculoskeletal

Chapter 39

PERCUTANEOUS ABLATION OF PAINFUL METASTASES INVOLVING BONE

Matthew R. Callstrom

J. William Charboneau

Skeletal metastases are commonly encountered in cancer patients and often result in great pain and morbidity (1). Autopsy studies have shown that in patients who die from breast, prostate and lung cancer, up to 85% have evidence of bone metastasis at the time of death (2). Severe pain and frequent fractures resulting from metastatic cancer reduce the patients' quality of life and often lead to depression and mood changes.

The current standard of care for cancer patients with localized bone pain is external beam radiation therapy (RT). While most patients experience a reduction of pain, 20% to 30% of patients do not have relief. A recent review of 1,016 patients treated by RT demonstrated complete relief in 53% and partial relief in 83% (3). Additionally, following treatment, there is usually a delay of 4 to 12 weeks before pain relief is achieved, and many patients will experience a return of significant pain within a few months (3). Other conventional therapies have specific, although

limited, usefulness for treating painful metastatic disease. Surgery is usually reserved for fixation of a recent or impending fracture. Chemotherapy is usually ineffective for reduction of bone pain, although bisphosphonate therapy is useful for metastatic breast and prostate cancers (4–7). Radiopharmaceuticals may be of value for treatment of some patients with diffuse bone metastases but is not used for patients with focal painful metastatic disease (8–10).

Because of the limitations of current therapies to provide effective durable palliation of painful metastatic disease, new approaches have emerged for the treatment of these patients. These methods are based on a percutaneous approach using imaging guidance to deliver local therapy in the form of energy deposition, causing local destruction of tissues. High-temperature treatment using radiofrequency ablation (RFA) and low-temperature treatment using cryoablation therapy are most commonly used. This chapter describes patient selection, ablation techniques and the results of both RFA and cryoablation for palliation of focal painful metastases (11–17).

PATIENT SELECTION FOR ABLATION

Patients are considered for local ablative therapy when: 1) Their worst pain on a numerical rating scale is 4 or more on a scale of 10 in a 24-hour period (0 is no pain and 10 is pain as bad as you can imagine). Patients with lower pain scores are not treated because it is difficult to improve on mild pain and because this type of pain can usually be adequately managed by oral analgesics. 2) Their focal pain is limited to one or two sites. Patients with numerous painful lesions are not treated with this technique because this type of pain is better treated with a systemic approach. In addition, pain due to multiple lesions is difficult to adequately localize for directed therapy. 3) The patient's painful metastatic lesion must be amenable to the use of ablative devices. Lesions that are amenable to ablative therapy are typically osteolytic or mixed osteolytic/ osteoblastic in nature or otherwise composed of soft-tissue.

Patients are usually excluded from local ablative therapy when 1) successful treatment would require treating a portion of the lesion located within 1 cm of the spinal cord, brain, aorta, inferior vena cava, bowel or bladder or, 2) there are numerous lesions, as described earlier, or the painful lesion is predominately osteoblastic. Treatment of osteoblastic lesions is technically possible using bone biopsy techniques or with a bone drill for access to the affected area. However, these are infrequently performed because of the difficult access through sclerotic bone and because sclerotic metastases are often multi-focal. Although cryoablation will effectively treat intact bone, RFA energy is poorly delivered into sclerotic bone.

RFA TECHNIQUE

RFA can be administered with either general anesthesia or moderate conscious sedation and patients are often observed overnight in the hospital. A general anesthetic is more commonly used because the level of local pain during the RFA treatment can be greater than most patients can tolerate, even with moderate conscious sedation, and because the procedures can be long – lasting longer than an hour depending on the size of the target lesion. In addition, the use of general anesthesia allows the procedure to be performed without the additional necessity of providing supportive care for the patient as is required with conscious sedation. Epidural spinal anesthesia or focal nerve blocks are often helpful to ease the pain during the immediate post-ablation period. If an epidural catheter is employed, the duration of use is typically for a 12- to 24-hour period following the RFA treatment. Prior to removal of the catheter, the medication delivery is halted for a trial period. If the patient's pain has returned to the pretreatment level or improved, the catheter is removed and the patient is usually discharged with oral opioid analgesics for mild to moderate discomfort or pain.

It is critically important to examine each patient prior to treatment to determine whether the patient's pain corresponds to an identifiable lesion on imaging (Figure 39.1). The targeted area of ablation must include the bone-tumor interface, rather than the central portions of the mass, in order to achieve destruction of likely sites of origin of the pain, including nerve endings and involved periosteum. Either multi-tined electrodes or cool-tip electrodes can be used, depending on physician preference. A single ablation is typically performed for lesions less than 3 cm in diameter, and the time of ablation is typically 5 to 10 minutes at the target temperature of 100°C or until tissue impedance limits energy delivery to the target tissue (Figure 39.2). For larger lesions, overlapping ablations are performed with the goal of treating the entire bone-tumor interface, with the time of

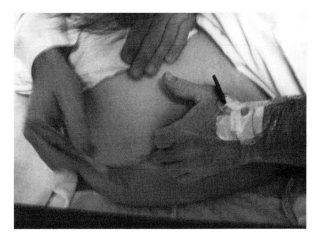

FIGURE 39.1. Patients are physically examined prior to the cryoablation procedure for careful identification of the area of focal pain. The area is marked on the skin and correlated with imaging findings prior to the cryoablation procedure. See Color Plate 33.

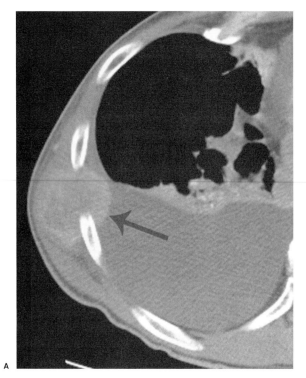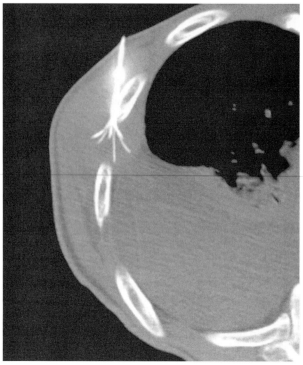

FIGURE 39.2. RFA of a painful metastatic renal cell carcinoma metastasis to a rib and body wall. (A) Contrast-enhanced CT scan demonstrates a 3-cm soft-tissue mass (*arrow*) in the intercostal space with involvement of the adjacent rib. (B) CT during RFA demonstrates the electrode deployed in the mass.

ablation again typically 5 to 10 minutes at the target temperature of 100°C or until tissue impedance limits energy delivery to the target tissue.

Various image-guided methods can be used to reduce the risk of collateral thermal damage to adjacent normal structures. For example, sterile water (usually D5W with the use of RFA to prevent the risk of conduction of energy with buffered fluids) can be injected through a spinal needle to displace loops of bowel away from a target lesion (Figure 39.3). Another method to help ensure safety and to provide feedback during an RFA procedure is to carefully place a temperature-sensing probe adjacent to a critical structure (Figure 39.4). Because the margin of the RFA cannot be accurately visualized with computed tomography (CT) or ultrasonographic (US) imaging (magnetic resonance imaging [MRI] may allow visualization), this thermal monitoring avoids unexpected elevations of temperature and potential injury to adjacent normal structures.

RFA RESULTS

A recent feasibility clinical trial and a subsequent international multicenter clinical trial of percutaneous RFA for treatment of painful metastatic lesions involving bone found that this procedure is safe and provides significant relief of pain (13–15, 17). These trials enrolled patients with persistent worst-pain scoring 4 or more on a scale of 10 in a 24-hour period who had failed to obtain pain relief with conventional treatments.

In the multicenter trial, 95% (59 of 62 patients) experienced a decrease in pain that was considered clinically significant using a predefined validated endpoint (at least a two-point drop in worst pain in a 24-hour period (Figure 39.5) (13). The various types of malignancies treated by RFA as part of this clinical trial are shown in Table 39.1. It is important to note that significant pain relief was obtained following treatment in spite of the fact that these patients had failed conventional therapies, including RT and chemotherapy. In addition to being significant, the duration of pain relief was long.

Patient response to treatment was not a function of the location of the painful lesion, although lesions at risk for impending fracture were not included in the trial. The majority of the treated tumors were located in the pelvis or sacrum, although many were located elsewhere in the body (Table 39.1). Notably, patients who have painful metastases involving the sacrum or presacral region have limited options for pain

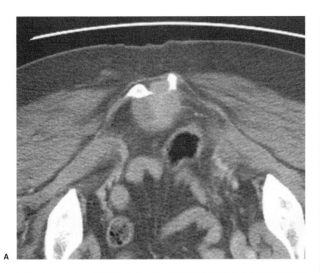

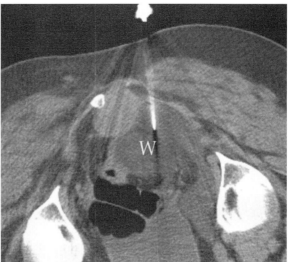

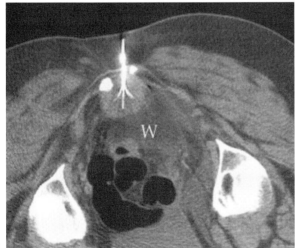

FIGURE 39.3. RFA of painful metastatic carcinoid tumor to sacrum. Water displaces bowel and prevents injury. (A) Prone CT demonstrates a 4-cm soft-tissue mass with associated destruction of the sacrum. A gas-filled loop of rectum is adjacent to the mass. (B) CT image shows needle in soft tissues; water (*W*) displaces rectum away from the tumor. (C) CT image shows RF electrode within tumor.

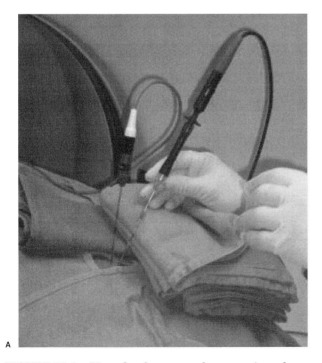

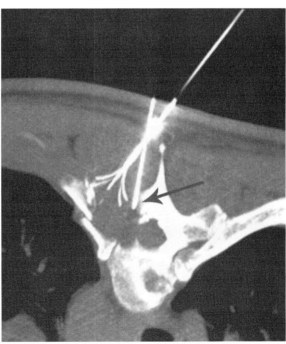

FIGURE 39.4. Use of a thermocouple to monitor elevation in tissue temperature from RFA treatment of a painful melanoma metastasis to the spine. (A) Photograph demonstrates thermocouple adjacent to RFA probe. (B) Prone CT image demonstrates osteolytic destruction of the pedicle of a thoracic vertebral body and adjacent rib, RFA probe in place and thermocouple (*arrow*) between the RFA electrode and the spinal canal.

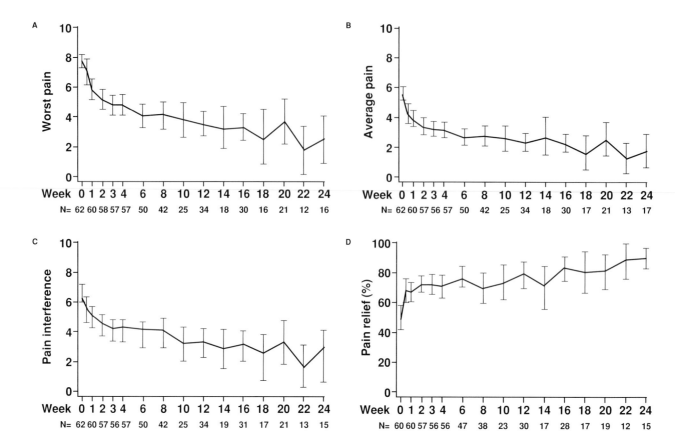

FIGURE 39.5.   Mean BPI pain scores over time for patients treated with RFA. (A) worst pain; (B) average pain; (C) interference of pain in daily activities; (D) pain relief from RFA and medications. Error bars represent the 95% confidence intervals. N = the number of patients completing BPI at each time point. (*From* Callstrom MR, Charboneau JW, Goetz P, et al. Image-guided ablation of painful metastatic bone tumors: A new and effective approach to a difficult problem. Skeletal Radiol 2006;35:1–15; with permission of Springer Science and Business Media.)

relief. These tumors are often secondary to locally recurrent metastatic rectal carcinoma, and unfortunately, the RT and surgical options are limited. RFA or cryoablation provide remarkable relief in most of these patients (Figure 39.6). Care should be taken to avoid ablation of the lumbosacral plexus and S1 nerve root to avoid injury of these important motor nerves. Additionally, bilateral ablation of the S2–S4 nerves must be avoided to prevent resultant incontinence of bladder or bowel function. Caution should be employed with unilateral ablation of the S2–S4 nerves in patients with prior RT to this area or in patients with poor bladder or bowel control.

Following RFA, significant adverse events in the multicenter trial were noted in 4 of 62 (6.5%) patients. Three patients experienced exacerbation of pre-existing tumor-cutaneous fistulas. These occurred when a clinically unrecognized tiny tumor-cutaneous fistula was present in patients with recurrences of mucinous-producing colorectal neoplasm in the presacral region. Following ablation, the increased volume of necrotic tissue was passed along the pre-

existing path of low resistance to the skin. One patient suffered a pathologic fracture after treatment of a large metastasis with involvement of the ilium, ischium and acetabulum. Currently, patients with metastatic lesions at risk for fracture in axial weight-bearing bone are treated with ablation followed by cementoplasty the following day to provide stabilization of the affected bone (Figure 39.7).

EMERGENCE OF PERCUTANEOUS CRYOABLATION

Although RFA is currently the most widely used of the percutaneous ablation methods, cryoablation has a long history of successful treatment of neoplasms, and recent technological advances have resulted in resurgence in its use. For many years, cryoablation has been used to successfully treat tumors of the prostate, kidney, liver and uterus (18–21). First-generation devices were limited to intraoperative use because of their large diameter, the use of liquid nitrogen for tissue cooling and the lack of well-insulated probes.

TABLE 39.1 Characteristics of Patients Treated with Radiofrequency Ablation in a Multicenter Trial

Number of patients	62	
Female	22	(35%)
Male	40	(65%)
Age (median)	64	(range 28–88)
Tumor type (number)		
Renal CA	14	
Colorectal CA	12	
Lung CA	4	
Breast	4	
Sarcoma	3	
Other	25	
Tumor size (longest diameter; cm)	6.3 cm	(range 1.0–18.0)
Tumor location		
Pelvis	19	
Sacrum	12	
Rib	6	
Vertebrae	4	
Other	21	
Prior radiation to treated site	44	(71%)
Concurrent opioid analgesics	52	(84%)

From Callstrom MR, Charboneau JW, Goetz P, et al. Image-guided ablation of painful metastatic bone tumors: A new and effective approach to a difficult problem. Skeletal Radiol, 2006; 35: 1–15; with permission of Springer Science and Business Media.

Current generation cryoprobes are well insulated and have diameters that range from approximately 11 to 17 gauge, allowing placement through the skin into tumors with image-guidance. These cryoprobes achieve tissue cooling by rapid expansion of pressurized room-temperature argon gas in the probe, resulting in rapid cooling, reaching –100°C within a few seconds. Active thawing of the resultant ice-ball is achieved by actively instilling pressurized helium gas, instead of argon gas, into the cryoprobes.

Cryoablation has several unique advantages over RFA for treatment of pain due to metastatic disease. Importantly, the zone of ablation is readily monitored with intermittent CT or MR imaging. The ice-ball that is generated appears as a low-attenuation region with a well-defined margin with both CT and MR imaging (Figure 39.8). The visualized outer edge of the ice-ball, which corresponds 0°C, defines the limits of the zone of ablation. Conversely, the zone of ablation produced by RF is not visible with CT imaging, although it can be estimated with temperature-sensitive MR pulse sequences. This limitation is important for two critical reasons: 1) treatment of lesions with RFA in close proximity to vital structures, including large nerves or the bowel or bladder, is difficult, and a large safety margin must be maintained to avoid injury, and 2) complete ablation of metastatic lesions is not readily achieved with RFA because the zone of ablation can only be estimated.

Cryoablation also allows the simultaneous use of multiple cryoprobes, which allows complete ablation of large lesions (up to approximately 8 cm diameter) in a single session while avoiding leaving residual neoplasm as is possible between sequential single overlapping ablations (Figure 39.8) (22). Although multiple RFA electrode and microwave generators are becoming available, simultaneous operation is limited by a lack of visualization of the ablation zone during the procedure using US or CT monitoring.

Treatment of metastatic lesions is often complicated by close proximity of adjacent normal structures. In order to achieve complete or sufficient

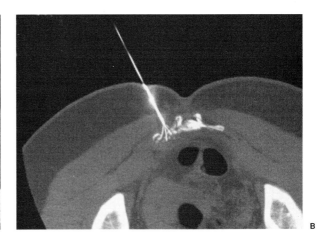

FIGURE 39.6. RFA of a painful sacral metastasis from urachal carcinoma. Patient experienced complete relief of pain following treatment for 3 years, until the time of her death. (A) Prone CT demonstrates osteolytic destruction of the lower aspect of a portion of the sacrum (*arrow*). (B) RFA electrode deployed in the tumor.

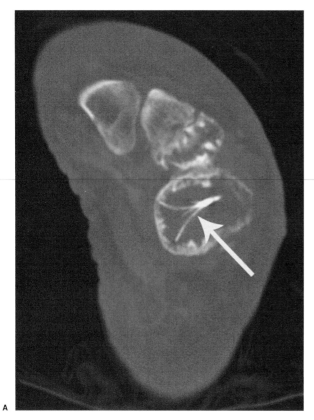

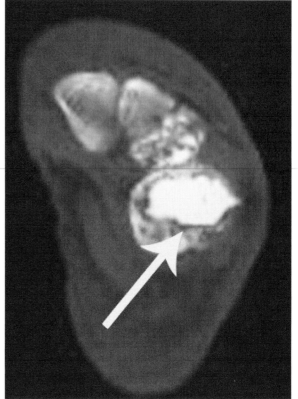

A

B

FIGURE 39.7. RFA and cementoplasty of a painful lung carcinoma metastasis to the cuboid. Patient had been unable to walk for several months prior to the procedure and had complete relief of pain and was able to resume walking without subsequent fracture of the treated site. **(A)** Axial CT image demonstrates RFA electrode (*arrow*) in the osteolytic cuboid metastasis. **(B)** Axial CT image demonstrates bone cement (*arrow*) filling the cuboid. The cementoplasty procedure was performed 1 day after the RFA procedure.

ablation of a target lesion, it is often necessary to displace these adjacent normal structures with sterile fluid or gas. However, these techniques do not always result in adequate displacement and, in the case of RFA, the treatment may fail to completely ablate the target lesion in order to avoid collateral damage to the adjacent normal tissues. In contrast, the cryoablation procedure is compatible with the use of tissue-displacement devices, such as balloons, that allow further safe displacement of adjacent structures with resultant safe complete ablation of the target lesion (Figure 39.9).

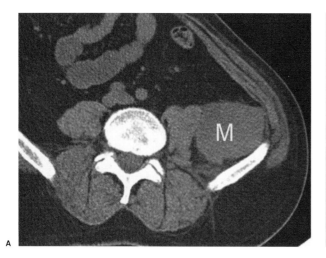

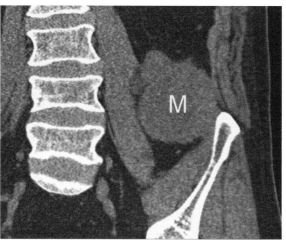

A

B

FIGURE 39.8. Cryoablation of a large retroperitoneal metastasis from thyroid carcinoma. **(A)** Axial and **(B)** coronal CT images demonstrate a 7-cm diameter metastasis (*M*) in the retroperitoneum anterior and superior to the left iliac bone.

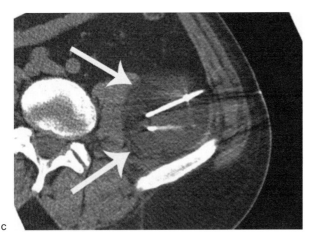

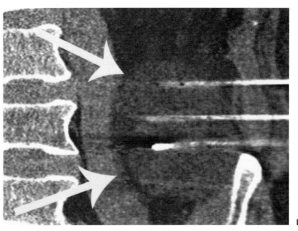

FIGURE 39.8. *(Continued)* **(C)** Axial and **(D)** coronal CT images during the cryoablation procedure demonstrate a large ice-ball (*white arrows*) surrounding the mass. A total of eight cryoprobes were operated simultaneously.

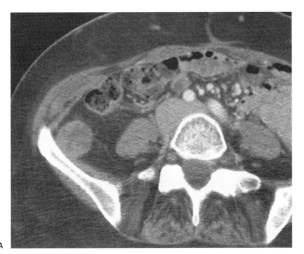

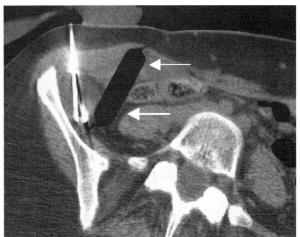

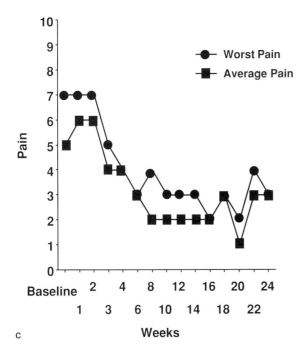

FIGURE 39.9. Metastatic ovarian cancer abutting the right iliac bone resulting in 7/10 worst pain in a 24-hour period prior to treatment. **(A)** Contrast-enhanced CT of the pelvis demonstrates a metastatic mass in the right pelvis. **(B)** Non-contrast CT of the pelvis showing two cryoprobes placed into the lesion, with an ice-ball encompassing the lesion. A balloon was deployed at the time of the procedure to displace the adjacent ascending colon (*arrows*). **(C)** Worst and average pain scores over a 24-hour period at baseline and over a 2-year follow-up period. (*From* Callstrom MR, Charboneau JW, Goetz P, et al. Image-guided ablation of painful metastatic bone tumors: A new and effective approach to a difficult problem. Skeletal Radiol, 2006; 35: 1–15; with permission of Springer Science and Business Media.)

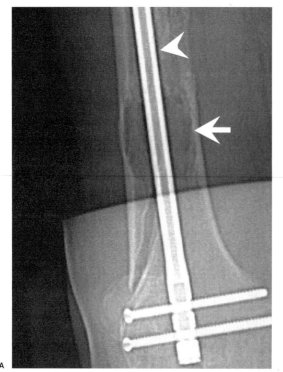
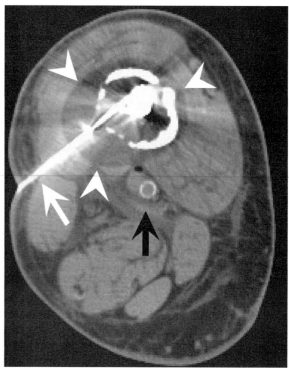

FIGURE 39.10. (A) Plain film radiograph of the right femur demonstrates an intramedullary rod (*arrowhead*) across an osteolytic destructive mid-diaphyseal metastasis (*arrow*) with a pathologic fracture. (B) Axial CT image demonstrates the ice-ball (*white arrowheads*) generated by the percutaneously placed probes (*white arrow*) encompasses the destructive lesion without involving the adjacent vessels and nerves (*black arrow*). The small amount of gas adjacent to the femoral vein resulted from instillation of a small amount of saline in this region. The patient was unable to walk more than a short distance with the assistance of a cane prior to the procedure, with worst pain of 8/10. Twelve weeks following cryoablation treatment, he was walking without a cane, with worst pain of 3/10. (*From* Callstrom MR, Charboneau JW. Percutaneous ablation: Safe, effective treatment of bone tumors. Oncology, 2005 Oct; 19(11 Suppl 4): 22–26; with permission.)

Most patients treated with RFA experience substantial pain during the procedure, which typically requires general anesthesia for adequate pain control. In addition, most of these patients experience a substantial increase in their typical pain for 8 to 12 hours post procedure. This pain is sufficiently great that intravenous opioid analgesia alone poorly controls the pain, and additional regional anesthesia, such as via epidural catheters and nerve blocks, is necessary for adequate pain control. In contrast, the cryoablation procedure can be performed with moderate conscious sedation without significant pain reported by the patient. Additionally, patients have improved or unchanged pain in the immediate post-cryoablation recovery period that is readily managed with intravenous analgesia (Figure 39.10).

The primary disadvantage of cryoablation is that the procedure requires greater time to perform than RFA. On average, a cryoablation treatment requires approximately 2 hours of procedural time. In our hands, this is approximately 30 to 60 minutes longer than what is needed for the same procedure to be performed with RFA, despite usually needing multiple overlapping ablations with RFA. This increased time is also despite the relatively rapid ablation portion of the procedure, which utilizes a single freeze-thaw-freeze cycle that is typically 10-5-10 minutes, respectively. The increased time of the cryoablation procedure is primarily due to the careful placement of multiple cryoprobes in a manner that allows complete or near-complete ablation of the target lesion. In addition, achieving local control of the target lesion is possible with cryoablation and, in these cases, ablation of the target lesion with a sufficient margin of normal tissue requires additional time for placement of the cryoprobes to achieve this goal. Another disadvantage of cryoablation is that the equipment is more cumbersome to use, with the need for placement of multiple probes adjacent to one another with the necessary connections to the cryoprobe controller. The cryoprobes are also one-time use only, and the use of multiple probes increases the

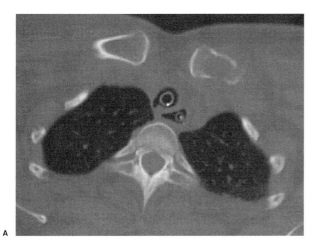

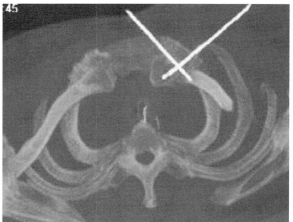

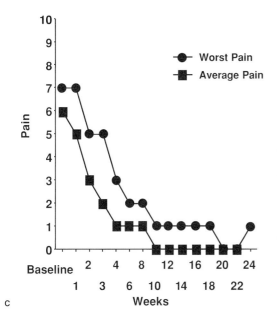

FIGURE 39.11. Metastatic paraganglioma involving the clavicular head treated with cryoablation. (A) Noncontrast CT demonstrates an osteolytic lesion involving the left clavicle. The lesion caused 7/10 worst pain in a 24-hour period prior to treatment. (B) 3D volumetric CT image showing two cryoprobes placed into the lesion. (C) Worst and average pain scores over a 24-hour period at baseline and over a 2-year follow-up period. (*From* Callstrom MR, Charboneau JW, Goetz P, et al. Image-guided ablation of painful metastatic bone tumors: A new and effective approach to a difficult problem. Skeletal Radiol, 2006; 35: 1–15; with permission of Springer Science and Business Media.)

cost of the procedure beyond the typical cost of the corresponding RFA procedure.

CRYOABLATION TECHNIQUE

Two vendors, Endocare Inc. (Irvine, CA) and Galil Medical (Plymouth Meeting, PA), produce 2.4-mm and 1.7-mm diameter (11- and 13-gauge) and 1.2-mm diameter (17-gauge) cryoprobes, respectively. Both products use argon gas expansion through an orifice located in the sealed needle to cause rapid cooling (Joule-Thompson principle). The size of the ice-ball that is generated varies depending on the length of uninsulated tip, the volume of gas passing through the probe and the time of freezing. Given relative cellular tolerance to freezing temperatures, complete cell death occurs within about 3 mm internal to the ice-ball margin (23, 24).

In most cases, the cryoprobes are placed in a parallel arrangement approximately 2 cm apart with probes on the periphery of the tumor 1 cm from the outer margin, with complete coverage of the soft-tissue/bone interface (Figure 39.8). In some cases, a perpendicular arrangement allows a more complete coverage of the area (Figure 39.11). US imaging can be used to guide cryoprobe placement for lesions that are superficially located. In most cases, CT imaging is then used for monitoring the formation of the ice-ball because only the most superficial margin of the ice is seen by US imaging due to an impenetrable acoustic shadow on the leading edge of the ice.

A single cryoprobe is placed for lesions of 3 cm or less in diameter. For larger lesions (greater than 5 cm in diameter), the entire lesion is often not completely treated; rather, ablation treatments are focused on the margin of the lesion involving bone with the goal of treating the soft-tissue/bone interface. A freeze-passive thaw-freeze cycle is performed for each lesion with a goal of 10-5-10 minutes, respectively, for the cycle. Shorter or longer freezing times are used depending on the adequacy of coverage of the lesion and the proximity of adjacent critical structures. Limited non-contrast CT imaging is performed as often as every 2 minutes throughout the freezing portions of the cycle, with body window and level settings

(W400, L40), to monitor the growth of the ice-ball. Following completion of the final freeze of the cryoablation, the cryoprobes are warmed with active heating via helium gas until the temperature(s) reach above 20°C. The cryoprobes are then withdrawn.

Cryoablation may also be used for the treatment of patients with painful metastases at risk for fracture in axial-loading locations such as a vertebral body or in the periacetabular region when the treated lesion is augmented with cementoplasty (Figure 39.12). In our

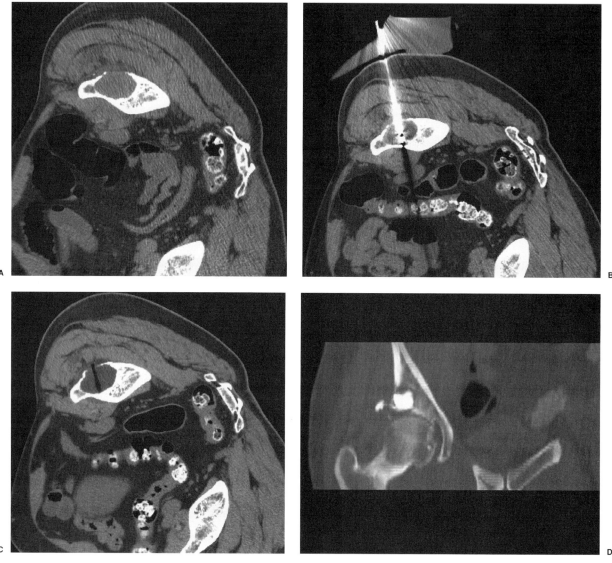

FIGURE 39.12. Pain palliation and stabilization of a non-small cell lung cancer metastatic lesion involving the periacetabular region using cryoablation followed by cementoplasty. **(A)** Non–contrast-enhanced CT of the pelvis demonstrates an osteolytic lesion in the left supra-acetabular region. The patient had difficulty walking without the use of a cane prior to the procedure. **(B)** Non-contrast CT of the pelvis showing two cryoprobes placed into the lesion. **(C)** Non-contrast CT of the pelvis immediately following removal of the cryoprobes (linear shows the low-attenuation ice-ball encompassing the malignant lesion). **(D)** 3D volumetric image showing methylmethacrylate cement filling the supra-acetabular defect. The patient also received 3000 cGy in 10 fractions. Patient continues to be pain-free and walking normally 11 months after the treatment. (*From* Callstrom MR, Charboneau JW, Goetz P, et al. Image-guided ablation of painful metastatic bone tumors: A new and effective approach to a difficult problem. Skeletal Radiol, 2006; 35: 1–15; with permission of Springer Science and Business Media.)

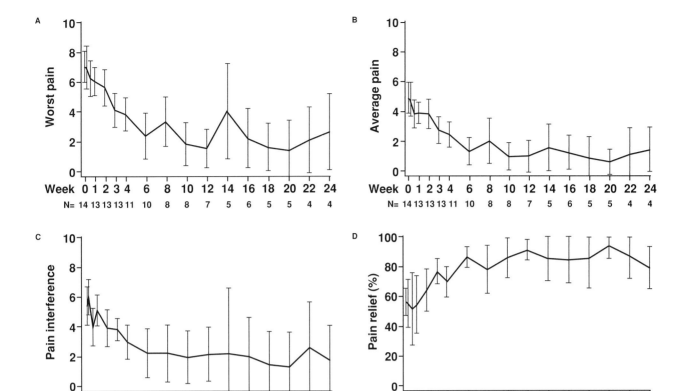

FIGURE 39.13. Mean BPI pain scores over time for patients treated with cryoablation. (A) worst pain; (B) average pain; (C) interference of pain in daily activities; (D) pain relief from cryoablation and medications. Error bars represent the 95% confidence intervals. N = the number of patients completing BPI at each time point. (*From* Callstrom MR, Atwell TD, Charboneau JW, et al. Painful metastases involving bone: Percutaneous image-guided cryoablation – prospective trial interim analysis. Radiology, 2006; 241: 572–580; with permission.)

practice, these procedures are performed on successive days. This 2-day treatment schedule is followed rather than performing the procedures serially on the same day for two reasons: 1) It takes approximately 30 minutes to 1 hour for the ice-ball to completely thaw, depending on the size of the treated lesion; and 2) we typically perform the cryoablation procedure with general anesthesia, and the cementoplasty procedure requires only minimal conscious sedation.

CRYOABLATION RESULTS

As part of an ongoing prospective clinical trial, we have used cryoablation to treat 14 patients with painful metastatic disease involving bone. An interim analysis of the patients treated to date found clinically significant reductions in pain (25). Prior to cryoablation, the mean score for worst pain in a 24-hour period was 6.7/10. Four, six and eight weeks following cryoablation, the mean score for worst pain in a 24-hour period dropped to 3.8/10, 2.5/10 and 3/10.

Four weeks following treatment, 7 of 11 patients (64%, exact binomial confidence interval: 31% to 89%) experienced at least a three-point decrease in worst pain (a two-point reduction in pain is considered clinically significant). Over the course of the follow-up period of 24 weeks, 12 of 14 patients (86%, exact 95% binomial confidence interval: 57% to 98%) reported at least a three-point drop in worst pain over the past 24-hour period (Figure 39.13).

The characteristics of this patient population and the response to therapy were similar to patients treated in the multicenter RFA trial described earlier. Although this study did not directly compare RFA and cryoablation methods for palliation of pain due to metastatic disease, patients' reported pain scores following cryoablation are statistically similar to pain scores found after RFA. Importantly, patients who participated in this trial also reported an improved quality of life following treatment. There were no significant adverse effects in these patients, and no patient required an epidural catheter for immediate post-procedural pain control.

CONCLUSION

It is clear that RFA and cryoablation are safe and effective treatments for the palliation of painful metastatic lesions refractory to standard therapies. Importantly, the quality of life for these patients is improved after therapy. A single ablation treatment is effective in most patients, is well tolerated and provides a long duration of pain relief.

REFERENCES

1. Mercadante S. Malignant bone pain: Pathophysiology and treatment. Pain, 1997: 1–18.
2. Nielsen OS, Munro AJ, and Tannock IF. Bone metastases: Pathophysiology and management policy. J Clin Oncol 1991; 9: 509–524.
3. Tong D, Gillick L, and Hendrickson FR. The palliation of symptomatic osseous metastases: Final results of the Study by the Radiation Therapy Oncology Group. Cancer, 1982 Sep 1; 50(5): 893–899.
4. Wong R and Wiffen PJ. Bisphosphonates for the relief of pain secondary to bone metastases. Cochrane Database Syst Rev, 2002(2): CD002068.
5. Fulfaro F, Casuccio A, Ticozzi C, et al. The role of bisphosphonates in the treatment of painful metastatic bone disease: A review of phase III trials. Pain, 1998; 78: 157–169.
6. Lipton A. Bisphosphonates and breast carcinoma. Cancer, 1997; 80: 1668–1673.
7. Yuen KK, Shelley M, Sze WM, et al. Bisphosphonates for advanced prostate cancer. Cochrane Database Syst Rev, 2006(4): CD006250.
8. Pons F, Herranz R, Garcia A, et al. Strontium-89 for palliation of pain from bone metastases in patients with prostate and breast cancer. Eur J Nucl Med, 1997; 24(10): 1210–1214.
9. Piffanelli A, Dafermou A, Giganti M, et al. Radionuclide therapy for painful bone metastases. An Italian multicentre observational study. Writing Committee of an Ad Hoc Study Group. Quarterly Journal of Nuclear Medicine, 2001; 45(1): 100–107.
10. Robinson RG, Preston DF, Schiefelbein M, et al. Strontium 89 therapy for the palliation of pain due to osseous metastases. JAMA, 1995; 274(5): 420–424.
11. Callstrom MR, Atwell TD, Charboneau JW, et al. Percutaneous image-guided cryoablation of painful metastases involving bone: Prospective trial interim analysis. Radiology, 2006 Nov; 241(2):572–580.
12. Callstrom MR and Charboneau JW. Percutaneous ablation: Safe, effective treatment of bone tumors. Oncology, 2005 Oct; 19(11 Suppl 4): 22–26.
13. Callstrom MR, Charboneau JW, Goetz MP, et al. Image-guided ablation of painful metastatic bone tumors: A new and effective approach to a difficult problem. Skeletal Radiol, 2006; 35: 1–15.
14. Callstrom MR, Charboneau JW, Goetz MP, et al. Painful metastases involving bone: Feasibility of percutaneous CT- and US-guided radio-frequency ablation. Radiology, 2002 Jul; 224(1): 87–97.
15. Goetz M, Rubin J, Callstrom M, et al. Percutaneous US and CT-guided radiofrequency ablation of painful metastases involving bone. ASCO, 2002 May 24–30: 1544.
16. Callstrom MR, Johnson CD, Fletcher JG, et al. CT colonography without cathartic preparation: Feasibility study. Radiology, 2001 Jun; 219(3): 693–698.
17. Goetz MP, Callstrom MR, Charboneau JW, et al. Percutaneous image-guided radiofrequency ablation of painful metastases involving bone: A multicenter study. J Clin Oncol, 2004 Jan 15; 22(2): 300–306.
18. Desai MM, Gill IS. Current status of cryoablation and radiofrequency ablation in the management of renal tumors. Curr Opin Urol, 2002 Sep; 12(5): 387–393.
19. Onik G. Image-guided prostate cryosurgery: State of the art. Cancer Control, 2001 Nov-Dec; 8(6): 522–531.
20. Zhou XD, Tang ZY. Cryotherapy for primary liver cancer. Semin Surg Oncol, 1998 Mar; 14(2): 171–174.
21. Cowan BD, Sewell PE, Howard JC, et al. Interventional magnetic resonance imaging cryotherapy of uterine fibroid tumors: Preliminary observation. Am J Obstet Gynecol, 2002 Jun; 186(6): 1183–1187.
22. Dodd GD, 3rd, Frank MS, Aribandi M, et al. Radiofrequency thermal ablation: Computer analysis of the size of the thermal injury created by overlapping ablations. AJR Am J Roentgenol, 2001 Oct; 177(4): 777–782.
23. Chosy SG, Nakada SY, Lee FT, Jr., et al. Monitoring renal cryosurgery: Predictors of tissue necrosis in swine. J Urol, 1998 Apr; 159(4): 1370–1374.
24. Campbell SC, Krishnamurthi V, Chow G, et al. Renal cryosurgery: Experimental evaluation of treatment parameters. Urology, 1998 Jul; 52(1): 29–33; discussion, 33–24.
25. Callstrom MR, Atwell TD, Charboneau JW, et al. Painful metastases involving bone: Percutaneous image-guided cryoablation – prospective trial interim analysis. Radiology, 2006 Nov; 241(2): 572–580.

Chapter 40

INTRA-ARTERIAL THERAPY FOR SARCOMAS

Mihkail C. S. S. Higgins

Michael C. Soulen

SCOPE

Soft-tissue sarcomas comprise roughly 1% of all malignant tumors and occur in about 8300 patients in the United States each year (1). In spite of progress in the diagnosis and treatment of sarcomas, still, more than 50% of patients die annually from this rare malignancy (2). Two thousand of these tumors arise in bone. The remainder mainly arise from mesodermal soft tissues anywhere in the body, with 60% of these soft-tissue sarcomas being found in the extremities. Most sarcomas are sporadic, but occasionally they are associated with trauma, foreign bodies, chemical carcinogens, radiation or genetic disorders such as neurofibromatosis, Gardner's syndrome, certain gene mutations or chromosomal abnormalities. A viral etiology exists for several animal sarcomas, with Kaposi's sarcoma being the most common virally induced sarcoma in humans.

At present, the relevant prognostic factors for soft-tissue sarcoma as defined in the stage classification system of the American Joint Committee on Cancer (AJCC) include grade, size and depth relative to the superficial investing muscular fascia (3). In addition to the aforementioned factors, large prospective databases relate the treatment and prognosis of soft-tissue sarcomas to location (4, 5), microscopic margin positivity (6), histopathologic subtype (7) and presentation status (primary tumor vs. local recurrence). Sarcomas are classified histologically as low or high grade, with high-grade tumors being more aggressive and therefore more likely to recur locally or distantly after resection of the primary. Tumors larger than 5 cm have a worse prognosis than tumors smaller than 5 cm.

Although local control of extremity and superficial trunk sarcomas can be rendered in more than 90% of treated patients with limb-sparing multimodal treatment regimens, sarcomas in other anatomic sites prove more difficult to control, particularly due to the delay in disease presentation and hence diagnosis, the presence of juxtaposing vital neurovascular or osseous structures and the violation of deep anatomic compartments, prohibiting wide excision (8). Positive microscopic resection margins markedly reduce the local recurrence-free survival rate for soft-tissue sarcomas, with the exception of primary fibrosarcoma and retroperitoneal sarcomas. The prognostic value of positive microscopic margins may be limited to anatomic primary tumor sites in the extremity. The cell type of the sarcoma is of some prognostic importance; synovial sarcoma and rhabdomyosarcomas are typically very aggressive, leiomyosarcoma and malignant peripheral nerve tumor pathology have been shown to be independent adverse prognostic factors for disease-specific survival, whereas extremity liposarcoma and fibrosarcoma tend to be less fatal, suggesting a more indolent pathology (7).

The initial assessment of grade, size and location determines the type of therapy appropriate for an individual patient. Small, low-grade tumors are well treated by wide surgical resection when their location permits. Excision with a 2-cm-wide negative margin is usually curative. Large, high-grade tumors have a 50% recurrence rate after excision alone. Because of this, amputation was the treatment of choice for many years. Amputation provides excellent local control but results in significant disability for the patient, many of whom will go on to die from distant metastases anyway. Over the past two decades, a multimodality approach that combines surgery with adjuvant or neoadjuvant radiation therapy or chemotherapy has evolved. The goals of the multimodality approach are three-fold: limb-sparing resection with preservation of function, prevention of local recurrence and control of distant metastases.

RADIOLOGICAL STAGING OF SARCOMAS

Proper staging and planning of multimodality therapy for sarcomas require assessment of the size and anatomic extent of the tumor relative to the affected tissue compartment, determination of involvement of adjacent neurovascular structures and regional nodes, evaluation for distant metastases and the histologic grading of the tumor. The latter is determined by biopsy, the former by magnetic resonance imaging and angiography (MRI/MRA) or enhanced computed tomographic (CT) examination. CT examination of the chest and a bone scan complete the metastatic work-up. Angiography is rarely required for diagnosis or staging.

Preoperative angiography is useful for large retroperitoneal or abdominal sarcomas when the organ of origin is uncertain and for assessing venous invasion (9). Defining the blood supply to the tumor can help distinguish a primary retroperitoneal mass from an adrenal or renal primary tumor. Retroperitoneal sarcomas are supplied by the lumbar arteries, but can also be fed by branches of the celiac, mesenteric and renal arteries. Retroperitoneal leiomyosarcomas can arise from the inferior vena cava primarily (5%) or involve the inferior vena cava (IVC) along with an extravascular mass (33%).

Primary and metastatic sarcomas of bone and soft tissue tend to be hypervascular, and a greater degree of hypervascularity correlates with higher histologic grade for some sarcomas. Preoperative angiography of extremity sarcomas is useful for planning intra-arterial therapy and surgical resection (10). Encasement of major vessels may require vascular bypass as part of the limb reconstruction or preclude limb-salvage surgery altogether. Patency of runoff vessels and of the palmar or pedal arches must be determined prior to resection of tibial or forearm arteries.

LIMB-SPARING RESECTION OF EXTREMITY SARCOMAS

Over the past 20 years, much progress has been made in the approach to soft-tissue sarcomas, with the emphasis being on streamlining treatment while preserving local control. Despite this, it has been difficult to recommend an evidence-based treatment plan due to the rarity of these tumors, the variation in their presentation, the diversity of tumor responsiveness and the varying therapeutic approach used among institutions. Modern surgical techniques, including bone and neurovascular grafts, homologous and prosthetic joints and vascularized plastic reconstructions, still permit resection with preservation of a functional limb in 85% to 95% of cases. However, there has been a move from aggressive limb resections to function-preserving surgery plus radiation for the majority of patients with localized tumors. Tumors that are high grade, larger than 5 cm and with margins less than 10 mm require adjuvant or neoadjuvant therapy to prevent local recurrence (6). Bulky tumors, in particular, tend to benefit from preoperative therapy that reduces the tumor size, therefore creating well-demarcated margins to aid in clear tumor excision.

Preoperative Radiation Therapy

Many treatment regimens aimed at local control of soft-tissue sarcomas employ surgical resection plus radiotherapy, with local control being achieved in 70% to 100% of patients at 2 to 10 years. In most series, local control is better than 90% except for large tumors with poor margins (11, 12). The major problems with preoperative radiotherapy are wound complications and limb dysfunction due to fibrosis or radionecrosis. Wound complications occur in 16% to 40% of patients, about one half of whom will require a second operation (13, 14). Secondary amputation or, rarely, death due to wound complications occur in 1% to 7% of patients. Predictive factors for wound complications are preoperative radiation dose and size of excision. Ten percent to 20 percent of salvaged limbs never regain function due to late effects of radiation (15). Reduction in preoperative radiation dose decreases complications at the expense of local control (16). Despite the local control promoted by adjuvant radiotherapy, attempts to identify subsets of patients who do not need radiation therapy are being made. This is due to the fact that radiation offers no survival benefit, and at the same time promotes significant short- and long-term risks such as edema, fibrosis and second malignancies. At present, patient groups possibly benefiting from surgery alone comprise those with T1a disease and those with T1b and T2(a and b) disease when microscopic margins are clearly negative and when tumor-free margins exceed 1 cm.

Preoperative versus Postoperative Radiation Therapy

Similar benefits have been seen from this multimodal approach whether radiation is given preoperatively or postoperatively. Typically, preoperative external-beam radiation is given in the range of 40 to 50 Gy, administered in 200-cGy daily fractions, followed in most patients by a postoperative boost to a total of 60 to 66 Gy, whereas postoperative external-beam radiation tends to be 60 to 66 Gy (17, 18). Because the goal of every therapy is to maximize local tumor control and optimize function, for external-beam treatment, preoperative radiotherapy warrants smaller field sizes and lower doses. Because reduced doses correlate with increased functional outcome, preoperative radiotherapy is often preferred in large high-grade tumors with poor margins. Due to the high percentage (35%) of wound complications (mostly acute and generally reversible) reported in patients receiving preoperative radiotherapy versus the wound complications (17%) reported in postoperative radiation procedures (mostly late and irreversible), sequencing recommendations remain complex (18). Because patients treated with preoperative radiation with upper extremity tumors (43%) have demonstrated fewer wound complications than those with lower extremity tumors, patients with an upper extremity tumor may be considered for preoperative radiation. Given the reduced likelihood of radiation-associated wound complications associated with upper extremity tumors and the lower risk of treatment-related edema and fibrosis associated with preoperative radiation, this recommendation is very attractive. Moreover, when dose and field issues are most critical, preoperative radiotherapy is often preferable, particularly in the arms, where, in addition to offering a low risk of wound

complications, it allows further protection to lung and joint tissue, while restricting radiation exposure to the skin and to vital structures such as the brachial plexus. In spite of varying reports of physical function and wound complications, preoperative and postoperative approaches demonstrate similar high levels of local control for extremity soft-tissue sarcoma without any marked variation in progression-free survival rates (18).

Intraoperative electron radiotherapy (IOERT) has recently emerged and is being used to treat surgical sites that may contain undiagnosed malignancy after limb-sparing surgical resection of extremity soft-tissue sarcomas. During limb-sparing surgery, it demonstrates an ability to allow for increases in radiation dose without 90-day or late wound complication rates when combined with preoperative or postoperative external-beam radiotherapy for patients with extremity soft-tissue sarcomas (19). By reducing early and late radiation-related morbidity through IOERT while maximizing residual occult tumor cell necrosis, the therapeutic gain for a multimodal approach using IOERT, limb-sparing surgery and external-beam radiation therapy for treatment of extremity soft-tissue sarcomas can be enhanced. In an effort to maintain local control, some centers have also evaluated preoperative chemotherapy, either combined with reduced radiation doses or in place of preoperative radiation. In one notable case, a randomized trial of the radiation sensitizer razoxane in 82 patients with locally advanced disease demonstrated increased response rates for radiotherapy paired with razoxane compared with photon irradiation alone (74% vs. 49%, respectively) in addition to higher rates of local control (64% vs. 30%, respectively; $p \leq 0.05$) (20).

Neoadjuvant Chemotherapy

High-grade soft-tissue sarcomas treated by surgery alone have local recurrence rates as high as 70% to 90% (21). Patients with high-grade soft-tissue sarcomas who are intended to receive adjuvant therapy could benefit from preoperative (neoadjuvant) therapy (16). Cytoreduction is thought to decrease the breadth of excision and hence the morbidity of the surgical procedure, in turn making limb salvage an option for patients with tumors otherwise treated by amputation. Preoperative chemotherapy also permits earlier initiation of systemic therapy, without the customary delay for wound healing after surgery. Blood supply to the periphery of the tumor is undisturbed, providing optimal delivery of chemotherapeutic drugs to the cells most likely to be responsible for local recurrence or dissemination during surgery. Unfortunately, response rates of sarcomas to systemic chemotherapy are only 15% to 30%, with relatively little tumor necrosis found on pathological examination after resection. Responses tend to be slow, requiring multiple courses of chemotherapy over months, with consequent delay of surgery. Preoperative administration of systemic chemotherapy has not significantly improved limb-salvage rates.

Because preoperative chemotherapy regimens have, in most cases, been given with radiation treatment, there has been much debate surrounding the relative contributions of one modality versus the other, thus making interpretation of results from these studies difficult. In a collaboration between the Radiation Therapy Oncology (RTOG) and the Massachusetts General Hospital (MGH), patients were given 2.5 g/m^2 of infusional ifosfamide daily for 3 days, 60 mg/m^2 doxorubicin and 675 mg/m^2 decarbazine (DTIC) every 3 weeks with split-course external-beam irradiation (4400 cGy, 2200 divided evenly between each of the first two cycles of chemotherapy) (22). Three rounds of an identical chemotherapy regimen were also administered postoperatively. Grade 4 toxicities (neutropenia, 66%; skin toxicity, 12%; thrombocytopenia, 29%), in addition to a 7% infection rate, were reported. Despite this, preoperative chemotherapy and radiotherapy were performed in 88% and 93% of patients, respectively, with wound healing in the absence of infection taking longer than expected in 26% of patients. Two-year survival was nearly 95%.

In a published report from the Mayo Clinic Group, neoadjuvant IMAP (ifosfamide, mitomycin, doxorubicin and cisplatin) + granulocyte macrophage-colony stimulating factor (GM-CSF) was administered to patients with large high-grade soft-tissue sarcomas (23). Patients were given 4500 cGy of external-beam irradiation along with reduced-dose chemotherapy and 1000 cGy of radiotherapy intraoperatively or postoperatively. Two-year freedom from metastases was roughly 85%, and 5-year survival was estimated at 80%.

Intra-arterial Chemotherapy

Experimental studies have shown that regional intra-arterial delivery of chemotherapeutic drugs to the limb increases tissue concentrations by a factor of 4 to 10 (24, 25). Cisplatinum, doxorubicin, and 5-fluorouracil do not undergo significant first-pass extraction in the extremities and therefore can be delivered regionally without sacrificing systemic levels. Transient balloon occlusion can increase local tissue levels by another order of magnitude (25).

Intra-arterial Chemotherapy for Osteosarcoma

At M.D. Anderson Cancer Center, 96 patients with osteosarcomas of the extremities were treated with intravenous (IV) doxorubicin (90 mg/m^2/96 hours) followed by intra-arterial (IA) cisplatin (120 to 160 mg/m^2/2 hours) (26). Cycles were repeated monthly for an average of four treatments. The limb-salvage rate increased from 8% to 80% with the use of regional therapy. Sixty-eight percent of the tumors had 90% or greater necrosis. The local recurrence rate was only 6%, less than the local failure rate after amputation. Five-year disease-free survival was about 60% overall; close to 80% among patients with a good pathologic response (≥90% necrosis), but only 30% among patients with less than or up to 90% tumor necrosis, despite the addition of high-dose methotrexate to the postoperative systemic chemotherapy regimens for patients with a poor response. Long-term survival in this series was similar to that seen with amputation and adjuvant chemotherapy, indicating no loss of survival with neoadjuvant therapy and limb-sparing resection.

At the Istituto Rizzoli in Italy, 144 patients were treated with IV methotrexate (8 gm/m^2/6 hours), IV doxorubicin (60 mg/m^2/8 hours), and IA cisplatin (120 mg/m^2/72 hours) for two cycles prior to resection (27).[27] All three drugs were continued systemically after surgery, with ifosfamide and etoposide (VP-16) added for patients with a poor pathologic response. Limb salvage increased from 4% without preoperative therapy to 91%, with a local recurrence rate of only 1.5%. Seventy-eight percent of tumors had at least 90% or better necrosis. Disease-free survival was over 80% at less than 3 years, median follow-up in this immature series.

At UCLA (28), 83 assorted skeletal sarcomas (57 osteosarcomas) were treated with 90 mg IA doxorubicin over 3 days followed by 3500 cGy in 10 fractions, and then resection 1 to 2 weeks later. IV doxorubicin and methotrexate were given postoperatively. Limb salvage was 100%, with two local recurrences (2.4%). Three-year survival for patients with osteosarcoma was 65%.

Kashdan et al. (29) delivered the entire preoperative dose of chemotherapy intra-arterially (doxorubicin 80 mg/m^2 + floxuridine 5 mg/m^2 over 10 days, with two 120 mg/m^2 boluses of cisplatin on day 4 and day 10) for one or two cycles with resection 3 to 6 weeks later. All patients received adjuvant doxorubicin, methotrexate, vinblastine, actinomycin-D and cyclophosphamide. Limb salvage was 89% with a 4% local recurrence rate. Cumulative survival was 82% at 2 years. Improvement in resectability or tumor necrosis with the intensified and prolonged intra-arterial regimen was not demonstrated in this small series.

Intra-arterial Chemotherapy for Soft-tissue Sarcomas

Four studies address the varying effects of neoadjuvant therapy used to treat soft-tissue sarcomas. The UCLA protocol used 3 days IA doxorubicin (90 mg/m^2) followed by a reduced dose of preoperative radiotherapy (30 to 40 cGy) for large (>5 cm) high-grade soft-tissue sarcomas (28, 30–32). Among 186 patients, limb-salvage surgery was possible in 95%, with a 2% local recurrence rate, but wound complications remained high at 20% to 40%. Median survival ranged from 76% at 32 months to 58% at 56 months. Reducing the preoperative radiation dose from 3500 cGy to 2800 cGy in a subsequent series led to a decrease in wound complications from 35% to 20% and a decrease in secondary amputations from 6% to none (16).

At the National Tumor Institute in Milan, Italy, 101 patients with large (mean 14 cm) soft-tissue sarcomas were treated with IA doxorubicin 100 mg/m^2 over 8 or 9 days for two cycles and then resected (33). Forty-five percent of these were patients with local recurrence after prior resection. Limb salvage was accomplished in 80%, but the local recurrence rate was high, at 29%. This largely reflected the high prevalence of inadequate margins in this series of very large high-grade and often recurrent tumors. Five-year survival was 54%.

Kónya and Vigváry (34) treated 51 patients with 129 short infusions (20 to 40 minutes) of cisplatin and doxorubicin, combining superselective infusion, chemoembolization, balloon occlusion-infusion and tourniquet infusion. There were three complete responses. Two patients were excluded when they developed distant metastases while on the neoadjuvant protocol. Limb salvage was possible in 43 of the remaining 46 patients (93%). Recurrence and survival rates were not reported.

Soulen et al. (35) reported on 15 patients with very large (mean 15 cm) high-grade sarcomas treated with a prolonged multi-drug IA chemotherapy regimen as outlined earlier for Kashdan's osteosarcoma series (29). Limb salvage was achieved in 87% with no wound complications. Eleven of fifteen tumors (73%) had 80% to 100% necrosis. Three-year survival was 67%. These limited series suggest that aggressive neoadjuvant chemotherapy can achieve limb salvage and local control rates similar to those reported with neoadjuvant radiation therapy, without the wound complications and limb dysfunction associated with radiotherapy.

In Europe, other strategies to enhance local control of soft-tissue sarcomas have been explored, with one of the most popular being isolated limb perfusion, which was in part proposed to address the in-transit metastasis confounding malignant melanoma pathology as well as the local control issue of satellitosis. In addition, because patients with non-resectable soft-tissue sarcomas of the extremities do not have increased survival if treated by amputation or disarticulation, isolated limb perfusion with tumor necrosis factor (TNF-α) + melphalan has emerged as a respectable limb-sparing neoadjuvant therapy. Reports reveal limb salvage rates in patients with unusually large (median, 16 cm) locally advanced soft-tissue sarcomas that were thought to be treatable only with amputation or functionally mutilating surgery of 82% (median follow-up, 2 years) when using an isolated limb perfusion with TNF-α + melphalan (36). While the utility of this technique is with patients with advanced metastatic disease and an uncontrollable, rapidly growing tumor threatening the limb, the disadvantage lies in the toxicity of TNF.

Adjuvant Chemotherapy

Due to the high risk of distant recurrence (>50%) in patients with high-grade large soft-tissue sarcomas, much research has centered on the effects of adjuvant chemotherapy (21). Adjuvant chemotherapy is currently the standard of care for select bone and soft-tissue sarcomas that most commonly occur in children, such as Ewing sarcoma, rhabdomyosarcoma and osteogenic sarcoma (37). It is also generally recommended for particular high-risk stage III soft-tissue sarcomas such as the less chemotherapy-sensitive subtypes (dedifferentiated liposarcoma) and the chemotherapy-sensitive subtypes (round cell liposarcomas and synovial sarcomas) (37). It is understood that adjuvant chemotherapy is not indicated for patients with low-grade soft-tissue sarcomas and those with small (T1) intermediate- or high-grade soft-tissue sarcomas (AJCC stages I and II). Although some trials demonstrate relatively higher overall survival rates with adjuvant therapy, no statistical significance between chemotherapy and no-chemotherapy groups was reported in these trials (38,39). In one trial of note in 2001, epirubicin and ifosfamide administered every 3 weeks for five cycles with granulocyte macrophage-colony stimulating factor (GM-CSF) for patients with large (>5 cm), high-grade soft-tissue sarcomas provided disease-free survival of 48 months in the treatment group versus 16 months in the control (no chemotherapy) group. An absolute overall survival benefit of 19% at 4 years was rendered, whereas overall survival was 75 months compared to 46 months. The 4-year metastasis-free survival was the same in both groups, which begs the question of whether local or distant recurrence is the therapeutic effect promoted (40). Still, these numbers show some benefit that in many ways is comparable to the use of adjuvant chemotherapy in the setting of breast or colorectal cancer. Generally speaking, the primary trend in response to adjuvant anthracycline-based chemotherapy seems not to be the prevention of metastatic disease but rather only a delay in the presence of diagnosable metastatic disease. For this reason, its routine use in patients with stage III disease has been generally discouraged. Presently, however, the role of anthracycline-based adjuvant chemotherapy in patients with localized soft-tissue sarcomas is still very much ill-defined.

TECHNIQUE AND COMPLICATIONS OF INTRA-ARTERIAL CHEMOTHERAPY IN THE EXTREMITIES

Safe performance of regional chemotherapy requires attention to detail in catheter placement and careful daily examination of the patient by the interventional radiologist. Initial diagnostic angiography should be performed via an access remote from the affected limb – femoral for upper extremity tumors, contralateral leg for lower extremity tumors – in order to evaluate completely the arterial supply to the lesion. If no blood supply from proximal branches is detected to tumors arising distal to the knee or elbow, subsequent catheterizations can be performed ipsilaterally in an antegrade fashion to allow the patient greater mobility. An axillary or brachial approach has been used for lower extremity infusions in order to permit ambulation, but this technique increases the chance of catheter tip migration. Retrograde catheterization for ipsilateral infusion should not be performed because of the risk of catheter dislodgment.

Once the tumor's blood supply is mapped, a 4F or 5F straight catheter should be placed as selectively as possible, with its tip proximal to the most proximal branches feeding the tumor. Patient motion due to drug-induced emesis is likely, so the catheter must be secured as stably as possible, preferably in a location that permits a few centimeters of tip migration without jeopardizing the infusion. Curved or angled catheter configurations should not be used unless absolutely necessary to achieve stable catheter positioning, in order to avoid migration of the catheter tip into a side branch with resultant local toxicity. Heparin-bonded catheters such as Anthron (Toray Industries, Tokyo, Japan) may help minimize pericatheter thrombosis, although this has not been proven.

After catheter placement, patients with a femoral catheter should be placed at strict bed rest with the hips and knees straight. Systemic heparinization and daily monitoring of the activated partial thromboplastin time (PTT) are recommended by some authors to minimize arterial and venous thromboembolism. While the benefit of heparin has not been rigorously proven, the risk of anticoagulation is low, and limb loss due to catheter-related arterial thromboembolism has been reported in the absence of adequate anticoagulation. The catheterization site and the extremity being infused should be inspected daily. Some centers use periodic fluorescein injection and a Wood's lamp to assess the territory infused by the catheter. Local erythema of the infused territory is normal, but focal painful myositis or dermatitis suggests migration of the catheter tip or streaming of the chemotherapy into a small branch vessel. If this occurs, the chemotherapeutic infusion should be halted immediately because local toxicity can cause skin and tissue necrosis. Arteriography should be performed and the catheter repositioned. Catheters can be safely withdrawn and resecured but should never be advanced, because bacterial colonization of the catheter and tract can cause sepsis. If advancement or exchange of the catheter is required, a fresh puncture should be made. Use of a pulsatile infusion pump can improve mixing of the drugs with the blood and minimize streaming. In addition to inspection of the infused territory, the puncture site and the arterial and venous system of the catheterized and infused extremities should be examined daily for evidence of bleeding, catheter dislodgment or thromboembolism.

Catheter-related complications increase with duration of infusion. In a series of 333 short (2- to 24-hour) cisplatin infusions, no catheter-related complication was reported (41). Among series using a 3-day IA doxorubicin protocol, Eilber (28) reported two arterial thromboses among 183 infusions. One was treated with thrombectomy, and the other led to amputation. No heparin was used in these patients. Wanebo (32) reported two arterial thromboses among 60 infusions, both associated with inadequate anticoagulation. The outcome in these two patients was not reported. Kashdan and Soulen (29, 35), among a total of 73 prolonged (≥10-day) multi-drug infusions, reported seven cases of arterial thrombosis requiring alteration of therapy. Five were treated with catheter removal followed by observation or prolongation of anticoagulation, one with thrombectomy, and one with thrombectomy and bypass. The latter patient developed intractable gangrene requiring amputation. Both patients requiring surgery had a subtherapeutic PTT. Twenty-four percent of 29 patients who had routine pull-out arteriograms before catheter removal had small (≤5 mm), non-occlusive, asymptomatic pericatheter or distal thrombi, irrespective of whether anticoagulation was therapeutic. Two additional patients developed deep vein thrombosis of the lower extremity despite therapeutic heparin infusions. Other complications included catheter dislodgment, catheter occlusion, focal skin necrosis due to local toxicity, fever requiring catheter removal and hemorrhage remote from the catheterization site in patients who were anticoagulated or thrombocytopenic. Azzarelli's report of more than 100 8- or 9-day IA doxorubicin infusions does not mention any complications (33).

INTRA-ARTERIAL THERAPY OF NON-EXTREMITY SARCOMAS

Sarcomas of the Axial Skeleton

Sarcomas arising in the pelvis or shoulder girdles are less amenable to resection with preservation of a func-

tional limb and are more likely to be unresectable than sarcomas arising in the extremities. IA chemoinfusion or chemoembolization can be performed either for palliation or to attempt to achieve sufficient tumor regression to permit resection. In small series employing IA cisplatin infusion or gelfoam chemoembolization, often combined with systemic chemotherapy and radiotherapy, partial responses were seen in about one half of patients and stabilization in most of the remaining patients (42, 43).

Gastrointestinal Sarcomas

Primary sarcomas of the gastrointestinal tract and abdomen are quite rare, and are best treated by resection. IA chemoinfusion or chemoembolization of unresectable tumors is possible if feeding vessels that are not also supplying the gut can be identified and superselectively catheterized (author's personal experience), but there is no broad experience with this technique.

Gastrointestinal and retroperitoneal sarcomas tend to metastasize to the liver. Liver metastases are treated by resection, when possible. Response rates of unresectable metastases to systemic chemotherapy are relatively poor. Chemoembolization is a well-established technique for treatment of hepatoma and has been applied to a variety of liver metastases. Experience with metastatic sarcomas is limited due to the rarity of the disease. The hypervascular nature of these tumors suggests that they may be sensitive to arterially directed therapy. M.D. Anderson Cancer Center reported on 14 patients treated with a combination of cisplatin and gelfoam chemoembolization followed by vinblastine chemoinfusion (44). Ten responded for a median duration of 12 months. Among 16 patients chemoembolized at the University of Pennsylvania with cisplatin/doxorubicin/mitomycin-C, iodized oil and polyvinyl alcohol particles, 13 regressed or stabilized. Three-year survival was 40% with a median of 20 months (45).

CONCLUSION

In the past decade, with the maturity of a number of trials looking at the efficacy of intra-arterial chemotherapy and radiotherapy for the treatment of soft-tissue sarcomas, therapeutic recommendations are now more evidence-based for patients suffering from these rare malignancies. Patients with sarcomas not amenable to cure by surgical resection alone because of the size, grade or location of their tumor can benefit from preoperative therapy. Regional intra-arterial chemotherapy permits limb-sparing resection in most of these patients, with less morbidity than is associated with preoperative radiation therapy. Neoadjuvant chemoinfusion and limb-salvage surgery enable patients to maintain a better quality of life than if they underwent amputation, with no detriment to local control or long-term survival. Regional infusion therapy requires scrupulous attention from the interventional radiologist to minimize complications. Although axial and gastrointestinal primary sarcomas are less amenable to catheter-directed therapies, metastases to the liver can achieve durable responses to chemoembolization.

REFERENCES

1. Khatri VP and Goodnight JE Jr. Extremity soft tissue sarcomas: Controversial management issues. Surg Oncol, 2005; 14: 1–9.

2. Weitz J, Antonescu CR, and Brennan MF. Localized extremity soft tissue sarcoma: Improved knowledge with unchanged survival over time. J Clin Oncol, 2003; 21: 2719–2725.

3. Soft tissue sarcoma, AJCC Cancer Staging Manual, 5th edition, pp. 140–146. Philadelphia: Lippincott Williams and Wilkins, 1998.

4. Deshmukh R, Mankin HJ, and Singer S. Synovial sarcoma: The importance of size and location for survival. Clin Orthop Relat Res, 2004; 419: 155–161.

5. Eilber FC, Rosen G, Nelson SD, et al. High-grade extremity soft tissue sarcomas: Factors predictive of local recurrence and its effect on morbidity and mortality. Ann Surg, 2003; 237: 218–226.

6. McKee MD, Liu DF, Brooks JJ, et al. The prognostic significance of margin width for extremity and trunk sarcoma. J Surg Oncol, 2004; 85: 68–76.

7. Koea JB, Leung D, Lewis JJ, et al. Histopathologic type: An independent prognostic factor in primary soft tissue sarcoma of the extremity? Ann Surg Oncol, 2003; 10: 432–440.

8. O'Sullivan B, Wylie J, Catton CN, et al. The local management of soft tissue sarcoma. Semin Radiat Oncol, 1999; 9: 328–348.

9. Hartman DS, Hayes WS, Choyke PL, et al: Leiomyosarcomas of the retroperitoneum and inferior vena cava: Radiologic-pathologic correlation. Radiographics, 1992; 12: 1203–1220.

10. Mitty HA, Hermann G, Abdelwahah IF, et al: Role of angiography in limb-tumor surgery. Radiographics, 1991; 11: 1029–1044.

11. Wilson AN, Davis A, Bell RS, et al: Local control of soft tissue sarcoma of the extremity: The experience of a multidisciplinary sarcoma group with definitive surgery and radiotherapy. Eur J Cancer, 1994; 30A: 746–751.

12. Pitcher ME, Fish S, and Thomas JM: Management of soft tissue sarcoma. Br J Surg, 1994; 81: 1136–1139.

13. Peat BG, Bell RS, Davis A, et al: Wound-healing complications after soft-tissue sarcoma surgery. Plast Reconstr Surg, 1994; 93: 980–987.

14. Bujko K, Suit HD, Springfield DS, et al: Wound healing after preoperative radiation for sarcoma of soft tissues. Surg Gynecol Obstet, 1993; 176: 124–134.

15. Keus RB, Rutgers EJT, Ho GH, et al: Limb-sparing therapy of extremity sarcomas: Treatment outcome and long-term functional results. Eur J Cancer, 1994; 30A: 1459–1463.

16. Huth JF, Eilber FR: Preoperative intraarterial chemotherapy. In: Pinedo HM, Verweij J, (eds.) Treatment of Soft Tissue Sarcoma, pp. 103–110. Boston: Kluwer Academic Press, 1988.

17. Spiro IJ, Rosenberg AE, Springfield D, et al. Combined surgery and radiation therapy for limb preservation in soft tissue sarcoma of the extremity: The Massachusetts General experience. Cancer Invest, 1995; 13: 86–95.

18. O'Sullivan B, Davis AM, Turcotte R, et al: Preoperative versus postoperative radiotherapy in soft tissue sarcoma of the limbs: A randomized trial. Lancet, 359: 2235–2241, 2002.

19. Kunos C, Colussi V, Getty P, et al: Intraoperative electron radiotherapy for extremity sarcomas does not increase acute or late morbidity. Clin Orthop Relat Res, 2006 May; 446: 247–252.

20. Rhomberg W, Hassenstein EO, and Gefeller D: Radio-therapy vs. radiotherapy and razoxane in the treatment of soft tissue sarcomas: Final results of a randomized study. Int J Radiat Oncol Biol Phys, 1996; 36: 1077–1084.

21. Spira AI and Ettinger DS: The use of chemotherapy in soft-tissue sarcomas. The Oncologist, 2002; 7: 348–359.

22. Kraybill WG, Spiro I, Harris J et al. Radiation Therapy Oncology Group (RTOG) 95–14: A phase II study of neoadjuvant chemotherapy (CT) and radiation therapy (RT) in high risk (HR), high grade, soft tissue sarcomas (STS) of the extremities and the body wall: A preliminary report. Proc Am Soc Clin Oncol, 2001: 1387a.

23. Edmonson JH, Petersen IA, Shives TC, et al. Chemotherapy, irradiation and surgery for function-preserving therapy of primary extremity soft tissue sarcomas: Initial treatment with ifosfamide, mitomycin, doxorubicin, and cisplatin plus granulocyte macrophage-colony stimulating factor. Cancer, 2002; 94: 786–792.

24. Benjamin RS: Regional chemotherapy for osteosarcoma. Semin Oncol, 1989; 16: 323–327.

25. Anderson JH, Gianturco C, and Wallace S: Experimental transcatheter intraarterial infusion-occlusion chemotherapy. Invest Radiol, 1981; 16: 496–500.

26. Benjamin RS, Chawla SP, Carrasco CH, et al: Preoperative chemotherapy for osteosarcoma with intravenous Adriamycin and intra-arterial cisplatinum. Ann Oncol, 1992; 3(Suppl II): 3–6.

27. Picci P, Bacci G, Ruggieri P, et al: The treatment of localized osteosarcoma of the extremities: The Italian experience. Ann Oncol, 1992; 3(Suppl II): 13–18.

28. Eilber FR, Morton DL, Eckardt J, et al: Limb salvage for skeletal and soft tissue sarcomas. Cancer, 1984; 53: 2579–2584.

29. Kashdan BJ, Sullivan KL, Lackman RD, et al: Extremity osteosarcoma: Intraarterial chemotherapy and

limb-sparing resection with 2-year follow-up. Radiology, 1990; 177: 95–99.

30. Goodnight JE, Bargar WL, Voegeli T, et al: Limb-sparing surgery for extremity sarcomas after preoperative intraarterial doxorubicin and radiation therapy. Am J Surg, 1985; 150: 109–113.

31. Hoekstra HJ, Koops HS, Molenaar WM, et al: A combination of intraarterial chemotherapy, preoperative and postoperative radiotherapy, and surgery as limb-saving treatment of primarily unresectable high-grade soft tissue sarcomas of the extremities. Cancer, 1989; 63: 59–62.

32. Wanebo HJ, Temple WJ, Popp MB, et al: Combination regional therapy for extremity sarcoma: A tricenter study. Arch Surg, 1990; 125: 355–359.

33. Azzarelli A, Quagliuolo V, Fissi S, et al: Intra-arterial induction chemotherapy for soft tissue sarcomas. Ann Oncol, 1992; 3(Suppl II): 67–70.

34. Kónya A and Vigváry Z: Neoadjuvant intraarterial chemotherapy of soft tissue sarcomas. Ann Oncol 1992; 3(Suppl II): 127–129.

35. Soulen MC, Weissmann JR, Sullivan KL, et al: Intraarterial chemotherapy and limb-sparing resection of large soft-tissue sarcomas of the extremities. J Vasc Intervent Radiol, 1992; 3: 659–663.

36. Eggermont AM, Schraffordt KH, Klausner JM, et al. Isolated limb perfusion with tumor necrosis factor and melphalan for limb salvage in 186 patients with locally advanced soft tissue extremity sarcomas. The cumulative multicenter European experience. Ann Surg, 1996; 224: 756–764.

37. Pisters P, O' Sullivan B, and Maki RG: Evidence-based recommendations for local therapy for soft tissue sarcomas. J Clin Oncol, 2007; 25: 1003–1008.

38. Frustaci S, De Paoli A, Bidoli E, et al: Ifosfamide in the adjuvant therapy of soft tissue sarcomas. Oncology, 65: 80–84, 2003.

39. Petrioli R, Coratti A, Correale P, et al: Adjuvant epirubicin with or without ifosfamide for adult soft tissue sarcoma. Am J Clin Oncol, 2002; 25: 468–473.

40. Frustaci S, Gherlinzoni F, De Paoli A, et al. Adjuvant chemotherapy for adult soft tissue sarcomas of the extremities and girdles: Results of the Italian randomized cooperative trial. J Clin Oncol, 2001; 19: 1238–1247.

41. Carrasco CH, Charnsangavej C, Raymond AK, et al: Osteosarcoma: Angiographic assessment of response to preoperative chemotherapy. Radiology, 1989; 170: 839–842.

42. Marangolo M, Tienghi A, Fiorentini G, et al: Treatment of pelvic osteosarcoma. Ann Oncol, 1992; 3(Suppl II): 19–22.

43. Fiorentini G, Dazzi C, Tienghi A: Chemofiltration and chemoembolization: New techniques in advanced pelvic bone malignancies. Ann Oncol, 1992; 3(Sugl II): 37–38.

44. Mavligit GM, Zukwiski AA, Ellis LM, et al. Gastrointestinal leiomyosarcoma metastatic to the liver. Durable tumor regression by hepatic chemoembolization infusion with cisplatin and vinblastine. Cancer, 1995; 75: 2083–2088.

45. Rajan DK, Soulen MC, Clark TW, et al. Sarcomas metastatic to the liver: Response and survival after cisplatin, doxorubicin, mitomycin-C, ethiodol, and polyvinyl alcohol chemoembolization. J Vasc Interv Radiol, 2001; 12: 187–193.

Prostate

Chapter 41

PROSTATE CRYOABLATION: A ROLE FOR THE RADIOLOGIST IN TREATING PROSTATE CANCER?

Gary Onik

Prostate cancer is third in incidence in the male population, just behind lung and colon cancer. With 250,000 cases diagnosed and an associated 40,000 deaths per year in the United States, prostate cancer represents a major development opportunity for the radiologist practicing interventional oncology. There are now low-morbidity image-guided treatment alternatives that are well suited to interventional radiologists committed to developing a patient-oriented practice.

With the decision of the Centers for Medicare and Medicaid Services (formerly the Health Care Financing Administration [HCFA]) in 1999 to approve prostate cryoablation for the treatment of primary prostate cancer, treatment options for patients were expanded (1). Despite decades of investigation and incremental improvements in both radical prostatectomy (RP) and radiation therapy, neither treatment modality has distinguished itself as the procedure of choice for treating primary prostate cancer. Both modalities have limitations in treating patients with

higher stage and Gleason grade disease. Also, the associated complications of RP and radiation therapy, although different in character, are not appreciably different in incidence, allowing one to definitively recommend one treatment over the other. As a result, each approach can be justifiably recommended as the procedure of choice. These options, along with "watchful waiting" (2) or, as it is now called, "active surveillance," as possible strategies for prostate cancer management have led to patient confusion and frustration. Adding cryoablation as still another treatment option to this already confusing environment further complicates patient choices. As we will see, however, there have been major improvements in cryosurgical results gained in recent years due to the basic understanding of the thermal destruction of tissue and the advances in cryosurgical technique and equipment. Add to this its unique inherent advantages of being able to treat extensive local disease, be repeated and form a platform for the focal therapy of prostate cancer, as well as its inherent low morbidity, and image-guided prostate cryosurgery (or perhaps another similarly image-guided ablative technology) has the potential to become the treatment of first choice for all stages and grades of localized prostate cancer.

BACKGROUND

The treatment of localized prostate cancer remains controversial. Although pathologic studies have shown that the prevalence of prostate cancer is high, many of these cancers are not clinically significant (3). In addition, even clinically significant cancers – generally accepted as those of a volume of 0.5 ml or greater – have a variable biologic behavior. On the other hand, the treatments for prostate cancer include a substantial risk of lifestyle-limiting morbidity. With some recent studies showing minimal survival benefit between no treatment and RP, the concept of "watchful waiting" – that is, not treating the primary tumor at all – has gained acceptance by some as a viable management alternative in certain patient populations. The decision to treat prostate cancer with a particular therapy or with "watchful waiting" requires a careful assessment of the risk versus benefit for that patient. Obviously, as the complications and lifestyle-limiting side effects of treatments are reduced, these decisions become easier.

The re-introduction of prostate cryosurgery using a percutaneous approach under ultrasound guidance was consistent with this concept of trying to decrease the morbidity of prostate cancer treatment. In 1966, Gondor et al. (4) first reported the concept of a cryosurgery procedure for the treatment of prostate disease. Subsequently, an open transperineal cryosurgery procedure was developed in which the freezing was carried out on the surface of the prostate with visual monitoring. Using this same approach, Bonney et al. (5) reported results in 229 patients followed for up to 10 years. A comparison of patients who underwent RP and radiation therapy showed equal survival between the two modalities. Although cryosurgery showed some advantages, such as being able to treat patients with large, bulky tumors, poor monitoring of the freezing process resulted in major complications such as urethro-cutaneous and urethro-rectal fistulas, thus limiting the acceptance of the procedure. In 1993, the first series of percutaneous ultrasound-guided and monitored prostate cryosurgery was reported by Onik et al.

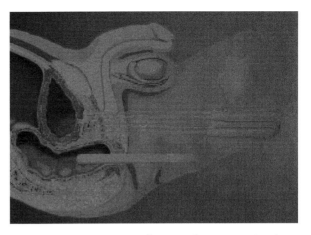

FIGURE 41.1.   Diagram showing the transperineal approach of prostate cryosurgery. The cryoprobes are placed percutaneously through the perineum using trans-rectal ultrasound for guidance. The approach is identical in concept to brachytherapy of the prostate. [Reproduced with permission from Endocare, Inc, Irvine, California (1-800-418-4677; http://www.endocare.com).] See Color Plate 34.

(6) (Figures 41.1 and 41.2), which stimulated a resurgence of interest in this treatment modality.

As with any new procedure, ultrasound-guided prostate cryosurgery went through a significant learning curve in which the goals of the procedure looked attainable but the reported results, in both cancer control and complications, were variable. A negative perception of the procedure was compounded by the fact that most early series predominantly treated patients in whom radiation therapy had failed, with these patients having higher complication rates, particularly incontinence, than those without a history of radiation therapy (73% vs. 3%) (7, 8). The situation

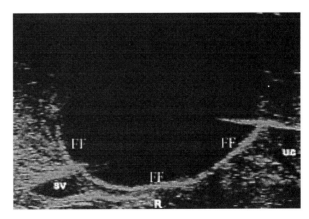

FIGURE 41.2.   US showing the ice as it extends toward the rectum. The freezing front (FF) is exquisitely seen as a hyperechoic (*white*) line extending toward the rectum (R). The seminal vesicle (SV) and urogenital diaphragm (UG) can be identified. The ability to visualize the freezing as it encompasses the prostate and approaches the rectum gives a "freezing radiation source" greater control than traditional brachytherapy.

was also exacerbated by a high urethral complication rate caused by the use of an ineffective urethral warming catheter (9).

Despite these early obstacles, the long-term results from multiple institutions were examined, and in 1999 the Centers for Medicare and Medicaid Services removed cryosurgery from the investigational category and included it with radiation and RP as a treatment for primary prostate cancer. A recently published article by Katz et al. (10) reviewed the 5-year biochemical disease-free survival of patients treated with brachytherapy, computed tomographic (CT) conformal radiation therapy, radical prostatectomy and cryoablation for every article published in the last 10 years. The results were stratified based on whether the patients were low, medium or high risk for biochemical failure. Based on this analysis, the range of results for cryoablation was equivalent to all other treatments in low- and medium-risk patients and appeared to be superior in high-risk patients. Overall complications rates were similar with all the modalities. The only article directly comparing cryoablation with radical prostatectomy, published by Gould et al. (11), showed cryoablation to be equivalent to RP in low-risk patients, but as patients' preoperative prostate-specific antigen (PSA) increased, cryoablation results were superior to RP. The basis for this apparent superiority in high-risk patients may be the ability of cryoablation to treat extra-capsular extension of cancer and to be repeated if needed. Based on these results, one can conclude that cryoablation is a safe and effective treatment for treating prostate cancer.

PATIENT SELECTION

The extent and pathologic character of the patient's disease are importance factors in choosing a proper therapy for prostate cancer. Treatments such as RP and brachytherapy (without external boosting) have higher recurrence rates as the extent and aggressiveness (Gleason score) of the disease increase. One of the great advantages of cryosurgery is the flexibility of the procedure to be tailored to treat both high- and low-risk patients, as well as patients in whom radiation therapy has failed.

Patients at High Risk for Local Recurrence

The use of cryosurgery for the treatment of solid organ cancers made a resurgence with the advent of ultrasound monitoring of hepatic cryosurgery, first proposed by Onik et al. in 1984 (12). Hepatic cryosurgery filled a unique place in the armamentarium of liver cancer treatment in that it successfully treated patients with multiple tumors or tumors that were unresectable due to proximity to major vasculature that could not be sacrificed (13, 14). Because of its target patient population of previously untreatable patients with an expected mortality of virtually 100%, imaging-guided hepatic cryosurgery was readily embraced by the surgical oncology community (15) at a time that was prior to the development of percutaneous cryoprobes that could be utilized by interventional oncologists.

The situation with prostate cancer is similar to liver cancer in that a significant portion of prostate cancer patients have a risk of positive margins, based on the high proportion of patients who have capsular penetration at the time of definitive treatment. However, efforts at preoperative staging have been inadequate to identify this patient population. The difficulty is further compounded by the fact that at the time of RP, the surgeon's ability to appreciate capsular penetration and involvement of the neurovascular bundles is inadequate. Vaidya et al. (16) reported virtually no correlation between the surgeon's determination of tumor penetration into the peri-prostatic tissue with involvement of the neurovascular bundle and actual pathologic confirmation. The result is that, in this study, as well as in other reports, positive margin rates of 30% associated with nerve-sparing RP are not uncommon. Using various clinical parameters such as Gleason score, clinical stage and PSA level, the statistical chance for capsular penetration can be reasonably predicted preoperatively (17, 18). This approach can lower the positive margin rate when rigorously applied, as demonstrated by Eggleston et al. (19). In actual clinical practice, however, most urologists believe that RP is still the "gold standard" of treatment. This leads to a natural reluctance, based on a statistical analysis, to deny a treatment that they believe may provide the best chance for cure. Based on the success of cryosurgery in treating unresectable liver cancer, it was hoped that the ability to freeze into the peri-prostatic tissue and encompass tumor capsular penetration could improve the treatment of prostate cancer patients at high risk of positive surgical margins. The preliminary data seem to support the potential success of this primary goal of prostate cryosurgery – improved treatment outcomes

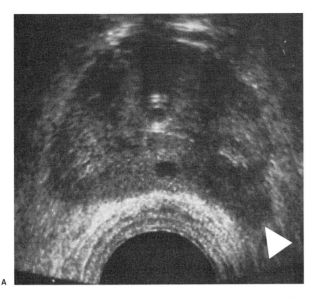
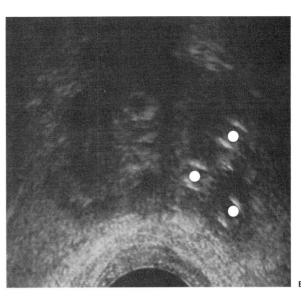

FIGURE 41.3. (A) Ultrasound shows gross extracapsular extension of tumor through the area of the left neurovascular bundle (*arrowhead*). (B) Three cryoprobes have been placed to cover the area and destroy the extra-capsular disease.

in patients at high risk of local recurrence. Numerous studies on ultrasound-guided prostate cryosurgery have demonstrated the ability of the procedure to successfully treat patients with stage T3 prostate cancer with demonstrated gross extra-capsular disease (20, 21) (Figure 41.3). Demonstration of this concept in patients with a "high likelihood" of capsular penetration, based only on statistical analysis, is more problematic given that the exact margin status of the patient is not known preoperatively or post-operatively following a cryosurgical procedure. There is, however, some evidence to support excel-lent results in patients at high risk for positive margins. Onik et al. (22) have shown that aggressive periprostatic freezing was facilitated by separating the rectum from the prostate at the time of the operation by a saline injection into Denonvilliers' fascia (Figure 41.4). No local recurrence was seen in 61 patients followed for up to 4 years despite the fact that 68% of the patients were considered at high risk of capsular penetration and local failure, based on the factors of Gleason score of 7 or greater, PSA greater than 10 ng/ml, already failed radiation or extensive bilateral disease based on preoperative biopsies. These results were

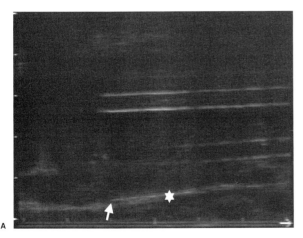
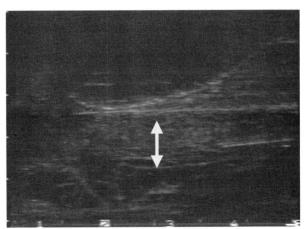

FIGURE 41.4. (A) US shows the tip of a needle placed into Denonvillier's fascia, which appears as a white line between the rectum and the prostate (*arrow*). The width of the fascia is indicated by the diamond shape. (B) US after injection of saline into Denonvillier's fascia. The double-headed arrow shows the increase in space between the prostate and the rectum. Downward traction on the rectum by the US probe keeps the space open.

confirmed by Bahn et al. (23) in which 7-year results in more than 500 patients showed that patients with medium and high risk had virtually identical results to low-risk patients (88% biochemical disease-free [BDF] using the American Society for Therapeutic Radiology and Oncology [ASTRO] criteria).

When cryosurgery is performed aggressively to achieve a negligible detectable PSA level, comparisons with RP should be possible. In the only published study comparing the outcomes between aggressive "total" cryosurgery and RP in one clinical practice (11), cryosurgery had a 23% greater chance of resulting in a PSA level of less than 0.2 ng/ml than did RP (96% vs. 73%). When a 0.0 PSA was used as the success criteria, cryosurgery maintained its approximately 20-percentage-point advantage over RP (66.9% vs. 48.2%). As patients became at greater risk for positive margins based on a PSA of 20 ng/ml or greater, cryosurgery maintained its results whereas the results of RP deteriorated further (86% vs. 36%). Although this study was retrospective and included a relatively small number of patients, its results are consistent with the original cryosurgical treatment rationale of destroying extracapsular cancer by treating the peri-prostatic tissues. In addition, these findings are consistent with the other studies showing success in treating T3 disease and other high-risk patients, as well as the unequivocally successful results seen in treating unresectable liver tumors. These results, together with the relatively low morbidity of the procedure and its ability to be performed in older patients and repeated when needed, we believe, make cryosurgery the procedure of choice in this patient population.

Adjuvant hormone therapy in high-risk patient populations is an important strategy. When combined with radiation, short-term hormone therapy appears to improve locoregional control and distant metastatis in patients with bulky tumors (T2–T4) (24). Long-term adjuvant hormonal therapy in addition to radiation appears to significantly affect the survival of patients having a Gleason score of greater than 7 (25). Because adjuvant therapy in these studies also had a significant effect on local control of tumor, the question of the importance of such control of tumor on the incidence of subsequent metastatic disease still needs investigation. Based on these concepts, we routinely place patients who are of medium to high risk of recurrence on 6 months of androgen ablation therapy prior to definitive cryosurgical treatment.

Patients with Organ-confined, Low-volume, Low Gleason Score Disease

Focal Cryosurgery: "The Male Lumpectomy"

The use of breast-sparing surgery lumpectomy to treat breast cancer revolutionized the local control of that disease. Lumpectomy experience showed that patient quality of life can successfully be integrated into the equation of cancer treatment without major effect on treatment efficacy (26). Men with prostate cancer face many of the same issues that breast cancer patients do. Focal therapy, in which just the known area of cancer is destroyed, appears to be a logical extension of the watchful waiting concept and very analogous to the lumpectomy in breast cancer. Focal therapy minimizes the risks associated with expectant management because the clinically threatening index cancer has been treated. Minimizing prostate trauma could, by treating only a portion of the prostate, decrease the risk of lifestyle-altering complications associated with morbid whole-gland treatments. In 2002, Onik et al. (27) published the first article on the focal treatment of prostate cancer using cryosurgical ablation. Nine patients were reported who had been followed for an average of more than 3 years; all patients were BDF, indicating that local control of prostate cancer was attainable with a focal approach. Morbidity was also low, with seven of the nine patients retaining potency and none experiencing incontinence. A follow-up article is now in press describing our further experience with focal cryoablation or "male lumpectomy" (28). In this paper, 51 patients, all of whom had at least 1-year follow-up, are reported, in whom the BDF rate using focal cryosurgery is 95%. In addition, no patient had evidence for a local recurrence in an area treated. Only 4 of the 51 patients had recurrences in areas not previously treated. All were re-treated and were subsequently free of disease. Local control of cancer was 100% despite the fact that 50% of the patients were medium to high risk for local recurrence. Once again, all patients were continent, and potency was maintained in 85% of patients (Figure 41.5).

The main conceptual objection to focal treatment of prostate cancer is that it is often a multi-focal disease. Prostate cancer, however, is a spectrum of diseases, some of which may be amenable to focal therapy. The prostate cancer pathology literature shows that a significant number of patients have a single-focus prostate cancer and that many others have

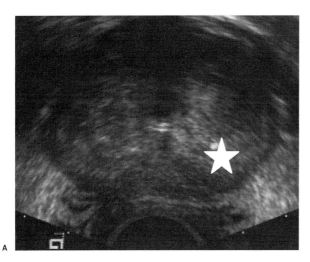
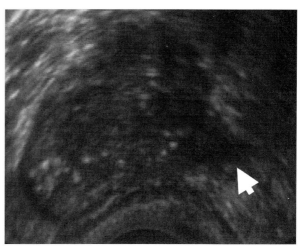

FIGURE 41.5. (A) US shows the prostate of a 60-year-old man. The star indicates where his biopsy was positive for a Gleason 6 carcinoma. He was treated with focal cryosurgery. He was continent and potent immediately after the proce- dure. (B) Two years post-cryosurgery, the US shows that the area of previous cryosurgery has contracted to a small scar (*arrow*). The patient's biopsies were negative, and his PSA level remains stable 6 years after the procedure.

additional cancer foci that may not be clinically significant (29–32). Until now, however, little attention has been paid in differentiating those patients with unifocal from multifocal disease because all treatments aimed at total gland removal or destruction.

In a study examining radical prostatectomy specimens, Djavan et al. (29) showed that patients with unifocal disease constituted nearly one third of the cases. In addition, Villers et al. (30) showed that 80% of multifocal tumors are less than 0.5 cc, indicating they may not be of clinical significance. This study was confirmed by Rukstalis et al. (31) and Noguchi et al. (32), in whose studies pathologic examination showed that unifocal tumors were present in 20% and 25% of patients, respectively, and, using the size criteria of 0.5 cc or less as an insignificant tumor, an additional 60% and 39% of patients might be candidates for a focal treatment approach. Based on this pathological evidence, a significant opportunity exists to investigate a focal treatment approach for prostate cancer.

Newer biopsy techniques now being used, in which the gland is biopsied transperineally every 5 mm using a brachytherapy-type grid, could have an impact on excluding patients with significant multifocal disease. A recent paper by Crawford et al. (33), using computer simulations on RP and autopsy specimens, demonstrated that transperineal prostate biopsies, spaced at 5-mm intervals through the volume of a patient's prostate, had a sensitivity of 95% in finding clinically significant tumors. Our results in 110 patients undergoing what we call 3D prostate mapping biopsies (3D-PMB), consistent with the

protocol Crawford investigated, showed that cancer could be demonstrated in 50% of patients who previously had negative biopsies in the previously uninvolved prostate lobe on transrectal ultrasound (TRUS) biopsy (34). 3D-PMB also provides superior localization of the tumor site than TRUS biopsies are able to provide. This information can therefore be used to guide the focally destructive agent to optimize destruction of the tumor while limiting the area that needs to be treated, hopefully minimizing the chance for side effects (Figure 41.6).

Focal cryoablation is a unique blend of an aggressive yet minimal procedure, which accounts for its combination of excellent cancer control and lack of complications. Extensive freezing of the periprostatic tissue can still be carried out on the side of the demonstrated tumor. In patients with a high Gleason score or in those with cancer demonstrated at the base of the gland, prophylactic freezing of the confluence of the seminal vesicles can also carried out. The expected incidence of urinary and rectal complications is lower than that of total cryosurgery, RP or brachytherapy. No patient in our series demonstrated persistent incontinence. Probably most important, however, is that an error in patient selection is correctable by re-treatment without added morbidity, a situation unique to cryosurgery.

Patients with Local Recurrence after Radiation Therapy

Patients who received a maximal dose of radiation but suffer a local recurrence without evidence

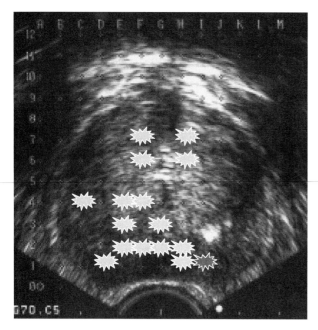

FIGURE 41.6. Ultrasound of a patient who presented with a single core positive, Gleason 6 on his TRUS biopsy on the left side of the gland. The starburst patterns indicate all the locations he was positive on his 3D-PMB. The pink starburst indicates an area of extra-capsular extension. See Color Plate 35.

of metastatic disease are still theoretically curable. Unfortunately, radiation destroys the tissue planes needed for a safe and effective attempt at salvage RP. RP in a salvage situation has demonstrated positive margins in 40% of patients (35) with prohibitive morbidity, demonstrating a 58% incontinence rate and an incidence of rectal injury as high as 15% (36). Consequently, salvage RP is rarely performed in this setting, with most patients being placed on palliative hormone ablation therapy. Based on the successful application of cryotherapy in patients with liver cancer, percutaneous prostate cryosurgery was immediately applied to this difficult-to-treat patient population. The treatment of patients for salvage after radiation therapy was not without difficulties. Early findings showed poor cancer control results, with fewer than 25% of patients reaching PSA levels of 0.2 ng/ml or less, and positive biopsy rates as high as 35%. Also, complications in this patient population could be significant. Whereas the incontinence rate for non-salvage cryosurgery patients is less than 2%, as many as 42% of radiation salvage patients can experience significant incontinence (37). Advances in cryosurgical technique have improved these results, with an article by de la Taille et al. (38) demonstrating a 60% success rate at providing an undetectable PSA. The associated incontinence rate was 9%. Based on

these results, cryosurgery was approved by The Centers for Medicare and Medicaid Services as the only treatment specifically approved for the indication of recurrent local cancer after radiation failure. We are just gaining experience with treating these patients with focal therapy, and although the cancer control rates are yet to be determined, it appears that the incidence of incontinence can greatly be reduced by this approach. We believe that, based on its potential for cure, cryosurgery has become the procedure of choice in this difficult-to-treat patient population.

TECHNICAL CONSIDERATIONS IN CRYOSURGERY

Saline Injection into Denonvilliers' Fascia

A major theoretical criticism of prostate cryosurgery involves the anatomy of the pelvis with the proximity of the prostate capsule to the rectal mucosa. Inadequate space between the prostate and the rectum can result in freezing the rectal mucosa, with resultant urethro-rectal fistula. Subsequently, fear of causing urethra-rectal fistula may result in stopping the freezing process prematurely and thus lead to a high incidence of tumor recurrence. Even for the experienced cryosurgeon, cryosurgery was, at times, a nerve-wracking balancing act between adequate treatment and rectal injury.

Probably the most important advance in the technique of prostate cryosurgery leading to the reproducibility of results involves the injection of saline into Denonvilliers' fascia at the time of freezing to temporarily increase the space between the rectum and prostate (Figure 41.3). The success of this maneuver is dependent on a downward traction of the rectum by the transrectal ultrasound probe to keep the space open once the injection has been made. We have now utilized this saline injection technique in more than 400 patients, demonstrating that this maneuver virtually eliminates the risk of rectal freezing and the complication of urethro-rectal fistula without increasing morbidity.

Temperature Monitoring in Critical Areas and Improved Cryosurgical Protocols

For reliable destruction of cancer by freezing, temperatures must reach certain critical limits. Recent in vitro and in vivo studies have shown that at least two freeze-thaw cycles with temperatures reaching

−35°C are needed to reliably destroy prostate cancer cells (39). Clinical studies have confirmed these parameters as well as the improvement that can occur in clinical results when temperature is monitored by thermocouples placed in critical areas in the prostate and two full freeze-thaw cycles are carried out. We routinely place thermocouples at the capsule in the known area of the tumor and at the apex of the gland when whole-gland destruction is being carried out. In general, thermocouples should be placed equidistant between cryoprobes at the theoretically warmest location, in order to not give misleading results. Thermocouples are also very useful in monitoring temperatures in critical locations to prevent complications. We routinely place a thermocouple into the area of the external sphincter to keep that structure above freezing temperatures and in the area of the neurovascular bundle when nerve sparing is being attempted.

Role of Ultrasound in Monitoring Prostate Cryosurgery

Modern cryosurgery would be impossible without transrectal ultrasonographic (US) monitoring. This imaging is needed to accurately place the probes and monitor the extent of freezing to prevent complication such as rectal freezing. Only a biplane transrectal probe should be used to monitor prostate cryosurgery. Most all of the monitoring of the freezing process should be carried out by the longitudinal linear array probe because of the shadowing effect caused by the ice. Use of a sector probe overestimates the extent of the freezing, obscuring the margins of the ice in the shadow created by the freezing front, given the margin of the freezing front is at 0°C. The freezing front will not represent the area of reliably destroyed tissue, hence the need for thermocouple monitoring.

Argon-based Cryosurgical Equipment

The original liquid nitrogen (LN2)-based freezing equipment has now been replaced by Joule-Thompson argon gas systems. These systems allow faster freezing rates, which improves the reliability of cancer destruction. The more precise control of the freezing process by gas systems also adds to the safety of the procedure by allowing the freezing process to be stopped in a more timely fashion. Increasing the number of probes from five to eight has allowed a more uniform freezing temperature to be achieved throughout the gland, which also improves

results. Increasing the number of probes beyond eight could have a potentially negative effect, however. A "cryoseed system" (Galil Medical Inc, Haifa, Israel) that utilizes 17-gauge needle probes to create a 1-cm-diameter ice-ball was not able to totally ablate the prostate gland based on reported PSA results (40). These poor results are probably the result of the short freezing length of these probes and the difficulty in accurately overlapping the freezing zones along the length of the gland. All of the data currently used to gain acceptance of cryosurgery were developed with cryosurgical probes that freeze the length of the gland in one freeze; departing from this concept jeopardizes much of what has been learned about how to obtain consistent results using cryosurgery.

FUTURE TECHNICAL IMPROVEMENTS

At the present time, the greatest improvements being made are those that have already been well established in the area of brachytherapy. Because the freezing capabilities of cryoprobes are predictable, planning software is already available to direct proper cryoprobe placement based on gland size and shape. Planning software has now been coupled to guidance software and hardware, which will simplify what was once a totally freehand approach to cryoprobe placement.

CONCLUSION

As we have seen, ultrasound-guided cryoablation holds a unique place among prostate cancer treatments. It has the advantage of extending efficacious treatment to patients who are at particularly high risk for local recurrence and who have failed radiation therapy. With the advent of the concept of focal therapy for prostate cancer, cryoablation may make its most important contribution to the care of the prostate cancer patient by offering excellent local tumor control without the attendant morbidity of previous whole gland treatments.

REFERENCES

1. Bagley GP. Health Care Financing Administration. Medicare coverage policy: Decisions. Cryosurgery ablation of the prostate (#CAG-00031). Available at: http://www.hcfa.gov/coverage/8b3-f1.htm. Accessed November 7, 2001.

2. George N. Therapeutic dilemmas in prostate cancer: Justification for watchful waiting. Eur Urol, 1998; 34(suppl 3): 33–36.

3. Villers A, McNeal JE, Freiha FS, et al. Multiple cancers in the prostate. Morphologic features of clinically recognized vs. incidental tumors. Cancer, 1992; 70: 2313–2318.

4. Gondor MJ, Soanes WA, and Shulman S. Cryosurgical treatment of the prostate. Invest Urol, 1966; 3: 372–378.

5. Bonney WW, Fallon B, Gerber WL, et al. Cryosurgery in prostatic cancer: Survival. Urology, 1982; 19: 37–42.

6. Onik GM, Cohen JK, Reyes GD, et al. Trans-rectal ultrasound guided percutaneous radical cryosurgical ablation of the prostate. Cancer, 1993; 72: 1291–1299.

7. Pisters LL, von Eschenbach AC, Scott SM, et al. The efficacy and complications of salvage cryotherapy of the prostate. J Urol, 1997; 157: 921–925.

8. Wong WS, Chinn DO, Chinn M, et al. Cryosurgery as a treatment for prostate carcinoma: Results and complications. Cancer, 1997; 79: 963–974.

9. Cespedes RD, Pisters LL, von Eschenbach AC, et al. Long-term followup of incontinence and obstruction after salvage cryosurgical ablation of the prostate: Results in 143 patients. J Urol, 1997; 157: 237–240.

10. Katz A and Rewcastle JC. The current and potential role of cryoablation as a primary treatment for prostate cancer. Current Oncology Reports, 2003; 5: 231–238.

11. Gould RS. Total cryoablation of the prostate versus standard cryoablation versus radical prostatectomy: Comparison of early results and the role of trans-urethral resection in cryoablation. J of Urol, 1999; 162: 1653–1657.

12. Onik G, Cooper C, Goldberg HI, et al. Ultrasonic characteristics of frozen liver. Cryobiology, 1984; 21: 321–328.

13. Onik G, Rubinsky B, Zemel R, et al. Ultrasound-guided hepatic cryosurgery in the treatment of metastatic colon carcinoma: Preliminary results. Cancer, 1991; 67: 901–907.

14. Ravikumar TS, Kane I, Cady B, et al. A 5-year study of cryosurgery in the treatment of liver tumors. Arch Surg, 1991; 126: 1520–1524.

15. Steele G Jr. Cryoablation in hepatic surgery. Semin Liver Dis, 1994; 14: 120–125.

16. Vaidya A, Hawke C, Tiguert R, et al. Intraoperative T staging in radical retropubic prostatectomy: Is it reliable? Urology, 2001; 57: 949–954.

17. Partin AW, Yoo J, Carter HB, et al. The use of prostate specific antigen, clinical stage and Gleason score to predict pathological stage in men with localized prostate cancer. J Urol, 1993; 150: 110–114.

18. Tewari A and Narayan P. Novel staging tool for localized prostate cancer: A pilot study using genetic adaptive neural networks. J Urol, 1998; 160: 430–436.

19. Eggleston JC and Walsh PC. Radical prostatectomy with preservation of sexual function: Pathological findings in the first 100 cases. J Urol, 1985; 134: 1146–1148.

20. Connolly JA, Shinohara K, and Carroll P. Cryosurgery for locally advanced (T3) prostate cancer. Semin Urol Oncol, 1997; 15: 244–249.

21. Miller RJ Jr, Cohen JK, Merlotti LA, et al. Percutaneous transperineal cryosurgical ablation of the prostate for the primary treatment of clinical stage C adenocarcinoma of the prostate. Urology, 1994; 44: 170–174.

22. Onik G, Narayan P, Brunelle R, et al. Saline injection into Denonvilliers' fascia during prostate cryosurgery. J Min Ther Relat Tech, 2000; 9: 423–427.

23. Bahn DK, Lee F, Bandalament R, et al. Seven-year outcomes in the primary treatment of prostate cancer. Urology, 2002 Aug; 60(2 Suppl 1): 3–11.

24. Pilepich MV, Winter K, John MJ, et al. Phase III radiation therapy oncology group (RTOG) trial 86-10 of androgen deprivation adjuvant to definitive radiotherapy in locally advanced carcinoma of the prostate. Int J Radiat Oncol Biol Phys, 2001; 50: 1243–1252.

25. Lawton CA, Winter K, Murray K, et al. Updated results of the phase III Radiation Therapy Oncology Group (RTOG) trial 85-31 evaluating the potential benefit of androgen suppression following standard radiation therapy for unfavorable prognosis carcinoma of the prostate. Int J Radiat Oncol Biol Phys, 2001; 49: 937–946.

26. Santiago RJ, Wu L, Harris E, et al. Fifteen-year results of breast-conserving surgery and definitive irradiation for Stage I and II breast carcinoma: The University of Pennsylvania experience. Int J Radiat Oncol Biol Phys, 2004 Jan 1; 58(1): 233–240.

27. Onik G, Narayan P, Vaughan D, et al. Focal nerve sparing cryoablation for the treatment of primary prostate cancer: A new approach to preserving potency. Urology, 2002; 60(1): 109–114.

28. Onik G, Vaughan D, Lotenfoe R, et al. "Male lumpectomy," focal therapy for prostate cancer using cryoablation. Urology, 2007 Dec; 70(6 Suppl): 16–21.

29. Djavan B, Susani M, Bursa B, et al. Predictability and significance of multi-focal prostate cancer in the radical prostatectomy specimen. Tech Urol, 1999; 5(3): 139–142.

30. Villers A, McNeal JE, Freiha FS, et al. Multiple cancers in the prostate: Morphologic features of clinically recognized vs. incidental tumors. Cancer, 1992; 70 (9): 2312–2318.

31. Rukstalis DB, Goldknopf JL, Crowley EM, et al. Prostate cryoablation: A scientific rationale for future modifications. Urology, 2002 Aug; 60(2 Suppl 1): 19–25.

32. Noguchi M, Stamey TA, McNeal JE, et al. Prognostic factors for multi-focal prostate cancer in radical prostatectomy specimens: Lack of significance of secondary cancers. J Urol, 2003; 170(2 pt1): 459–463.

33. Crawford ED, Wilson SS, Torkko KC, et al. Clinical staging of prostate cancer: A computer-simulated study of transperineal prostate biopsy. BJU Int, 2005 Nov; 96(7): 999–1004.

34. Onik GM. 3D global mapping biopsies. A more efficacious method of determining the extent of prostate cancer. Presented at Consensus Conference on Focal Therapy of Prostate Cancer. Orlando, Florida, February 24, 2006.

35. Neerhut GJ, Wheeler T, Cantini M, et al. Salvage radical prostatectomy for radiorecurrent adenocarcinoma of the prostate. J Urol, 1988; 140: 544–549.

36. Rainwater LM and Zincke H. Radical prostatectomy after radiation therapy for cancer of the prostate: Feasibility and prognosis. J Urol, 1988; 140: 1455–1459.

37. Bales GT, Williams MJ, Sinner M, et al. Short-term outcomes after cryosurgical ablation of the prostate in men with recurrent prostate carcinoma following radiation therapy. Urology, 1995; 46: 676–680.

38. de la Taille A, Hayek O, Benson MC, et al. Salvage cryo-therapy for recurrent prostate cancer after radiation therapy: The Columbia experience. Urology, 2000; 55: 79–84.

39. Tatsutani K, Rubinsky B, Onik GM, et al. Effect of thermal variables on frozen human primary prostatic adenocarcinoma cells. Urology, 1996; 48: 441–447.

40. Moore Y and Sofer P. Successful treatment of locally confined prostate cancer with the seed net system: Preliminary multi-center results. Clinical Application Notes Feb 2001. Available through Galil Medical, Haifa, at http://Galilmedical.com. Accessed November 7, 2001.

PART IV

SPECIALIZED INTERVENTIONAL TECHNIQUES IN CANCER CARE

Chapter 42

VASCULAR ACCESS: VENOUS AND ARTERIAL PORTS

Thierry de Baère

Eric Desruennes

Externalized central venous catheters and totally implantable central venous access port systems are widely used to improve venous access reliability in patients receiving prolonged courses of cytotoxic therapy, anti-infectious chemotherapy or long-term parenteral nutrition. Totally implantable venous access port systems have several advantages over externalized catheters, including reliable venous access, low incidence of infection, absence of maintenance and fewer restrictions on activities such as bathing and sports. Ports are usually inserted by surgeons, anesthesiologists or radiologists in order to gain direct access to the central circulation as well as the hepatic artery to deliver cytotoxic drug directly to the liver. At the current time, minimally invasive techniques provided by interventional radiologists allow placement of catheter or port systems for intra-arterial hepatic chemotherapy (IAHC) without the need for open surgery or repeated catheterization.

Other directed intra-arterial therapies have been used, namely in the pelvis, but will not be described in this chapter, which will deal with central venous catheter and port placement for hepatic intra-arterial therapy.

VENOUS PORTS

Description

These devices consist of a port made of titanium or plastic with a self-sealing septum, accessible by percutaneous needle puncture, and a radiopaque catheter usually made in a well-tolerated long-term substance – silicone or polyurethane. Most ports are single lumen, but there are others with two lumens for separate administration of incompatible drugs. The connection between the catheter and the port can either be sealed during the manufacturing process or made at the time of placement.

Indications

The main indications for port insertion are cytotoxic chemotherapy for solid tumors and long-term antibiotic therapy, whereas externalized catheters are used in hematologic diseases and long-term parenteral nutrition. Blood sampling is possible with ports provided copious flushing is completed after sampling.

Preoperative Assessment

Platelet count should be more than 50,000/mm^3, white cells more than 1000 and international normalized ratio (INR) less than 1.5. A preoperative chest radiograph is not mandatory but useful in cases of pulmonary disease, lymphoma and ear-nose-throat (ENT) tumors. In such cases and when a mediastinal invasion, compression or thrombosis is suspected, a chest computed tomographic (CT) scan is necessary to verify the absence of superior vena cava occlusion or partial thrombosis.

Vitamin K antagonists should be replaced by low-molecular-weight heparin (LMWH). A reduced dose of LMWH should be administered the day before implantation and none the morning of the implantation. Ticlopidine, clopidogrel and other anti-platelet agents should be discontinued 5 days before implantation. There is no need to stop low-dose aspirin as well as non-steroid anti-inflammatory drugs.

Access Route

The percutaneous subclavian access is the first described and the most well-known. Access to the subclavian vein is easy and rapid because there are reliable anatomical landmarks, especially the bones. It can be approached by an infra- or supraclaviclar route. The two main drawbacks are the practically non-reducible incidence of pneumothoraces (1% to 5%) and, for long-term catheters and ports placed via the infraclavicular route, the risk of compression between the clavicle and first rib (pinch-off syndrome). Pinch-off syndrome occurs in 1% of cases (1, 2) and may lead to the fracture of the catheter (Figure 42.1) and the embolization of a catheter fragment in the cardiac chambers or the pulmonary arteries. For these reasons, subclavian access is not the best route for long-term central venous access unless the

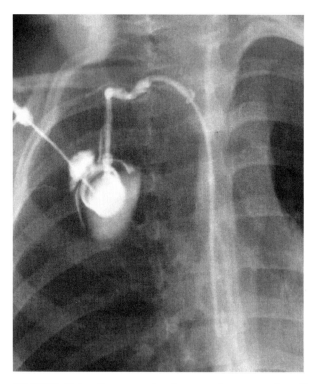

FIGURE 42.1. Fracture of catheter and extravasation of contrast in the costoclavicular space of an 18-month-old infant (pinch-off syndrome).

vein is punctured lateral to the mid-clavicular line or via a supraclavicular route. For both of these cases, access should be performed using ultrasound-guided technique.

The percutanous access of the **internal jugular vein** has gained popularity because of the absence of pneumothoraces and pinch-off syndrome. The relatively high rate of inadvertent carotid puncture becomes irrelevant (incidence close to zero) when using ultrasound (3). In our institution (1700 ports and tunnelized catheters implanted each year), 75% of the ports are placed using an internal jugular access. The right internal jugular vein is in direct line with the superior vena cava and the right auricle and is ideally suited for long-term access. On the other hand, the aesthetic aspect is not always perfect because the catheter is sometimes clearly visible around the neck area. For aesthetic reasons, the best approach for jugular vein catheterization is probably the posterior approach behind the clavicular head of the sternocleidomastoid muscle.

The external jugular vein is not used very often because its junction with the brachiocephalic trunk is sometimes acute and will not always allow the passage of the catheter.

The cutdown approach of the **cephalic vein** is often used by surgeons. Here, an aesthetic advantage is evident, particularly in women, but it also has some disadvantages such as 5% to 10% failures because the vein is either too small or sinuous to be catheterized, thereby causing more venous thromboses than when using the other methods.

The **forearm veins** are sometimes used for venous access, either via a cut-down approach or through a percutaneous vein puncture guided by venography or ultrasound.

The percutaneous access of the **femoral vein** has specific indications such as mediastinal compression or invasion of the superior vena cava in lung cancer or lymphoma, superior vena cava thrombosis, impossibility to puncture neck or chest veins due to local tumor invasion, infection, and post-radiation therapy stenosis. Provided that the technique is well applied and the tip of the catheter is close to the right atrium, infectious and thrombotic complications are comparable to those seen after subclavian or jugular access (4, 5). Because of the frequency of lung cancer and mediastinal location of lymphoma, femoral access should represent 5% to 10% of all implanted ports (Figure 42.2).

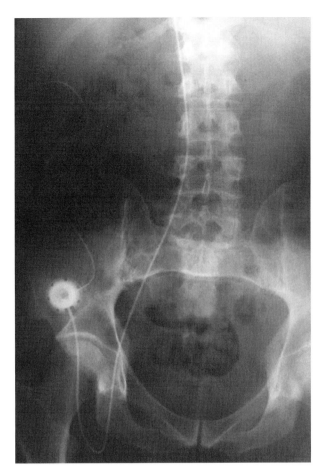

FIGURE 42.2. Femoral long-term access; the port is implanted on the abdominal wall in front of the iliac bone.

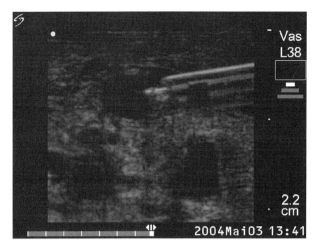

FIGURE 42.3. Ultrasound image perpendicular to the internal jugular vein demonstrating the needle entering the vein.

Ultrasound Use

In a meta-analysis published in 2003, Hind et al. compared guidance using real-time two-dimensional ultrasonography with the anatomical landmark method of puncture. He demonstrated that catheterization under ultrasound guidance is quicker and safer than the landmark method in both adults and children (3). In our institution, ultrasound imaging of the targeted vein is systematically used to located the target before puncturing the internal jugular and femoral veins in adults and children. Then, when ultrasound screening reveals difficulties, including small veins, cervical nodes or anatomical abnormalities, or in cases of previous failures and in small infants, the probe is sterilely dressed for real-time guidance (Figure 42.3).

Catheter Tip Location

All recent studies have shown that the position of the tip of central venous devices is a significant factor for predicting catheter dysfunction and catheter-related venous thrombosis. When the tip is located

in the last third of the superior vena cava or the right atrium, the rate of venous thrombosis is between 3% and 5%, compared with 42% 46% when the tip lies in the proximal third of the vena cava or in the brachiocephalic veins (6, 7). Recommendations from these studies are that the optimal tip position for central venous catheters and ports should be the distal third of the superior vena cava or the proximal right atrium. This last position does not conform to manufacturer and Food and Drug Administration guidelines, although no complications have been observed in long-term central venous lines, the tips of which lay in the right atrium.

Update on Vein Thrombosis Prophylaxis and Treatment

The presence of mediastinal lymph nodes has been shown to be a risk factor for catheter-related venous thrombosis (8), and one should carefully examine the chest CT scan before implanting a central venous device in patients suffering from lung cancer, lymphoma and other diseases, including advanced ENT or thyroid cancer, for example. Patients with catheters that are too short, gastrointestinal cancers or extended metastatic diseases have a higher risk of deep vein thrombosis as well.

For patients with catheter-related deep vein thrombosis and cancer, treatment with LMWH for at least 3 to 6 months is recommended (9). If the tip of the catheter is in the correct location and the port is functioning well, it is possible to keep it in place and to avoid retrieving it.

Recent studies failed to show any benefit from prophylaxis with warfarin or LMWH compared with placebo for the prevention of catheter-related thrombosis (10, 11). Based on these findings, the American College of Chest Physicians Conference on Antithrombotic and Thrombolytic Therapy recently suggested that the risk of clinically important catheter-related venous thrombosis may be too low to warrant routine prophylaxis and recommended that clinicians do not routinely use prophylaxis in cancer patients (12).

Catheter-related Infection

Minor temporary local infection should be treated with local antiseptics and possibly oral antibiotics. Nevertheless, the port should be explanted in case of local swelling or purulent drainage.

Systemic infection is defined as fever, chills and a positive blood culture. Methods of diagnosing catheter-related infection without removing the catheter consist of comparison of paired blood cultures drawn simultaneously via the port and from a peripheral venous site. Quantitative blood cultures or measurement of differential time to germ growth are used for this purpose (13). After a port infection has been proved, the port should be removed in the presence of severe neutropenia or septic shock, or when *Staphylococcus aureus*, *Pseudomonas* and *Stenotrophomonas* or *Candida* species are isolated from blood cultures. Parenteral then oral antibiotic therapy should be prescribed for at least 10 days in case of bacteremia. Antibiotic-lock technique without removing the port is a possible alternative when *Staphylococcus epidermidis*, *Escherichia coli* or other digestive microorganisms are isolated (14). Local antibiotic locks consist of 2 ml of highly concentrated amikacin or vancomycin (15 mg/ml) that are changed every day for at least 10 days, after which blood cultures should be performed a few days after the end of the treatment to confirm the success or the failure of this treatment.

Image-guided Interventions for Port Dysfunction

The technical aspects, feasibility, safety and efficacy of endovascular management of mechanical complications related to implanted central venous devices are described in a recent paper (15). Three procedures are commonly used: retrieval of a fractured and embolized catheter, repositioning of the migrated catheter tip and fibrin-sheath stripping.

Retrieval of the embolized catheter is performed with loop snares. These snares can be custom made using a 7F to 9F catheter (Cook, Bjaeverskov, Denmark) with a 3-m, 0.018 to 0.021 guidewire folded in (B. Braun, Melsungen, Germany). However, in pediatric patients or when the central venous device (CVD) catheter has to be snared in the heart or the pulmonary artery, a ready-to-use nitinol snare measuring 15 to 30 mm in diameter is usually preferred (Amplatz goose neck, Microvena corp, White Bear Lake, MN). The CVD catheter is retrieved via the puncture site with or without the need for an introducer. When the embolized catheter is initially located in the heart or the pulmonary artery, it might be useful to reposition the catheter in the vena cava before snaring it, namely when no catheter free end can be grasped with the loop-snare. In such cases, a 6F angled pig-tail catheter is placed alongside the embolized catheter and repeatedly rotated until it enfolds the embolized catheter. The pig-tail catheter is then gently withdrawn and repositioned in a location where it would be easy to snare. The catheter is then released by rotating the pig-tail catheter in the opposite direction

Replacement of migrated distal tips is usually achieved with a 5F or 6F pig-tail catheter using the same technique as that described for repositioning of embolized catheters before snaring.

Fibrin sheath stripping is performed with a nitinol loop snare. The snare is inserted via the femoral vein and opened beyond the tip of the catheter. It is then advanced to encircle the distal tip of the malfunctioning catheter. The snare is closed around the most proximal part of the catheter, and mild to moderate tension is exerted while slowly pulling the snare toward the distal tip of the catheter. This maneuver is repeated until contrast medium injected through the port flows normally through the distal tip of the catheter.

Feasibility of retrieval is 95%, and retrieval must always be attempted due to the significant risk of leaving a migrated catheter in the venous circulation (16–18). When a catheter tip has migrated, the catheter must not be used because the risk of infusion into the wrong veins can result in major complications (19–21). Repositioning is easy to perform; however, only about 50% of migrations are definitively resolved, mostly because migration often occurs because the catheter is too short. Replacing it may prove pointless as it is simply too short to be used and will invariably migrate again. It is therefore probably advisable to reserve endovascular repositioning for port catheters that are cumbersome to exchange, and to replace simple catheters that can be more easily exchanged than port catheters.

Hepatic Intra-arterial Port

Indications

Because IAHC is a local treatment, it is most often used in cases of liver cancer without extra-hepatic disease, and less frequently in patients with liver predominant disease. It is often used as rescue after failure of intravenous therapies for metastases and has shown high response rates even when drugs that were or became ineffective with intravenous administration were used. Because it is highly efficient, IAHC might also be used as inductive therapy in chemonaive patients with nearly resectable liver metastases to give the patient the best chance to become a surgical candidate, and as adjuvant treatment after curative hepatectomy, namely, patients with high risk of intra-hepatic recurrences (high number of liver metastases, elevated stage of the primary tumor). For primary tumors, and especially hepatocellular carcinoma (HCC), the use of IAHC is less common due to the high efficacy of trans-arterial chemoembolization (TACE). Indications could include patients who did not respond to TACE or are not candidates for TACE due to portal vein thrombosis or advanced liver insufficiency (22, 23).

Rationale

Colorectal cancer is the most common cancer in the Western world, and the most common cause of death from this cancer is due to hepatic metastases. Hepatic metastases will occur in 50% to 75% of patients during the disease. Twenty percent are present at the time of diagnosis, and 30% to 50% will appear later. Even if surgery is the best treatment option for liver metastases, it will only be possible in 20% of patients. Furthermore, 70% of patients who undergo surgery will develop new liver metastases. Consequently, there is a large place for chemotherapy in order to treat liver metastases. Despite real increases in response rates to systemic chemotherapy, from 10% to 20% receiving 5-fluorouracil (5-FU) alone to 16% to 40% with combination of 5-FU and folinic acid, and even better results with last-generation regimens including 5-FU + oxaliplatin and 5-FU + irinotecan, there are still

a number of non-responders who could benefit from IAHC, which has been shown to provide responses in non-responders to previously mentioned systemic chemotherapy regimens. IAHC has the main advantage of increasing drug concentrations in tumors, thus resulting in a significant increase in response rates because many tumors display a steep dose-response curve. The advantage for such an intra-arterial route is proportional to first-pass extraction of the drug by the liver and inversely proportional to body clearance of the drug. Consequently, the choice of the drug is of utmost importance. Floxuridine (FUDR) has been extensively used for IAHC because it is extracted by the liver at more than 95% during the first pass, with an increase in exposure to the liver ranging from 100 to 300 times over that achieved with a systemic administration. When compared with intravenous perfusion, the estimated increase in liver exposure by IAHC is 20-fold for tetrahydropyranyl (THP) doxorubicin (Adryamicin), 5- to 10-fold for 5-FU, 4- to 7-fold for cisplatin, 6- to 8-fold for mitomycin, 4-fold for oxaliplatin, and only 2-fold for doxorubicin. All clinical trials using 5-FU or FUDR have demonstrated better response rates for IAHC than for intravenous treatments. However, only a few trials have demonstrated a survival benefit (24, 25). Intra-arterial chemotherapy was more or less abandoned at the time intravenous irinotecan and oxaliplatin proved to give equivalent response rates to intra-arterial 5-FU. However, recently, a French multicentric trial has used these new drugs intra-arterially with IAHC, using 100 mg/m² of oxaliplatin repeated every second week, with overall response rates of 64% (95% CI: 44% to 81%) in heavily pretreated patients (26). In addition, new drug combinations, including IAHC with irinotecan plus intravenous oxaliplatin, allowed as high as 88% of tumor response (27).

Adjuvant postoperative IAHC after liver resection has been demonstrated to increase survival (28). In the past, implantation of ports for intra-arterial hepatic chemotherapy required a laparotomy. Recently, a laparoscopic approach has been reported in a small series (29). In the past, the percutaneous approach has been used to place the catheter in the hepatic artery for chemotherapy, with the need for repeated peripheral arterial access and hepatic artery catheterization for each subsequent chemotherapy delivery (30). Today, minimally invasive technique perfected by interventional radiology allows placement of a catheter linked to a port for IAHC without the need for open surgery or repeated catheterization.

Technique

Access Route

The catheter is usually introduced through the axillary or femoral arteries (31–33). The intercostal artery route was reported in only one series (34). Since the first report by Arai et al. in 1982, the axillary route is utilized much more commonly than the femoral route. This approach is preferred because its allows easier insertion of the catheter in the hepatic artery due to the usually descending orientation of the initial part of the celiac trunk, thus avoiding the sharp angulation encountered when using femoral access. Disadvantages of the axillary route are a higher rate of overall and severe complications, including up to 3% of aneurysms requiring arterial stent for treatment, which, in turn, can cause axillary artery thrombosis (33), and .05% to 1% incidence of stroke (30, 32). Aneurysms are due to the difficulty of access and manual compression of the axillary artery, which lead some teams to access the axillary artery through surgical exposure and cut-down of a small branch – namely, the thoracic-acromial artery (32). Strokes are caused by emboli induced by the body of the catheter lying in front of the arising of the left vertebral artery and, for some authors, retrieval or exchange of such catheters is risky enough to make them recommend that such maneuvers should be performed through a femoral access, if possible (32). Using the femoral artery for catheter port insertion is technically more challenging but can be achieved nowadays in the vast majority of patients due to improvements in endovascular material design. Furthermore, a femoral access will most often be needed for endovascular flow remodeling, even if the indwelling catheter is inserted through the axillary route.

Arterial Flow Remodeling

Flow remodeling is nearly always needed before indwelling catheter insertion (Figure 42.4), because IAHC requires the perfusion of chemotherapy in the complete liver and only in the liver through a single artery. First, replaced hepatic arteries should be occluded proximally with stainless steel coils, reproducing by endovascular techniques a surgical ligation, in order to allow perfusion of the complete liver

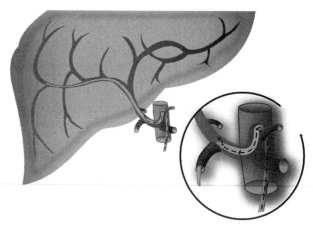

FIGURE 42.4. Schematic drawing of an intra-arterial catheter implantation.

through a single artery and then a single catheter (Figures 42.5, 42.6 and 42.7). Second, arteries not feeding the liver but feeding the stomach, the duodenum or the pancreas, which arise between the perfusion hole in the catheter (Figure 42.8) and the liver should be occluded to avoid the toxicity caused by extra-hepatic drug distribution. In clinical practice, the gastroduodenal artery and the right gastric artery are the more common arteries requiring endovascular occlusion because it is rarely possible to place the perfusion hole of the catheter downstream of them

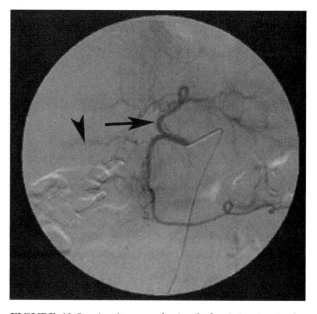

FIGURE 42.5. Angiogram obtained after injection in the middle hepatic artery showing feeding of the left lobe of the liver (*arrow*) and the gastroduodenal artery. The right gastric artery can be faintly seen (*arrowhead*).

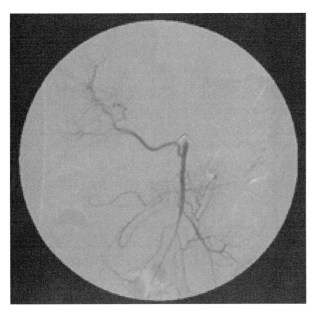

FIGURE 42.6.   Angiogram obtained after injection in the superior mesenteric artery showing a replaced right hepatic artery.

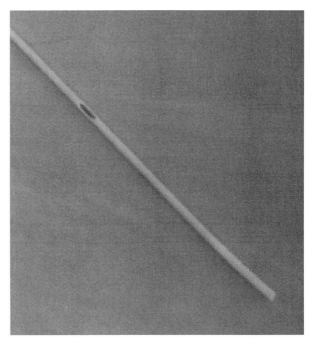

FIGURE 42.8.   Close-up view of the distal part of the 5F indwelling catheter demonstrating a side hole 7 cm from the tip.

(Figure 42.9). Occlusion of the right gastric artery (Figure 42.5) is a key factor to lower toxicity of infused drugs to the liver, as discussed in the results section. The right gastric artery occlusion is probably the most technically challenging part of IAHC catheter insertion. First, it is sometimes difficult to see it on the hepatic artery angiogram; second, it can arise

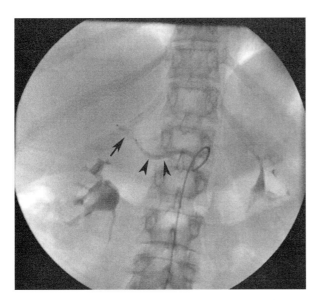

FIGURE 42.7.   Angiogram obtained in the main hepatic artery after occlusion of the replaced hepatic artery with an endovascular occluding device (*arrow*). The contrast medium is seen in the distal branches of the replaced right hepatic artery due to proximal shunting between the main and replaced hepatic artery (*arrowheads*).

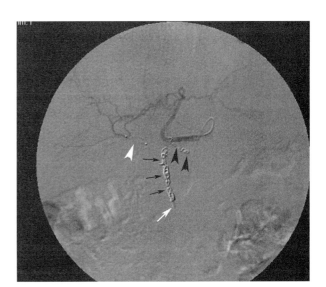

FIGURE 42.9.   The right gastric artery has been occluded with coils (*black arrowheads*), and the tip of the indwelling catheter (*white arrow*) has been placed in the gastroduo-denal artery, which has also been occluded with coils (*black arrows*). Injection of contrast medium in the femoral implanted port opacifies the complete hepatic vasculariza-tion and only hepatic arteries through the side hole within the catheter. Note the collateral arterial pathways through the liver hilum that supply the right hepatic artery distal to the occluding device (*white arrowhead*).

anywhere between the common hepatic artery and the distal part of the left branch of the hepatic artery. When its origin cannot be seen on the hepatic artery angiogram, it is often useful to perform a selective angiogram of the left gastric artery. In most instances, retrograde injection into the right gastric artery will be seen, which will help determine the location of the origin of the right gastric artery from the hepatic artery. Sometimes it will be possible to perform hyperselective catheterization of the left gastric and then retrograde catheterization of the right gastric to perform coil embolization of its origin. The absence of reported toxic effect on the gallbladder makes it unnecessary to systematically occlude its feeding vessels; however, a very large cystic artery should probably be occluded.

Catheter Positioning

The IAHC catheter can be placed floating in the hepatic artery lumen or can be fixated into the gastroduodenal artery. Fixation of the catheter tip is obtained by inserting the catheter deeply in the gastroduodenal artery and placing coils or cyanoacrylate glue around it, in order to provide both fixation of the catheter and occlusion of the gastroduodenal artery. In such fixated catheters, a side hole is created a few centimeters from the tip to allow drug delivery through the side hole, which is placed in the hepatic artery upstream of the gastroduodenal artery take off. The distal portion of the lumen catheter, between the side hole and the distal hole, will spontaneously occlude within a few minutes to a few hours due to clotting. In practice, after the initial angiogram and occlusion of the replaced hepatic artery and right gastric artery have been performed, the gastroduodenal artery is catheterized as distally as possible down to the distal right epiploic artery. Then, the 5F diagnostic catheter is exchanged over a stiff 0.018-inch guidewire for the indwelling catheter with a side hole placed in the distal common hepatic artery. If catheterization of the distal gastroduodenal artery is not possible with a 5F catheter, catheterization can be obtained with a microcatheter with a 0.025 lumen that will allow the exchange over a stiff 0.025 guidewire. Indwelling catheters tapered from 5F to 2.7F dedicated to IAHC (Celsite ST 305C, B/Braun, Chasneuil, France) are now commonly available in Europe and the United States. Then, the gastroduodenal artery will be occluded around the indwelling catheter. This occlusion can be obtained with a second catheter introduced through a contralateral (left) femoral puncture. More interestingly, the side hole in the indwelling catheter can be used to insert a microcatheter through it. This microcatheter will then be used for occlusion of the gastroduodenal artery (GDA) with 0.018 coils. At last, if catheterization of the GDA is not possible at all, a free-floating catheter can be placed in the hepatic artery. In this setting, 5F indwelling catheters can be used. After angiographic control of the correct location of the catheter, providing complete and unique liver perfusion, the catheter is tunnelized and linked to a port placed either on the chest wall or the pelvic wall according to the selected access route. Catheter maintenance means flushing with heparin solution (500 UI/10 ml) after completion of chemotherapy until the next course. Angiographic or radionuclide control is performed routinely, every two courses, to check for patency and perfusion territory of the catheter.

In our center, we use oxaliplatin (100 mg/m^2) delivered intra-arterially over 2 hours combined with intravenous folinic acid (40 mg/m^2) and 5-FU bolus at day 1, extended with 5-FU (1200 mg/m^2) over 48 hours.

Contraindications

Obviously, the hepatic artery must be patent to allow for IAHC, and occlusion or severe stenosis of the hepatic artery constitutes contraindications to IAHC. In the same manner, retrograde flow due to severe stenosis of the celiac trunk does not allow for port-catheter placement. The artery chosen for access (femoral or axillary) must be patent and free of any stenosis or severe atherosclerotic disease in order to avoid thrombosis after insertion of the indwelling catheter. Because material will be implanted, in order to avoid local sepsis, the patient must not have local or general sepsis before catheter placement. Patency of the portal system is not mandatory, but one should be aware that, in cases with compromised portal vein patency, there is a risk of hepatic necrosis if the indwelling catheter induces hepatic artery thrombosis.

Results

Technical success of catheter insertion is very high, close to 100% in our experience and in most series, including the most recently and largest reported (32). Even if it is more time-consuming, catheter fixation technique should be preferred to a free-floating catheter due to the risk of tip dislodgment in up to

20% of cases with free catheters (35). Thrombosis of the hepatic artery is rare and seems to be related to the size of the indwelling catheter – namely, when catheters larger than 5F are placed in the hepatic artery. The largest series of percutaneous implantation reports patency of 91%, 81% and 58% at 6 months, 1 and 2 years, respectively, allowing 3 to 102 courses of chemotherapy per catheter (mean = 35) (32). In the only comparative study between percutaneously and intraoperatively placed ports, intraoperatively placed ports allowed a greater number of chemotherapy courses than percutaneously placed ports, 4.3 ± 3.4 versus 6.5 ± 4.2, respectively (36). This is probably explained by an overall incidence of device-related complications causing temporary or definitive suppression of IAHC in 42.7% of percutaneously placed and 7.1% of surgically placed ones. Rates of complication were the same if the 35.7% of tip migration in the percutaneous group were not taken into account. Indeed, such migration would have not occurred had the catheter tips been fixated in the gastroduodenal artery instead of being free floating in the hepatic artery. Obviously, hospital stay and analgesic requirements were significantly lower in the percutaneous group – 1.8 ± 0.7 days and 2 ± 0.9 doses respectively – than in the surgical group – 8.2 ± 22 days and 9.7 ± 3.2 doses. Interestingly, gastroduodenal complications related to chemotherapy toxicity in cases of extra-hepatic diffusion were lower in the percutaneous group (7.1%) than in the surgical group (17.8%). It is worth emphasizing that no instance of cholecystitis was reported in three series, including 153 patients altogether, with percutaneously implanted catheters or ports, including only eight cholescystectomized patients (31, 33, 36). This is despite cholecystectomy being described in the surgical literature as a necessary step to prevent cholecystitis due to drug diffusion to the gallbladder through the cystic artery arising usually downstream of the catheter infusion hole.

The rate of reintervention to maintain functionality of the port catheter system is variable from one study to another and was estimated to be as high as 37% in our experience (37). Most of the reinterventions were due to gastric pain, resulting in the need for embolization of a previously non-occluded right gastric artery or occlusion of a collateral vessel to an occluded right gastric. The main complication of IAHC through percutaneously implanted ports is gastric ulceration occurring in patient in whom the right gastric artery could not be occluded. A rate of 36% of acute gastric mucosal lesions has been reported in patients who had undergone IAHC without embolization of the right gastric artery, but this rate decreased to 3% in patients with embolized right gastric artery (38). We recorded similar results in our center, with 30% and 5% rates of ulceration, respectively.

In our experience, IAHC with oxaliplatin combined with systemic 5-FU + folinic acid, demonstrated 11 partial responses among 16 patients who had been non-responders to previous systemic chemotherapy (26, 39).

CONCLUSION

With the advent of percutaneous catheter implantation, thereby avoiding surgery, and because of the increasing use of new drug regimens delivered intra-arterially, such as oxaliplatin and irinotecan, there is a new interest in IAHC in an attempt to increase resectability of initially unresectable liver tumors. In addition, other products such as chemo-immunotherapy (40), vasopressors such as nor-epinephrine (41), or antiangiogenic therapies could constitute exciting new therapeutic paradigms and provide new hope for intra-arterial therapy.

REFERENCES

1. Aitken DR and Minton JP. The "pinch-off sign": A warning of impending problems with permanent subclavian catheters. Am J Surg 1984; 148: 633–636

2. Ouaknine-Orlando B, Desruennes E, Cosset MF, et al. The pinch-off syndrome: Main cause of catheter embolism. Ann Fr Anesth Reanim 1999; 18: 949–955.

3. Hind D, Calvert N, McWilliams R, et al. Ultrasonic locating devices for central venous cannulation: Meta-analysis. BMJ 2003; 327: 361.

4. Bertoglio S, Disomma C, Meszaros P, et al. Long-term femoral vein central venous access in cancer patients. Eur J Surg Oncol 1996; 22: 162–165.

5. Wolosker N, Yazbek G, Munia MA, et al. Totally implantable femoral vein catheters in cancer patients. Eur J Surg Oncol 2004; 30: 771–775.

6. Cadman A, Lawrance JA, Fitzsimmons L, et al. To clot or not to clot? That is the question in central venous catheters. Clin Radiol 2004; 59: 349–355.

7. Luciani A, Clement O, Halimi P, et al. Catheter-related upper extremity deep venous thrombosis in cancer patients: A prospective study based on Doppler US. Radiology 2001; 220: 655–660.

8. Labourey JL, Lacroix P, Genet D, et al. Thrombotic complications of implanted central venous access devices: Prospective evaluation. Bull Cancer 2004; 91: 431–436.

9. Buller HR, Agnelli G, Hull RD, et al. Antithrombotic therapy for venous thromboembolic disease: The Seventh ACCP Conference on Antithrombotic and Thrombolytic Therapy. Chest 2004; 126: 401S–428S.

10. Couban S, Goodyear M, Burnell M, et al. Randomized placebo-controlled study of low-dose warfarin for the prevention of central venous catheter-associated thrombosis in patients with cancer. J Clin Oncol 2005 Jun 20; 23(18): 4063–4069.

11. Reichardt P, Kretzschmar A, Biakhov M, et al. A phase III randomized double-blind, placebo-controlled study evaluating the efficacy and safety of daily low-molecular-weight heparin (dalteparin sodium, fragmin) in preventing catheter-related complications in cancer patients with central venous catheters. Ann Oncol 2006; 17: 289–296.

12. Geerts WH, Pineo GF, Heit JA, et al. Prevention of venous thromboembolism: The Seventh ACCP Conference on Antithrombotic and Thrombolytic Therapy. Chest 2004; 126: 338S–400S.

13. Blot F, Nitenberg G, Chachaty E, et al. Diagnosis of catheter-related bacteraemia: A prospective comparison of the time to positivity of hub-blood versus peripheral-blood cultures. Lancet 1999; 354: 1071–1077.

14. Messing B, Peitra-Cohen S, Debure A, et al. Antibiotic-lock technique: A new approach to optimal therapy for catheter related sepsis in home-parenteral nutrition patients. J Parenter Enteral Nutr 1988; 12: 185–189.

15. Bessoud B, De Baere T, Kuoch V, et al. Experience at a single institution with endovascular treatment of mechanical complications caused by implanted central venous access devices in pediatric and adult patients. AJR Am J Roentgenol 2003; 180: 527–532.

16. Kock H, Pietsch M, Krause U, et al. Implanted vascular access systems: Experience in 1500 patients with totally implanted central venous port systems. World J Surg, 1998; 22: 12–16

17. Mahon T and Lawrence D, Sr. Technical report: An injection technique for repositioning subclavian catheters. Clin Radiol, 1991; 44: 197–198.

18. Roizenthal M and Hartnell G. The misplaced central venous catheter: A long loop technique for repositioning. JVIR, 1995; 6: 263–265.

19. Currarino G. Migration of jugular or subclavian venous catheters into inferior tributaries of the brachiocephalic veins or into the azygos vein, with possible complications. Pediatr Radiol, 1996; 26: 439–449.

20. Haskal Z, Leen V, Thomas-Hawkins C, et al. Transvenous removal of fibrin sheaths from tunneled hemodialysis catheter. J Vasc Interv Radiol, 1996; 7: 513–517.

21. Knelson M, Hudson E, Suhocki P, et al. Functional restoration of occluded central venous catheter: New interventional techniques. J Vasc Interv Radiol, 1995; 6: 623–627.

22. Seki H, Kimura M, Yoshimura N, et al. Hepatic arterial infusion chemotherapy using percutaneous catheter placement with an implantable port: Assessment of factors affecting patency of the hepatic artery. Clin Radiol, 1999; 54: 221–227.

23. Hwang JY, Jang BK, Kwon KM, et al. Efficacy of hepatic arterial infusion therapy for advanced hepatocellular carcinoma using 5-fluorouracil, epirubicin and mitomycin-C. Korean J Gastroenterol, 2005; 45: 118–124.

24. Meta-Analysis Group in Cancer. Reappraisal of hepatic arterial infusion in the treatment of nonresectable liver metastases from colorectal cancer. J Natl Cancer Inst, 1996; 252–258.

25. Kemeny NE, Niedzwiecki D, Hollis DR, et al. Hepatic arterial infusion versus systemic therapy for hepatic metastases from colorectal cancer: A randomized trial of efficacy, quality of life, and molecular markers (CALGB 9481). J Clin Oncol, 2006; 24: 1395–1403.

26. Boige V, Lacombe S, and de Baere T. Hepatic arterial infusion of oxaliplatin combined with 5FU and folinic acid in nonresectable liver metastasis of colorectal cancer: A promising option for failures to systemic chemotherapy. Proceedings of ASCO 2003. J Clin Oncol, 2003; 22: 291.

27. Kemeny N, Jarnagin W, Paty P, et al. Phase I trial of systemic oxaliplatin combination chemotherapy with hepatic arterial infusion in patients with unresectable liver metastases from colorectal cancer. J Clin Oncol, 2005; 23: 4888–4896.

28. Kemeny N, Huang Y, Cohen A, et al. Hepatic arterial infusion of chemotherapy after resection of hepatic metastases from colorectal cancer. N Engl J Med 1999; 341: 2039–2048.

29. Franklin M and Gonzales J. Laparoscopic placement of hepatic artery catheter for regional chemotherapy infusion. Surg Laparosc Endosc Percutan Tech, 2002; 12: 398–407.

30. Habbe TG, McCowan TC, Goertzen TC, et al. Complications and technical limitations of hepatic arterial infusion catheter placement for chemotherapy. J Vasc Interv Radiol, 1998; 9: 233–239.

31. Herrmann KA, Waggershauser T, Sittek H, et al. Liver intraarterial chemotherapy: Use of the femoral artery for percutaneous implantation of catheter-port systems. Radiology, 2000; 215: 294–299.

32. Tanaka T, Arai Y, Inaba Y, et al. Radiologic placement of side-hole catheter with tip fixation for hepatic arterial infusion chemotherapy. J Vasc Interv Radiol, 2003; 14: 63–68.

33. Zanon C, Grosso M, Clara R, et al. Combined regional and systemic chemotherapy by a mini-invasive approach for the treatment of colorectal liver metastases. Am J Clin Oncol, 2001; 24: 354–359.

34. Castaing D, Azoulay D, Fecteau A, et al. Implantable hepatic arterial infusion device: Placement without laparotomy, via an intercostal artery. J Am Coll Surg, 1998; 187: 565–568.

35. Grosso M, Zanon C, Zanon E, et al. The percutaneous placement of intra-arterial catheters with "reservoirs" for subcutaneous infusion: The technique and preliminary results. Radiol Med (Torino), 1997; 94: 226–232.

36. Aldrighetti L, Arru M, Angeli E, et al. Percutaneous vs. surgical placement of hepatic artery indwelling catheters for regional chemotherapy. Hepatogastroenterology, 2002; 49: 513–517.

37. de Baere T, El Fassy E, Lapeyre M, et al. Intra-arterial hepatic (IAH) oxaliplatinum through ports implanted percutaneously in the femoral artery. J Vasc Interv Radiol, 2004; 15 (Abstr): S226.

38. Inaba Y, Arai Y, Matsueda K, et al. Right gastric artery embolization to prevent acute gastric mucosal lesions in patients undergoing repeat hepatic arterial infusion

chemotherapy. J Vasc Interv Radiol, 2001; 12: 957–963.

39. Ducreux M, Ychou M, Laplanche A, et al. Hepatic arterial oxaliplatin infusion plus intravenous chemotherapy in colorectal cancer with inoperable hepatic metastases: A trial of the gastrointestinal group of the Federation Nationale des Centres de Lutte Contre le Cancer. J Clin Oncol, 2005; 23: 4881–4887.

40. Okuno K, Yasutomi M, Kon M, et al. Intrahepatic interleukin-2 with chemotherapy for unresectable liver metastases: A randomized multicenter trial. Hepatogastroenterology, 1999; 46: 1116–1121.

41. Shankar A, Loizidou M, Burnstock G, et al. Noradrenaline improves the tumour to normal blood flow ratio and drug delivery in a model of liver metastases. Br J Surg, 1999; 86: 453–457.

Chapter 43

GASTROINTESTINAL STENTING

Todd H. Baron

Endoscopic palliation of biliary and luminal obstruction can be achieved with the use of gastrointestinal stents. Although rigid esophageal stents were initially employed for palliation of dysphagia, self-expandable stents (plastic and metal) are almost exclusively used currently. Self-expandable metal stents (SEMS) are used for palliation of malignant gastroduodenal and colonic obstruction and can be deployed as far distally or proximally in the gastrointestinal tract as can be reached with long-length endoscopes passed orally or rectally, respectively. The use of biliary stents for malignant biliary obstruction is discussed in Chapter 31. This chapter will outline the use of stents in the gastrointestinal tract to provide endoluminal palliation.

BASIC PRINCIPLES

SEMS are composed of a variety of metal alloys with varying shapes and sizes depending on the individual manufacturer and organ of placement (1). SEMS are preloaded in a collapsed (constrained) position, mounted on a small-diameter delivery catheter. A central lumen within the delivery system allows for passage over a guidewire. Once the guidewire has been advanced beyond the obstruction, the constrained stent is passed over the guidewire and positioned across the stricture. The constraint system is released or withdrawn, which allows radial expansion of the stent and of the stenosed lumen during deployment. The radial expansile forces and degree of shortening differ between stent types (2). Metal SEMS may also have a covering membrane (covered stents) to prevent tumor ingrowth through the mesh wall and to close fistulas. SEMS produce imaging artifacts on both computed tomography (CT) and magnetic res-

onance imaging (MRI), which may hinder accurate interpretation of pathology in and around the SEMS. Although most SEMS materials appear to be safe for MRI, specific stent shape, orientation to the magnetic field and type of alloy composition influence signal intensity in vitro. Therefore, this information should be obtained before an MRI is performed in a patient who has undergone SEMS placement (3, 4).

Tissue reactions to metal SEMS are known based on animal data (5) and autopsy and surgical findings in humans (6). The uncovered portion of the stent becomes incorporated into both the tumor and surrounding tissue by pressure necrosis. In the areas uninvolved by tumor above and below the stenosis, the stent incorporates deeply into the wall of the organ. This reaction allows anchoring of the stent and helps to prevent stent migration. Covering of the stent prevents integration into the wall and promotes stent migration, especially when fully covered. Therefore, partially covered stents are used in which the mid-portion is covered and the ends are uncovered to allow anchoring of the stent. Stent embedment is essential for anchoring but accounts for some of the adverse effects seen when the pressure from expansion causes stent material to erode through the esophageal wall, resulting in tracheoesophageal fistula and bleeding from erosion into vascular structures. The one commercially available plastic stent does not imbed into tissue.

PALLIATION OF MALIGNANT DYSPHAGIA

In patients with advanced disease, the focus of care shifts to improving or preserving quality of life.

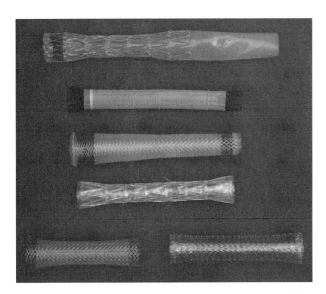

FIGURE 43.1. Various commercially available esophageal stents in their fully deployed state. The uppermost stent has an anti-reflux valve. See Color Plate 36.

Obstruction of the esophageal lumen by tumor leads to dysphagia and poor nutritional status. Such patients are also at risk for aspiration pneumonia.

Endoscopically placed stents apply internal radial forces to the esophagus, mechanically widening the esophageal lumen (Figure 43.1). Stents are useful in palliating malignant dysphagia resulting from both intrinsic tumors (Figure 43.2) of the esophagus and from extrinsic malignant processes causing compression of the esophagus, such as extra-esophageal cancers and lymphadenopathy.

Endoscopically placed stents provide an alternative to surgery for the palliation of inoperable cancers involving the esophagus or gastric cardia. Unlike feeding tubes, the use of stents can result in palliation of dysphagia, allowing peroral nutrition. Covered metal stents allow closure of tracheoesophageal fistulas (Figure 43.3) (7).

SEMS have largely replaced conventional rigid plastic stents, which required aggressive dilation of the stricture to allow placement and carried increased risk of perforation (8). SEMS have the advantages of a thin wall and collapsed design, allowing expansion to a larger, suitable diameter after deployment. The lower cost of plastic stents may make them preferred in areas of the world where resources are limited (9).

Efficacy of SEMS for Malignant Dysphagia

Dysphagia has been shown to be effectively and reliably relieved after insertion of SEMS. For example, in a review of 121 patients with SEMS for malignant esophageal obstruction, dysphagia scores improved in 95% (10). Complications include food impaction, bleeding, stent migration and tumor ingrowth and overgrowth (11).

Dysphagia from cancers at the gastroesophageal junction (GEJ) can be effectively managed with SEMS that traverse the GEJ. Their placement results in free reflux of stomach contents into the esophagus, placing these patients at high risk for reflux esophagitis and aspiration. Proton pump inhibitors are administered to these patients, although they do not provide

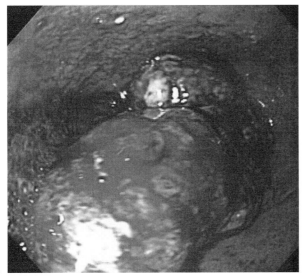
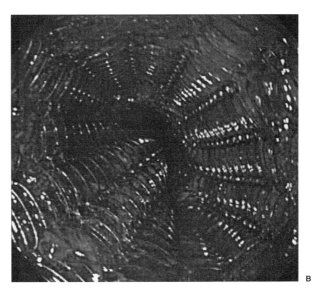

FIGURE 43.2.   Palliation of esophageal obstruction. (A) Endoscopic view of obstructing tumor. (B) Immediately after placement of partially covered stent. See Color Plate 37.

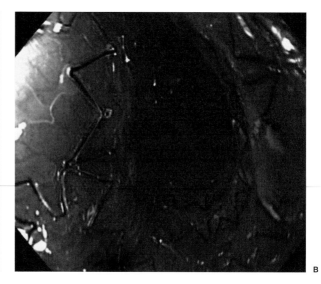

FIGURE 43.3.   Closure of tracheoesophageal fistula. (A) Endoscopic view of fistula: Note guidewire is in esophageal lumen. (B) Immediately after placement of covered stent. See Color Plate 38.

a barrier to reflux or regurgitation of gastric contents. Anti reflux valves have been added to combat this problem (Figure 43.1) (12, 13).

Early complications after esophageal stent placement may include perforation, aspiration, chest pain and malpositioning of the stent. Perforation is usually related to use of excessive force in dilation or guidewire trauma and can usually be managed non-operatively. Transient (up to 1 week) chest pain is expected and is treated with narcotic analgesics. More prolonged or severe, intractable chest pain may occur following uncomplicated stent placement, but an evaluation to exclude a procedural-related complication should be instituted. Airway obstruction can occur in the presence of a large mediastinal mass that impinges upon an area at or near the trachea or tracheal bifurcation. It can be managed with emergent stent removal or with mechanical intubation and subsequent airway stent placement (14).

Late esophageal complications may occur as a result of SEMS placement (Table 43.1) (15). These may include gastroesophageal reflux and aspiration if the stent traverses the gastroesophageal junction. As mentioned, such patients should be placed on high-dose proton pump inhibitor therapy indefinitely. Additional precautions should be taken, such as elevating the head of the bead and avoiding recumbency within 3 hours of a meal. Chest pain may result from gastroesophageal reflux. Stent occlusion may result from an impacted food bolus, which can be dislodged endoscopically. Tissue-related stent occlusion may be due to tumor ingrowth, tumor overgrowth or

tissue hyperplasia. Treatment options to restore luminal patency usually involve placement of a new stent through the previous stent. Covered metal stents are associated with less tumor ingrowth than uncovered stents but are more prone to migration (16). Major bleeding can result from erosion of the stent through the esophagus and into a major vessel such as the aorta. Tracheoesophageal fistula can result from stent erosion into the respiratory tree.

Types of Stents

A variety of Food and Drug Administration-approved stents are available for palliation of malignant dysphagia (Figure 43.1) (17). The few published comparative

TABLE 43.1 Complications of Expandable Metal Esophageal Stents

Early
Perforation
Chest pain
Bleeding (mild)
Airway obstruction
Aspiration

Late
Perforation
Tracheoesophageal fistula
Obstruction: tumor ingrowth, overgrowth, tissue
    hyperplasia
Food impaction
Reflux with aspiration, esophagitis
Bleeding (often massive)
Migration

studies suggest there is little difference in clinical outcomes among metal stents (18–20).

Self-expandable Plastic Stent

Recently, a self-expandable plastic stent has been developed for relief of malignant dysphagia. The potential advantages of the stent over SEMS are its removability, avoidance of erosive complications (fistula) and decrease in tissue hyperplasia. Two single-arm studies from outside the United States suggest that this stent is useful for palliation of malignant dysphagia (21, 22), but a randomized trial comparing this stent with SEMS showed equal palliation of dysphagia although with significantly more complications, especially late stent migration (23).

Chemoradiation Therapy and Stent Placement

The safety of placing SEMS after previous administration of radiation or chemotherapy is controversial (24–26). In one study of 200 patients, the incidence of complications and outcome after SEMS placement were not affected by prior radiation or chemotherapy (27). However, in another study of 116 patients, prior chemoradiotherapy was the only independent predictive factor of post-procedure major complications, with an odds ratio of 5.6 (28). In contrast, there is little information about the effect of concomitant radiation and stent placement (29). A theoretical disadvantage of stent placement and concomitant chemotherapy is the potential increased risk of stent migration.

MALIGNANT GASTRIC OUTLET OBSTRUCTION

Malignant gastric outlet obstruction (GOO) produces post-prandial abdominal pain, early satiety, vomiting and intolerability of oral intake. SEMS for GOO was first described in 1992 (30). Since that time, numerous publications have described the efficacy of SEMS for palliating GOO. The types of stents and technique for placement have been described elsewhere (31). In a systematic review of 32 case series, including 10 prospective series, the efficacy of SEMS for gastroduodenal malignancies was reported (32). The majority of malignancies included were gastric and pancreatic in origin. In all, 606 patients underwent attempted stent placement.

Technical success, defined as successful stent placement and deployment, was achieved in 589 (97%). Technical failure was attributed to severe obstruc-

TABLE 43.2 Complications of Enteral Stents

	Gastroduodenal (%)	Colonic (%)
Migration	25	12
Obstruction	17	7
Perforation		4
Bleeding	1	
Tenesmus, incontinence and pain (distal rectal placement)		

tion, difficult anatomy, malpositioning and one failed delivery. Clinical success, defined as relief of symptoms and improved oral intake, occurred in 89% of the technical successes. Clinical failures were due to early stent migration (20%) and disease progression (61%), and procedural complications (15%) such as malpositioned stent or partially expanded stent. Severe complications included bleeding (1%). There were no procedure-related deaths. Non-severe complications occurred in 27% of attempted stent placements. The most commonly reported non-severe complication was stent occlusion (17%), primarily due to tumor growth or obstruction away from the stent. Late migration occurred in 5% of patients, generally managed with additional stent placement. Pain was reported in 2% of subjects. Evidence of biliary obstruction after stent placement was noted in 1% of subjects. The mean survival was 12.1 weeks. In summary, severe complications occurred in 1.2%, non-severe complications occurred in 27%. Most non-severe complications were related to stent obstruction. Complications related to gastroduodenal stenting (11) are seen in Table 43.2.

It is important to note the need to consider prophylactic biliary stent placement prior to gastroduodenal stent placement if there is concern for future biliary obstruction, as the papilla may become inaccessible once the gastroduodenal stent has been placed (Figure 43.4).

Surgical gastroenterostomy has been compared to endoscopic SEMS for palliation of unresectable malignant antro-pyloric stenosis (33). In a small, randomized prospective trial of 18 patients, stent placement was successful in 100%. Mean time to oral intake was 6.3 days for surgical patients and 2.1 days for stent treatment (p ≤ 0.0001). Median duration of hospital stay was longer in the surgical group, 10 days, compared with 3.1 days in the stent group. Mean

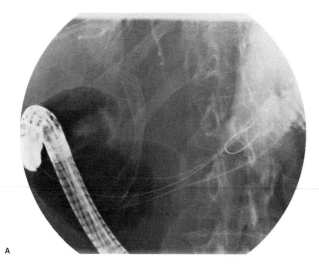

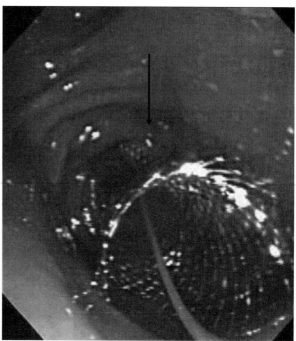

FIGURE 43.4. Double stenting of pancreatic cancer. (A) Radiograph taken immediately after deployment of biliary SEMS and duodenal SEMS. (B) Endoscopic view of both duodenal stent and biliary stent (*arrow*) immediately after deployment. See Color Plate 39.

procedure time was twice as long compared to the endoscopy group. One major complication occurred in the stent and surgery groups – stent dislocation and postoperative hemorrhage, respectively. No difference in morbidity or mortality was seen.

Other retrospective studies have shown similar results. Time to ingestion of both liquids and light-consistency diet and post-procedure duration of hospital stay are significantly shorter in the endoscopic stent group compared with surgical groups. Post-procedural and procedural costs are higher in the gastrojejunostomy groups (34). These findings favor endoscopic placement of expandable metal stents rather than open or laparoscopic gastrojejunostomy for palliation of malignant gastric outlet obstruction on the basis of effectiveness, fewer complications, reduced cost and earlier resumption of oral intake.

COLONIC OBSTRUCTION

The mortality associated with acute colonic obstruction is high, and colonic obstruction due to malignancy is the number one cause of emergency large-bowel surgery (35).

Endoscopically placed stents are placed for several indications in patients with obstructive colorectal malignancies (36). The methods of colorectal stent placement have been described in detail elsewhere

(36). Stents can be used for temporary decompression prior to resection of operable colonic tumors. This decompression may permit a one-stage bowel resection operation, versus a two-stage operation for an unprepared colon. The two-stage operation includes resection of involved bowel and the creation of a colostomy, followed by colostomy takedown and reanastomis of colon, which is necessary if the colon has not been cleansed. Secondly, stents can be used for palliation of inoperable obstructive colorectal malignancies (Figure 43.5). Extrinsic compression from pelvic malignancies and lymphadenopathy may also be palliated with stents. Finally, a covered stent can be placed in the rectum to seal fistulas to the vagina and bladder (37).

Sebastian et al. (38) published a comprehensive report on the efficacy and safety of SEMS for malignant colorectal obstruction based on studies published from 1990 to 2003. No randomized trial was identified. Fifty-four case series comprising 1198 patients were included in this pooled analysis; 791 of the patients had undergone stent placement for palliation. In the remaining patients, stenting was performed as a bridge to surgery. Of the patients treated palliatively, technical success in stent placement was achieved in 93%, and clinical success was achieved in 91% (cumulative rates). Perforations, predominately in the rectosigmoid region, occurred in 3.8% of patients. Of those, 64% required emergency

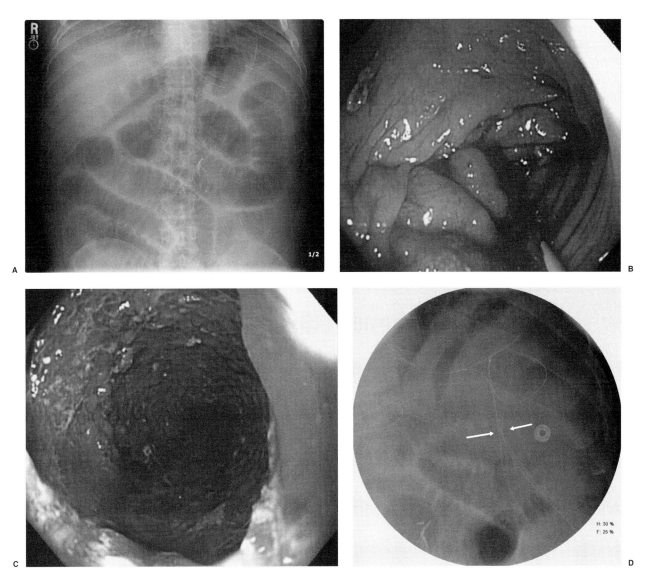

FIGURE 43.5. Palliative stent placement for obstructing mass near splenic flexure. (A) Plain radiograph showing dilated small bowel and colon to the splenic flexure. (B) Endoscopic view of obstructing mass. (C) Endoscopic view of Wallstent immediately after deployment. (D) Radiographic view immediately after successful deployment. Note waist in midportion (*arrows*) corresponding to obstructing mass. See Color Plate 40.

surgery. In 17.7% of perforations, pre-dilation was thought to be a causative factor. The use of laser therapy in the pre-stent setting was also thought to contribute to perforation in a few cases. Perforations were attributed to balloon dilation, stent wires and guidewires. Migration in technically successful stent placements occurred in 11.8% of cases, two-thirds of which occurred within the first week. Most migration was distal (94.7%). Fifteen percent of the palliative stents migrated compared with only 3.9% of the stents used as bridge to surgery. The cumulative procedure-related mortality rate for all stent placements was 0.58%. Most of these deaths were patients receiving palliative therapy. Re-obstruction was noted in 7.3% of patients at a median time of

24 weeks. Re-obstruction was due to tumor ingrowth in most cases. Other causes of obstruction, such as fecal impaction, mucosal prolapse, tumor overgrowth and peritoneal seeding, occurred less frequently. Laser, argon plasma coagulation, stent replacement and surgery were among the modalities used to treat re-obstruction. It is important to note that stent placement in the right colon is also effective (39). Complications of gastroduodenal/colonic (enteral) SEMS are listed in Table 43.2.

CONCLUSION

Endoluminal palliation of the esophagus can be achieved with placement of expandable plastic and metal stents. Stents are widely available for this use. SEMS placement is the only endoscopic management option that restores luminal continuity in patients with malignant gastroduodenal and colonic obstruction. In the colon, stents can be used to restore luminal patency both preoperatively and for palliation in order to avoid colostomy.

REFERENCES

1. Baron TH. Expandable gastrointestinal stents. Gastroenterology, 2007; 133: 1407–1411.
2. Chan AC, Shin FG, Lam YH, et al. A comparison study on physical properties of self-expandable esophageal metal stents. Gastrointest Endosc, 1999; 49: 462–465.
3. Taal BG, Muller SH, Boot H, et al. Potential risks and artifacts of magnetic resonance imaging of self-expandable esophageal stents. Gastrointest Endosc, 1997; 46: 424–429.
4. Nitatori T, Hanaoka H, Hachiya J, et al. MRI artifacts of metallic stents derived from imaging sequencing and the ferromagnetic nature of materials. Radiat Med, 1999; 17: 329–334.
5. Silvis SE, Sievert CE Jr, Vennes JA, et al. Comparison of covered versus uncovered wire mesh stents in the canine biliary tract. Gastrointest Endosc, 1994; 40: 17–21.
6. Bethge N, Sommer A, Gross U, et al. Human tissue responses to metal stents implanted in vivo for the palliation of malignant stenoses. Gastrointest Endosc, 1996; 43: 596–602.
7. Papachristou GI and Baron TH. Use of stents in benign and malignant esophageal disease. Rev Gastroenterol Disord, 2007 Spring; 7(2): 74–88.
8. De Palma GD, Di Matteo E, Romano G, et al. Plastic prosthesis versus expandable metal stents for palliation of inoperable esophageal thoracic carcinoma: A controlled prospective study. Gastrointest Endosc, 1996; 43(5): 478–482.
9. Szentpali K, Palotas A, Lazar G, et al. Endoscopic intubation with conventional plastic stents: A safe and cost-effective palliation for inoperable esophageal cancer. Dysphagia, 2004; 19(1): 22–27.
10. O'Sullivan GJ and Grundy A. Palliation of malignant dysphagia with expanding metallic stents. J Vasc Interv Radiol, 1999; 10(3): 346–351.
11. Baron TH. Minimizing endoscopic complications: Endoluminal stents. Gastrointest Endosc Clin North Am, 2007; 17: 83–104, vii.
12. Dua KS, Kozarek R, Kim J, et al. Self-expanding metal esophageal stent with anti-reflux mechanism. Gastrointest Endosc, 2001; 53(6): 603–613.
13. Laasch HU, Marriott A, Wilbraham L, et al. Effectiveness of open versus antireflux stents for palliation of distal esophageal carcinoma and prevention of symptomatic gastroesophageal reflux. Radiology, 2002; 225(2): 359–365.
14. Sihoe AD, Wan IY, and Yim AP. Airway stenting for unresectable esophageal cancer. Surg Oncol, 2004 Jul; 13(1): 17–25.
15. Wang MQ, Sze DY, Wang ZP, et al. Delayed complications after esophageal stent placement for treatment of malignant esophageal obstructions and esophagorespiratory fistulas. J Vasc Interv Radiol, 2001 Apr; 12(4): 465–474.
16. Vakil N, Morris AI, Marcon N, et al. A prospective, randomized, controlled trial of covered expandable metal stents in the palliation of malignant esophageal obstruction at the gastroesophageal junction. Am J Gastroenterol, 2001; 96(6): 1791–1796.
17. Baron TH. A practical guide for choosing an expandable metal stent for GI malignancies: Is a stent by any other name still a stent? Gastrointest Endosc, 2001; 54(2): 269–272.
18. Sabharwal T, Hamady MS, Chui S, et al. A randomised prospective comparison of the Flamingo Wallstent and Ultraflex stent for palliation of dysphagia associated with lower third oesophageal carcinoma. Gut, 2003; 52(7): 922–926.
19. Siersema PD, Hop WC, van Blankenstein M, et al. A comparison of 3 types of covered metal stents for the palliation of patients with dysphagia caused by esophagogastric carcinoma: A prospective, randomized study. Gastrointest Endosc, 2001; 54(2): 145–153.
20. Riccioni ME, Shah SK, Tringali A, et al. Endoscopic palliation of unresectable malignant oesophageal strictures with self-expanding metal stents: Comparing Ultraflex and Esophacoil stents. Dig Liver Dis, 2002; 34(5): 356–363.
21. Dormann AJ, Eisendrath P, Wigginghaus B, et al. Palliation of esophageal carcinoma with a new self-expanding plastic stent. Endoscopy, 2003; 35(3): 207–211
22. Costamagna G, Shah SK, Tringali A, et al. Prospective evaluation of a new self-expanding plastic stent for inoperable esophageal strictures. Surg Endosc, 2003; 17(6): 891–895.
23. Conio M, Repici A, Battaglia G, et al. A randomized prospective comparison of self-expandable plastic stents and partially covered self-expandable metal stents in the palliation of malignant esophageal dysphagia. Am J Gastroenterol, 2007 Dec; 102(12): 2667–2677.
24. Kinsman KJ, DeGregorio BT, Katon RM, et al. Prior radiation and chemotherapy increase the risk of life-threatening complications after insertion of metallic stents for esophagogastric malignancy. Gastrointest Endosc, 1996; 43: 196–203.
25. Siersema PD, Hop WC, Dees J, et al. Coated self-expanding metal stents versus latex prostheses for esophagogastric cancer with special reference to prior radiation and chemotherapy: A controlled, prospective study. Gastrointest Endosc, 1998: 47: 113–120.
26. Bartelsman JF, Bruno MJ, Jensema AJ, et al. Palliation of patients with esophagogastric neoplasms by insertion of a covered expandable modified Gianturco-Z endoprosthesis: Experiences in 153 patients. Gastrointest Endosc, 2000; 51: 134–138.
27. Homs MY, Hansen BE, van Blankenstein M, et al. Prior radiation and/or chemotherapy has no effect on the outcome of metal stent placement for esophagogastric carcinoma. Eur J Gastroenterol Hepatol, 2004; 16: 163–170.
28. Lecleire S, Di Fiore F, Ben-Soussan E, et al. Prior chemoradiotherapy is associated with a higher life-threatening complication rate after palliative insertion of

metal stents in patients with oesophageal cancer. Aliment Pharmacol Ther, 2006; 23: 1693–1702.

29. Ludwig D, Dehne A, Burmester E, et al. Treatment of unresectable carcinoma of the esophagus or the gastroesophageal junction by mesh stents with or without radiochemotherapy. Int J Oncol, 1998; 13: 583–588.

30. Truong S, Bohndorf V, Geller H, et al. Self-expanding metal stents for palliation of malignant gastric outlet obstruction. Endoscopy, 1992; 24(5): 433–435.

31. Baron TH, Schofl R, Puespoek A, et al. Expandable metal stent placement for gastric outlet obstruction. Endoscopy, 2001; 33(7): 623–628.

32. Dormann A, Meisner S, Verin N, et al. Self-expanding metal stents for gastroduodenal malignancies: Systematic review of their clinical effectiveness. Endoscopy, 2004; 36(6): 543–550.

33. Fiori E, Lamazza A, Volpino P, et al. Palliative management of malignant antro-pyloric strictures. Gastroenterostomy vs. endoscopic stenting. A randomized prospective trial. Anticancer Res, 2004; 24(1): 269–271.

34. Mittal A, Windsor J, Woodfield J, et al. Matched study of three methods for palliation of malignant pyloroduodenal obstruction. Br J Surg 2004; 91(2): 205–209.

35. Baron TH. Benign and malignant colorectal strictures. In: Waye JD, Rex DK, Williams CB, eds. Colonoscopy: Principles and Practice, 1st edition, pp. 611–623. Massachusetts: Blackwell Publishing, 2003.

36. Baron TH, Rey JF, and Spinelli P. Expandable metal stent placement for malignant colorectal obstruction. Endoscopy, 2002; 34(10): 823–830.

37. Repici A, Reggio D, Saracco G, et al. Self-expanding covered esophageal ultraflex stent for palliation of malignant colorectal anastomotic obstruction complicated by multiple fistulas. Gastrointest Endosc, 2000; 51(3): 346–348.

38. Sebastian S, Johnston S, Geoghegan T, et al. Pooled analysis of the efficacy and safety of self-expanding metal stenting in malignant colorectal obstruction. Am J Gastroenterol, 2004; 99(10): 2051–2057.

39. Repici A, Adler DG, Gibbs CM, et al. Stenting of the proximal colon in patients with malignant large bowel obstruction: Techniques and outcomes. Gastrointest Endosc, 2007; 66: 940–944.

Chapter 44

DIAGNOSIS AND MANAGEMENT OF SUPERIOR VENA CAVA SYNDROME

Robert J. Lewandowski

Bassel Atassi

Riad Salem

BACKGROUND

Superior vena cava (SVC) syndrome, first described in 1757 by William Hunter (1), refers to a constellation of clinical symptoms caused by obstruction of the SVC. This obstruction is nearly always (>85%) attributable to advanced malignancy (2, 3), most commonly lung cancer. In fact, SVC syndrome affects 3% to 4% of patients with bronchogenic cancer (4). Other primary thoracic malignancies, lymphoma and metastatic disease (particularly from breast and testicular primaries) have also been implicated in SVC syndrome either secondary to extrinsic compression of the SVC or due to direct tumor invasion (2). Benign causes of SVC syndrome include venous stenoses, thrombosis (secondary to vascular access catheters and invasive monitoring devices), extrinsic compression from thoracic aortic aneurysms and mediastinal fibrosis from granulomatous disease (5).

The diagnosis of SVC syndrome is initially made clinically. SVC syndrome is characterized by congestion and swelling of the face and upper thorax, with distended superficial chest veins. Other associated symptoms include dyspnea, hoarseness, dysphagia, severe headache and cognitive dysfunction (6, 7). The most severe complications of SVC syndrome include glottic edema and venous thrombosis in the central nervous system (venous stroke).

Contrast-enhanced computed tomography (CT) of the chest with vascular reconstruction images should be obtained in these patients, as it can both confirm the site of SVC obstruction as well as delineate the cause of the obstruction (8). Alternatively, magnetic resonance imaging (MRI) can be obtained in those patients with contraindications to CT. The gold standard for diagnosing SVC syndrome is venography.

Medical management of SVC syndrome includes bed rest, head elevation, steroids, diuretics and, possibly, systemic anticoagulation. These strategies have limited clinical benefit and do not treat the underlying abnormality (9, 10). External-beam radiation with or without chemotherapy is the traditional first-line therapy for acute SVC syndrome (11–16); however, time is required for radiation to take effect, with clinical benefit often not becoming evident for 3 to 4 weeks. Furthermore, radiation therapy can produce side-effects such as dysphagia, nausea and vomiting, and tumor edema from radiation injury may actually worsen the clinical symptoms. Radiation is also less successful when used to treat those with non-small cell cancers or those with recurrent disease. Surgery for patients with SVC syndrome is rarely indicated secondary to its invasiveness and the complexity of the mediastinal venous system. Palliative surgery involves a sternotomy and venous bypass between either the left brachiocephalic or jugular vein and the right atrial appendage (17). These patients typically have a poor overall prognosis secondary to their advanced malignancy.

The use of expandable metallic stents for the treatment of SVC stenosis was first described in animals in 1986 (18) with clinical reports appearing by 1992 (19–22). Since that time, there have been many reports in the literature supporting endovascular therapy of SVC syndrome (23–45). Stents have now arguably become the standard of care for patients presenting with clinical sequelae of chronic SVC obstruction (14, 29), as stenting the SVC is less invasive than surgical bypass, as well as less cytotoxic than external-beam radiation. Stenting has proved to be safe and effective while providing rapid relief of symptoms. Furthermore, SVC stenting does not preclude additional oncology therapies.

INDICATIONS

Metallic stents for SVC syndrome are typically reserved for patients with malignant obstruction (>85% of patients with SVC syndrome). Placing metallic stents in patients with benign disease is controversial given patients' long life expectancy. There is a risk that the metallic stents could develop neointimal hyperplasia and subsequently occlude over time, with the return of symptoms.

Although treatment for SVC syndrome should be done in a timely manner, it is no longer considered a medical emergency (46, 47). The exception is patients who present with dyspnea, depressed central nervous system or sinus thrombosis. These patients should have stents placed expeditiously in order to re-establish venous flow.

CONTRAINDICATIONS

There are no absolute contraindications to metallic stent therapy for SVC syndrome. Relative contraindications include a severe, uncorrectable coagulopathy and severe cardiac disease. As with all endovascular procedures, a severe, uncorrectable coagulopathy poses increased risk to the patient for bleeding complications. Patients with severe cardiac disease are at increased risk for cardiac failure or pulmonary edema secondary to hemodynamic changes following relief of their SVC obstruction. These changes are the

result of increased venous return to the right atrium. Patients at such risk may require smaller-diameter stents or post-procedure medications such as diuretics and dopamine (48). The role of SVC stenting in young patients with long life expectancy remains controversial. An extended life expectancy, although not a contraindication, should be factored into the decision-making process, as the long-term sequelae of neointimal hyperplasia and life-long intervention will undoubtedly play a role in stent management.

TECHNIQUE

Informed consent is obtained prior to the procedure. The patients receive intravenous (IV) conscious sedation with continuous physiologic monitoring. Many advocate the use of intraprocedural anticoagulation.

The initial step is to perform superior vena cavography. This defines extent of disease and the presence of thrombus within the venous system. The femoral and jugular veins are the conventional access sites, although the basilic and subclavian veins have been used (32). These latter two access sites may be particularly useful when the obstructive process involves the brachiocephalic veins. Based on information from the venogram and pre-procedure cross-sectional imaging, a decision must be made whether thrombolysis should be performed. Mechanical or pharmacologic thrombolysis can both reduce the length of obstruction requiring stenting, and the subsequent risk of pulmonary emboli (24–26, 33, 34). Thrombolysis may be considered in patients with SVC syndrome from acute thrombosis.

Following venography, the obstruction must be crossed. This is typically facilitated with a combination of selective catheters (e.g., angled-glide catheter) and hydrophilic guidewires (e.g., glidewire). Once the lesion is traversed, the hydrophilic guidewire should be exchanged for an exchange-length stiff guidewire. This wire will serve as the working wire over which stenting will be performed. Road-map or fluoro-fade imaging techniques are helpful for proper stent placement. Angioplasty without stenting does not appear to have a significant role in treating this disease given the high recurrence rate following balloon angioplasty alone (49, 50). However, angioplasty may be necessary to facilitate the stent deployment device across the stenosis. The literature does not demonstrate a significant difference between

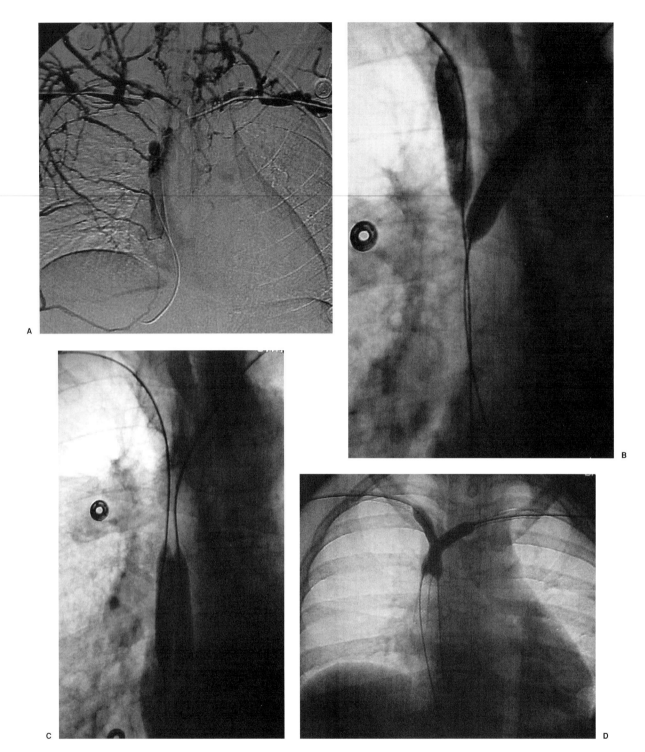

FIGURE 44.1.   70-year-old man with bronchogenic carcinoma and acute SVC syndrome. (A) Central venogram
obtained by bilateral basilic vein access demonstrates occlusion at the confluence of the brachiocephalic veins and SVC
with tremendous collateralization. Guidewires have crossed
the lesions bilaterally. (B and C) 10-mm angioplasty balloons
were used to allow delivery of stent deployment system. (D)
Kissing 10-mm Wallstents were placed and dilated. These
stents were dilated with a 10-mm balloon.

using one of the three most commonly used stents:
Wallstent (Schneider Stent Inc., USA), the Palmaz
stent (Johnson & Johnson, Warren, NJ) and the
Gianturco Z-stent (Cook Inc., Bloomington, IN)
(Figures 44.1 and 44.2) (26, 28, 30, 31, 36). Self-

expanding stents are often favored given their greater
length and ability to mold into the shape of the vessel into which they are deployed. However, balloon-
expandable stents offer greater precision in placement
and may be useful when the obstructive lesion is near

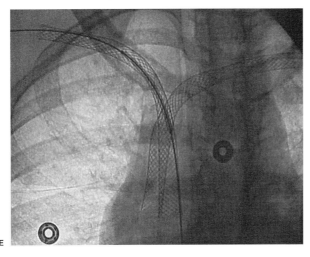

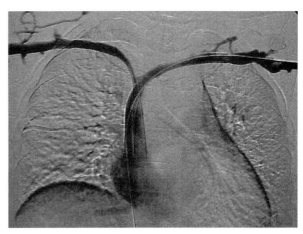

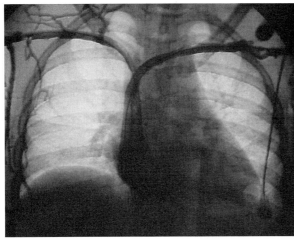

FIGURE 44.1. (*Continued*) **(E) Balloon expandable stent was necessary to reinforce the right-sided stent. (F and G) Post-procedure venograms demonstrate patency of the central veins and stents with marked reduction in collateral vessels.**

the brachiocephalic veins. However, caution should be exercised when deploying ballon expandable stents for SVC obstruction: "watermelon seeding" of the stent into the right atrium has been observed (Figure 44.3). Given the knowledge that such a complication might occur, it is even more important to maintain wire access through the stents at all times until the procedure is completed satisfactorily.

There also may be a role for covered stents, particularly when intracaval tumor is present (31). Intracaval tumor can prevent correct endothelialization of the stent, and the tumor might grow beyond the stent struts on an uncovered stent (51). In essence, the stent should of sufficient length to cover the occlusion with at least 10 mm free at both ends of the occlusion. The stent ideally does not cover the brachiocephalic veins. If the obstructive process involves these veins, some authors advocate stenting both brachiocephalic veins into the SVC ("kissing stents") whereas others have had success relieving only one side (preferably the right side). This method of stenting the right side

only has been found to relieve the most distressing symptoms and allows the existing collateral veins on the unstented side to drain more effectively (14, 29). Also, these authors concluded that those with bilateral stents had more complications than those with unilateral stent placement. Following stent deployment, a balloon dilatation is undertaken to ensure full stent deployment. A completion venogram is performed to confirm stent position and assess for complications (Figure 44.4).

PATIENT MANAGEMENT

SVC stenting may be performed on an outpatient basis. Patients should be observed for at least 2 to 6 hours following the procedure. Hemodynamic monitoring is typically performed every 15 minutes for the first hour and every 30 minutes for the second hour (52). Patients are then discharged either to their home or hospital bed if they are stable and meet institution-specific discharge criteria. The role of long-term

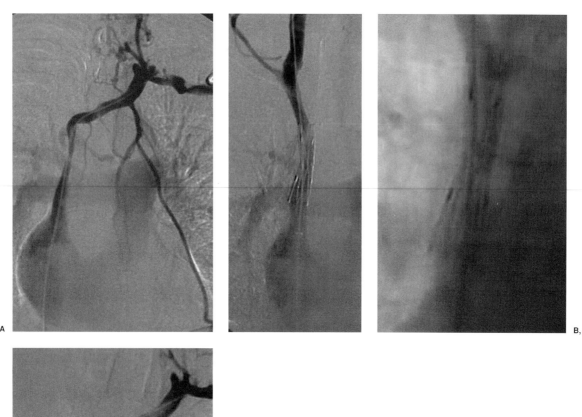

FIGURE 44.2. 56-year-old woman with lymphoma. (A) Venogram via the left basilic vein demonstrates severe stenosis of SVC. Note that this stenosis does not extend to the confluence of the brachiocephalic veins. (B) The right internal jugular (IJ) vein was accessed, and a Gianturco Z-Stent was deployed across the stenosis. This venogram performed via the right IJ demonstrates patency of the stent and SVC. (C) Close-up view of Z-stent. (D) Post-procedure left basilic vein venogram demonstrates patency of the stent, SVC, and left brachiocephalic vein. This stent, placed appropriately in the SVC, does not "jail" either of the brachiocephalic veins.

anticoagulation to maintain stent patency remains controversial. Whereas some authors support fully anticoagulating these patients (24, 30, 38), others have favored only anti-platelet regimens (29, 39).

Most patients are seen in follow-up by the referring physician. As interventional radiologists develop more clinical focus, patients are often seen in interventional radiology clinics as well. There is no standard imaging protocol for these patients. Chest radiographs (frontal and lateral) are initially obtained to assess stent expansion and serve as a baseline to monitor for future stent migration (29–31). If clinical symptoms recur, further imaging with CT, MRI, or venography can be performed.

OUTCOMES

The technical and clinical success rates of SVC stenting compare favorably with traditional first-line therapies for SVC syndrome (53). The technical success rate of SVC stenting is greater than 95%, and the clinical success is 80% to 95%. In general, facial edema resolves within the first 24 hours of stenting and upper extremity swelling resolves within 72 hours.

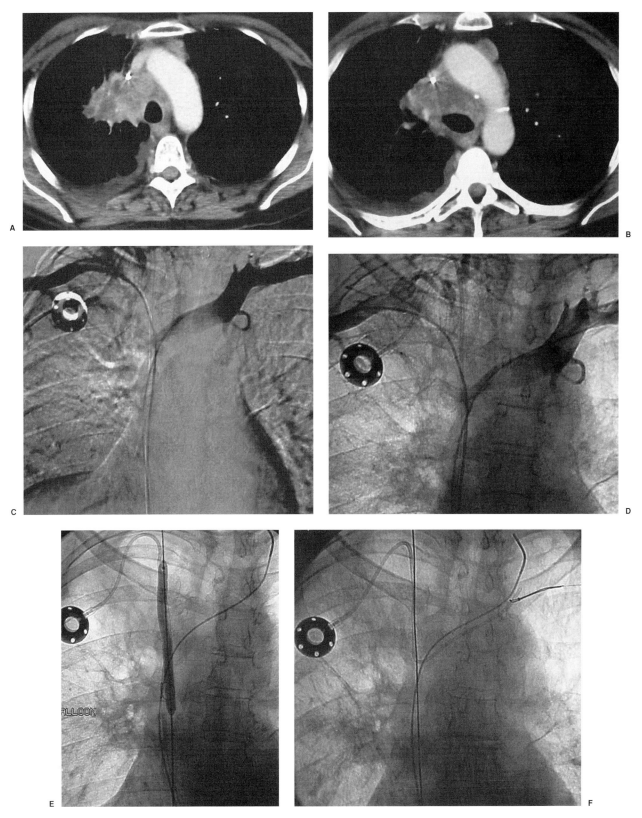

FIGURE 44.3. 56-year-old woman with breast cancer. (A and B) CT images of the chest show a large heterogenous mass compressing the SVC. Note the white catheter tip from patient's chest port. (C and D) Central venograms via bilateral basilic vein access demonstrate occlusion of the SVC, extending to the brachiocephalic veins. (E) Access was obtained from the right IJ and right common femoral vein. Angioplasty performed via right internal jugular (IJ) with 6-mm balloon. (F) A snare passed from left basilic vein was used to remove the chest port catheter tip from the SVC in preparation for SVC stent placement.

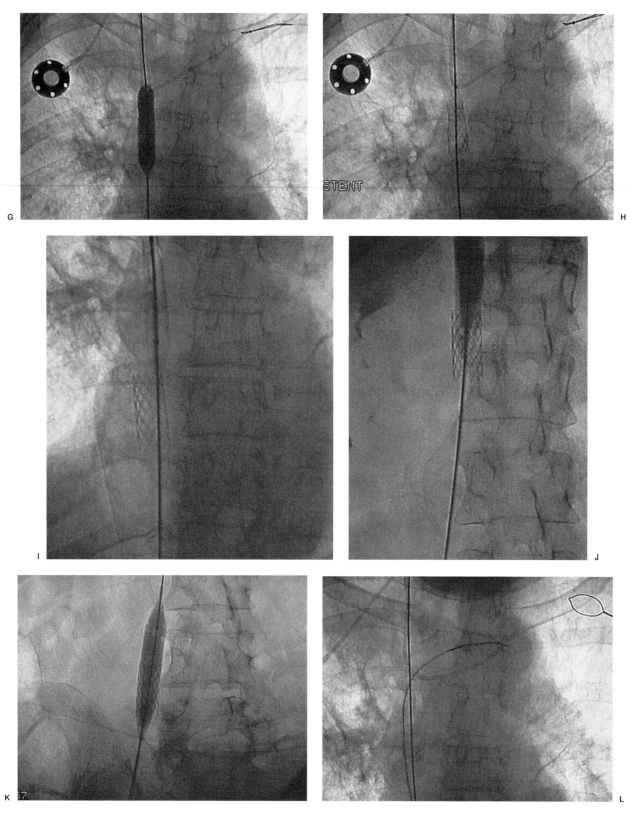

FIGURE 44.3. (*Continued*) (G and H) Balloon expandable stent placement. (I) The stent migrated ("watermelon seed") into the right atrium with subsequent balloon dilatation attempts. (J and K) The stent was pulled into the right common iliac vein in preparation for deployment in the right common iliac vein. (L) The chest port catheter tip was then snared from the right common femoral vein access and brought back into the SVC.

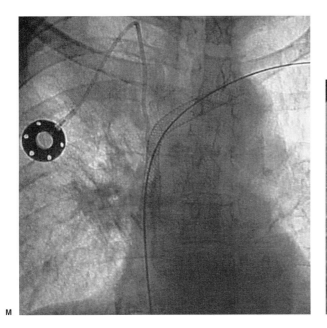

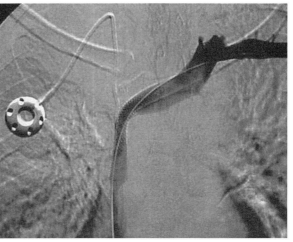

FIGURE 44.3. (*Continued*) (M) A Wallstent was placed via the left side, extending from the left brachiocephalic vein and into the SVC. (N) Post procedure, left central venogram demonstrates patency of the stent, left brachiocephalic vein, and SVC. The patient's symptoms resolved following this intervention.

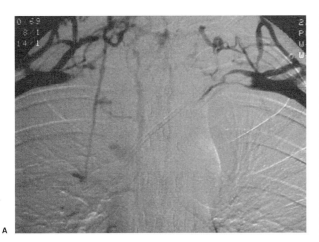

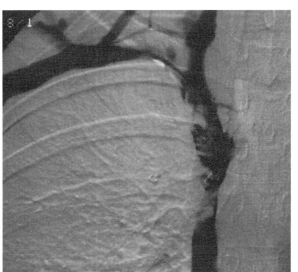

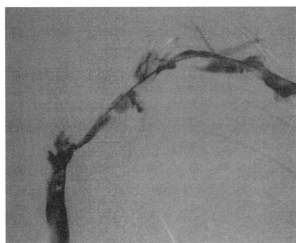

FIGURE 44.4.   49-year-old woman with bilateral subclavian vein occlusions secondary to port placement for chemotherapy. (A) Central venogram via bilateral basilic vein access demonstrates bilateral subclavian vein occlusion. (B and C) Following pharmacologic thrombolysis, flow is reestablished. Note the residual thrombus.

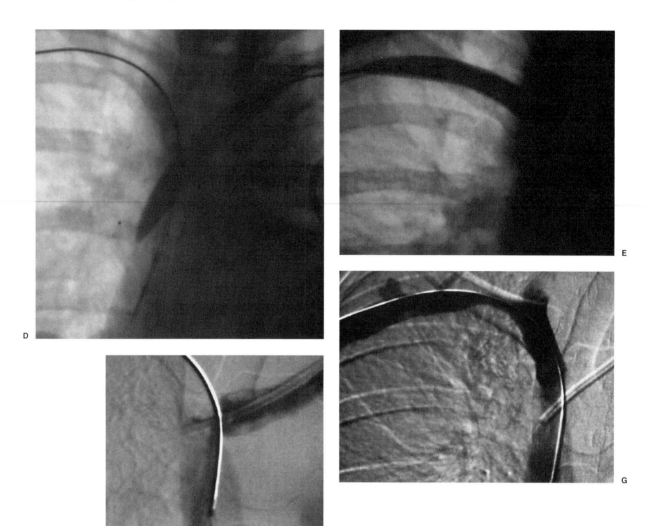

FIGURE 44.4. (*Continued*) (D–F) Angioplasty and mechanical maceration of the residual thrombus. (G) Subsequent right basilic venogram demonstrates restored patency of central veins without the need for stenting in this patient with benign disease.

Most other symptoms typically resolve within this 24- to 72-hour window. Dyspnea appears to be the most persistent symptom, but the etiology of dyspnea is often multi-factorial. Symptoms were found to recur in 0% to 40% of patients when followed for up to 8 months; however, re-intervention is often successful at re-establishing stent patency (23–45).

COMPLICATIONS

The complication rate of SVC stenting compares favorably with traditional first-line therapies for SVC syndrome (53). Complication rates range from 0% to 23% in the published literature (23–45). These complications include fever with mild elevation in white blood cell count, back pain following stent deployment, acute or chronic occlusion of the stent, stent migration (54), stent fracture, access site hematoma, cardiac failure, pulmonary edema, pulmonary emboli, SVC rupture with the potential for pericardial tamponade (55), hemorrhage, hemoptysis, epistaxis and recurrent laryngeal nerve palsy.

REFERENCES

1. Hunter WH. History of aneurysm of the aorta with some remarks on aneurysm in general. Medical Observations and Inquiries, 1757; 1: 323.
2. Shimm DS, Logue GL, and Rigsby LC. Evaluating the superior vena cava syndrome. JAMA, 1981; 245(9): 951–953.

3. Ostler PJ CD, Watkinson AF, and Gaze MN. Superior vena cava obstruction: A modern management strategy. Clin Oncol, 1997; 14: 338–351.

4. Zollikofer CL, Antonucci F, Stuckmann G, et al. Historical overview on the development and characteristics of stents and future outlooks. Cardiovasc Intervent Radiol, 1992; 15(5): 272–278.

5. Chen JC, Bongard F, and Klein SR. A contemporary perspective on superior vena cava syndrome. Am J Surg, 1990; 160(2): 207–211.

6. Stanford W, Jolles H, Ell S, et al. Superior vena cava obstruction: A venographic classification. AJR Am J Roentgenol, 1987; 148(2): 259–262.

7. Rosenblom S. Superior vena cava obstruction in primary cancer of the lung. Ann Intern Med, 1949; 31: 470–478.

8. Bechtold RE, Wolfman NT, Karstaedt N, et al. Superior vena caval obstruction: Detection using CT. Radiology, 1985; 157(2): 485–487.

9. Escalante CP. Causes and management of superior vena cava syndrome. Oncology (Williston Park), 1993; 7(6): 61–68; discussion, 71–72, 75–77.

10. Baker GL and Barnes HJ. Superior vena cava syndrome: Etiology, diagnosis, and treatment. Am J Crit Care, 1992; 1(1): 54–64.

11. Howard N. Factors affecting prognosis in superior vena caval obstruction due to bronchial carcinoma. Clin Radiol, 1961; 12: 295–298.

12. Perez CA PC, van Amburg AL. Management of superior vena cava syndrome. Semin Oncol, 1978; 5: 123–124.

13. Urban T, Lebeau B, Chastang C, et al. Superior vena cava syndrome in small-cell lung cancer. Arch Intern Med, 1993; 153(3): 384–387.

14. Nicholson AA, Ettles DF, Arnold A, et al. Treatment of malignant superior vena cava obstruction: Metal stents or radiation therapy. J Vasc Interv Radiol, 1997; 8(5): 781–788.

15. Wurschmidt F, Bunemann H, and Heilmann HP. Small cell lung cancer with and without superior vena cava syndrome: A multivariate analysis of prognostic factors in 408 cases. Int J Radiat Oncol Biol Phys, 1995; 33(1): 77–82.

16. Davenport D, Ferree C, Blake D, et al. Radiation therapy in the treatment of superior vena caval obstruction. Cancer, 1978; 42(6): 2600–2603.

17. Doty DB and Baker WH. Bypass of superior vena cava with spiral vein graft. Ann Thorac Surg, 1976; 22(5): 490–493.

18. Charnsangavej C, Carrasco CH, Wallace S, et al. Stenosis of the vena cava: Preliminary assessment of treatment with expandable metallic stents. Radiology, 1986; 161(2): 295–298.

19. Zollikofer CL, Antonucci F, Stuckmann G, et al. Use of the Wallstent in the venous system including hemodialysis-related stenoses. Cardiovasc Intervent Radiol, 1992; 15(5): 334–341.

20. Irving JD, Dondelinger RF, Reidy JF, et al. Gianturco self-expanding stents: Clinical experience in the vena cava and large veins. Cardiovasc Intervent Radiol, 1992; 15(5): 328–333.

21. Rosch J, Uchida BT, Hall LD, et al. Gianturco-Rosch expandable Z-stents in the treatment of superior vena cava syndrome. Cardiovasc Intervent Radiol, 1992; 15(5): 319–327.

22. Solomon N, Wholey MH, and Jarmolowski CR. Intravascular stents in the management of superior vena cava syndrome. Cathet Cardiovasc Diagn, 1991; 23(4): 245–252.

23. Carrasco CH, Charnsangavej C, Wright KC, et al. Use of the Gianturco self-expanding stent in stenoses of the superior and inferior venae cavae. J Vasc Interv Radiol, 1992; 3(2): 409–419.

24. Stock KW, Jacob AL, Proske M, et al. Treatment of malignant obstruction of the superior vena cava with the self-expanding Wallstent. Thorax, 1995; 50(11): 1151–1156.

25. Tanigawa N, Sawada S, Mishima K, et al. Clinical outcome of stenting in superior vena cava syndrome associated with malignant tumors. Comparison with conventional treatment. Acta Radiol, 1998; 39(6): 669–674.

26. Kee ST, Kinoshita L, Razavi MK, et al. Superior vena cava syndrome: Treatment with catheter-directed thrombolysis and endovascular stent placement. Radiology, 1998; 206(1): 187–193.

27. Antonucci F, Salomonowitz E, Stuckmann G, et al. Placement of venous stents: Clinical experience with a self-expanding prosthesis. Radiology, 1992; 183(2): 493–497.

28. Furui S, Sawada S, Kuramoto K, et al. Gianturco stent placement in malignant caval obstruction: Analysis of factors for predicting the outcome. Radiology, 1995; 195(1): 147–152.

29. Lanciego C, Chacon JL, Julian A, et al. Stenting as first option for endovascular treatment of malignant superior vena cava syndrome. AJR Am J Roentgenol, 2001; 177(3): 585–593.

30. Hennequin LM, Fade O, Fays JG, et al. Superior vena cava stent placement: Results with the Wallstent endoprosthesis. Radiology, 1995; 196(2): 353–361.

31. Kishi K, Sonomura T, Mitsuzane K, et al. Self-expandable metallic stent therapy for superior vena cava syndrome: Clinical observations. Radiology, 1993; 189(2): 531–535.

32. Miller JH, McBride K, Little F, et al. Malignant superior vena cava obstruction: Stent placement via the subclavian route. Cardiovasc Intervent Radiol, 2000; 23(2): 155–158.

33. Crowe MT, Davies CH, and Gaines PA. Percutaneous management of superior vena cava occlusions. Cardiovasc Intervent Radiol, 1995; 18(6): 367–372.

34. Edwards RD and Jackson JE. Case report: Superior vena caval obstruction treated by thrombolysis, mechanical thrombectomy and metallic stents. Clin Radiol, 1993; 48(3): 215–217.

35. Smayra T, Otal P, Chabbert V, et al. Long-term results of endovascular stent placement in the superior caval venous system. Cardiovasc Intervent Radiol, 2001; 24(6): 388–394.

36. Elson JD, Becker GJ, Wholey MH, et al. Vena caval and central venous stenoses: Management with Palmaz balloon-expandable intraluminal stents. J Vasc Interv Radiol, 1991; 2(2): 215–223.

37. Oudkerk M, Kuijpers TJ, Schmitz PI, et al. Self-expanding metal stents for palliative treatment of superior vena caval syndrome. Cardiovasc Intervent Radiol, 1996; 19(3): 146–151.

38. Urruticoechea A, Mesia R, Dominguez J, et al. Treatment of malignant superior vena cava syndrome by endovascular stent insertion. Experience on 52 patients with lung cancer. Lung Cancer, 2004; 43(2): 209–214.

39. Gross CM, Kramer J, Waigand J, et al. Stent implantation in patients with superior vena cava syndrome. AJR Am J Roentgenol, 1997; 169(2): 429–432.

40. Watkinson AF and Hansell DM. Expandable Wallstent for the treatment of obstruction of the superior vena cava. Thorax, 1993; 48(9): 915–920.

41. Chin DH, Petersen BD, Timmermans H, et al. Stent-graft in the management of superior vena cava syndrome. Cardiovasc Intervent Radiol, 1996; 19(4): 302–304.

42. Dyet JF, Nicholson AA, and Cook AM. The use of the Wallstent endovascular prosthesis in the treatment of malignant obstruction of the superior vena cava. Clin Radiol, 1993; 48(6): 381–385.

43. Gaines PA, Belli AM, Anderson PB, et al. Superior vena caval obstruction managed by the Gianturco Z Stent. Clin Radiol, 1994; 49(3): 202–206; discussion, 207–208.

44. Thony F, Moro D, Witmeyer P, et al. Endovascular treatment of superior vena cava obstruction in patients with malignancies. Eur Radiol, 1999; 9(5): 965–971.

45. Wilkinson P, MacMahon J, and Johnston L. Stenting and superior vena caval syndrome. Ir J Med Sci, 1995; 164(2): 128–131.

46. Schraufnagel DE, Hill R, Leech JA, et al. Superior vena caval obstruction. Is it a medical emergency? Am J Med, 1981; 70(6): 1169–1174.

47. Gauden SJ. Superior vena cava syndrome induced by bronchogenic carcinoma: Is this an oncological emergency? Australas Radiol, 1993; 37(4): 363–366.

48. Yamagami T, Nakamura T, Kato TI, et al. Hemodynamic changes after self-expandable metallic stent therapy for vena cava syndrome. AJR Am J Roentgenol, 2002; 178(3): 635–639.

49. Davidson CJ, Newman GE, Sheikh KH, et al. Mechanisms of angioplasty in hemodialysis fistula stenoses evaluated by intravascular ultrasound. Kidney Int, 1991; 40(1): 91–95.

50. Kovalik EC, Newman GE, Suhocki P, et al. Correction of central venous stenoses: Use of angioplasty and vascular Wallstents. Kidney Int, 1994; 45(4): 1177–1181.

51. Rosch J, Putnam JS, and Uchida BT. Modified Gianturco expandable wire stents in experimental and clinical use. Ann Radiol (Paris), 1988; 31(2): 100–103.

52. Uberoi R. Quality assurance guidelines for superior vena cava stenting in malignant disease. Cardiovasc Intervent Radiol, 2006; 29(3): 319–322.

53. Rowell NP and Gleeson FV. Steroids, radiotherapy, chemotherapy and stents for superior vena caval obstruction in carcinoma of the bronchus: A systematic review. Clin Oncol (R Coll Radiol), 2002; 14(5): 338–351.

54. Entwisle KG, Watkinson AF, and Reidy J. Case report: Migration and shortening of a self-expanding metallic stent complicating the treatment of malignant superior vena cava stenosis. Clin Radiol, 1996; 51(8): 593–595.

55. Brown KT and Getrajdman GI. Balloon dilation of the superior vena cava (SVC) resulting in SVC rupture and pericardial tamponade: A case report and brief review. Cardiovasc Intervent Radiol, 2005; 28(3): 372–376.

Chapter 45

PALLIATIVE CARE AND SYMPTOM MANAGEMENT

Drew A. Rosielle

David E. Weissman

William S. Rilling

PALLIATIVE CARE AND COMMUNICATION WITH CANCER PATIENTS

Overview of Palliative Care

The World Health Organization defines palliative care as care *[T]hat improves the quality of life of patients and their families facing the problems associated with life-threatening illness, through the prevention and relief of suffering by means of early identification and impeccable assessment and treatment of pain and other problems, physical, psychosocial and spiritual* (1). Medical care is focused on symptom relief and maximizing patient function, without necessarily impacting the natural history of the underlying illness. The **unit of care** is defined as the patients, along with their loved ones, and bereavement support is integral to its mission. Palliative care is interdisciplinary, involving not only nurses and physicians but also chaplains, psychologists, social workers, and speech, physical, occupational and other therapists. Although palliative care has historic roots in the terminal care of dying cancer patients, its scope encompasses a wide variety of patients with non-malignant diseases. These include dementia and other neurodegenerative disorders; advanced organ disease such as lung, heart, liver and kidney failure; and critically ill patients in medical, neurological, surgical and trauma criti-cal care units (2, 3). Ideally, palliative care is provided to patients with severe illnesses early in the course of their disease, alongside disease-modifying or curative therapy. As an illness progresses, and as disease-modifying or even life-prolonging interventions become less available, a patient's entire care may become palliative focused. Although much of the care of patients with life-threatening illness can be described as palliative, many patients will not require specialist palliative care, and basic competency in palliative care is important for clinicians across a variety of specialties and practice types (4).

Palliative medicine describes the physician's role in the aforementioned care model. Besides expert symptom assessment and treatment, palliative medicine physicians offer expertise in determining prognosis and communication encounters with patients and families involving breaking bad news, establishing goals of medical care and planning for the future in light of a life-threatening illness. The scope of practice of palliative medicine physicians varies by location and institution. Common settings include inpatient consultative palliative care services, acute inpatient palliative care wards, outpatient palliative care clinics, cancer pain and symptom management clinics, nursing home palliative care services and hospice settings. Palliative care services are increasingly being developed for children (5).

Hospice care is related to but distinct from palliative care. Their underlying philosophies and interdisciplinary approach to care are identical. Hospice, however, has a distinct model of care and reimbursement system that is largely defined by the Medicare Hospice Benefit (MHB) in the United States. Medicaid and private insurers generally provide similar benefits. The MHB requires physician certification that a patient has an expected prognosis of 6 months or less if the disease runs its expected course. Patients can continue to receive hospice care beyond 6 months as long as their anticipated life expectancy remains less than 6 months. The vast majority of hospice care is provided in patients' homes or is provided to patients within long-term care facilities where the facility is considered the patient's "home." The MHB provides payment for skilled nursing, home health aide and volunteer visits; durable medical equipment and medications related to the terminal diagnosis; respite care; physical and occupational therapy; social work and chaplaincy services; and bereavement follow-up (6). Medicare-certified hospice agencies must be able to provide acute, inpatient level care for severe symptom control or imminent death. The MHB does not cover room and board fees for long-term care facilities, including residential hospices.

Communication with Cancer Patients

Cancer is a terrifying, often life-threatening diagnosis, and cancer treatments are often toxic, complicated and difficult to understand. In fact, it has been shown that many advanced cancer patients do not understand that their cancer is incurable, or that their treatment is not intended to cure them (7). Strong emotions and intra-family conflicts are common, making communication about important issues difficult for patient and clinician alike. This section will highlight important elements of communication with cancer patients by discussing the science and art of prognostication and breaking bad news.

Prognostication

For patients with advanced cancer, discussing prognosis and breaking bad news can be particularly challenging. The first step is for the clinician to establish a prognosis based on current best evidence. Prognostication in advanced cancer – as with any illness – is inexact, but a substantial amount of research is available for guidance. For cancers that are not advanced, disease-specific factors such as the type of cancer,

its stage and histologic grade and early responses to chemotherapy are important for determining a broad prognostic range. As cancer progresses, patient factors, particularly functional status, become important for prognostication. **Functional status**, also known as **performance status**, is a global measure of a patient's mobility and ability to care for him- or herself. As a patient becomes more debilitated from her or his advancing cancer, performance status and duration of survival diminish. The Karnofsky Performance Status (KPS) is a reliable and widely used scale to measure functional status (8–10). It rates a patient's functional status from 0 (dead) to 100 (no disease-related symptoms) (see Table 45.1). Prognosis with the KPS has been studied across multiple cohorts of terminally ill cancer patients, with overall consistent results. Patients with a KPS of 40 have a median life expectancy of approximately 2 to 3 months; expected survival decreases rapidly with poorer performance status (10–13). A good way to assess performance status is to ask the patient how much of the day she or he spends in bed or in a chair; more than 50% of the day indicates substantial disability and a prognosis of less than 3 months for most patients. Functional status is also strongly correlated with survival in patients in Phase I chemotherapy trials (14).

Other factors that influence prognosis include age and symptom burden. Younger individuals tend to decline less quickly than the elderly, although this protective effect is lost as disability progresses (13). The onset of certain symptoms in advanced cancer portends a worse prognosis. Cognitive impairment, xerostomia, dysphagia, anorexia and weight loss and dyspnea have all been individually and independently associated with a decreased survival (9, 12–15). Median survival is only 1 to 2 months after the onset of hypercalcemia of malignancy, except for tumors that readily respond to treatment such as early breast cancer or myeloma (16–18). Median survival with untreated brain metastases is 1 month; it improves to 3 to 6 months with treatment (19).

Despite relatively well-established prognostic guidelines, physicians are generally poor prognosticators. Most studies have shown that physicians often overestimate prognosis of terminally ill cancer patients by a factor of three to five (11, 20, 21). In addition, physicians often deliberately disclose an overly optimistic prognosis to terminally ill cancer patients (22), usually in an attempt to not "take away hope" from a patient. It has not been shown that empathetic

TABLE 45.1 Karnofsky Performance Status Scale

Condition	Performance Status %	Comments
Able to carry on normal activity and to work. No special care is needed.	100	Normal. No complaints. No evidence of disease.
	90	Able to carry on normal activity. Minor signs or symptoms of disease.
	80	Normal activity with effort. Some signs or symptoms of disease.
Unable to work. Able to live at home, care for most personal needs. A varying degree of assistance is needed.	70	Care of self. Unable to carry on normal activity or to do active work.
	60	Requires occasional assistance but is able to care for most of own needs.
	50	Requires considerable assistance and frequent medical care.
Unable to care for self. Requires equivalent of institutional or hospital care. Disease may be progressing rapidly.	40	Disabled. Requires special care and assistance.
	30	Severely disabled. Hospitalization is indicated although death not imminent.
	20	Hospitalization necessary, very sick; active supportive treatment necessary.
	10	Moribund. Fatal processes progressing rapidly.
	0	Dead.

Originally published by the American Society of Clinical Oncology. Schag CC, Heinrich RL, Ganz PA. J Clin Oncol 1984; 2(3): 187–193; with permission.

disclosure of prognosis causes patient harm by taking away hope or, for that matter, helps patients by improving the quality of terminal care (12). There is a large amount of heterogeneity in patients' reports of what they want to know from prognostic disclosures. Generally, patients want honest, straightforward information presented compassionately, but individual exceptions to this abound (23, 24). When discussing prognosis, it is recommended to give accurate but general ranges, such as "2 to 4 weeks," or "3 to 5 months" (25). It is also important to share prognostic uncertainty with patients, preparing them for the best as well as the worst. An example would be saying: "Because of all the things we have spoken about, I think you have 1 to 2 months to live. It is important for you to know that doctors are often wrong when we predict time. Some people live longer than we think they will and some people live a lot shorter than we predict. I do not know what will happen in your case."

In a sense, prognostic disclosures can be viewed as any other medical intervention, presenting a balance of risks and benefits. Risks include emotional harm to a patient and its consequences. Potential benefits include allowing patients to make appropriate future plans, to identify life and treatment priorities given how short or long their prognosis is and to more fully weigh burdens and benefits of future medical care in light of their prognosis. For clinicians, the impetus for a prognostic disclosure sometimes goes beyond a

desire for honesty and respecting patient autonomy and is part of an effort to help frame a patient's overall clinical picture and suggest certain treatment options. In these situations, if a patient does not want frank disclosure, it is often possible to frame prognosis vaguely, while still providing sufficient information to a patient to allow him or her to make appropriate decisions. An example of language to use in this situation is: "I agree with you that only God can truly know how long you will live. However, I no longer have any treatments left that are able to stop or slow down your cancer, and I am worried that time is short. In light of this, I want to talk with you about the best way to care for you in the future."

Breaking Bad News

Breaking bad news is emotionally difficult for patients and clinicians. No approach to breaking bad news can or should ameliorate fully the bad news' psychic impact on a patient or a family – however, certain approaches can reduce further harm. Much individual variation exists among patients regarding how they want to hear bad news, but generally they want information offered in an honest and simple manner, for a loved one to be present and for there to be ample time for questions (24). It can be helpful to consider four elements or steps to breaking bad news: preparation, content, patient's response and close (Table 45.2) (11, 26, 27). In preparation, it is helpful to arrange a

TABLE 45.2 Four Elements of an Approach to Delivering a Prognosis

Tasks	Possible Ways to Express It
Preparation	
Research the patient's condition to determine prognostic parameters with and without therapy, both "life-prolonging" and "palliative."	
Arrange meeting in private place with ample time, seating, tissues, and no interruptions (e.g., telephones, pagers, staff).	
Alert the patient ahead of time that you need to discuss important aspects of his or her health. Suggest that the patient bring a person important in his or her life to the meeting.	"The next time we meet, we will be reviewing important test results regarding your illness. I think it is important that you bring with you someone who is important to you."
At the meeting, first establish how the patient is feeling, identifying symptoms that can be the later focus of discussion of palliative therapies. Establish current level of debilitation (i.e., performance status).	"First, I'd like to find out how you are feeling right now." "Do you have any pain or other symptoms from the illness?" "How are you spending your days?" "Are you able to wash up?" "Who's doing the cooking and cleaning now?" "How much of the day do you think you are in bed or on the couch?"
Establish the patient's understanding of his or her illness. Ask what the patient hopes you will be able to do.	"I wonder what your current understanding of your illness is and what you hope we can do for you."
Finally, establish what the patient wishes to know from you about their illness.	"Some people want to know everything possible about their illness and others prefer to know very little. How much about your illness do you want to know from me today?"
Content	
Tell the patient that you have bad news to share ("Give a warning shot").	"I am sorry to say that I have bad news to share today."
State the news clearly, simply and sensitively.	"It appears that the cancer has spread to your bones, which means that it is no longer curable."
Provide information in small amounts at a time.	
Make optimistic statements that are truthful.	"I am very hopeful that with medicine we can control your bone pain."
Anchor the survival estimate you communicate in previously published data and modify it by the patient's current clinical status.	"On average, patients with stage IV gastric cancer live 4 months. One-quarter of patients will live 1.5 months or less, and one-quarter live 8 months or more. While I do not know for sure where you are in that group, the fact that you are feeling so poorly right now and in bed most of the time makes me concerned that you may not live longer than the average 4 months."
Patient's response	
Acknowledge the patient's affect and express empathy.	"I can tell how very difficult it is for you to hear this bad news."
Assure the patient of your continued involvement in his or her medical care. Squarely address the issue that forgoing chemotherapy does not create a therapeutic void; patients often conflate "doing something" with chemotherapy	"Although we cannot cure or shrink your cancer with chemotherapy, we certainly can continue to take care of you and treat you with medicines for any symptoms that the cancer may cause. There is always something that we can do to help you."
Close	
Summarize the new news sensitively and outline a short-term plan of care.	"What we have discussed is that your cancer has progressed to involve your bones, which has caused the calcium in your blood to become dangerously high. What I recommend we do next is to focus on returning the calcium level to normal and strengthening the bone around the tumor by adding a new medicine that is given by vein every month. I recommend that you get the first dose today in our office."
Arrange a follow-up visit (even if the patient is being referred for hospice care) since it is a tangible example of your continued commitment to the patient.	
Offer to discuss the news with people important to the patient who are not present.	
Provide the patient with a means of contacting you or your team in an emergency.	

quiet environment with minimal chance of interruption, and to make sure the patient has an opportunity to invite loved ones they want to be present. Additionally, it is important to be prepared for questions regarding the patient's past care, prognosis and treatment options. Prior to delivering bad news, it is recommended to ask the patient what she or he understands about his or her disease; its treatment; what she or he foresees in the future; and what the patient wants to know. This way the clinician can establish how much and what sort of information she or he needs to share. For example, a clinician will need to present information to a terminally ill patient differently if the patient states, "I know I have incurable cancer and that I've been getting sicker," versus, "I've been having a rough time but I have faith that I'm going to beat this no matter what."

Prior to delivering the content of the bad news, the clinician should gently issue a warning that bad news is forthcoming. Next, the news should be delivered clearly, in straightforward, unadorned language, avoiding medical terminology and complicated statistics. If a patient wants detailed medical explanations he or she will generally tell you. If it is believed the patient is dying, and especially if the patient's knowledge of this is important for planning appropriate future care, it should be stated explicitly. For example, one might say, "You have received several chemoembolization treatments for your liver cancer. The first one seemed to help you – the cancer shrank and you felt better for a while. However, after the last two treatments, the cancer did not shrink and you have been getting sicker, and are now so weak that you are spending most of the day on the couch. Unfortunately, these are indications that more treatments are not going to help you live longer or feel better. I wish it was not this way, but you are dying from the cancer."

After delivering the bad news, it is important to stop and allow the patient and family to respond, even if there is a period of silence. Patients may express grief, despair, anger, guilt or other strong emotions. Some patients may express relief at knowing what is going on. Regardless, it is important to empathetically acknowledge the patient's emotions and to allow the patient time to present them, as well as any questions, before moving forward. The close of the interaction will depend on the nature of the news. Patients and families will generally want to know what the news means for the future, such as the availability and types of future treatments. If the bad news marks a distinct turn in the focus of a patient's care (i.e., from curative to non-curative, or from life-prolonging to palliative), the patient's own goals for the future – both personal and medical – should be assessed (28). One can ask, "In light of this information, I would like to discuss what is important for you in the future, in regard to both your personal life and your future medical care." This allows the patient opportunity to bring up personal, spiritual and familial goals and concerns, as well as opens discussion between patient and clinician about the best way to meet those goals given what is medically available and feasible. For some patients, a change in treatment focus can be quite traumatic. In this case, it is important to stress that despite this apparent change, the focus has been on and continues to be providing the patient the best possible care, even if aspects of that care now are different.

Interventional oncologists are often referred patients with advanced disease who have failed multiple prior medical or surgical treatments. Careful evaluation of the patient's performance status, patient and family goals and understanding of the disease, available treatment options and risks and benefits of treatment are required prior to recommending a treatment plan. For many of these patients, even minimally invasive treatments are not indicated and will only decrease their quality of life. Prospectively identifying these patients can be challenging, and patients and families often have unrealistic expectations. Nevertheless, it is important to consider and discuss not performing any further interventional therapy in patients with advanced disease.

MEDICAL SYMPTOM MANAGEMENT

Much of the clinical practice of symptom management for cancer patients is based on decades of clinical experience rather than well-controlled clinical trials. Despite this, experience has shown that most cancer-related symptoms can be effectively treated to the point of an acceptable patient-defined quality of life. General principles of symptom management are listed below.

1. Consider a wide differential diagnosis and pursue a problem-focused evaluation. New or progressive symptoms in the cancer patient most likely arise as direct effects of the cancer, but medication side effects, medical comorbidities, psychological

processes and paraneoplastic syndromes may be the primary reason for a new symptom, or may be adding additional distress to cancer-related symptoms.

2. Reconsider a diagnosis if a symptom is not responding or progressing as expected. Develop a treatment plan that involves frequent assessment of the patient's response to therapy as well as any adverse effects. If the patient has an inadequate response to a drug, consider either dose escalation or addition or substitution of a second agent, preferably one that modulates the symptom in a new way. An example of this would be adding a serotonin antagonist to a dopamine antagonist for refractory nausea.

3. Arrange close follow-up after every change in the treatment plan. Many cancer patients are elderly and should always be screened for polypharmacy and drug-drug interactions.

4. Employ non-pharmacologic and complementary interventions alongside of pharmacological treatment.

5. Prompt referral of patients to specialist providers is recommended when routine treatments fail to provide adequate symptom relief. Palliative medicine physicians, pain specialists and mental health professionals are available at many institutions.

This section will discuss the medical management of the most common and disturbing symptoms the cancer patient faces, including pain, nausea, constipation, diarrhea, anorexia, fatigue, ascites, pruritus, depression, anxiety and insomnia.

Pain

At least one-third of cancer patients will experience pain while undergoing treatment, and at least three fourths of end-stage cancer patients will experience significant pain (29). The vast majority of patients' pain can be effectively treated with conscientious and aggressive management (30). This section will review the evaluation and treatment of cancer pain, reviewing opioid, non-opioid and adjuvant analgesics, as well as highlighting pain management issues for bone metastases.

Pain is categorized as either nociceptive or neuropathic in origin. Nociceptive pain refers to pain generated by the afferent neural pathways, which respond to tissue damage, whether from tumor infiltration, infection, infarction, distension or other unwelcome stimuli. It is divided into two subtypes: somatic and visceral. Somatic pain arises from the skin, muscles, bones and connective tissues. Arthritic pain, fractures and osseous metastases are common examples of somatic pain. It is usually described as dull, achy and well localized (31). Visceral pain arises from the abdominal and thoracic organs and is often described as deep, poorly localized, but sharp. It can be referred, such as shoulder pain referred from metastases causing liver capsular distension. When caused by distension of hollow organs such as bowel, gallbladder or ureter, visceral pain is typically described as crampy or colicky. Neuropathic pain describes pain generated by damaged or dysfunctional neural tissue within the central or peripheral nervous system. It can be localized to a single nerve or nerve root, as in a radiculopathy, or more diffusely to distal nerve fibers as in diabetic or chemotherapy-induced peripheral neuropathy. Neuropathic pain is frequently described as burning, shooting or numb, and is often associated with changes in pain perception such as allodynia or hyperesthesia. It is estimated that approximately 40% of cancer patients with pain have a neuropathic component (31). Common scenarios include radicular pain from vertebral metastases impinging on nerves as they exit the spinal cord or Herpes zoster infection (shingles).

Table 45.3 outlines key features of a comprehensive pain assessment. Necessary elements include a thorough physical examination and evaluation of the location and radiation of the pain; temporal aspects of the pain; its severity – typically measured by one of several pain scales (e.g., 0 to 10); pain quality (e.g., dull or sharp) to assess for somatic versus visceral versus neuropathic origin; aggravating and alleviating factors; and the use of medications and non-medical treatments and their effects. Particular attention should be paid to the limitations in function brought about by the pain (e.g., with sleep, eating, movement and mood), as well as specific goals the patient has, such as improved sleep or going back to work. Finally, a thorough pain assessment includes discussion of social, psychological and spiritual factors that may be contributing to or affected by the pain (32).

Consideration should be given to a broad differential diagnosis of new or worsening pain in the cancer patient, as not all pain is the direct result of tumor-associated tissue damage. For instance, back pain in a

TABLE 45.3 Elements of a Comprehensive Pain Assessment

Domain	Aspects of the Domain to Assess
Location	Superficial vs. deep; localized or diffuse or radicular radiation pattern
Temporality	Onset, duration, constant vs. intermittent, diurnal variation, tempo of progression
Severity	Current, worst, best, average severity; rated on 0–10 scale
Quality	Sharp, dull, aching, burning, throbbing, numb
Aggravating and alleviating factors	Change with position, certain movements and activities
Treatments	Drug and non-drug, including complementary and alternative; over-the-counter and prescription; efficacy of treatments; adverse effects of treatments
Functional limitations	Pain impact on ability to move, breathe, talk, eat, social interaction, recreational and vocational activities
Concurrent symptoms	Insomnia, anorexia, nausea, dyspnea, anxiety, mood disturbance
Psychosocial aspects of pain	Effect on relationships with family and friends; meaning of pain to the patient; spiritual and existential effects of the pain
Treatment goal	Severity level and functional goal (improved sleep, back to work, etc.)

cancer patient may represent benign chronic or acute musculoskeletal back pain; vertebral metastases causing bony pain or compressing a nerve root, causing neuropathic pain; vertebral compression fractures; epidural metastases; referred pain from abdominal or retroperitoneal tumor; or muscle spasm from psychological stress or pain elsewhere.

Treatment: Non-drug Therapy

All patients should be evaluated for the potential use of non-drug therapies. These include education and counseling, relaxation techniques, physical modalities and physical/occupational therapy. Patient education by itself is an analgesic intervention. Patients feel a greater sense of control and empowerment when they understand the cause and potential treatment options. Simple counseling interventions include reframing and normalization, along with bedside imagery and relaxation techniques. Physical modalities include application of heat, cold and massage, which are simple and cost-efficient analgesic modalities suitable for most patients. Finally, physical or occupational therapy can be a useful adjunct for many pain conditions. The role of complementary and alternative medicine treatments for cancer pain is less clear (33, 34). It is reasonable to use them as determined by safety, patient interest, affordability and local availability.

Treatment – Drug Therapy

Non-opioid Analgesics

Non-opioid analgesics include acetaminophen, non-steroidal anti-inflammatory drugs (NSAIDs) and tramadol. Unlike opioids, all have dose-limiting side effects and analgesic ceiling effects. NSAIDs, such as ibuprofen, diclofenac, etodolac, naproxen and related drugs, work by inhibiting cyclo-oxygenase in damaged tissues, thereby decreasing tissue levels of inflammatory and pain-provoking arachidonic metabolites (35). They all can worsen renal and heart failure, inhibit platelet aggregation and promote gastrointestinal bleeding, which limits their use in many cancer patients. When used safely, they are believed to act synergistically with opioid analgesics in alleviating visceral and somatic pain (30) and can limit opioid dose escalation (36). Newer, selective cyclo-oxygenase-2 inhibitors (e.g., celecoxib) have moderately lower gastrointestinal toxicity than traditional NSAIDs but are otherwise no safer or more efficacious and have no particular role in treating cancer pain (37). Acetaminophen's mechanism of action remains unclear. It is often used in combination products with opioids. Its dose is limited to approximately 4 g daily in healthy patients due to a hepatotoxic metabolite. Tramadol has complicated pharmacodynamics: it is a weak opioid agonist that also modulates norepinephrine and serotonin. It has been shown to be effective for mild to moderate cancer pain from a variety of sources but is inappropriate for severe pain (38). Side effects include nausea, dizziness, sweating and lowering of the seizure threshold; compared with opioids, it is less sedating and constipating (38).

Opioid Analgesics

Opioids are analgesics derived from the opium poppy plant – or their synthetic analogs – which agonize

TABLE 45.4 Commonly Used Opioid Preparations (United States)

Opioid	Major Routes	Combination Product	Long-acting Product
Codeine	PO	Acetaminophen	No
Fentanyl	TD, oral transmucosal	No	TD
Hydrocodone	PO. Anti-tussive elixir available in combination with an antihistamine	*Only* available as combination product with acetaminophen or ibuprofen	No
Hydromorphone	PO, PR, IV, SC	No	Not available in the US
Methadone	PO, PR, IV, elixir	No	See text
Morphine	PO, PR, IV, SC, elixir	No	Yes, dosed q8 to q24 hours depending on formulation
Oxycodone	PO, PR, elixir	Yes, with acetaminophen and NSAIDs	Yes, dosed q8 to q12 hours

Abbreviations: PO = by mouth; PR = by rectum; IV = intravenous; SC = subcutaneous; TD = transdermal.

opioid receptors. Opioids are the standard for treatment of moderate to severe cancer pain (39). They are most effective for somatic or visceral pain; neuropathic pain is often more difficult to relieve with opioids, but a therapeutic trial is usually appropriate (31). Opioids are available in myriad dosing formulations and by multiple routes, including oral, rectal, buccal, transdermal, intravenous, subcutaneous, intramuscular, nasal, nebulized, epidural and intrathecal. Opioids have no ceiling dose; their use is mainly limited by side effects.

Several principles apply to the use of opioids for cancer pain.

1. Oral morphine is considered the opioid of choice due to its effectiveness, familiarity, ease of administration and low cost (39). There is no evidence that any one opioid provides superior analgesia, although patients may idiosyncratically have fewer adverse effects with some opioids than others.

2. There is no role for partial-opioid agonists such as pentazocine or nalbuphine for cancer pain: they provide no therapeutic or safety benefit over pure opioid agonists and can precipitate withdrawal in patients currently on opioid agonists (40).

3. Meperidine and propoxyphene should be avoided. They have no analgesic benefit and are prone to severe neuroexcitatory side effects, especially in the elderly and those with renal insufficiency (41).

4. When available, the oral route is preferred, although most opioids can be given by multiple routes. Intramuscular injections are unnecessarily painful and offer no benefit over less painful subcutaneous injections and should be avoided (31).

5. Patients with continuous moderate to severe pain are best managed by a combination of both short- and long-acting opioids. Short-acting formulations are used for breakthrough pain to supplement the long-acting opioid.

A variety of short-acting oral opioids are available in the United States (Table 45.4) as either pure opioid formulations or in combination with a non-opioid such as acetaminophen or an NSAID. Combination products have a ceiling dose due to the non-opioid. All short-acting oral opioids have an onset of analgesia in 30 minutes, with peak effect at 60 to 90 minutes, providing 3 to 4 hours of analgesia (31). Oral transmucosal fentanyl, an ultra-short acting opioid, is absorbed through the buccal mucosa. It has unique pharmacokinetic and dosing properties compared with other short-acting opioids, providing an onset of analgesia in 5 to 10 minutes (42).

Five long-acting opioid preparations are available in the United States: sustained-release morphine, oxycodone, and oxymorphone, a transdermal fentanyl patch and methadone. Sustained-release morphine and oxycodone are dosed every 8 to 12 hours, are well tolerated and are the first choice for continuous moderate to severe cancer pain. There are also two long-acting morphine preparations that can be dosed once daily. The transdermal fentanyl patch is applied once every 72 hours and is indicated for continuous moderate to severe cancer pain in patients with swallowing impairment or who are intolerant of other long-acting opioids. Due to its long half-life, this product should not be dose escalated more frequently than every 3 days and thus is most appropriate for opioid-tolerant patients on relatively stable opioid doses. Methadone is a unique opioid; with chronic use it can be dosed every 8 to 12 hours and it may be particularly effective for neuropathic pain compared with other opioids (43). However, it has an extremely long elimination half-life – up to 130 hours – making dose adjustments complicated (44). Methadone's potency relative to other opioids increases as the dose of other opioids increases, making switching to and from methadone problematic. For these reasons, it is recommended that initial dosing and titration be managed by experienced pain management practitioners (31).

The frequency of dose adjustments depends on the opioid product in use. Short-acting opioids can be dose escalated every 2 to 4 hours; long-acting oral opioids every 24 hours; and the fentanyl patch or methadone every 72 hours (45). For patients with inadequately controlled pain, it is generally recommended to increase their opioid dose from 25% to 50% for ongoing mild to moderate pain and 50% to 100% for moderate to severe pain, irrespective of starting dose (45). Patients with severe or rapidly escalating pain are best managed in the inpatient hospital setting, where rapid opioid titration can be performed under controlled conditions.

Patients and practitioners frequently have concerns about opioid safety and toxicity – concerns that often result in inadequate dosing and undertreatment of pain. Fortunately, patients usually become tolerant to many opioid side effects, allowing ongoing upward titration of opioids for pain (46). Central nervous system (CNS) depression is a particularly feared side effect. It manifests first as sedation and somnolence and only later as respiratory depression. Risk factors for respiratory depression include opioid naiveté, advanced age, use of other CNS-depressant medications, rapid intravenous bolus dosing, deteriorating renal or liver function and poor respiratory reserve (46). Ongoing pain directly counteracts CNS depression (30), and tolerance to opioids' CNS-depressant effects rapidly develops, limiting the risk of respiratory depression (30). Constipation, nausea and pruritus are also common side effects of opioids and are addressed individually later in this chapter. Morphine and hydromorphone are metabolized in the liver to renally excreted active metabolites, many of which have unwelcome neuroexcitatory side effects, including hyperalgesia (47). It is believed that fentanyl, methadone and perhaps oxycodone are safer to use in renal failure, although this has not been clinically tested (37).

Practitioners and patients alike frequently have concerns about opioid tolerance and addiction (48). Opioid *tolerance* describes the need for a higher dose of an opioid in order to achieve a similar effect. Although tolerance develops to many adverse effects of opioids (nausea, CNS depression), it rarely occurs with its analgesic effects (31, 49). Typically, patients' requirements for increased opioid amount reflect a worsening of their underlying cancer, not tolerance (30, 50). The term *addiction*, often used synonymously with *psychological dependence*, describes the "aberrant use of a substance in a manner characterized by loss of control, compulsive or escalating use, preoccupation, and continued use despite harm" (51). It is different from *physical dependence*, which is defined by an abstinence, or withdrawal, syndrome, which occurs following discontinuation or dose reduction of the drug, or administration of a pharmacologic antagonist. Physical dependence is a predictable and expected phenomenon after ongoing opioid use and should not be confused with psychological dependence, which is defined *behaviorally*. Although it is unclear which percentage of the cancer population has substance-abuse problems, evidence overwhelmingly supports the fact that psychological dependence is rarely induced by the use of opioids when used to treat pain (52, 53). Reluctant patients need education and support to encourage opioid use. Patients with past or current substance-abuse problems are best managed together with a pain management or addiction specialist (51).

Adjuvant Analgesics

Adjuvant analgesics refers to a heterogeneous group of drugs, typically used in addition to opioids and non-opioids to treat neuropathic pain and other pain syndromes that do not respond well to conventional analgesics. Anticonvulsant and antidepressant agents are the most commonly used and best studied classes of adjuvants. Other classes of drugs are more rarely used and will not be fully discussed here. These include gamma-aminobutyric acid (GABA) agonists such as baclofen, benzodiazepines, glucocorticoids, the anesthetic agents lidocaine and ketamine and clonidine.

Anticonvulsants have long been used for chronic neuropathic pain syndromes such as post-herpetic neuralgia, trigeminal neuralgia and diabetic neuropathy (54). Initially, it was felt these were suited only for pain with a lancinating or paroxysmal component, but this assumption has not withstood scrutiny, and

TABLE 45.5 Dosing Guidelines for Second-generation Anticonvulsants as Adjuvant Analgesics

Drug	Starting Dose	Usual Effective Dose
Gabapentin	100 mg tid or 300 qhs	900–3,600 mg daily divided bid-tid
Pregabalin	150 mg daily	150–300 mg bid
Lamotrigine	25–50 mg daily	200–400 mg daily
Topiramate	25 mg daily	100–200 mg bid
Oxcarbazepine	75–150 mg bid	150–800 mg bid
Tiagabine	4 mg qhs	4 mg tid
Levetiracetam	250–500 mg bid	500–1,500 mg bid
Zonisamide	100 mg daily	100–200 mg bid

From McDonald AA, Portenoy RK. How to use antidepressants and anticonvulsants as adjuvant analgesics in the treatment of neuropathic cancer pain. J Supp Oncol, 2006; 4: 43–52. Copyright 2006, with permission from Elsevier.

TABLE 45.6 Dosing and Titration of Gabapentin for Neuropathic Pain*

Starting Dose	
Routine	100–300 mg bid
Elderly, medically frail	100–300 mg qhs
Renal insufficiency (CrCl <60 ml/min, >15 ml/min)	100–200 mg qhs
Renal failure (CrCl <15 ml/min)	100 mg qhs
Dose increments	
Routine	50%–100% every 3 days
Elderly, medically frail	Slower titration
Renal insufficiency/failure	Slower titration
Usual effective dose	
Routine	900–3,600 mg in 2–3 divided doses
Elderly, medically frail	300–1,800 mg in 2–3 divided doses
Renal insufficiency (CrCl <60 ml/min, >15 ml/min)	300–1,800 mg in 2–3 divided doses
Renal failure (CrCl <15 ml/min)	100–300 mg qhs

*Goal of titration: Continue dose escalation until treatment-limiting side effects (ineffective therapy) or until dose increment yields no additional benefit (maximal benefit).

CrCl = creatinine clearance.

From McDonald AA, Portenoy RK. How to use antidepressants and anticonvulsants as adjuvant analgesics in the treatment of neuropathic cancer pain. J Supp Oncol, 2006; 4: 43–52. Copyright 2006, with permission from Elsevier.

anticonvulsants are used widely for all types of neuropathic pain (29). Newer, second-generation anticonvulsants are preferred for their more desirable side-effect profiles and ease of use (see Table 45.5). Gabapentin is considered the first-line anticonvulsant for neuropathic pain for several reasons. It is better tolerated than other anticonvulsants, has been studied extensively for neuropathic pain, including cancer pain, and has almost no drug-drug interactions (55, 56). Common side effects include somnolence, ataxia and edema; doses should be started low, increased slowly and adjusted for renal function (see Table 45.6). Pregabalin is a newer agent with pharmacodynamics and side effects similar to gabapentin. It has greater oral bioavailability, undergoes hepatic metabolism and requires less dose titration than gabapentin.

Antidepressants are also well established in the treatment of neuropathic pain (54). Tricyclic antidepressants such as amitriptyline, nortriptyline and desipramine all have analgesic effects distinct from their antidepressant effects (see Table 45.7). However, their use is limited by side effects, including somnolence, orthostatic hypotension, delirium, cardiac conduction abnormalities and constipation (29). These are most problematic for the elderly and medically frail. Because of this, they are not considered good first-line agents, except for younger people for whom nocturnal sedation is desirable. Some newer antidepressants have analgesic properties (see Table 45.7). Venlafaxine and duloxetine have the most evidence supporting their use in neuropathic pain syndromes

TABLE 45.7 Dosing Guidelines of Antidepressants as Adjuvant Analgesics

Drug	Starting Dose	Usual Effective Dose
Tricyclic antidepressants		
Amitriptyline	10–25 mg nightly	50–150 mg nightly
Nortriptyline	10–25 mg nightly	50–150 mg nightly
Desipramine	10–25 mg nightly	50–150 mg nightly
SSRIs		
Paroxetine	10–20 mg daily	20–40 mg daily
Citalopram	10–20 mg daily	20–40 mg daily
Others		
Venlafaxine	50–75 mg daily	75–225 mg daily
Bupropion	100–150 mg daily	150–450 mg daily
Duloxetine	60 mg daily	60 mg daily

SSRIs = selective serotonin reuptake inhibitors.

From McDonald AA, Portenoy RK. How to use antidepressants and anticonvulsants as adjuvant analgesics in the treatment of neuropathic cancer pain. J Supp Oncol, 2006; 4: 43–52. Copyright 2006, with permission from Elsevier.

(56). Newer antidepressants are far better tolerated than tricyclic antidepressants, although their comparative efficacy has not been evaluated.

Bone Metastases

Painful bone metastases are common in many cancers and offer unique pain management challenges. Bone metastases need close assessment and management to avoid complications such as reduced mobility, fracture, spinal cord compression and hypercalcemia. Acutely, most pain from bone metastases responds to opioids and anti-inflammatory agents, including NSAIDs and corticosteroids (35, 57). Several interventions exist for more long-term and definitive treatment of painful bony metastases. Bisphosphonates reduce osteoclast activity at the tumor site, leading to analgesia after approximately a month of use. There is good evidence these improve quality of life and reduce pain in lung, prostate and renal cancers. Their role for pain relief in other cancers, as well as how long to use them, remains controversial (37). Radiation remains the gold standard for treatment of painful bone metastases; virtually all patients with painful bone metastases should be referred to a radiation oncologist for evaluation. External-beam radiation provides pain relief in up to 90% of patients, with approximately 50% achieving complete relief in 1 to 2 months (58). The systemic administration of radioisotopes such as ^{89}Sr is used for diffuse, painful osseous metastases that cannot be treated solely by external-beam radiation. Pain relief occurs in up to 70% of patients, starting within 1 to 4 weeks after radioisotope administration and can last for over a year (59). Myelosuppression is the most common limiting side effect. Additional interventional techniques are being used to palliate metastases (60), as are kyphoplasty, vertebroplasty and related procedures for malignant vertebral compression fractures (61). Early studies have shown that percutaneous radiofrequency ablation can be used to palliate bone metastases, and can be effective in treating patients who have failed radiation therapy or have already received maximal radiation doses to a particular region (62, 63).

Refractory Pain

A minority of cancer patients will not achieve acceptable analgesia with the appropriate use of conventional drug and non-drug therapies. The first steps in approaching patients with inadequately controlled pain or pain not following an expected course are 1) complete a thorough multidimensional pain assessment or reassessment to explore the reason for refractory pain, remembering that psychological and spiritual issues are common in cancer patients and may be expressed as an increase in pain; 2) ensure that sufficient opioid, non-opioid and adjuvant analgesics have been tried; and 3) seek consultation from a clinician with pain management or palliative care expertise. A variety of invasive procedures is available to meet the wide range of difficult pain management problems. These include epidural or intrathecal administration of drugs through implanted catheters or pumps; neurolytic procedures to destroy autonomic afferent or autonomic nerves, such as intercostal, celiac or hypogastric plexus blocks; or neurosurgical procedures to interrupt pain pathways to the brain such as a cordotomy (64, 65). The success of these procedures depends to a large extent on a thorough and accurate assessment of pain etiology combined with the technical skills of the practitioner.

Nausea and Vomiting

Up to 60% of patients with advanced cancer will experience nausea, and one-half of these, vomiting (66). Despite advances in the prevention and treatment of chemotherapy-related nausea, patients still rate nausea as one of the primary detriments to quality of life while undergoing cancer therapy (67). Nausea and vomiting may aggravate weight loss, can lead to aspiration pneumonia and electrolyte disturbances, and can interfere with timely cancer treatment.

The biochemistry and pathophysiology of nausea and vomiting are complex physiologic processes coordinated in the brainstem vomiting center (VC). The VC lies in the nucleus tractus solitarius, which receives input primarily from the chemoreceptor trigger zone (CTZ) located rostral to the VC at the base of the fourth ventricle. The CTZ is outside the blood-brain barrier and acts as a sampling port for emetogenic toxins in the blood and cerebrospinal fluid. Nausea from chemotherapy, opioids, renal failure and other metabolic disturbances are all mediated, in part, through this mechanism. Dopamine, serotonin and neurokinin-1 receptors are important in nausea-related signaling in the CTZ. Afferent neural input to the CTZ comes from several sources. Gastrointestinal afferent input, such as from distension or inflammation, is mediated by the vagus nerve. Afferent input from the cerebral cortex is involved in anticipatory or

TABLE 45.8 Causes of Nausea and Vomiting in the Cancer Patient

Drugs
  Opioids
  Chemotherapeutic agents
  Digoxin
  Antidepressants
  NSAIDs
  Antibiotics
  Iron

Gastrointestinal causes
  Esophagitis, reflux
  Gastritis, peptic ulcer disease
  Gastroparesis
  Constipation, ileus
  Bowel obstruction
  Biliary obstruction
  Pancreatitis

Metabolic
  Uremia
  Hypercalcemia
  Adrenal insufficiency

Central nervous system
  Elevated intracranial pressure (e.g., tumor metastases)
  Meningitis
  Vestibular disease

anxiety-related nausea. Finally, the vestibular apparatus sends input to the CTZ in motion-related and some cases of opioid-induced nausea; acetylcholine and histamine receptors are particularly important in this system. Because of these multiple potential causes of nausea, it is important to consider a wide differential diagnosis and pursue appropriate diagnostic work-up that is focused on the most likely cause (see Table 45.8).

Two causes of nausea deserve special mention in the cancer patient: chemotherapy- and opioid-induced. Acute chemotherapy-induced nausea occurs within the first 24 hours after receiving emetogenic chemotherapy – usually within the first few hours. It has been studied extensively and has well-established prophylactic drug regimens. Most regimens use a combination of dexamethasone and an antagonist of the serotonin receptor subtype-3 (5HT3) such as ondansetron, granisetron, dolasetron or others. The 5HT3 inhibitors have generally replaced dopamine antagonist-based therapies, due to increased efficacy and a better side-effect profile (68). More recently, the neurokinin-1 receptor antagonist aprepitant has become available for moderate to highly emetogenic chemotherapy (69). Delayed chemotherapy-induced

nausea and vomiting occurs for several days after the initial chemotherapy dose and is more common with certain chemotherapy agents (e.g., cisplatin) than others. It responds less well to serotonin antagonists (68), but glucocorticoids and aprepitant have demonstrated some efficacy (69–71).

Nausea is a normal response to opioid use; it is not an allergic reaction (72, 73). Opioid-induced nausea occurs at the initiation of therapy or – less commonly – following a dose increase. Some patients idiosyncratically have more nausea with certain opioids and less with others. Among the opioids, morphine and codeine appear to be the most emetogenic (72). For most patients, nausea resolves within a few days, and no dose or drug adjustment is necessary. For a small percentage of patients, nausea continues, and alternative opioids should be tried. Treatment is empiric, and antidopaminergic antiemetics (e.g., prochlorperazine) are a reasonable first choice. Ondansetron has shown some efficacy in postoperative opioid-induced nausea (74), but this has not been demonstrated in the treatment of cancer pain (73).

Table 45.9 lists commonly used antiemetic agents. Dopamine antagonists are a good first choice due to cost, availability and side-effect profile. Metoclopramide is perhaps the most well studied and has shown efficacy in managing non-specific nausea associated with advanced cancer (75–77). It is a gastrointestinal prokinetic agent, making it particularly useful in the setting of gastroparesis. Metoclopramide is effective for chemotherapy-induced nausea, but its use has largely been supplanted by newer agents (78). Other agents in this class include prochlorperazine, haloperidol, droperidol and chlorpromazine. Of these, haloperidol has been studied the most (79). Droperidol is available intravenously but can cause prolongation of the QT interval and should be used cautiously in the setting of cardiac conduction abnormalities. Chlorpromazine is a powerful anticholinergic, and it is best used as an antiemetic when sedation is also a goal (75). Newer, atypical antipsychotic agents such as olanzapine probably have antiemetic activity (80–82), although it is unclear that they offer any benefit over other antidopaminergic agents (66). Promethazine has some antidopaminergic effects but is also a powerful antihistamine and anticholinergic and is not generally indicated for the cancer patient. All the dopamine antagonists can cause extrapyramidal reactions, as well as sedation, xerostomia and orthostasis.

TABLE 45.9 Common Antiemetic Agents

Class	Common Dosing	Comments
Dopamine antagonists		
Prochlorperazine	5–10 mg PO tid–qid; 25 mg PR	Available PO, IV and PR.
Metoclopramide	5–10 mg PO tid–qid; best given before meals. Up to 120 mg/day has been used.	Prokinetic. PO, IV, SC and PR routes available.
Chlorpromazine	10–25 mg PO qid	PO, IV, PR and SC. Very sedating.
Haloperidol	0.5–2 mg PO q4h	PO, PR and IV available.
Droperidol	0.625–1.25 mg IV q3–4h	IV only. Risk of QT prolongation; ECG recommended for extended dosing.
Serotonin antagonists		Indicated for prophylaxis of chemotherapy-induced nausea and vomiting.
Ondansetron	4–8 mg PO qid; 24–32 mg prior to chemotherapy	IV and orally disintegrating tablet available.
Granisetron	1–2 mg PO daily	IV available.
Dolasetron	12.5–100 mg PO	IV available. Extended dosing has not been described.
Cannabinoids		
Dronabinol	2.5–5 mg PO q2–4h	Limited by CNS side effects.
Neurokinin-1 antagonists		
Aprepitant	125 mg PO once, then 80 mg daily	Unknown efficacy except as part of a regimen for chemotherapy-induced nausea.
Glucocorticoids		
Dexamethasone	2–4 mg q6h	PO, IV, SC and PR.

IV = intravenous; PR = per rectum; SC = subcutaneous; PO = orally; CNS = central nervous system.

Antihistamines have a limited role in cancer-related nausea, except for those patients with a vestibular component or for whom sedation is desirable. Anticholinergic agents such as scopolamine or glycopyrrolate have particular usefulness in managing nausea, secretions and colic related to bowel obstruction, but as single agents they are weak antiemetics (66). These agents also diminish oropharyngeal, pulmonary and gastrointestinal secretions and can be tried for patients for whom nausea is exacerbated by excessive secretions. Scopolamine is available as a transdermal patch but can cause delirium. Glycopyrrolate, a quarternary amine that does not cross the blood-brain barrier and therefore causes less delirium, can be used intravenously, orally or subcutaneously.

The role of 5HT-3 antagonists outside of chemotherapy-induced nausea is not clear, although available evidence and clinical experience suggest they can be effective antiemetics in multiple clinical scenarios (77, 83). These agents are generally well tolerated; headache, constipation and dizziness are the most common side effects. Dolasetron can cause cardiovascular conduction abnormalities so should be used cautiously in this setting.

Cannabinoids are effective for chemotherapy-induced nausea and vomiting, although probably not for highly emetogenic chemotherapy (84). Their usefulness for other causes of nausea is unclear, and their effectiveness is strongly limited by CNS side effects such as dizziness and sedation. Psychotomimetic side effects are also common, particularly in the elderly (85). Dronabinol is the only cannabinoid available in the United States. The glucocorticoid dexamethasone is a well-established antiemetic for chemotherapy-induced nausea. Additionally, it is often used as part of a regimen for terminally ill people with refractory nausea associated with advanced cancer and can be particularly useful for relieving symptoms associated with bowel obstruction (75–77). Nausea from cerebral edema will respond rapidly to dexamethasone. Glucocorticoids are associated with serious side effects: delirium, gastric ulceration, osteoporosis, insomnia, glucose intolerance, peripheral edema, myopathy and immunosuppression. Accordingly, their use is best limited to the short term. Benzodiazepines are effective for anticipatory nausea related to chemotherapy but have not shown efficacy in other conditions (86). Acupuncture and acupressure point stimulation are at best modestly effective for chemotherapy-induced nausea, as adjuvants to pharmacologic agents (87, 88).

Constipation

Constipation is a common and distressing symptom in cancer patients. Estimates of rates of constipation range from 40% to 90%, and its prevalence increases as cancer advances (89, 90). Constipation, as a subjective complaint of inadequate passage of stool, can reflect a patient's perception of increased hardness of stool, decreased size or frequency of stools, or both. Besides causing discomfort, constipation can lead to obstipation and bowel obstruction and contribute to anorexia, weight loss and delirium in the elderly and medically frail (91).

The consistency and frequency of stooling represent a complex balance of multiple external and internal factors. These include the amount and type of oral intake, gastrointestinal electrolyte and fluid transport, bowel motility and interactions among the sympathetic, parasympathetic and somatic nervous systems. Any or all of these may contribute to a patient's constipation and add to the challenge of its evaluation and treatment. Constipation should be considered not only in patients with actual complaints of constipation but also in those with a variety of other symptoms, including nausea, anorexia, abdominal pain or bloating, delirium and genitourinary complaints. Diarrhea, especially in previously constipated patients, should raise concern for overflow diarrhea, in which fecal material liquefies proximal to a mass of constipated stool and escapes around it. In addition to a careful history and physical examination, plain-film radiography of the abdomen can be helpful to confirm a diagnosis of constipation, establish its extent, and rule out bowel obstruction (89).

Table 45.10 lists common causes of constipation in cancer patients. Opioid-induced constipation deserves special mention. More than one-half of all opioid-treated patients will report constipation (92), and it is noted with intravenous, transdermal and spinal opioid use (89). There is some evidence that transdermal fentanyl is less constipating than oral opioids (93). Opioids reduce gastrointestinal motility via directly inhibiting peristalsis and increasing sphincter tone; they also decrease gastrointestinal secretions.

TABLE 45.10 Common Causes of Constipation in Cancer Patients

Drugs
  Opioids
  Serotonin antagonists (e.g., ondansetron)
  Anticholinergic agents (e.g., tricyclic antidepressants, antisecretory drugs)
  Antacids (calcium or aluminum containing)
  Chemotherapeutic agents (particularly vinca alkaloids)
  Iron
  NSAIDs
  Antihypertensive agents (e.g., calcium channel blockers, beta-adrenergic blockers, diuretics)

Metabolic factors
  Hypercalcemia
  Uremia

Mechanical
  Bowel obstruction
  Bowel strictures
  Fecal impaction

Other
  Poor oral intake of solids or liquids
  Patient inactivity
  Inability to reach or use commode
  Spinal cord compression/cauda equina syndrome

Treatment of constipation is largely empiric and the best therapy is prophylaxis. Most agents have some efficacy across a variety of causes of constipation. There are four major categories of pharmacological treatments: stimulants, bulk-forming agents, osmotics and surfactant laxatives (see Table 45.11). Decisions about which agents to use should be based on rapidity of desired effect and severity of constipation. Generally, if a patient is responding inadequately to one class of laxative, a second class should be added. Doses should be started low, then titrated upward to avoid cramping and diarrhea. Commonly used agents for prophylaxis include mild stimulants (e.g., senna) or saline laxatives (e.g., milk of magnesia). Surfactant laxatives are not effective prophylactic agents.

Bulk-forming agents such as fiber and psyllium have a limited role for the cancer patient. They increase stool mass and water content but do not promote motility and so are ineffective for opioid-induced constipation and should not be used as monotherapy (92). Additionally, they work best when taken with large amounts of water, which is often impractical for the medically ill (94). Stimulant laxatives such as senna and bisacodyl stimulate the myenteric plexus and increase forward peristalsis and so are particularly effective for opioid-induced constipation.

TABLE 45.11 Commonly Used Laxatives

Drug	Dosing	Onset of Action
Stimulant laxatives		
Senna	8.6–68.8 mg daily, divided bid	6–12 hours
Bisacodyl	5–30 mg daily; oral or rectal	6–12 hours
Surfactant laxatives		
Docusate	100–500 mg daily, divided up to qid	24–72 hours
Mineral oil	15–45 ml, divided	6–8 hours
Saline osmotic laxatives		
Magnesium citrate (1.745 g/30 ml)	150–300 ml daily	0.5–3 hours
Magnesium hydroxide	30–60 ml daily, may divide bid	0.5–3 hours
Polyethylene glycol	17 g daily, taken in water	24 hours
Carbohydrate osmotic laxatives		
Lactulose (10 g/15 ml liquid)	15–60 ml daily, divided up to tid	24–48 hours
Sorbitol 70% solution	30–150 mg daily or bid	24–48 hours

Onset of action data from Fallon M, O'Neill B. ABC of palliative care: Constipation and diarrhoea. BMJ, 1997; 315: 1293–1296, and Mancini I, Bruera E. Constipation in advanced cancer patients. Supp Care Cancer, 1998; 6: 356–364.

Indeed, many recommend initiating scheduled senna at the same time as scheduled opioids are prescribed as prophylaxis (92). Historic concerns about colonic damage from long-term stimulant laxative use have not been substantiated (94).

Surfactant laxatives work by increasing water and oil penetration into stool and lubricating its passage. Oil-based lubricants such as mineral oil are effective but poor long-term choices as they can lead to fat-soluble vitamin deficiencies. Additionally, they can lead to a severe chemical pneumonitis if aspirated. Osmotic laxatives contain poorly absorbable salts or carbohydrates, which osmotically retain fluid in the intestinal lumen, causing laxation. Saline osmotic laxatives usually contain a magnesium salt. In higher doses, these can have cathartic effects, but in lower doses can be used safely long-term. For opioid-induced constipation, they can be a helpful addition to a stimulant laxative. They should be used cautiously in renal failure due to concern for hypermagnesemia. Carbohydrate laxatives such as lactulose or sorbitol can also have cathartic effects at higher doses. Lactulose, although effective, is limited by cost and its poorly tolerated, sickly sweet taste. All oral laxatives can cause cramping, bloating, nausea and flatulence, as well as diarrhea and concomitant electrolyte disturbances.

Rectal therapies (enemas or suppositories) are best reserved for refractory constipation. All enemas cause colonic distension, which stimulates rectal contraction and fecal evacuation. Electrolyte-containing enema solutions increase water retention in the rectum and thus stool volume and softness. Suppositories have either a stimulant (e.g., bisacodyl) or surfactant (e.g., glycerin) effect. Impaction should be treated mechanically with manual disimpaction and with large-volume enemas and stool softeners, along with attention to pain management as the procedure can be quite distressing.

Opioid antagonists have been used successfully to treat opioid-induced constipation (5, 96). In particular, a newer agent – methylnaltrexone – appears very promising in clinical trials (89).

Diarrhea

Chronic diarrhea is reported in only 10% of cancer patients (90, 97), but when present can have a dramatic impact on a patient's quality of life. Drugs and infections are major culprits; however, many other causes should be considered, including the effects of abdominal or pelvic radiation, pancreatic insufficiency, graft-versus-host disease, co-existing inflammatory bowel disease and short-bowel syndrome (98). Laxatives, antibiotics and chemotherapeutic agents – particularly fluorouracil, irinotecan and cisplatin – are common drug causes (99). Opioid withdrawal can cause severe diarrhea. Acute infectious diarrhea is also a possibility, and *Clostridium difficile* diarrhea, in particular, needs to be considered for patients with recent hospitalizations or antibiotic use. More chronic infectious causes such as *Cryptosporidium*, as well as viral etiologies, should be considered in chronically immunocompromised patients.

Pharmacologic treatment of diarrhea is empiric; no single agent has shown to be superior. Intraluminal agents such as the adsorbent kaolin and bismuth subsalicylate have efficacy for traveler's diarrhea but do not play a particular role for cancer-associated problems. Opioid anti-motility agents such as loperamide, diphenoxylate and codeine are all effective for drug-induced and chronic diarrhea. Antimotility therapy is contraindicated for suspected *C. difficile*-related diarrhea. In this case, cholestyramine, the bile acid sequestrant, is a safe choice for symptom relief while awaiting the effects of definitive therapy. Octreotide dramatically reduces gastrointestinal secretions and can be used in extreme cases of chronic diarrhea. It can be of particular help for refractory treatment-associated diarrhea (99). Any patient who does not respond to conservative treatment or who encounters medical or lifestyle complications as a result of their diarrhea should immediately be referred for specialist evaluation.

Constitutional Symptoms

The constitutional symptoms of fatigue, anorexia and weight loss are common and disturbing manifestations of cancer for the patient, family and caregivers. Lack of appetite and weight loss are cardinal symptoms of an advanced cancer, especially in the last 3 months of life. Anorexia occurs in up to 70% of cancer patients (100), and at least one-half will experience weight loss in the course of their disease (101). Patients and families usually find anorexia and weight loss particularly distressing. They are "cancer stigmata" (101), and conflict between family members, or family members and the health care team, over issues of nutrition and oral intake occur commonly. Education and emotional support provided by the health care team are important in alleviating fears of starvation. Health professionals can assist conflicted families by focusing "blame" for the anorexia on the cancer and not the patient. Nutritional counseling is reasonable, especially if poor caloric intake is suspected, although it has not shown any significant long-term benefit (102).

The cancer anorexia-cachexia syndrome, characterized by anorexia, early satiety, weight loss, muscle wasting, debilitation and asthenia, is very common as cancer progresses. Cancer-induced derangements in the production of inflammatory cytokines, such as

TABLE 45.12 Potentially Treatable Causes of Anorexia and Weight Loss

Oral
    Oropharyngeal mucositis
    Xerostomia
    Thrush
    Treatment-related changes in smell and taste
    Poor dentition, ill-fitting dentures

Gastrointestinal
    Esophagitis
    Dysphagia
    Nausea, vomiting
    Gastroparesis
    Proximal gastrointestinal obstruction (tumor-related, stricture)
    Constipation
    Diarrhea, steatorrhea

Psychosocial
    Depression
    Anxiety
    Inability to shop for, pay for or prepare food

tumor necrosis factor-alpha, interleukin-6 and others, are believed to underlie the syndrome. In contrast to starvation, in which bodily energy consumption is conserved and fat is preferentially consumed due to a caloric deficit, in cancer cachexia, bodily energy consumption increases and fat and muscle tissues are mobilized equally, even without a caloric deficit (102, 103). Unfortunately, this means that increasing caloric consumption in cancer cachexia, whether by hyperalimentation or appetite stimulation, has little impact on lean body mass, quality of life or longevity. Indeed, it is not clear that treating cancer anorexia-cachexia with currently available therapies is of any meaningful benefit except psychologically to the patient and family (102).

The cancer patient who begins to lose weight or is complaining of anorexia should be evaluated for potentially reversible causes (see Table 45.12). Orexigenic therapy can be successful in increasing a patient's appetite and caloric intake. It can also increase weight, although only by increasing fat mass. Several classes of orexigenic agents have been studied. Progesterones, particularly megestrol and medroxyprogesterone acetate, are the most closely studied. Megestrol is an effective appetite stimulant at doses between 480 and 800 mg/day. Medroxyprogesterone acetate can lead to weight gain at doses of 500 mg twice daily (104). Both can aggravate edema and elevate the risk of thromboembolic events. Survival and quality of life have not been shown to improve with either agent (100, 105). Glucocorticoids are also effective but have not been studied long term and have severe, limiting side effects (100). The cannabinoid dronabinol can improve appetite and weight at a dose of 2.5 mg given one hour after meals (85). However, its use is limited by disturbing psychotomimetic side effects. Androgens have not shown any efficacy (105). There is ongoing study into modulating the inflammatory substrate of anorexia-cachexia with agents such as omega-3 fatty acids, thalidomide, amino acids, pentoxifylline, NSAIDs and novel agents (100, 102, 103). None has yet shown strong promise clinically.

Fatigue shares much in common with cancer-related anorexia and weight loss, and some argue that they all are part of the same pathophysiologic processes of inflammation and neurohormonal disruption that accompany cancer (106, 107). It is generally the most frequently cited symptom associated with cancer and its treatment, occurring in virtually 100% of patients (90, 108, 109). Fatigue can persist for years beyond curative treatment (106). Cancer-related fatigue is distinct from exercise-induced fatigue (110). It is disproportionate to activity and poorly relieved by rest and sleep. Patients feel globally limited – not only physically but emotionally, mentally, vocationally and socially.

Although frequently due to the cancer itself, other causes include effects of chemotherapy or radiotherapy, weight loss, depression, anxiety, poor sleep, poorly controlled pain, anemia and major organ failure (heart, liver, lung or kidney). Medication side effects, particularly from opioids and other psychotropic drugs, often contribute as well. Treatment of fatigue starts with addressing underlying causes that are amenable to intervention, such as anemia or depression. Anemia is well studied and worth investigating and treating in the fatigued cancer patient. Generally, the goal is to keep the hemoglobin level above 11 g/dl (111). Erythropoietin is routinely used to prevent and treat anemia in the cancer patient and has been shown to reduce transfusions and improve fatigue and quality of life in patients undergoing cancer treatment (112–114). In advanced cancer patients and the terminally ill, anemia and its correction play a much smaller role in impacting fatigue, as other factors become more important (115, 116). Psychostimulants such as methylphenidate have been used successfully for severe fatigue in patients with advanced cancer (117).

Education and support should be offered to all patients complaining of fatigue. Inquiring about specific activities that are limited by the fatigue can allow for troubleshooting and goal setting, even if the fatigue itself cannot be ameliorated. For patients who are able, moderate aerobic exercise is recommended, as it paradoxically improves fatigue in patients undergoing treatment and helps prevent further deconditioning (118–120). It is unclear whether energy conservation – resting to "store-up" energy for important activities – is helpful (113).

Ascites

Approximately 10% of all cases of ascites are due to malignancy (121), most commonly due to genitourinary or gastrointestinal cancers (122). Malignant ascites is usually secondary to peritoneal carcinomatosis, although a minority of patients will have some element of portal hypertension from either massive hepatic tumor infiltration or underlying cirrhosis (123). Chylous ascites is a rare occurrence, usually from lymphoma. As in the general population, nephrosis, congestive heart failure, biliary or pancreatic ductal leakage and thrombotic events can also cause ascites. In cirrhosis, the cause of ascites is portal hypertension, leading to splanchnic vasodilation and salt and fluid retention (124). The pathophysiology of ascites from peritoneal carcinomatosis is poorly understood but is believed to be due to direct fluid efflux from tumor implants as well as impaired fluid resorption across the peritoneum (125). Cirrhotic ascites alone has a very high mortality – up to 50% in 2 years (126). Mean survival from the onset of malignant ascites is about 20 weeks (122).

Management of ascites differs based on its cause. Salt restriction and diuresis are the mainstays of therapy for portal hypertensive ascites. Patients should be instructed to consume a low-sodium diet (less than 2000 mg daily). Most patients with cirrhosis and ascites respond well to oral diuretics, usually spironolactone alone or in combination with a loop diuretic such as furosemide. Patients should be started on moderate doses (50 mg to 100 mg of spironolactone and 20 mg to 40 mg of furosemide), which can then be titrated upward until effective (124). Gynecomastia can be an intolerable side effect of spironolactone; amiloride can be substituted in this case. Overly aggressive diuresis can have serious complications, including acid-base and electrolyte imbalance as well as renal failure. Hypokalemia and metabolic alkalosis are both risk factors for developing hepatic encephalopathy, so frequent monitoring of electrolytes and renal function is wise (127). For patients without peripheral edema, weight loss should be limited to 500 g/day while undergoing diuresis to prevent these complications (126). Supportive measures should be undertaken to prevent the more severe complications of liver failure, such as spontaneous bacterial peritonitis, hepatic encephalopathy and gastrointestinal bleeding.

Treatment of malignant ascites is aimed at the underlying cancer. Unfortunately, many patients will have advanced cancer that is poorly responsive to oncologic therapies. In these cases, management is empiric and should be based on patients' overall prognosis and how symptomatic they are from the ascites. Because there is no physiologic derangement of salt and fluid retention, the benefit of salt restriction and diuretics is unclear (125). No study has been performed to clarify their role. In patients for whom an element of portal hypertension is suspected, a trial of salt restriction and diuresis is reasonable. Otherwise, the management of malignant ascites is drainage, usually via large-volume paracentesis of up to 6 L at a time (121). More durable interventions such as peritoneovenous shunting and peritoneal drainage catheters can be immensely helpful in select patients (121). For all patients, attention should be given to assessing and treating symptoms associated with ascites, such as pain, dyspnea and nausea.

Pruritus

Pruritus is a common and perplexing symptom in cancer patients, occurring in about 30% (128). It has a wide variety of causes and treatments, and this section will discuss only diffuse pruritus as a result of cancer and other systemic illnesses. Itching can have dozens of causes in the cancer patient, including cutaneous tumor involvement, paraneoplastic syndromes, drug effects, iron deficiency and cholestasis. It is a classic symptom of hematologic malignancies, particularly Hodgkin's disease. Opioid analgesics, particularly when delivered spinally, are commonly pruritogenic. Simple causes also occur in the cancer patient, such as dry skin, eczema and cutaneous allergies. Additionally, at least one-half of patients receiving hemodialysis will suffer from pruritus (129).

The pathophysiology of pruritus is poorly understood. Peripherally, itching is mediated by C-type afferent neurons, which are anatomically similar to, but functionally distinct from, nociceptive fibers.

Serotonin, histamine, acetylcholine, prostaglandins, substance P and related neuropeptides, cytokines and opioids have all been implicated in the peripheral generation of pruritus (128, 130). Centrally, opioids, GABA and serotonin play a role in its mediation (131, 132).

Perhaps as a result of these heterogeneous causes, a panoply of treatments has been investigated for pruritus. Regardless of etiology, patients should be instructed to avoid scratching and to prevent dry skin (133). Antihistamines are clearly effective for pruritus with a strong histaminergic cause, such as urticaria or insect bites; otherwise, their efficacy is limited. Cimetidine, a histamine antagonist, can be quite effective for pruritus associated with hematologic malignancies (134). Recently, certain antidepressants have been studied for refractory pruritus; 20 mg/day of paroxetine daily has been shown to be modestly effective for pruritus from a variety of systemic causes (130).

Cholestatic pruritus is common in advanced gastrointestinal cancer patients. Relief of biliary obstruction by surgery, stenting or drainage is preferable but sometimes impossible or impractical. Cholestyramine binds bile acids in the lumen of the gastrointestinal tract, thereby decreasing bile acid resorption and ameliorating cholestatic itch. Daily doses of up to 12 g are usually needed, but many patients cannot tolerate this dose due to its grainy, unpalatable consistency (132). Rifampin, dosed at 150 mg twice daily, is believed to increase hepatic clearance of pruritogenic substances in cholestasis (133,135). It can cause liver failure, so it needs to be used cautiously in cholestasis. Opioid antagonists have been shown to be quite effective for cholestatic itch. Indeed, there are reports of opioid withdrawal-like syndromes in opioid-naïve people given opioid antagonists for cholestatic pruritus, suggesting a role for increased production of endogenous opioids in its generation (134). Naloxone is effective but needs to be given intravenously; naltrexone can be given orally and has been shown to be effective in doses as low as 50 mg/day (132, 136). The use of these agents is limited for patients who require opioids for pain, as opioid withdrawal can be precipitated. Androgens, glucocorticoids, lidocaine, phenobarbital, midazolam and serotonin antagonists have all been studied for cholestasis, with variable results (128, 133, 137–139).

Opioid-induced pruritus is an idiosyncratic nonallergic reaction and not a contraindication to continued use. If possible, switching to another opioid is recommended as the itching often disappears with the new drug. Opioid antagonists effectively relieve itching but need to be used with caution to prevent withdrawal; expert consultation is recommended (140). Ondansetron, a 5HT-3 antagonist, has shown some promise in the treatment of opioid-induced and cholestatic pruritus, although data are limited (134).

Psychiatric Symptoms

Psychiatric symptoms are common, underdiagnosed and yet treatable in cancer patients. This section will focus on the assessment and management of depression, anxiety and insomnia in cancer patients.

Depression

Depressive symptoms are more common in cancer patients than in the general population (107). Most estimates of rates of major depressive disorder (MDD) are between 10% and 25% of patients with cancer, compared with fewer than 5% of the general population (107, 141, 142). Depressive symptoms (including diminished mood, anhedonia, feelings of guilt and sadness, fatigue, weight loss, sleep disturbance and memory problems) are more common than rates of MDD and may be due to the underlying cancer, co-existing medical disease, expected feelings of loss and sadness that accompany a cancer diagnosis or an adjustment disorder. Nevertheless, depression is not an inevitable or normal part of having cancer. By definition, MDD interferes with a patient's quality of life and functioning (143). Indeed, MDD is associated with worse overall and cancer-related mortality, and evidence suggests it interferes with appropriate cancer evaluation and treatment (144–146). Therefore, early and aggressive identification and management of depression are mandatory.

Depression is underrecognized by most care providers of cancer patients (147). Diagnosis of depression is notoriously complicated in cancer due to overlap of the somatic symptoms of depression with common somatic complaints in cancer (fatigue, anorexia and weight loss, sleep disturbances and sexual dysfunction). Additionally, feelings of grief, sadness and loss, as well as thoughts about dying, are common in cancer patients and not necessarily pathologic. Assessment of depression should take these difficulties into account, giving less emphasis to somatic symptoms and more to psychiatric ones (mood, interest in previously pleasurable activities and social withdrawal). Persistent feelings of guilt, shame, worthlessness and hopelessness, and suicidality are not characteristic of the expected emotional adjustments to a potentially life-threatening diagnosis, and are strongly suggestive of depression (see Table 45.13) (148). A simple bedside tool – asking, "Have you been feeling down, depressed or hopeless most of the time over the past two weeks?" – has shown excellent sensitivity and specificity in screening cancer patients for depression, although it has yet to be fully validated in a range of populations (149, 150).

Both pharmacologic and non-pharmacologic therapies for depression are helpful (151, 152). Indeed, psychotherapy together with pharmacotherapy of depression is considered to be more efficacious than either alone (153). Once depression is identified, immediate involvement of a patient's primary physician or referral to appropriate professionals is important. Many institutions have mental health professionals with specific training in cancer care. Additionally, many palliative care teams are able to provide these services. As with all psychological problems, unwelcome somatic symptoms such as pain or nausea will worsen depression and need to be aggressively managed.

Three main classes of pharmacologic agents are available: 1) tricyclic (and related) antidepressants;

TABLE 45.13 Differentiating Depression from Expected Sadness and Grief in Cancer

Patient Characteristics Less Suggestive of Depression	Patient Characteristics More Suggestive of Depression
Sadness, grief, and guilt that is intermittent and about specific losses and limitations	Pervasive feelings of grief, guilt and shame that are generalized to all aspects of life
Accepting and appreciative of support offered by family, caregivers	Feels worthless, not deserving of offered help
Recognizes that he or she can control many aspects of life	Feels helpless, out of control, unable to effect any meaningful change
Feels hope about controllable aspects of the future	Feels hopeless about most aspects of the future
States that he or she has periods of sadness and grief	States "I am depressed."
Ability to enjoy aspects of day to day personal, work, and family life despite limitations and some "bad days"	Persistent anhedonia; mood does not lift when around loved ones or when performing previously enjoyable activities
Thoughts about mortality and death	Thoughts about suicide; an active desire for death

TABLE 45.14 Commonly Used Antidepressants

Class	Common Dosing	Comments
Tricyclic (and related)		
Amitriptyline	25–150 mg at night. 10 mg is starting dose in elderly	Cardiac conduction delays and anticholinergic side effects often limit their use. Sedating.
Nortriptyline	25–150 mg at night. 10 mg is starting dose in elderly.	Some efficacy for neuropathic pain. Start with low doses and increase slowly,
Desipramine	25–200 mg/day. May divide bid. 10 mg is starting dose in elderly.	particularly in elderly.
Selective serotonin reuptake inhibitors		
Paroxetine	20–50 mg daily. 10 mg is starting dose in elderly.	May have particular benefit in anxiety disorders.
Fluoxetine	20–60 mg QAM	Activating. Long half-life.
Sertraline	25–200 mg daily	
Citalopram	20–60 mg daily	
Escitalopram	10–20 mg daily. Start with 5 mg in elderly.	
Selective serotonin and norepinephrine reuptake inhibitors		
Bupropion	100 mg bid to150 mg tid	Available in sustained-release form.
Venlafaxine	37.5–75 mg bid to tid	Available in sustained-release form. May have particular benefit in anxiety disorders and neuropathic pain.
Mirtazapine	15–45 mg QHS	Associated with sedation and weight gain.
Duloxetine	20–60 mg daily or bid	Effective for neuropathic pain.
Psychostimulants		
Methylphenidate	Start 2.5–5 mg in AM and at noon.	Available in sustained-released form. Unclear what the maximum effective dose is in depression.
Dextroamphetamine	Start 2.5–5 mg in AM	

2) newer, selective neurotransmitter reuptake inhibitors; and 3) psychostimulants (see Table 45.14). Given the prevalence of depressive symptoms in the cancer population, surprisingly little cancer-specific research has been performed. What has been completed confirms that cancer patients respond to antidepressant therapy and, as in the general population, no class of antidepressants has superior efficacy (142). Choice of antidepressant should be based on patient comorbidity, preference and cost. With the exception of psychostimulants, all antidepressants take 2 to 8 weeks to ameliorate mood; however, the side effects are immediate. Counseling patients regarding this is important to prevent premature treatment discontinuation. All antidepressants should be started at low doses and titrated upward until therapeutic effect is obtained or side effects limit further use. The antibiotic linezolid is a monoamine oxidase inhibitor and is relatively contraindicated for patients on antidepressants; prompt consultation with a psychiatrist is warranted in this setting (154). Antidepressants should be gradually tapered when stopping to avoid a discontinuation syndrome.

Tricyclic (and related) antidepressants such as amitriptyline, nortriptyline and desipramine have significant anticholinergic side effects such as orthostatic hypotension, xerostomia, dizziness, constipation, urinary retention, sedation and delirium. In addition, they can cause cardiac conduction abnormalities such as atrioventricular nodal block and QT prolongation. They should be used with extreme caution in the elderly and medically frail. Tricyclic antidepressants are helpful for the treatment of neuropathic pain, usually at doses lower than what is needed to treat depression (29).

Newer agents include selective serotonin reuptake inhibitors (SSRIs) such as fluoxetine, paroxetine, sertraline and citalopram, as well as novel agents that selectively and variably modulate adrenergic and dopaminergic reuptake along with serotonin.

These include bupropion, venlafaxine, mirtazapine and duloxetine. Gastrointestinal upset, sexual dysfunction and xerostomia are common side effects of all these agents. Seizures, serotonin syndrome and a short-lived paradoxical increase in anxiety and suicidality are rare but should be considered. SSRIs are associated with a small increased risk of bleeding and should be used cautiously in those with thrombocytopenia (155). Fluoxetine can be quite activating and is best avoided in patients with prominent anxiety or insomnia. Emerging evidence suggests that venlafaxine or duloxetine may be efficacious in treating neuropathic pain as well as chronic pain associated with depression (156, 157). Mirtazapine can cause weight gain as well as improve sleep and thereby may be of particular use in cancer patients with prominent weight loss or insomnia (158). Fluoxetine, sertraline, citalopram and escitalopram are available as solutions suitable for feeding tubes; mirtazapine is available as an orally disintegrating tablet.

Psychostimulants such as methylphenidate and dextroamphetamine are useful in patients with prominent symptoms of psychomotor retardation (159). They usually begin alleviating depressive symptoms within 2 days and therefore can be particularly helpful in patients with short life expectancies (143). Generally, they are dosed twice daily, in the early morning and again at noon, to avoid nocturnal insomnia. Dose adjustments can be made every 2 to 3 days.

Anxiety

Anxiety occurs commonly in cancer patients; estimates of prevalence are between 30% and 50% (160–162). An unclear percentage of cancer patients, perhaps around 10%, will have a primary anxiety disorder (panic disorder, phobias or generalized anxiety disorder) (141). Temporary anxiousness around specific events (e.g., awaiting test results, before clinic visits or procedures) is common and not pathologic. However, when anxiousness becomes pervasive or limits a patient's ability to participate in daily activities or necessary medical care, it should be treated. Anxiety may be secondary to a variety of conditions, including drug effects (especially glucocorticoids and antidopaminergic agents), drug or alcohol withdrawal, uncontrolled pain or dyspnea and depression.

Anxiety responds well to cognitive or psychotherapeutic interventions (152), and prompt referral for more challenging situations is important. Complementary interventions such as aromatherapy, massage, progressive muscle relaxation and guided-imagery therapy can be helpful (163, 164). Pharmacologic treatment of anxiety is used for temporary, incidental anxiety and for chronic, pervasive symptoms. Incidental anxiety – such as before a procedure – best responds to cognitive interventions; however, pre-treatment with short-acting benzodiazepines is the pharmacologic mainstay. Longer-term treatment of anxiety is more complicated and best performed in conjunction with a patient's primary provider or a mental health professional. Scheduled, low-dose, long-acting benzodiazepines (e.g., clonazepam or sustained-release alprazolam) are effective but run the risk of excessive sedation, tolerance and abuse. Buspirone is a non-benzodiazepine anxiolytic that has minimal abuse potential but, like SSRIs used for depression, takes several weeks to be effective (165). SSRIs – particularly escitalopram, paroxetine and sertraline – are effective for generalized anxiety disorder (166). SSRI dosing for anxiety is similar to that for depression.

Insomnia

Insomnia is a symptom of poor quality or quantity of sleep. It occurs in about one-half of cancer patients and adversely affects quality of life (167,168). The causes of insomnia in the cancer patient are legion. These include other physical symptoms (pain, dyspnea, hot flashes, night sweats, nausea); psychiatric disorders (depression, anxiety, adjustment disorders); drug effects (e.g., glucocorticoids, antidepressants, beta-adrenergic agonists, alcohol, caffeine, nicotine, psychostimulants); drug withdrawal and primary sleep disorders (primary insomnia, restless leg syndrome or obstructive sleep apnea) (169). Treatment of insomnia should be directed at the underlying cause, when possible. Offending drugs should be tapered, or changed to morning dosing if feasible. All patients should be instructed in the basics of sleep hygiene: avoiding daytime napping; using the bedroom only for sleep and intimate activities; avoiding stimulants, alcohol and exercise in the evening; and keeping a regular sleep schedule (167, 170). Pharmacologic treatment of insomnia is best reserved for short-term treatment, and concomitant behavioral interventions are important for any patient for whom ongoing sleep disturbances are expected. Residual daytime somnolence, rebound insomnia and tolerance all limit the long-term effectiveness of hypnotic agents, especially benzodiazepines. Newer, non-benzodiazepine hypnotics (zolpidem, zaleplon and eszopiclone) have shorter half-lives and less hang-over effect and abuse potential. Nevertheless, rebound insomnia and tolerance are quite common with these agents.

COORDINATING CARE IN PATIENTS WITH ADVANCED CANCER

Patients with advanced cancer and multiple cancer-related symptoms require coordinated multidisciplinary management to optimize care. As one of the many specialists who will be involved in the care of these patients, interventional oncologists have an opportunity and responsibility to help coordinate care. Many different practice models exist, and the specialists involved will vary from patient to patient. In some patients, such as those with end-stage hepatocellular carcinoma, the interventional oncologist may be the patient's primary physician coordinating care. In others, the palliative care physician, medical oncologist, surgical oncologist or hepatologist may be coordinating care with the interventional oncologist in a consultant role. Whatever the role assumed in a particular patient, communication among the managing physicians is critical.

CONCLUSION

As stated earlier, palliative care is focused on symptom relief and maximizing patient function, without necessarily impacting the natural history of the underlying disease. As the field of interventional oncology matures, interventional radiologists caring for patients with advanced cancer will need to be comfortable with the management of common clinical problems encountered in this patient population. Interventional radiologists will need to feel comfortable with communicating prognosis and other critical information to patients and their families. Working in concert with colleagues in other clinical cancer specialties, interventional oncologists will be able to offer therapeutic options that will maximize quantity and quality of life and help to optimally manage the many common symptoms in this challenging and rewarding patient population.

REFERENCES

1. World Health Organization. WHO definition of palliative care. Available at: http://www.who.int/cancer/palliative/definition/en. Accessed April 1, 2006.
2. Mosenthal AC and Murphy PA. Trauma care and palliative care: Time to integrate the two? J Am Coll Surg, 2003; 197: 509–516.
3. Curtis JR and Rubenfeld GD. Improving palliative care for patients in the intensive care unit. J Palliat Med, 2005; 8: 840–854.
4. von Gunten CF. Secondary and tertiary palliative care in US hospitals. JAMA, 2002; 287: 875–888.
5. Himelstein BP, Hilden JM, Boldt AM, et al. Pediatric palliative care. N Engl J Med, 2004; 350:1752–1762.
6. Morrison RS and Meier D. Palliative care. N Engl J Med, 2004; 350: 2582–2590.
7. Craft PS, Burns CM, Smith WT, et al. Knowledge of treatment intent among patients with advanced cancer: A longitudinal study. Eur J Cancer Care, 2005; 14: 417–425.
8. Schag CC, Heinrich RL, and Ganz PA. Karnofsky performance status revisited: Reliability, validity, and guidelines. J Clin Oncol, 1984; 2: 187–193.
9. Vigano A, Dorgan M, Jeanette B, et al. Survival prediction in terminal cancer patients: A systematic review of the medical literature. Palliat Med, 2000; 14: 363–374.
10. den Daas N. Estimating length of survival in end-stage cancer: A review of the literature. J Pain Symptom Manage, 1995; 10: 548–555.
11. Lamont EB and Christakis NA. Complexities in prognostication in advanced cancer. "To help them live their lives the way they want to." JAMA, 2003; 290: 98–104.
12. Maltoni M, Pirovano M, Scarpi E, et al. Prediction of survival of patients terminally ill with cancer. Results of an Italian prospective multicentric study. Cancer, 1995; 75: 2613–2622.
13. Reuben DB, Mor V, and Hiris J. Clinical symptoms and length of survival in patients with terminal cancer. Arch Intern Med, 1988; 148: 1586–1591.
14. Janisch L, Mick R, Schilsky RL, et al. Prognostic factors for survival in patients treated in phase I clinical trials. Cancer. 1994; 74: 1965–1973.
15. Maltoni M, Caraceni A, Brunelli C, et al. Prognostic factors in advanced cancer patients: Evidence-based clinical recommendations – a study for the steering committee of the European Association for Palliative Care. J Clin Oncol, 2005; 23: 6240–6248.
16. Ralson SH, Gallacher SJ, Patel U, et al. Cancer-associated hypercalcemia: Morbidity and mortality. Clinical experience in 126 treated patients. Ann Intern Med, 1990; 112: 499–504.
17. Iwase M, Kurachi Y, Kakuta S, et al. Clin Oral Investig, 2001; 5: 194–198.
18. Siddiqui F and Weissman DE. Fast facts and concepts #151; Hypercalcemia of malignancy. February 2006. End-of-Life Physician Education Resource Center. www.eperc.mcw.edu.
19. Khuntia D, Brown P, Li J, et al. Whole-brain radiotherapy in the management of brain metastasis. J Clin Oncol, 2006; 24: 1295–1304.
20. Glare P, Virik K, Jones M, et al. A systematic review of physicians' survival predictions in terminally ill cancer patients. BMJ, 2003; 327: 195–201.
21. Christakis NA and Lamont EB. Extent and determinants of error in doctors' prognoses in terminally ill patients: Prospective cohort study. BMJ, 2000; 320: 469–473.
22. Lamont EB, Christakis NA. Prognostic disclosure to patients with cancer near the end of life. Ann Intern Med, 2001; 134: 1096–1105.
23. Hagerty RG, Butow PN, Ellis PM, et al. Communicating prognosis in cancer care: A systematic review of the literature. Ann Oncol, 2005; 16: 1005–1053.

24. Randall TC and Wearn AM. Receiving bad news: Patients with haematological cancer reflect upon their experience. Palliat Med, 2005; 19: 594–601.

25. Weissman DE. Fast facts and concepts #13; Determining prognosis in advanced cancer, 2nd edition. July 2005. End-of-Life Palliative Education Resource Center. www.eperc.mcw.edu.

26. Ambuel B and Weissman DE. Fast facts and concepts #6; Delivering bad news: part 1, 2nd edition, July 2005. End-of-Life Palliative Education Resource Center. www.eperc.mcw.edu.

27. Ambuel B and Weissman DE. Fast facts and concepts #11; Delivering bad news; part 2, 2nd edition. September 2005. End-of-Life Palliative Education Resource Center. www.eperc.mcw.edu.

28. Weissman DE. Decision making at a time of crisis near the end of life. JAMA, 2004; 292: 1738–1743.

29. Lussier D, Huskey AF, and Portenoy RK. Adjuvant analgesics in cancer pain management. The Oncologist, 2004; 9: 571–591.

30. Mercadante S and Portenoy RK. Opioid poorly-responsive cancer pain: Part 1: Clinical considerations. J Pain Symptom Manage, 2001; 21: 144–150.

31. Thomas JR and von Gunten CF. Pain in terminally ill patients. Guidelines for pharmacological management. CNS Drugs, 2003; 17: 621–631.

32. Cherny NI. Cancer pain: Principles of assessment and syndromes. In: Berger AM, Portenoy RK, Weissman DE (eds). Principles and Practice of Palliative Care and Supportive Oncology, 2nd edition, pp. 3–52. New York: Lippincott Williams and Wilkins, 2002.

33. Menefee LA and Monti DA. Nonpharmacologic and complementary approaches to cancer pain management. J Am Osteopath Assoc, 2005; 105: S15–20.

34. Hillard RE. Music therapy in hospice and palliative care: A review of the empirical data. eCAM, 2005; 2: 173–178.

35. Mercadante S, Casuccio A, Agnello A, et al. Analgesic effects of nonsteroidal anti-inflammatory drugs in cancer pain due to somatic or visceral mechanisms. J Pain Symptom Manage, 1999; 17: 351–356.

36. Mercadante S, Fulfaro F, and Casuccio A. A randomized controlled study on the use of anti-inflammatory drugs in patients with cancer pain on morphine therapy: Effects on dose-escalation and a pharmacoeconomic analysis. Eur J Cancer, 2002; 38: 1358–1363.

37. Davis MP, Walsh D, Lagman R, et al. Controversies in pharmacotherapy of pain management. Lancet Oncol, 2005; 6: 696–704.

38. Leppert W and Luczak J. The role of tramadol in cancer pain treatment – a review. Supp Care Cancer, 2005; 13: 5–17.

39. Hanks GW, de Conno F, Cherny N, et al. Morphine and alternative opioids in cancer pain: The EAPC recommendations. Br J Cancer, 2001; 84: 587–593.

40. Gutstein, HB, Akil H. Opioid analgesics. In: Hardman JG, Limbird LE (eds). Goodman and Gilman's: The Pharmacological Basis of Therapeutics, 10th edition, pp. 569–619. New York: McGraw–Hill, 2001.

41. Weissman DE. Fast facts and concepts #71; Meperidine for pain: What's all the fuss? June 2002. End-of-Life Physician Education Resource Center. www.eperc.mcw.edu.

42. Aranoff GM, Brennan MJ, Douglas PD, et al. Evidence-based oral transmucosal fentanyl citrate (OTFC) dosing guidelines. Pain Med, 2005; 6: 305–314.

43. Ripamonti C, Zecca E, and Bruera E. An update on the clinical use of methadone for cancer pain. Pain, 1997; 70: 109–115.

44. Bruera E and Sweeney C. Methadone use in cancer patients with pain: A review. J Palliative Med, 2002; 5: 127–138.

45. Gordon DB and Weissman DE. Fast facts and concepts #70; PRN range analgesic orders. June 2002. End-of-Life Physician Education Resource Center. www.eperc.mcw.edu.

46. Quigley C. The role of opioids in cancer pain. BMJ, 2005; 331: 825–829.

47. Dean M. Opioids in renal failure and dialysis patients. J Pain Symptom Manage, 2004; 28: 497–504.

48. Paice JA, Toy C, and Shott S. Barriers to cancer pain relief: Fear of tolerance and addiction. J Pain Symptom Manage, 1998; 16: 1–9.

49. Sloan P and Melzack R. Long-term patterns of morphine dose and pain intensity among cancer patients. Hosp J, 1999; 14: 35–47.

50. Collin E, Poulain P, Gauvain-Piquard A, et al. Is disease progression the major factor in morphine 'tolerance' in cancer pain treatment? Pain, 1993; 55: 319–326.

51. National Cancer Institute. Substance Abuse Issues In Cancer (PDQ). Available at: http://www.cancer.gov/cancertopics/pdq/supportivecare/substanceabuse/health professional. Accessed April 1, 2006.

52. Schug SA, Zech D, Grond S, et al. A long-term survey of morphine in cancer pain patients. J Pain Symptom Manage, 1992; 7: 259–266.

53. Aronoff GM. Opioids in chronic pain management: Is there a significant risk of addiction? Curr Rev Pain, 2000; 4: 112–121.

54. Management of chronic pain syndromes: Issues and interventions. Pain Med, 2005; 6: S1–S21.

55. Caraceni A, Zecca E, Bonezzi C, et al. Gabapentin for neuropathic cancer pain: A randomized controlled trial from the gabapentin cancer pain study group. J Clin Oncol, 2004; 22: 2909–2917.

56. McDonald AA and Portenoy RK. How to use antidepressants and anticonvulsants as adjuvant analgesics in the treatment of neuropathic cancer pain. J Supp Oncol, 2006; 4: 43–52.

57. Hanks GW. The pharmacological treatment of bone pain. Cancer Surv, 1988; 7: 87–101.

58. Pinski J and Dorff TB. Prostate cancer metastases to bone: Pathophysiology, pain management, and the promise of targeted therapy. Eur J Cancer, 2005; 41: 932–940.

59. Finlay IG, Mason MD, and Shelley M. Radioisotopes for the palliation of metastatic bone cancer: A systematic review. Lancet Oncol, 2005; 6: 392–400.

60. Posteraro AF, Dupuy DE, and Mayo–Smith WW. Radiofrequency ablation of bony metastatic disease. Clin Radiol, 2004; 59: 803–811.

61. Hacein-Bey L, Baisden JL, Lemke DM, et al. Treating osteoporotic and neoplastic vertebral compression fractures with vertebroplasty and kyphoplasty. J Palliat Med, 2005; 8: 931–938.

62. Callstrom MR and Charboneau JW. Percutaneous ablation: Safe, effective treatment of bone tumors. Oncology, 2005; 19(Suppl 4): S22–S26.

63. Posteraro AF, Dupuy DE, and Mayo-Smith WW. Radiofrequency ablation of bony metastatic disease. Clin Radiol, 2004; 59: 803–811.

64. Elkersh MA, Simopoulos TT, and Bajwa ZH. Fundamentals of interventional pain medicine. The Neurol, 2005; 11: 285–293.

65. Wong GY, Schroeder DR, and Carns PE. Effect of neurolytic celiac plexus block on pain relief, quality of life, and survival in patients with unresectable pancreatic cancer. A randomized controlled trial. JAMA, 2004; 291: 1092–1099.

66. Davis MP and Walsh D. Treatment of nausea and vomiting in advanced cancer. Support Care Cancer, 2000; 8: 444–452.

67. de Boer-Dennert M, de Wit R, Schmitz PI, et al. Patient perceptions of the side-effects of chemotherapy: The influence of 5HT3 antagonists. Br J Cancer, 1997; 76: 1055–61.

68. Aapro M. 5-HT3-receptor antagonists in the management of nausea and vomiting in cancer and cancer treatment. Oncology, 2005; 69: 97–109.

69. Olver IN. Update on anti-emetics for chemotherapy-induced emesis. Intern Med J, 2005; 35: 478–481.

70. Hesketh PJ, Grunberg SM, Gralla RJ, et al. The oral neurokinin-1 antagonist aprepitant for the prevention of chemotherapy-induced nausea and vomiting: A multinational, randomized, double-blind, placebo-controlled trial in patients receiving high-dose cisplatin – the Aprepitant Protocol 052 Study Group. J Clin Oncol, 2003; 21: 4077–4080.

71. Herrstedt J, Muss HB, Warr DG, et al. Efficacy and tolerability of aprepitant for the prevention of chemotherapy-induced nausea and emesis over multiple cycles of moderately emetogenic chemotherapy. Cancer, 2005; 104: 1548–1555.

72. Campora E, Merlini L, Bruzzone M, et al. The incidence of narcotic-induced emesis. J Pain Symptom Manage, 1991; 6: 428–430.

73. Hardy J, Daly S, McQuade B, et al. A double-blind, randomised, parallel group, multinational, multicentre study comparing a single dose of ondansetron 24 mg p.o. with placebo and metoclopramide 10 mg t.d.s. p.o. in the treatment of opioid-induced nausea and emesis in cancer patients. Support Care Cancer, 2002; 10: 231–236.

74. Chung F, Lane R, Spraggs C, et al. Ondansetron is more effective than metoclopramide for the treatment of opioid-induced emesis in post-surgical adult patients. Ondansetron OIE Post-Surgical Study Group. Eur J Anaesthesiol, 1999; 16:669–677.

75. Glare P, Pereira G, Kristjanson LJ, et al. Systematic review of the efficacy of antiemetics in the treatment of nausea in patients with far-advanced cancer. Supp Care Cancer, 2004; 12: 432–440.

76. Bruera E, Seifert L, Watanabe S, et al. Chronic nausea in advanced cancer patients: A retrospective assessment of a metoclopramide-based antiemetic regimen. J Pain Symptom Manage, 1996; 11: 147–153.

77. Mystakidou K, Befon S, Liossi C, et al. Comparison of the efficacy and safety of tropisetron, metoclopramide, and chlorpromazine in the treatment of emesis associated with far advanced cancer. Cancer, 1998; 83: 1214–1243.

78. Sorbe BG, Hobgerg T, Glimelius B, et al. A randomized, multicenter study comparing the efficacy and tolerability of tropisetron, a new 5-HT3 receptor antagonist, with a metoclopramide-containing antiemetic cocktail in the prevention of cisplatin-induced emesis. Cancer, 1994; 73: 445–454.

79. Critchley P, Plach N, Grantham M, et al. Efficacy of haloperidol in the treatment of nausea and vomiting in the palliative patient: A systematic review. J Pain Symptom Manage, 2001; 22: 631–634.

80. Passik SD, Lundbert J, and Kirsh KL. A pilot exploration of the antiemetic activity of olanzapine for the relief of nausea in patients with advanced cancer and pain. J Pain Symptom Manage, 2002; 23: 526–532.

81. Passik SD, Kirsh KL, Theobald DE, et al. A retrospective chart review of the use of olanzapine for the prevention of delayed emesis in cancer patients. J Pain Symptom Manage, 2003; 25: 485–488.

82. Navari RM, Einhorn LH, Passik SD, et al. A phase II trial of olanzapine for the prevention of chemotherapy-induced nausea and vomiting: A Hoosier Oncology Group study. Supp Care Cancer, 2005; 13: 529–534.

83. Currow DC, Coughlan M, Fardell B, et al. Use of ondansetron in palliative medicine. J Pain Symptom Manage, 1997; 13: 302–307.

84. Tramer MR, Carroll D, Campbell FA, et al. Cannabinoids for control of chemotherapy induced nausea and vomiting: Quantitative systematic review. BMJ, 2001; 323: 1–8.

85. Walsh D, Nelson KA, and Mahmoud FA. Established and potential therapeutic applications of cannabinoids in oncology. Supp Care Cancer, 2003; 11: 137–143.

86. Malik IA, Khan WA, Qazilbash M, et al. Clinical efficacy of lorazepam in prophylaxis of anticipatory, acute, and delayed nausea and vomiting induced by high doses of cisplatin: A prospective randomized trial. Am J Clin Oncol, 1995; 18: 170–175.

87. Ezzo J, Vickers A, Richardson MA, et al. Acupuncture-point stimulation for chemotherapy-induced nausea and vomiting. J Clin Oncol, 2005; 23: 7188–7198.

88. Roscoe JA, Morrow GR, Hickok JT, et al. The efficacy of acupressure and acustimulation wrist bands for the relief of chemotherapy-induced nausea and vomiting. A University of Rochester Cancer Center Community Clinical Oncology Program multicenter study. J Pain Symptom Manage, 2003; 26: 731–742.

89. Mancini I and Bruera E. Constipation in advanced cancer patients. Supp Care Cancer, 1998; 6: 356–364.

90. Homsi J, Walsh D, Rivera N, et al. Symptom evaluation in palliative medicine: Patients report vs systematic assessment. Supp Care Cancer, 2006; 14: 444–453.

91. Fallon M and O'Neill B. ABC of palliative care: Constipation and diarrhoea. BMJ, 1997; 315: 1293–1296.

92. Tamayo AC and Diaz-Zuluaga PA. Management of opioid-induced bowel dysfunction in cancer patients. Supp Care Cancer, 2004; 12: 613–618.

93. Allan L, Richarz U, Simpson K, et al. Transdermal fentanyl versus sustained release oral morphine in strong-opioid naïve patients with chronic low back pain. Spine, 2005; 30: 2484–2490.

94. Muller-Lissner SA, Kamm MA, Scarpignato C, et al. Myths and misconceptions about chronic constipation. Am J Gastroenterol, 2005; 100: 232–242.

95. Meissner W, Schmidt U, Hartmann M, et al. Oral naloxone reverses opioid-associated constipation. Pain, 2000; 84: 105–109.

96. Sykes NP. An investigation of the ability of oral naloxone to correct opioid-related constipation in patients with advanced cancer. Palliat Med, 1996; 10: 135–44.

97. Cherny NI. Taking care of the terminally ill cancer patient: Management of gastrointestinal symptoms in patients with advanced cancer. Ann Oncol, 2004; 15: S205–S213.

98. Cascinu S. Management of diarrhea induced by tumors or cancer therapy. Curr Opinion Oncol, 1995; 7: 325–329.

99. Ippoliti C. Antidiarrhea agents for the management of treatment-related diarrhea in cancer patients. Am J Health Syst Pharm, 1998; 55: 1573–1580.

100. Yavuzsen T, Davis MP, Walsh D, et al. Systematic review of the treatment of cancer-associated anorexia and weight loss. J Clin Oncol, 2005; 23: 8500–8511.

101. Body JJ. The syndrome of anorexia-cachexia. Curr Opin Oncol, 1999; 11: 225–260.

102. MacDonald N. Is there evidence for earlier intervention in cancer-associated weight loss? J Supp Oncol, 2003; 1: 279–286.

103. Wilcock A. Anorexia: A taste of things to come? Palliat Med, 2006; 20: 43–45.

104. Simons JP, Schols AM, Hoefnagels JM, et al. Effects of medroxyprogesterone acetate on food intake, body composition, and resting energy expenditure in patients with advanced, nonhormone-sensitive cancer: A randomized, placebo-controlled trial. Cancer, 1998; 82: 553–560.

105. Desport JC, Gory-Delabaere G, Blanc-Vincent MP, et al. Standards, options, and recommendations for the use of appetite stimulants in oncology (2000). Br J Cancer, 2003; 89: S98–S100.

106. Sood A, Moynihan TJ. Cancer-related fatigue: An update. Curr Oncol Rep, 2005; 7: 277–282.

107. Raison CL and Miller AH. Depression in cancer: New developments regarding diagnosis and treatment. Biol Psychiat 2003; 54: 283–294.

108. Hickok JT, Roscoe JA, Morrow GR, et al. Frequency, severity, clinical course, and correlates of fatigue in 372 patients during 5 weeks of radiotherapy for cancer. Cancer, 2005; 104: 1772–1778.

109. Ahlberg K, Ekman T, Gaston-Johansson F, et al. Assessment and management of cancer–related fatigue in adults. Lancet, 2003; 362: 640–650.

110. Adamsen L, Midtgaard J, and Andersen C, et al. Transforming the nature of fatigue through exercise: Qualitative findings from a multidimensional exercise programme in cancer patients undergoing chemotherapy. Eur J Cancer Care, 2004; 13: 362–370.

111. Glaspy J. Anemia and fatigue in cancer patients. Cancer, 2001; 92: S1719–S1724.

112. Patrick D, Gagnon DD, Zagari MJ, et al. Assessing the clinical significance of health-related quality of life (HRQoL) improvements in anaemic cancer patients receiving epoetin alfa. Eur J Cancer, 2003; 39: 335–345.

113. Mock V. Evidence-based treatment for cancer-related fatigue. J Natl Cancer Inst Monograph, 2004; 32: 112–118.

114. Smith RE. Erythropoietic agents in the management of cancer patients. Part 1: Anemia, quality of life, and possible effects on survival. J Supp Oncol, 2003; 1: 249–258.

115. Munch TN, Zhang T, Wiley J, et al. The association between anemia and fatigue in patients with advanced cancer receiving palliative care. J Palliat Med, 2005; 8: 1144–1149.

116. Monti M, Castellani L, Berlusconi A, et al. Use of red blood cell transfusions in terminally ill cancer patients admitted to a palliative care unit. J Pain Symptom Manage, 1996; 12: 18–22.

117. Bruera E, Driver L, and Barnes EA. Patient–controlled methylphenidate for the management of fatigue in patients with advancer cancer: A preliminary report. J Clin Oncol, 2003; 21: 4439–4443.

118. Schwartz AL, Mori M, Gao R, et al. Exercise reduces daily fatigue in women with breast cancer receiving chemotherapy. Med Sci Sports Exerc, 2001; 33: 718–723.

119. Dimeo FC, Stieglitz RD, Novelli-Fischer U, et al. Effects of physical activity on the fatigue and psychologic status of cancer patients during chemotherapy. Cancer, 1999; 85: 2273–2277.

120. Iop A, Manfredi AM, and Bonura S. Fatigue in cancer patients receiving chemotherapy: An analysis of published studies. Ann Oncol, 2004; 15: 712–720.

121. Covey AM. Management of malignant pleural effusions and ascites. J Supp Oncol, 2005; 3: 169–176.

122. Garrison RN, Kaelin LD, Galloway RH, et al. Malignant ascites. Clinical and experimental observations. Ann Surg, 1986; 203: 644–651.

123. Runyon BA, Hoefs JC, and Morgan TR. Ascitic fluid analysis in malignancy–related ascites. Hepatol, 1988; 8: 1104–1109.

124. Gines P, Cardenas A, Arroyo V, et al. Management of cirrhosis and ascites. N Engl J Med, 2004; 350: 1646–1654.

125. Lee CW, Bociek G, and Faught W. A survey of practice in management of malignant ascites. J Pain Symptom Manage, 1998; 16: 96–101.

126. Saravanan R and Cramp ME. Investigation and treatment of ascites. Clin Med, 2002; 2: 310–313.

127. Marrero J, Martinez FJ, and Hyzy R. Advances in critical care hepatology. Am J Respir Crit Care Med, 2003; 168: 1421–1426.

128. Lidstone V and Thorns A. Pruritus in cancer patients. Cancer Treat Rev, 2001; 27: 305–312.

129. Lugon JR. Uremic pruritus: A review. Hemodial Intl, 2005; 9: 180–188.

130. Zylicz Z, Kragnik M, van Sorge AA, et al. Paroxetine in the treatment of severe non-dermatological pruritus: A randomized, controlled trial. J Pain Symptom Manage, 2003; 26: 1105–1112.

131. Prommer E. Re: pruritus in patients with advanced cancer. J Pain Symptom Manage, 2005; 30: 201–202.

132. Twycross R, Greaves MW, Handwerker H, et al. Itch: Scratching more than the surface. Q J Med, 2003; 96: 7–26.

133. Bosonnet L. Pruritus: scratching the surface. Eur J Cancer Care. 2003; 12: 162–165.

134. Krajnik M and Zylicz Z. Understanding pruritus in systemic disease. J Pain Symptom Manage, 2001; 21: 151–168.

135. Price TJ, Patterson WK, and Olver IN. Rifampicin as treatment for pruritus in malignant cholestasis. Supp Care Cancer, 1988; 6: 533–535.

136. Terg R, Coronel E, Sorda J, et al. Efficacy and safety of oral naltrexone treatment for pruritus of cholestasis, a crossover, double blind, placebo-controlled study. J Hepatol 2002; 37: 717–722.

137. Prieto LN. The use of midazolam to treat itching in a terminally ill patients with biliary obstruction. J Pain Symptom Manage, 2004; 28: 531–532.

138. Villamil AG, Bandi JC, Galdame OA, et al. Efficacy of lidocaine in the treatment of pruritus in patients with chronic cholestatic liver disease. Am J Med, 2005; 118: 1160–1163.

139. PorzioG, Aielli F, Narducci F, et al. Pruritus in a patient with advanced cancer successfully treated with continuous infusion of granisetron. Supp Care Cancer, 2004; 12: 208–209.

140. Friedman JD and Dello Buono FA. Opioid antagonists in the treatment of opioid-induced constipation and pruritus. Ann Pharmacol, 2001; 35: 85–91.

141. Aass N, Fossa SD, Dahl AA, et al. Prevalence of anxiety and depression in cancer patients seen at the Norwegian Radium Hospital. Eur J Cancer, 1997; 33: 1597–604.

142. Pirl WF. Evidence report on the occurrence, assessment, and treatment of depression in cancer patients. J Natl Cancer Inst Monograph, 2004; 32: 32–39.

143. Stiefel F, Trill MD, Berney A, et al. Depression in palliative care: A pragmatic report from the Expert Working Group of the European Association for Palliative Care. Supp Care Cancer, 2001; 9: 477–488.

144. Ebmeier KP, Donaghey C, and Steel JD. Recent developments and current controversies in depression. Lancet, 2006; 367: 153–167.

145. Goodwin JS, Zhang DD, and Ostir GV. Effect of depression on diagnosis, treatment, and survival of older women with breast cancer. J Am Geriatr Soc, 2004; 52: 106–111.

146. Hjerl K, Andersen EW, Keiding N, et al. Depression as a prognostic factor for breast cancer mortality. Psychosomat, 2003; 44: 24–30.

147. Passik SD, Dugan W, McDonald MV, et al. Oncologists' recognition of depression in their patients with cancer. J Clin Oncol, 1998; 16: 1594–1600.

148. Periyakoil VJ. Fast facts and concepts #43; Is it grief or depression? Second edition. August 2005. End-of-Life Physician Education Resource Center. www.eperc.mcw.edu.

149. Chochinov HM, Wilson KG, Enns M, et al. "Are you depressed?" Screening for depression in the terminally ill. Am J Psychiatry, 1997; 154: 674–676.

150. Arnold RA. Fast fact and concept #146; Screening for depression in palliative care. December 2005. End-of-Life Physician Education Resource Center. www.eperc.mcw.edu.

151. Holland JC, Morrow GR, Schmale A, et al. A randomized clinical trial of alprazolam versus progressive muscle relaxation in cancer patients with anxiety and depressive symptoms. J Clin Oncol, 1991; 9: 1004–1011.

152. Sheard T and Maguire P. The effect of psychological interventions on anxiety and depression in cancer patients: results of two meta-analyses. Br J Cancer. 1999; 80: 1770–1780.

153. Thase ME, Greenhouse JB, Frank E, et al. Treatment of major depression with psychotherapy or psychotherapy-pharmacotherapy combinations. Arch Gen Psychiatry, 1997; 54: 1009–15.

154. Clark DB, Andrus MR, and Byrd DC. Drug interactions between linezolid and selective serotonin reuptake inhibitors: Case report involving sertraline and review of the literature. Pharmacotherapy, 2006; 25: 269–276.

155. Weinrieb RM, Auriacombe M, Lynch KG, et al. Selective serotonin re-uptake inhibitors and the risk of bleeding. Expert Opin Drug Safety, 2005; 4: 337–344.

156. Kroenke K, Messina N, Benattia I, et al. Venlafaxine extended release in the short-term treatment of depressed and anxious primary care patients with multisomatoform disorder. J Clin Psychiatry, 2006; 67: 72–80.

157. Raskin J, Pritchett YL, Wang F, et al. A double-blind, randomized multicenter trial comparing duloxetine with placebo in the management of diabetic peripheral neuropathic pain. Pain Med, 2005; 6: 346–356.

158. Theobald DE, Kirsh KL, Holtsclaw E, et al. An open-label, crossover trial of mirtazapine (15 and 30 mg) in cancer patients with pain and other distressing symptoms. J Pain Symptom Manage, 2002; 23: 442–447.

159. Pereira J and Bruera E. Depression with psychomotor retardation: Diagnostic challenges and the use of psychostimulants. J Palliat Med, 2001; 4: 15–21.

160. Burgess C, Cornelius V, Love S, et al. Depression and anxiety in women with early breast cancer: Five year observational cohort study. BMJ, 2005; 330: 702.

161. Hipkins J, Whitworth M, Tarrier N, et al. Social support, anxiety and depression after chemotherapy for ovarian cancer: A prospective study. Br J Health Psychol, 2004; 9: 569–581.

162. Fowler JM, Carpenter KM, Gupta P, et al. The gynecologic oncology consult: Symptom presentation and concurrent symptoms of depression and anxiety. Obstet Gynecol, 2004; 103: 1211–1217.

163. Fellowes D, Barnes K, and Wilkinson S. Aromatherapy and massage for symptom relief in patients with cancer. Cochrane Database Syst Rev, 2004; (2): CD002287.

164. Sloman R. Relaxation and imagery for anxiety and depression control in community patients with advanced cancer. Cancer Nurs, 2002; 25: 432–435.

165. Bottomley A. Anxiety and the adult cancer patient. Eur J Cancer Care, 1998; 7: 217–224.

166. Goodman WK. Selecting pharmacotherapy for generalized anxiety disorder. J Clin Psychiatry, 2004; 65: S8–S13.

167. Graci G. Pathogenesis and management of cancer-related insomnia. J Supp Oncol, 2005; 3: 349–359.

168. Theobald DE. Cancer pain, fatigue, distress, and insomnia in cancer patients. Clin Cornerstone, 2004; 6: S15–S21.

169. Miller M and Arnold RM. Fast facts and concepts #101; Insomnia: Patient assessment. November 2003. End-of-life Physician Education Resource Center. www.eperc.mcw.edu.

170. Miller M and Arnold RM. Fast facts and concepts #104: Non-pharmacologic therapy for insomnia. January 2004. End-of-Life Physician Education Resource Center. www.eperc.mcw.edu.

Chapter 46

COMPLICATIONS OF THERAPEUTIC ENDOVASCULAR PROCEDURES IN MALIGNANT LIVER DISEASES

José I. Bilbao

José J. Noguera

In recent years, intra-arterial treatment has become one of the first options in the therapeutic approach to primary and metastatic liver tumors. In spite of having good results, these endovascular procedures are not exempt of complications that have to be understood and promptly recognized in order to decrease their morbidity and mortality. The most common complications are described subsequently and distributed in three main groups. First, the complications arising from embolization of liver tumors, with reference to systemic toxicities (post-embolization syndrome [PES], hepatic insufficiency and changes in portal pressure), local complications (rupture of hepatocarcinoma [HCC] and biliary complications) and distant complications (pulmonary embolism of lipiodol or particles and metastatic spread of disease in the lungs). Secondly, the complications related to chemotherapy administered directly from the hepatic artery are then discussed, with mention of the complications caused by the catheter (migration and arterial obstruction), and complications associated with drug infusion in the extra-hepatic arteries. Finally, the complications of radioembolization, a relatively new approach that is performed with microspheres loaded with ^{90}Ytrium (^{90}Y) are also discussed.

EMBOLIZATION OF HEPATIC TUMORS

Systemic Toxicities

Post-embolization Syndrome

PES is characterized by a set of signs and symptoms occurring after embolization. Some of them are subjective and hard to quantify, which include nausea, vomiting, abdominal pain, fever and hypertransaminasemia, lasting a maximum of 7 to 10 days (1, 2) with variable incidence according to the diagnostic criteria (15% to 90%). Paye (3) and Wigmore (4) define PES as the presence of a temperature of over 38.5°C or cytolysis, defined by an increase in alanine aminotransferase (ALT) greater than 100 U/L or over twice the level prior to the embolization. Of these two main criteria for PES (temperature and cytolysis), the most common is hypertransaminasemia, and it could be said that "there is no fever without cytolysis" (3), which suggests that cytolysis might be the most accurate definition of PES. It was originally attributed to tumor necrosis induced by the intra-arterial treatment (2–4) and was therefore regarded as a sign of response to therapy. However, it was later shown by two studies that the factor responsible for hypertransaminasemia and fever was not tumor lysis, but the damage caused to the hepatic parenchyma that is not affected by the tumor (3, 4). In the first of these investigations, a lower incidence of PES was found in cirrhotic patients than in patients with hepatic fibrosis alone (3). In the former, as the percentage of healthy hepatocytes is lower, the hypertransaminasemia induced by cytolysis is less acute. Another study later reported that patients develop PES irrespective of whether the tumor is a primary neoplasm or a metastasis (4). Cytolysis of HCC causes hypertransaminasemia, whereas cytolysis of a hepatic metastasis cannot deliver transaminases into the general circulation. Nonetheless, the hypertransaminasemia induced in both types of tumors is similar, which indicates that hypertransaminasemia is due to lysis of the non-diseased tissue. Although PES is self-limiting and requires no treatment other than hydration and antiemetics (2), its importance lies in the need for hospitalization after the procedure and prolongation of the hospital stay (2). It is therefore necessary to know the risk factors and means of prevention. The risk factors for PES are high doses of chemotherapy (2) and the absence of cirrhosis (3). Moreover, it is noteworthy that the frequency of PES gradually declines in successive treatments (1, 2). Administration of corticoids before intra-arterial treatment reduces the incidence, intensity and duration of PES (5, 6).

Liver Failure

There are no clear diagnostic criteria for liver malfunction after chemoembolization. Chan (7) defines liver failure as the appearance of one of the following: development of encephalopathy; increasing ascites; increase in the prothrombin time (PTT) by more than 3 seconds over the level before embolization; or increase in the serum bilirubin level to twice the upper level of normal or basal level, depending whether it is normal or abnormal before the treatment. Other authors add worsening in the Child-Pugh stage in the definition of liver failure (1, 8).

This malfunction lasts for a maximum of 3 weeks (1, 7) and is irreversible in around 3% of the cases. This absence of clear diagnostic criteria means that the frequency of liver malfunction after chemoembolization seems to be very variable (2% to 60%) (8). Liver ischemia plays a major role in the development of liver insufficiency after chemoembolization, as it is more likely to happen in patients with portal vein obstruction (1).

This liver failure may be predicted in some patients, as there is a set of risk factors for developing liver malfunction, practically all of which are related to the state of hepatic function before treatment (1, 7–10). The patients with the greatest risk are those with analytical abnormalities before treatment (higher bilirubin, PT and transaminases) and patients with cirrhosis, who have a greater risk of developing irreversible hepatic failure. In addition, there is a positive correlation between the frequency of hepatic malfunction and the dose of chemotherapy administered (7).

The monoethylglycinexylidide (MEGX) test (11), which studies the hepatic metabolic reserve, can predict the occurrence of hepatic insufficiency after chemoembolization. A cut-off point of 26 ng/ml on the MEGX test is a highly sensitive and specific predictor of hepatic failure after treatment (8). It is thus possible to identify patients with less hepatic reserve, who are at greatest risk of developing an episode of hepatic failure after embolization (7).

Changes in Portal Pressure

Embolization of liver tumors causes alterations in the portal hemodynamics (12, 13), the explanation of which is based on various observations. First, the occlusion of some non-tumor portal branches has been described during embolization with lipiodol. The oily contrast acts as a "particle" that passes through presinusoidal arterio-portal 40- to 50-μm shunts, a phenomenon that increases the presinusoidal portal pressure. In addition to this, a reparative hypermetabolic state that appears after embolization initiates a regulation of portal and arterial flow mediated by adenosine, increasing the hepatic blood supply (12). This means that a reduction in arterial supply secondary to embolization causes a compensatory increase in portal flow, and vice versa (14). It has been reported that the increase in the portal flow rate (in both the embolized and non-embolized lobes) causes a rise in pressure in the esophageal varices (13). This alteration in portal hemodynamics justifies the cases that have been described, albeit infrequently, concerning the rupture of esophageal varices after hepatic chemoembolization (12). In patients with gastro-esophageal varices, it is therefore recommended that possible bleeding from ruptured varices should be borne in mind; some such patients may benefit if specific treatment is given for the varices before embolization (15).

Local Complications

Rupture of HCC

One well-known complication of HCC is spontaneous rupture, which is described as having a frequency of up to 15% (16–18). On some occasions, rupture may be induced by the administration of intra-arterial treatment, although this occurs in fewer than 1% of cases (15, 16), and its pathophysiology is unclear. Several hypotheses have been published (15–17), such as mechanical stimulation by the catheter and reparative processes and angiitis caused by contamination or by chemotherapy drugs, resulting in the formation of pseudoaneurysms, which may or may not be reversible (15).

The rupture manifests as hemoperitoneum and anemia, which may occur during or after treatment. This complication has a poor prognosis because patients with HCC are mostly cirrhotic, with underlying hemorrhagic disorders. Moreover, patients subjected to endovascular treatments are initially unoperable, so any bleeding complication is unlikely to be treated by surgery (15, 16). Another possible consequence of extrahepatic rupture of HCC is peritoneal dissemination of the tumor (19), with an adverse effect in patient survival, although cases of extrahepatic rupture have been described with no evidence of tumor spread years after hemoperitoneum caused by intra-arterial treatment (18).

When the hemorrhage is intra-tumoral, which may be manifest in only a slight hypertransaminasemia, the clinical prognosis is not as poor as in cases of extrahepatic rupture (17), as the surrounding hepatic parenchyma facilitates hemostasis.

Biliary Complications

Biliary complications can be divided into two groups: those affecting the gallbladder and those concerning the bile ducts. The latter are subdivided into those of the small peripheral bile ducts (collections from the bile duct, also known as bilomas; Figure 46.1), and those of the major central bile ducts, which manifest as stenoses.

The bile ducts are vascularized exclusively by the hepatic artery, which makes it extremely sensitive to ischemic complications when hepatic arterial embolization is performed. The largest series reports a 4% incidence of such complications (15, 20). Risk factors exist that predispose patients to developing ischemic biliary complications (15), such as previous

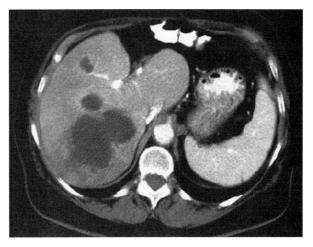

FIGURE 46.1. A 62-year-old patient with liver metastases from a neuroendocrine tumor was treated with bland embolization of the right lobe. Particles were 150-μ spheres; 15 days after the procedure he came with abdominal pain without fever. A CT was performed that showed an intrahepatic fluid collection, without signs of infection. The diagnosis of "biloma" was established, and patient recovered with conservative treatment.

dilation and stenosis of the bile duct, too proximal embolization in the hepatic artery, repeated treatment over a short period of time and chemotherapy added to the embolic particles.

Furthermore, the size and type of the tumor influence the incidence of biliary complications. Compared with liver metastases, HCC is, in most cases, a highly hypervascular tumor with large feeding arteries. This fact facilitates an increase in the tumoral uptake of the embolizing material and the chemotherapy drug, which means that the non-diseased parenchyma around the tumor receives smaller quantities of the drug. In patients with HCC, bilomas thus appear less frequently than in cases of metastases (3.6% as compared with 9.6%) (21). Moreover, HCC mainly occurs in cirrhotic patients, in whom arterio-portal shunts are frequently found that can reduce the damage to non-tumor parenchyma (22). The tumor size has an influence similar to the histological type: larger nodules take in a larger quantity of drugs than smaller ones, so bilomas develop more easily in patients with smaller tumors (21), since theoretically the non-tumor parenchyma around the lesion receives the embolizing material and chemotherapy drugs that the small nodule has not taken in.

In a series reported by Kim (20), the most common finding (70% of all biliary complications) is the development of subcapsular bilomas. These originate in microvascular damage to the peribiliary capillary plexus, resulting in necrosis of the peripheral bile ducts with leakage and subsequent development of the biloma (21).

The development of hepatic abscess (due to super-infection of a biloma) is a very rare complication (less than 1%) of endovascular treatment for hepatic tumors (7, 9, 15, 22, 23). As is the case with bilomas, the incidence of abscesses depends on the histological type, being less common after embolization of HCC than metastatic disease (24) because of the differences in vascular supply to these tumors noted earlier. Among the risk factors for superinfection of a biloma and the consequential development of a hepatic abscess, obstruction of the portal vein and the coexistence of previous disease of the bile duct have been described (15, 23). Patients with abscesses may manifest clinically with fever, abdominal pain (as in PES) and leukocytosis. The diagnosis is performed with ultrasound (US) or computed tomography (CT). The treatment includes the administration of antibiotics and the placement of a percutaneous drainage catheter if deemed necessary (15, 23).

Another extremely rare complication of chemoembolization of the liver is arterio-biliary fistula (25), caused by ischemic damage and subsequent necrosis of the bile duct, putting it in contact with arterial branches so that hemobilia, anemia, cholestatic syndrome and cholangitis may occur.

Ischemic damage to the major bile ducts may cause biliary stenosis, which is found in large series in fewer than 1% of cases (20, 26). Special mention should be made of fluxoridine, an anti-metabolite used in the treatment of inoperable metastases of colon cancer. The complications that have been described for this drug include disorders of liver function and the bile duct, which occur at a frequency that is far from inconsiderable (5% to 29%), and which are similar to sclerosing cholangitis, with jaundice and cholangitis (27). Cholangiographic studies show complete obstructions or stenosis of the intra- or extrahepatic bile duct, or dilations of the bile ducts with no obvious points of obstruction.

Undetected embolization of the gallbladder is relatively common; however, it is clinically relevant in fewer than 1% of patients (7, 15, 26), in whom it may cause cholecystitis (28). The infusion of particles and chemotherapy into the cystic artery can be due, mainly, to two reasons. First, the wide range of anatomical variations in its origin, sometimes difficult to identify, and second, reflux of the embolizing material during its infusion even when the tip of the catheter is placed distal to the origin of the artery (15). Most of these patients can be given conservative treatment, although some may require percutaneous cholecystostomy or cholecystectomy in cases of gangrenous or emphysematous cholecystitis, or if there is perforation (15).

Distant (Pulmonary) Complications

Pulmonary complications of intra-arterial hepatic treatment occur very infrequently (fewer than 1%) (7, 15, 29). Both lipiodol, which is given with chemotherapy, and embolizing material can reach the pulmonary circulation. The presence of arteriovenous shunts (AVS) plays a key role in the development of lung complications (29, 30), especially if the inferior phrenic artery is the afferent vessel for treatment (31).

Lipiodol, which is deposited in the pleura and lung, can cause consolidation, pleural effusion and patchy or scattered deposits in the parenchyma (Figure 46.2). Most of these (95%) are asymptomatic and are mainly situated in the posterior regions of the right lower lobe, although when large AVS are present, they may be found throughout the organ (31). Lipiodol increases the patency of pulmonary vessels and exerts a toxic effect directly on the alveolus. This effect seems to be dose dependent: Chung (30) observed that patients with symptomatic embolism had received doses greater than 20 ml of lipiodol.

The ability of *spheres* to migrate to the pulmonary circulation depends both in the presence of AVS and on their caliber, and cases have been described of fatal pulmonary embolism caused by 40- to 120-μm spheres (29). One feature common to these cases is that the first clinical manifestation is oxygen desaturation of unexplained origin, which is why it is advisable to stop the procedure if desaturation of this kind occurs. The possible alternatives are embolization using larger spheres or, alternatively, use of other percutaneous ablative techniques. In the fatal cases reported, hemodynamic disorders were described, such as pulmonary arterial hypertension (caused by occlusion of the pulmonary arteries by the spheres) and arterial hypotension (due to the reduction in blood returning to the left heart from the pulmonary circulation) (29).

The relationship between hepatic chemoembolization and its influence on the appearance of pulmonary metastases (32, 33) is controversial. It has been argued that there is a greater risk of pulmonary

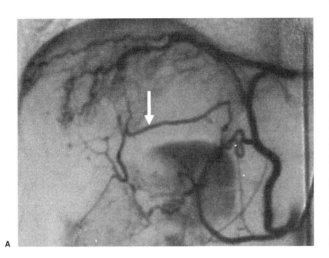

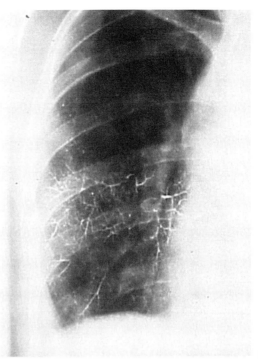

FIGURE 46.2. Patient with HCC, embolized with 10 ml of lipiodol. The treatment was performed from the right inferior phrenic artery (RIPA): (A) RIPA arteriogram which partially vascularizes the tumor (*arrow*). (B) Posteroanterior chest radiograph: Hyperdense images in a branching pattern corresponding to lipiodol migrated into pulmonary arteries.

metastases after chemoembolization on the basis that the latter causes an increase in the activity of degrading enzymes and a reduction in the activity of the tumor invasion inhibiting factor, as well as an architectural disorder resulting from ischemic necrosis (33). All these factors can facilitate the movement of tumor cells into the blood flow and their migration toward the lung; however, an open debate still rages about the viability of these tumor cells that lodge in the lung and their ability to form metastatic nodules. In any case, the risk factor for the occurrence of pulmonary metastases acknowledged by most authors is the size of the liver tumor (32, 33).

CHEMOTHERAPY INFUSION

Obstruction and Migration of the Catheter

Permanent catheters attached to peripheral infusion devices (subcutaneous ports), with access via the subclavian or femoral arteries, allow multiple sessions of intra-arterial chemotherapy to be given to the liver, while avoiding the need to repeat the procedure in each cycle of treatment. Perfusion systems were classically inserted by open surgery, involving cannu-

lation of the gastroduodenal-hepatic artery (GDA), fixing the cannula to the artery and connecting the proximal end of the cannula to a peripheral infusion device.

Later, percutaneous techniques were developed, allowing the doctor to place, from a subclavian or femoral approach, a catheter in the selected hepatic artery with its proximal end attached subcutaneously to the port. The procedure was complemented with the occlusion (embolized with coils) of the GDA to prevent leakage of the chemotherapy agent through extrahepatic arteries (34). However, this technique has the drawback that the tip of the catheter may move, which means that it could migrate, for example to the splenic artery. Yamagami modified this technique (35, 36) by inserting the tip of the catheter in the GDA, occluding its distal end with a microcoil and fixing the catheter to the artery with coils or N-butyl cyanoacrylate (NBCA). Thus, the drug, which reaches the common hepatic artery via a lateral orifice in the catheter, does not progress through the gastroduodenal artery or the right gastric artery, which is also occluded with coils. It has been shown that fixing the distal end of the catheter reduces the incidence of migrations and obstructions (36). The lower rate of obstructions in the form of thrombosis has been attributed to the reduction of the stimulus exerted by the tip of the catheter on the wall of the artery when it is in a stable position in the GDA (37). In fact, it has also been shown that fixing with NBCA and coils results in a lower rate of re-patency than if coils alone are used (0.7% compared with 4.2%) (36). Also, fixation prevents hepatic arterial occlusion, diminishing the rates of thrombosis from 22% without fixation to 5.3% to 8.8% when fixation is used (33–35).

Extrahepatic Complications

Administration of chemotherapy through the hepatic artery can cause extrahepatic lesions to occur as the drug passes through collateral vessels originating in the hepatic artery itself or its distal branches. Such vessels, which supply extrahepatic tissues, normally originate in the left and proper hepatic arteries, whereas scarcely 3% of them come from the right hepatic artery (38). The arteries involved in this type of complication are the right gastric and left accessory, the falciform, the posterosuperior pancreatoduodenal and the inferior right phrenic arteries. Drug infusion through the gastric arteries and superoinferior pancreato-duodenal arteries is perceived clinically as epigastric pain, nausea and fever (39) as a consequence of gastroduodenitis, gastroduodenal ulcers (38) and even pancreatitis (40). If the drug reaches the falciform artery, it can cause a supra-umbilical skin rash (38), whereas the presence of the drug in the inferior right phrenic artery causes the lung disorders that were described earlier.

Embolization of the GDA has been shown to limit the frequency of gastroduodenal lesions (40). But this reduction in the incidence of damage to the gastrointestinal mucosa is still more marked when embolization of the right gastric artery is added (39). On occasions, direct embolization of the right gastric artery is not technically possible because of its small caliber and the angulation at its origin. In such cases, there is the option of gaining access to the right gastric artery through the left gastric artery, which allows a higher percentage of successful embolizations in the first session (41), although it also suffers from one limitation: sometimes there is no anastomosis between the two gastric arteries or, if there is, it is so narrow in caliber that it does not technically permit embolization through the left gastric artery.

The possibility of producing splenic infarction due to reflux of embolic agents into the splenic artery during chemoembolization of the hepatic artery deserves special mention. Some predisposing factors have been identified, such as the celiac stenosis with reversal flow in the common hepatic artery, increased blood flow through the splenic artery (because of cirrhosis or splenomegaly) and catheter-induced spasm of the hepatic artery (42).

LIVER RADIOEMBOLIZATION

Liver Failure after Radioembolization

Treatment with ^{90}Y is based on the selective endovascular administration of a high dose of radiation to have a tumoricidal effect on primary and secondary hepatic tumors (120 to 155 Gy) (43–47) without crossing the threshold of a total hepatic dose of 30 to 40 Gy, in excess of which radiation-induced hepatitis has been described (43, 47–49).

The mechanism through which the radiation can provoke hepatic failure is still unclear. Fajardo (50) described that it could be based on endothelial vascular damage, as this is the most radiation-vulnerable cellular line of mesenchymal tissues (51). This damage affects mainly the centrilobular veins and, often, the adjacent sinusoids (50). This will cause fibrin deposition. Afterward, fibrin would be replaced by collagen, causing fibrous occlusion of the vein.

Treatment with interstitial hepatic radiotherapy using ^{90}Y can cause damage to the liver that is often slight and transitory (44,47). This is mainly evidenced in abnormal blood test findings (bilirubin, transaminases, PT). Carr (44) describes how almost 100% of his patients were found to have a raised PT, although none had more than twice the normal maximum. In other series, roughly one-third of patients were found to have hyperbilirubinemia higher than twice the normal maximum (44, 47, 48). The hepatitis caused by radiation, which can simulate veno-occlusive disease (52), is part of a syndrome that begins 2 to 24 weeks after the exposure to ionizing radiation. Other features of this are an increase in weight and abdominal perimeter due to ascites, an increase in alkaline phosphatase to over twice the normal maximum, with slight hyperbilirubinemia and hypertransaminasemia. In short, this syndrome could be defined as **anicteric ascites** (52).

Once more, it can be seen that, in addition to the total dose given, the hepatic functional reserve is an important predictor of hepatic malfunction as a result of treatment, as it can be observed that the patients who develop major analytical disorders are those who have higher total bilirubin before commencing treatment (47).

Extrahepatic Complications after Radioembolization

Lung

Radiation pneumonitis is caused by migration of particles loaded with ^{90}Y to the pulmonary circulation via hepatopulmonary shunts (HPS). According to data from the results obtained with external-beam radiotherapy, radiation pneumonitis occurs very rarely below total doses of 20 Gy to the lung but is quite common at doses of over 60 Gy (53). The shunt must be quantified before any treatment is planned, by administering macroaggregates of albumin loaded with ^{99}Tc m into the hepatic artery, and measuring the proportion of macroaggregates that reach the lung out of the total quantity administered.

The incidence reported over the last series is very low, because patients with HPS of over 13% to 20% (43, 44, 53–55), or estimated pulmonary doses of over 30 Gy in a single treatment, or 50 Gy in successive treatments, are excluded from treatment. A protocol of reduced doses can also be calculated for shunts between 10% and 20% (55). The ^{90}Y particles that reach the pulmonary circulation are more likely to settle in arterial branches of the first order, at intra- and extra-vascular sites and, in the latter case, phenomena such as phagocytosis and foreign-body reactions set in. Pathology studies show type II hyperplasia of the pneumocytes, hyaline membranes and fibrosis occupying the air space (53). This means that the areas of radiation pneumonitis show radiologically as zones of peripheral condensation, which characteristically do not affect the subpleural regions, so that their outer limit is parallel to the pleura and the fissures. CT is able to detect these signs at an earlier stage (between the first and second week) than simple radiography (between two and four months). Fibrosis is evident from a restrictive pattern in respiratory function tests (53).

It might seem logical that embolization of the HPS before treatment with ^{90}Y should reduce the incidence of radiation pneumonitis, but Leung (53) observed that embolization of these shunts using particles did not prevent radiation pneumonitis from developing in patients with shunts of more than 15%. He advances three possible reasons for this: 1) the particles prevent the passing of albumin microaggregates, but not that of spheres loaded with ^{90}Y, 2) there may be different rheological behavior between the macroaggregates and the spheres and 3) after embolization of the HPS with particles, collateral circulation may develop that perpetuates the HPS.

Gallbladder

The migration of spheres to the gallbladder can produce cholecystitis (44, 52) or even gallbladder necrosis (56). The alteration is produced by the mechanical occlusion of the vessels by the spheres and the damage that direct radiation causes to the vessels and extravascular tissue (56). As in the case of other endovascular techniques, it is recommended (if technically possible) to place the tip of the catheter distally to the origin of the cystic artery and to perform a meticulous vascular study.

Gastrointestinal Tract

Radioactive spheres deposited in the gastrointestinal tract can cause a range of manifestations, from slight nausea, vomiting and abdominal pain (43, 46, 54) to bleeding gastroduodenal ulcers (45, 52, 54, 57). These ulcers are radiation induced, have an insidious evolution, are usually larger and may be life-threatening (48). Their management is frequently difficult, and sometimes surgical management is needed (54, 57).

Others

Cases of myelotoxicity have been described, caused by the migration of radioactive spheres to the bone marrow (58). This complication is now very uncommon (43, 45, 46, 52, 59). In any case, it is interesting to note that Carr (44) observed a drop of over 50% in the white blood cell count in more than 80% of his patients, although this finding had no clinical repercussions. Moreover, slight granulocytopenia and low platelet count accompanied this. Deposits of ^{90}Y-charged spheres have also been found in the skin (45), and ulcers developed in the areas of the deposit.

REFERENCES

1. Caturelli E, Siena DA, Fusilli S, et al. Transcatheter arterial chemoembolization for hepatocellular carcinoma in patients with cirrhosis: Evaluation of damage to nontumorous liver tissue – long-term prospective study. Radiology, 2000; 215: 123–128.

2. Leung DA, Goin JE, Sickles C, et al. Determinants of postembolization syndrome after hepatic chemoembolization. J Vasc Interv Radiol, 2001; 12: 321–326.

3. Paye F, Farges O, Dahmane M, et al. Cytolysis following chemoembolization for hepatocellular carcinoma. Br J Surg, 1999; 86: 176–180.

4. Wigmore SJ, Redhead DN, Thomson BN, et al. Postchemoembolisation syndrome – tumour necrosis or hepatocyte injury? Br J Cancer, 2003; 89: 1423–1427.

5. Bissler JJ, Racadio J, Donnelly LF, et al. Reduction of postembolization syndrome after ablation of renal angiomyolipoma. Am J Kidney Dis, 2002; 39: 966–971.

6. Feng YL, Ling CQ, Zhu DZ, et al. Ginsenosides combined with dexamethasone in preventing and treating postembolization syndrome following transcatheter arterial chemoembolization: A randomized, controlled and double-blinded prospective trial. Zhong Xi Yi Jie He Xue Bao, 2005; 3: 99–102.

7. Chan AO, Yuen MF, Hui CK, et al. A prospective study regarding the complications of transcatheter intraarterial lipiodol chemoembolization in patients with hepatocellular carcinoma. Cancer, 2002; 94: 1747–1752.

8. Huang YS, Chiang JH, Wu JC, et al. Risk of hepatic failure after transcatheter arterial chemoembolization for hepatocellular carcinoma: Predictive value of the monoethylglycinexylidide test. Am J Gastroenterol, 2002; 97: 1223–1227.

9. Llovet JM, Real MI, Montana X, et al. Arterial embolisation or chemoembolisation versus symptomatic treatment in patients with unresectable hepatocellular carcinoma: A randomised controlled trial. Lancet, 2002; 359: 1734–1739.

10. Carr BI. Hepatic artery chemoembolization for advanced stage HCC: Experience of 650 patients. Hepatogastroenterology, 2002; 49: 79–86.

11. Oellerich M, Burdelski M, Ringe B, et al. Lignocaine metabolite formation as a measure of pre-transplant liver function. Lancet, 1989; 1: 640–642.

12. Spahr L, Becker C, Pugin J, et al. Acute portal hemodynamics and cytokine changes following selective transarterial chemoembolization in patients with cirrhosis and hepatocellular carcinoma. Med Sci Monit, 2003; 9: CR383–388.

13. Okada K, Koda M, Murawaki Y, et al. Changes in esophageal variceal pressure after transcatheter arterial embolization for hepatocellular carcinoma. Endoscopy, 2001; 33: 595–600.

14. Jacobson ED and Pawlik WW. Adenosine regulation of mesenteric vasodilation. Gastroenterology, 1994; 107: 1168–1180.

15. Sakamoto I, Aso N, Nagaoki K, et al. Complications associated with transcatheter arterial embolization for hepatic tumors. Radiographics, 1998; 18: 605–619.

16. Liu CL, Ngan H, Lo CM, et al. Ruptured hepatocellular carcinoma as a complication of transarterial oily chemoembolization. Br J Surg, 1998; 85: 512–514.

17. Choi JH, Kim JH, Won JH, et al. Spontaneous intratumoral hemorrhage into hepatocellular carcinoma during transcatheter arterial embolization: A case report. J Korean Med Sci, 2004; 19: 895–897.

18. Bilbao JI, Ruza M, Longo JM, et al. Intraperitoneal hemorrhage due to rupture of hepatocellular carcinoma after transcatheter arterial embolization with lipiodol. A case report. Eur J Radiol, 1992; 15: 68–70.

19. Yeh CN, Chen HM, Chen MF, et al. Peritoneal implanted hepatocellular carcinoma with rupture after TACE presented as acute appendicitis. Hepatogastroenterology, 2002; 49: 938–940.

20. Kim HK, Chung YH, Song BC, et al. Ischemic bile duct injury as a serious complication after transarterial chemoembolization in patients with hepatocellular carcinoma. J Clin Gastroenterol, 2001; 32: 423–427.

21. Sakamoto I, Iwanaga S, Nagaoki K, et al. Intrahepatic biloma formation (bile duct necrosis) after transcatheter arterial chemoembolization. AJR Am J Roentgenol, 2003; 181: 79–87.

22. Haratake J, Hisaoka M, Yamamoto O, et al. Morphological changes of hepatic microcirculation in experimental rat cirrhosis: A scanning electron microscopic study. Hepatology, 1991; 13: 952–956.

23. Huang SF, Ko CW, Chang CS, et al. Liver abscess formation after transarterial chemoembolization for malignant hepatic tumor. Hepatogastroenterology, 2003; 50: 1115–1118.

24. Inoue H, Hori A, Satake M, et al. Liver abscess formation after treatment of liver cancer by arterial injection using adriamycin/mitomycin C oil suspension (ADMOS). Nippon Igaku Hoshasen Gakkai Zasshi, 1992; 52: 155–163.

25. Chen JH, Ho YJ, and Shen WC. Asymptomatic arteriobiliary fistula after transarterial chemoembolization of metastatic liver tumors. Hepatogastroenterology, 2001; 48: 842–843.

26. Tarazov PG, Polysalov VN, Prozorovskij KV, et al. Ischemic complications of transcatheter arterial chemoembolization in liver malignancies. Acta Radiol, 2000; 41: 156–160.

27. Aldrighetti L, Arru M, Ronzoni M, et al. Extrahepatic biliary stenoses after hepatic arterial infusion (HAI) of floxuridine (FUdR) for liver metastases from colorectal cancer. Hepatogastroenterology, 2001; 48: 1302–1307.

28. Takayasu K, Moriyama N, Muramatsu Y, et al. Gallbladder infarction after hepatic artery embolization. AJR Am J Roentgenol, 1985; 144: 135–138.

29. Brown KT. Fatal pulmonary complications after arterial embolization with 40- to 120-μm tris-acryl gelatin microspheres. J Vasc Interv Radiol, 2004; 15: 197–200.

30. Chung JW, Park JH, Im JG, et al. Pulmonary oil embolism after transcatheter oily chemoembolization of hepatocellular carcinoma. Radiology, 1993; 187: 689–693.

31. Tajima T, Honda H, Kuroiwa T, et al. Pulmonary complications after hepatic artery chemoembolization or infusion via the inferior phrenic artery for primary liver cancer. J Vasc Interv Radiol, 2002; 13: 893–900.

32. Liou TC, Shih SC, Kao CR, et al. Pulmonary metastasis of hepatocellular carcinoma associated with transarterial chemoembolization. J Hepatol, 1995; 23: 563–568.

33. Lin SC, Shih SC, Kao CR, et al. Transcatheter arterial embolization treatment in patients with hepatocellular carcinoma and risk of pulmonary metastasis. World J Gastroenterol, 2003; 9: 1208–1211.

34. Cosin O, Garrido F, Gil R, et al. Intra-arterial hepatic reservoir for chemotherapy. Percutaneous placement in left subclavian artery. Radiologia, 2005; 47: 329–334.

35. Yamagami T, Nakamura T, Yamazaki T, et al. Catheter-tip fixation of a percutaneously implanted port-catheter system to prevent dislocation. Eur Radiol, 2002; 12: 443–449.

36. Yamagami T, Kato T, Iida S, et al. Value of transcatheter arterial embolization with coils and n-butyl cyanoacrylate for long-term hepatic arterial infusion chemotherapy. Radiology, 2004; 230: 792–802.

37. Seki H, Kimura M, Yoshimura N, et al. Hepatic arterial infusion chemotherapy using percutaneous catheter placement with an implantable port: Assessment of factors affecting patency of the hepatic artery. Clin Radiol, 1999; 54: 221–227.

38. Song SY, Chung JW, Lim HG, et al. Nonhepatic arteries originating from the hepatic arteries: Angiographic analysis in 250 patients. J Vasc Interv Radiol, 2006; 17: 461–469.

39. Inaba Y, Arai Y, Matsueda K, et al. Right gastric artery embolization to prevent acute gastric mucosal lesions in patients undergoing repeat hepatic arterial infusion chemotherapy. J Vasc Interv Radiol, 2001; 12: 957–963.

40. Chuang VP, Wallace S, Stroehlein J, et al. Hepatic artery infusion chemotherapy: Gastroduodenal complications. AJR, 1981; 137: 347–350.

41. Yamagami T, Nakamura T, Iida S, et al. Embolization of the right gastric artery before hepatic arterial infusion chemotherapy to prevent gastric mucosal lesions: Approach through the hepatic artery versus the left gastric artery. AJR Am J Roentgenol, 2002; 179: 1605–1610.

42. Chung JW, Park JH, Han JK, et al. Hepatic tumors: Predisposing factors for complications of transcatheter oily chemoembolization. Radiology, 1996; 198: 33–40.

43. Lau WY, Ho S, Leung TW, et al. Selective internal radiation therapy for nonresectable hepatocellular carcinoma with intraarterial infusion of 90Yttrium microspheres. Int J Radiat Oncol Biol Phys, 1998; 40: 583–592.

44. Carr BI. Hepatic arterial 90Yttrium glass microspheres (TheraSphere) for unresectable hepatocellular carcinoma: Interim safety and survival data on 65 patients. Liver Transpl, 2004; 10: S107–110.

45. Herba MJ and Thirlwell MP. Radioembolization for hepatic metastases. Semin Oncol, 2002; 29: 152–159.

46. Salem R, Lewandowski R, Roberts C, et al. Use of Yttrium-90 glass microspheres (TheraSphere) for the treatment of unresectable hepatocellular carcinoma in patients with portal vein thrombosis. J Vasc Interv Radiol, 2004; 15: 335–345.

47. Goin JE, Salem R, Carr BI, et al. Treatment of unresectable hepatocellular carcinoma with intrahepatic yttrium 90 microspheres: Factors associated with liver toxicities. J Vasc Interv Radiol, 2005; 16: 205–213.

48. Geschwind JF, Salem R, Carr BI, et al. Yttrium-90 microspheres for the treatment of hepatocellular carcinoma. Gastroenterology, 2004; 127: S194–205.

49. Ho S, Lau WY, Leung TW, et al. Internal radiation therapy for patients with primary or metastatic hepatic cancer: A review. Cancer, 1998; 83: 1894–1907.

50. Fajardo LF and Colby TV. Pathogenesis of veno-occlusive liver disease after radiation. Arch Pathol Lab Med, 1980; 104: 584–588.

51. Fajardo LF and Berthrong M. Vascular lesions following radiation. Pathol Annu, 1988; 23(Pt 1): 297–330.

52. Murthy R, Nunez R, Szklaruk J, et al. Yttrium-90 microsphere therapy for hepatic malignancy: Devices, indications, technical considerations, and potential complications. Radiographics, 2005; 25 Suppl 1: S41–55.

53. Leung TW, Lau WY, Ho SK, et al. Radiation pneumonitis after selective internal radiation treatment with intraarterial 90Yttrium-microspheres for inoperable hepatic tumors. Int J Radiat Oncol Biol Phys, 1995; 33: 919–924.

54. Stubbs RS, Cannan RJ, Mitchell AW. Selective internal radiation therapy with 90Yttrium microspheres for extensive colorectal liver metastases. J Gastrointest Surg, 2001; 5: 294–302.

55. Murthy R, Xiong H, Nunez R, et al. Yttrium 90 resin microspheres for the treatment of unresectable colorectal hepatic metastases after failure of multiple chemotherapy regimens: Preliminary results. J Vasc Interv Radiol, 2005; 16: 937–945.

56. Thamboo T, Tan KB, Wang SC, et al. Extra-hepatic embolisation of Y-90 microspheres from selective internal radiation therapy (SIRT) of the liver. Pathology, 2003; 35: 351–353.

57. Shepherd FA, Rotstein LE, Houle S, et al. A phase I dose escalation trial of yttrium-90 microspheres in the treatment of primary hepatocellular carcinoma. Cancer, 1992; 70: 2250–2254.

58. Mantravadi RV, Spigos DG, Tan WS, et al. Intraarterial yttrium 90 in the treatment of hepatic malignancy. Radiology, 1982; 142: 783–786.

59. Sato K, Lewandowski RJ, Bui JT, et al. Treatment of unresectable primary and metastatic liver cancer with yttrium-90 microspheres (TheraSphere): Assessment of hepatic arterial embolization. Cardiovasc Intervent Radiol, 2006; 29: 522–529.

Index

Page numbers followed by "*f*" indicate figures, and page numbers followed by "*t*" indicate tables.